Mosby's
Comprehensive Review
of Practical Nursing
for
Exa

17
EDITION

Mosby's Comprehensive Review of Practical Nursing for the NCLEX-PN® Examination

Mary O. Eyles, PhD, RN
Consultant and Instructor
Hunterdon County PolyTech Career and Technical School
Flemington, New Jersey;
Consultant/Director of Education
National Association for Practical Nurse Education and Service, Inc. (NAPNES)
Alexandria, Virginia;
Member Nursing Advisory Committee
Practical Nurse and Health Occupations Program
Middlesex County Vocational Technical School
Piscataway, New Jersey

ELSEVIER

3251 Riverport Lane
St. Louis, Missouri 63043

MOSBY'S COMPREHENSIVE REVIEW OF PRACTICAL   ISBN: 978-0-323-08858-9
NURSING FOR THE NCLEX-PN® EXAMINATION

Notices

Knowledge and best practice in this field are constantly changing. As new research and experience broaden our
understanding, changes in research methods, professional practices, or medical treatment may become necessary.

Practitioners and researchers must always rely on their own experience and knowledge in evaluating and
using any information, methods, compounds, or experiments described herein. In using such information or
methods they should be mindful of their own safety and the safety of others, including parties for whom they
have a professional responsibility.

With respect to any drug or pharmaceutical products identified, readers are advised to check the most
current information provided (i) on procedures featured or (ii) by the manufacturer of each product to be
administered, to verify the recommended dose or formula, the method and duration of administration, and
contraindications. It is the responsibility of practitioners, relying on their own experience and knowledge of
their patients, to make diagnoses, to determine dosages and the best treatment for each individual patient, and
to take all appropriate safety precautions.

To the fullest extent of the law, neither the Publisher nor the authors, contributors, or editors, assume any
liability for any injury and/or damage to persons or property as a matter of products liability, negligence or otherwise,
or from any use or operation of any methods, products, instructions, or ideas contained in the material herein.

Library of Congress Cataloging-in-Publication Data
Mosby's comprehensive review of practical nursing for the NCLEX-PN(R) examination. – 17th ed. / [edited by]
Mary O. Eyles.
    p. ; cm.
Comprehensive review of practical nursing for the NCLEX-PN(R) examination
Includes bibliographical references and index.
ISBN 978-0-323-08858-9 (pbk.)
I. Eyles, Mary O. II. Title: Comprehensive review of practical nursing for the NCLEX-PN(R) examination.
[DNLM: 1. Nursing, Practical–Examination Questions. 2. Nursing, Practical–Outlines. WY 18.2]
RT62
610.73'076–dc23

                                                                                    2013012046

Executive Content Strategist: Kristin Geen
Content Manager: Jamie Randall
Publishing Services Manager: Jeff Patterson
Project Manager: Megan Isenberg
Design Direction: Karen Pauls

Printed in the United States of America

Last digit is the print number: 9   8   7   6   5   4   3   2   1

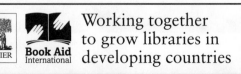

This text is dedicated to the loving memory of my husband,
Robert J. Eyles, Jr.,
whose love and support continue to give me strength
and courage to meet the challenges of the future.

Additionally, I wish to take this opportunity
to thank all of the Men and Women of the Armed Forces
for their continuing efforts to protect the freedoms
we are so privileged to enjoy.
May God Bless America!

CONTRIBUTORS

G. Constance Butherus, MA, RN
Chair, Human Rights Committee
Hunterdon Developmental Center
Clinton, New Jersey;
Chair, Council of Practical Nursing Education
National Association of Practical Nurse Education and Service
Alexandria, Virginia

Sally Flesch, PhD, RN
Professor Emerita
Black Hawk College
Moline, Illinois

Patricia M. Jacobson, MSN, BSN
Retired Nursing Instructor
Bullard Havens, Connecticut Technical High School
Bridgeport, Connecticut

Virginia Lester, MSN, RN
Assistant Professor
Angelo State University
San Angelo, Texas

Patricia B. Lisk, BSN, RN
Instructor, Practical Nursing (Ret)
Department Chairperson of PCA (Ret)
Augusta Technical College
Augusta, Georgia

Kelly Ann Pike, MS, BSN, RN, CHES
Program Coordinator
Practical Nurse and Health Occupations Program
Middlesex County Vocational Technical School
Piscataway, New Jersey

Sharon Powell-Laney, EdD, MSN, RN
Adjunct Professor
Liberty University Online
Lynchburg, Virginia;
Staff Nurse, Intensive Care Unit
Punxsutawney Area Hospital
Punxsutawney, Pennsylvania

REVIEWERS

Janis Baker, BSN, RN
Lead Instructor
Valley Baptist School of Vocational Nursing
Harlingen, Texas

Rebecca Michelle Barton, MSN, BSN, RN
Assistant Professor
University of Cincinnati-Blue Ash
Fairborn, Ohio

Terry Bichsel, BSN, RN
Practical Nursing Coordinator
Moberly Area Community College
Moberly, Missouri

Patricia L. Clowers, MSN
Director of Nursing and Allied Health
East Mississippi Community College
Mayhew, Mississippi

Mattie D. Davis, DNP, MSN, RN
Nursing Instructor
JF Drake State College
Huntsville, Alabama

Kathy A. Dillard, BSN, RN
Child Care Health Consultant
School Nurse, Former Licensed Practical Nursing
    Instructor
Bossier Parish School Board
Benton, Louisiana

Kimberly Forst, MSN, RN
Instructor of BSN Nursing
Saint Francis University
Loretto, Pennsylvania

Daneen Jeppson, FNP, MSN
Assistant Professor of Nursing
University of Montana
College of Technology
Missoula, Montana

Linda Johnson, DHA (c), MSN, PHN, RN
Los Medanos College
Pittsburg, California

Christina D. Keller, MSN, RN
Instructor
Radford University
Clinical Simulation Center
Radford, Virginia

T. Camille Lindsey Killough, BSN, RN
Pearl River Community College
Hattiesburg, Mississippi

Cathy Sermon Maddry, MSN, RN
Health Occupations Department Head
Northwest Louisiana Technical College
Minden, Louisiana

Helena J. Moissant, MSN, PHN, RN
Providence Medical Center
Medford, Oregon

Martha Olson, MS, BSN, RN, BSN
Associate Professor of Nursing
Iowa Lakes Community College
Emmetsburg, Iowa

Roni Paul, BSN, RN, CEN
ER Nurse Practical Nursing Instructor
FTCC and Womack Army Medical Center
Fayetteville, North Carolina

Jennifer Ponto, BSN, RN
Faculty, Vocational Nursing Program
South Plains College
Levelland, Texas

Russlyn A. St. John, MSN, RN
Coordinator, Practical Nursing/ Professor
St. Charles Community College
Cottleville, Missouri

Claudia Stoffel, MSN, RN, CNE
Practical Nursing Program Coordinator
West Kentucky Community and Technical College
Paducah, Kentucky

Monna L. Walters, MSN, RN
Director of Vocational Nursing Program
Lassen Community College
Susanville, California

Monica N. Warburton, BSN, RN
Assistant Professor of Nursing
Ellsworth Community College
Iowa Falls, Iowa

Elise Webb, MSN, RN
Nursing Instructor and CE Health Program Coordinator
Wilson Community College
Wilson, North Carolina

Karen Winsor, MSN, ACNS-BC
Advanced Practice Nurse for Orthopedic Trauma
University Medical Center at Brackenridge
Austin, Texas

Peggy Valentine, MSNc, BSN, RN
Director of Nursing
Skyline College
Roanoke, Virginia

Preface

Mosby's Comprehensive Review of Practical Nursing for the NCLEX-PN® Examination has been developed to provide individuals preparing for entry or reentry into nursing at the practical/vocational nurse level with a dependable source of information as they move toward their goal of becoming valued members of today's health care team. The editor and contributors of this text have the utmost respect for and recognize the licensed practical nurse/licensed vocational nurse (LPN/LVN) as a valued and much-needed member of today's health care team, providing high-quality nursing care to patients nationwide in a variety of health care settings. It is because of this respect and recognition that this text has been developed.

This seventeenth edition of *Mosby's Comprehensive Review of Practical Nursing for NCLEX-PN® Examination* addresses the basic practical/vocational nursing curriculum—from concepts basic to all levels of nursing to the complexities of specialty areas—all while incorporating the nursing process throughout. This text also refers to the approved listing of NANDA International Nursing Diagnoses. Although the LPN/LVN is not solely responsible for formulating a nursing diagnosis, the LPN/LVN does assist the registered professional nurse by collecting data essential to the formulation of a nursing diagnosis.

The text contains 10 chapters, with Chapters 1 through 4 covering the basic content found in the NCLEX-PN® Examination:

- Chapter 1 reviews important details of the latest NCLEX-PN® Test Plan, offers tips to improve study habits, reviews each of the testing formats that are used on the examination, and provides examples of each format along with test-taking skills that will help the test-taker identify the correct response from the given options. This chapter also has a special section for foreign-educated nurses who are preparing to begin the certification process necessary to take the NCLEX-PN® Examination.
- Chapter 2 covers the basics and includes the history of practical/vocational nursing, the functions of its professional organizations, and the basic concepts of effective nursing care while focusing on professional obligations and patient rights. This chapter also discusses the changing trends in nursing and health care and how these trends affect the role of the practical/vocational nurse.
- Chapter 3 covers the administration of medications and the pharmacological aspects of nursing care and incorporates the nursing process as it relates to these specific areas. This chapter reviews the major classifications of drugs along with their actions and adverse effects, and it presents the role of the LPN/LVN in the administration of medications.
- Chapter 4 covers the importance of nutrition in the life cycle and the critical role the nurse plays in assisting patients to maintain adequate nutritional status, especially during stressful periods of illness.

Chapters 5 through 10 cover the more complex nursing concepts encountered in the various specialty areas, such as medical-surgical nursing, mental health nursing, obstetrics, pediatrics, nursing care of the aging adult, and disaster preparedness (emergency nursing):

- Chapter 5 covers the nursing assessment of medical-surgical conditions and is presented according to body systems. Selected groups of major diagnoses, medical management, and nursing care are presented in this chapter.
- Chapter 6 presents the basic mental health nursing principles necessary for nurses to understand patients' physical and social responses to disease.
- Chapter 7 presents essential information necessary for planning the nursing assessment and analyzing the nursing needs of the childbearing family.
- Chapter 8 presents the care of both well and sick children from infancy through adolescence and covers both preventive health care and restorative nursing measures.
- Chapter 9 focuses on aging as a normal process and strives to increase the practitioner's knowledge and understanding of this stage of life. This chapter presents the reader with the physiological, psychological, economic, and role changes that occur and discusses how such changes affect nursing care.
- Chapter 10 emphasizes the nursing assessments and interventions that are critical to caring for victims in an emergency or during and after a disaster, such as a weather-related incident.

For the sake of clarity and consistency, the word *nurse* is used to indicate a practical/vocational nurse. The recipient of care is termed the *patient* to provide consistency as well, although we acknowledge that the term *client* may be preferred and, in some cases, used within this text.

The most current, up-to-date developments in health care and in the field of practical/vocational nursing are incorporated in this text. This edition has been thoroughly reviewed to ensure the most current and accurate content is provided. The content of each chapter is organized in a concise outline format to enhance study. New Critical Thinking Challenges have been added to help students learn important decision-making skills. Review questions at the end of each chapter help the reader determine what he or she learned in a particular subject area and what areas need additional work. Answers and rationales for correct and incorrect answer options follow the review questions.

Two comprehensive examinations are included—one at the end of the text, and one additional examination on the Evolve website (http://evolve.elsevier.com/Mosby/comprehensivePN/). Each examination contains 250 questions and follows the format of the NCLEX-PN® Examination. The correct answer and rationales for both correct and incorrect answer options are provided after each examination.

This edition of *Mosby's Comprehensive Review of Practical Nursing for the NCLEX-PN® Examination* includes more questions than ever. The Evolve website contains all the questions from the text as well as more than 2500 bonus test items that are *not* found in the text, bringing the total number of practice questions to more than 4000. All alternate item formats are found in the book or online, including the newest audio and graphic option types. The website provides review and test modes of content-specific or comprehensive examinations. To reinforce study and build confidence, it is highly recommended that students practice answering questions on a computer to simulate the NCLEX-PN computer adaptive test (CAT).

As coordinating editor, I would like to thank all of those individuals who have worked so diligently in preparing this text—all of the contributors and item writers, as well as those at Elsevier, especially Kristin Geen, Jamie Randall, and Megan Isenberg—without whom this text would not have been possible. I would also like to acknowledge the memory of my loving husband, Robert, who lost his long-standing battle with cancer 6 years ago. Although he is no longer with me in a physical sense, he continues to provide that special support that serves to guide our efforts during the revision process.

To those who will use this text, we wish you the very best as you enter into a service that will offer you both challenge and satisfaction, the greater of which is the satisfaction of extending care and a helping hand—your hand—to those in need.

Welcome to the caring profession—*welcome to nursing.*

Mary O. Eyles, PhD, RN

Contents

Preparing for the Licensure Examination

The practice of nursing is regulated by law in each state; the District of Columbia; and the U.S. possessions of Guam, Puerto Rico, the Virgin Islands, American Samoa, and the Northern Mariana Islands for the express purpose of protecting the public. The state board of nursing in each of these jurisdictions is charged with upholding the regulation of such law. To do so, each state board of nursing requires that qualified individuals take a licensing examination developed and prepared by the National Council of State Boards of Nursing (NCSBN or The National Council). The examination, known as the National Council Licensure Examination for Practical Nurses (the NCLEX-PN® examination), is available in the previously named jurisdictions and only in English. Puerto Rico has developed its own licensing examination that is available in Spanish; however, the content covered in the examination closely parallels that of the NCLEX-PN examination. This text serves as a valuable review tool regardless of the licensure examination taken by an individual.

First and foremost, all candidates must register to take the NCLEX-PN examination. Because the registration process may differ from state to state, you should contact the State Board of Nursing in the state in which you want to become licensed for detailed information on the process. There are several ways you can register (online, by telephone, or by mail). It is critical that you follow the registration instructions precisely because improperly completed forms or those not accompanied by the appropriate fees will be returned, thus delaying the overall registration process.

Once eligibility to test has been determined, you will receive an *Authorization to Test (ATT)* form. You can now proceed to schedule an appointment to take the NCLEX-PN examination at a Pearson VUE Professional Center (www.vue.com/nclex). The ATT form is an essential document; it contains your test authorization number, your candidate identification number, and an expiration date. It is important that you note the expiration date on the form because you must take the NCLEX-PN examination *before the date listed on the form.* Do not misplace this document; you will need it to be admitted to the examination.

If you must cancel or reschedule the date for your examination, you can do so up to 24 hours before your scheduled testing date. Although it is possible to cancel or reschedule, you will forfeit fees already paid, and your ATT form will become invalid.

A special section later in this chapter details issues that foreign-educated nurses face when preparing for licensure in the United States.

The NCLEX-PN examination covers all areas of the practical/vocational nursing curriculum and has been designed to test "the knowledge, skills, and abilities that are essential for the entry-level practical/vocational nurse to meet the needs of patients who require the promotion, maintenance, or restoration of health" (NCSBN, 2011). Periodic revision of the examination test plan can be expected because of the continually changing face of nursing. Nevertheless, such changes do not compromise use of this text when preparing for the licensing examination. This chapter is essential as you begin your preparation because it reviews any changes in the examination test plan and provides details and examples of the new testing formats that will be part of the examination.

WHY REVIEW?

The practical/vocational nurse uses "specialized knowledge and skills which meet the health needs of people in a variety of settings under the direction of qualified health professionals" (National Federation of Licensed Practical Nurses [NFLPN], 2003). "Competency implies knowledge, understanding and skills that transcend specific tasks and is guided by a commitment to ethical/legal principles" (National Association for Practical Nurse Education and Service [NAPNES], 2007). The licensure examination assesses entry-level competencies using a variety of testing formats that analyze an individual's use of the clinical problem-solving process (the nursing process) to gather relevant health care data, assist in identifying patient needs at various periods during an individual's life span from birth through the elder years, and contribute to team (interdisciplinary) efforts in a variety of settings.

The purpose of this text is threefold: (1) to assist you in identifying areas of specific strengths and weaknesses in your nursing knowledge and skills, (2) to increase your understanding of nursing knowledge through additional study, and (3) to increase your familiarity with and ability to respond to written test questions and corresponding clinical situations similar to those presented in the NCLEX-PN examination.

The National Council's test plan for the NCLEX-PN examination consists of one essential content dimension or framework: *client need.* This framework provides a structure that is universal in defining the actions and competencies necessary to provide safe and effective nursing care to patients in various health care settings. Therefore the dimension of *client need* is critical to ensure the overall intent of the examination: *to protect the public through safe practitioners.* A more detailed description of the 2011 NCLEX-PN Test Plan and the distribution of content for the examination are provided in Box 1-1.

The 2011 revision encompassed minor changes to the four major *client needs* categories, and two of the four categories are further divided into subcategories as was done

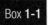 **Box 1-1**   Test Plan for the National Council of State Boards of Nursing Licensure Examination for Practical/Vocational Nurses: Major Client Need Categories, Related Concepts, and Distribution of Content

---

SAFE AND EFFECTIVE CARE ENVIRONMENT

Coordinated Care   13%-19% of items
Includes all collaborative efforts with other members of the health care team necessary to facilitate delivery of effective patient care

Safety and Infection Control   11%-17% of items
Includes all means taken to protect patients, families, and health care personnel from health and environmental hazards

HEALTH PROMOTION AND MAINTENANCE   7%-13% of items
Includes efforts to provide patient care, while incorporating prevention and early detection of disease, throughout the expected stages of growth and development from conception through advanced old age

PSYCHOSOCIAL INTEGRITY   7%-13% of items
Includes efforts to provide care, assisting with promotion and support of the emotional, mental, and social well-being of patients

PHYSIOLOGICAL INTEGRITY

Basic Care and Comfort   9%-15% of items
Includes all means to provide comfort to patients and assist them in the performance of activities of daily living

Pharmacological and Parenteral Therapies   11%-17% of items
Includes all means by which to provide care specific to administering medication and monitoring patients receiving parenteral therapies

Reduction of Risk Potential   9%-15% of items
Includes all measures taken to reduce the patient's potential for development of complications or health problems relative to treatments, procedures, or existing conditions

Physiological Adaptation   9%-15% of items
Includes all participatory efforts taken to provide care to patients with acute, chronic, or life-threatening physical health conditions

INTEGRATED PROCESSES

Integrated throughout the four patient needs categories and subcategories are additional concepts and processes that are essential to the safe and effective practice of entry-level practitioners. These concepts and processes are clinical problem solving (nursing process), caring, communication and documentation, and teaching and learning. Entry-level scope of practice is determined by the laws and statutes of each jurisdiction or state.

Modified from National Council of State Boards of Nursing: *The NCLEX-PN® examination test plan for the national council licensure examination for practical nurses*, Chicago, April 2011. Detailed information about the NCLEX-PN Test Plan and the NCLEX Examination Candidate Bulletin is available from the National Council of State Boards of Nursing on their website: www.ncsbn.org.

---

in the 2003 revision; however, two of the four categories became separate entities in 2005. The 2011 changes included revision of the percentage of test items in all categories and subcategories, except for the category of Health Promotion and Maintenance, which remains at 7% to 13%. Possible changes in the 2014 revision of the NCLEX-PN Test Plan may include slight increases or decreases in the percentage of items from each category and subcategory, as well as minor changes in related content for each category and subcategory. These anticipated changes are based on a review of the changes that have occurred in the 2013 NCLEX-RN Test Plan. Please note that although the test plan may undergo change every 3 years to remain current and reflect updated entry-level practice, all content and related concepts will remain critical components of the NCLEX-PN examination.

EFFECTIVE STUDY AND USE OF THIS TEXT

The key to effective study and use of this text can be determined *only by you*. This review is presented in a manner that is easily adaptable to various forms of study habits and familiarizes you with timed tests or examinations.

Each chapter outlines a specific content area within the practical/vocational nurse curriculum, followed by a set of questions relative to that particular content area. The answers and the rationales for both the correct and incorrect responses are found at the end of the chapter. Rationales for all four answer choices are provided for each question. The rationale for the correct answer is listed first, followed by rationales for the incorrect responses.

The questions in this text have been classified to reflect those of the NCLEX-PN examination—*cognitive level, nursing process (integrated process), client need,* and *level of difficulty*. These classifications follow the question number in the Answers and Rationales portion of the chapter:

1. First classification or word—the cognitive level of the question
   Knowledge, comprehension, application, or analysis
   The practical/vocational nurse requires skill in all levels of cognitive ability; however, the majority of the test items for the NCLEX-PN examination are written at the application or analysis level of cognitive abilities.
2. Second classification or word—phase of the nursing process (integrated process)
   Assessment, planning, implementation, or evaluation

3. Third classification or word(s)—one of the four client need categories
   Safe and effective care environment
   Health promotion and maintenance
   Psychosocial integrity
   Physiological integrity
   (See Box 1-1 for a more detailed outline of client need categories and related concepts.)
4. Letters in parentheses—the difficulty of the question
   The letter (a) signifies that more than 75% of students should answer the question correctly.
   The letter (b) signifies that 50% to 75% of students should answer the question correctly.
   The letter (c) signifies that 25% to 50% of students should answer the question correctly.

You may want to start your study process with the chapter questions first to determine areas in which you need more study time and then return to review the outline of that particular chapter in its entirety. Once you have completed review of the chapter, return to the questions and review a second time. Concentrate study efforts on those areas in which you scored low during your first assessment of the chapter questions. Should you need more in-depth study, you may refer to texts from the Bibliography found at the end of each chapter, your own nursing texts, or current nursing journals.

Once you have completed the content review and corresponding chapter questions, you are ready to take the comprehensive examination found in the text, which consists of two parts, each containing 125 questions and taking approximately 2 hours to complete. An additional comprehensive examination, also consisting of two parts, each containing 125 questions and taking approximately 2 hours to complete, is found on the accompanying CD. Time yourself or have someone else monitor your time. Although you are given 5 hours to complete the NCLEX-PN examination, practicing time management skills during your review sessions promotes self-confidence and should decrease extreme anxiety during the actual examination.

In April 1994 the National Council began administering the NCLEX-PN examination by means of computerized adaptive testing (CAT), a definite change from the traditional paper-and-pencil method of testing. CAT allows candidates to take the examination at their own pace. No set minimum amount of time has been established for the examination; however, a maximum time period of 5 hours is available to all candidates. Each candidate's examination is essentially unique to him or her because it is created interactively as the candidate progresses through the examination.

To effectively use this text in preparation for CAT, we suggest that, using a pencil or pen with erasable ink, you darken your answer choice on the chapter review questions and the comprehensive examination questions. Marking your answers in this manner allows you to concentrate on answering the questions much as you would during the actual examination.

Even though time may no longer be a major concern, becoming more proficient in time management will be to your advantage during the actual examination. The review process, which includes proper use of this text, increases not only your nursing knowledge, but also your self-confidence in that knowledge and in your test-taking abilities.

The Evolve website (http://evolve.elsevier.com/Mosby/comprehensivePN/) offers the student three modes from which to choose: *Study, Exam, and Comprehensive Examination.* In the study and exam modes, categorized questions help the student identify areas of strength and weakness by classification. To achieve this, the questions are divided into the following 9 categories:
- Nursing Concepts, the Nursing Process, and Trends in Nursing
- Pharmacology
- Nutrition
- Medical-Surgical Nursing
- Mental Health Nursing
- Maternity Nursing
- Pediatric Nursing
- Nursing Care of the Aging Adult
- Emergency Preparedness

The Comprehensive Examination mode consists of two 250-question comprehensive examinations; students can choose to take Comprehensive Examination 1, Comprehensive Examination 2, or a random selection with questions from each of the comprehensive examinations.

Remember that intelligence plays a vital role in your ability to learn. However, being *smart* involves more than just intelligence. Being practical and applying common sense are also part of the learning experience.

Regardless of how you choose to study, you may find the *tips to improve study habits* in Box 1-2 helpful as you develop your study plan.

A word of warning: *do not* expect to achieve the maximum benefits of this review text by cramming a few days before the examination. *It doesn't work!* Instead, organize planned study sessions in an environment that you find relaxing, free of stress, and supportive of the learning process.

Box 1-2   Tips to Improve Study Habits

1. Establish your study priorities and the goals by which to achieve these priorities. Write them out and review the goals during each of your study periods to ensure focused preparation efforts.
2. Enhance your organizational skills by developing a checklist and creating ways to improve your ability to retain information, such as using index cards with essential data, which are easy to carry and review whenever you have a spare moment.
3. Enhance your time-management abilities by designing a study program that best suits your needs and current daily routines by considering issues such as the following:
   a. Amount of time needed
   b. Amount of time available
   c. "Best" time to study
   d. Time for emergencies and relaxation
4. Prepare for study by reflecting on the following:
   a. An environment that is conducive to learning
   b. The appropriate study material
   c. Planned study sessions alone, with a friend, or with a group
   d. A formal review course

ITEM FORMATS

By now you more than likely have been exposed to a variety of testing in both the objective and subjective formats. The licensing examination primarily contains the objective type, better known as the *multiple-choice* form of testing. The multiple-choice question by now is one with which you are most familiar. Each multiple-choice question contains a stem (the main intent of the question) followed by four plausible answers or alternatives that either complete a statement or answer the question. Only one of the alternatives is the *best* answer; the remaining three alternatives are known as *distracters,* so named because they are written in such a way that they could be the correct answer and thus distract you to a certain degree.

However, since April 2003 alternate and more innovative item formats have been added to the examination. These new formats include *multiple response, fill in the blank* (i.e., calculation), *drag and drop/ordered response, hot spot* (i.e., identifying an area on a picture or graphic), *chart/exhibit* (i.e., reading information in a chart or exhibit to solve a problem), *graphic* (i.e., multiple-choice question with graphic answer options instead of text), and *sound (audio)* or *video.* All item formats, including the standard multiple-choice format, could have charts, tables, or graphic images. *Do not panic!* At some point in your nursing program, you will have been exposed to all of the previously named formats. Samples of these formats appear in Boxes 1-3 to 1-10.

TEST-TAKING SKILLS

Whether these testing formats are familiar to you or not, the following *common sense* pointers will help you to avoid some common test-taking errors:

1. Listen to the examiner and follow directions carefully. All candidates are given a short training session, which includes a keyboard tutorial complete with a practice session. Prior computer experience is not necessary. Should you have any questions specific to directions given, ask the examiner for clarification.

Box 1-3 **Multiple Choice**

While doing prenatal teaching with a patient, the nurse includes the many body changes that occur during pregnancy. The patient asks the nurse what hormonal changes she might expect, especially during the early months of her pregnancy. Which hormone would the nurse be correct in telling the patient is secreted only during early pregnancy?

1. Estrogen
2. Progesterone
3. Follicle-stimulating hormone (FSH)
4. Human chorionic gonadotropin (hCG)

Answer: 4

hCG is produced early in pregnancy by trophoblastic tissue; it stimulates progesterone and estrogen production by the corpus luteum to maintain pregnancy until the placenta takes over; it also is used in pregnancy tests to determine pregnancy. Progesterone and estrogen are also essential in pregnancy, as they are during a woman's childbearing years. FSH is one of the hormones responsible for maturation of the ovarian follicle during the follicular phase of the ovarian cycle.

Reference: Leifer G: *Maternity nursing: an introductory text,* ed 11, St Louis, 2012, Saunders.

Box 1-4 **Multiple Response**

A newly admitted 16-year-old who sustained a head injury in a bicycle accident has orders for seizure precautions. Of the following nursing interventions, select all that apply for these precautions.

1. Provide a barrier-free environment.
2. Encourage a noise-free setting.
3. Protect patient from falling.
4. Avoid restraining patient.
5. Assess character of seizure.

Answer: 1, 2, 3

In a multiple-response question you are asked to select all options that apply to the situation, which in this case involves seizure precautions. The first three options apply to interventions that are precautionary in nature, whereas the last two options apply to interventions that are used during the actual seizure.

Box 1-5 **Fill in the Blank**

The physician orders diazepam (Valium), 7.5 mg IM 2 times daily for a patient experiencing acute agitation from alcohol withdrawal. Diazepam is supplied in a 10-mg (2-mL) Bristojet container. How many milliliters should the nurse administer per dose?

Answer: 1.5 mL

In this question you are asked to calculate the correct dose of the medication to be given. The following formula is used to determine the correct dose:

$$\frac{\text{Desired dose [D]} \times \text{Quantity [Q]}}{\text{Dose on hand [H]}} = \text{Amount given}$$

Once you have determined the dose, you will be asked to type your answer in the appropriate space. You will be able to use the on-screen calculator on the computer to determine your answer.

Reference: Asperheim Favaro MK, Favaro J: *Introduction to pharmacology,* ed 12, St Louis, 2012, Mosby.

---

2. Answer the question that is asked. Read the situation and the question carefully, looking for key words or phrases. Do not read anything into the question or apply what you did in a similar situation during one of your clinical experiences. Think of each question as being an ideal, yet realistic, situation.
3. Have confidence in your initial response to an item because it more than likely is the correct answer. If you are unable to answer a multiple-choice question immediately, eliminate the alternatives that you know are incorrect and proceed from that point. The same goes for a multiple-response question that requires you to choose two or more of the given alternatives. If a fill-in-the-blank question poses a problem, read the situation and essential information carefully and then formulate your response. Although a time factor is not involved, do not spend an excessive amount of time on any one question. One minute—60 or possibly 70 seconds—is the recommended time allotted to any one question, but not all questions will take even a full minute; some may take only 20 to 30 seconds to read and answer.

Box 1-6   Drag and Drop/Ordered Response

The nurse is preparing to pour and administer oral medications. Prioritize the following guidelines in proper order when administering oral medications.

Answer:
1. Wash hands
2. Identify patient

UNORDERED RESPONSE

Wash hands

Identify patient

Make sure patient swallows pills

ORDERED RESPONSE

Compare drug label with medication administration record (MAR)

Pour pills into lid of vial

Document on MAR

This question asks you to place the specific nursing actions necessary for administration of oral medications in proper order. Follow the directions on the computer screen to guide you in responding to this type of question. Essentially you would use the mouse to drag and drop the unordered responses (those in the left column) where you think they belong in the ordered response (right) column. The key is to move all options from the left column to the right column as appropriate and in proper order for the procedure in question.

3. Compare drug label with medication administration record (MAR)
4. Pour pills into lid of vial
5. Make sure patient swallows pills
6. Document on MAR

Reference: Asperheim Favaro MK, Favaro J: *Introduction to pharmacology,* ed 12, St Louis, 2012, Mosby.

It is important to note that, with CAT, skipping questions or going back to review and/or change a response is not possible. You must answer the question on the screen because you will not be able to continue with the examination until you have done so.

4. Avoid taking a wild guess at an answer. However, should you feel insecure about a question, eliminate the alternatives that you believe are definitely incorrect, and reread the information given to make sure you understand the intent of the question. This approach increases your chances of randomly selecting the correct answer or getting a clearer understanding of what is being asked. Although there is no penalty for guessing on the NCLEX-PN examination, the subsequent question will be based, to an extent, on the response you give to the question at hand; that is, if you answer a question incorrectly, the computer will adapt the next question accordingly based on your knowledge and skill performance on the examination up to that point.

5. Candidates receive information before the examination and a tutorial the day of the examination. Additional information can be obtained by logging onto the Pearson VUE website, www.vue.com/nclex, or the website for the NCSBN, www.ncsbn.org.

6. Above all, begin with a positive attitude about yourself, your nursing knowledge, and your test-taking abilities. A positive attitude is achieved through self-confidence gained by effective study. This means (a) answering questions (assessment), (b) organizing study time (planning), (c) reading and further study (implementation), and (d) answering questions (evaluation).

EMOTIONAL PREPAREDNESS

Being emotionally prepared for an examination is key to your success. Proper use of this text over an extended period of time (at least 4 to 6 months before the actual examination) ensures your understanding of the mechanics of the examination and increases your confidence about your nursing knowledge. Your lifelong dream of becoming a nurse is now within your reach! You are excited, yet anxious. This feeling is normal. A little anxiety can be good because it increases awareness of reality; but excessive anxiety has the opposite effect, acting as a barrier and keeping you from reaching your goal. Your attitude about yourself and your goals will help keep you focused, adding to your strength and inner conviction to achieve success.

What happens if you find yourself in a slump over the examination? Take a time-out to refocus and reenergize! Talk to friends and family who support your efforts in achieving one of your major accomplishments in life. This effort will help you regain confidence in yourself and get you back on track toward the realization of your long-anticipated goal.

"There are two ways to face the future. One way is with apprehension; the other is with anticipation."

Jim Rohn

Practicing a few relaxation techniques may also prove helpful, especially on the day of the examination. Relaxation techniques such as deep breathing, imagery, head rolling, shoulder shrugging, rotating and stretching of the neck, leg lifts, and heel lifts with feet flat on the floor can effectively reduce tension

Box **1-7**	Hot Spot

A nurse is teaching a group of nursing assistants basic first aid and is reviewing pressure points and various techniques used to control bleeding. Identify the pressure points labeled *A, B, C, D,* and *E* in the illustration by placing the correct letter next to the appropriate name of the pressure point in the blank provided.

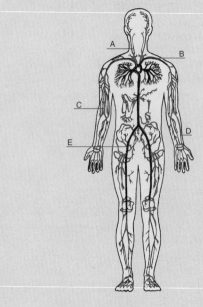

_____ Femoral artery
_____ Radial artery
_____ Brachial artery
_____ Carotid artery
_____ Subclavian artery
Answer: E, D, C, A, B

In this type of question, you are asked to identify specific areas on the illustration. In this case you are asked to identify five pressure points on a given figure. In some instances you may be asked to identify only one item on the illustration; however, you will also be asked to use the computer mouse to "point and click" on a specific area on the illustration.

Figure modified from Kidd PS, Stuart PA: *Mosby's emergency nursing reference,* St Louis, 1996, Mosby. Reference: Christensen B, Kockrow E: *Foundations of nursing,* ed 6, St Louis, 2011, Mosby.

while causing little or no distraction to those around you. It is recommended that you practice one or two of these techniques intermittently to avoid becoming tense. The more anxious and tense you become, the longer it will take you to relax.

TEST-WISE CUES

Before you begin your review, consider the following guidelines because they may prove quite helpful when preparing for the examination and during the examination itself.

Multiple-Choice Items (Box 1-3)
- Many times the correct answer is the longest alternative given, but do not count on it. NCLEX item writers (those who write the questions) are also aware of this and attempt to avoid offering you such *helpful hints.*
- Avoid looking for an answer pattern or code. There may be times when four or five consecutive questions have the same letter or number for the correct answer.

Box **1-8**	Chart/Exhibit Item

The nurse administrator of an assisted-living facility asks the nurse manager to determine which of the last 6 months (January through June) was the most active relative to admission of new residents to the facility. Review the information given below to determine which month was most active relative to resident admissions.

1. January
2. February
3. March
4. April
5. May
6. June

EXHIBIT

Resident Admissions: January-March

January: 6
February: 4
March: 2

Resident Admissions: April-June

April: 7
May: 3
June: 9

For this item the exhibit contains two tabs, each containing the number of admissions for three of the 6 months in question. The situation asks you to determine the month in which the most admissions took place. This will be done by reviewing the tabs in the chart/exhibit, then selecting the correct response. The month in which the most admissions were realized was June (noted in tab 2), making June the correct option.

Box **1-9**	Audio

In this item you are provided an audio clip to listen to and are asked to select the option that correctly answers the question.
   Place headset on.
   Click the "play" button below to listen to the audio clip.
   Adjust volume as appropriate.
   Click "play" to repeat.

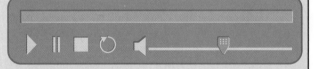

Identify the lung sound heard on the audio clip.
1. Stridor
2. Low-pitched crackles
3. Low-pitched wheeze
4. Pleural friction rub
   The lung sound heard on this audio clip is low-pitched crackles (2). Be sure to visit http://evolve.elsevier.com/Mosby/comprehensivePN to practice some audio questions.

Box 1-10 Graphic

The nurse is to give a patient a cleansing enema before a diagnostic procedure. Which position is the most appropriate for administering the enema?

1.

2.

3.

4.

Answer: 2
The left Sims position is the preferred position for giving an enema, be it a cleansing enema or low volume enema.

Figures 1 and 4 from Sorrentino SA, Remmert LN: *Mosby's textbook for nursing assistants,* ed 8, St Louis, 2012, Mosby; Figure 2 from Frank ED, Long BW, Smith BJ: *Merrill's atlas of radiographic positioning and procedures,* ed 12, St Louis, 2012, Mosby; Figure 3 from deWit SC: *Fundamental concepts and skills for nursing,* ed 3, St Louis, 2009, Saunders.

- Key words or phrases in the stem of the question such as *first, primary, early,* or *best* are also important. Similarly, words such as *only, always, never,* and *all* in the alternatives are frequently evidence of a wrong response. As in life, no real absolutes exist in nursing; however, every rule has its exceptions, so answer with care.
- Be alert for grammatical inconsistencies. If the response is intended to complete the stem (an incomplete sentence) but makes no grammatical sense to you, it might be a distracter rather than the correct response. Again, item writers try to eliminate these inconsistencies.
- Look for options that are similar in nature. If all are correct, either the question is poor or all options are incorrect, the latter

of which is more likely. *Example: If the answer you are seeking is directed to a specific treatment and all but one option deal with signs and symptoms, you would be correct in choosing the treatment-specific option.*

- Identify option components as correct or incorrect. This may help you identify a wrong answer. Example: If you are being asked to identify a diet that is specific to a certain condition, your knowledge about that condition would help you choose the correct response (e.g., cholecystectomy = low-fat, high-protein, low-calorie diet).
- Identifying content and what is being asked about that content is critical to your choosing the correct response. Be alert for words in the stem of the item that are the same or similar in nature to those in one or two of the options. Example: If the item relates to and identifies stroke rehabilitation as its focus and only one of the options contains the word stroke in relation to rehabilitation, you are safe in identifying this choice as the correct response.
- Be alert for details. Details provided in the stem of the item, such as *behavioral changes* or *clinical changes* (or both) *within a certain time period,* can provide a clue to the most appropriate response or, in some cases, responses.
- You have at least a 25% chance of selecting the correct response in multiple-choice items. If you are uncertain about a question, eliminate the choices that you believe are wrong and then call on your knowledge, skills, and abilities to choose from the remaining responses. *Keep in mind that you must answer the question on the screen before you can proceed with the examination.*

Alternate-Format Items—A Closer Look
Multiple-Response Item (Box 1-4). Be alert for details about what you are being asked to do. In this item you are asked to select all options that apply to a given situation. All options likely relate to the situation, but only some of the options relate directly to the situation. In the example all options relate to seizures, but only three are preventive actions, the focus of the situation.

Fill-in-the-Blank Item (Box 1-5). Items that ask you to fill in the blank require you to calculate an answer in response to a given situation. An on-screen calculator will be available for you to determine your response, which you will then type in the provided space.

Drag-and-Drop/Ordered Response Item (Box 1-6). In this item you are asked to prioritize (put in order) the options presented. For example, you might be asked the steps of performing a nursing action or skill such as those involved in medication administration. Because you will be using a computer, you will be asked to use the mouse in a drag-and-drop manner (you will be provided a tutorial on how to do this) to put the steps in order. *Please note: In this written text you will be asked to prioritize in numerical order, thus providing you with the experience of prioritizing steps involved with various skills.*

Hot Spot Item (Box 1-7). In this type of item, you are asked to identify various points on a figure or graphic.

Chart/Exhibit Item (Box 1-8). In an exhibit item you are asked a question relating to a given situation and an exhibit. The exhibit will consist of several tabs, each containing information necessary to answer the question. Once you have viewed the information in each tab, you can then indicate your answer by choosing the correct response from the options that appear to the left of the exhibit.

Audio or Video Clip (Box 1-9). In this item you are asked to respond to a specific question after listening to an audio clip or viewing a video clip. Directions to access the audio or video clip are provided as part of the item.

Graphic (Box 1-10). In this item you will be asked a question with graphics as options instead of text.

Please note: Additional examples of item formats can be found at www.ncsbn.org and are available to all candidates preparing to take the NCLEX-PN examination.

Throughout the Examination

Throughout the entire examination, please keep the following in mind:

- *Read every word of each question and option before responding to the item.* Glossing over the questions just to get through the examination quickly can cause you to misread or misinterpret the real intent of the question.
- Be aware that information from previously asked questions may help you respond to other examination questions.
- *Above all, do not panic!* Panic will only increase your anxiety. *Stop for a moment, close your eyes, take a few deep breaths, and resume review of the question.*
- Equally important is the amount of time you take to read an item. *The maximum amount of time you should spend on an item is 60 to 70 seconds.* Spending more time on an item can lead to overanalyzing, thereby losing sight of the intent of the question.

THE NCLEX-PN EXAMINATION

The NCLEX-PN examination is administered by means of CAT. The examination is assembled interactively as the candidate responds to items presented, making each examination unique to the candidate's knowledge, skills, and abilities. All successful candidates will answer no fewer than 85 questions or a maximum of 205 questions within the 5-hour allotted time frame, 25 of which are pretest items that are not scored. Rest periods, all of which are optional according to the 2011 NCLEX-PN Test Plan, and the computer tutorial are included as part of the 5-hour testing session. Once the candidate has answered the minimum number of items, testing stops "when the candidate's ability is determined to be either above or below the passing standard with 95% certainty" (2011 NCLEX-PN Test Plan).

Initially the computer asks a relatively easy question; if it is answered correctly, the candidate receives a more difficult question to answer. Questions continue to become more difficult until such time as the candidate answers incorrectly; then the questions become less difficult. This process continues until the computer can identify, with 95% certainty, that the candidate's ability is clearly above or below the passing standard. Once the candidate has answered the minimum number of questions, the computer compares his or her ability level with the standard required for passing. Candidates above the passing standard pass, whereas those below the passing standard do not pass. If the candidate's ability level is close to the passing standard but questionable, the computer continues the process until it has

enough information to make a proper pass-fail determination. At this point the examination ends.

Please note that both those who pass and those who fail do answer 50% of the questions correctly, simply because the computer chooses questions based on an individual candidate's ability.

In some instances candidates' ability level is so close to the passing standard that all items in the item pool may not provide adequate information to ascertain their ability level. In these instances the candidates will complete the maximum number of items, and the computer will make a pass or fail decision based on equating the final ability level.

The candidate who passes the examination earns the license to practice as a licensed practical nurse/licensed vocational nurse (LPN/LVN). A candidate who fails receives a diagnostic profile, which helps the individual to focus further study efforts for retaking the examination.

The examination has been developed with the basic knowledge necessary for the practice of practical/vocational nursing. Test items reflect the cognitive levels of knowledge, comprehension, application, and analysis, with many of the items having been written specifically to the application and analysis levels.

Although the test plan focuses on one major dimension, that of client need, keep in mind that the processes of *clinical problem solving (nursing process), caring, communication and documentation,* and *teaching and learning* are integrated throughout each of the categories and subcategories relative to client need (see Box 1-1).

Please note that the NCLEX-PN examination contains test items (questions) that are being validated for future NCLEX-PN examinations. These items are not identifiable to the test taker. Whether candidates answer these questions correctly or incorrectly, they will not gain or lose points. These are simply questions that are being validated (tested) for possible use in future examinations.

Once again, the NCLEX-PN examination is individualized based on the candidate's knowledge, skills, and ability level while meeting test plan requirements.

ESSENTIAL REMINDERS

The night before the examination you may wish to review some key concepts that you believe need additional time, but then relax and get a good night's sleep. Remember to set your alarm, allowing yourself plenty of time to dress comfortably (preferably in layers, depending on the weather), have a good breakfast, and arrive at the testing site at least 15 to 30 minutes early. Personal belongings, electronic devices (including watches), and food or drink are not permitted in the computer area (test room). Be sure you know how to get to the testing site, where to park, and where the test will be given. If the testing site is in an unfamiliar area, consider a test run 1 week before the date of your examination. In addition, remember to take eyeglasses (if needed); your ATT form; and two additional forms of identification such as a driver's license, passport, or voter ID.

At the testing center a digital fingerprint, signature, and photograph will be taken, which will serve as additional means of identification specific to you. This information will then accompany your NCLEX-PN examination results.

Listen to the testing center staff carefully during orientation, and make sure that you completely understand the instructions you are given. Ask for clarification of any information or instructions you do not fully understand.

Being prepared reduces your stress or tension level and helps you remember that *positive attitude.*

"What the mind can conceive and believe, the mind can achieve."
Napoleon Hill

A SPECIAL NOTE TO FOREIGN CANDIDATES

This section provides the foreign-educated nurse with information specific to the certification process necessary to sit for the NCLEX-PN examination. Because requirements may differ from state to state, it is important that you contact the board of nursing in the state in which you plan to work (obtain licensure) as an LPN or LVN. This information is available on the NCSBN website (www.ncsbn.org) or may be obtained by writing to the NCSBN at 111 E. Wacker Drive, Suite 2900, Chicago, IL 60601.

Because security is critical, immigration law in the United States requires health care professionals to successfully undergo a screening program to obtain a *VisaScreen certificate* before receiving an occupational visa per Section 343 of the Illegal Immigration Reform and Immigration Responsibility Act (IIRIRA) of 1996. The Commission on Graduates of Foreign Nursing Schools (CGFNS) offers the federal screening program; and the International Commission on Health Care Professions, a division of CGFNS, administers the VisaScreen, which includes an educational analysis, a license verification, an assessment of proficiency in the English language, and an examination of nursing knowledge. Detailed information specific to VisaScreen certification can be obtained through the CGFNS website at www.cgfns.org.

Educational analysis involves submission of (1) proof of secondary school education, (2) proof of completion of a government-approved health care program at least 2 years in length, and (3) proof of successful completion of the minimum number of required theoretical and clinical clock and/or credit hours required by the program.

Verification of licensure requires that the applicant submit copies of all current and past licenses held for review.

Proficiency in the use of the English language is also essential; the applicant is required to submit proof of a passing score on an approved U.S. Department of Education and Health and Human Services English language proficiency examination (Box 1-11).

Testing an applicant's knowledge of nursing is done through a 1-day qualifying examination that is administered as part of the process for obtaining a CGFNS certificate, required in most states of the United States as one of the eligibility requirements to take the NCLEX-PN examination.

In addition to the CGFNS certificate, other state requirements include the following:
1. Proof of citizenship or lawful alien status.
2. Official transcripts of education credentials, which must be sent directly to the board of nursing in the state in which the applicant selects to be licensed. These documents must be sent by the school of nursing, not the applicant.
3. Proof of classroom instruction and clinical practice in a variety of nursing areas, including medical/surgical nursing, maternity nursing, pediatric nursing, and mental health nursing.

Box 1-11	English Language Proficiency Examination and Testing Organizations

TESTS ADMINISTERED BY THE EDUCATIONAL TESTING SERVICE (ETS) WORLDWIDE
Test of English as a Foreign Language (TOEFL)
Test of English for International Communication (TOEIC)
Contact Information
Educational Testing Service (ETS)
PO Box 6151
Princeton, NJ 08541-6151
Telephone: (609) 771-7100
Email: toefl@ets.org
Website: www.ets.org or www.toefl.org

INTERNATIONAL ENGLISH LANGUAGE TESTING SYSTEM (IELTS), JOINTLY MANAGED BY THE BRITISH COUNCIL AND IELTS AUSTRALIA
Contact Information
International English Language Testing System (IELTS)
IELTS Administrator
Cambridge Examinations and IELTS International
100 East Corson Street, Suite 200
Pasadena, CA 91103
Telephone: (626) 564-2954
Email: ielts@ceii.org
Website: www.ielts.org

4. Copy of nursing license and/or diploma.
5. Proof of proficiency in the use of the English language.
6. Recent photograph of the applicant.
7. Appropriate application fees.

The certification program offered by the CGFNS is specifically for nurses educated and licensed outside the United States. It ensures eligibility and the applicant's qualifications to meet licensure and practice requirements in the United States and also predicts success on the NCLEX-PN examination.

The three parts of the CGFNS certification process are (1) the credentials review (educational analysis); (2) the 1-day qualifying examination, which tests nursing knowledge; and (3) the English Language Proficiency Examination.

In some cases applicants may be exempt from the English language proficiency requirement if their native language is English; if their nursing education was received in Australia, Canada (except Quebec), New Zealand, or the United Kingdom; or if their nursing education was received in Trinidad and Tobago with English as the language of instruction along with textbooks written in English.

Once the applicant has successfully fulfilled these eligibility requirements, he or she is ready to take the NCLEX-PN examination. The examination will take place at Pearson VUE Professional Testing Centers (Box 1-12). The NCLEX-PN candidate website is www.vue.com/nclex and has step-by-step registration instructions and forms that must be completed by all applicants.

With testing sites for the NCLEX-PN examination in the countries mentioned previously, licensed nurses interested in obtaining licensure in the United States have the opportunity to take and pass the NCLEX-PN examination even before traveling to the United States.

Box **1-12** Pearson VUE Professional Testing Centers	
United States	India
American Samoa	Japan
Australia	Mexico
Canada	Northern Mariana Islands
England	Philippines
Germany	Puerto Rico
Guam	Taiwan
Hong Kong	Virgin Islands

The opportunity to obtain licensure in the United States provides a challenge to the foreign-educated nurse, one that requires commitment, dedication, and patience. Once eligibility requirements have been met, it is recommended that, just like the United States–educated nurse, the foreign-educated nurse review content and answer practice questions in preparation for the final step of the process, the NCLEX-PN examination.

In 2011 (January through December), 755 foreign-educated nurses took the NCLEX-PN examination for the first time. Of those, fewer than 50% (45.56%) passed the examination. In addition, 855 foreign-educated nurses repeated the examination, and 18.42% of those passed the examination. In 2010 (January through June), 932 foreign-educated nurses took the NCLEX-PN examination for the first time. Of those, 48.18% passed the examination. In addition, 964 foreign-educated nurses repeated the examination, and 21.37% of those passed the examination. Therefore, based on these figures provided, it is critical that foreign-educated nurses review and be well prepared for the NCLEX-PN examination.

CONCLUSION

You started preparation for the licensing examination the day you began your nursing program. Every lecture, quiz, examination, term paper, and clinical experience had definite purpose and meaning. This seventeenth edition of *Mosby's Comprehensive Review of Practical Nursing for the NCLEX-PN® Examination* has been developed as a culmination of this preparation process. Success is now in your hands because only your persistence and commitment will motivate you to achieve your long-awaited goal.

"Part of success is preparation on purpose."

Jim Rohn

Bibliography

Asperheim Favaro MK, Favaro J: *Introduction to pharmacology*, ed 12, St Louis, 2012, Saunders.

Christensen B, Kockrow E: *Foundations and adult health nursing*, ed 6, St Louis, 2010, Mosby.

Leifer G: *Maternity nursing: an introductory text*, ed 11, St Louis, 2012, Saunders.

National Association for Practical Nurse Education and Service (NAPNES): *Standards of practice for LP/VNs*, Silver Spring, MD, 2007, NAPNES.

National Council of State Boards of Nursing: *NCLEX® examination candidate bulletin*, Chicago, 2012, National Council of State Boards of Nursing.

National Council of State Boards of Nursing: *Test plan for the National Council licensure examination for practical/vocational nurses*, Chicago, 2011, National Council of State Boards of Nursing.

National Federation of Licensed Practical Nurses (NFLPN): *Nursing practice standards for the licensed practical/vocational nurse*, Raleigh, NC, 2003, NFLPN.

Rohn J: *Excerpts from the treasury of quotes*, Southlake, TX, 2002, Jim Rohn International.

Silvestri L: *Saunders comprehensive review for the NCLEX-PN® examination*, ed 4, St Louis, 2010a, Saunders.

Silvestri L: *Saunders strategies for test success: passing nursing school and the NCLEX exam*, ed 2, St Louis, 2010b, Saunders.

Online References

Commission on Graduates of Foreign Nursing Schools (CGFNS): www.cgfns.org.

Educational Testing Service (ETS), Princeton, NJ: www.ets.org.

International English Language Testing System (IELTS): www.ielts.org.

National Association for Practical Nurse Education and Service (NAPNES): www.napnes.org.

Pearson VUE Testing Centers: http://vue.com.

National Council of State Boards of Nursing (NCSBN): www.ncsbn.org.

Nursing Concepts, the Nursing Process, and Trends in Nursing

Objectives

After studying this chapter, the student should be able to:

1. Recognize the psychological, social, and environmental factors that shape patient individuality.
2. Discuss factors contributing to health and illness.
3. Use critical thinking skills to solve patient problems.
4. Demonstrate correct techniques for performing various nursing skills.
5. Discuss the importance of the history of the nursing profession to today's nurses.
6. Verbalize the ethical and legal aspects of rendering nursing care.

Nursing is an ongoing relationship with patients in various stages of development and at different points on the health-illness continuum. This chapter reviews the history of practical/vocational nursing and the functions of its professional organizations; discusses the basic concepts of effective nursing care, while focusing on professional obligations and patient rights; and outlines changes in the health care delivery system and how these changes relate to the practice of licensed practical nursing/licensed vocational nursing.

HEALTH AND ILLNESS

HEALTH DEFINED

A. According to the World Health Organization (WHO), health is "a state of complete physical, mental, and social well-being and not merely an absence of disease or infirmity."
B. According to Abraham H. Maslow, health exists when all human needs are satisfied.
C. According to Hans Selye, health exists when an individual is in a relative state of adaptation to his or her environment.
D. In 1990, *Healthy People 2000: National Health Promotion and Disease Prevention Objectives* was published in an effort to reduce preventable diseases, disabilities, and deaths. In 2000 these objectives were reevaluated, and *Healthy People 2010* was formulated with two main goals: to increase life expectancy for people of all ages while improving their quality of life and reducing health disparities.
E. *Healthy People 2020* has four overarching goals: to attain high-quality, longer lives free of preventable disease, disability, injury, and premature death; to achieve health equity, eliminate disparities, and improve the health of people in all groups; to create social and physical environments that promote good health for all; and to promote quality of life, healthy development, and healthy behaviors across all life stages.

ILLNESS DEFINED

A. No single definition exists.
B. Illness exists when disease is present, when an individual believes that he or she is ill (subjective symptoms), or when

objective signs of illness are detected by the individual or the professional.
C. Illness exists when all basic human needs are not satisfied.
D. Illness is a state of disturbance in the homeostasis of the body, either of body structure and function or of emotional or sociologic functioning.

HEALTH-ILLNESS CONTINUUM

A. An individual is rarely totally healthy or totally ill.
B. The individual's position is constantly changing in the balance between health and illness.
C. The individual's position on the continuum is determined by need satisfaction, the stage of disease progression, and his or her perception of relative health or illness.

VARIABLES INFLUENCING HEALTH BELIEFS AND PRACTICES

A. Many variables influence a person's perception of health and illness.
B. Internal variables include the patient's developmental stage, knowledge level, perception of functioning, emotional factors, and religious or spiritual views.
C. External variables include the patient's family practices, socioeconomic status, and cultural practices.

TRENDS IN NURSING

PRACTICAL/VOCATIONAL NURSING IN THE UNITED STATES

History

A. Practical/vocational nursing evolved to provide better use of nursing personnel and ease the shortage of nurses.
B. The first school to train practical/vocational nurses was the Ballard School in New York City, founded in 1893. This 3-month program taught care of chronic invalids, older persons, and children. Graduates of this program were referred to as *Attendant Nurses.*

C. In 1907 the Thompson School was founded in Brattleboro, Vermont. The Household Nursing Association School of Attendant Nursing was founded in Boston in 1918.

D. In the 1940s approximately 50 approved programs were in existence; during the 1950s the number of schools of practical/vocational nursing grew. Most programs were extended to 12 months, placing emphasis on integrating class instruction with clinical experience.

E. In 1956 Public Law 911 appropriated millions of dollars for improving and expanding practical/vocational nurse training. The U.S. Office of Education established a practical nurse education service.

F. Today more than 1200 practical/vocational nursing schools are located in hospitals, colleges, and vocational-technical schools, providing instruction to more than 50,000 students each year.

G. Approximately 500,000 practical/vocational nurses are licensed in the United States and five U.S. territories (American Samoa, Guam, Northern Mariana Islands, Puerto Rico, and the Virgin Islands).

Education

A. Practical/vocational nursing programs must meet requirements and be approved by the state board of nursing.

B. Practical/vocational nursing schools of high standards may voluntarily apply for national accreditation by the National League for Nursing Accrediting Commission (NLNAC).

C. Admission requirements of practical/vocational nursing programs vary, but, in general, applicants must:
1. Be at least 17 years of age
2. Have a high school diploma or equivalent
3. Have good physical and mental health
4. Be of good moral character

D. The curriculum incorporates content and concepts from the biological and physical sciences, behavioral sciences, and principles and practices of nursing.

E. The curriculum includes nursing theory and clinical practice, which provide the students with learning opportunities to meet physical and psychosocial needs of mothers and infants, children, medical-surgical patients, older adults, and patients with long-term illnesses.

F. Graduates receive a diploma or certificate and are eligible to take the National Council Licensure Examination for Practical Nurses licensing examination (the NCLEX-PN examination).

G. Practical/vocational nursing is the entry level into the practice of nursing.

Role Responsibilities

A. The licensed practical nurse/licensed vocational nurse (LPN/LVN) has a vital and effective role as a member of the health care team.

B. The LPN/LVN provides direct nursing care to patients whose conditions are stable under the supervision and direction of a registered nurse (RN) or physician.

C. The LPN/LVN assists the RN with the care of patients whose conditions are unstable or complex.

D. The LPN/LVN, adhering to the nursing process, observes, assesses, records, reports, and performs basic therapeutic, preventive, and rehabilitative procedures.

E. LPN/LVNs work in acute- and long-term care hospitals, nursing homes, physicians' offices, ambulatory care

---

Box 2-1 Practical/Vocational Nursing Program Standards

The "Standards of Practice" of the National Association for Practical Nurse Education and Service (NAPNES) have been revised and expanded and are now entitled "Educational Competencies of Graduates of Practical/Vocational Nursing Programs."

These competencies encompass the following:
1. Professional behaviors
2. Communication
3. Assessment and evaluation
4. Planning
5. Caring interventions
6. Management of care

Because of the detail and expanded nature of the competencies, please refer to Appendix A, pp. 569–571 of this text. It is essential that all those reviewing for the NCLEX-PN examination be aware of these competencies and what they entail because several questions on the examination may be directly or indirectly based on these behaviors and responsibilities.

These competencies are intended as a road map for scope and content of practical/vocational nursing educational programs. The guidelines will assist the following:
1. Educators, in development, implementation, and evaluation of practical/vocational nursing curricula.
2. Students, in understanding expectations of their competencies on completion of the educational program.
3. Prospective employers, in appropriate use of the practical/vocational nurse.
4. Consumers, in understanding the scope of practice and level of responsibility of the practical/vocational nurse.

---

facilities, home health agencies, community agencies, schools, and industries.

F. The need for LPN/LVNs has increased in long-term care and decreased in acute-care hospitals.

G. To identify the abilities of the beginning practitioner in practical/vocational nursing, see Box 2-1 and Appendix A.

Continuing Education

A. Each LPN/LVN is responsible for maintaining competency and increasing his or her level of knowledge.

B. The rapid growth of nursing and medical knowledge and advances in technology require nurses to keep up-to-date.

C. The LPN/LVN must take advantage of learning opportunities through in-service programs where employed; attending seminars and workshops available through institutions and school, official, or voluntary organizations; and reading professional journals.

D. Membership in nursing organizations provides continuing education opportunities, usually at a lower cost to members.

E. Some states now require continuing education credits for LPNs/LVNs.

Health Care Team

A. Members of the health care team vary, depending on the patient's needs and goals.

B. Constant team members are as follows:
1. Physicians: diagnose and prescribe.
2. Nurses: plan and carry out nursing care.
3. Patient and family: participate in planning care.

C. Other team members include certified nursing assistants (CNAs), unlicensed assistive personnel (UAPs), physical therapists, social workers, speech therapists, occupational therapists, respiratory therapists, dietitians, and clergy.

D. Successful nursing care depends on the interaction and co-operation of all members of the team.

E. The LPN/LVN collaborates with team members.

LPN/LVN ROLE IN LEADERSHIP

A. Leadership has been defined as the use of one's individual skills to influence others to work or perform to the best of their ability.

B. The number of LPN/LVN positions in extended-care facilities is increasing. LPN/LVNs are being placed in the role of charge nurse, responsible for assigning CNA and UAP job tasks.

C. Assigning is within the scope of practice of the LPN/LVN and involves allotting tasks that are in the job description of CNAs and UAPs.

D. The LPN/LVN must know agency policy and job descriptions of CNAs and UAPs before assigning tasks.

E. Tasks assigned may include assistance with activities of daily living (ADLs) and uncomplicated tasks. See the Critical Thinking Challenge box for an exercise dealing with the issue of task assignment.

[?] Critical Thinking Challenge

Task Assignment

A nurse has the following set of tasks to complete during the next 8 hours:

> Complete assessments of four patients, and electronically chart the assessments
> Obtain vital signs of four patients
> Administer narcotics to a postoperative patient
> Bathe an unresponsive patient
> Complete Accu-Cheks on three patients

The nurse would like to assign some of these tasks to a UAP. Which of the tasks should she assign? What will she want to know about the UAP who is working with her? How will she hold the UAP accountable?

The nurse will want to know the competency level of the UAP who is working with her. If the UAP is new to the facility, the nurse may not assign as many tasks as she would if the UAP and the UAP's competency level were known.

The nurse should assign the UAP to obtain vital signs of patients who have had stable vital signs. The UAP can also bathe the unresponsive patient and complete Accu-Cheks on the diabetic patients. The nurse should tell the UAP when the tasks will need to be completed and that a report on the activities will be needed at a specified time. The nurse can then be free to assess her patients and administer narcotics as needed to the postoperative patient.

F. The LPN/LVN provides clear, concise descriptions of what tasks are to be accomplished; a time frame; and feedback and praise for staff members' efforts.

G. The LPN/LVN is legally liable for improperly assigning tasks.

Delegation

A. Many states are debating the issue of delegation as it pertains to the LPN/LVN scope of practice.

B. Bernhard and Walsh (1995) define delegation as the process of assigning part of one person's responsibility to another qualified person, with the person's consent. Delegation is a transfer of responsibility and authority while maintaining accountability.

C. LPN/LVNs must ensure that the nurse practice act of their state permits delegation. The nurse practice act should authorize specific tasks to be delegated.

D. The LPN/LVN must ensure that the delegate has demonstrated the appropriate level of competency to perform the delegated task.

Conflict Resolution

A. Conflict results when one person's expectations or rights cross those of another person.

B. LPN/LVNs in leadership roles need to become accustomed to resolving conflicts.

C. The steps in conflict resolution include recognition, clarification, negotiation (compromise), and decision making.

D. In addition to conflict resolution, LPN/LVNs must address common individual problems. See Box 2-2 for examples of some of those employee problem areas.

E. LPN/LVNs have an ethical and legal responsibility to report substance abuse among peers. See the Critical Thinking Challenge box for an exercise involving peer substance abuse. Drug addiction among nurses tends to be greater than among the general population, although exact figures are difficult to determine.

[?] Critical Thinking Challenge

Recognizing Substance Abuse in a Peer

You have been working with Rob for 6 months on a busy medical-surgical floor. Lately Rob has been coming to work a little tardy, his scrubs and appearance are disheveled, and he sometimes looks as though he is not focused on his tasks. You have found many times that Rob's patients still complain of pain even after having been medicated with pain medication. You suspect that Rob may have a substance abuse problem. What should you do?

Start with your nurse manager. Share your concerns with the nurse manager (you are probably not the only one who has noted these behaviors). Patient safety is the highest priority. Once Rob has been investigated, you can be there for him emotionally and help support his decision to seek counseling for his problem. This does not have to be the end of his nursing career; your state has a peer assistance program.

F. Most states have impaired professional rehabilitation programs to help rehabilitate health care personnel addicted to drugs and/or alcohol.

Box 2-2 **Employee Problem Areas**

- Excessive tardiness or absence
- Excessive use of telephone for personal calls
- Negative attitudes; not being a team player
- Poor quality of work
- Substance abuse

LEGISLATION RELATED TO PRACTICE OF LICENSED PRACTICAL/VOCATIONAL NURSING

Nurse Practice Act

A. Nursing is subject to laws passed by the state legislature.

B. Laws pertaining to nursing are in the state nurse practice act.

C. The nurse practice act varies from state to state. Some states define the practice of nursing, whereas others describe what a nurse may or may not do in the practice of nursing.

D. The nurse practice act also provides for some type of nursing board to regulate nursing practice and procedures regarding the following:
1. Approval of nursing schools and curriculum requirements
2. Licensure and renewal
3. Grounds for suspension and revocation of licensure

E. The LPN/LVN must practice nursing within the legally defined scope of his or her state nurse practice act.

State Boards of Nursing

A. State boards of nursing administer the state nurse practice act.

B. Membership on the board varies from state to state, usually consisting of RNs, LPN/LVNs, and consumers appointed by the governor.

C. In most states both professional and practical/vocational nursing practices are under the same board; some states have two boards, one for each.

D. Functions of the state board of nursing
1. Enforces established educational requirements of schools of nursing
   a. Surveys program to determine if preestablished standards are being met
   b. Approves new programs that meet standards
   c. Withholds or withdraws approval from programs that do not meet standards
2. Controls licensure
   a. Grants license to applicants who have passed the National Council of State Boards of Nursing (NCSBN) licensing examination
   b. Renews license
   c. Denies, suspends, or revokes license for cause
3. Conducts investigations and hearings relating to charges of unsafe nursing practice
4. Interprets the nurse practice act based on past practice, standard of care, and information from other states

Licensure

A. Licensure protects the public from unqualified practitioners.

B. A license is mandatory to practice nursing.

C. Licensure permits use of the title *licensed practical nurse* (LPN) or *licensed vocational nurse* (LVN).

D. Qualifications vary from state to state, but most states require the following for licensure:
1. Graduation from an approved program in practical/vocational nursing
2. Proof of moral character
3. Minimum score on the nationally administered examination

E. License must be renewed for a small fee at regular intervals.

F. Many states require LPN/LVNs to submit proof of continuing education before license is renewed.

G. The license may be revoked or suspended for acts of misconduct or incompetence, such as those associated with drug addiction, or conviction of a felony.

H. Licensure by endorsement occurs when a state board of nursing reviews the credentials of a nurse licensed in another state and determines that the nurse meets the qualifications of the state.

Examination

A. As of 1994 the NCSBN examination is given to all qualified applicants via computerized adaptive testing (CAT). This test, the NCLEX-PN examination, is used to determine whether the LPN/LVN candidate is prepared to practice nursing safely. The examination tests knowledge of nursing care and ability to apply that knowledge in a clinical situation with beginning competence.

B. Testing takes place in more than 1200 computer testing sites throughout the United States. Candidates schedule a test date after graduation. Testing occurs throughout the year, 6 days per week, 15 hours per day. Each examinee sits at an individual computer terminal and answers questions on the screen. The candidate's answer to each question determines the next question to be presented. No two persons receive the same test.

C. The test stops when the candidate's ability level has been estimated at a predetermined degree of accuracy. The minimum number of test items that must be answered is 85; the maximum number of items is 205. The maximum time allotment for the test is 5 hours; most candidates complete the test in less than 5 hours.

ETHICAL PRINCIPLES: CODE OF ETHICS

A. A code of ethics lists principles established by a professional group as a means of self-regulation.

B. Each LPN/LVN is responsible for upholding the professional standards of conduct and ethics.

LEGAL IMPLICATIONS FOR THE LICENSED PRACTICAL NURSE/LICENSED VOCATIONAL NURSE

Responsibilities

A. To function within the scope of the state nurse practice act

B. To maintain standards of care

C. To function according to employer or agency policy

D. To apply the skills and knowledge that a prudent LPN/LVN with comparable training would apply in a similar situation

E. To maintain complete and accurate patient records

F. To maintain confidentiality

Delivery of Nursing Care

A. Functional method: each nursing team member is assigned specific tasks (e.g., obtaining and recording all vital signs, administering all medications).

B. Team nursing: a group of patients is cared for by a team consisting of professional nurses, practical/vocational nurses, nurses' aides, and at times student nurses.

C. Primary nursing
1. One nurse assigned to patient from admission to discharge, usually an RN
2. Total responsibility for care on all shifts
3. Coordinates care with other health workers (e.g., LPN/LVN, nurses' aide)

Illegal Actions

A. Torts—civil law
1. An act or wrong committed by one person against another that results in injury or damage
2. Can be either the commission or omission of an act
3. Acts of negligence include:
   a. Professional misconduct
   b. Incorrect performance of care
   c. Illegal or immoral conduct
   d. Examples include:
      (1) Administration of wrong medication.
      (2) Administration of medication or treatment to wrong patient.
      (3) Failure to ensure safety through use of side rails or restraints as ordered by the physician.
      (4) Failure to prevent injury while applying heat.
      (5) Gross negligence: Patient's life is endangered or lost—often results in criminal action.
B. Intentional torts
1. Legal liability exists even if no damage occurs to the other person
2. May not be covered by malpractice insurance
3. Assault and battery
   a. Assault
      (1) Definition: threat or attempt to make bodily contact with another person without that person's consent, with intent to injure
      (2) Example: threatening to restrain or physically punish patient if he or she does not cooperate
   b. Battery
      (1) Definition: act of making unauthorized contact.
      (2) Example: Nurse actually restrains the patient.
4. False imprisonment
   a. Definition: unwarranted restriction of another person by force or threat of force.
   b. Examples: detaining patient in hospital against his or her will; unwarranted use of restraints.
   c. Patient who wishes to leave hospital against advice of the physician may be asked to sign a release; patient cannot be detained if he or she refuses to sign.
5. Invasion of privacy
   a. Definition: unauthorized disclosures about a patient even if information is true
   b. Examples include:
      (1) Release of patient's medical information
      (2) Exposure of patient during procedures or transportation
6. Defamation
   a. Definition: attack on the name, business, or professional reputation of another through false and malicious statements to a third person
   b. Types
      (1) Slander: oral statement
      (2) Libel: written statement

Other Legal Aspects

A. Good Samaritan laws
1. These laws give certain persons legal protection when giving aid at the scene of an accident; not all states cover nurses.
2. Their purpose is to encourage people to give assistance at the scene of an emergency.
3. These laws do not make it legally necessary for a nurse to assist.
4. When nurses do assist, they are expected to use good judgment in deciding whether an emergency exists.
5. The LPN/LVN is expected to exercise a standard of care that a reasonable LPN/LVN with comparable training would exercise in similar circumstances.
B. Child abuse
1. All states have laws that require reporting of known or suspected cases of child abuse.
2. The laws grant immunity from civil suits to individuals who are required to report child abuse.
C. Narcotics
1. The Controlled Substances Act of 1970 is a federal law that regulates the manufacture, sale, prescription, and dispensing of narcotics and other harmful drugs.
2. Violation of the law by a nurse is a felony and will result in revocation of the LPN/LVN license.
D. Wills
1. A will is a legal declaration of how a person (testator) wishes to dispose of his or her property after death.
2. For a will to be valid, the testator must be of sound mind and acting without force.
3. No legal reason exists for the nurse not to witness a will; the witness is witnessing only the person's signature, not the contents of the will.
4. A beneficiary of the will must not witness the signing.
E. Advance directives: documents in which an individual can specify his or her wishes regarding end-of-life care
1. Durable power of attorney for health care—the individual appoints someone to make health care decisions if the patient himself or herself is unable to do so; may be the patient's lawyer or an impartial friend. The power of attorney for health care should not be the patient's physician or a family member who benefits from the will.
2. Living will—a document that specifies the patient's wishes regarding health care decisions. The document usually states that the patient's wishes should be followed when "no reasonable chance for recovery" exists.
3. The Patient Self-Determination Act ensures that all individuals are aware of their rights with regard to advance directives when they are admitted to any acute-care hospital that receives federal funding.
F. Malpractice insurance
1. Professional liability policies cover liability arising out of the rendering of or failure to render professional service.
2. The policy is a safeguard against suits for damages; proving innocence can be expensive.
3. The policy can be purchased from nursing organizations, bargaining organizations, and private insurance companies.
4. Malpractice insurance provides monetary award of damages within specified limits of the policy and legal fees, court costs, and payment of bond.
5. Employer's insurance protects the employee only while he or she is on duty.

PATIENTS' RIGHTS

Bill of Rights

A. Patients have the right to courteous, individual care given without discrimination as to race, color, religion, gender, marital status, national origin, or ability to pay.

B. A patient's bill of rights, also known as a "patient care partnership," is a statement of what the patient can expect from the institution.

C. The following is paraphrased from the Patient's Bill of Rights adopted by the American Hospital Association. The patient should:
   1. Be given considerate and respectful care.
   2. Obtain from the physician complete current information concerning diagnosis, treatment, and prognosis in terms that the patient can be reasonably expected to understand.
   3. Receive from the physician information necessary to give informed consent before the start of any procedure or treatment.
   4. Be allowed to refuse treatment to the extent permitted by law and be informed of the medical consequences of that action.
   5. Be given every consideration of privacy concerning his or her medical care program.
   6. Expect that all communications and records pertaining to his or her care be treated as confidential.
   7. Expect that, within its capacity, a hospital must respond reasonably to the request of a patient for services.
   8. Obtain information concerning any relationships of the patient's hospital to other health care and educational institutions insofar as his or her care is concerned.
   9. Be advised if the hospital proposes to engage in or perform human experimentation affecting the patient's care or treatment.
   10. Expect reasonable continuity of care.
   11. Examine and receive an explanation of the bill, regardless of the source of payment.
   12. Know what hospital rules and regulations apply to the patient's conduct.

Standard of Care

A. Patients are entitled to a safe, competent standard of nursing care, no matter who administers it (RN, LPN/LVN, student).

B. The LPN/LVN is accountable for his or her own actions and must ensure that the patient receives qualified care.

C. If the LPN/LVN thinks that the patient assignment is beyond his or her ability, he or she must discuss the matter with the RN before carrying out the assigned tasks.

D. Standard of care is established by:
   1. State nurse practice act.
   2. Job description provided by the institution.
   3. Hospital policies and procedures.
   4. Patient's nursing care plan.

Patient Advocate

A. An advocate acts on behalf of another person and stands up or speaks up on behalf of that person.

B. The patient has the right to information needed to make informed decisions freely and without pressure.

C. The responsibility of the LPN/LVN is to:
   1. Maintain standard of care.
   2. Support patients in the decisions they make.
   3. Inform physician when the patient apparently does not understand what is going to happen to him or her.
   4. Observe and speak out regarding instances of incompetent, unethical, or illegal practice by any member of the health care team.

5. Know hospital policy regarding the procedure to follow when patients' rights are being violated.

D. Many hospitals employ a patient representative who serves as a liaison between the patient and the institution and who has the power to act to resolve patients' problems.

Informed Consent

A. Before any invasive procedure can be performed, the patient must give written consent, except in extreme emergency when failure to treat may be considered negligence.

B. The patient must be fully informed of the extent of the proposed procedure, risks and benefits, alternatives, and their consequences.

C. Consent must be obtained by the physician, whose duty it is to advise the patient.

D. This consent must be obtained while the patient is of sound mind; it should be signed before administration of any preoperative narcotic medications.

E. Consent may be withdrawn by the patient before the procedure.

Patient Medical Records: The Chart

A. The chart is a legal document, in either paper or electronic form.

B. The chart provides an account of the patient's hospitalization.

C. The chart may be used as evidence in courts of law and records only information related to the patient's health problem.

D. The Health Insurance Portability and Accountability Act of 1996 (HIPPA) has four objectives:
   1. Ensures health insurance portability when workers change jobs
   2. Reduces health care fraud and abuse
   3. Enforces standards for health information
   4. Guarantees security and privacy of health care (information contained in records must be held in confidence)

E. Only authorized persons should have access to patient records.

F. Most states consider medical records the property of the hospital, and the contents the property of the patient.

NURSING ORGANIZATIONS

A. Membership
   1. The LPN/LVN has the responsibility to join a professional organization and support practical/vocational nursing by becoming an active member.
   2. Membership provides:
      a. Fellowship and interaction with other LPN/LVNs.
      b. Opportunity to enhance and strengthen the role of LPN/LVNs.
      c. Means to keep current on issues relating to practical/vocational nursing.
      d. A voice in planning policies of the association.
      e. Continuing education opportunities.

B. National Association for Practical Nurse Education and Service (NAPNES) (www.napnes.org)
   1. NAPNES was organized in 1941 to promote the development of sound practical/vocational nursing education and to promote advancement and recognition of the LPN/LVN as a member of the health team.
   2. Membership includes:
      a. Regular members: LPN/LVNs, practical nursing educators, other RNs, general educators, physicians,

hospital and nursing home administrators, practical/vocational nursing students, and interested laypersons.
  b. Student members: students in state-approved schools of practical/vocational nursing.
  c. Agency members: hospitals, nursing homes, schools of practical/vocational nursing, alumni groups, civic organizations, and other institutions or groups in harmony with NAPNES objectives.
  3. Functions and activities listed by NAPNES
   a. Serves as clearinghouse for information about practical/vocational nursing, including information about functions and roles of LPN/LVNs
   b. Publishes *Journal of Practical Nursing* quarterly
   c. Prepares publications useful to faculties in schools of practical/vocational nursing
   d. Sponsors workshops and seminars for LPN/LVNs and practical nursing educators in conjunction with state LPN/LVN associations, universities, and national organizations
   e. Engages in activities aimed at protecting and strengthening position of LPN/LVNs and cooperates with state LPN/LVN associations in activities of this kind
   f. Provides consultation to state LPN/LVN constituencies on matters relating to their organization and programs
   g. Sponsors "national certification" in pharmacology and long-term care for LPN/LVNs
C. National Federation of Licensed Practical Nurses (NFLPN) (www.nflpn.org)
  1. NFLPN was organized in 1949 to foster high standards in practical nursing and promote practical nursing.
  2. Membership is limited to LPN/LVNs and student practical/vocational nurses.
  3. Affiliate membership is available to individuals who are not LPN/LVNs or students but are interested in the work of NFLPN.
  4. Many state associations exist.
  5. Functions of the NFLPN
   a. Provides leadership for LPN/LVNs employed in the United States
   b. Fosters high standards of practical/vocational nursing education and practice
   c. Encourages every LPN/LVN to make continuing education a priority
   d. Achieves recognition for LPN/LVNs and advocates the effectiveness of LPN/LVNs in every type of health care facility
   e. Interprets the role and function of the LPN/LVN for the public
   f. Represents practical/vocational nursing through relationships with other national nursing, medical, and allied health organizations; legislators; government officials; health agencies; educators; and other professional groups
   g. Serves as the central source of information on the new and changing aspects of practical/vocational nursing education and practice
D. National League for Nursing (NLN) (www.nln.org)
  1. The NLN was organized in 1952 by the combination of the National League for Nursing Education and six other national nursing organizations.

  2. Membership includes:
   a. Individual membership: anyone interested in nursing: RNs, LPN/LVNs, student nurses, consumers.
   b. Agency membership: hospitals, nursing homes, public health agencies, schools of nursing.
  3. Functions
   a. Defining and furthering good standards for all nursing service
   b. Defining and promoting good standards for institutions giving nursing education on all levels
   c. Helping to extend facilities to meet these services when necessary
   d. Helping in proper distribution of nursing education and nursing service
   e. Working to improve organized nursing services in hospitals, public health agencies, nursing homes, and other agencies; accrediting community public health nursing services; and developing criteria and other self-evaluation tools
   f. Working to improve nursing education programs; NLNAC acts as an accrediting agency for all levels of nursing education
   g. Constructing, processing, and providing preadmission, achievement, and qualifying tests
   h. Gathering and publishing information about trends in nursing, personnel needs, community nursing services, and schools of nursing
  4. The official journal is *Nursing and Health Care.*
  5. In 1982 (reaffirmed in 1987 and currently relevant as an archived document), the NLN Council of Practical Nursing Programs adopted a resolution in support of practical/vocational nursing (Box 2-3). In 1984 the Council recognized the NFLPN as the official organization for LPN/LVNs.
E. NCSBN (www.ncsbn.org)
  1. Established in 1978 to strengthen and coordinate the credentialing of nurses nationally
  2. Membership open to any state board of nursing; presently composed of 53 state boards
  3. Maintains a liaison with national organizations that represent nursing
  4. Controls the NCLEX examination process that prepares the LPN/LVN and RN licensure examinations
F. American Nurses Association (ANA) (www.ana.org)
  1. National organization for RNs formed in 1896 as the Nurses Association Alumnae; renamed American Nurses Association in 1911
  2. Concerned with standard of nursing practice and promoting general welfare of the professional nurse
  3. Limits membership to RNs
  4. Publishes *American Journal of Nursing,* a monthly magazine
G. Alumni associations
  1. Organization of graduates from the LPN/LVN's respective school
  2. Membership provides a means of:
   a. Keeping informed of school's progress.
   b. Offering suggestions to improve programs.
   c. Providing continuing education.
   d. Facilitating social activities with classmates and other graduates.
   e. Offering scholarships to future students.

Box 2-3   National League for Nursing Statement Supporting Practical/Vocational Nursing and Practical/Vocational Nursing Education*

The Executive Committee of the Council of Practical Nursing Programs of the National League for Nursing believes that practical/vocational nursing is a vital component of the occupation of nursing and supports individuals who elect practical/vocational nursing as a permanent career choice. The minimum educational credential for entry into practical/vocational nursing is a diploma or certificate.

Nursing is an occupation that exists on a continuum, and education for nursing can be developed at different levels of knowledge and skills required to fulfill identified yet different nursing roles. The nursing profession has an obligation to society to develop sound and efficient patterns for nursing education that meet the varied nursing needs of society and permit educational options for persons who wish them.

Practical/vocational nurses are involved in the nursing process. With the supervision and direction of a registered nurse or physician, they use the nursing process to give direct care to patients whose conditions are considered to be stable. This care encompasses observation, assessment, recording, and reporting to appropriate persons; and performing basic therapeutic, preventive, and rehabilitative procedures. When patients' conditions are unstable and complex, the practical/vocational nurse assists and collaborates with the registered nurse in the provision of care.

The practical/vocational nurse is prepared for employment in health care settings in which the policies and protocols for providing patient care are well defined and in which supervision and direction by a registered nurse or physician are present. These settings may be acute- or long-term care hospitals, nursing homes, home health agencies, and ambulatory care facilities.

Practical/vocational nurses function within the definition and framework of the regulations set forth by the nurse practice act of the state in which they are employed. The practice of practical/vocational nursing requires licensure, which is the responsibility of the board of nursing in each state, to protect the public and safeguard nursing practice.

Education of the practical/vocational nurse is characterized by its consistent emphasis on the clinical practice experience necessary to meet common nursing problems. The curriculum—based on concepts from the physical and biological sciences that underlie nursing measures and the behavioral science concepts necessary to individualize care—is a planned sequence of correlated theory and clinical experience.

After completing the program of study in practical/vocational nursing, the graduate demonstrates the specific competencies related to assessment, planning, implementation, and evaluation of nursing care as identified by the Council of Practical Nursing Programs.

The licensed practical nurse/licensed vocational nurse is responsible for maintaining and updating her or his competencies. Adequate orientation and continuing in-service education are responsibilities of the employing agency. However, the practical/vocational nurse must take advantage of other opportunities for continuing self-improvement and, if desired, career advancement.

Opportunities for career mobility without undue penalty must exist in the system of nursing education to provide for changing career goals.

* Issued in 1982, reaffirmed in 1987, currently relevant as an archived document.

TRENDS IN DELIVERY OF HEALTH CARE

A. Traditionally the health care focus was on diagnosis and treatment of disease.
B. Trends
  1. Emphasis on prevention of illness and maintenance of health
  2. Decrease in length of hospital stay
  3. Rise in home health care
C. Reason for changes in delivery of health care
  1. Technological advances: Scientific knowledge has provided early diagnosis and effective treatment of diseases.
  2. Consumer movement: The public has exerted pressure for the right to health at an affordable price through legislative action.
  3. Population change: Life expectancy has significantly increased, with an increase in the number of older adults and a declining birth rate.
  4. Nature of disease pattern is changing: decrease in acute diseases with an increase in chronic and degenerative diseases.
  5. Health care costs continue to be scrutinized.
D. Related health problems
  1. Growing technology and use of complex scientific equipment has caused:
    a. Increase in cost of health care; even a short hospitalization can be financially crippling.
    b. Fragmentation of care caused by increased number of health workers required by technology.
  2. Increased population has caused health problems related to air, noise, and water pollution with overcrowding and unsanitary living conditions.
  3. Aging population: The likelihood for older persons to become ill and develop chronic and degenerative diseases increases.
  4. Uneven distribution of health care facilities and resources available to:
    a. Elderly, poor, and minority populations.
    b. Rural areas and inner cities.
  5. Cost capitation is a managed care strategy that provides a fixed payment for all members (patients) for each pay period (usually 1 year). Profit is attained by keeping patients out of expensive care settings. It focuses on health promotion for cost containment; risk for patient is related to denied payment for expensive, high-tech treatments.
  6. Core measures is a program developed by Medicare/Medicaid to ensure that important aspects of care are carried out for all members of society.
E. Caring: the heart of nursing practice
  1. Caring behaviors are actions or responses by nurses when providing patient services.
  2. The most frequently described caring behaviors include attentive listening, honesty, responsibility, comforting, patience, provision of information, sensitivity, respect, touch, and addressing the patient by his or her given name (Venes, 2010).

3. The nurse must use caring behaviors during patient contact in light of recent technological advances, the more businesslike atmosphere of the health care industry, and the current nursing shortage.

DISEASE PREVENTION AND MAINTENANCE OF HEALTH

Handwashing

Handwashing is the single most important task done by health care workers to decrease the spread of disease (Box 2-4).

Levels of Health Care

A. Primary
  1. Promotion of health and prevention of disease, including:
     a. Immunization against infectious diseases
     b. Health education such as nutrition counseling
     c. Physical fitness program
     d. Research to find cause of disease
  2. Takes place in prenatal centers, well-baby centers, schools, and health maintenance organizations (HMOs)

Box **2-4** Overview of Centers for Disease Control and Prevention (CDC) Hand Hygiene Guidelines

The Centers for Disease Control and Prevention (CDC) recently released new recommendations for hand hygiene in health care settings. *Hand hygiene* is a term that applies to handwashing with soap and water, use of an antiseptic alcohol-based hand rub, or surgical hand antisepsis (water and antiseptic agent). Evidence suggests that hand antisepsis—the cleansing of hands with an antiseptic hand rub—is more effective in reducing health care–associated infections than washing the hands with soap and water.

FOLLOW THESE GUIDELINES IN THE CARE OF *ALL* PATIENTS
- Continue to wash hands with either a nonantimicrobial soap and water or an antimicrobial soap and water whenever the hands are visibly soiled.
- Use an alcohol-based hand rub to routinely decontaminate the hands in the following clinical situations. (*Note:* If alcohol-based hand rubs are not available, the alternative is hand hygiene with soap and water.)
  - Before and after direct patient contact
  - After contact with a patient's intact skin (e.g., when taking a pulse or blood pressure or lifting and moving a patient)
  - Before donning sterile gloves when inserting central intravascular catheters
  - Before performing invasive procedures (e.g., urinary catheter insertion, nasotracheal suctioning) that do not require surgical asepsis
  - After contact with blood, body fluids, excretions or other potentially infectious materials, mucous membranes, nonintact skin, and wound dressing
  - If hands will be moving from a contaminated body site to a clean body site during patient care
  - After contact with inanimate objects (including medical equipment) in the immediate vicinity of the patient
  - After removing gloves
- Before and after eating and after using a restroom, wash hands with a health care facility–approved alcohol-based hand rub or soap and water.
- Antimicrobial-impregnated wipes (i.e., towelettes) are not a substitute for using an alcohol-based hand rub or antimicrobial soap.
- If contact with spores (e.g., *Clostridium difficile* or *Bacillus anthracis*) is likely to have occurred, hands must be washed with soap and water. The physical action of washing and rinsing hands is recommended because alcohols, chlorhexidine products, iodophors, and other antiseptic agents have poor activity against spores.

- Do not wear artificial fingernails or extensions if duties include direct contact with patients at high risk for infection and associated adverse outcomes (e.g., those in intensive care units or operating rooms).

METHOD FOR DECONTAMINATING HANDS
When using an alcohol-based hand rub, apply product to palm of one hand and rub hands together, covering all surfaces of hands and fingernails, until hands are dry. Follow the manufacturer's recommendations regarding the volume of product to use. Note how many applications of the product are permitted before handwashing with soap and water must be performed. Most products state no more than five applications before washing the hands with soap and water.

FOLLOW THESE GUIDELINES FOR SURGICAL HAND ANTISEPSIS
- Surgical hand antisepsis reduces the resident microbial count on the hands to a minimum.
- The CDC recommends use of an antimicrobial soap and scrubbing of the hands and forearms up to the elbows for the length of time recommended by the manufacturer, usually 2 to 5 minutes. Refer to agency policy for time required.
- When using an alcohol-based surgical hand scrub product with persistent antimicrobial activity, follow the manufacturer's instructions. Before applying the alcohol solution, prewash hands and forearms with a nonantimicrobial soap, clean under the nails, and rinse and dry hands and forearms completely. After application of the alcohol-based product as recommended, allow hands and forearms to dry thoroughly before donning sterile gloves.

GENERAL RECOMMENDATIONS FOR HAND HYGIENE
- Use hand lotions or creams to minimize the occurrence of irritant contact dermatitis associated with hand antisepsis or hand hygiene.
- Do not wear artificial fingernails or extenders when having direct contact with patients at high risk (e.g., those in intensive care units or operating rooms).
- Keep natural nail tips less than ¼ inch long.
- Wear gloves when contact with blood, body fluids, or other potentially infectious materials, mucous membranes, and nonintact skin could occur.
- Remove gloves after caring for a patient. Do not wear the same pair of gloves for the care of more than one patient, and do not wash gloves between uses with different patients.

Adapted from deWit: *Fundamental concepts and skills for nursing,* ed 3, St Louis, 2009, Saunders. Modified from Centers for Disease Control and Prevention: *Standard precautions, 2007.* Retrieved March 23, 2010 from www.cdc.gov/hicpac/2007IP/2007isolationPrecautions.html.

B. Secondary
1. Early diagnosis and treatment to stop the progress of disease
2. Prevention of complications
3. The largest and most expensive segment of the health care delivery system
4. Usually takes place in hospitals but also in clinics and physicians' offices
C. Tertiary
1. Rehabilitation after illness to return the patient to a level of maximum functioning
2. Involves assessing patient's strengths and weaknesses, assisting the patient to increase strengths and cope with limitations, assisting with rehabilitation measures, and encouraging self-care
3. Agencies providing tertiary care: rehabilitation hospitals, skilled nursing homes, and hospices
4. Other groups involved with rehabilitation: special interest groups such as Alcoholics Anonymous and Reach to Recovery

Barriers to Preventive Health Care
A. High cost
1. Preventive measures are not always covered under insurance plan.
2. Lower socioeconomic groups are unable to finance cost.
B. Inconvenience
1. Clinics are usually open only during the day.
2. Getting an appointment with a physician can be difficult.
C. Unpleasantness of diagnostic or treatment measures; fear of pain
D. Fear of findings; many seek care only after symptoms are acute

Role of the Licensed Practical Nurse/Licensed Vocational Nurse
A. To act as a role model by promoting personal health
1. Assess own health status through regular physical and dental examinations.
2. Observe basic principles of personal hygiene and avoid products known to be harmful to health such as tobacco and drugs.
3. Provide for adequate rest, sleep, and nutrition.
4. Participate in primary care programs.
5. Obtain treatment for any infection or injury.
B. LPN/LVN functions within the health care system
1. Promote health: providing patient teaching
2. Prevent disease: providing safe environment for patients; encouraging and participating in screening programs
3. Discovery and treatment of disease: assisting physician with patient's physical examination, making observations, collecting specimens and data, and performing procedures as ordered
4. Rehabilitation: assisting patients with rehabilitation procedures

Health Care Agencies
A. The LPN/LVN should know what resources are available, what services they provide, and how to make use of the services.
B. International agency

1. WHO is an agency of the United Nations established in 1948.
2. WHO assists nations to strengthen and improve their health services by providing advisory service in disease control.
C. Official agencies in the United States—federal, state, and local—are supported by tax dollars and are accountable to the public.
1. U.S. Department of Health and Human Services (USDHHS)
a. Administration of federal programs relating to health is under the jurisdiction of the USDHHS.
b. The USDHHS has four major divisions:
(1) Social Security Administration (SSA): administers the national system of health, old age, survivor, and disability insurance
(2) Health Care Financing Administration (HCFA): created in 1977 to oversee the Medicare and Medicaid programs
(3) Office of Human Development Services: administers programs on aging, children, youth and families, and Native Americans
(4) Public Health Service (PHS): involved with improving and protecting the health and environment of the United States; major components include:
(a) Centers for Disease Control and Prevention (CDC)
(b) Food and Drug Administration (FDA)
(c) Health Resources and Services Administration (HRSA)
(d) National Institutes of Health (NIH)
(e) Substance Abuse, and Mental Health Services Administration (SAMHSA)
(f) Administration for Children and Families (ACF)
2. State health departments
a. Supported by tax funds from the state
b. Functions vary among the states; usually responsible for licensing of hospitals, nursing homes, and undertakers; health education materials; vital statistics; and communicable disease control
3. Local health department functions also vary; the general functions include:
a. Keeping vital statistics
b. Reporting communicable diseases
c. Providing maternal and child health services
d. Providing environmental sanitation; inspecting food establishments
D. Voluntary agencies
1. Depend on voluntary contributions for funds
2. Are concerned with prevention and solution of specific health problems
3. Provide funds for research and educational projects
4. National organizations that function through state or local chapters
5. Examples of voluntary agencies include:
a. American Cancer Society
b. American Diabetes Association
c. American Heart Association
d. American Red Cross
e. National Society for the Prevention of Blindness

E. Health service providers: Presently a realignment of services is shifting care from acute hospital settings to ambulatory and home care.
  1. Hospitals
     a. Short-term facilities provide acute care for patients undergoing treatment for health problems.
     b. Long-term facilities provide service over an extended period for patients with chronic or long-term health problems; rehabilitation and recreational and occupational therapy are stressed.
  2. Nursing homes, also called *long-term* or *extended-care facilities;* two categories established by the federal government:
     a. Skilled nursing facility (SNF), which provides 24-hour nursing service for the recuperating resident who no longer needs intensive nursing but still requires skilled nursing
     b. Intermediate-care facility (ICF), which provides regular nursing care, but not around the clock, for residents not capable of living by themselves
  3. Hospices
     a. Care is provided to assist the terminally ill patient to achieve the highest possible quality of life.
     b. The goal is to maintain the patient in his or her own environment.
     c. Care is provided in the home by home-care nurses.
  4. Home care
     a. Continuity and comprehensive health service are provided for individuals who do not need to be hospitalized but who require more than ambulatory care.
     b. Services provided vary from homemaker services to skilled nursing care.
     c. Estimated skilled nursing care may be provided at one third of the cost of hospitalization.
  5. Ambulatory care: care provided on outpatient basis
  6. Geriatric day-care centers: patients cared for during the day at the center and return home during the evening
F. Financing health care
  1. HMOs
     a. Provide comprehensive health services to participants on a prepaid basis
     b. Emphasize primary care to prevent costly illness and hospitalization
     c. Do not cover illness outside service area
  2. Related health insurance plans and organizations
     a. Preferred provider organization (PPO): network of health care agencies that offer insurance plan enrollees services at reduced rates; cost is higher for medical service from outside providers
     b. Exclusive provider organization (EPO): PPO insurance plan that does not reimburse for services of providers outside the network
     c. Point of service (POS): plan that uses a primary care physician to refer patients to additional services within the plan; unauthorized use of services costs more
  3. Medicare and Medicaid: government-supported health insurance programs created in 1965 by an amendment to the Social Security Act
     a. Medicare, Title XVIII, provides medical care to older adults receiving Social Security benefits regardless of their need, to people with permanent disabilities, and to those with end stages of renal disease.
     b. Medicaid, Title XIX, was designed to defray expenses that Medicare did not provide for older adults in need. It also provides services for the poor. The program is jointly sponsored with matching funds from federal and state governments. Today the states contribute a larger share than the federal government.
  4. Diagnosis-related groups (DRGs) and managed care
     a. DRGs were established to determine Medicare reimbursement. Costs of care are averaged based on diagnosis. DRGs are being phased out because of managed care systems.
     b. Managed care encompasses various methods for financing and organizing the delivery of health care in which costs are lowered by controlling the provision of services.
     c. Both DRGs and managed care have resulted in early discharges, decreased acute-care census, and reevaluation of need for in-hospital care for many diagnoses.

FACTORS INFLUENCING HEALTH AND ILLNESS

GROWTH AND DEVELOPMENT OF THE ADULT

A. Growth is change in physical size and functioning.
B. Development is change in psychosocial functioning.
C. Growth and development progress from the simple to the complex and in orderly sequences.
D. Individuals grow and develop at different rates.
E. Most growth has occurred by adulthood.
F. Certain tasks must be accomplished in each stage of development.
G. Stages cannot be skipped; each must be accomplished before the next.
H. Stages and tasks of adult development
  1. Young adulthood (18 to 40 years)
     a. Characteristics
        (1) The "prime" of biological life
        (2) Reproductive capacity at its height
        (3) A generally healthy period of life
     b. Tasks
        (1) Developing a set of personal moral values
        (2) Establishing a personal identity and lifestyle
        (3) Establishing intimate relationships outside the family
        (4) Establishing own family or support unit
        (5) Establishing a career: a field of work
        (6) Achieving independence
  2. Middle adulthood (40 to 65 years)
     a. Characteristics
        (1) Physical changes that develop gradually: diminishing strength, energy, and endurance; wrinkles; graying and loss of hair; changes in vision; menopause; and increased weight
        (2) Beginning of chronic illnesses: cancer and heart disease
        (3) Decreased demands of parenthood, with children achieving independence
        (4) Increased demands of elderly parents
        (5) Expected period of work and financial success
        (6) A period sometimes involving crisis: the "empty nest," realization that lifelong dreams are yet unmet

b. Tasks
(1) Adjusting to changes: physical, family, and social
(2) Recognizing own mortality
(3) Developing concern beyond the family: future generations and society in general
3. Older adulthood (older than 65 years)
a. Characteristics
(1) Many variations exist in levels of functioning and health.
(2) Retirement often brings fixed income.
(3) Most older adults are undergoing the normal physical changes of the aging process; most maintain active lifestyles.
b. Tasks
(1) Adjusting to loss of friends and family members
(2) Adapting to the physical changes of the aging process
(3) Adapting to psychosocial changes: relationships with children, retirement, and housing
(4) Reviewing life and preparing for death
4. Development of the family
a. Understanding the patient's role in the family, the influence of the family on the patient, and the developmental stage of the family helps to better understand the patient and his or her feelings and needs.
b. Characteristics
(1) Traditional: wife, husband, and perhaps children
(2) Nontraditional but common
(a) Single parent (usually the mother) as a result of death, divorce, or never having been married
(b) Communal: unrelated adults with or without children in a group setting
c. Stages and tasks
(1) Marriage
(a) Establishing a home
(b) Establishing individual responsibilities
(c) Establishing a gratifying sexual relationship
(d) Establishing good communication
(2) Child-rearing stage
(a) Taking on new responsibilities (e.g., financial) and maintaining an optimal atmosphere for growth and development
(b) Making continuing efforts to maintain communication among all family members
(c) Adapting to changes that occur as children become independent
(3) Postparental stage
(a) A crisis period caused by lifestyle changes
(b) A relaxed period with fewer parental demands
(c) More time available for hobbies and personal pleasures

ENVIRONMENTAL (EXTERNAL) FACTORS

A. Physical agents
1. Heat: may lead to heat exhaustion or heat stroke
2. Ultraviolet rays of the sun: produce sunburn
3. Cold: may cause hypothermia, frostbite, or even death, especially in very young or very old people
4. Electric current: may cause shock, burns, or death
B. Chemical agents
1. Taken accidentally or intentionally

2. Taken by ingestion, such as medicine overdose
3. Inhaled, such as gases, insecticidal sprays, and factory emissions
C. Cultural background: the beliefs and practices common to a group of people and passed down from generation to generation
1. Cultural practices influence food habits, reactions to illness, family interactions, and health practices.
2. The nurse needs to be aware of the patient's cultural practices and beliefs to meet needs in a way most beneficial to the patient.
D. Religious background
1. Religious practices may affect health practices.
2. Complying with a patient's religious practices may help reduce anxiety during illness.
3. The nurse must be aware of the patient who may follow all, some, or none of the practices of their religion and may turn to or completely away from them while ill.
4. The nurse must know the practices of the major religions and learn about others when the occasion arises to best meet the patient's needs (Table 2-1).
E. Socioeconomic level
1. Economic level may influence accessibility of health care.
2. Lack of social and economic resources may contribute to disturbed mental health.
3. Substandard living accommodations and sanitation may predispose to diseases such as tuberculosis (TB).
F. Infectious agents
1. Microorganisms: small living organisms that can be seen only with a microscope
a. Pathogens: disease-producing organisms
b. Nonpathogens: organisms that do not usually cause disease
c. Normal flora: microorganisms that normally live on or in an individual's body
2. Types of microorganisms
a. Bacteria
b. Viruses
c. Fungi
d. Protozoa
e. Rickettsia

INTERNAL FACTORS

A. Congenital factors
1. Defined as being present at birth
2. May be hereditary, caused by malformation during intrauterine life, or a result of birth injuries
3. Often caused by maternal infections such as German measles during the first trimester of pregnancy
4. Certain drugs, including alcohol, implicated in congenital defects
B. Hereditary factors
1. Defined as being transmitted by the genes from parents to offspring
2. Can produce conditions such as phenylketonuria, hemophilia, or sickle cell disease
C. Body defense mechanisms
1. Methods used by the body to protect itself from invasion by disease-producing substances.
2. First barriers are unbroken skin and mucous membranes.
3. Tears wash foreign particles, including some microorganisms, from the eyes.

Table 2-1 **Common Religious Practices**

RELIGION	CLERGY	SABBATH	PRACTICES
Judaism Reform Conservative Orthodox	Rabbi	Sundown Friday to sundown Saturday	Kosher laws observed Meat and dairy products not served at the same meal No pork products Only fish with scales and fins may be eaten Male child circumcised Excused from dietary practices when ill
Protestantism Episcopal Methodist Presbyterian Baptist Others	Priest Minister	Sunday	Sacraments of baptism and communion
Catholicism Roman Others	Priest	Sunday	Sacraments of baptism, confession, communion, confirmation, marriage, holy orders, sacrament of the sick (last rites) Critically ill infants may be baptized by the nurse Abstention from meat on Ash Wednesday and Fridays during Lent (40 days from Ash Wednesday to Easter) Some still abstain from meat on all Fridays Catholics attend mass each week either on Saturday evening or Sunday morning; communion can be administered at the bedside
Jehovah's Witnesses	Every member is a minister	Sunday	Do not accept blood or blood products
Seventh-Day Adventist Church	Elder	Sundown Friday to sundown Saturday	Abstain from pork and pork products
Islam	Imam	Friday	Alcohol and pork products forbidden
The Church of Jesus Christ of Latter-Day Saints (Mormons)	Elder	Sunday	Abstain from tobacco, coffee, tea, colas, and alcohol

4. The normally acid secretions of the vagina usually destroy pathogens.
5. Cilia (hairlike projections) in the nose, trachea, and bronchi sweep pathogens out of the respiratory tract.
6. Reflexes such as coughing and sneezing rid the body of pathogens.
7. Inflammatory reaction
   a. A local reaction that occurs when tissue is injured by physical agents, chemical agents, or microorganisms.
   b. Signs are redness, heat, pain, swelling, limited movement.
   c. After an injury the inflammatory process begins: Blood flow to the area increases; leukocytes move out of capillaries to the area; phagocytes begin to engulf and digest bacteria; pus forms from dead pathogens and dead tissue; healing begins.
   d. Conditions caused by inflammation commonly end with the suffix "itis" (e.g., vaginitis, cystitis).
8. Immune response
   a. The response of the body to the invasion of foreign protein substances: bacteria, viruses, foods, chemicals, tissue.

   b. An antigen is any invading substance that can trigger the immune response.
   c. Antibodies are proteins (gamma globulins) produced by the body to defend against the invading antigen.
D. Immunity
   1. The state of being resistant to a particular pathogen.
   2. Active immunity: occurs when the individual produces his or her own antibodies.
      a. It results naturally after an individual has had a specific disease such as chickenpox.
      b. It is acquired after the administration of:
         (1) Vaccines made of living or killed organisms such as the measles vaccine.
         (2) Toxoids made of neutralized toxins (poisons) produced by bacteria such as tetanus.
   3. Passive immunity: results from receiving antibodies developed by another source (animal or human).
      a. It is received naturally by fetus from mother: lasts only approximately 6 months.
      b. It is acquired from the administration of:
         (1) Immune serum, usually from animals: provides short-term immunity to a specific organism such as that causing rabies.

(2) Gamma globulin, usually from humans: also provides short-term immunity to a specific organism such as hepatitis.
4. Autoimmunity
   a. Antibodies are produced by the body against its own tissues.
   b. Autoimmunity is thought to be a factor in diseases such as rheumatoid arthritis and rheumatic fever.
E. Fluid and electrolyte balance
   1. Body fluids make up 50% to 60% of adult body weight.
   2. Body fluids make up 75% to 80% of a young child's weight.
   3. Body fluids consist mostly of water.
   4. Electrolytes are substances that, when dissolved in water, become electrically charged ions (Table 2-2).
   5. Amounts of fluids and electrolytes must be normal at all times for the body to be in homeostasis (a state of equilibrium).
   6. Fluids and electrolytes are present in "compartments" but constantly flow between the compartments to maintain balance (Figure 2-1).
F. Tissue and wound healing
   1. Healing is affected by a person's general condition, age, and nutritional status; the blood supply to the area; and the extent of the injury.
   2. Many injured tissues are repaired by cell regeneration: cells are replaced by identical or similar cells.
      a. Tissues of the skin and digestive and respiratory tracts and bone regenerate well.
      b. Nervous, muscle, and elastic tissues have little ability to regenerate.
   3. When regeneration cannot take place, granulation tissue is formed, which eventually becomes a scar.
   4. Formation of scar tissue often leaves disfigurement (e.g., after burns) or diminished function (e.g., in heart tissue after myocardial infarction).
   5. Types of wounds
      a. Incision: clean wound made by sharp instrument
      b. Contusion: closed wound; bruise; made with blunt force; underlying tissue damaged
      c. Abrasion: rubbed or scraped-off skin or mucous membrane
      d. Puncture: small opening or hole made by a pointed instrument
      e. Laceration: tear or rip leaving jagged edges
   6. Wound healing is classified as first, second, or third intention (Table 2-3).

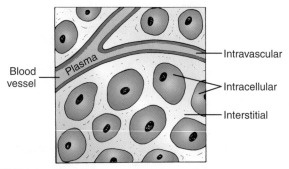

FIGURE 2-1 Body fluid compartments. Intracellular, inside the cells; extracellular, outside the cells. Extracellular compartments may be either interstitial (between the cells) or intravascular (in the vessels).

Table 2-3	**Wound Healing**	
TYPE OF HEALING	**TYPE OF WOUND**	**HOW HEALING OCCURS**
First intention	Minimum tissue damage	Without infection
	Simple incision	No separation of wound edges
		Results in minimum scar
Second intention	Decubitus or pressure ulcer	Wound edges do not join
	Severe burn	Spaces between wound edges fill with granulation tissue
		Results in scar
Third intention	Dehisced suture line	Wound edges come together at first and then reopen
		Results in scar and possibly contraction of surrounding tissue

CONCEPTS BASIC TO NURSING

REDUCING THE SPREAD OF MICROORGANISMS
A. Infectious disease chain
   1. Presence of pathogenic organisms
   2. A susceptible host; susceptibility affected by:
      a. Nutritional status
      b. Age

Table 2-2	**Principal Electrolytes**			
PRINCIPAL ELECTROLYTES	**NORMAL SERUM VALUE***	**PROBLEMS ASSOCIATED WITH EXCESS**		**PROBLEMS ASSOCIATED WITH DEFICIT**
Na⁺ (sodium)	134-145 mEq/L	Dry mucous membranes, thirst, restlessness, hypertension, hypernatremia		Confusion, weakness, coma (hyponatremia)
K⁺ (potassium)	3.6-5 mEq/L	Nausea, vomiting, diarrhea, irritability, cardiac standstill (hyperkalemia)		Weakness, cardiac arrhythmias (hypokalemia)
Ca⁺⁺ (calcium)	9-11 mg/dL	Nausea, vomiting, muscle weakness (hypercalcemia)		Muscle cramps, tetany, convulsions (hypocalcemia)

* Norms vary by institution. These numbers are generalized norms.

c. Personal health habits
d. Medical treatments in progress (radiation therapy and bone marrow–depressing drugs)
e. Trauma
f. Chronic illness
g. Stress
h. Fatigue

3. Portal of entry to the body: break in skin or mucous membrane, vaginal opening, respiratory tract, urethra, or blood
4. Reservoir: microorganisms that multiply and increase in number in the bladder, lungs, or throat
5. Modes of transmission (movement or spread) of microorganisms
   a. By contact (excreta, used tissues)
   b. By air, on droplets (sneezing, coughing)
   c. On fomites (books, stethoscopes)
   d. In food or water
   e. By vectors (animals, insects)
6. Portal of exit from the body: mouth, nose, rectum, skin, blood, or reproductive tract

B. Measures to reduce the spread by breaking the chain (interrupting the process)
1. Handwashing: most important measure
2. Medical asepsis: practices that limit the numbers, growth, and spread of microorganisms (clean technique)
   a. Linens: no shaking or holding against uniform
   b. Use of antiseptics and disinfectants
   c. Not using anything that touches the floor
3. Surgical asepsis: practices that eliminate microorganisms and their spores from sterile items or areas (sterile technique)
   a. Used during operative procedures, in delivery room, and while caring for patients with breaks in skin and for procedures in which sterile body cavities (e.g., bladder, lung, vein) are entered
   b. General principles
      (1) Sterile items become nonsterile (contaminated) when touched by anything that is not sterile.
      (2) Sterile field that becomes wet is considered nonsterile.
      (3) Sterile items out of eyesight or below waist level are considered nonsterile.
      (4) Nurses need to develop a sterile conscience (self-judgment of whether aseptic practices have been broken) and act accordingly.
   c. Means of sterilization
      (1) Steam under pressure: autoclave
      (2) Boiling
      (3) Liquid chemicals
      (4) Gas
4. Isolation and barrier techniques (protective asepsis): practices that limit the transfer of microorganisms either from the infected person or to a highly susceptible person
   a. Disease-specific isolation: each disease receives its specific protective measures—historically used for TB, not used much anymore
   b. Transmission-based precautions: isolation determined by mode of transmission
      (1) Airborne—used for patients who have serious illness transmitted by airborne droplet nuclei (e.g., TB, measles, varicella)
      (2) Droplet—used for patients known or suspected to have serious illness transmitted by large-particle droplets (e.g., diphtheria, meningitis, influenza, mumps, rubella)
      (3) Contact isolation—used for patients with serious illness transmitted by direct patient contact (e.g., wound infections)
      (4) TB isolation—use of negative-airflow rooms and special filters; practiced for all patients with known or suspected TB
      (5) Immunocompromised—used for patients who require protective isolation because of low leukocyte counts
   c. Standard Precautions: guidelines recommended by the CDC to control and reduce the risk of transmission of bloodborne and other pathogens; a combination of Universal (Blood and Body Fluid) Precautions and body substance isolation; apply to all patients receiving care regardless of diagnosis or presumed infection status; apply to blood, all body fluids, nonintact skin, and mucous membranes

C. Types of infections
1. Nosocomial: acquired as a result of hospitalization
2. Local: confined to a relatively small, specific area (e.g., a wound)
3. Systemic: infection spreads throughout body
4. Methicillin-resistant *Staphylococcus aureus* (MRSA): caused by *S. aureus* that has become resistant to all antibiotics but vancomycin
5. Vancomycin-resistant enterococci (VRE): a virtual "superbug" microorganism that is resistant to all antibiotics
6. Colonization: state in which an individual has MRSA or VRE within his or her body without creation of an infectious situation but should still be isolated from the general acute-care population

BODY MECHANICS

A. Good body mechanics is defined as efficient use of the structure and muscles of the body.
B. Use applies to both patients and nurses.
C. Use helps to prevent injuries, conserve energy, and prevent fatigue.
D. Principles of good body mechanics
1. Maintain proper alignment (posture): Head, neck, and spine should be in a straight line, with feet 10 to 12 inches (25 to 31 cm) apart and pointed straight ahead and knees slightly flexed (Figure 2-2).
2. Maintain a wide base of support; keep feet separated to provide balance (see Figure 2-2).
3. Keep center of gravity directly above the base of support (see Figure 2-2).

E. Points to remember
1. Use largest and strongest muscles (legs, arms, shoulders) when moving or lifting heavy objects (Figure 2-3).
2. Do not let your back do the work.
3. Roll, slide, push, or pull an object rather than lifting it.
4. Keep objects close to your body when lifting or moving; avoid reaching, twisting, or bending unnecessarily.
5. Point feet in the direction of movement.
6. Use devices whenever possible: patient lifters, trapeze, turning sheets, and rolling carts.
7. Obtain assistance when necessary.
8. Have the patient help as much as possible when he or she is being moved or lifted.

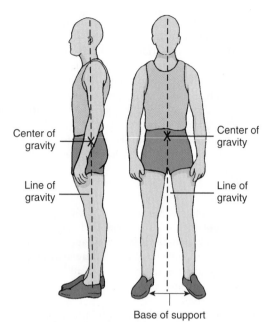

FIGURE 2-2 Body alignment. Good position for body mechanics: chin is high and parallel to the floor, abdomen is tight in and up with gluteal muscles tucked in, and feet are spread apart for a broad base of support. (From Potter PA, Perry AG, Stockert P, Hall A: *Fundamentals of nursing,* ed 8, St Louis, 2013, Mosby.)

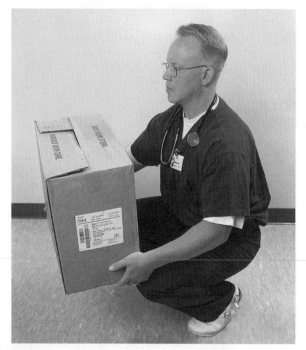

FIGURE 2-3 Proper method for lifting using leg muscles with object being lifted close to body. (From deWit SC: *Fundamental concepts and skills for nursing,* ed 3, St Louis, 2009, Saunders.)

COMMUNICATION

A. Definition: exchange of messages between two or more people, including information, thoughts, and feelings
B. Purposes in nursing
   1. To establish a meaningful, helping relationship between nurse and patient
   2. To transmit information among health care workers

C. Means
   1. Verbal
   2. Written
   3. Nonverbal
   4. Electronic
D. Guidelines
   1. Verbal communication
      a. Introduce self, stating name and title.
      b. Be sincerely interested in the patient.
      c. Be an attentive, active listener.
      d. Stand or sit close to the patient.
      e. Allow the patient to express thoughts and feelings freely without fear of being judged.
      f. Clarify what has been said to ensure understanding.
      g. Ask open-ended questions rather than questions resulting in yes or no answers: "What has happened to change your mind?"
      h. Use incomplete sentences: "You are afraid that…"
      i. Report information accurately and thoroughly.
      j. Report abnormal findings immediately.
      k. Maintain confidentiality.
   2. Written communication
      a. Record information clearly, concisely, and accurately.
      b. Nurses' notes are part of a legal document.
         (1) Use a pen.
         (2) Use only standard abbreviations.
         (3) Do not erase or obliterate errors (Figure 2-4).
         (4) Leave no blank spaces.
         (5) Sign the note at the time it is written.
         (6) Note the date and time on each entry.
      c. Formats for nurses' notes
         (1) SOAP: subjective data, objective data, assessment, plan (Figure 2-5, *A*)
         (2) Narrative: in paragraph form (Figure 2-5, *B*)
         (3) PIE: problem, intervention, evaluation
         (4) Focus charting: data (assessment); action (planning, implementation); response (evaluation) (Figure 2-5, *C*)
         (5) Charting by exception: used with flow sheets and electronic charting; pertinent data charted at beginning of shift, only changes in treatments or patient condition noted after that; must include details on patient status for accurate monitoring
   3. Nonverbal communication
      a. Exchanging messages by body posture, movements, gestures, and touch
      b. Often a more accurate expression of what is being thought or felt than verbal expression
   4. Communicating patient problems to other health care workers; use of SBAR format to improve effectiveness of communication efforts
      S—Situation: Communicate why you are calling or notifying the primary care provider; provide information concerning the problems such as vital signs and other assessment findings.

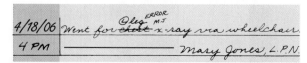

FIGURE 2-4 Correcting an error in a nurse's note.

A

4/18/06	PROBLEM #6 – Drainage on Cast. Ⓛ
4 PM	—— lateral aspect of knee ——
	S – "I have no pain or numbness." —
	O – Toes pink, warm, mobile. VS stable.
	A – Normal postoperative drainage. —
	P – Mark area of drainage. Reassess
	patient and cast q ½ hr. ——
	—— Elaine Stevens, L.P.N.

B

000-123
Doe, Jane Room 348^A
Female - 60
Dr. Pearson-Bennett

ADDRESSOGRAPH

NURSE'S RECORD

Code: ✓ = Yes	0 = No	Ⓧ = Refer to Nurse's Notes

DATE: 12/4/94   /

CODE for 23:00 to 7:00   A = Awake   S = Sleeping   C = Comatose

23:00 A	24:00 S	1:00 S	2:00 S	3:00 A	4:00 S	5:00 S	6:00 A

DIET Cl Liq   APPETITE

B Cl Liq		100%
D		
S		
G = Good F = Fair		P = Poor

OBSERVATIONS:	23-7	7-15	15-23
CardioVascular, Regular	✓	✓	
G.I., soft	✓	✓	
G.U., voiding	✓	Ⓧ	
Catheter care	0	0	
Neuro., no deficit	✓	✓	
Resp., Regular	✓	✓	
Skin Assessment	✓	✓	
O₂	0	0	
Telemetry	0	0	

SYSTEMS

ROUTINE			
Bath	0	BB	
Oral Care	✓	✓	
Back Care	✓	✓	
Side Rails up	✓	✓	
Call Light in reach	✓	✓	
Bed in Lo Position	✓	✓	
Turn every 2°	✓	✓	
Safety Reminder Device	0	0	

IVs	RT Hand	RT Hand	
Location			
Site Care	✓	✓	
Tubing Change	✓	✓	
Site Evaluation q 8 hours	✓	✓	
Labels Dated	✓	✓	
Flow Meter	✓	✓	
Discontinued	0	0	
Site Change	0	0	
IV to Heparin Lock	IV	IV	

OTHER	
Egg Crate	

INITIALS: FE / FE / JC / JC

NURSE'S NOTES:

0600 awake and alert. Skin pink, warm and dry. T-tube draining dark green liquid. IV infusing in lt. antecubital area @ 20 gtts/minute. No evidence of erythema or edema. Sleeping well for 2 hour intervals. Has obtained relief from pain since 11p.m. medication. Ambulated to bathroom, voided 100 mL of dark amber urine c/o slight vertigo and assisted to bed. Dressings dry and intact. ～～～ F Ellefson RN

0700-1100   0700   alert and oriented x3. Skin pink, warm, and dry. 99⁸-88-22. Denies incisional discomfort. Coughs well c̄ splinting of incision. Cough non-productive, lungs clear, bowel sounds hyperactive. Abdominal dressing dry and intact. T-tube draining dark green liquid, 30 mL drainage in bag. IV infusing @ 20 gtts/minute in lt. antecubital space, no erythema or edema @ site
～～～ J. Christensen, LPN

0900   ambulated to bathroom with 1 assist. c/o burning on urination. Ⓧ Voided 100 mL of dark, amber, cloudy urine. T. 101² (0), c/o feeling hot and flushed.
～～～ J. Christensen, LPN

1100 Dr. Pearson-Bennett notified. Fluids encouraged. #16 Fr. Catheter inserted s̄ difficulty. 300 mL of dark, amber, cloudy urine obtained. Specimen to laboratory for C & S. IV antibiotic started after catheterization by G. Johnston RN. Oral fluids taken well. A bd. dressings changed-incision approximated. Staples intact, no erythema noted. T-tube in place. T. 100 (0). Resting comfortably.
～～～ J. Christensen, LPN

SIGNATURES: G. J. Garnet Johnston, RN   FE Francis Ellefson RN
J. C. Jessica Christensen, LPN

FIGURE 2-5 **A,** Nurse's note in SOAP format. **B,** Narrative charting.

Continued

DATE	12/7	
TIME	FOCUS	NURSES NOTES
1400	post-op pain	Ambulating in hall c̄ moderate assist. I.V. infusing ~~~~~
		@ 20 gtts/min. Still feels warm, main concern is ~~~~~
		incisional pain, splinting is helpful. Positioned in ~~~~~
		bed c̄ pillows for support. Medicated for pain. ~~~~~
		Practiced relaxation breathing exercises. *J. Christensen, LPN*
1400	pain/fever	States, "I am more comfortable and relaxed now." Skin warm ~~~~~
		and dry. T. 99 ⁶ (0). c/o some burning on urination, ~~~~~
		less than in a.m. Taking fluids well. Urine light ~~~~~
		yellow and less cloudy. ~~~~~ *J. Christensen, LPN*

C

FIGURE 2-5, cont'd C, Focus charting nurse's notes.

B—Background: Include the status of the patient; give specifics about what is different about the patient based on assessment findings.

A—Assessment: Communicate what you think the problem may be or that you do not know what the problem is but that the patient appears to be deteriorating in some way.

R—Recommendation: Offer suggestions that you may have regarding diagnostic tests that may be recommended or changes in treatments or orders.

5. Electronic communication: via email, written nurses' notes on electronic charts. Make sure that you read electronic messages before sending them. Older-generation individuals may not be accustomed to emails and messages. Most employers have the ability and the legal right to monitor electronic communication.

BASIC HUMAN NEEDS

A. Definition: described by the psychologist Abraham Maslow as needs that must be met for humans to function at their highest possible level

B. Used by many nurses as a systematic guide for assessment

C. Premises
1. The hierarchy of needs—lower-level needs must be met before higher-level ones can be addressed.
2. People are usually able to meet their own needs.
3. When people are unable to meet their own needs, intervention is required.

4. In caring for the whole person, the nurse is involved in helping to meet the basic needs and dealing with signs and symptoms of disease.

5. Chronological age is not a variable in ascending the hierarchy of needs.

D. Hierarchy of needs (Figure 2-6)
1. Physiological: oxygen, water, food, elimination, rest and sleep, activity, sexuality, and relief of pain
2. Safety and security: protection from injury, maintenance of body defenses, structure and order in both the environment and relationships, and freedom from anxiety
3. Love and belonging: not just romantic love but a feeling of affection (the need for caring relationships)

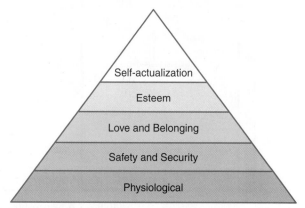

FIGURE 2-6 Hierarchy of basic human needs as described by Maslow.

4. Esteem: a feeling of worth and value to both self and others
5. Self-actualization: reaching one's fullest potential

NURSING PROCESS

A. Definition: a set of predetermined steps that nurses use to identify and help solve patient problems
B. Purposes
   1. To provide planned, coordinated, and individualized patient care
   2. To communicate problems and approaches among all individuals providing patient care
C. The process: names of steps differ slightly according to various sources but include:
   1. Assessment: gathering and organizing of data; statement of patient problems (unmet needs); the nursing diagnosis
   2. Planning: setting goals to be accomplished, and constructing a plan of action to accomplish the goals
   3. Implementation: carrying out the nursing actions to accomplish the goals and solve the problem (meet the need)
   4. Evaluation: determining whether the goal was accomplished and the problem solved

ASSESSMENT: A CONTINUOUS PROCESS

A. Sources of data
   1. Patient
   2. Family or significant others
   3. Patient's chart
      a. Physician's order sheet
      b. Nurses' notes
      c. Laboratory reports
         (1) Blood chemistry
            (a) Electrolytes: see Fluid and electrolyte balance, p. 24
            (b) Creatinine: assesses kidney function
         (2) Complete blood count (CBC): assesses adequacy of the various blood cells—red cells, white cells, platelets
         (3) Blood sugar (BS) or glucose: fasting blood sugar (FBS) or postprandial blood sugar (after meals) or hemoglobin A_{1c} (HgbA$_{1c}$) 3-month gauge of glucose levels in the body
      d. X-ray reports
         (1) Chest x-ray examination: assesses condition of lungs and size of heart
         (2) Upper gastrointestinal (UGI) series: assesses condition of esophagus, stomach, and duodenum with barium sulfate used as the contrast medium; can also diagnose dysphagia
         (3) Barium enema (BaE): assesses condition of colon with barium sulfate used as the contrast medium
         (4) Gallbladder series (GBS): assesses condition of the gallbladder with radiopaque dye
      e. Electrocardiogram (ECG) reports: assess the electrical activity of the heart
      f. Biopsy reports: assess a tissue specimen for cell changes
      g. Progress notes of other health care workers
         (1) Physician
         (2) Social worker
         (3) Dietitian
         (4) Physical therapist
         (5) Occupational therapist
         (6) Respiratory therapist
   4. Nursing report
B. Subjective versus objective data
   1. Subjective data
      a. Information reported by the patient
      b. Information that is not observable by another person
         (1) Pain
         (2) Nausea
         (3) Anxiety
         (4) Dizziness
         (5) Ringing in the ears (tinnitus)
         (6) Numbness
   2. Objective data
      a. Information gathered through the senses: sight, hearing, smell, and touch
      b. Information gathered with a measuring instrument: thermometer, sphygmomanometer, scale
         (1) Vital signs
         (2) Weight, height
         (3) Hematuria
         (4) Wheezing
         (5) Edema
         (6) Cyanosis
C. Methods of gathering data
   1. Formal interviewing (communication with patient and family or significant others): usually on patient's admission to the hospital
      a. Gather data on age, occupation, and reason for hospitalization; medications; allergies; previous hospitalizations; previous illnesses; prostheses; valuables; and special diet.
      b. Gather data on difficulty with ADLs, sleep, elimination, activity, eating, and any special needs.
   2. Listening
   3. Observing the patient and attached equipment
      a. Use an orderly approach.
         (1) Head-to-toe format
         (2) System-by-system format
         (3) Basic human needs
      b. Look for signs and symptoms of disease (variations from normal or from patient's usual baseline).
   4. Performing a physical examination
      a. Methods
         (1) Inspection
         (2) Palpation
         (3) Percussion
         (4) Auscultation
      b. Assisting with the physical examination
         (1) Be sure that the patient understands the examination and why it is being done.
         (2) Gather equipment.
         (3) Position patient appropriately (Figure 2-7).
         (4) Drape covers to provide for privacy.
         (5) Collect patient data using:
            (a) Interviewing.
            (b) Auscultation.
            (c) Inspection.
            (d) Palpation.
            (e) Examination.

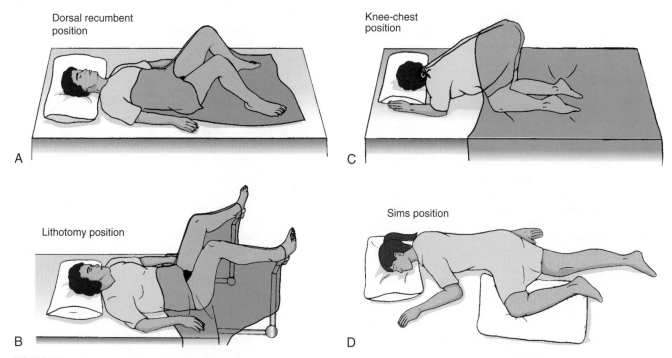

Dorsal recumbent position

Knee-chest position

Lithotomy position

Sims position

A

B

C

D

FIGURE 2-7 Positioning and draping for the physical examination. **A,** Dorsal recumbent position. **B,** Lithotomy position. **C,** Knee-chest position. **D,** Sims position. (Adapted from deWit SC: *Fundamental concepts and skills for nursing,* ed 3, St Louis, 2009, Saunders.)

(6) After the examination make the patient comfortable and safe, following orders, if any.

(7) Chart the procedure and patient's reactions; note specimens obtained.

c. The practical nurse's role in assisting with diagnostic examinations

(1) Explain procedure to the patient.

(2) Explain and carry out specific requirements.

(a) Nothing by mouth (NPO) or special meals

(b) Clothing

(c) Positioning

(d) Medications

(3) Chest x-ray examinations: No metal objects (zippers, bra fastenings, necklaces, pins) should be in view of radiograph.

(4) Blood studies: See agency procedure manual for requirements of various studies.

(5) UGI series: Give nothing by mouth after midnight (NPO p̄ MN); medication or enema to eliminate barium after the x-ray examination.

(6) BaE: Give low-residue meal evening before; NPO p̄ MN; medications or enema to clear colon before and after x-ray examination.

(7) Excretory urogram or intravenous pyelogram (IVP): NPO p̄ MN, medications to clear colon before x-ray examination; use iodine-based dye to diagnose conditions of the kidney, ureters, bladder; notify physician if patient is allergic to iodine or shellfish.

(8) GBS: Give fat-free meal evening before, NPO p̄ MN, oral ingestion of dye tablets; dye is iodine-based; check patient for iodine or shellfish allergy.

(9) Lumbar puncture: Signed consent form is required; empty bladder and bowel before procedure; patient lies curled on side with head

almost touching knees; nurse faces patient holding shoulders and knees; patient remains flat in bed after procedure.

(10) Arteriogram: Visualization of an artery after injection of a radiopaque dye; patient stays still for a period because of chance of bleeding at puncture site.

(11) Bronchoscopy: Visualization of the bronchi using a scope; patient's throat is usually anesthetized; check for a gag reflex after procedure before fluids are given.

(12) Magnetic resonance imaging (MRI): Patients must have no metal implanted in their body or metal pins, barrettes, or jewelry on while they are in the MRI machine.

(13) Colonoscopy, sigmoidoscopy: In general, patient is sedated lightly before procedure; cleansing enemas are required before the procedure.

(14) Papanicolaou (Pap) test: Cells are taken from cervix of female and "fixed" onto a slide before being sent to the laboratory; it is often an uncomfortable procedure; patient should void before this procedure and receive emotional support.

5. Measuring vital signs: to assess functioning of cardiovascular and respiratory systems

a. Temperature

(1) Normal adult ranges

(a) Axillary: 96° to 98° F (35.56° to 36.67° C)

(b) Oral: 97° to 99° F (36.11° to 37.22° C)

(c) Rectal: 98° to 100° F (36.67° to 37.78° C)

(d) Tympanic: 97° to 99° F (36.11° to 37.22° C)

(e) Temporal: 97° to 99° F (36.11° to 37.22° C)

(2) Oral temperature

(a) Mercury thermometer is left in place 2 to 4 minutes or according to agency policy.

Although mercury thermometers have been phased out in most facilities, they are still used in some isolated situations.

(b) Electronic thermometer is left in place until final reading is indicated.

(c) Wait 10 minutes if the patient has been eating, smoking, drinking a hot or cold beverage, or chewing gum.

(d) Contraindications to oral temperatures
- Patient is receiving oxygen.
- Patient is irrational or unconscious.
- Patient is younger than 5 years of age.
- Patient is breathing through the mouth.
- Patient is prone to seizures.
- Patient recently had oral surgery or mouth trauma.
- Patient is on suicide precautions.

(3) Rectal temperature

(a) Mercury thermometer is held in place 3 to 4 minutes or according to agency policy. Mercury thermometers may still be used in some situations.

(b) Electronic thermometer is held in place until final reading is indicated.

(c) Lubricate before inserting; insert 1 to 1½ inches (3.75 cm).

(d) Contraindications to rectal temperatures
- Rectal or perineal surgery
- Diseases of the rectum
- Diarrhea
- Use with caution in patients with cardiovascular disease.
- Use with caution in restless or combative patients.

(4) Axillary temperature

(a) Mercury thermometer is held in place 10 minutes. See (3)(a).

(b) Electronic thermometer is held in place until final reading is indicated.

(c) Pat the axilla dry before inserting; hold arm close to side.

(5) Tympanic temperature

(a) Press "on" button and apply disposable cover on probe tip.

(b) Seal ear opening with probe; seal outer ear opening in infants.

(c) Press "scan" button and read temperature after beeper has sounded.

(d) Discard probe cover and replace thermometer in recharger.

(e) Contraindications
- Recent exposure to cold air
- Inflammatory ear condition
- Excessive cerumen accumulation

(6) Temporal

(a) Press button to scan.

(b) Swipe probe over patient forehead, and then rest temporal on carotid artery.

(c) Wait for beeps to subside, then read temperature.

b. Pulse: the beat of the heart heard at the apex or felt at specific sites as a wave of blood flows through an artery

(1) Observe rate, rhythm, and strength.

(2) Normal adult range: 60 to 100 beats/min; varies greatly among individuals; rate more rapid for children.

(3) If rate or rhythm is irregular, take pulse apically and count for 1 full minute.

(4) Variations

(a) Bradycardia: slow heart rate—under 60 beats/min

(b) Tachycardia: fast heart beat—over 100 beats/min

(c) Irregular: uneven intervals between beats

(d) Thready: weak pulse—easily obliterated

(e) Bounding: very strong pulse—difficult to obliterate

(5) Sites: felt with fingertips at places where an artery crosses over muscle or bone close to the skin and at the apex of the heart

(a) Temporal

(b) Carotid

(c) Brachial

(d) Radial

(e) Femoral

(f) Popliteal

(g) Pedal

(h) Apical: heard with stethoscope over the fifth intercostal space, midclavicular line

(6) Apical-radial pulse: to detect a difference between rates at the two sites (the pulse deficit)

(a) Requires two people: one taking the radial pulse and one taking the apical pulse.

(b) Must be counted simultaneously for 1 full minute.

(c) Apical rate can never be lower than the radial rate.

c. Respiration: the process of inhaling and exhaling air into and out of the lungs. One inhalation plus one exhalation equals one respiration.

(1) Observe rate, rhythm, and depth; normal adult range is 14 to 20 respirations per minute; varies greatly with activity level; rate is higher for children.

(2) Patient must not be aware that respirations are being observed.

(3) Variations

(a) Apnea: absence of breathing

(b) Tachypnea: rapid breathing

(c) Stertorous breathing: noisy breathing; snoring

(d) Cheyne-Stokes respirations: rhythmic repeated cycles of slow shallow respirations increasing in depth rate and then gradually becoming slower and shallower, followed by a period of apnea; often precede death

(e) Dyspnea: difficulty breathing

(f) Orthopnea: breathing possible only while in an upright position

(g) Kussmaul respirations: paroxysms of dyspnea often preceding diabetic coma or other acidotic conditions

(4) Count respirations for 1 full minute if rate is abnormal or rhythm is irregular.

d. Blood pressure (BP): force exerted by the blood against the walls of the arteries (measured in millimeters [mm] of mercury [Hg])

(1) Normal adult range is 60 to 80 mm Hg diastolic, 90 to 120 mm Hg systolic; levels vary among individuals and with activity.

(2) BP can be measured at brachial artery or popliteal artery: ensure that arrow on cuff lines up with area where artery is palpated most clearly.

(3) Be sure that cuff is proper size for the individual.

(4) Terminology

(a) Systolic: pressure in the arteries during contraction of the heart

(b) Diastolic: pressure in the arteries during relaxation of the heart

(c) Hypotension: lower than normal BP—under 100/60 mm Hg—can occur with many conditions

- Symptomatic hypotension: patient becomes dizzy
- Orthostatic hypotension: dizziness caused by a sudden change in BP created by rising to a standing position quickly

(d) Hypertension: higher than normal BP—140/90 mm Hg

(e) Pulse pressure: difference between systolic and diastolic pressures

e. Pulse oximetry: noninvasive continuous monitor of blood oxygen saturation

(1) Normal adult range is 95% to 100%.

(2) Report readings under 90%, which indicate hypoxia. Oxygen saturation in the arterial blood (SaO_2) under 70% is life-threatening.

(3) Clip-on or adhesive probe attaches to finger, toe, earlobe, or bridge of nose.

(4) Uses light for reading; do not block light on probe. Area being assessed should be clean, dry, and without nail polish.

(5) Rotate clip every 4 hours (q4h)—check for proper clip position with alarms.

(6) Check abnormal readings with arterial blood gases.

6. Measuring weight and height

a. Weight

(1) Should be measured before breakfast

(2) Should be measured in same amount of clothing each day

(3) Can use results in establishing medication dosages, gain or loss of body fluid, and nutritional status

(4) Can use standing, chair, or stretcher scale; be sure that scale is balanced

b. Height

(1) Have patient stand on a paper towel in bare feet.

(2) Have patient stand tall.

(3) Height can be used in determining some medication dosages and anesthesia requirements.

7. Collecting specimens

a. General guidelines

(1) Follow agency procedure for collection, container, labels, requisitions, and recording.

(2) Label all specimen containers correctly, and send with a laboratory requisition.

(3) Send specimens to the laboratory promptly.

(4) Wear protective gloves.

(5) Wash hands thoroughly after handling specimen.

(6) Generally a specimen should be obtained before any antibiotic administration.

b. Urine specimens

(1) Urinalysis: routine examination of urine

(a) Only the patient and container need be clean.

(b) Specimens are often collected as part of admission procedure.

(2) Culture and sensitivity

(a) Clean-catch, midstream: Genitalia and meatus are cleansed. Specimen is taken after stream has started but before voiding is completed.

(b) Catheterized specimen: Sample is obtained by using sterile technique and equipment.

(3) 24-hour specimens: First voiding is discarded and time is noted. All urine for the next 24 hours is collected. See agency policy for type of container and storage methods. Collection is normally done to determine creatinine clearance levels.

(4) Sugar and acetone testing

(a) Urine should be obtained 30 to 60 minutes before meal or at a designated time.

(b) Double-voided specimen gives more accurate results.

- Have patient empty bladder.
- Collect specimen as soon as patient can void again.
- Additional fluids may be needed to produce specimen.

(c) Test specimen with Tes-Tape, Clinitest, Clinistix, or Keto-Diastix; follow manufacturer's directions precisely for accurate results.

(d) Report results immediately to medication nurse.

(e) Record results in proper place.

(5) Specimens from indwelling catheter

(a) Closed drainage system must be maintained.

(b) Specimens must be obtained from specimen "port" with needle and syringe by sterile technique.

c. Stool specimens

(1) Collect in clean bedpan.

(2) Use tongue depressor or wooden spatula to transfer stool to specimen container.

(3) Types of testing

(a) For blood: Occult (guaiac, Hematest); patient must be on a red meat–free diet 3 days before test.

(b) For culture and sensitivity: Use sterile container.

(c) For ova and parasites: Stool must still be warm when it reaches the laboratory.

d. Sputum specimens

(1) Specimen is best collected in the morning before breakfast.

(2) Patient first rinses mouth with water.

(3) Instruct patient to take deep breath, cough deeply, and expectorate into container.

(4) Specimen must be from the lung, not just mouth saliva.

e. Blood specimen: capillary puncture (e.g., blood glucose testing). It may be a finger stick for child or adult, heel stick for infant. Agency certification may be required.

(1) Explain procedure to patient; warn that it does hurt.

(2) Assemble equipment: gloves, alcohol swab, lancet, collector, gauze or cotton ball, and adhesive bandage.

(3) Wash hands; don gloves.

(4) Enhance blood supply by applying warmth; do not milk site.

(5) Puncture side of nondominant finger or side of heel.

(6) Puncture with lancet; wipe away first drop of blood; collect sample.

(7) Apply pressure to site; apply bandage.

f. Blood specimen: venipuncture; requires puncture of vein for collection of several milliliters of blood for variety of laboratory tests. Agency certification is usually required.

(1) Explain procedure to patient; warn that it may hurt.

(2) Assemble equipment: gloves, tourniquet, alcohol swabs, sterile gauze pads, tape, a sharps container, appropriate vacuum tubes, vacuum adapter, and double-ended needle.

(3) Wash hands; don gloves.

(4) Hyperextend arm for ease of access to antecubital vein; apply tourniquet; have patient make fist.

(5) Clean site with alcohol; pull skin taut from below site; insert needle (bevel up) at 5-degree angle.

(6) Once needle "pops" into vein, slide vacuum tube onto needle; remove and replace tubes as each fills; remove tourniquet after last tube is filling.

(7) Remove final tube; lay gauze over puncture site, remove needle, and apply pressure to site for at least 5 minutes.

(8) Immediately discard needle into sharps container; label tubes before leaving patient's side.

g. Other specimens

(1) Vomitus: may be tested for blood

(2) Gastric analysis: examination of stomach contents; obtained by aspirating from nasogastric tube

(3) Wound drainage: if infection is suspected

D. Statement of patient problems requiring nursing intervention

1. Identifying unmet basic human needs resulting in a problem for the patient

2. Identifying problems arising from the patient's signs and symptoms

3. Actual problems: those that the patient is currently having

4. Potential problems: those that may develop and should be prevented from occurring

E. Nursing diagnosis: The LPN/LVN assists the RN in formulating nursing diagnosis.

PLANNING PATIENT CARE

A. Definition: process of setting priorities, determining patient-centered goals, and deciding on nursing actions to achieve the goals; ends with writing of the nursing care plan

B. Setting priorities

1. Problems that are life-threatening are of highest priority—use Maslow's hierarchy of needs.

2. When no single problem seems more important than the others, the patient may help determine priorities.

C. Determining goals or expected outcomes

1. Goals or outcomes are stated in terms of patient behavior so achievement can be evaluated easily.

2. Whenever possible, patients should be involved in setting goals.

3. Long-term goals are those hoped for in the future, usually set by the RN.

4. Short-term goals are those sought immediately or in the near future.

D. Decisions about which nursing measures to use are based on sound knowledge of current nursing practice, principles, rationales, and judgment.

E. A written nursing care plan or concept map provides continuity of patient care.

IMPLEMENTATION OF NURSING MEASURES

A. Principles

1. Preparation

a. Nurse must know how, when, and why measure is to be performed, checking for a physician's order when necessary.

b. Patient and family or significant others

(1) To reduce anxiety, patients need to know what measure is to be performed, why it is necessary, and what is expected of them.

(2) A specific measure may need special preparation such as positioning, medications, and attire.

c. Have all necessary equipment ready and in working order.

2. Performance

a. The nurse must have knowledge of and ability to perform the measure and seek help when necessary.

b. Medical asepsis is always followed; surgical asepsis and Standard Precautions are followed as required.

c. Work must be organized to conserve nurse's and patient's energy and to meet patient's need for security.

d. Assessment of patient's response to the measure is ongoing.

3. Aftercare

a. Patient is made safe and comfortable.

b. Equipment is cleaned and returned to proper place or disposed of properly.

c. Results of the measure and whether it helped achieve the goal are evaluated.

4. Reporting and recording: Significant observations are reported immediately; the date and time the measure was performed and the results of the measure are recorded.

EVALUATION OF PLAN OF CARE

A. Criteria for evaluation
   1. Has the need been met?
   2. Is the problem solved or being solved?
   3. Has the goal or expected outcome been achieved?
B. Revision of the nursing care plan
   1. Revision is based on evaluation of effectiveness.
   2. The LPN/LVN collaborates with the RN in revising problem list, goals, and nursing measures.

MEASURES TO MEET OXYGEN NEEDS

A. Assessment: Color of skin or oral mucosa, level of consciousness, vital signs, presence of cough (productive or nonproductive), nature of sputum (amount, consistency, color), energy level, and pulse oximetry reading are assessed. Baseline assessment should be completed at beginning of shift and every 4 hours thereafter.
B. General measures
   1. Encourage exercise and activity to help expand lungs, providing better oxygenation.
   2. Turn and position bedridden patients every 2 hours (q2h) to prevent pooling of secretions in the lungs and capillary congestion that may lead to decubitus ulcer formation because of tissue hypoxia.
   3. Encourage coughing and deep breathing at least every 2 hours for inactive or bedridden patients to help with oxygenation and bringing up secretions.
   4. Ensure adequate fluid intake to keep secretions thin, thus making it easier for the patient to expectorate.
C. Use of nebulizer (aerosol)
   1. The nebulizer is a method of delivering medications directly to the respiratory tract.
   2. It breaks liquids into a mist of droplets, which are inhaled.
D. Incentive spirometer: to improve inspiratory volume
   1. With lips sealed around a mouthpiece, the patient takes a deep breath, holds it for 3 seconds, and slowly exhales.
   2. The spirometer indicates, by a light or small plastic balls reaching an indicated level, whether the patient has inhaled the desired volume.
E. Intermittent positive pressure breathing (IPPB) therapy
   1. IPPB forces the patient to inhale more deeply, allowing better oxygenation and loosening of secretions.
   2. Apparatus may be attached to oxygen or compressed air.
   3. Humidity is provided, usually by normal saline solution.
   4. Medications may be added.
   5. Patient should be sitting up during treatment and encouraged to cough up secretions after treatment.
F. Chest physical therapy
   1. Postural drainage uses various positions so gravity can assist in removal of secretions (Figure 2-8).
   2. Percussion is a manual technique of striking the chest wall over the affected area with cupped hands in a rhythmical motion.

3. Vibration is a manual compression and tremorlike motion with hands or a mechanical device against the chest wall of the affected area done during exhalation.
4. Nurse positions the patient so affected areas are vertical and gravity can assist in drainage.
5. Position also depends on diagnosis and condition.
6. Schedule before or at least 2 hours after meals. Provide emesis basin and tissues and oral hygiene after treatment.
7. This therapy is contraindicated in patients with lung abscess or tumors, pneumothorax, and diseases of the chest wall.
G. Suctioning: oral, nasopharyngeal, or tracheal
   1. It is performed to remove accumulated secretions blocking airway or to obtain a sputum specimen.
   2. It is usually a sterile procedure.
   3. Introduce catheter gently; do not apply suction while introducing catheter.
   4. Suction intermittently for no more than 10 seconds.
   5. Slowly withdraw catheter with a rotating motion while suctioning continues.
   6. Unless copious amounts of secretions are present, wait 30 seconds between suctionings.
   7. Repeat procedure until all excess secretions have been removed.
   8. Administer oxygen before and between suctionings if needed.
H. Administration of oxygen
   1. Safety precautions
      a. Caution patients and visitors that smoking is prohibited.
      b. Post warning sign on door or bed: "NO SMOKING—OXYGEN IN USE."
      c. Do not use heating pads, electric blankets, or electric razors.
      d. Do not use woolen blankets.
      e. Secure oxygen tanks so they do not tip over.
   2. Physician's order is required for method of administration, rate of oxygen flow, and concentration.
   3. Oxygen must always be humidified.
   4. Nasal cannula prongs fit into nares; oxygen is ordered as liters per minute.
      a. Turn oxygen on and check flow through prongs before positioning on patient.
      b. Adjust strap after placing cannula on patient.
      c. Periodically check for sufficient water in humidity source.
      d. Periodically check patient's nares and behind ears for pressure.
      e. Periodically assess patient's oxygen saturation and for changes in condition.
   5. Oxygen by mask: simple mask; Venturi mask (delivers oxygen in precise concentrations) is ordered as percentage of oxygen delivered: (e.g., 40%, 50%) or as liters per minute.
      a. Proceed as with nasal cannula.
      b. Fit mask snugly to face, and adjust strap.
      c. Periodically assess patient and equipment as with nasal cannula.
      d. If condition warrants, an order may be obtained to change mask to nasal cannula for mealtime.
I. Care of patient with a tracheostomy
   1. Tracheotomy is the creation of an opening into the trachea.

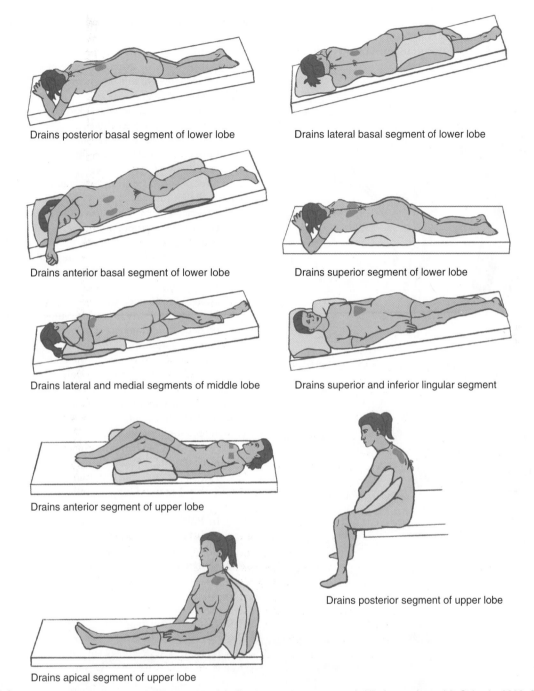

Drains posterior basal segment of lower lobe

Drains lateral basal segment of lower lobe

Drains anterior basal segment of lower lobe

Drains superior segment of lower lobe

Drains lateral and medial segments of middle lobe

Drains superior and inferior lingular segment

Drains anterior segment of upper lobe

Drains posterior segment of upper lobe

Drains apical segment of upper lobe

FIGURE 2-8 Positions for postural drainage. (From deWit SC: *Fundamental concepts and skills for nursing,* ed 3, St Louis, 2009, Saunders.)

2. Tracheostomy is the creation of a tracheal opening for insertion of a tracheal tube.
3. Tube is either metal or plastic; it is usually cuffed (Figures 2-9 and 2-10).
4. Tube is held securely in place with cotton ties around the neck (Figure 2-11).
5. Ties are changed with extreme caution to prevent patient from coughing out tube.
6. A gauze dressing is placed under the tube to absorb secretions; dressing must be changed every shift.
7. Inner cannula is removed, cleaned with peroxide and pipe cleaners, and rinsed with normal saline at least once per shift by sterile technique; commercially prepared kits are available.
8. Skin around stoma is cleansed with normal saline or sterile water and patted dry and assessed at least once per shift.
9. Tube must be suctioned frequently. Patient is often apprehensive and needs frequent reassurance; have pad and pencil nearby for communication purposes.
10. Patient may take oral feedings if ordered; cuff must be inflated at all times.

J. Medication classifications: Refer to Chapter 3 for more detailed information on drugs that affect the respiratory system.

1. Respiratory stimulants
2. Respiratory depressants
3. Medications acting on mucous membranes: administered orally or as spray or vapor
   a. Mucolytics
   b. Expectorants
4. Bronchodilators

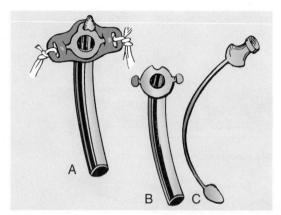

FIGURE 2-9 Metal tracheostomy tube. **A,** Outer cannula. **B,** Inner cannula. **C,** Obturator. (From Harkness GA, Dincher JR: *Medical-surgical nursing: total patient care,* ed 10, St Louis, 2000, Mosby.)

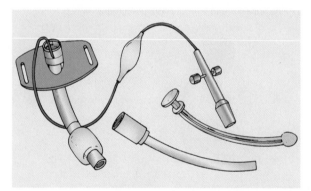

FIGURE 2-10 Cuffed tracheostomy tube. (From Harkness GA, Dincher JR: Medical-surgical nursing: total patient care, ed 10, St Louis, 2000, Mosby.)

MEASURES TO MEET FLUID NEEDS

A. Assessment: daily weights, comparison of intake and output, appearance of urine, presence of edema, fluid preferences, moistness of mucous membranes, skin turgor
B. Fluid excess (edema)
   1. Associated with heart and kidney disease: body unable to rid itself of excess fluid
   2. Can result from excessive intravenous (IV) fluids
   3. Observed as edema, weight gain, and reduced urine output
   4. Sites of edema: eyes, fingers, ankles, sacral area
C. Fluid deficit (dehydration)
   1. Associated with inadequate fluid intake, diarrhea, excessive perspiration, vomiting, bleeding, and increased urine output
   2. Observed as dry skin and mucous membranes, thick mucus, poor skin turgor, behavioral changes, or changes in vital signs
D. Measuring intake and output
   1. Measure all fluids taken: IV fluids; tube feedings; and obvious fluids such as water, milk, ice cream, gelatin, custard, and soup.
   2. Measure all fluids leaving the body: urine, vomitus, diarrhea, gastric secretions, fluids from surgical drains, and blood.
   3. Know capacity of agency fluid containers.
   4. Set measuring containers on level surface to read measurements accurately.
   5. Record and total amounts in appropriate places.
E. Administering IV fluids
   1. Assess site of needle insertion.
      a. Infiltration: Fluid is entering subcutaneous tissues instead of vein; area is pale, cool, and swollen.
      b. Phlebitis: Vein is inflamed; area is red, warm, and swollen.
   2. Assess tubing: there are no kinks; there is no leakage along entire length of tubing; tubing should be labeled and changed every 48 to 72 hours or per agency policy.
   3. Assess rate of flow.

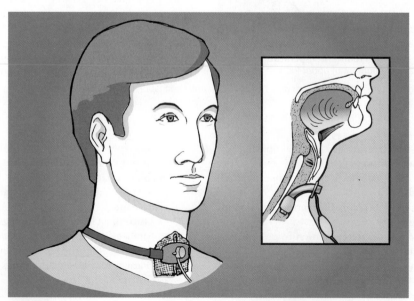

FIGURE 2-11 Tracheostomy tube in place. (From Harkness GA, Dincher JR: *Medical-surgical nursing: total patient care,* ed 10, St Louis, 2000, Mosby.)

4. Assess IV fluids.
   a. The IV fluid hanging must match physician's order.
   b. Check that the amount administered is on schedule.
F. Medication classifications—diuretics: Refer to Chapter 3 for more detailed information.

MEASURES TO MEET NUTRITIONAL NEEDS

A. Assessment: weight/height ratio, weight changes, skin and mucous membranes, food preferences, meal patterns, ability to eat, appetite
B. Preparing for meals
  1. Environment
    a. Control odors, noise, and unpleasant sights; remove soiled equipment and linens.
    b. Avoid stressful situations before and during mealtime.
  2. Patient
    a. Provide opportunity for elimination before tray arrival.
    b. Allow patient to wash hands and complete oral hygiene before meal.
    c. Position comfortably, preferably in sitting position.
  3. Meal tray
    a. Ensure correct tray for correct patient.
    b. Arrange tray to be accessible to patient.
    c. Assist in opening containers, removing covers, and cutting and preparing food.
    d. Serve trays first to patients who are able to feed themselves.
C. Assisting the patient to eat
  1. Place napkin across patient's chest.
  2. Explain what foods and liquids are on the tray.
  3. Prepare foods and feed in order of patient's preference.
  4. Encourage the patient to assist as much as possible.
  5. Do not rush; allow patient time to chew and swallow.
  6. Talk with the patient during meal.
  7. Provide opportunity for handwashing and oral care.
D. Gastric gavage (tube feeding)
  1. Gastric gavage is used when patient is unable to eat, swallow, or take in adequate quantities of food.
  2. Blended foods and fluids (commercially or agency prepared) are passed to the stomach through a nasogastric tube, either intermittently or by slow continuous drip.
  3. Check amount, frequency, and type ordered by physician.
  4. Feeding must be at room temperature before administering.
  5. Placement of tube must be checked before feeding begins.
    a. Nasogastric or nasoduodenal tubes
      (1) Begin by aspirating stomach contents with a syringe.
      (2) Inject 10 mL of air into large-bore feeding tube while simultaneously listening with a stethoscope over the stomach to hear a whooshing sound.
      (3) Obtain radiographic confirmation of small-bore feeding tube before beginning feeding.
    b. Gastrostomy or jejunostomy tubes
      (1) Aspirate stomach contents with a syringe.
      (2) Measure, record, and return aspirated contents.
  6. Place patient in sitting position.
  7. Aspirate tube for stomach contents. Hold feeding if more than 100 mL of residual material is obtained.

8. Administer feeding slowly: 200 mL during 30- to 45-minute period.
9. Feeding should be followed by ordered amount of water.
10. Clamp tube after completion of feeding to prevent air entering stomach.
11. If nausea, vomiting, diarrhea, or cramps occur, rate may be too fast, patient may be intolerant of feeding or volume, or the feeding may be too concentrated.
12. Tube may be left in place between feedings or removed after each feeding as ordered by physician.
13. Have patient remain in sitting position for 45 minutes to help prevent aspiration and facilitate digestion.
E. Medication classifications: Refer to Chapter 3 for more detailed information.
  1. Vitamin supplements
  2. Mineral supplements

MEASURES TO MEET URINARY ELIMINATION NEEDS

A. Assessment: intake/output ratio; color, odor, amount, and consistency of urine; frequency of urination; continence
B. Common problems of urination
  1. Incontinence: inability to control voiding
    a. Requires frequent skin care and linen change
    b. May be reduced with scheduled toileting
    c. May be secondary to medications (diuretics)
  2. Retention: inability to void
    a. If adequate amounts of fluid have been taken in, no more than 8 hours should pass between voidings, except during sleeping hours.
    b. Palpation of bladder can determine distention of full bladder.
    c. Bladder scans can be useful in detecting bladder volume.
  3. Anuria: no urine being produced by the kidneys
  4. Dysuria: difficult or painful urination ("burning")
C. Assisting with urination
  1. Offer bedpan or urinal at regularly scheduled times.
  2. Keep bedpan or urinal and toilet tissue within easy reach for patients who can assist themselves.
  3. Keep call signal within easy reach.
  4. Provide privacy.
  5. Hearing the sound of running water or having warm water poured over the perineum may induce voiding.
  6. Provide opportunity for handwashing after urination.
D. Care of patient with retention catheter
  1. Presence of indwelling catheter greatly predisposes patient to urinary tract infection.
  2. Opening a closed urinary system is to be avoided.
  3. Drainage container must be kept below level of the bladder but must not touch the floor.
  4. Drainage tubing must be free of kinks; catheter should be taped to patient's leg, allowing for slack.
  5. Drainage container is emptied at end of shift or if container becomes nearly full; urine is measured and assessed and the amount recorded.
  6. Catheter care is given at least once per shift and after every bowel movement.
    a. Meatus and catheter are cleansed with soap and water, from meatus down catheter and away from body.

b. Removal of crusts and secretions from meatus and catheter may require use of hydrogen peroxide.

c. A bacteriostatic ointment is often ordered to be applied to the meatus.

7. Unless contraindicated, fluid intake should reach 2000 to 3000 mL/24 hr.

E. Catheterization

1. "Straight": Catheter is removed at end of procedure (intermittent catheterization). Procedure is often ordered to relieve urine retention (common after surgery or childbirth), obtain a sterile urine specimen, or measure residual urine after voiding.

2. Indwelling, retention, or Foley: Catheter is left in place in bladder.

3. Assemble equipment: sterile catheterization tray or disposable kit containing catheter, basin, container with lid (for specimen, if ordered), cotton balls, antiseptic solution, lubricant, sterile gloves, and drape.

4. For indwelling catheterization, add Foley catheter, syringe, solution for inflating balloon, drainage bag with tubing, and tape for securing catheter.

5. After explaining procedure to patient and ensuring privacy, place female patient in dorsal recumbent position and male patient in supine position.

6. Place equipment on an over-the-bed table or between patient's legs; using sterile technique, open package, don gloves, and place drape.

7. For female patient, while holding labia apart, cleanse vulva and meatus well, going from front to back toward vagina; use cotton ball for one stroke only before discarding.

8. For male patient cleanse around penis from meatus toward base using each cotton ball once around.

9. Insert catheter into meatus (3 to 4 inches [7.5 to 10 cm] in female patient and 6 to 8 inches [15 to 20 cm] in male patient) until urine flows. Advance catheter 1 inch more and drain urine (no more than 750 mL at one time to prevent hypovolemic shock). Remove catheter ("straight") or inflate balloon and connect drainage tubing (indwelling).

F. Intermittent bladder irrigation (hand bladder irrigation)

1. To rid bladder and catheter of clots or mucus; to instill antibiotic or other solutions

2. Open technique

a. Assemble equipment: sterile solution (type and amount as ordered), sterile container for solution, bulb syringe, and basin for return flow.

b. Disconnect catheter from drainage tube over empty basin; protect ends from contamination.

c. Allow solution to flow in by gravity or gentle pressure; drain by gravity or gentle suction; repeat until returns are clear or ordered amount of solution has been used.

d. Subtract amount of solution used from amount of returns; record output.

3. Closed technique

a. Assemble equipment: 20- to 30-mL syringe with needle, alcohol swabs, solution ordered, and clamp.

b. Draw solution into syringe by sterile technique.

c. Clamp tubing distal to needle entry point.

d. Cleanse resealable rubber entry port on drainage tubing with alcohol swab.

e. Insert needle into port.

f. Inject fluid into catheter.

g. Remove needle.

h. Release clamp and allow fluid to drain into drainage bag.

i. Observe fluid return.

j. Repeat until ordered amount of solution has been used.

k. Empty drainage bag, subtracting amount of irrigant from total; record urine output.

G. Continuous bladder irrigation (through-and-through or three-way irrigation)

1. To prevent clot formation, reduce obstruction of catheter, and circulate antibiotic or other solutions continuously in bladder.

2. Equipment: Patient has three-way catheter or needs sterile Y-tube connector attached to drainage channel of the regular two-way catheter; large bottle or bag of solution with tubing attached hanging from IV pole.

3. With three-way catheter: Using sterile technique

a. Remove plug from irrigating channel; protect plug and tubing from contamination.

b. Insert solution tubing into irrigating channel.

4. With two-way catheter: Using sterile technique

a. Attach single end of sterile Y-tube connector to catheter.

b. Attach drainage tubing to one end of Y.

c. Attach solution tubing to other end of Y.

5. Start solution flow at rate ordered by physician.

6. Observe fluid return through drainage tubing.

7. Replace solution bottle or bag when it becomes nearly empty.

8. Empty drainage container when it becomes nearly full and when solution container is replaced.

9. Subtract amount of irrigant solution from total amount of drainage to record actual urine output.

H. Removal of indwelling catheter

1. Assemble equipment: syringe without needle, underpad, basin, urinal or bedpan, toilet tissue, and protective gloves.

2. After explaining procedure and ensuring privacy, place pad under patient.

3. Remove tape from catheter and patient's leg.

4. Put on protective gloves.

5. Place basin under patient's meatus.

6. Insert syringe into balloon channel; fluid will return on its own.

7. After all fluid has returned, gently pull on catheter to remove it.

8. If resistance is met, stop and obtain assistance from the RN.

9. Help patient wash perineum.

10. Teaching

a. Patient should continue to drink fluids.

b. Burning on urination may occur during first few voidings.

c. Complete continence and normal voiding pattern may take time to return.

d. Instruct patient to void into bedpan or urinal so the color, consistency, and amount of urine can be assessed.

11. Encourage relaxation: anxiety may inhibit ability to void.

12. Continue to assess bladder distention, intake/output ratio, and patient complaints until normal patterns of elimination have been achieved.

I. Straining urine for calculi—patients who have suspected renal calculi should have each urine specimen strained for the presence of stones. Use small-gauze filter and send any material retrieved to the laboratory.

J. Medication classifications
   1. Cholinergics: to induce bladder contraction (bethanechol [Urecholine], neostigmine [Prostigmin])
   2. Anticholinergics: to reduce bladder spasms and urinary frequency (tolterodine [Detrol], flavoxate hydrochloride [Urispas])

MEASURES TO MEET BOWEL ELIMINATION NEEDS

A. Assessment: the patient's pattern of elimination; amount, color, consistency, odor, and shape of stool; patient's activity level; amount and type of food and fluid intake; passage of flatus; abdominal distention

B. Common problems of elimination
   1. Constipation: passage of dry, hard feces
   2. Diarrhea: frequent passage of liquid or unformed stools
   3. Impaction: formation of a hardened mass of stool in the lower bowel, forming an obstruction to the passage of normal stool; often characterized by the frequent seepage of small amount of liquid stool
   4. Abdominal distention: swollen abdomen caused by retention of flatus in the intestines; generally accompanied by a lack of bowel sounds (peristalsis); sometimes referred to as an *ileus* or *paralytic ileus*

C. General nursing measures
   1. Encourage intake of roughage in the diet: fresh fruits and vegetables and whole grain breads and cereals.
   2. Encourage intake of adequate amounts of fluids unless contraindicated: 2000 to 3000 mL/day.
   3. Encourage maximum amount of physical activity.
   4. Encourage patient to respond to the urge to defecate.
   5. Position patient comfortably and provide adequate time and privacy for elimination.
   6. Provide access to call signal and toilet tissue.
   7. Provide opportunity for handwashing after elimination.

D. Rectal tube
   1. Rectal tube is used to assist in expelling flatus.
   2. Assemble equipment: rectal tube with flatus bag or waterproof pad, lubricant, glove, and tape.
   3. After explaining procedure and providing privacy, position patient in left lateral (Sims) position.
   4. With gloved hand, insert lubricated tube 2 to 4 inches (5 to 10 cm) into rectum.
   5. Tape tube to patient's buttock and leave in place no longer than 20 to 30 minutes.
   6. Note passage of flatus or stool; report and record findings.

E. Rectal suppository
   1. Rectal suppositories are used to stimulate peristalsis and aid stool elimination, soothe painful rectum or anus, and administer medications.
   2. Assemble equipment: suppository as ordered, glove, lubricant, bedpan, toilet tissue.
   3. Suppository begins to melt at room temperature, providing its own lubrication.
   4. Separate buttocks and with gloved, lubricated index finger insert pointed end of suppository into anus.
   5. Gently insert 3 to 4 inches (7.5 to 10 cm) into rectum.
   6. Hold buttocks together until initial urge to defecate has passed.
   7. Best results occur within 30 minutes.

F. Commercially prepared prefilled enema
   1. Commercially prepared prefilled enemas are used to promote bowel or flatus movement.
   2. Assemble equipment: enema (usually 120 mL), underpad, bedpan, toilet paper, gloves.
   3. After explaining procedure and providing privacy, place patient in left lateral (Sims) position.
   4. With gloved hand, insert prelubricated tip of enema to the hub and squeeze container until most of solution is instilled.
   5. Encourage patient to retain solution until urge to defecate is felt.
   6. Place call signal, bedpan, and toilet tissue within easy reach.
   7. If patient uses toilet, instruct not to flush so results can be assessed.

G. Oil-retention enema
   1. Oil-retention enemas are used to soften and lubricate stool, promoting easier passage.
   2. Oil-retention enemas are often followed by cleansing enema.
   3. Equipment and administration are the same as those for previously mentioned commercially prepared enema.
   4. Encourage patient to retain oil 30 to 60 minutes.

H. Cleansing enemas
   1. Cleansing enemas are used to relieve constipation or flatus or to cleanse the bowel before diagnostic procedures, surgery, or childbirth.
   2. Solutions are used as ordered by physician.
      a. Tap water: can cause fluid and electrolyte imbalance.
      b. Soap solution: 5 mL of liquid soap to 1000 mL of water; can irritate mucous membranes of bowel.
      c. Saline solution: can cause fluid and electrolyte imbalance.
   3. Assemble equipment: disposable enema kit containing enema bag, tubing with clamp, liquid soap, and lubricant; waterproof underpad; solution at a temperature no greater than 105° F (40.56° C); bedpan and toilet tissue; IV pole; protective gloves.
   4. After explaining procedure and providing privacy, place patient in left lateral (Sims) position.
   5. Put on protective gloves.
   6. Insert lubricated tubing about 3 to 5 inches (7.5 to 12.5 cm) into rectum.
   7. With bottom of enema bag hanging 12 inches (30 cm) above anus or 18 inches (45 cm) above mattress, slowly administer 500 to 1000 mL of solution.
   8. If patient complains of cramping or has difficulty retaining solution:
      a. Slow administration rate by lowering bag, or temporarily stop flow.
      b. Encourage slow, deep breathing through the mouth.
   9. After fluid has been administered, assist patient to bathroom or onto bedpan or commode; instruct patient not to flush toilet so results can be assessed.

10. If enemas are ordered "until clear," repeat procedure until returns are clear of stool (or barium-after-barium enema).
11. Observe patient during procedure for signs of weakness or fatigue, which would necessitate stopping the procedure to allow rest.

I. Digital removal of fecal impaction
1. Digital removal of fecal impaction is used for breaking up the hard fecal mass and removing it.
2. Assemble equipment: gloves, waterproof underpad, lubricant, bedpan.
3. Liberally lubricate gloved index finger.
4. With patient in left lateral (Sims) position, gently insert finger into hardened mass of stool.
5. Gently break off small pieces of the stool, bringing them out and placing them in the bedpan.
6. Assess patient for signs of weakness and fatigue; this is an uncomfortable, tiring procedure and may need to be stopped intermittently.
7. Assist patient to bedpan: disimpaction may induce defecation.

J. Colostomy irrigation
1. Colostomy irrigation is used to regulate the discharge and drainage of fecal contents and flatus.
2. Time of irrigation depends on physician's order and patient's own established routine; when colostomy has become regulated, irrigation may only be done every other day; some patients never irrigate their colostomy.
3. Assemble equipment:
   a. Irrigating appliance (types vary)
   b. Irrigating container (enema bag)
   c. Tubing and catheter (may be part of enema kit)
   d. Irrigating solution: usually 500 to 1000 mL of tap water or physiological saline solution at 100° F (37.78° C)
   e. Lubricant
   f. Drainage bag (may be part of irrigating appliance) and bedpan if not using on toilet
   g. Waterproof underpad if being performed in bed
   h. Fresh colostomy appliance, dressing, or stoma pad
   i. IV pole
   j. Protective gloves
4. After explaining procedure and ensuring privacy, place patient on toilet (most convenient) or in bed in left lateral (Sims) position.
5. Put on protective gloves.
6. Raise irrigation container 18 inches (45 cm) above stoma, clear catheter of air, lubricate catheter, introduce it through irrigating appliance, and insert it into stoma 2 to 6 inches (5 to 15 cm); do not advance if resistance is met.
7. Allow solution to flow slowly and remove catheter; return is usually completed within 45 to 60 minutes.
8. When return is completed, remove irrigating appliance; wash and dry abdomen; and apply fresh colostomy appliance, dressing, or stoma pad as indicated.
9. Record character and amount of returns, patient's tolerance, and degree of assistance provided by patient.

K. Medication classifications: Refer to Chapter 3 for more detailed information on drugs that affect the gastrointestinal (GI) system.
1. Stool softeners
2. Laxatives, cathartics
3. Antidiarrheals

MEASURES TO MEET REST AND SLEEP NEEDS

Rest and sleep are necessary for restoring physical and mental well-being, reducing stress and anxiety, and maintaining the ability to attend to and concentrate on activities of life.

A. Assessment: normal number of hours of sleep, usual bedtime, usual bedtime habits or practices, sleep difficulties, daytime fatigue, usual methods of obtaining rest, sleep medications being used
B. Physician's orders for rest must be clarified: Is bed rest ordered to provide rest for a damaged heart, the entire body, or an injured part such as a foot?
C. Providing for rest and sleep
1. Promote relaxation: Provide diversions, pain relief, clean and wrinkle-free bed, a noise-free and odor-free room, and easy access to bedside equipment and call signal; give a relaxing back rub. Measures such as meditation and yoga can promote relaxation and sleep.
2. Reduce patient's anxiety level by allowing time for him or her to talk about stressful or fear-producing situations.
3. If possible, position patient in usual sleeping position with amount of covers desired.
4. Plan and organize care to allow patient uninterrupted rest and sleep periods.
5. Give sleeping medication or herbal preparations if ordered and if required by patient.
D. Sleep disturbances
1. Sleep apnea: a disorder that occurs when an individual sleeps, characterized by periods of apnea (absence of spontaneous respiration) during sleep that cause daytime tiredness and fatigue
2. Narcolepsy: a disorder that involves the patient falling asleep while performing activities, which can be dangerous
E. Medication classifications: Refer to Chapter 3 for more detailed information.
1. Sedatives: to reduce anxiety
2. Hypnotics: to induce sleep

MEASURES TO MEET ACTIVITY AND EXERCISE NEEDS

Physical activity is necessary for proper functioning of all body systems and promotion of emotional well-being; immobility can lead to physical and emotional disability.

A. Assessment: posture, ability to walk, ability to turn and move in bed, usual activity level, skin condition
B. Patient's activity and exercise levels are ordered by the physician.
1. Bed rest (BR): Patient is confined to bed.
2. Bathroom privileges (BRP): Although confined to bed, patient may perform urinary and bowel elimination in the bathroom.
3. May dangle: Although confined to bed, patient may sit on edge of bed with legs and feet hanging down over side of bed and supported by footstool.
   a. Order is often accompanied by orders for frequency and duration of dangling time (e.g., dangle every shift for 10 minutes).

b. Provide footstool.

c. Assess vital signs.

d. Stay with patient to assess tolerance and assist back to bed.

4. Allow to chair: Although patient may sit in chair, he or she is not permitted to ambulate any farther.

5. Out of bed (OOB) ad lib: Patient can and should perform as much activity out of bed as desired.

6. Encourage patient to perform as many activities as orders permit.

C. Dangers of immobility

1. Atelectasis: collapse of lung caused by reduced depth and rate of respirations or obstruction of lungs by excessive secretions

2. Hypostatic pneumonia: caused by pooling of lung secretions and the resulting congestion and infection

3. Thrombus formation: caused by reduced rate of blood flow through the veins and prolonged coagulation time

4. Constipation: caused by slowed peristaltic action

5. Contractures: permanent shortening of muscles, leading to joint immobility

6. Skin breakdown and decubitus ulcer formation: caused by prolonged pressure and reduced circulation to an area

7. Urinary tract infections and kidney stones: caused by stasis of urine and demineralization of bones

D. Measures to prevent dangers of immobility

1. Coughing and deep breathing

a. Measures are performed every 2 hours.

b. Patient should be in semi-Fowler position and take 10 deep breaths followed by deep cough to raise secretions.

2. Turning and repositioning every 2 hours

3. Range-of-motion (ROM) exercises: to maintain full range and flexibility of joint movement

a. Performed 8 to 10 times on each joint at least once every day.

b. Passive range of motion (PROM): performed for the patient.

c. Active range of motion (AROM): performed by the patient.

d. Each joint is put through all of its possible movements (Figure 2-12).

4. Maintaining adequate fluid intake (2000 to 3000 mL/day)

5. Providing for adequate nutritional intake

6. Performing frequent skin care; keeping skin clean, dry, and lubricated

E. Devices used to help prevent dangers of immobility

1. Footboard: prevents plantar flexion (foot drop).

a. Soles of patient's feet are flat against board and in proper alignment.

b. Board should be padded.

2. Bed cradle: keeps weight of bed covers off a body part.

3. Alternating pressure mattress: changes pressure on body parts in contact with the mattress.

a. Only one layer of loosely pulled linen should be between mattress and patient.

b. Keep pins and other pointed objects away from this mattress.

4. Sheepskin: provides a soft surface, reducing skin abrasion.

5. Special beds such as the CircOlectric: allow patient's position to be changed more readily.

6. Sequential compression devices prevent thrombophlebitis. Other terms are *sequential TED hose, Venodynes*.

7. Antiembolism stockings.

8. Canes: are used for extra stability, support, and balance; should be used in the hand opposite the affected extremity and advanced at the same time as that extremity.

9. Crutches: are useful in assisting with the mobility needs of patients with disorders of the lower extremities; several crutch gaits can be used.

a. For balance: Crutches can be used as a source of balance when patient has full weight bearing on both legs.

b. For mobility: When patient has partial weight bearing on one extremity, the opposite crutch is advanced at the same time as that extremity so weight can be born on the crutch instead of the extremity.

c. Rules for crutches: Length is very important. The crutch should come within two fingerbreadths of the axilla of the individual. Weight is distributed on the handgrips, not the axillary area. Physical therapy teaches crutch walking, but nurses must reinforce teaching.

10. Walkers: are used for stability, mostly in the older population. Proper technique for using a walker should be taught and reinforced.

a. Push up from a seated position without using the walker; the walker may tip if the patient pulls himself or herself to a standing position with the walker.

b. The height of the walker should be such that the patient has a 30-degree bend to the arm while ambulating.

c. The patient should place his or her weight on the walker if he or she has compromised strength or mobility in one of the extremities.

MEASURES TO MEET PAIN RELIEF NEEDS

Individuals (including nurses) vary in their perception of and response to pain. Pain is often intensified in the presence of anxiety and fatigue and the absence of distraction.

A. Assessment: intensity, onset, duration, quality, and location of pain; patient's nonverbal responses to pain—behavior, change in vital signs, nausea; factors associated with the pain—activity and visitors; pain relief measures. Nurses should use a scale of 1 to 10 to gauge intensity of pain. Level 1 would be very little pain; level 10 would signify excruciating pain.

B. Therapeutic relationship may help reduce anxiety, thus reducing pain level.

C. Alter contributing factors: Relieve constipation and nausea; eliminate environmental disturbances such as bright lights, odors, and noise.

D. Provide diversional activities: television, radio, and visitors.

E. Reposition, give back rub, and tighten linens.

F. Apply heat or cold if ordered.

G. Encourage relaxation.

1. To reduce muscle tension

2. First need:

a. A comfortable position

b. A quiet environment

c. A focus on something outside the body such as a word to repeat, an object to examine, or something to imagine

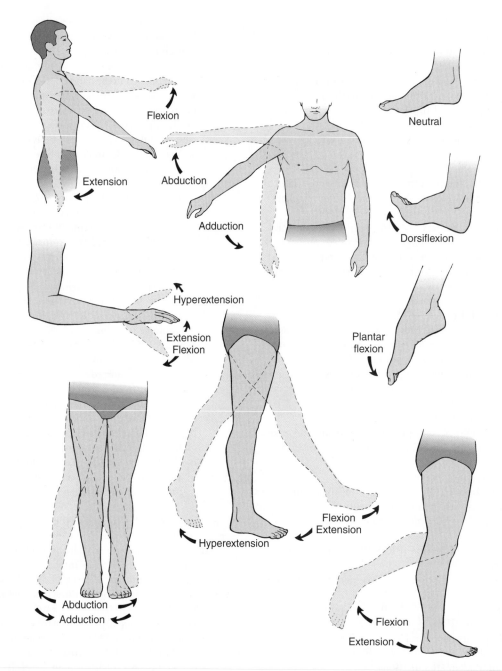

FIGURE 2-12 Range of joint motions. (From Beare PG, Myers JL: *Adult health nursing,* ed 3, St Louis, 1998, Mosby.)

3. Techniques
   a. Exercises in which various muscle groups are alternately tensed and relaxed
   b. Exercises in which various muscle groups are alternately stretched and relaxed
   c. Breathing techniques similar to those used in the Lamaze method of childbirth (controlled and focused)
   d. Biofeedback: learning to control normally autonomic body functions
      (1) Muscle tension is monitored.
      (2) Subject receives feedback about the success of attempts to control functions.
   e. Massage therapy: effective complementary and alternative therapy, especially for muscle tension
   f. Meditation and yoga: complementary therapies that are successful in decreasing some patients' pain perceptions
H. Transcutaneous electrical nerve stimulation (TENS) is a method in which a small, battery-operated device provides continuous mild electric current to skin.
   1. Clean skin with alcohol before applying electrodes on or around pain site.
   2. No tingling indicates that controls are too low; pain or muscle spasm indicates that controls are too high.
I. Medication classifications: Refer to Chapter 3 for more detailed information.
   1. Placebo: inactive substance administered to satisfy the patient's need for a drug

a. Pain relief after administration is probably a result of anxiety reduction.

b. Relief felt after administration of a placebo does not mean that pain did not exist.

2. Analgesics

a. Narcotics

b. Nonnarcotics

MEASURES TO MEET SAFETY AND HYGIENE NEEDS

Although individuals are usually capable of meeting safety and hygiene needs themselves, in strange environments and times of stress and illness, help is often needed. Individuals need protection from injury, maintenance of intact skin and mucous membranes and of body alignment, and structure and order in their environment.

A. Assessment

1. Protection from injury: level of consciousness, ability to move, and knowledge of environment, equipment, and patient's medications

2. Maintenance of intact skin and mucous membranes and alignment: personal hygiene; condition of skin, mucous membranes, joints, and posture

3. Structure and order in the environment: arrangement of personal belongings, cleanliness of patient's unit, environmental conditions, potential hazards

B. Measures to protect from injury

1. Bed side rails: use whenever bed is above its lowest level; use for patients who are unconscious, sedated with narcotics, disoriented, confused, or children; may need a physician's order because side rails are considered a restraint.

2. Call signal: should always be within patient's reach; patient should know how to use it.

3. Restraints (patient protectors or patient protective devices)

a. Restraints require physician's order to place and remove unless an emergency exists and patient is in immediate need of protection.

b. Restraints are used to restrict movement of the individual or of one or more extremities.

c. Explain to patient and family why restraint is being used.

d. Remain quiet and calm while applying restraint to reduce patient's fear and stress.

e. Apply restraint securely enough to provide protection but loosely enough to permit circulation and lung expansion.

f. Periodically check pulses and skin integrity distal to the restrained extremity (radial, pedal pulses).

g. Continue to provide patient with all necessary nursing care, including turning, fluids, hygiene, and opportunity for elimination.

h. Secure restraint to bed frame rather than to bed rail.

i. Types of restraints

(1) Sheet around waist to secure patient in chair

(2) Jacket or vest, mitts, ankle and wrist restraints

(3) Safety belts

j. Measures to avoid restraints

(1) Reorientation measures

(2) Alarms and monitors

(3) Specialized chairs

4. Reduce environmental hazards.

a. Proper care of hospital equipment

(1) Equipment should be stored properly.

(2) All apparatus, equipment, and furnishings should be kept in good repair.

(3) All apparatus, equipment, and furnishings should be used correctly.

b. Prevention of fire

(1) Properly care for and use electrical equipment.

(2) Prohibit smoking in bed.

(3) Observe oxygen safety measures.

(4) Use RACE acronym if fire occurs.

R—Rescue anyone closest to the fire.

A—Pull alarm or notify the operator.

C—Confine the fire, shut doors, and block off fire.

E—Extinguish the fire using a fire extinguisher aimed at the base of the flames.

c. Prevention of accidents

(1) Keep floor dry, clean, and free of litter.

(2) Place rubber tips on crutches, canes, and walkers.

(3) Dispose of dressings and needles properly.

(4) Have frequent fire drills.

(5) Lock wheels on beds, wheelchairs, and stretchers.

(6) Maintain good lighting.

d. Protection from microorganisms and pests

(1) Use proper handwashing and maintain medical asepsis.

(2) Disinfect and sterilize properly.

(3) Minimize food storage in patient unit.

5. Transferring patient from bed

a. Protect from falling by using transfer belt and having patient wear sturdy shoes rather than slippers.

b. Two or three people may be required to transfer helpless or heavy patients.

c. Be sure that bed and stretcher wheels and wheelchairs are in locked position.

d. Make use of lifting devices such as Hoyer lift.

e. Use good body mechanics.

C. Measures to promote and maintain intact skin and mucous membranes

1. Bed making: dry, tight, wrinkle-free bed helps maintain skin integrity and provide for comfort.

a. Assemble equipment: sheets, spread, blanket, pillow, and pillow covering.

b. Care of soiled linens

(1) Always place on a surface above floor or in individual laundry bags.

(2) Deposit in linen hamper (disposable "linens" are available and used especially for patients with communicable diseases).

c. Types of bed making

(1) Closed bed is made in preparation for new patient.

(2) Open bed is occupied, but patient is out of bed.

(3) Occupied bed is made with patient in it.

(4) Fracture or orthopedic bed is made from head to foot.

(5) Postanesthetic or recovery bed is made to receive patient easily from stretcher (Figure 2-13).

d. Bed positions

(1) Low Fowlers: Head is raised (gatched) 18 to 20 inches (45 to 50 cm) above flat bed level.

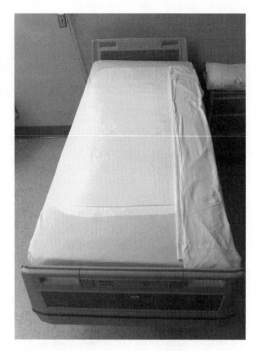

FIGURE 2-13 Postanesthesia unit ready to accept patient. (From Sorrentino SA, Remmert L, Gorek B: *Mosby's essentials for nursing assistants*, ed 4, St. Louis, 2010, Mosby.)

    (2) Semi-Fowlers: Head is raised 45 degrees, and knee is gatched 15 degrees.

    (3) High Fowler: Head of bed is raised to a 90-degree angle.

    (4) Trendelenburg: Head is lower than the level of the feet (no gatch).

2. Daily bath
   a. Clean, dry, intact, and healthy skin and mucous membranes are first line of defense against microorganisms.
   b. Bath time is also important for establishing relationship with patient and for assessment.
   c. Some patients do not desire, need, or require complete bath each day.
   d. Bed bath is given to the patient who is restricted to bed or helpless to bathe self.
   e. Assisted bath: Patient bathes as much of self as possible; may need assistance with back, feet, legs, and perineum.
   f. Tub bath or shower is for patient who is capable of doing so; a physician's order is required.
   g. Commercial sponge bath packets contain moisturizing cleansing agent; they are warmed in microwave and decrease heat loss, skin drying, exposure, and task time.

3. Skin care
   a. Use soap sparingly; rinse well with warm water; pat skin dry.
   b. Lotions prevent dry skin.
   c. Gently massage bony prominences with lotion to promote circulation.
   d. Use deodorant or antiperspirant as necessary.
   e. Avoid heavy use of powder, which can cake, causing skin irritation.

4. Mouth care
   a. Routine mouth care involves use of toothbrush, mouthwash, or substitutes.
   b. Special mouth care involves more frequent routine care plus the judicious use of glycerin and lemon swabs or hydrogen peroxide if ordered.
   c. Unconscious patient
      (1) Have suction at the bedside.
      (2) Turn the patient on his or her side with head up and to the side.
      (3) Use soft Toothettes to clean mouth.
      (4) Make sure that all liquid is drained or suctioned from mouth to decrease chance of aspiration.
   d. Care of dentures
      (1) Clean dentures over towel-lined basin of water to reduce chance of breakage if dropped.
      (2) Hold dentures with gauze or cloth to prevent dropping.
      (3) Clean with tepid water; hot water may change shape.
      (4) Store dentures in clearly marked denture cup with tepid water in drawer of bedside stand when not in patient's mouth.

5. Hair care
   a. Comb or brush daily; groom as desired.
   b. If tangled:
      (1) Use 95% alcohol for oily hair.
      (2) Use mineral oil for dry hair.
      (3) Start at ends, working toward scalp.
      (4) Hold hair close to head to prevent pulling.
   c. Braid long hair if not objectionable to patient.
   d. Shampoo as often as necessary and as patient's condition permits.
   e. Give pediculosis (lice) treatment as ordered by physician.
      (1) Commercial preparations are available.
      (2) Use fine-toothed comb to remove nits (eggs).
      (3) Patient may be isolated to avoid spread.

6. Nail care: Perform daily and as indicated; physician's order is necessary to cut nails; extreme care must be used for patients with diabetes or circulatory problems.
   a. Scrub under nails as necessary.
   b. Cut nails even with tips of fingers and toes.
   c. Round fingernails to curve with fingertips.
   d. Cut toenails straight across.

7. Shaving: Male patients may want to shave while they are in the hospital.
   a. Check with RN to make sure that patient can be shaved with a razor; if he is taking anticoagulants or has a bleeding disorder, shaving may be contraindicated.
   b. Soften beard with a warm washcloth.
   c. Apply shaving lotion.
   d. Shave in the direction of hair growth.
   e. Cleanse face with warm washcloth after completion.

8. Decubitus (pressure) ulcer care: Assess areas over all bony prominences such as sacrum, heels, elbows, hips, and shoulder blades, and along edges of casts and braces.
   a. Contributing factors
      (1) Crumbs or food particles in the bed
      (2) Exposure to moisture such as urine
      (3) Wrinkles in sheets

(4) Unrelieved pressure for longer than 2 hours

(5) Conditions that restrict movement

(6) Poor nutritional, circulatory, or fluid balance status

b. Treatment

(1) "An ounce of prevention is worth a pound of cure"—turn and reposition every 2 hours.

(2) Identify high-risk patients.

(3) Report and initiate care for beginning signs of redness, whiteness, or breaks in skin.

(4) Use devices such as sheepskin, egg-crate mattress, alternating-pressure mattress, water mattress, or Clinitron bed.

(5) Avoid using waterproof underpads.

(6) Use special cleansing agents and dressings as ordered by physician or as indicated by agency policy.

9. Use turning sheet to move and turn patient with minimum of friction, which may cause abrasions.

D. Measures to maintain body alignment

1. Encourage good posture while sitting, standing, and lying.

2. Bed-lying positions

a. Supine: lying on back

b. Prone: lying on abdomen with head turned to the side

c. Side-lying (Sims): lying on side with upper hip and knee sharply flexed

3. Reposition patient at least every 2 hours.

4. Guidelines for proper positioning

a. Normal body curves must be supported by small pillows or pads; use "bridging" techniques.

b. Joints that are normally flexed need support.

c. Bony prominences need to be protected from pressure; place pillows between knees in Sims position.

d. Use devices such as sandbags or rolls to keep joints and body parts positioned.

e. Periodically check patient for discomfort or difficulties.

f. Ensure that patient can reach call signal.

E. Measures to promote structure and order in the patient's environment

1. Physical factors

a. Lighting

(1) Lighting should be indirect except for reading or for procedures.

(2) General lighting should be diffused.

(3) Sunlight promotes healing and feeling of well-being.

b. Waste disposal: Trash, human excretions, and soiled dressings and linens should be discarded according to agency procedures.

2. Alternative and complementary therapies

a. Sound

(1) Music therapy promotes rest and relaxation.

(2) Noise causes fatigue and anxiety.

b. Décor

(1) Pastel colors (yellow or pink) are soothing and relaxing.

(2) Harsh colors (red or black) overstimulate senses.

(3) Flowers and pictures enhance environment.

c. Odors

(1) Foul or strong odors should be eliminated by means of room deodorizer or removal of causative agent.

(2) Mild, fragrant odors reduce antiseptic smell and patient embarrassment.

d. Privacy: Curtains, screens, and proper draping should be used as indicated to reduce embarrassment and protect patient dignity.

3. Care of the environment: varies according to agency policy

a. Responsibilities of housekeeping and ancillary services (central supply and maintenance)

(1) Daily damp dusting and floor cleaning

(2) Scrubbing, disinfecting, sterilizing, and storing of equipment after patient transfer, discharge, or death

(3) Repairing or replacing defective equipment or furnishings

b. Responsibilities of the nursing personnel

(1) Place bedside table, call signal, telephone, and personal articles within patient's reach.

(2) Straighten and damp dust bedside unit (includes care of flowers).

(3) Care for patient belongings (clothing, valuables, glasses, dentures, prostheses).

(4) Prevent cross-infection between patients.

OTHER THERAPEUTIC NURSING MEASURES

WOUND CARE

A. Cleaning the wound: if a wound culture is ordered, always obtain the specimen before cleansing.

1. Commonly used antiseptics

a. 70% alcohol

b. Povidone-iodine (Betadine)

2. Hydrogen peroxide is used to remove dry and crusted secretions.

3. Always clean from innermost to outermost aspect of wound.

B. Wound irrigation

1. Wound irrigation is used to remove secretions or excessive discharge from surfaces or body cavities or to apply moist heat. Remove dead tissue to clean wound (débride).

2. Clean or sterile technique may be used, depending on area to be irrigated.

3. Assemble equipment: may vary according to area to be irrigated (disposable kits are available).

a. Container to hold irrigating solution

b. Container for return flow of solution

c. Irrigating solution

d. Irrigator: usually bulb syringe or large plunger-type syringe

e. Protection for patient and linens; may use waterproof disposable pads

f. Gloves, masks, and goggles if needed

g. Replacement dressing if indicated

C. Dressing changes

1. Dressing: material placed on a wound or incision to protect, absorb drainage, or promote healing

2. Dressings classified by method of application

a. Clean

b. Sterile

c. Moist or dry

3. Disposable kits or hospital-assembled kits
4. Types of dressing material
   a. Gauze
   b. Petrolatum gauze
   c. Telfa
5. Material for securing dressings
   a. Tape: in various widths
      (1) Adhesive
      (2) Paper
      (3) Nonallergenic
   b. Montgomery straps
   c. Bandages and binders
6. Nurse may be responsible for changing dressing or assisting physician in changing dressing.
7. Initial change of postoperative dressing is done by physician unless an order specifies otherwise.
8. Dressings that are not to be changed should be reinforced with additional material if drainage seeps through.

D. Care of patient with wound infection
1. Infection may be local (confined to wound) or systemic (generalized throughout body), often depending on the causative organism.
2. Signs of local infection result from increased circulation and accumulation of waste in the area.
   a. Redness, heat, pain, and swelling
      (1) Dehiscence: The wound edges have pulled apart, and wound approximation is lacking.
      (2) Evisceration: The wound edges are apart, and organs (viscera) are protruding through the wound; apply moist saline-soaked gauze until physician arrives.
   b. Purulent drainage
   c. Loss of function
   d. Changes in vital signs
3. Signs of systemic infection
   a. Increase in temperature, pulse, and respirations (TPR); possible decrease in BP
   b. Nausea and vomiting
   c. General malaise
   d. Loss of appetite
4. Basic principles of treatment
   a. Physical and mental rest
   b. Rest and elevation of infected limb (if applicable)
   c. Application of heat or cold
5. Special treatment may include:
   a. Medications (sulfonamides, antibiotics)
   b. Incision and drainage of wound
   c. Débridement: removal of foreign, infected, or necrotic tissue
6. Infection control committee investigates and follows up on infections occurring in an agency.

BANDAGES

A. Bandages are applied to give support, immobilize a part, apply pressure, or hold dressings.
B. Types of bandages
1. Strips or rolls of gauze, cotton flannel, or elastic material
2. Variable widths, depending on purpose and part to be bandaged
C. Types of basic turns in bandaging
1. Circular
2. Spiral
3. Spiral reverse
4. Recurrent
5. Figure-of-eight
D. Safety factors
1. Apply in direction from distal to proximal.
2. Apply tightly enough to serve purpose but loosely enough to permit circulation (presence of pulse).
3. Do not fasten over bony prominence, area of pressure, or a wound.
4. The part being bandaged should remain in functional position.
5. Triangular bandage, cravat, or sling is used for fractured wrists, arms, and shoulders. The tie of the cravat should be on the side of the patient's neck, not the back. The patient's wrist should be slightly higher than the elbow. Manufactured slings are available.

BINDERS

A. Purposes
1. For support: abdomen or chest
2. To hold dressings in place
3. To apply pressure
B. Types
1. Straight
2. Tailed: T-binder, four-tailed, or Scultetus (many-tailed)

ANTIEMBOLISM STOCKINGS

A. Purposes
1. To help maintain circulation
2. To prevent thrombi or phlebitis formation, especially if patient is unable to undergo early ambulation after surgery
B. Application and maintenance
1. Exact size is obtained by measuring calf or leg length and circumference.
2. Be sure that legs are clean and dry before applying.
3. Apply with patient lying down; stockings should fit evenly and smoothly; no wrinkles.
4. Periodically check foot and leg for redness, irritation, swelling, and presence of pulse.
5. Stockings should be removed daily for bathing and skin inspection purposes; in most cases, stockings are removed at night, laundered, and put on in the morning before the patient gets out of bed.

APPLICATION OF HEAT AND COLD

A. Physiological principles
1. Cold applications (by constricting blood vessels) prevent or reduce swelling, stop bleeding, decrease suppuration, and reduce pain.
2. Heat applications (by dilating blood vessels) increase supply of oxygen and nutrients to body cells and increase amount of toxins and excess fluids carried away.
B. Types of cold applications
1. Dry: ice bag, ice cap, ice collar, hypothermic devices
2. Moist: cold packs and compresses
C. Nursing observations
1. White, mottled skin
2. Frostbite
3. Numbness
4. Lowered body temperature
D. Guidelines
1. Caps and bags are two-thirds filled, and air is removed.
2. Containers are closed securely.
3. Caps and bags are always covered.
4. Application is removed every 30 minutes for 1 hour.

5. Ice is replaced frequently.
6. These treatments are contraindicated or used only with great care in patients with poor circulation or impaired sensation.
7. Physician's order is always required.

E. Types of heat applications
1. Dry: hot water bottle, sunlight, heating pad, and incandescent, ultraviolet, and infrared lights
2. Moist: warm compresses, hot soaks, hot packs, and K-pad units

F. Nursing observations
1. Redness
2. Swelling
3. Pain
4. Change in vital signs
5. Loss of function in part

G. Guidelines
1. Physician's order is always required.
2. Carefully observe body parts that are very sensitive and burn easily (eyes, neck, inner aspect of arm).
3. Bottles and pads are always covered.
4. Never allow patient to lie on heating device.
5. Check for faulty electrical wiring.
6. Never use safety pins with electric devices.
7. Check body temperature frequently.
8. Check distance of heating bulbs from body area; bulbs should be at least 18 inches (45 cm) away.
9. Wring out compresses well to prevent burn; if area is infected, use compresses only once and discard.
10. Agency policy may require application of a thin layer of petrolatum to area receiving heat.

H. Special baths
1. Hot (sitz) or cold (Figure 2-14)
2. Medicated

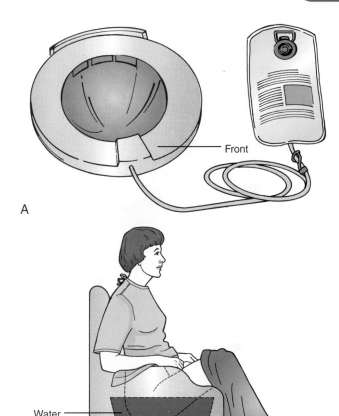

FIGURE 2-14 Sitz baths. **A,** Disposable. **B,** Built-in. (Adapted from Sorrentino SA: *Mosby's textbook for nursing assistants,* ed 6, St Louis, 2004, Mosby.)

MEASURES FOR EYE, EAR, AND THROAT DISORDERS

EYE TREATMENTS

A. Hot compresses
1. Assemble equipment: sterile basin of solution as ordered, gauze pad, heating device, paper bag, and protective gloves.
2. Put on protective gloves.
3. Apply thin layer of petrolatum over lid.
4. Wring out gauze pad with hands (if clean technique) or with two pairs of forceps (if sterile technique) and allow pad to stop steaming. Apply compress slowly until patient is accustomed to heat or allow patient to apply compress if able.
5. Try to keep compress on eyelid only. If lid is inflamed, compress may be placed on lid and cheek; if eyeball is inflamed, compress may be placed on lid and brow.
6. Change compresses every 30 to 60 seconds for 15 to 20 minutes as ordered.
7. If discharge is present, use clean pad each time compress is applied.
8. Use two sets of equipment if both eyes are involved.

B. Irrigation
1. Assemble equipment: basin of sterile solution as ordered at 95° to 100° F (35° to 37.78° C), medicine dropper or ear syringe, basin for return flow, cotton balls to protect uninvolved eye and dry treated eye,

and face towel to protect bed; separate irrigating tip is needed for each eye.
2. Direct flow of solution into conjunctival sac from inner angle to outer angle of eye; position patient toward affected side (Figure 2-15).

EAR TREATMENT: IRRIGATION

A. Assemble equipment: sterile ear syringe, solution as ordered at 105° (40.56° C) to 108° F (42.2° C), basin for return flow, and towel to protect bed.
B. Position patient: Patient may lie down, but sitting position is preferred, with head tilted slightly so affected ear is downward. Patient may hold basin for return flow if able.
C. Retract pinna, in direction according to age, to expose orifice of external canal. Direct flow gently against side of canal. Interrupt irrigation if pain or dizziness occurs, and notify physician.

THROAT TREATMENTS

A. Throat swab
1. Assemble equipment: sterile applicators, tongue blade, medication as ordered, tissue wipes, flashlight, and paper bag.
2. When swabbing throat, avoid stimulating gag reflex by not touching uvula.

B. Throat culture
1. Assemble equipment: sterile culture tube, applicator, tissue wipes.

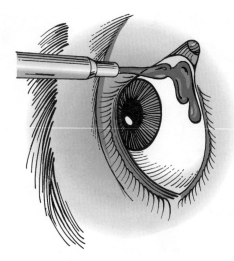

FIGURE 2-15 Irrigation of the eye. The nurse turns the patient's head toward the eye that is to be irrigated. Solution flows from the inner canthus to the outer canthus of the eye. The irrigator is held less than 4 inches (10 cm) away from the eye. The patient may assist by retracting the lower eyelid and collecting irrigating solution with absorbent material. (From Perry AG, Potter PA, Elkin MK: *Nursing interventions and clinical skills,* ed 5, St Louis, 2012, Mosby.)

2. After touching sides and back of throat with applicator, put applicator in culture tube without contaminating inside of tube by breaking off top of applicator that was touched by fingers.

C. Throat irrigation
   1. Assemble equipment: irrigating container, solution as ordered at 110° F (43.33° C), tubing with rubber tip on end, tissue wipes, basin for return flow, towel to protect patient, protective gloves.
   2. Put on protective gloves.
   3. Have patient tilt head forward over basin and breathe through nose; discourage deep breathing.
   4. Have patient do treatment if able.
   5. Hold container slightly above patient's mouth; direct flow toward affected area.
      a. Irrigation may be interrupted for patient's comfort.
      b. Flow should not be directed toward uvula or base of tongue.
   7. Tilt patient's head to one side and then the other to facilitate results.

MEASURES FOR GASTROINTESTINAL DISORDERS

GASTRIC INTUBATION
A. Purposes
   1. To administer gavage feedings
   2. To obtain specimens (gastric analysis, cytology)
   3. To irrigate or cleanse (lavage)
   4. For decompression (suction)
B. Tube locations
   1. Nose to stomach: nasogastric
   2. Mouth to stomach: orogastric
   3. Artificial opening into stomach: gastrostomy
C. Insertion of tube
   1. This procedure is not always the responsibility of the LPN/LVN; refer to agency policy.

2. Assemble equipment: flashlight, tongue blade, stethoscope, cup of water, irrigating syringe, water-soluble lubricant, 12- to 18-gauge French tube, gloves, towel to protect patient's clothing.
   3. If rubber tube is used, it should be chilled first.
   4. Place patient in semi-Fowler position with towel protecting clothing.
   5. Approximate distance of tube insertion is the length from tip of nose to earlobe to xiphoid process; may use a piece of tape to mark measurement.
   6. Apply water-soluble lubricant to tip of tube; if intubation is for cytology study, tube is lubricated with water or saline solution.
   7. With gloved hands, hold tube 3 inches (7.5 cm) from tip, place into nostril or mouth, and advance.
   8. Have patient flex neck and take repeated shallow breaths when tube passes into pharynx (approximately 3 inches [7.5 cm]).
   9. Have patient swallow while tube is advanced.
D. Checking placement of tube
   1. Check back of throat with tongue blade and flashlight to see if coiling has occurred.
   2. Aspirate stomach contents; may need to advance tube if no stomach contents are obtained. Check the pH of the stomach contents—should be 2 to 4 on the pH scale.
   3. While injecting 5 mL of air, use stethoscope to listen for air entering stomach.
   4. Observe patient's respirations and note ability to speak; respirations may be labored, or patient will be unable to speak if tube is in trachea or lungs.
   5. If possible, obtain chest radiograph to check placement, especially of small-bore feeding tubes.
E. Securing tube (Figure 2-16)
   1. Anchor with strip of tape. Secure to nose and cheek if nasogastric tube is used. Avoid resting tube on side of nares to avoid irritation or necrosis.

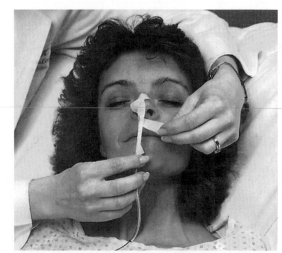

FIGURE 2-16 Securing the nasoenteral tube. A length of adhesive tape is partially split for use in anchoring the tube to the nostril. The unsplit portion is affixed to the nose; one of the split portions is wrapped around the tube, then the other portion is wrapped around the tube. A narrow strip of tape may be used to secure the tube. The tube is then taped to the nostril and cheek and clamped or connected to suction. (From Potter PA, Perry AG: *Fundamentals of nursing,* ed 7, St Louis, 2009, Mosby.)

2. Tube should be secured in some manner, either looped through a rubber band and attached to the patient's gown with a safety pin or with the use of a manufactured tube-tape device.
F. Removing tube
   1. Clamp tube.
   2. Remove anchoring tape.
   3. Put on protective gloves.
   4. Draw tube through towel to wipe off secretions.
   5. Have patient inhale and exhale slowly.
   6. Pull tube with one continuous, rapid motion.
   7. Have basin ready in case patient vomits.

SUCTION AND IRRIGATION

A. Nasogastric or GI tubes (Levin, Cantor, Miller-Abbott, or Salem Sump) may be connected to mechanical suction apparatus.
B. Suction
   1. Rate is ordered by physician or according to agency policy.
   2. Suction may be intermittent or continuous.
   3. Collection container is emptied and rinsed; amount of drainage is measured and recorded at end of shift and when container becomes nearly filled.
   4. Turn off or clamp off suction when assessing for bowel sounds. Suction may mimic the sounds of peristalsis.
C. Irrigation
   1. Check orders for frequency, solution type, amount, and method of aspiration (force or gravity).
   2. Assemble equipment: solution as ordered, container for solution, basin for return flow, irrigating syringe (bulb or plunger type), protective pad.
   3. Check placement of tube.
   4. Fill syringe and free it of air.
   5. Instill solution into tube slowly and gently.
   6. Allow solution to return by aspiration or by gravity.
   7. Remove syringe and reconnect to suction if ordered.
D. Patients with indwelling tubes should be given frequent mouth and nose care.
E. Accurate measurement of intake and output (subtracting irrigating solution) is essential.

MEASURES FOR VAGINAL CARE

PERINEAL CARE

A. Assemble equipment: solution as ordered, cotton balls (or washcloth) for cleansing and drying, gloves, perineal pad with belt, bedpan.
B. With gloved hands, put patient on bedpan; pour solution over vulva, clean with cotton balls or washcloth; dry vulva; make patient comfortable.
C. If using bottle method, fill bottle with warm water and squeeze solution over vulva; dry, wiping from urinary meatus toward anus and wiping only once with each cotton ball.

VAGINAL IRRIGATION (DOUCHE)

A. Assemble equipment: irrigating container with solution as ordered, tubing with douche tip, clamp, cotton balls for drying, gloves, perineal pad with belt, bedpan, bed protection.
B. Have patient void; place patient on bedpan, or patient may administer to self in bathroom if able.
C. Insert tip down and back into vagina.
D. Irrigate under low pressure. Have solution flowing before insertion of douche tip. Rotate douche tip until prescribed amount is used.
E. If patient is on bedpan, raise head of bed slightly to allow fluid to drain into bedpan.

MEASURES FOR PATIENTS UNDERGOING SURGERY

PREOPERATIVE PREPARATION

A. Psychosocial aspects
   1. Nurse assesses patient's knowledge and expected results of surgery.
   2. Anxiety may interfere with preoperative teaching.
   3. Extremely frightened patients may respond poorly to surgery.
   4. Planned, individualized, simple explanations enhance patient cooperation and reduce anxiety.
   5. Nurse assesses and responds to patient's religious needs.
   6. Common preoperative fears
      a. Fear of mutilation
      b. Fear of death
      c. Fear of change in family role
      d. Fear of pain
   7. Family or significant others must understand measures taken to prepare patient.
   8. Family or significant others should participate in explanations and encouragement.
B. Physical preparation
   1. Explain preoperative tests (CBC, ECG, urinalysis, x-ray examinations).
   2. Explain, demonstrate, and have patient practice any special postoperative exercises that will need to be done (turning, deep breathing, pumping feet).
   3. Follow preoperative orders as prescribed by physician (enema, diet, medications).
   4. Prepare appropriate skin area (refer to agency procedure manual).
   5. Care for valuables.
   6. Follow and complete the preoperative checklist.
      a. Informed consents for surgery and anesthesia signed and witnessed
      b. Nail polish, prostheses, jewelry, and makeup removed
      c. Patient dressed in hospital gown only
      d. Hygienic measures performed (bath with mouth care and voiding or catheterization)
      e. Vital signs collected and recorded and abnormalities reported
      f. Identification and allergy bracelets put in place
C. Record observations and procedures.
D. After patient leaves for operative procedure, prepare postoperative bed and unit.

POSTOPERATIVE CARE

A. Immediate care
   1. Ensure and maintain patent airway.
   2. Maintain adequate circulation.
   3. Observe for complications at operative site and in general (hemorrhage, shock, swelling, severe pain). Carefully observe dependent areas of the body for concealed hemorrhage.

4. Assess and secure dressing, drainage, and IV tubing.
5. Assess mental status (orientation).
6. Position patient properly; keep patient warm.
7. Assess vital signs as often as ordered or more frequently as condition warrants. Decreased BP, tachycardia, confusion, and restlessness are signs of shock.
8. Follow physician's orders.
9. Report signs of restlessness, excessive drainage, or abnormal reactions.
10. Support patient and family or significant others by briefly answering questions and offering explanations.

B. Routine care
1. Follow physician's orders.
2. Assess and record vital signs frequently during first 24 hours; report changes immediately.
3. Assess dressing or surgical site frequently.
4. Give oral hygiene as needed.
5. Have patient turn, deep breathe, and, unless contraindicated, cough and exercise legs at least every 2 hours. Patient should try to pump ankles (alternately dorsiflex and plantarflex the feet) to decrease chance of thrombus formation.
6. Assess and record intake and output (patient may need order for catheterization if he or she does not void within 6 to 8 hours after surgery).
7. Assist patient with passive or active exercises unless contraindicated.
8. Encourage and help patient to ambulate as much as orders permit, which decreases chance for thrombus formation and pneumonia and alleviates gas pains from decreased peristalsis.
9. Care for any drains the patient may have.
   a. Penrose: large, "noodlelike" drain that drains onto a sterile dressing
   b. Jackson-Pratt: "grenadelike" drain that needs to be emptied periodically; drain then reconstituted by squeezing it and applying a plug; negative pressure used to drain the surgical site
   c. Hemovac, Urevac: drains blood or urine through use of negative pressure
10. Perform daily assessment.
    a. Lungs: breath sounds and cough
    b. Circulation: color, temperature, capillary refill of extremities; pain in legs or chest and IV site
    c. GI tract: nausea, vomiting, distention, bowel sounds, passage of flatus
    d. Urine: amount, color, odor, frequency
    e. Mental status: withdrawal, confusion, anxiety, restlessness
11. Offer pain medication.

MEASURES RELATED TO RADIATION THERAPY

A. Radiation
1. Radiate: to send out rays (light, heat, or roentgen)
2. Radiation used in diagnosis and therapeutic treatment of various conditions (especially for malignancies)
3. Types of radiation
   a. Alpha rays: harmless; do not travel far
   b. Beta rays: more penetrating; stop at person's body surface
   c. Gamma rays: very penetrating

B. Types of therapy
1. Infrared lamp
2. Ultraviolet
3. Diathermy
4. Roentgen ray (x-ray; low voltage, external)
5. Betatron, cobalt, cesium (high voltage, external)
6. Internal radiation
   a. Implants (skin surface, intratumor, intracavitary)
   b. Liquid forms of radioisotopes
   c. Injection (intracavitary, systemic)

C. Radiation therapy and the nurse
1. Internal implant
   a. Explain procedure and precautions to patient and family or significant others.
      (1) Patient needs to know that he or she will be in isolation and how many days isolation is likely to last.
      (2) Patient should know that nursing personnel and visitors will be spending a minimum amount of time at the bedside and yet will be available when needed.
   b. Ensure good fluid intake unless contraindicated.
   c. Have patient move about as little as possible.
   d. Assess for signs of radiation reactions (nausea, vomiting, skin irritation).
   e. Communicate frequently with patient from doorway without entering room.
   f. Use precautions at all times.
2. Radiation precautions with implant
   a. "RADIATION IN USE" sign with directions is posted on patient's door.
   b. No staff member or visitor spends more than 1 hour per day with patient; care must be well organized.
   c. Pregnant women and children should not enter the patient's room.
   d. Check placement of implant every 4 hours.
   e. Wear gown and gloves while handling excreta, secretions, and utensils. Excreta may need to be double flushed in toilet; know agency policy.
   f. Wash contaminated gloves with soap and water before removing.
   g. Wash hands with soap and water.
   h. If implant becomes dislodged, call radiologist immediately—do not touch implant.
3. Nursing care for specific situations
   a. Therapy involving mouth
      (1) Oral hygiene with brushing teeth (or dentures) should be done three times per day (tid).
      (2) Smoking should be discouraged.
      (3) Teeth should be assessed for change in condition; if changes observed, notify physician.
      (4) Male patient should not shave if jaw is being treated.
   b. Uterine therapy
      (1) Bed rest is maintained to prevent displacement of implant.
      (2) Bedpan is inspected for loss of implant before contents are discarded.
      (3) Foley catheter with continuous irrigation may be ordered to reduce bladder irritation.
      (4) Vaginal irrigation may be ordered after removal of implant.

c. Radioactive gold administered intraperitoneally
  (1) Leakage on dressings appears bright red and may be confused with blood.
  (2) Dressings should be wrapped in newspaper and disposed of in special container.
4. External radiotherapy
  a. Explain procedure to patient and family or significant others.
  b. Never remove skin markings.
  c. Avoid washing the marked area.
  d. Do not apply ointments, creams, or powders to marked area.
  e. Encourage good fluid intake and nutrition.
  f. Observe for radiation reactions.

MEASURES CONCERNING PATIENT'S DEPARTURE

A. Transferring patient
  1. Patient may be transferred from one service to another, from one floor to another, or from one agency to another.
  2. Physician's order is required.
  3. Transfer patient by wheelchair or on stretcher; follow agency policy.
  4. Explain transfer to patient; be sure that all personal belongings are transferred with patient.
  5. Avoid transferring during mealtime or change of shift to reduce confusion.
  6. Make proper charting notations; notify family or significant others.
B. Discharging patient
  1. Written or electronic order by physician is required unless patient has signed out against medical advice.
  2. Nurse's responsibilities
    a. Gather and check all personal belongings with patient.
    b. Make sure that patient understands all instructions regarding diet, medications, treatments, and follow-up appointments.
    c. Notify family or significant others as necessary.
    d. Accompany patient to exit.
    e. Make proper charting notations.
  3. Discharge planning
    a. Planning begins after initial nursing assessment and is included on care plan.
    b. Nursing interventions are directed toward eventual discharge of patient.
    c. Planning consists of teaching patient and family or significant others.
      (1) Cause of illness
      (2) Drugs, treatments, diet
      (3) Health care follow-up
      (4) Functions within limitations

CARING FOR THE DYING

A. Signs of approaching death
  1. Patient is pale, with pinched expression of anxiety.
  2. Eyes are glazed and dull; pupils do not react to light.

3. Mouth remains partially open unless patient attempts to speak; speech is mumbled and often confused.
4. Muscle tone becomes flaccid.
5. Skin is cool and clammy and may be mottled; this is caused by diminished circulation; body temperature is often elevated.
6. Respirations are rapid and shallow, often progressing to Cheyne-Stokes respirations.
7. Pulse becomes weak and thready.
8. Patient may be diaphoretic, thirsty, and incontinent of urine and feces.
B. Five stages in the process of reaction to a terminal illness or dying: Refer to Chapter 6 for more detailed information regarding death and dying.
  1. Denial
  2. Anger
  3. Bargaining
  4. Grief or depression
  5. Acceptance
C. Nursing care of dying patient
  1. Provide symptomatic nursing care. Palliative care is comfort care. Nurse and physician attempt to increase patient comfort by performing certain actions. Surgery and medications may be a form of palliative care.
  2. Provide good personal hygiene.
  3. Turn patient frequently.
  4. Provide treatments and medications as long as possible or until discontinued.
  5. Carry out desires of patient and family or significant others as far as possible; be sensitive to religious or cultural beliefs.
  6. Be available to provide emotional support and privacy to patient and family or significant others.
  7. Remember that hearing may be the last sense to fail.
D. Spiritual needs of patient
  1. Fulfill needs as requested by patient and family or significant others.
  2. Continue to adhere to patient's individual religious beliefs.
E. Care of body after death (postmortem care): Physicians pronounce death in most cases. RNs may pronounce death (in some states) in acute care facilities (a recent change as of 2012) and also under special circumstances (hospice patients).
  1. Lower head of bed.
  2. Leave one pillow under head to prevent congestion of blood in vessels of face.
  3. Close eyes.
  4. Place dentures in mouth immediately and close mouth.
  5. Clean body; follow agency policy for removal of drains, IV needle and tubing, dressings, and tubes.
  6. Straighten body and place in natural position.
  7. Allow viewing of body by family or significant others if they desire.
  8. Wrap in shroud and label with tags according to agency policy.
  9. Gather, pack, label, and care for patient's personal belongings.
  10. Record observations, procedures, disposition of valuables, and time of death; complete records.

Bibliography

Chitty KK, Black BP: *Professional nursing: concepts and challenges*, ed 6, St Louis, 2011, Saunders.

Christensen BL, Kockrow EO: *Foundations of nursing*, ed 6, St Louis, 2010, Mosby.

deWit SC: *Fundamental concepts and skills for nursing*, ed 4, St Louis, 2014, Saunders.

Edmunds MW: *Introduction to clinical pharmacology*, ed 7, St Louis, 2013, Mosby.

Emergency Nurse's Association: *Sheehy's manual of emergency care*, ed 7, St Louis, 2013, Mosby.

Herlihy B, Maebius NK: *Human body in health and illness*, ed 4, Philadelphia, 2011, Saunders.

Hill SS, Howlett HS: *Success in practical/vocational nursing*, ed 7, St Louis, 2013, Saunders.

Linton AD: *Introduction to medical-surgical nursing*, ed 5, St Louis, 2012, Mosby.

Morrison-Valfre M: *Foundations of mental health care*, ed 5, St Louis, 2013, Mosby.

Nix S: *Williams' basic nutrition and diet therapy*, ed 14, St Louis, 2013, Mosby.

Perry AG, Potter PA, Elkin MK: *Nursing interventions and clinical skills*, ed 5, St Louis, 2012, Mosby.

Potter PA, et al: *Basic nursing: a critical thinking approach*, ed 7, St Louis, 2011, Mosby.

Potter PA, et al: *Fundamentals of nursing*, ed 8, St Louis, 2013, Mosby.

Sorrentino SA, Remmert L, Gorek B: *Mosby's essentials for nursing assistants*, ed 4, St. Louis, 2010, Mosby.

Venes D: *Taber's cyclopedic medical dictionary*, ed 21, Philadelphia, 2010, FA Davis.

Wold GH: *Basic geriatric nursing*, ed 5, St Louis, 2012, Mosby.

REVIEW QUESTIONS

1. A patient is being prepared for sealed internal radiation therapy for cervical cancer. Which information, when given to the patient by the nurse, would best help reduce the patient's anxiety concerning this procedure?
   1. Pain medication will be offered regularly.
   2. Visitors will be limited during this treatment.
   3. The nurse will be available whenever needed.
   4. The patient will not be radioactive during this treatment.
2. HIPPA guidelines preserve the patient's right to:
   1. Refuse treatment.
   2. Maintain privacy.
   3. Litigation.
   4. Assisted suicide.
3. A nurse is instructing a student in the proper method for obtaining a throat culture. The student asks why she should swab the sides of the throat before the back of the throat. The nurse responds that this method will:
   1. Delay stimulating the gag reflex.
   2. Stimulate production of secretions.
   3. Avoid contamination of the culture site.
   4. Obtain adequate specimens for culture.
4. One hour after the nurse applies an elastic bandage to a patient's sprained ankle, the patient complains of tingling and burning in the toes. The nurse should:
   1. Palpate for pedal pulses.
   2. Reapply the bandage less snugly.
   3. Instruct her to elevate the affected foot.
   4. Encourage her to wiggle her toes every 2 hours.
5. The nurse performs all of the following when performing a wound irrigation. Which would do the most to decrease the risk of contamination?
   1. Raising the bed to a workable height.
   2. Explaining the procedure to the patient.
   3. Handwashing before and after the procedure.
   4. Donning appropriate personal protective equipment.
6. Which patient is most at risk for decubitus ulcer formation?
   1. A 20-year-old patient with a lumbar-4 injury confined to a wheelchair
   2. A 6-year-old patient in skeletal traction for a fractured right femur
   3. An ambulatory 90-year-old patient with Alzheimer disease
   4. A 75-year-old patient on bed rest after total knee replacement
7. A patient is 1-day postoperative after gastric resection. The patient has a nasogastric tube attached to low-intermittent suction and complains of severe thirst. The nurse's next course of action is to:
   1. Call the physician for an order allowing ice chips.
   2. Instill approximately 100 mL of normal saline into his tube.
   3. Explain that he must remain NPO until the tube is removed.
   4. Assist the patient in brushing his teeth and rinsing his mouth.
8. A patient who is receiving external radiation treatments asks the nurse if he can remove the ink on his skin. Which is the best answer by the nurse?
   1. "No, I am sorry, we need you to leave those on so we know where to point the radiation next time."
   2. "I will need to get some adhesive remover to get the ink off."
   3. "I will need to consult with the physician about this."
   4. "No, we need to make sure that we irradiate the tumor in the exact spot as the last time."
9. A patient had a urethral retention catheter removed 6 hours ago and has not yet voided. What should be the nurse's next course of action? Select all that apply.
   _____ 1. Assess the patient's abdomen for distention.
   _____ 2. Catheterize the patient with a straight catheter.
   _____ 3. Assess volume of urine in the bladder with a bladder scanner.
   _____ 4. Ambulate the patient to the bathroom so he can try again.
10. A patient has returned to the unit after a transurethral resection of the prostate (TURP). The nurse notes that the bedside drainage unit is filled with red urine and numerous large clots. The abdomen is distended, and the bladder can be palpated above the symphysis pubis. What is the nurse's first course of action?
    1. Change the patient's position.
    2. Notify the surgeon of your findings.
    3. Check the chart for bladder irrigation orders.
    4. Document your observations on the flow sheet.
11. A patient who has been on bed rest attempts to stand and walk without dangling first. If the patient becomes dizzy and weak, he is most likely experiencing:
    1. Anemia.
    2. Postural hypotension.
    3. Hypoxia.
    4. Hypertension.

12. A patient who is 1-day postoperative after abdominal hysterectomy has a urinary catheter, a Penrose drain, and an IV of dextrose 5% in Ringer's lactate infusing at 100 mL/hr. The patient is complaining of a sense of urinary urgency and lower abdominal pressure and requests an injection of meperidine hydrochloride (Demerol). What is the nurse's first course of action?
    1. Check when this patient was last medicated for pain.
    2. Request that the physician change the IV flow rate order.
    3. Determine that urine is draining into the bedside drainage unit.
    4. Assure the patient that catheters often cause this type of discomfort.

13. The nurse is planning to irrigate the colostomy of a patient. The patient asks why the colostomy is being irrigated. The nurse's best explanation is that irrigation helps to:
    1. Control constipation.
    2. Cleanse the bowel.
    3. Regulate the discharge of feces.
    4. Eliminate the need for stool softeners.

14. Which tasks would be appropriate for an LPN/LVN to assign to a UAP? Select all that apply.
    _____ 1. Feeding a patient with a CVA
    _____ 2. SOAPIE charting
    _____ 3. Assisting with a shower for a patient who is paralyzed
    _____ 4. Administering 6:00 PM medications
    _____ 5. Wound dressing for a patient with a decubitus ulcer
    _____ 6. Passing 10:00 PM snacks

15. The physician has ordered a patient's IV to infuse at 100 mL/hr. The IV was started at 7:00 PM. When the nurse does rounds at 11:00 PM, 200 mL of fluid has infused into the patient. The nurse's initial course of action is to:
    1. Notify the physician that the IV has infiltrated.
    2. Note the amount on the patient's intake and output record.
    3. Check the tubing and infusion site for possible obstructions.
    4. Change the rate of flow until the correct amount has infused.

16. Which nursing measure would best address the communication needs of a patient with a newly inserted tracheostomy tube?
    1. Providing a pad and pencil within reach
    2. Having tissues easily available to the patient
    3. Reassuring the patient that nurses are always nearby
    4. Arranging to have telephone service discontinued temporarily

17. The nurse has been assigned to perform colostomy care for a patient who has had a recent hemicolectomy. The nurse can best determine how the patient tolerated the procedure by:
    1. Noting all objective signs and symptoms during the procedure.
    2. Asking the patient if anything is bothering him during the procedure.
    3. Questioning the patient regarding his well-being at the end of the treatment.
    4. Observing the patient's verbal and nonverbal actions throughout the procedure.

18. A patient who has just returned from having a bronchogram asks the nurse if he can have a drink of water. Which is the best response by the nurse?
    1. "Sure, just let me get your vital signs."
    2. "We need to wait until you wake up a little more."
    3. "I need to check your gag reflex first."
    4. "You should chew on some ice first."

19. Which nursing diagnosis is most pertinent for a patient who has had diarrhea for 3 days?
    1. Impaired skin integrity
    2. Imbalanced nutrition: less than body requirements
    3. Deficient knowledge
    4. Risk for imbalanced fluid volume

20. A patient with heart failure is beginning a treatment regimen that includes diuretic medications. Which instructions regarding obtaining weights should the nurse reinforce to the patient?
    1. Weigh each morning on arising.
    2. Weigh 1 hour after taking medication.
    3. Weigh each time a medication is omitted.
    4. Weigh only when shortness of breath develops.

21. The nurse notes the following orders on the care plan of a patient with a decubitus ulcer who is on enteric isolation. Which order would the nurse question?
    1. Use a mask when changing heavily soiled dressings.
    2. Teach self-care of the wound.
    3. Limit visitors.
    4. Measure wound once per week.

22. An elderly patient required a Foley catheter after hip surgery. Laboratory tests now indicate that the patient has developed a *Pseudomonas aeruginosa* urinary tract infection. In light of this patient's medical history, the nurse would suspect that this is a(n):
    1. Superinfection.
    2. Nosocomial infection.
    3. Autoimmune response.
    4. Antibiotic resistance response.

23. A gown should be removed by:
    1. Touching the outside of the gown only.
    2. Removing the gown outside the patient's room.
    3. Allowing another individual to remove it for you.
    4. Touching the inside of the gown only.

24. For which reason should the nurse question a patient's cultural practices when obtaining a health history?
    1. Cultural practices may affect how the patient views the health care team.
    2. It determines whether the patient should receive last rites.
    3. Certain cultures offer social supports to ill members.
    4. The patient may wish to have family members with him or her during examinations.

25. The nurse is caring for a patient with a white blood count (WBC) of 0.2×10^9 L. The patient has been undergoing chemotherapy for 3 months for prostate cancer. What special precautions need to be implemented for this patient? Select all that apply.
    _____ 1. Protective isolation precautions.
    _____ 2. Patient should wear a mask when being transported through the hospital.
    _____ 3. The patient should not receive any injections during this time.
    _____ 4. No raw fruits and vegetables or cut flowers should be allowed in the room.

26. Licensing laws regulate the practice of nursing to:
    1. Protect the public from injury.
    2. Guarantee the best possible nursing care.
    3. Ensure that every nurse has good moral character.
    4. Support nurse employment by limiting the competition.
27. The nurse is bandaging a patient's elbow. Into which position should the elbow be placed before it is bandaged?
    1. Rotation
    2. Extension
    3. Slightly flexed
    4. Slightly hyperextended
28. The nurse is instructed to bandage a patient's lower extremity with an elastic wrap. The leg is extremely edematous. What should the nurse do first?
    1. Elevate the extremity for 15 to 20 minutes before wrapping
    2. Wrap from the most distal to the proximal end of the extremity
    3. Ensure that the elastic wrap is smooth and free of wrinkles
    4. Check distal pulses every 15 minutes
29. Which would best reduce the chance of infection during the bed bath procedure?
    1. Thoroughly rinsing and drying all skinfolds
    2. Applying clean gloves before beginning the bath
    3. Using separate washcloth sections for each eye
    4. Changing the bath water after bathing each extremity
30. A nurse is applying a triangular bandage to elevate a patient's arm. Where should the knot be tied during this procedure?
    1. Near the patient's elbow
    2. At the side of the neck
    3. Toward the back of the patient's head
    4. Wherever the patient wants it tied
31. An elderly patient has arrived at the physician's office complaining of ear pain, vertigo, and impaired hearing. The physician has ordered a normal saline ear irrigation to loosen embedded earwax. After this procedure, the nurse would take care to:
    1. Retract the pinna of the ear.
    2. Determine the patient's tolerance of movement.
    3. Encourage the patient to remain supine for several hours.
    4. Thoroughly dry the ear canal with cotton-tipped applicators.
32. A female patient has been admitted to the hospital unit with a fever of unknown origin. The physician has ordered urine and blood specimens for culture and a broad-spectrum antibiotic. The nurse should:
    1. Obtain the specimens before beginning antibiotic therapy.
    2. Ask the physician to clarify which procedure should be performed first.
    3. Begin the antibiotic therapy immediately, before obtaining the specimens.
    4. Obtain the blood, start the medication, and tell the patient to call when she is able to void.
33. A postoperative patient has all of the following signs and symptoms. Which is most indicative that the patient may have thrombophlebitis?
    1. Pain in the foot and ankle
    2. Fever and dry skin

3. Pain in the calf when the foot is flexed
4. One leg much cooler than the other

34. Which observations would indicate that the nurse should withhold a tube feeding? Select all that apply.
    _____ 1. Oozing at the gastrostomy site
    _____ 2. Absence of bowel sounds
    _____ 3. Presence of more than 100 mL of residual feeding
    _____ 4. Absence of residual feeding when the gastrostomy tube is suctioned
35. If a patient complains of the urge to defecate after the nurse begins to administer a tap-water enema, the nurse should:
    1. Adjust the tube location while maintaining fluid flow.
    2. Lower the enema bag while instructing the patient to breathe deeply.
    3. Reassure the patient that the discomfort should pass in a few minutes.
    4. Immediately discontinue the procedure to allow patient bowel evacuation.
36. A nursing assistant asks why the operating room nurse must clip or shave hair from a surgical site. What is the nurse's best explanation for this procedure?
    1. The physician would otherwise have difficulty suturing the site.
    2. The procedure is done to reduce the number of microorganisms on the patient's skin.
    3. The patient will experience less discomfort after surgery.
    4. The dressings will not adhere if the hair is not removed.
37. Which preoperative order would most help prevent postoperative nausea and vomiting?
    1. Cleansing enemas
    2. NPO for 6 to 12 hours
    3. Teaching coughing and deep-breathing exercises
    4. Lactated Ringer's solution IV at 40 mL/hr
38. A nurse is changing a patient's decubitus ulcer dressing using sterile technique. Which step in the procedure is incorrect?
    1. Remove old dressing with sterile gloves.
    2. Irrigate the wound from top to bottom.
    3. Pack the wound using a sterile cotton swab.
    4. Tape the dressing to allow for patient movement.
39. A patient returns from surgery with a Jackson-Pratt (JP) in place. The JP is used to:
    1. Dress the operative site.
    2. Hold the dressing in place.
    3. Clean the surgical site.
    4. Drain the operative site.
40. What should the nurse carefully document after a surgical dressing change? Select all that apply.
    _____ 1. The specific location of the wound
    _____ 2. The characteristics of the suture line
    _____ 3. The type of antibiotic cleansing solution
    _____ 4. The patient's emotional response to the surgical procedure
41. The nurse is collecting a blood specimen. To minimize risk to the patient, the nurse should release the tourniquet:
    1. As soon as an appropriate vein is palpated.
    2. Before withdrawing the needle from the patient's vein.
    3. After applying a bandage to the venipuncture site.
    4. As soon as blood begins flowing into the specimen tube.

42. Placing the patient's arm in a downward position during venipuncture helps to:
    1. Dilate blood vessels for better access.
    2. Diminish patient discomfort during the procedure.
    3. Prevent backflow of any chemical additives in the blood tubes.
    4. Prevent any unnecessary arm movement during the procedure.

43. A patient's abdominal incision is no longer approximated, and the nurse observes viscera protruding from the incision. The nurse should immediately:
    1. Attempt to replace the viscera back in the incision.
    2. Call the physician.
    3. Place a saline-soaked sterile dressing over the wound.
    4. Place the patient in the shock position.

44. A patient returns from the postanesthesia care unit after a cholecystectomy with the following vital signs: T, 98.6° F (37° C); P, 72; R, 20; BP, 120/64. Fifteen minutes after the patient arrives on the unit, the following vital signs are collected: T, 98.6° F (37° C); P, 128; R, 30; BP, 98/48. What might the change in vital signs indicate?
    1. Infection
    2. Dehiscence
    3. Thrombophlebitis
    4. Hemorrhage

45. Which nursing intervention would best prevent the complication of thrombophlebitis?
    1. Early ambulation
    2. Sequential antiembolic devices
    3. Coughing and deep breathing
    4. Incentive spirometry

46. A nurse is teaching a patient who has terminal cancer and is scheduled to have a colostomy. What should be included in the patient's teaching?
    1. "This surgery should cure your cancer."
    2. "Hopefully this procedure will alleviate some of your symptoms."
    3. "This procedure might be able to be reversed."
    4. "This surgery should help us diagnose you better."

47. A patient has just died. When is the best time for the nurse to perform postmortem care?
    1. Before family viewing of the body.
    2. After transport of the body to the morgue.
    3. As quickly as possible to decrease tension on the unit.
    4. After allowing the family the opportunity to view the body.

48. A postoperative patient who has been on bed rest since his surgery 5 days ago makes the following statements. Which statement may indicate that a postoperative complication may be developing?
    1. "I wish I could eat pizza without getting nauseous."
    2. "I need someone to rub my leg; it's swollen and sore."
    3. "The only way to get rid of this gas is to drink ginger ale."
    4. "I feel the need to have lots of salt on my fruit."

49. A patient wants to know why wet-to-dry dressings are being used to treat his stasis leg ulcer. The nurse's best response would be that this treatment:
    1. Increases circulation to the wound.
    2. Cleans the wound by removing dead tissue and debris.
    3. Promotes the absorption of drainage by capillary action.
    4. Decreases pain by lowering edema along wound edges.

50. A postoperative patient who had an appendectomy complains of gas pains. Which suggestion from the nurse would best alleviate this problem?
    1. "Why don't you try taking a walk?"
    2. "I'll get you a rectal tube."
    3. "I'll get you some Mylicon."
    4. "Why don't you drink some milk?"

51. While assisting an elderly nursing home resident with a bath, the nurse observes that the skin is dry and the resident has been scratching. A priority nursing diagnosis would be:
    1. Excess fluid volume.
    2. Impaired tissue integrity.
    3. Chronic confusion.
    4. Impaired skin integrity.

52. Before beginning a new tube feeding through a nasogastric tube, the nurse must first:
    1. Measure and replace any residual feeding.
    2. Warm the feeding to approximately 105° F (40.55° C).
    3. Check for correct tube placement in the stomach.
    4. Dislodge encrusted formula with a warm water flush.

53. The nurse has requested a UAP to assist in moving a paralyzed patient up in bed. What is an appropriate instruction to the UAP for this procedure?
    1. Stand one step back from the bed while lifting.
    2. Keep your back straight and your knees flexed.
    3. Keep your knees straight and your back flexed.
    4. Keep your feet close together for balance.

54. A patient is 10 hours postoperative after an abdominal hysterectomy. What assessment information would alert the nurse that normal postoperative progression is not occurring?
    1. The patient has serosanguineous drainage on her dressing.
    2. The patient splints her incision when coughing and deep breathing.
    3. The patient has not voided since the surgery.
    4. The patient is reluctant to ambulate because of incisional pain.

55. A nurse is assisting a physician in obtaining a Pap smear. What must the nurse do to the specimen before sending it to the laboratory?
    1. "Fix" it to the slide.
    2. Refrigerate it.
    3. Stain it.
    4. Place it on ice.

56. A nurse has discontinued an IV infusion and IV catheter. The patient asks why the nurse is applying pressure to the site. What is the nurse's best explanation?
    1. "I need to make sure that a clot develops at the spot."
    2. "You could bleed out if I don't hold pressure!"
    3. "I may need to apply pressure for up to 5 minutes to make sure a clot has formed."
    4. "Because you are on blood thinner, I need to hold it longer."

57. What is the correct sequence of events to follow if a fire occurs in a facility?
    1. Notify the switchboard, extinguish flames, close doors, and remove persons.
    2. Call for help, remove persons, confine the fire, and extinguish any flames present.
    3. Rescue persons, activate the alarm, confine the fire, and extinguish any flames present.
    4. Activate the alarm, confine the fire, remove any persons present, and use fire extinguisher.

58. Which action is appropriate for a nurse to correct a mistaken entry made in charting?
    1. Use an eraser to remove the entry.
    2. Put a line through the entry, and date and initial it.
    3. Recopy the entry and destroy the original sheet.
    4. Paint over the entry using white correction fluid.

59. A nurse is preparing a patient who is to undergo magnetic resonance imaging (MRI). Which questions would be important for the nurse to ask? Select all that apply.
    _____ 1. "Are you allergic to iodine?"
    _____ 2. "Are you claustrophobic?"
    _____ 3. "Do you have any metal in your body?"
    _____ 4. "Do you have a pacemaker?"
    _____ 5. "Can you give yourself an enema?"

60. A patient has a nasogastric tube inserted to receive supplemental feedings before surgery. The patient asks what the purpose of the tube is. Which response by the nurse is correct?
    1. "The tube is meant to assist your bowels to move."
    2. "Fluids and gas will be removed from your GI tract."
    3. "This will allow us to give you feedings and build up your strength."
    4. "The tube will speed your healing time after the surgery."

61. A nursing assistant asks why a cholangiogram is done. What is the correct information to give the assistant?
    1. "It is used to detect kidney damage."
    2. "It is a generalized liver test."
    3. "It can diagnose heart problems."
    4. "It can tell us if the gallbladder is working correctly."

62. The nurse is instructing a UAP to place an ostomy appliance on a patient, ensuring that the appliance fits snugly. The UAP inquires as to why the ostomy appliance must be so tight. The nurse's best response is:
    1. "The appliance must stay on a long time because they are expensive."
    2. "The appliance has to stay on when the patient takes a bath or shower."
    3. "The appliance may leak if it's loose, causing the skin to become excoriated."
    4. "If the appliance stays on well, the smell of the drainage can be better contained."

63. A patient is scheduled for abdominal surgery. The nurse is planning the patient's care and is aware that the reason for an NPO order before an operation is:
    1. Anesthesia stops the digestive process.
    2. Energy from food is not needed during surgery.
    3. Vomiting occurs normally in the recovery phase.
    4. An empty stomach reduces the chance for aspiration of stomach contents.

64. A nurse is suctioning secretions from a patient's nasal artificial airway. The nurse applies suction for no longer than:
    1. 3 seconds.
    2. 10 seconds.
    3. 30 seconds.
    4. 1 minute.

65. A patient is admitted with pancreatitis. Which diagnostic examination would the nurse expect to be performed on the patient?
    1. A magnetic resonance imaging (MRI) examination
    2. Endoscopic retrograde cholangiopancreatography (ERCP)
    3. An arteriogram
    4. A sigmoidoscopy

66. A thoracentesis is planned for a patient. The nurse should position the patient to allow access for drainage from the:
    1. Peritoneal cavity.
    2. Ascitic cavity.
    3. Pericardial sac.
    4. Pleural cavity.

67. A co-worker approaches a nurse with concerns that a small-bore feeding tube may not be properly placed. The co-worker reports that she did not hear the characteristic "whoosh" when she instilled air in the tube. Which method should the nurse advise the co-worker to use to establish placement of the tube?
    1. Obtain an order for a chest radiograph.
    2. Attach the chest tube to suction.
    3. Irrigate the tube with 30 mL of sterile saline.
    4. Place the end of the tube in a glass of water and watch for bubbles.

68. The nurse is interviewing a 52-year-old patient who has come to the physician's office complaining of feelings of hopelessness and depression. Which patient statement would reflect life changes common to this age-group?
    1. "I can't imagine starting my life over again."
    2. "My lifestyle will change so much after my retirement."
    3. "My kids have all left home, and I feel so depressed now."
    4. "The prospect of all this time on my hands is driving me crazy."

69. The nurse is planning an exercise program for a group of elderly individuals who have a history of cardiopulmonary disease. Which activity would best meet the exercise needs of these individuals?
    1. Jogging
    2. Walking
    3. Skiing machines
    4. Rowing machines

70. A patient of the Jehovah's Witness faith is scheduled for surgical repair of a hip fracture. Which preoperative order may conflict with this patient's religious practices?
    1. Incentive spirometry every 4 hours while awake
    2. Coughing, deep breathing, and leg exercises every 2 hours
    3. Type and cross-match for two units of packed red blood cells
    4. Magnetic resonance imaging of the right hip region

71. What is the best way for the nurse to position a bedpan for a patient who is able to help with the procedure?
    1. Ask the patient to raise his buttocks off the bed while the nurse slides the bedpan under him.
    2. Help the patient to a sitting position on the bedpan on the side of the bed.
    3. Ask the patient to roll over and position the bedpan on his buttocks and have him roll over onto it.
    4. Ask the patient to get out of bed and use a bedside commode.

72. If a nurse is allowed to clip a patient's toenails, which technique is recommended?
    1. Clip nails as short as possible.
    2. Clip nails with square corners.
    3. Round off the edges of the nails.
    4. Clip the nails straight across.

73. A patient with a healing stage III decubitus ulcer asks the nurse if the ulcer will leave a scar once it has healed. Which response by the nurse is most correct?
    1. "Sometimes there is a scar, and sometimes there isn't."
    2. "I don't think you should worry about that right now."

3. "Usually there is a scar present with this type of healing."
4. "I think you should ask your doctor about that tomorrow."

74. A patient has an indwelling urinary retention catheter. The nurse is instructed to obtain a sterile urine specimen from the patient. To accomplish this task, the nurse should:
1. Remove the patient's catheter and have him or her void.
2. Remove the urine from the balloon port with a syringe.
3. Collect the specimen from the sampling port on the drainage tube with a syringe.
4. Disconnect the catheter from the drainage tubing and let urine drain into the specimen container.

75. While transporting a patient to the radiology department in a wheelchair, the nurse should place the urinary drainage bag from her retention catheter:
1. On the patient's lap
2. Clipped to patient's front robe pocket
3. On the IV pole that is attached to the wheelchair
4. Hung from the side rail or back rail of the wheelchair that is below hip level

76. A nurse is providing denture care for a patient. What should be done when storing the dentures?
1. Place the patient's name on the denture cup.
2. Line the denture cup with a paper towel.
3. Place a cleansing tablet in the denture cup first.
4. Place adhesive grip on the patient's dentures.

77. Which statement made by a patient going for a colonoscopy indicates that further teaching is needed?
1. "Thank goodness I will be put out for the procedure!"
2. "I will have to have cleansing enemas beforehand."
3. "I hope my rectum doesn't hurt too much afterward."
4. "My doctor may be able to see where my bleeding is coming from."

78. A hospitalized patient has complained of insomnia to the nurse. Which action should be included in this patient's plan of care?
1. Open the patient's door to give him a sense of security.
2. Leave the television on all night long.
3. Allow the patient to exercise before going to bed.
4. Give the patient a backrub with warm lotion before the patient goes to bed.

79. A nurse is applying a bandage to a patient's foot, ankle, lower leg, and knee. Where should the nurse begin bandaging the extremity?
1. At the foot
2. At the knee
3. At the ankle
4. At the middle of the leg

80. In an emergency situation, what is the first priority of patient care?
1. Obtaining the victim's medical history
2. Controlling bleeding from a compound fracture
3. Maintaining an open airway for adequate oxygenation
4. Performing a survey at the scene of the victim's accident

81. A nurse is assessing vital signs of a patient who has had a right mastectomy. Where should the nurse measure the patient's blood pressure (BP)?
1. On the patient's lower forearm
2. On the patient's left arm
3. Over the popliteal artery
4. On the patient's lower leg

82. A patient is ordered Tylenol gr. X every 6 hours p.r.n. for headache. The patient requests the Tylenol, which is delivered as a 325-mg tablet. How many tablets should the nurse give the patient?
Answer: ____ tablet(s)

83. Which assessment data should be reported immediately after having been obtained?
1. A newborn with a respiratory rate of 32 breaths/min
2. A 30-year-old athlete with a pulse rate of 58 beats/min
3. An 87-year-old patient with Alzheimer disease with a respiratory rate of 20 breaths/min
4. A 40-year-old postthyroidectomy patient with a pulse rate of 120 beats/min

84. A nurse needs to obtain a sputum specimen from a patient. At which time of day would it be easier for the nurse to obtain the specimen?
1. After a meal
2. Between meals
3. In the morning
4. In the evening

85. In teaching a patient about respiratory care, which measure would the nurse recommend to prevent respiratory secretions from becoming thick and difficult to expectorate?
1. Adequate sleep
2. Regular exercise
3. A nourishing diet
4. A generous fluid intake

86. What would indicate to the nurse that a patient may need sputum suctioned from his respiratory tract?
1. A respiratory rate of 22 breaths/min
2. A heart rate that is tachycardic
3. A gurgling noise in his airway
4. Expectoration of a large amount of green mucus

87. The nurse is speaking with a family concerning hospice care for an elderly relative. The nurse advises the family that one of the basic goals of hospice care is that:
1. The patient will not have to pay for his medications.
2. Hospice nurses will try to make the patient as comfortable as possible.
3. Care will be provided in a hospital or SNF.
4. The family will provide most skilled care.

88. The nurse learns that a patient has an advance directive. This document ensures that:
1. Only lifesaving heroic measures will be used.
2. The patient's right to make decisions about his death will be honored.
3. The physician will not attempt to dissuade the patient from any treatment plans.
4. The family's rights to make final decisions concerning the care of the terminally ill patient will be honored.

89. When should the nurse begin preparing for a patient's discharge?
1. When the patient is admitted to the hospital
2. After the physician writes the discharge instructions
3. During the patient's last 2 or 3 days of hospitalization
4. After procedures take place that may necessitate a convalescent period

90. Which nursing action is performed on patients with known or suspected renal calculi?
1. Flank massage
2. Urine reductions
3. Straining of all urine
4. Restriction of fluid intake

91. While collecting a 24-hour urine specimen, the nurse should:
    1. Send each void to the laboratory immediately.
    2. Place the specimens in the refrigerator.
    3. Make sure that every other void is sent to the laboratory.
    4. Keep all urine on ice for the entire 24 hours.

92. A postoperative patient is complaining of "gas pains." Which nursing intervention would aid in relieving the patient's discomfort?
    1. Maintaining the patient on bed rest
    2. Contacting the physician for medication
    3. Inserting a rectal tube for 30 minutes
    4. Encouraging the use of straws for drinking liquids

93. A nurse is instructed to perform chest physiotherapy (CPT) on a patient with bronchitis. What is the correct rationale for this procedure?
    1. Moves residual air from the patient's lungs
    2. Prevents pneumonia from developing
    3. Forces the patient to take deep breaths
    4. Breaks up and mobilizes secretions

94. Which patient is most at risk for developing a decubitus ulcer?
    1. A patient with a urinary tract infection
    2. A patient with chronic obstructive pulmonary disease
    3. A patient with cholecystitis
    4. A patient who is constipated

95. When the integrity of the skin has been damaged or broken as in an abrasion or decubitus ulcer, the body loses some of its ability to:
    1. Resist infections.
    2. Produce antibodies.
    3. Eliminate waste products.
    4. Maintain correct body alignment.

96. An obese postoperative patient asks the nurse why the physician wants her to wear an abdominal binder. What is the best statement from the nurse?
    1. "Because you are so large, the incision might break open."
    2. "The binder will help reduce the stress on your suture line."
    3. "You will be able to walk better if you wear it."
    4. "It will decrease your incisional pain."

97. A nurse has been asked to shave a male patient. Which laboratory values would the nurse recognize as a contraindication to shaving the patient?
    1. WBC of 14.8
    2. INR of 3.1
    3. Hemoglobin level of 17
    4. BUN of 91

98. The nurse is performing mouth care on an unconscious patient. In which position should the nurse place the patient?
    1. Prone, with head turned to one side
    2. Supine, with suction equipment nearby
    3. Semi-Fowler, with a towel under the chin
    4. Side-lying, with head turned to the side

99. During a preoperative assessment of a patient, the nurse finds that the patient experiences sleep apnea. The nurse recognizes sleep apnea as a:
    1. Problem caused by snoring or overeating.
    2. Problem that is increased if the patient is overly nervous or upset.
    3. Syndrome that is transitory and not considered dangerous.
    4. Syndrome that can cause symptoms of daytime tiredness and fatigue.

100. What is the best way for the nurse to assess the intensity of a patient's pain?
    1. Ask the patient how long he or she has been experiencing the pain
    2. Ask the patient to point to the location of the pain that he or she is feeling
    3. Ask the patient to rate the pain on a scale of 1 (mild) to 10 (severe)
    4. Ask the patient to gauge the pain using words such as "bad" or "severe"

101. A patient is learning to walk with crutches. After traveling down the hallway, the patient complains of numbness in his axilla and tingling of his fingers. The nurse should:
    1. Switch the patient to a walker.
    2. Notify the physician of possible nerve damage to the arm.
    3. Adjust the crutch length and review appropriate crutch technique with the patient.
    4. Provide padding to the patient's axilla and assist in doing range-of-motion exercises.

102. A patient has right-sided weakness from the effects of a cerebrovascular accident. The patient begins to use a cane. The nurse instructs the patient to use the cane in the left hand and move it simultaneously with:
    1. Both arms.
    2. Both feet.
    3. The left leg.
    4. The right leg.

103. A nurse is assessing an individual on bed rest for possible edema. Where might the nurse find edema in a patient who is confined to bed?
    1. Feet
    2. Hands
    3. Calves
    4. Sacrum

104. A nurse is instructing a UAP to administer a nonmedicated vaginal douche to an elderly patient. Which statement made by the UAP signifies understanding of the procedure?
    1. "The patient should wait to void until after the douche is given."
    2. "The douche tip should be inserted, and then instillation of fluid can begin."
    3. "The fluid should be already flowing when I place the tip into the vagina."
    4. "The fluid should be instilled using lots of pressure to make sure that the vagina gets clean."

105. Which vital signs collected by the nurse from adult patients are considered abnormal and need to be reported?
    1. Oral temperature 99° F (37.22° C), pulse 68, respirations 20, blood pressure (BP) 122/80
    2. Rectal temperature 102° F (38.89° C), pulse 100, respirations 22, BP 118/50
    3. Axillary temperature 97.8° F (36.56° C), pulse 88, respirations 20, BP 138/70
    4. Tympanic temperature 98.5° F (37° C), pulse 74, respirations 16, BP 120/84

106. A patient who is on a 1000 mL/day fluid restriction because of renal insufficiency is observed to be consuming a large amount of water from the water faucet in her room. The nurse estimates that she may have consumed more than 3000 mL in a short period. The nurse should expect that the patient's weight will:
    1. Increase.
    2. Decrease.
    3. Remain the same; the patient will just rid herself of excess fluid.
    4. Remain the same; the patient needed the water because of her dehydrated state.

107. A patient is being monitored by pulse oximetry via a clip-on probe. The machine alarm sounds, and the oxygen saturation reads 60%. The patient is sitting up in bed and talking with his family. What is the nurse's first course of action?
    1. Call the physician immediately.
    2. Begin oxygen therapy at 3 L/min via nasal cannula.
    3. Adjust the clip-on probe on the finger or move it to another finger.
    4. Remove family members from the room to better deal with this emergency.

108. A nurse is caring for a patient who is on bed rest. The time is 8:50 AM. The patient will need to be transferred at 9:00 AM to the x-ray department by stretcher for an abdominal flat plate. Place the following skills in the correct sequence from beginning to end.
    1. Make the patient's bed.
    2. Have the patient void.
    3. Assist the patient in moving onto the stretcher.
    4. Elevate the patient's head for comfort.

109. A patient receiving oxygen therapy asks why the nurse takes a pulse oximetry measurement each shift. What is the correct explanation by the nurse?
    1. "This number is the amount of oxygen you have in your blood."
    2. "It helps us determine if you are receiving enough oxygen."
    3. "It allows the physician to determine the amount of oxygen ordered."
    4. "It is an important vital sign for any person on oxygen."

110. A nurse is packing a surgical incision with a 2 × 2 gauze pad soaked in saline solution. The nurse drops the wet gauze pad on the edge of the sterile field. What should the nurse do next?
    1. Pick up the gauze pad and put it in the wound.
    2. Leave the gauze where it fell and prepare a new one.
    3. Pick up the gauze and rinse it out in the saline solution before using.
    4. Begin anew, with a new sterile tray, dressings, and gloves.

111. A patient is receiving 75% humidified oxygen by means of a tracheostomy collar. The patient requires suctioning. Which action should the nurse perform that will be safe for the patient?
    1. Restrain the patient.
    2. Administer supplemental oxygen to the patient.
    3. Apply suction while carefully advancing the catheter.
    4. Use a rotating motion while carefully advancing the catheter.

112. Which fluids should be measured and factored in a patient's fluid output? Select all that apply.
    _____ 1. Vomitus
    _____ 2. Urine output
    _____ 3. Diarrhea
    _____ 4. Tube feedings

113. Which action would best assist in reducing the incidence of aspiration in a patient receiving a tube feeding?
    1. Clamp tube after feeding has infused.
    2. Flush tube with water after each feeding.
    3. Dilute feedings to half-strength solutions.
    4. Have patient remain in an upright position for 45 minutes after feeding.

114. The nurse is inserting a nasogastric tube into a patient. What would indicate that the tube is in the patient's trachea?
    1. The patient is unable to speak.
    2. The nurse cannot see the tube in the back of the throat.
    3. The patient blows his nose, and blood is present on the tissue.
    4. The nurse notes that the tube has a return of light green drainage.

115. A hospitalized patient is ordered both an oil-retention enema and a cleansing enema. Which statement correctly explains the rationale for administering these enemas?
    1. The enemas work together to stimulate peristalsis.
    2. The oil-retention enema softens the stool, and the cleansing enema stimulates peristalsis.
    3. If the oil-retention enema does not work to evacuate the bowel, the cleansing enema can be given.
    4. The cleansing enema is generally given to soften the stool 30 minutes before the oil-retention enema.

116. A nurse has made a mistake in a nursing entry. The nurse meant to write that the vomitus amount was 75 mL. However, she mistakenly entered 175 mL. How should the nurse correct the error?
    1. Use a white-out pen to cover up the 1 in the 175.
    2. Rewrite the nurse's note using a new patient progress note.
    3. Erase the entry, and rewrite the correct figure.
    4. Draw a line through the error, and write the correct amount above and initial the entry.

117. A patient visits a physician's office with complaints of constipation for 6 days. The information in which patient statement made during the taking of the health history may be contributing to the constipation?
    1. "I exercise almost every day."
    2. "I eat plenty of raw vegetables."
    3. "I am not a big water drinker."
    4. "I go to the bathroom when I feel the need."

118. A nurse has inserted a urethral retention catheter, and 750 mL of urine quickly collects in the drainage bag. What is the nurse's next course of action?
    1. Clamp the Foley catheter for 20 minutes.
    2. Send a specimen to the laboratory.
    3. Increase the patient's IV fluid flow rate.
    4. Remove the catheter.

119. A UAP asks why a patient's arm is contracted into a flexed position. Which statement is the best response by the nurse?
    1. "A physical therapy consultation is needed to help this patient."
    2. "The muscles of the arm must have been damaged in some way."

3. "The muscles are permanently shortened because of the effects of immobility."

4. "The arm is just temporarily frozen; range-of-motion (ROM) exercises should restore it."

120. An elderly postoperative patient has an order to ambulate a few hours after surgery. The patient becomes upset with the nurse and wants to know why he should ambulate so soon after surgery. Which is the best response by the nurse?

1. "You know what they say, if you don't use it, you might lose it."

2. "Please get out of bed now. You can ask your doctor in the morning."

3. "Your doctor always orders his patients out of bed right after surgery."

4. "Walking will keep the fluids in your lungs moving so bacteria will not grow."

121. A nurse is applying antiembolic stockings on a patient before surgery. The patient asks why the stockings need to be so snug. The nurse responds that snugness is needed because:

1. "They do not do their job if they are too loose."

2. "The stockings pool blood in your legs during surgery."

3. "They are meant to exercise the muscles of the legs while you are in surgery."

4. "They help to prevent blood clots from developing by pushing blood toward the heart."

122. Which would be an appropriate short-term nursing goal (surgical day 1) for a patient with pain secondary to post-ORIF (open reduction internal fixation) of the left hip?

1. Patient will have decreased need for pain medication.

2. Patient will have decreased pain 30 minutes after meperidine (Demerol) 50 mg IM is given.

3. Patient will walk length of hallway three times per day.

4. Patient will participate in physical therapy sessions.

123. A nurse working in a skilled nursing facility is admitting a patient with Alzheimer disease. The family reports that the patient frequently becomes agitated late in the evening. What should be included in this patient's plan of care?

1. Encourage the patient to attend an aerobic class each evening.

2. Encourage the patient to watch old war movies in the evening.

3. Engage the patient in social hour.

4. Provide for quiet time for the patient in the evening.

124. A patient returns from surgery with a large abdominal dressing in place. As the evening progresses, the nurse notes that some drainage has seeped through the dressing. What is the nurse's best course of action?

1. Change the dressing.

2. Reinforce the dressing with additional gauze.

3. Remove the dressing and leave the wound open to air.

4. Remove the dressing and send it to the laboratory for culture.

125. A patient has consumed the following foods for lunch. What is the patient's intake?

5 oz of cranberry juice

120 mL of ice cream

8 oz of milk

1 cup of cream of tomato soup

4 oz of pudding

Answer: _____ mL

126. A nurse is applying heat to the leg of a patient with cellulitis of the leg. Which of the following facts in the patient's medical history necessitates special precautions on the part of the nurse?

1. Blindness

2. Paraplegia

3. Hypertension

4. Diabetes mellitus

127. When the nurse auscultates the lungs of a patient who is on bed rest, she hears diminished sounds with some rhonchi. Which nursing actions may clear the patient's lung sounds? Select all that apply.

_____ 1. Encourage use of incentive spirometer

_____ 2. Have patient perform coughing and deep-breathing exercises

_____ 3. Have patient ambulate

_____ 4. Administer pain medication

_____ 5. Administer oxygen therapy

128. A nurse is assessing a patient's incision line. Which of the following may indicate infection?

1. The area surrounding the sutures is red and swollen.

2. Some of the sutures have fallen out of the incision line.

3. There is no drainage around the sutures; the surrounding skin is pink.

4. Sutures are all intact; a small amount of serosanguineous drainage is present.

129. A 50-year-old woman visits the physician's office for a routine physical. The health history indicates that the patient has never had a mammogram. The nurse teaches the patient that mammograms:

1. Are done when breast cancer is suspected.

2. Should be done every 1 to 2 years as a routine screening examination.

3. Are not necessary if the woman does not have a history of breast cancer in the family.

4. Are difficult for the woman to undergo and therefore are recommended only every 5 to 10 years.

130. A nurse is assisting a UAP in setting up a footboard on a patient's bed. The UAP asks the nurse why a footboard would be used. The nurse's best response is:

1. "A footboard will assist in maintaining good abduction."

2. "It will prevent the patient from developing thrombophlebitis."

3. "It will keep the foot from developing plantar flexion."

4. "The patient will be able to use the board to help push herself up in bed."

131. A nurse is making the decision to purchase liability insurance. He should keep in mind that professional liability coverage:

1. Costs the same in all health care settings.

2. Protects the nurse from prosecution for criminal acts.

3. Does not cover acts outside the scope of nursing practice.

4. Provides coverage to the nurse for his or her entire professional career.

132. A nurse overhears a terminally ill patient with cancer state to his family members, "If I get over this cancer thing, I will travel with the church's missionary to South Africa next spring." Which stage of the dying process is this patient exhibiting?

1. Anger

2. Denial

3. Bargaining

4. Depression

133. A nurse is caring for a patient with a paralytic ileus. What assessment data are most important for this patient?
    1. Lung sounds
    2. Bowel sounds
    3. Peripheral pulses
    4. Neurological examination findings

134. The nurse is performing a 24-hour creatinine clearance test on a patient with possible renal failure. The test is scheduled from 6 AM on Thursday until 6 AM on Friday. The patient voids at 6 AM on Friday. What should the nurse do with this last void?
    1. Discard the urine.
    2. Add it to the collection container.
    3. Send the urine for culture.
    4. Send the urine for a routine urinalysis.

135. A patient has continuous bladder irrigation. He has a total urine output of 1100 mL for an 8-hour period. The continuous bladder irrigation has been instilling at 60 mL/hr. What is his true urine output?
    Answer: _____ mL

136. The UAP has collected a stool specimen from a patient suspected of having pinworms. She asks the nurse what to do with the specimen. How should the nurse direct the UAP?
    1. "Take it to the laboratory immediately."
    2. "Put it in the fridge, and the laboratory can pick it up at the end of the shift."
    3. "Place it on the counter, and call the laboratory to come pick it up."
    4. "Transfer the stool to a sterile specimen cup for transfer to the laboratory."

137. A patient complains of low back pain during a nursing home health visit. Which are appropriate nursing actions at this time? Select all that apply.
    _____ 1. Gather assessment data concerning the pain.
    _____ 2. Call the physician to increase the dosage of the patient's pain medication.
    _____ 3. Report the complaint to the RN supervisor.
    _____ 4. Offer to make the patient an appointment at the pain clinic.

138. The nurse needs to assess the following individuals. Which patient should the nurse see first?
    1. A patient who is receiving chest percussion from a respiratory therapist
    2. A patient who is being fed by a nursing assistant
    3. A patient who had a hypoglycemic episode last shift
    4. A patient who has just been medicated for pain

139. A patient has been diagnosed with dehydration. Which symptom would confirm the diagnosis?
    1. Hematuria
    2. Polyuria
    3. Enuresis
    4. Oliguria

140. Which tasks could the LPN/LVN safely assign to a UAP? Select all that apply.
    _____ 1. Monthly vital signs on a resident
    _____ 2. Feeding an elderly patient
    _____ 3. Transporting a patient to physical therapy
    _____ 4. Collecting a clean-catch urine specimen
    _____ 5. Administering a soap suds enema

141. A nurse is preparing to collect a specimen for an HgbA$_{1c}$. Which technique will be used for collecting the specimen?
    1. Venipuncture
    2. Palpation
    3. Percussion
    4. Auscultation

142. A patient with a tracheostomy wants to eat lunch orally. What is the correct sequence of events (from earliest to latest) to ready the patient for his meal?
    1. Provide the lunch.
    2. Inflate the balloon on the tracheostomy cuff.
    3. Suction the tracheostomy.
    4. Provide mouth care.

143. A nurse is measuring the urine output of a patient with an indwelling urinary catheter. How should the volume of urine be measured?
    1. Estimate the amount and mark it on the intake/output record.
    2. Empty the contents into a bedpan for measurement.
    3. Drain the catheter bag into a graduated cylinder for measurement.
    4. Measure the urine from the markings on the bag.

144. Two nurses are assessing an apical-radial pulse rate. One nurse reports the apical rate to be 72, and the other nurse reports the radial pulse as 80. Which best describes the activity?
    1. The pulse deficit was assessed correctly.
    2. The patient's radial pulse cannot be higher than the apical pulse; the assessment should be done again.
    3. The nurses should report the pulse deficit as 8.
    4. The nurses need to enlist the help of an RN in assessing the pulses.

145. A nurse is preparing to insert a urethral retention catheter into a patient. Place the following steps in order starting with the earliest (first) step to the latest (last) step.
    1. Document catheter size, tolerance, and urine return.
    2. Cleanse the perineum from pubis to rectum.
    3. Instill sterile water to inflate the balloon.
    4. Insert the catheter into the urethra until urine flow is established.
    5. Put on sterile gloves.
    6. Check the physician's order.

146. A patient of the Islamic faith refuses to eat a hot dog on his tray because he is afraid that it may contain pork products. What is the best response by the nurse?
    1. "I'm sure they are all-beef hot dogs."
    2. "So you don't want anything to eat, then?"
    3. "Would you like me to get a substitution from the kitchen?"
    4. "I don't understand why that should make a difference."

147. A patient who has consented to surgery tells the nurse that he now refuses that same surgery. Which is the best response by the nurse?
    1. "What has happened to change your mind?"
    2. "I will need to call your family about this."
    3. "You already signed the consent. I think you have to have the surgery."
    4. "Should I call the physician so you can talk to him?"

148. Place an X on the area of the chest where you will best hear a patient's apical pulse.

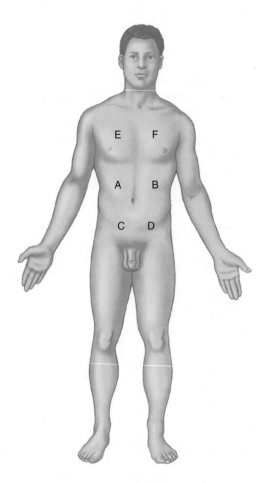

149. The nurse is preparing to irrigate an eye. What is the correct technique for performing the procedure?
    1. Keep patient's head in a neutral position, pouring solution in a downward manner above patient's eye.
    2. Turn patient's head away from the injured eye, pouring solution from the outer to inner canthus of the eye.
    3. Turn patient's head toward the injured eye, pouring solution from the inner to outer canthus of the eye.
    4. Maintain patient's head in a neutral position, swabbing the injured eye from inner to outer canthus.

150. Place an X on the letter where the nurse will begin to cleanse a midline abdominal incision.

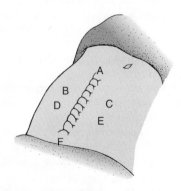

ANSWERS AND RATIONALES

1. Analysis, implementation, psychosocial integrity, (b).
    3. This statement reduces fear of abandonment and alleviates fear of needs not being met.
    1. Pain medication is not commonly needed during this procedure.
    2. Limiting visitors increases anxiety and causes feelings of isolation.
    4. The patient and secretions are radioactive during treatment.

2. Application, planning, safe and effective care environment, (c).
    2. The HIPPA guidelines are designed to streamline health care and preserve the patient's right to privacy.
    1. Patients always have the right to refuse treatment.
    3. Suing for malpractice or negligence is the right of an individual.
    4. No current guidelines exist in the United States to preserve a patient's right for assisted suicide.

3. Application, implementation, physiological integrity, (b).
    1. Stimulating the gag reflex may result in vomiting.
    2. Secretions do not originate in the throat area.
    3. Contamination of the culture site is not of primary consideration.
    4. The size of the specimen is not a concern with a throat culture.

4. Application, assessment, physiological integrity, (c).
    1. This intervention gathers more information before determining course of action.
    2. This may not be the course of action; more data are needed.
    3. Elevating the foot reduces edema, but it does not address the numbness and tingling.
    4. Wiggling her toes will not alleviate the numbness and tingling.

5. Application, implementation, safe and effective care environment, (a).
    4. This action best protects the nurse against the specific dangers of wound irrigation such as splashing or spraying of blood and body fluids.
    1. Common knowledge states that the bed should be at a workable height for all procedures.
    2. Explaining the procedure alleviates patient anxiety; it does not protect the nurse.
    3. Handwashing is indicated before and after all patient procedures.

6. Comprehension, planning, physiological integrity, (c).
    4. Older individuals with orthopedic injuries experience immobility complicated by impaired sensory function.
    1. Patients with a vertebral injury can still assist with relieving pressure.
    2. Patients in skeletal traction can still assist in relieving pressure.
    3. Ambulatory patients are at low risk for decubitus ulcer formation.

7. Analysis, planning, physiological integrity, (b).
    4. Mouth care relieves the discomfort related to the mouth dryness caused by mouth breathing.
    1. This is unwarranted; this situation does not warrant immediate medical attention.

2. This causes a potential for electrolyte imbalance.

3. This response does not address patient discomfort.

8. Application, implementation, physiological integrity, (c).

   4. *This answer gives a brief, reasonable answer to meet the patient's needs.*

   1. This answer is a little too graphic or alarming for the patient.

   2. The ink should not be removed.

   3. No reason exists to consult the physician when the nurse can give the appropriate response.

9. Application, planning, physiological integrity, (c).

   X   1. *The nurse can discern if the patient has a full bladder by this method, which will dictate further action.*

   _____ 2. This may be the eventual outcome of this scenario, but it is not the nurse's first course of action.

   X   3. *The nurse can discern if the patient has a full bladder by this method, which will dictate further action. Bladder scanners may not be readily available in all facilities.*

   _____ 4. This may be part of the nurse's plan; however, it is not the first course of action.

10. Application, planning, physiological integrity, (c).

    3. *The assessment data signify a catheter blockage that may be alleviated with bladder irrigation.*

    1. Position changes will not relieve an obstructed catheter.

    2. The assessment data can be expected; nurse can proceed within scope of practice without notifying the physician.

    4. The nurse should act on these observations, not document them.

11. Application, assessment, physiological integrity, (b).

    2. *Patients who have been on bed rest may have a drop in blood pressure arising or getting up quickly, which can be alleviated by dangling a few minutes at the bedside.*

    1. Anemia does cause dizziness; however, the question does not indicate that this is a problem.

    3. Hypoxia may cause this problem, but no indications exist that the patient has a respiratory disorder.

    4. Hypertension generally manifests with nosebleeds and headaches.

12. Application, assessment, physiological integrity, (c).

    3. *Urinary urgency and lower abdominal pressure are symptoms of a full bladder; the catheter may be malfunctioning or blocked.*

    1. The cause of the pain must first be determined.

    2. This is not related to the patient's physical discomfort.

    4. This response fails to address the patient's discomfort.

13. Application, implementation, physiological integrity, (c).

    3. *This is the primary purpose for irrigating a colostomy.*

    1. Although this is an outcome for the procedure, it is not the primary purpose.

    2. This is the purpose for enemas; however, it does not address why it is being done.

    4. Depending on the type of ostomy, stool softeners may or may not be needed.

14. Application, planning, safe and effective care environment, (c).

    X   1. *This action is normally assigned to a UAP.*

   _____ 2. This action requires a higher level of skill and is not within the UAP's scope of practice.

   X   3. *This action is normally assigned to a UAP.*

   _____ 4. This action requires a higher level of skill and is not within the UAP's scope of practice.

   _____ 5. This action requires a higher level of skill and is not within the UAP's scope of practice.

   X   6. *This action is normally assigned to a UAP.*

15. Application, evaluation, physiological integrity, (c).

    3. *A delayed infusion of IV solution is often caused by obstruction of the rate of flow; the action allows for further assessment of the problem.*

    1. Not enough data have been collected to make this assumption.

    2. These data indicate further action on the nurse's part.

    4. Changing the rate of flow places the patient at risk for injury.

16. Application, implementation, psychosocial integrity, (b).

    1. *This enables the patient to communicate his or her needs.*

    2. This is a secondary comfort measure; communication of needs would be a primary patient concern.

    3. The presence of the nurse is more important than reassurances.

    4. This does not address the patient's comfort.

17. Analysis, evaluation, physiological integrity, (b).

    4. *A full assessment includes both subjective and objective data.*

    1. Objective signs do not address cues that the patient himself can provide when evaluating progress.

    2. Limiting data collection to subjective information ignores the observable, measurable symptom not offered by the patient.

    3. Data must be gathered throughout the procedure to fully determine their effects on the patient.

18. Application, implementation, physiological integrity, (b).

    3. *This answers the patient's question correctly and addresses the patient's need.*

    1. This is not the appropriate response and can pose a hazard.

    2. This may be true but is not the correct way of responding.

    4. The patient should be NPO until the gag reflex has been assessed.

19. Analysis, planning, physiological integrity, (c).

    4. *This is the potential problem with the most serious consequences as indicated by Maslow's hierarchy of needs.*

    1. This may be a problem, especially if the patient is incontinent.

    2. No indications have been given that the individual is having difficulty obtaining nutrition.

    3. Deficient knowledge is not indicated in the question.

20. Analysis, implementation, physiological integrity, (b).

    1. *Weight should be measured at the same time each day and with the patient wearing the same clothing.*

    2. The patient should be weighed one time each day; the patient may be taking medication several times each day at different intervals.

    3. Medication should never be omitted; a more accurate measurement is weighing each morning.

    4. This is a symptom of advanced heart failure; daily weights indicate early symptoms.

21. Application, implementation, safe and effective care environment, (b).
    3. No reason exists for limiting visitors, provided they take the appropriate Contact Precautions.
    1. This is commonly part of Contact Isolation, and physicians do not frequently order this.
    2. This would be done no matter what type of isolation the patient was assigned.
    4. This is generally a normal nursing measure.

22. Analysis, evaluation, safe and effective care environment, (b).
    2. A nosocomial infection is an infection acquired during the course of a hospital stay or as a result of a medical treatment (urinary catheter).
    1. A superinfection is an illness produced by growth of a resistant organism during antimicrobial therapy.
    3. An autoimmune response is the immune reaction of the body against its own tissues.
    4. Antibiotic resistance is the continued growth of pathogenic organisms during antibiotic therapy.

23. Application, implementation, safe and effective care environment, (b).
    4. The nurse should remove the gown by shrugging it off the shoulders and rolling it up with the gloves by touching the inside of the gown only.
    1. Touching the outside of the gown would contaminate the nurse's hands.
    2. This practice is not carried out unless the patient is in reverse isolation.
    3. This would contaminate the other individual.

24. Analysis, assessment, psychosocial integrity, (b).
    1. Cultural beliefs influence the patient's choice of treatment and his or her perception of health care workers.
    2. Administration of last rites is a religious practice limited to the Roman Catholic religion.
    3. This is not the primary reason for gathering this information; the nurse needs to understand the patient's health practice beliefs to plan care.
    4. The nurse collects data concerning culture to formulate the patient's plan of care.

25. Application, planning, safe and effective care environment, (b).
    _X_ 1. The patient's WBC count is dangerously low, and the patient needs to be placed in Protective Isolation to decrease any chances for the patient to develop infection.
    _X_ 2. The patient should wear a mask for his own protection when traveling to different areas of the hospital for diagnostic examinations.
    _____ 3. This would be part of hemorrhagic precautions.
    _X_ 4. Fresh (raw) fruits, vegetables, and flowers may also increase the risk of infection for this patient.

26. Comprehension, implementation, safe and effective care environment, (b).
    1. Licensing laws are public safety measures.
    2. Licensing laws establish minimum standards.
    3. Moral character is a subjective measure that can be only minimally established by licensing law.
    4. Licensing laws do not limit the number of applicants to nursing practice.

27. Application, planning, safe and effective care environment, (b).
    3. The part being bandaged should remain in a functional position, which for the elbow is a slightly flexed position. This position is also more comfortable for the patient than any other position noted.
    1. Rotation is not a functional position for the elbow.
    2. Extension is not a functional position for the elbow.
    4. Hyperextension of the elbow is not the normal functional position for this joint.

28. Application, implementation, physiological integrity, (b).
    1. The patient's extremity should be elevated to decrease the amount of swelling before the wrap is placed. If the wrap is placed on an edematous extremity, skin breakdown may occur, or the wrap will fall off when the swelling decreases.
    2. This is the proper procedure, but it should be done after edema decreases in the leg.
    3. This is correct, but it is not the first course of action.
    4. This would be performed after the area has been wrapped.

29. Application, implementation, physiological integrity, (b).
    3. Using separate washcloth sections for each eye prevents the spread of organisms from one eye to the other.
    1. Rinsing and drying skinfolds reduces skin irritation.
    2. The use of clean gloves is a protective mechanism and part of standard precautions.
    4. Changing bath water to maintain the warmth of the water may be needed, but not necessarily after bathing each extremity.

30. Comprehension, implementation, physiological integrity, (b).
    2. This prevents pressure at the back of the neck and secures the cravat correctly.
    1. The knot would not secure the elbow if it were tied in this spot.
    3. This puts pressure on the patient's neck.
    4. Although it is good to give control to the patient, the patient may not have the correct knowledge to make this decision.

31. Application, implementation, physiological integrity, (c).
    2. Vertigo is a common side effect of this treatment.
    1. The pinna of the ear is retracted during the procedure.
    3. Most patients can resume activity shortly after treatment.
    4. Use of cotton-tipped applicators in the ears can lead to injury.

32. Application, implementation, physiological integrity, (b).
    1. Culture specimens can be inaccurate if obtained while the patient is receiving antibiotics.
    2. No clarification is necessary; this is a standard nursing function.
    3. Antibiotics interfere with microbial growth on the specimen cultures.
    4. Antibiotics interfere with microbial growth on the urine culture.

33. Application, assessment, physiological integrity, (b).
    3. The most common signs and symptoms of thrombophlebitis are pain in the calf on dorsiflexion of the foot.

1. Pain in the foot and ankle may be caused by other problems related to immobility, but pain in the calf is the most prominent symptom.
2. Fever and dry skin are symptoms of dehydration.
4. Temperature changes may occur with thrombophlebitis but are not a common symptom.

34. Application, assessment, physiological integrity, (c).

_____ 1. Gastrostomy site oozing is a common occurrence that requires skin integrity measures, but it does not indicate a need to withhold feedings.

__X__ 2. *This may indicate delayed gastric emptying; further feedings can induce vomiting.*

__X__ 3. *This may indicate delayed gastric emptying; further feedings can induce vomiting.*

_____ 4. No residual feeding return usually indicates full absorption of the feeding.

35. Application, implementation, physiological integrity, (b).

2. This may delay the patient's urge to defecate.

1. Maintaining fluid flow will increase the patient's urge to defecate.
3. This is untrue; the patient is likely to lose control of his bowels if the nurse does not adjust the flow rate.
4. The nurse would do this only if the prescribed amount of fluid has been given.

36. Application, implementation, physiological integrity, (b).

2. This is the correct rationale for this procedure.

1. The physician would not have difficulty. This is untrue.
3. Clipping hair has no outcome on patient pain perception.
4. Although it is more difficult to apply tape over hair, this is not the primary purpose.

37. Application, evaluation, physiological integrity, (c).

2. By having nothing in the stomach before surgery, the patient is less likely to have nausea and vomiting after surgery.

1. Cleansing enemas would help decrease problems after abdominal surgeries.
3. This decreases the chance for respiratory compromise after surgery.
4. This hydrates the patient before, during, and after surgery and replaces vital electrolytes lost during surgery.

38. Application, implementation, safe and effective care environment, (c).

1. The old dressing should be removed with clean gloves, not sterile.

2. This is the proper method for irrigation.
3. If packing is appropriate and ordered, sterile cotton swabs can be used.
4. This is always indicated.

39. Comprehension, implementation, physiological integrity, (b).

4. A JP is a type of grenade drain used to remove blood and fluid from the operative site.

1. A JP is not a type of dressing.
2. The JP does not hold dressings in place; it is a drain.
3. This is not the correct description of a JP.

40. Application, evaluation, safe and effective care environment, (b).

__X__ 1. *The nurse documents the exact location and size of the wounds.*

__X__ 2. *The nurse documents the characteristics of the suture line.*

_____ 3. The nurse does not need to address this area unless a specific problem exists.

_____ 4. The nurse does not need to address this area unless a specific problem exists.

41. Analysis, implementation, physiological integrity, (b).

4. Once blood begins to enter the specimen tube, the tourniquet is released to allow unrestricted blood flow.

1. Releasing the tourniquet causes the veins to recede, hindering access.
2. Keeping the tourniquet on during the blood draw lengthens the procedure and promotes venospasm.
3. This would promote bruising at the venipuncture site.

42. Comprehension, implementation, physiological integrity, (c).

1. Placing the arm in a downward position dilates the blood vessels for access.

2. The nurse's skill level influences patient discomfort.
3. Additives do not flow back into the blood tubes; they are already in the tubes.
4. The nurse restricts arm movement by holding the patient's arm.

43. Application, implementation, physiological integrity, (c).

3. This action keeps the viscera moist until the surgeon arrives to correct the problem.

1. This should never be done; the nurse may further compromise the patient.
2. This should be done after the saline-soaked gauze has been applied.
4. This may be contraindicated by the patient's condition.

44. Analysis, evaluation, physiological integrity, (c).

4. These vital signs should lead the nurse to believe that the patient is experiencing hemorrhagic shock.

1. The patient's temperature is normal, which would rule out infection.
2. Vital signs would not immediately alert the nurse to dehiscence.
3. Vital signs would not immediately alert the nurse to the complication of thrombophlebitis.

45. Comprehension, evaluation, physiological integrity, (c).

1. Early ambulation provides the most venous return, decreasing venous stasis, and is the best method for preventing this complication.

2. These devices do minimize thrombophlebitis, but early ambulation is the best method.
3. This practice does not prevent thrombophlebitis.
4. This practice does not prevent thrombophlebitis.

46. Application, assessment, physiological integrity, (c).

2. This is the proper rationale. The surgery is a palliative treatment.

1. The patient is terminally ill. The colostomy will not cure the cancer.
3. It is unlikely that this would be reversed when the purpose of the surgery is palliative.
4. The patient's diagnosis has already been made.

47. Application, implementation, psychosocial integrity, (a).

1. Cleansing and preparing the body before family viewing decreases the stress of the situation.

2. Postmortem care is always completed before the body is moved.
3. Family and patient needs are the priority of unit function.
4. The family will be less stressed if the patient's body is clean and has a more normal appearance.

48. Analysis, evaluation, physiological integrity, (c).
    2. *These statements indicate that the patient may be developing thrombophlebitis.*
    1. The expectation is that a solid food such as pizza would make a person nauseated at this time.
    3. This is a true statement, and a small amount of gas is expected to develop.
    4. The patient may have lost some sodium during surgery, but this does not indicate a problem.

49. Comprehension, planning, physiological integrity, (b).
    2. *The drying and subsequent removal of wet-to-dry dressings create mechanical débridement of wounds.*
    1. This is not the chief effect of this wound treatment; application of moist heat or increased patient activity would increase circulation.
    3. Wet-to-damp dressing promotes absorption of wound secretions.
    4. Wet-to-dry dressings have no effect on wound edema.

50. Application, implementation, physiological integrity, (b).
    1. *Walking assists in removing gas from the intestines.*
    2. This would be indicated only if the patient were not able to walk.
    3. This is a physician-ordered medication. Walking may alleviate the gas without medication.
    4. Milk does not assist the patient with removing gas, and the patient may not be on a full-liquid diet yet.

51. Analysis, planning, health promotion and maintenance, (b).
    4. *This condition will result unless corrective action is taken by the nurse.*
    1. There is no assessment information given to indicate an alteration in fluid status.
    2. Tissue integrity may be altered if the patient's skin integrity is breached, but it is not a pertinent diagnosis at this time.
    3. There are no assessment data given to indicate that the resident is confused.

52. Comprehension, implementation, physiological integrity, (b).
    3. *Because of the danger of aspiration, fluids should not be introduced into a nasogastric tube until correct placement has been verified.*
    1. Although this is a part of the procedure, the primary step is verification of tube location.
    2. The feeding need only be room temperature.
    4. Fluid should never be introduced into a nasogastric tube until placement in the stomach is verified.

53. Application, implementation, safe and effective care environment, (b).
    2. *This position relieves strain on back muscles and uses the strongest muscles for lifting.*
    1. To prevent injury, personnel must stand close to the object being lifted.
    3. This puts undue strain on the back muscles.
    4. This causes a narrow base of support; a wide base of support is needed for stability.

54. Analysis, evaluation, physiological integrity, (c).
    3. *The nurse should take action if the patient's status is 10 hours postoperative and the patient has not voided. Anesthesia may be causing retention of urine.*
    1. A small amount of bloody drainage should be expected after surgery.
    2. This is a normal method for decreasing incisional pain after surgery.
    4. Most patients are reluctant to ambulate immediately after surgery.

55. Analysis, planning, physiological integrity, (b).
    1. *The nurse must make sure that the specimen has adhered to the slide before sending it to the laboratory.*
    2. There is no need to refrigerate the slide, and doing so may change results.
    3. Staining is a method done in the laboratory to diagnose bacteria.
    4. Blood for arterial blood gas analysis must be placed on ice.

56. Analysis, implementation, physiological integrity, (b).
    3. *This is the correct response; it provides facts without alarming the patient.*
    1. More information is needed here. The patient may think he has a blood clot.
    2. This is alarming and most likely untrue.
    4. This may be true if we knew that the patient was taking an anticoagulant.

57. Application, planning, safe and effective care environment, (a).
    3. *Taking people out of harm's way is always the first step in the event of fire.*
    1. This sequence of events does not put the patient's safety first.
    2. This sequence does not place the patient's safety first.
    4. Preserving the safety of the patient is always the first step in the event of a fire.

58. Application, implementation, safe and effective care environment, (b).
    2. *If a line is made through the entry, others may still read the original entry; dating and initialing it is the proper procedure that signifies accountability.*
    1. This is improper and does not allow others to see the original mistake.
    3. This would be destroying property belonging to the hospital; it is considered falsifying records.
    4. Using correction fluid does not allow others to see the original message.

59. Application, implementation, physiological integrity, (c).
    _____ 1. Iodine is a nonmetallic element and is used as a contrast agent for blood vessels in computed tomography scans, not in MRI.
    __X__ 2. *Most MRI units are enclosed. Knowing if the patient has claustrophobia would be important.*
    __X__ 3. *Patients cannot have any metal on or in their body when undergoing an MRI test.*
    __X__ 4. *Patients cannot have any metal on or in their body when undergoing an MRI test.*
    _____ 5. Enemas are not given before an MRI; thus this information is not needed.

60. Application, implementation, physiological integrity, (b).
    3. Supplemental feedings are necessary to prepare the patient for the surgical procedure as indicated in this situation.
    1. Increasing peristalsis is not the action that the nasogastric tube is performing.
    2. A nasogastric tube inserted to decompress the stomach will result in removal of fluids and gas.
    4. This response does not answer the patient's question concerning the purpose of the tube.

61. Comprehension, implementation, physiological integrity, (c).
    4. This is the correct use of the information derived from a cholangiogram.
    1. An intravenous pyelogram is most useful in diagnosing kidney damage.
    2. Liver function tests are useful in diagnosing liver damage.
    3. A cardiac catheterization, a type of angiogram, is useful in the diagnosis of cardiac disease.

62. Application, implementation, physiological integrity, (b).
    3. The major reason for ostomy pouches to fit snugly is to prevent excoriation of the surrounding skin by the drainage.
    1. Although this is a true statement, this is not the major reason for a snug-fitting appliance.
    2. Normally pouches can be removed when the patient takes a bath; this is not the major reason for a snug-fitting appliance.
    4. Although this is true, it is not the major reason for a snug-fitting appliance.

63. Comprehension, planning, physiological integrity, (b).
    4. An NPO order ensures that the stomach will be empty, therefore decreasing the chance for aspiration if the patient vomits after surgery.
    1. Anesthesia does slow down the digestive process, but it does not stop it.
    2. The energy needs of a surgical patient increase, not decrease.
    3. Vomiting does not normally occur; and, if the stomach is empty, aspiration is less likely to occur.

64. Application, implementation, physiological integrity, (b).
    2. This period allows the nurse to remove secretions effectively and not interrupt the patient's normal breathing pattern for too long.
    1. This is not an adequate period to remove secretions.
    3. Thirty seconds is too long to keep a patient from his or her normal breathing patterns.
    4. The patient is not able to breathe during the suctioning; and this period is too long an interruption of normal breathing patterns.

65. Analysis, planning, physiological integrity, (b).
    2. ERCP is a procedure used to evaluate the pancreatic, hepatic, and gallbladder duct.
    1. An MRI is not likely to be ordered for this patient because it would not provide the most detailed information.
    3. An arteriogram is used to diagnosis arterial problems.
    4. A sigmoidoscopy is useful in diagnosing problems of the colon.

66. Application, implementation, physiological integrity, (c).
    4. This is the correct location to perform a thoracentesis.
    1. An abdominocentesis would be performed on the peritoneal cavity.

2. No such cavity exists. Ascites is edema in the peritoneal cavity.
3. The pericardial sac is around the heart. The procedure for removal of fluid is a pericardiocentesis.

67. Application, planning, physiological integrity, (c).
    1. The proper method for establishing the patency of a small-bore feeding tube is to obtain a chest radiograph, which must be ordered by the patient's physician.
    2. If the tube is in the patient's respiratory tract, the suction may cause damage to the mucosa.
    3. This can cause aspiration if the tube is in the respiratory tract.
    4. This method may not work; given the small bore of the feeding tube, a chest radiograph is a more exact way of establishing patency.

68. Analysis, assessment, health promotion and maintenance, (a).
    3. This statement reflects some of the developmental changes that occur in middle-age patients (empty-nest syndrome).
    1. Although this is a personal statement, it can be made by people in a variety of age groups.
    2. Most individuals retire in their 60s, and this patient would not typically have this concern yet.
    4. This is an ambiguous statement that requires further investigation.

69. Application, planning, health promotion and maintenance, (a).
    2. Walking is a nonstressful, pleasant activity that is especially beneficial for individuals who have chronic health problems; it also preserves the joints of elderly individuals.
    1. Jogging may be too stressful for older adults, especially those with cardiopulmonary disease.
    3. Ski machines may be too vigorous an activity and place undue strain on joints.
    4. Rowing machines may also be too vigorous, especially for patients with cardiopulmonary disease.

70. Application, evaluation, psychosocial integrity, (b).
    3. Individuals of the Jehovah's Witness faith do not accept blood or blood products and may question why a type and cross-match would be done.
    1. This is normal preoperative teaching that does not conflict with this particular religion's beliefs.
    2. Coughing, deep-breathing, and leg exercises should not conflict with this particular religion's beliefs.
    4. This noninvasive procedure does not conflict with Jehovah's Witness beliefs.

71. Application, implementation, physiological integrity, (b).
    1. This is the best method for assisting an individual who is able to help himself or herself.
    2. This may cause a break in skin integrity and would probably be uncomfortable.
    3. This is effective but is not the easiest method for assisting an individual who can help.
    4. The question refers to helping a patient onto a bedpan.

72. Application, planning, physiological integrity, (b).
    4. This method is appropriate and reduces the incidence of ingrown toenails.
    1. This may be painful and compromises skin integrity.
    2. Sharp corners will catch on bed linens.
    3. This would predispose the patient to ingrown toenails.

73. Application, implementation, physiological integrity, (b).
    3. The ulcer will fill in from the inside and upward, which leaves a scar.
    1. This is a flip response that demeans the individual.
    2. This response does not recognize the needs of the patient.
    4. The physician may be consulted, but the question is asked of the nurse who has the ability to answer it.

74. Application, implementation, physiological integrity, (a).
    3. By using a syringe and withdrawing the urine using the provided sampling port, the nurse can obtain a sterile specimen without breaking the continuity of the system.
    1. This action would not produce a sterile specimen and would necessitate putting the catheter back in the patient.
    2. Water, not urine, should come out of the balloon port on the catheter; this action would deflate the catheter balloon, causing dislodgement.
    4. Urine is no longer sterile after it has been sitting in the bottom of the drainage bag; a sterile urine specimen is needed.

75. Application, implementation, physiological integrity, (b).
    4. This placement ensures that the tubing will be below the urinary bladder; therefore the urine will not travel back up the drainage tube, an action that can result in a urinary tract infection.
    1. This position may result in urine traveling back up the drainage tubing, potentially causing a urinary tract infection.
    2. This position may result in urine traveling back up the drainage tubing back to the bladder.
    3. This position is also too high, resulting in urine traveling back up the drainage tubing.

76. Application, planning, physiological integrity, (b).
    1. This ensures that the dentures will not get lost and is the only correct answer.
    2. This is unnecessary.
    3. The patient may not want to use a denture-cleansing tablet.
    4. The patient may not want to use adhesive on the dentures.

77. Analysis, assessment, psychosocial integrity, (c).
    1. Most patients receive light sedation during the procedure; it is unlikely that the person will undergo general anesthesia.
    2. This is correct; the colon must be clean for visualization.
    3. The patient may have some discomfort from the procedure.
    4. Correct statement; the physician may be able to visualize an area of injury.

78. Application, implementation, physiological integrity, (b).
    4. A warm backrub may help relax the individual enough to fall asleep.
    1. This would allow hall noise to interfere with the patient's rest.
    2. Although this is done by some people, this action would be indicated only if the patient is used to falling asleep with the television on at home.
    3. Exercise increases epinephrine release, making falling asleep more difficult for the patient.

79. Application, implementation, physiological integrity, (b).
    1. The nurse bandages the extremity from the foot upward, facilitating venous return and reducing the incidence of swelling caused by the bandaging.
    2. If the nurse bandages from the knee down to the foot, venous return is compromised, and swelling of the foot may occur.
    3. If the nurse begins bandaging at the ankle, swelling of the foot may occur, and this technique does not facilitate venous return to the heart.
    4. Bandaging from the middle of the leg, either upward or downward, will not facilitate venous return and may cause swelling above and below the bandage.

80. Comprehension, planning, physiological integrity, (b).
    3. Adequate oxygenation is always the first priority in any emergency situation.
    1. Although important, this cannot be accomplished unless a patent airway is established.
    2. A victim's airway must be established before bleeding is controlled.
    4. This is not a priority nursing action and may be performed by ancillary personnel.

81. Application, implementation, physiological integrity, (b).
    2. The nurse reduces the chance of edema formation and nerve compression by checking the BP on the side opposite the mastectomy.
    1. This would be contraindicated on the right side and unnecessary on the left arm.
    3. This would be unnecessary unless both arms were compromised.
    4. Auscultating the BP in this area is difficult and unnecessary.

82. Comprehension, planning, physiological integrity (c).
    Answer: 2 tablets
    Two tablets can be given safely.
    Desired dose/Dose on hand × Quantity
    1 grain/65mg × 10 grains/X mg
    X=650mg=2 tablets

83. Application, evaluation, physiological integrity, (c).
    4. This patient is postoperative, a situation that would necessitate reporting the heart rate caused by a possible hemorrhage.
    1. This is a normal newborn respiratory rate.
    2. For athletic individuals to have low resting pulse rates is not uncommon.
    3. This is a normal respiratory rate for this age group.

84. Application, planning, physiological integrity, (b).
    3. Sputum specimens are more easily collected in the morning because secretions have been lying in the bronchial tubes during the night.
    1. A patient may have emesis or become ill if the nurse tries to obtain a sputum culture at this time.
    2. A patient may have emesis or become ill if the nurse tries to obtain a sputum culture at this time.
    4. Obtaining sputum specimens at night is more difficult because the patient has mobilized and coughed up secretions during the day.

85. Application, implementation, physiological integrity, (b).
    4. A generous fluid intake liquefies secretions, allowing them to be more easily expectorated.
    1. Adequate sleep is important in any treatment plan; however, it does not keep secretions from becoming thick.

2. Although important, regular exercise does not directly liquefy secretions.

3. A nourishing diet is important in the treatment plan but does not directly liquefy secretions.

86. Application, assessment, physiological integrity, (c).

   3. The gurgling noise signifies that the patient is unable to control his secretions and should be assisted by suctioning.

   1. Although this is a rapid respiratory rate, many individuals with a respiratory ailment are tachypneic, which does not indicate that suctioning is needed.

   2. When patients need suctioning, their heart rate normally increases; however, this is not itself an indicator for suctioning.

   4. If the patient is able to expectorate his mucus, he does not need to be suctioned.

87. Application, implementation, safe and effective care environment, (b).

   2. Hospice nurses try to make the patient comfortable for as long as he or she lives.

   1. Although this is true, it is not the primary purpose of hospice care.

   3. This is not always the case; many hospice patients are cared for at home.

   4. Most skilled care is performed by hospice personnel; however, the family is instrumental in providing for the basic care of the patient.

88. Comprehension, planning, safe and effective care environment, (b).

   2. An advance directive ensures that the patient or designee can make decisions concerning treatment before death.

   1. The patient or patient advocate will dictate which measures will be used as death approaches.

   3. The physician must uphold the patient's wishes; however, the physician has the right to advise the patient concerning a treatment plan.

   4. The patient designates a patient advocate to make end-of-life decisions; these decisions are based on the patient's wishes, not the family's.

89. Comprehension, planning, safe and effective care environment, (b).

   1. Planning for discharge should begin on the day of admission to the hospital.

   2. This does not give adequate time to organize community resources if the patient needs them.

   3. Predicting when a patient will be discharged is difficult; planning should begin well before discharge.

   4. The plan of care for the patient should be evaluated each day, making changes based on the procedures or treatments that the patient has.

90. Application, implementation, physiological integrity, (b).

   3. Urine is strained for patients with known or suspected calculi, to collect stones for evaluation.

   1. Flank massage is not indicated for patients with renal calculi.

   2. Urine reductions are indicated for patients with diabetes mellitus.

   4. Fluids are generally encouraged in patients who have suspected renal calculi.

91. Comprehension, implementation, physiological integrity, (b).

   4. For the proper laboratory tests to be completed, all voided urine must be collected and placed on ice until sent to the laboratory.

   1. In a 24-hour urine specimen, all urine that the patient voids in a 24-hour period is collected and placed in a brown container that is taken to the laboratory at the end of the 24 hours.

   2. The urine is kept on ice for the 24-hour period.

   3. All urine is collected for the 24-hour specimen.

92. Analysis, implementation, physiological integrity, (b).

   3. Inserting a rectal tube will stimulate peristalsis and relieve the abdominal pain and pressure.

   1. Normally, if activity is possible, it will help relieve the pain of flatus.

   2. Nonpharmaceutical interventions can usually alleviate this type of discomfort.

   4. This action decreases the amount of additional gas buildup but does not relieve the immediate discomfort.

93. Application, evaluation, physiological integrity, (b).

   4. The CPT breaks up the patient's secretions so they can be expectorated.

   1. This procedure is used to visualize secretions.

   2. CPT may assist in this, but it is not the primary purpose.

   3. Incentive spirometry is more useful for initiating deep breathing.

94. Analysis, assessment, physiological integrity, (c).

   2. A patient who has chronic obstructive pulmonary disease is reluctant to move from a position of comfort, which is usually an orthopneic position that puts much pressure on the coccygeal area.

   1. If the patient is ambulatory, a urinary tract infection should not predispose him or her to an ulcer.

   3. A patient with gallbladder disease is usually ambulatory and therefore is at low risk.

   4. A constipated patient should be at no further risk unless another problem is present.

95. Knowledge, planning, physiological integrity, (b).

   1. The skin is the first line of defense for the body, and a break in this defense reduces the ability of the body to resist infections.

   2. A break in the skin does not necessarily decrease the ability of the body to produce antibodies.

   3. Although the skin assists in eliminating perspiration, a break in the skin does not reduce this substantially.

   4. The ability to maintain correct body alignment should not be affected by a break in the skin.

96. Application, implementation, physiological integrity, (b).

   2. This is the correct, sensitive response to the patient's question.

   1. This is insensitive although true.

   3. This may or may not be the case for this individual.

   4. This may or may not be true.

97. Analysis, evaluation, physiological integrity, (c).

   2. An elevated INR indicates a possible bleeding disorder, and the nurse should not shave the patient.

   1. An elevated WBC is indicative of infection, which would not preclude the nurse from shaving the patient.

3. An elevated hemoglobin indicates a possible clotting disorder and would not preclude the nurse from shaving the patient.

4. An elevated BUN is indicative of renal disease and would not preclude the nurse from shaving the patient.

98. Application, implementation, physiological integrity, (b).

4. If possible, the patient should be placed on the side with head turned to the side; this facilitates removal of secretions and decreases the chance of aspiration.

1. This position is too difficult for an unconscious patient, although it would facilitate secretion drainage.

2. The patient should be placed so secretions naturally fall from the mouth; suction is an appropriate device that should be near.

3. The patient needs to be flat and side-lying; this position does not facilitate secretion drainage.

99. Comprehension, planning, physiological integrity, (b).

4. Sleep apnea is a disorder that results in frequent waking during the night, causing daytime fatigue.

1. This disorder is not normally caused by snoring or overeating.

2. Sleep apnea is not increased if the patient is nervous or upset.

3. Individuals with sleep apnea can have the disorder for a long time.

100. Comprehension, assessment, physiological integrity, (b).

3. This allows the patient to easily describe the intensity of the pain to the nurse and allows for evaluation of treatment options.

1. This will not assess the intensity of the pain, only the duration.

2. This response allows the patient to locate the pain but does not describe intensity.

4. These words are too subjective; the word "bad" may have different meanings to the nurse and patient.

101. Application, implementation, physiological integrity, (b).

3. The crutch length is too long, causing compression of the nerves in the axilla; adjusting the crutches and teaching the patient to place weight on his hands will alleviate the problem.

1. No indication has been found that the patient needs a walker instead of a crutch.

2. The pain and tingling are most likely caused by compression of a nerve, not nerve damage.

4. This does not correct the problem, which is improper crutch length and technique.

102. Comprehension, implementation, physiological integrity, (b).

4. The patient should use the cane to take weight off of her weak extremity, the right side.

1. This does not assist the patient in walking.

2. This may confuse the patient and does not effectively limit weight bearing on the right side.

3. Holding the cane in the left hand and moving it with the left leg does not limit weight bearing on the right side.

103. Analysis, assessment, physiological integrity, (b).

4. Patients on bed rest normally have their feet and head elevated; therefore excessive tissue fluid would fall into the sacral area.

1. Individuals who are ambulatory are most likely to notice edema of the feet.

2. Individuals who are bedfast may eventually develop edema of the hands; however, initially edema is normally found in the sacral area.

3. As the edema progresses, calves may become edematous; however, calf edema is more common in the ambulatory individual.

104. Application, implementation, safe and effective care environment, (b).

2. This response signifies a correct step in the procedure for administering a vaginal douche.

1. The patient should be encouraged to void before the douche is instilled.

3. The fluid should not be flowing as the douche tip is placed in the vagina.

4. Low pressure is used when instilling the fluid, to decrease tissue trauma.

105. Analysis, evaluation, physiological integrity, (b).

2. These vital signs are abnormal, signifying a fever, and should be reported.

1. All vital signs are normal for adult patients.

3. Axillary temperatures may be unreliable; however, all of these vital signs are within normal limits.

4. All vital signs are within normal limits.

106. Analysis, evaluation, physiological integrity, (b).

1. Because of the patient's inability to excrete fluids, his or her weight will likely increase because of the excess fluid.

2. The patient's weight will not decrease because the excess fluid will not be able to be eliminated.

3. Because of the patient's diagnosis, she will not be able to rid herself of the fluid.

4. The patient is most likely hypervolemic and not dehydrated.

107. Analysis, assessment, physiological integrity, (b).

3. If the patient's oxygen saturation were truly 60%, he or she would be in distress; the more likely cause for the alarm is that the probe has become dislodged.

1. The need for this action has not been established.

2. The nurse would need to report to the physician and receive orders to complete this task.

4. No need for this action exists at this time.

108. Analysis, planning, physiological integrity, (b).

Correct order: 2341.

2. Have the patient void.

3. Assist the patient in moving onto the stretcher.

4. Elevate the patient's head for comfort.

1. Make the patient's bed.

If this sequence is followed, the patient will be comfortable for the examination, and the nurse will conserve energy by waiting for the patient to leave before making the bed. This sequence anticipates the patient's needs and manages the nurse's time effectively.

109. Application, implementation, physiological integrity, (c).

2. This is the best of the four given responses; it accurately addresses the patient's concerns.

1. This information is inaccurate.

3. Although the pulse oximetry reading is important for monitoring, an arterial blood gas analysis will more fully allow the physician to determine the appropriate amount.

4. Although this is true, it does not give any rationale to the patient.

110. Application, implementation, safe and effective care environment, (b).
   2. **This choice allows the nurse to maintain sterility and reduce cost to the patient.**
   1. This would be unsanitary; the gauze was wet and was not entirely on the sterile field, which may not be waterproof.
   3. The gauze pad became contaminated when it was on the edge of the sterile field, and rinsing it in saline solution will not resterilize it.
   4. Beginning again is unnecessary; the situation can be resolved without the additional expense to the patient of beginning again.

111. Application, implementation, physiological integrity, (b).
   2. **The patient needs to have oxygen supplemented; the patient is accustomed to oxygen and must have it supplied in increased amounts before the suctioning procedure; failure to do so may cause hypoxia.**
   1. No indication exists that restraints are needed.
   3. Suction is never applied when the catheter is advanced.
   4. The patient needs to have oxygen before the suction catheter is advanced.

112. Comprehension, implementation, physiological integrity, (a).
   __X__ 1. **A patient's emesis should be measured and added to the output for that period.**
   __X__ 2. **A patient's urine output should be measured and added to the output for that period.**
   __X__ 3. **A patient's diarrhea should be measured and added to the output for that period.**
   _____ 4. The volume of tube feedings is added to a patient's intake.

113. Application, implementation, physiological integrity, (b).
   4. **By having the patient remain in an upright position, the feeding is less likely to flow back into the esophagus and be aspirated by the patient.**
   1. This is a common practice; however, it does not assist in reducing the risk of aspiration.
   2. This is a highly appropriate action but does not reduce the risk for aspiration.
   3. This may cause the patient to lose calories and should not be done unless ordered by the physician; it has no bearing on aspiration.

114. Application, implementation, physiological integrity, (b).
   1. **If the tube is in the patient's trachea, air will not flow to vibrate the vocal cords, and the patient will be unable to speak.**
   2. This signifies that the tube is still in the nasal cavity.
   3. A small amount of blood indicates tissue trauma from insertion of the tube.
   4. This signifies that the tube is in the stomach.

115. Comprehension, planning, physiological integrity, (b).
   2. **This statement correctly explains the actions of each enema.**
   1. Although both enemas may stimulate peristalsis somewhat, the cleansing enema is designed for this purpose.
   3. The oil-retention enema is given to soften stool and not specifically to evacuate the bowel.
   4. The oil-retention enema is the enema given to soften the stool and is normally given before the cleansing enema.

116. Comprehension, implementation, safe and effective care environment, (b).
   4. **The incorrect entry should be drawn through (so the error can still be read), the correct amount should be inserted, and the nurse should initial above the correction.**
   1. It is never permissible to white out any entry in a legal chart.
   2. This would be considered tampering with a written entry and is also illegal.
   3. The correction must be made so that everyone can read the mistaken entry.

117. Analysis, assessment, physiological integrity, (b).
   3. **The patient may not be drinking enough fluids, which may have contributed to the problem.**
   1. Exercise assists in establishing normal bowel function.
   2. Vegetables supply fiber, which should assist in establishing normal bowel patterns.
   4. Defecating as soon as the need is felt is important.

118. Application, implementation, physiological integrity, (b).
   1. **The patient is at risk for hypovolemic shock. The nurse should clamp the catheter immediately.**
   2. No reason is given to do this unless a specimen has been ordered.
   3. Although this would counteract the fluid loss, it cannot be done without a physician's order.
   4. This would not correct the problem, given that it has already occurred. Clamping the catheter delays emptying the bladder of any more urine.

119. Comprehension, implementation, safe and effective care environment, (b).
   3. **This response is the definition of a contracture; the muscle is permanently shortened because of the effects of immobility.**
   1. This does not address the UAP's question.
   2. An injury may have precipitated the decreased mobility, but the contracture is the direct result of the effects of immobility.
   4. Once contracted, the arm will remain this way permanently, and ROM exercises will not restore it.

120. Analysis implementation, physiological integrity, (b).
   4. **This is the most correct and most appropriate response by the nurse because it addresses the patient's question.**
   1. Although humorous, this answer is demeaning and does not answer the question.
   2. This response belittles the patient and shifts responsibility for explanation to another person.
   3. The patient wants to know why he needs to get out of bed; this response does not answer that question.

121. Application, implementation, physiological integrity, (a).
   4. **This is the most logical response to the question and describes the action of the stockings.**
   1. This does not tell the patient why the stockings are needed or why they should be snug.
   2. This is not the purpose for the stockings.
   3. Although the stockings compress the muscles of the legs, the reason they need to be snug is so blood is pushed back toward the heart.

122. Analysis, planning, safe and effective care environment, (b).
   2. **This is a short-term, easily measurable goal for this patient.**

1. This is an example of a long-term goal, not easily attainable on the first day after surgery.
3. This could be considered a long-term goal, not attainable on the first day after surgery.
4. This is an example of a long-term goal.

123. Application, planning, psychosocial integrity, (b).
    4. Patients are generally calmer when they are in a quiet, stress-free environment; pastel shades of carpeting and wall decorations are also calming.
    1. Although exercise is important, a lot of physical activity may overstimulate the patient.
    2. This may cause the patient to become overstimulated.
    3. These activities may overly stimulate the patient.

124. Application, implementation, physiological integrity, (b).
    2. The first surgical dressing should be changed by the surgeon; therefore the dressing should be reinforced until further orders can be obtained.
    1. The nurse is unsure of what is under the dressing; changing a fresh postoperative dressing requires a physician's order.
    3. Removing the dressing would require a physician's order.
    4. Dressings are not routinely sent to the laboratory, and no order has been given to change the dressing.

125. Analysis, implementation, physiological integrity, (b).
    Answer: 870 mL
    5 oz = 150 mL + 120 mL + 8 oz = 240 mL + 1 cup = 240 mL + 4 oz = 120 mL = 870 mL

126. Application, implementation, physiological integrity, (b).
    2. The patient who has decreased sensation to extremities is at increased risk for injury as a result of the application of heat.
    1. As long as the nurse explains the entire procedure to the patient, special precautions do not need to be taken for patients who are blind.
    3. Patients with hypertension are not at increased risk from the effects of the heat application.
    4. Although patients with diabetes mellitus may have neuropathy, which would place them at risk, the paraplegic individual remains the person at greatest risk from the heat application.

127. Application, planning, physiological integrity, (c).
    ___X___ 1. **This action helps to mobilize the patient's secretions so he can effectively expectorate them.**
    ___X___ 2. **This action helps to mobilize the patient's secretions so he can effectively expectorate them.**
    ___X___ 3. **This action will help mobilize the patient's secretions so he can effectively expectorate them.**
    _____ 4. This may further depress the patient's respirations.
    _____ 5. This will not assist the patient to clear his airway.

128. Application, assessment, physiological integrity, (b).
    1. The presence of redness and swelling indicates that infection may be present in the incision line.
    2. This does not directly indicate infection.
    3. These are normal assessment findings and indicate adequate healing.
    4. At times a small amount of bloody drainage may be observed in a new incision line; this does not indicate infection.

129. Application, implementation, health promotion, and maintenance, (b).
    2. Most physicians recommend that women over the age of 40 years undergo mammograms every 1 to 2 years.
    1. Mammograms are screening examinations and are done on women over age 40 years, despite any suspicions of cancer.
    3. All women should receive mammograms; women with strong family histories may be screened as often as every 6 months.
    4. Mammograms are not difficult for women, although they may be embarrassing to some women; mammograms are recommended every 1 to 2 years after age 40.

130. Application, implementation, physiological integrity, (b).
    3. The footboard is used to keep the feet in proper alignment and decrease the incidence of plantar flexion.
    1. An abductor pillow assists in maintaining an abducted state of the legs.
    2. Antiembolic stockings are better able to keep the patient from developing thrombophlebitis, although a footboard can be used to do pedal pushes, thereby exercising the calf muscles.
    4. This may be true but is not the purpose of the board.

131. Comprehension, planning, safe and effective care environment, (b).
    3. Liability insurance covers the nurse only while performing professional duties.
    1. Malpractice insurance costs vary from agency to agency.
    2. Malpractice insurance protects the nurse from financial damages.
    4. Malpractice insurance must be renewed periodically.

132. Comprehension, assessment, psychosocial integrity, (b).
    3. The patient is bargaining with God for his life.
    1. No evidence of anger is found in his statement.
    2. The patient accepts his diagnosis; he just wishes to change it.
    4. The patient does not appear depressed at this time.

133. Analysis, assessment, physiological integrity, (b).
    2. Given the patient's diagnosis, bowel sounds are the most important assessment criteria.
    1. Although lung sounds are important, bowel sounds are the most important assessment data for this patient.
    3. The patient's bowel sounds are of paramount importance.
    4. No indication can be found that a neurological examination is warranted for this patient; bowel sounds remain the top priority.

134. Application, planning, physiological integrity (b).
    2. The proper method for measuring a 24-hour urine is to collect all urine in that 24-hour period.
    1. All urine for this time period must be collected, or the test results will not be valid.
    3, 4. The nurse would need a physician's order to send the specimen for culture or for a routine urinalysis; the urine needs to be added to the collection container.

135. Application, implementation, safe and effective care environment, (a).
    Answer: 620 mL

1100 mL total urine output; continuous bladder irrigation infusing at 60 mL/hr for 8 hours, or a total of 480 mL. True urine output is 620 mL (1100 mL − 480 mL = 620 mL).

136. Application, implementation, safe and effective care environment, (b).
    1. **Specimens for ova and parasites must be examined immediately while they are still warm.**
    2. The stool must be warm for detection of the presence of ova and parasites.
    3. The sample must be sent to the laboratory immediately.
    4. There is no need for a sterile specimen cup. The sample will have cooled considerably after this action.

137. Application, planning, physiological integrity, (b).
    __X__ 1. **Data on the pain must first be gathered.**
    _____ 2. This action may be justified based on assessment data gathered and consultation with physician and RN, but it is not the LPN/LVN's priority action.
    __X__ 3. **The RN supervisor should be notified.**
    _____ 4. This action may be justified based on assessment data gathered and consultation with the physician and RN, but it is not the LPN/LVN's priority action.

138. Analysis, planning, physiological integrity, (c).
    3. **This patient needs to be evaluated first. He may be alone, and the nurse will want to make sure that he has had no ill effects from the hypoglycemic episode.**
    1. This patient is with a respiratory therapist and is receiving a treatment.
    2. The nursing assistant would alert the nurse to any potential problems.
    4. The nurse has most likely been in the room to medicate the patient. The patient should be evaluated in 15 to 30 minutes for effectiveness.

139. Analysis, assessment, physiological integrity, (c).
    4. **Oliguria, or scanty urine output, would be a sign of dehydration. The urine would be concentrated.**
    1. Hematuria is a problem associated with kidney or bladder dysfunction.
    2. Polyuria would be found in a patient with hypervolemia.
    3. Enuresis is bed-wetting, a common problem in hospitalized children, but it is not a sign of dehydration.

140. Application, planning, safe and effective care environment, (b).
    __X__ 1. **This action could be assigned. It is of a nonemergent nature in patients who are not acutely ill.**
    __X__ 2. **This action could be assigned. It is of a nonemergent nature in patients who are not acutely ill.**
    __X__ 3. **This action could be assigned. It is of a nonemergent nature in patients who are not acutely ill.**
    __X__ 4. **This action could be assigned. It is of a nonemergent nature in patients who are not acutely ill.**
    _____ 5. An enema is a treatment and medication. Because there are too many variables involved in giving an enema, the nurse needs to complete the procedure.

141. Application, planning, physiological integrity, (b).
    1. **Venipuncture is the only way to procure a blood sample for determining HgbA$_{1c}$.**
    2. Palpation is useful in assessing pulses and deformities.
    3. Percussion is useful in assessing tympanitis or areas of consolidation.
    4. Lung sounds and bowel sounds can be assessed with auscultation.

142. Application, planning, physiological integrity, (c).
    Correct order: 4321.
    4. **Provide mouth care.**
    3. **Suction the tracheostomy**
    2. **Inflate the balloon on the tracheostomy cuff.**
    1. **Provide the lunch.**
    This sequence of events will prepare the patient for his lunch. Providing mouth care increases saliva for the patient and cleanses the mouth; suctioning the tracheostomy reduces the amount of coughing and secretions that may develop during the meal; inflating the cuff keeps food from falling into the trachea, thus decreasing the chance for aspiration.

143. Application, planning, safe and effective care environment, (a).
    3. **This method ensures proper measurement of the urine.**
    1. Estimating is not an accurate measurement of the urine.
    2. The markings on the bedpan may not be accurate.
    4. The markings on the catheter bag are not considered to be accurate.

144. Application, implementation, physiological integrity, (b).
    2. **The radial pulse cannot be higher than the apical pulse; the nurses should assess for pulse deficit again.**
    1. The pulse deficit was not done correctly.
    3. The pulse deficit is not 8 and should not be recorded. We do not know what the actual deficit is from the information given.
    4. This is a skill that is perfectly within the scope of practice of the LPN/LVN.

145. Application, planning, physiological integrity (c).
    Correct order: 652431.
    6. **Check the physician's order.**
    5. **Put on sterile gloves.**
    2. **Cleanse the perineum from pubis to rectum.**
    4. **Insert the catheter into the urethra until urine flow is established.**
    3. **Instill sterile water to inflate the balloon.**
    1. **Document catheter size, tolerance, and urine return.**
    This is the proper method for inserting the catheter that maintains sterile technique.

146. Application, implementation, psychosocial integrity, (b).
    3. **This is the only response that addresses the patient's needs.**
    1, 2, 4. These responses belittle the patient's needs and question his faith.

147. Comprehension, planning, physiological integrity, (c).
    1. **This is an open-ended question that will allow the nurse to gather information before contacting the surgeon.**
    2. This does not address the needs of the patient.

3. This is an untrue statement and appears to be bullying the patient. The patient may be afraid, and this statement could be perceived as a threat.
4. The physician will need to speak with the patient after the nurse has contacted the physician.

148. Knowledge, assessment, physiological integrity, (b).
    B. The X is placed at the fifth intercostal space, mid-clavicular line (see below).

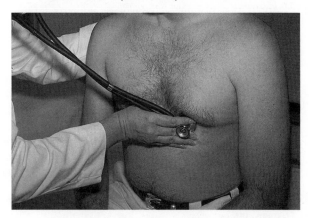

149. Application, implementation, physiological integrity, (a).
    3. The patient's head should be turned toward the eye that is injured. The irrigant solution should flow from the inner to the outer canthus, which reduces the risk of infection of the good eye.

1. This is incorrect because it would increase risk of infection and be uncomfortable for the patient.
2. This is also incorrect, increasing risk of infection to the good eye.
4. Swabbing is not considered part of the irrigation technique.

150. Knowledge, implementation, physiological integrity, (b).
    The nurse should begin at the top of the incision and work down (number 1, Illustration B) and then outward (number 1, Illustration A), using a new swab after each pass of the incision.

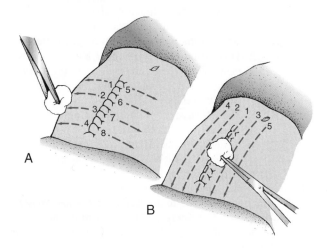

Pharmacology

Objectives

After studying this chapter, the student should be able to:

1. Verbalize the importance of using all aspects of the nursing process in the administration of medications.
2. Demonstrate correct technique in administering medication safely.
3. Correctly calculate appropriate doses of medications.
4. Describe a beginning understanding of major drug classifications, including actions, side effects, and nursing considerations.
5. Discuss the importance of continuing his or her education in the field of pharmacology.

This chapter covers two major areas: (1) administration of medications and (2) pharmacological aspects of nursing care. The nursing process as it applies to drugs and drug administration is explained and integrated throughout the text.

Calculation of dosage and intravenous (IV) infusion rate, principles of medication administration, procedures and sites for medication administration, blood transfusion administration, and pediatric drug administration are reviewed.

The major classifications of drugs are presented with their actions, adverse effects, and nursing process applications. Commonly used clinical drugs are listed with generic and brand names.

Today more than ever nurses have a responsibility to stay current with changes in pharmacology. Consumers have become more and more sophisticated and have a wide variety of resources available to them as well.

The role of the licensed practical/vocational nurse (LPN/LVN) in the administration of medications is determined by the state nurse practice acts and agency policy. However, knowledge of drugs has a significant impact on the quality of nursing care provided to each patient by the LPN/LVN. The LPN/LVN has a legal and moral responsibility to use the nursing process in the administration of medications.

Key drugs are identified by an asterisk (*).

PHARMACOLOGY AND THE NURSING PROCESS

A. Assessment: a systematic collection of subjective and objective data about the patient, drug, and environment
B. Planning: prioritizes the nursing diagnosis and specifies the goals and outcome criteria and the time in which these should be achieved
C. Implementation: consists of initiation and completion of the nursing care plan as defined by the nursing diagnosis and outcome criteria
D. Evaluation: an ongoing monitoring of the patient's response to drug therapy

ASSESSMENT

A. Assessing the patient
   1. Variables

   a. Growth and development related to age
   b. Body build—many antibiotics (particularly IV antibiotics), narcotics, and vasoactive drugs are ordered based on patient's weight and build
   c. Past and present medical history
   d. Nutritional practices
   e. Allergies
   f. Sociocultural beliefs—how this person's culture views medication and the health care system
   g. Knowledge of disease and drugs
   h. Cognitive function—the person's ability to understand the drug regimen
   i. Physical challenges—eyesight, hearing, weakness in extremities
   j. Physical assessment: vital signs, height, weight, laboratory results, results of diagnostic tests

   Additional detailed discussion of variables appears in the Pharmacokinetics section, p. 79.
   2. Medication history
   a. Over-the-counter (OTC) medications—an increasing number of medications have changed from prescription to OTC. The LPN/LVN has a responsibility to educate the patient on the dangers of self-medicating. Long-term use of OTC medications may mask symptoms of a more serious disorder.
   b. Prescription medications
   c. Substance abuse, including street drugs, smoking, alcohol, caffeine, food
   d. Problems with drug therapy in the past (e.g., allergies, adverse effects, noncompliance)
   e. Cultural variables—some medications have differing effects on individual groups. Some medications may not be allowed in certain cultures.

B. Assessing the drug
   1. Medication order
   a. From a physician, dentist, or nurse practitioner (if permitted by state law)
   b. Contains patient's name, date order was written, name of medication, dosage (size, frequency, number of doses), route, signature of health care provider

c. Accuracy, legibility, need for clarification

d. Incorrect, inappropriate, or illegible orders must be clarified before administration.

2. Types of medication orders

a. Routine or standard

b. *Pro re nata* (p.r.n.) order: given on a "when necessary" basis

c. Single order: to be given only once

d. Stat order: to be given only once and immediately

e. Standing order: established for all patients with a specific condition

f. Verbal order: must be written and signed within a specified time limit

g. Telephone order—emergency situations only: follow hospital policy concerning who is allowed to accept. In many states LPN/LVNs have special restrictions. They are allowed to follow only physician orders that are co-signed by a registered nurse (RN)

h. To decrease medication errors, The Joint Commission (TJC) no longer recommends that a nurse use "q" or "qod" for "every day" or "every other day."

C. Institutional-level management: drug distribution systems

1. Floor stock

2. Individual patient medication system: a supply of medication that is dispensed and labeled for a particular patient

3. Unit dose: individual doses of each medication ordered

4. Computerized or automatic drug dispensing system

5. Pyxis is an automated system that uses barcodes to ensure adequate medication dispensing.

6. The nurse must be aware of federal and state agency policy regarding the storage and dispensing of controlled substances.

PLANNING

A. Establish priorities: weigh the importance of one problem against another

B. Set goals: objective, measurable, and realistic with an established time period for achievement of the outcome

C. Outcome: should reflect expected changes through nursing care

D. Outcome criteria: provide a standard of measure that can be used to move toward the goal

See Critical Thinking Challenge box.

? Critical Thinking Challenge

A patient arrives at the walk-in clinic complaining of a headache, runny nose, and swollen glands. The patient is 54 years old and states that she never had allergies until she was 50 years old. While the nurse was taking a patient history, it was discovered that the patient had had no medical care since the birth of her last child at the age of 32. Before the patient is seen by a physician, what information would be essential for the nurse to obtain that would better assist the physician in meeting the needs of this patient?

Basic assessment data would include vital signs, height and weight, and questions concerning family history, any known allergies, including food allergies, over-the-counter medication history, including herbal supplements, and specific lifestyle questions specific to exercise and dietary patterns.

The patient should then be referred to the appropriate clinic physician and be encouraged to begin regular medical care. Patient responses to questions asked during the initial assessment help guide physician diagnosis as well as govern the choice of medication prescribed by the physician for this patient.

IMPLEMENTATION

A. Requires constant communication with patient and health care team

B. Requires proper administration of medication

1. Approach to patient

a. "Therapeutic use of self" attitude of nurse

b. Consistency of approach

c. Informed consent for patients

d. Compliance and right to refuse

2. Uses the six rights

a. Right drug

b. Right dose

c. Right time

d. Right route

e. Right patient

f. Right documentation

Please note that it is required procedure in many institutions for the nurse to open the medication at the patient's bedside.

3. Uses measures to support the therapeutic or desired effect—nursing actions can complement drug therapy or minimize unpleasant adverse reactions.

4. Observes for desired therapeutic effect

a. Establish baseline data for all medications.

b. Establish observational parameters (vital signs, diagnostic test results and laboratory data, pain assessment scales) to evaluate effectiveness of medications.

C. Teaches patients

1. Explain drug, dose, side effects, food-drug interactions, time schedule, method of administration, and so on.

2. Identify need for teaching.

3. Establish realistic teaching goals.

4. Select teaching methods—the method chosen should be individualized to fit the patient's needs.

5. Implement teaching.

6. Evaluate effectiveness.

D. Document accurately (form is set by agency policy)—some institutions consider this right the sixth right.

1. Information must be complete and accurate.

2. Documentation must be done immediately after administration.

3. Legal implications—if drug administration is not documented, the assumption is that the drug has not been administered.

4. Data should include:

a. Observations relevant to therapeutic effects.

b. Actions taken to prevent or treat adverse reactions.

c. Time when a drug is discontinued.

d. Reason or reasons for discontinuation of drug.

e. Reasons for refusal or noncompliance of patient.

f. It is no longer recommended that drugs be disposed of in the sink or the toilet.

(1) At home, patients should crush oral forms of medications, place in original containers, black out information, place in another container in a brown bag, and place in the trash.

(2) Syringes should be placed in a glass jar until full and then placed in a paper bag and disposed of in the trash. Nurses should follow agency policy.

(3) Patients should contact health care providers if they have any questions.

E. Dosage forms
   1. Factors influencing route of administration
      a. Specific chemical and physical properties of the drug
      b. Pathological condition of the patient
      c. Adequacy of medication compliance
   2. Dose: amount of drug to be given at one time
   3. Dosage: regulation of the frequency, size, number of doses
   4. Dosage form: final product administered to the patient
      a. Preparations for oral use
         (1) Liquids
            (a) Aqueous solutions: substances dissolved in water and syrups
            (b) Aqueous suspensions: solid particles suspended in liquid
            (c) Syrup: medication dissolved in a concentrated solution of a sugar to which flavors may have been added
            (d) Emulsions: fats or oils suspended in liquid with an emulsifier
            (e) Spirits: alcohol solution
            (f) Elixir: aromatic sweetened alcoholic and water solution
            (g) Tincture: alcoholic extract of plant or water solution
            (h) Fluid extract: concentrated alcoholic extract of plant or vegetables
            (i) Extract: syrup or dried form of pharmacologically active drug
         (2) Solids
            (a) Capsules—soluble case (usually gelatin) that contains liquid, dry, or beaded particles. Capsules may be timed release or sustained action (slow, continuous dissolution for an extended period).
            (b) Tablets: compressed powdered drug or drugs in small disks
               • Enteric-coated tablets: coated with a second layer of material to prevent dissolution in stomach; disintegrate in small intestine to prevent stomach irritation
               • Press-coated or layered tablets: contain a second layer of material pressed on or around them, which allows incompatible ingredients to be separated and to dissolve at different rates
               • Troches or lozenges: medicated tablets that dissolve slowly in the mouth
            (c) Powders or granules: loose or molded drug substances for drug administration with or without liquids
      b. Preparations for parenteral use
         (1) Ampules: sealed glass containers for liquid injectable medications; for single-dose use
         (2) Vials: glass containers with a rubber stopper, usually for multiple doses; contain liquid or powdered medications
         (3) Cartridge or Tubex: a single-dose unit of parenteral medication to be used with a specific injecting device
         (4) Patients with specific conditions (e.g., diabetes or chronic pain) may self-administer regulated doses of medication.
         (5) IV solutions: must be sterile and particle free
            (a) Continuous infusion may be used for fluid replacement with or without medication.
            (b) Intermittent—runs as a secondary administration set (piggyback) hung separately from the primary set by means of a secondary tubing
            (c) Heparin lock (PRN lock) or angiocatheter: a port site for direct administration of intermittent IV medications without the need for a primary IV solute
         (6) Certain medications (i.e., lidocaine) may be used subcutaneously to provide local anesthesia
      c. Preparations for topical use
         (1) Lotions: liquid suspensions that can be protective, emollient, cooling, astringent, pain relieving, antipruritic, cleansing, and so on
         (2) Ointments: semisolid medicines in a base for local use—protective, soothing, astringent, topical pain relieving
         (3) Paste: thick ointments used primarily for skin protection
         (4) Creams: emulsions that contain aqueous and oily bases
         (5) Aerosols: fine powders or solutions in volatile liquids that contain a propellant
         (6) Transdermal patches: patches containing medication that is absorbed continuously through the skin and acts systemically (primarily pain relief and the relief of vasoconstriction)
         (7) Powders: finely ground drugs or combinations of drugs
      d. Preparations for use on mucous membranes
         (1) Drops are aqueous solutions with or without a gelling agent (to increase retention time in the eye). Drops can be used for eyes, ears, or nose.
         (2) An aqueous solution of medications is topically administered, usually for topical action but occasionally used for systemic effects, including enemas, douches, mouthwashes, throat sprays, gargles.
         (3) Aerosol sprays, nebulizers, and inhalers deliver aqueous solutions of medication in droplet form to the target membrane such as the bronchial tree (bronchodilators).
         (4) Foams such as vaginal foams for contraception are powders or solutions of medication in volatile liquids with a propellant.
         (5) Suppositories usually contain medicinal substances mixed in a firm but malleable base to facilitate insertion into a body cavity (e.g., rectal, vaginal); can be used for local or systemic effects.
      e. Miscellaneous drug delivery systems
         (1) Intradermal implants are pellets containing a small deposit of medication that are inserted in a dermal pocket; usually used to administer hormones such as testosterone or estradiol.
         (2) Micropump system is a small external pump, attached by belt or implanted, that delivers medication by way of a needle in a continuous, steady dose. Examples include insulin, anticancer chemotherapy, opioids.

F. Dosage route: means of access to the site of action or systemic circulation; divided into three classifications
  1. Enteral: drug is administered directly into gastrointestinal (GI) tract.
    a. Oral: Drug is ingested and absorbed from stomach or small intestine. Route is convenient and economical. Drug can irritate stomach; it may be destroyed by digestive juices.
    b. Rectal: Drug is inserted into rectum and absorbed through mucous membrane. Route may be used in unconscious or vomiting patient.
  2. Parenteral: In practice, *parenteral* means administration by means of a needle; drugs must be sterile, and aseptic technique must be used.
    a. Intradermal: Drug is injected directly under the skin. Amount of drug is small, and absorption is slow. Examples of use include allergy testing, tuberculosis (TB) testing, administering small amounts of anesthesia.
    b. Subcutaneous: Drug is injected under the skin into subcutaneous fascia. Ideally solutions are limited to no more than 1 mL of solution. Examples of use include insulin, heparin, and morphine.
    c. Intramuscular: Drug is injected into muscle mass. Relatively rapid absorption is the result of good blood supply. Larger volumes up to 5 mL can be given.
    d. Intravenous: Drug is injected into the vein for immediate effect. Route permits direct control of blood drug concentrations. It is used when an immediate effect is desired; can be given by injection or infusion; and is useful in emergency situations. Precautions must be taken to avoid infiltration. Follow institution policy for the time required to stay with a patient after the initiation of a transfusion.
    e. Epidural (administration by this route is performed by a physician; however, the nurse is responsible for assisting and monitoring sites and effects): A catheter is implanted beneath the skin with its tip in the epidural space; the drug diffuses into the central spinal fluid, bypassing the blood-brain barrier; route is frequently used in the management of acute and chronic pain.
    f. Intraarterial (administration by this route is performed by a physician; however, the nurse is responsible for assisting and monitoring sites and effects): Drug is injected directly into an artery.
    g. Intraarticular (administration by this route is performed by a physician; however, the nurse is responsible for assisting and monitoring sites and effects): Drug is injected directly into a joint.
    h. Intraspinal (administration by this route is performed by a physician; however, the nurse is responsible for assisting and monitoring sites and effects): Drug is injected directly into spinal canal.
  3. Percutaneous: Medications are applied through or into the skin or mucous membranes. These medications may be used for local or systemic effects; an example would be local anesthetics.
    a. Sublingual: Drug is dissolved under tongue and absorbed rapidly through mucous membrane of mouth. It can irritate oral mucosa. The number of drugs given this way is limited; nitroglycerin is primary example.
    b. Buccal: Drug is dissolved between cheek and gum and absorbed through mucous membrane of the mouth.
    c. Lungs: Drug is inhaled as a gas or aerosol. Route is useful for drugs intended to act directly on the lungs.
    d. Vaginal: Drug is inserted into the vagina and absorbed through the mucous membrane.
    e. Ophthalmic: Drug is applied to the eye in form of drops or ointments; they must be sterile.
    f. Otic or aural: Drug is applied in the ear.
    g. Nasal: Drug is applied to the nasal cavity via a dropper or atomizer.
    h. Transdermal: Patch applied to skin provides controlled release of medication.

EVALUATION

A. Therapeutic goals: evaluate therapeutic effectiveness of drugs
B. Diagnostic goals: observe for potential adverse reactions
C. Teaching goals: verify patient's knowledge of drug or ability to perform a skill necessary for administration of the drug
D. Patient compliance: evaluates patient adherence to a prescribed plan of treatment; therapeutic blood levels checked with many medications to determine effectiveness

SOURCES OF DRUGS

A. Animals
B. Plants
C. Microorganisms
D. Synthetic chemical substances—the major source of drugs
E. Food substances

DRUG NAMES

A. Generic: the official, established nonproprietary name assigned to a drug; drug licensed under its generic name and often less expensive than brand-name drugs
B. Brand (trademark): a name assigned to a drug by its manufacturer; use of this name restricted to the specific manufacturer by the trademark
C. Chemical: the exact designation of the chemical structure as determined by the rules of accepted systems of chemical nomenclature
D. Prescription drug: a legal prescription is required for the drug to be dispensed; nonprescription or OTC drug may be purchased without a prescription

DRUG LEGISLATION

A. Food, Drug, and Cosmetic Act of 1938 (amended 1952, 1962)
  1. Contains detailed regulations to ensure that drugs meet standards of safety and effectiveness
  2. Requires physician's prescription for legal drug purchase
B. Controlled Substances Act of 1970
  1. Defines drug dependency and drug addiction
  2. Classifies drugs according to potential abuse and medical usefulness
  3. Establishes methods for regulating manufacture, distribution, and sale of controlled substances
  4. Establishes education and treatment programs for drug abuse

C. Controlled substances schedule
1. Schedule I: drugs that have a high potential for abuse and are not approved for medical use in the United States (e.g., cocaine)
2. Schedule II: drugs that have a high potential for abuse but are currently approved for medical use in the United States; possible severe psychological or physical dependence (e.g., morphine sulfate) with abuse
3. Schedule III: drugs that have a lower potential for abuse than those in Schedules I and II; possible high psychological or low-to-moderate physical dependence with abuse (e.g., aspirin [Empirin] with codeine)
4. Schedule IV: drugs that have some potential for abuse; possible limited psychological or physical dependence (e.g., diazepam [Valium]) with abuse
5. Schedule V: drugs that have the lowest potential for abuse; products that contain moderate amounts of controlled substances; may be dispensed by the pharmacist without a physician's prescription but with some restrictions such as amount, record keeping, and other safeguards (e.g., Robitussin A-C)
D. Drug Regulating Reform Act—shortens the drug investigation process to release drugs sooner to the public
E. Orphan Drug Act—encourages drug companies, through grants from the federal government, to investigate rare conditions
F. Needle Safety Act of 2000—requires hospitals to have a program regarding needlestick prevention

PRINCIPLES OF DRUG ACTION

A. The physiological means by which a drug exerts its desired effects
B. Examples: include increasing or decreasing the rate at which a cell or tissue functions or replacing something that is needed by the body

PHARMACOKINETICS

A. The study of what actually happens to a drug from the time it enters the body until it leaves the body
B. Includes onset, peak, and duration of the drug

MECHANISMS OF DRUG THERAPY

A. Dissolution: disintegration of dose form; dissolution of an active substance
B. Absorption: the process that occurs between the time a substance enters the body and the time it enters the bloodstream
C. Distribution: the transport of drug molecules within the body to receptor sites
D. Metabolism: biotransformation—the way in which drugs are inactivated by the body
E. Excretion: elimination of a drug from the body

VARIABLES THAT AFFECT DRUG ACTION

A. Dosage
B. Route of administration
C. Drug-diet interactions: Food slows absorption of drugs. Some foods containing certain substances react with certain drugs (e.g., antidepressants can cause adverse reactions if eaten with certain types of food, including cheese and red wine).
D. Weight: many antibiotics, particularly IV antibiotics, are ordered based on patient's weight.
E. Drug-drug interactions
1. Additive effect: occurs when two drugs with similar actions are taken together
2. Synergism (potentiation): a total effect of two similar drugs that is greater than the sum of the effects if each is taken separately
3. Interference: when one drug interferes with the metabolism or elimination of a second drug, resulting in intensification of effects of the second drug
4. Displacement: when one drug is displaced from a plasma protein-binding site by a second, causing an increased effect of the displaced drug
5. Antagonism: a decrease in the effects of drugs caused by the action of one on the other
F. Age
1. Fetus: metabolism and elimination mechanisms immature
2. Newborn: organ systems not fully developed
3. Children: depends on age and developmental stage
4. Elderly adults: Physiological changes may alter the actions of a drug in the body. Elderly patients often take more than one medication; therefore the chances for interactions are increased.
G. Body weight: affects drug action mainly in relation to dosage
H. Pregnancy: Many medications cross the placental barrier and can be harmful to the fetus.
I. Pathological condition: Disease processes are capable of altering drug mechanisms (e.g., patients with kidney disease have increased risk of drug toxicity because they have difficulty eliminating the medication; patients with liver disease have difficulty metabolizing medications).
J. Psychological considerations: Attitudes and expectations influence patient response (e.g., anxiety can decrease effect of analgesics).

Common Responses to Medications

A. Desired or therapeutic effect is the reason why a medication is administered.
B. Side effects are usually predictable secondary effects produced by the medication; they may be desirable or undesirable.
C. Adverse effects are more severe symptoms or problems that arise because of the medication. The nurse must be alert to reports of any adverse effects after the administration of medications.

Adverse Reactions to Drugs

A. Idiosyncratic reaction: unusual, unexpected reaction, usually the first time a drug is taken
B. Paradoxical effect: reactions opposite of what would be expected
C. Allergic reactions: stimulate antibody reactions from immune system of body
1. Urticaria (hives)
2. Anaphylaxis: severe allergic reaction involving cardiovascular and respiratory systems; may be life-threatening
D. GI effects
1. Anorexia
2. Nausea, vomiting
3. Constipation

4. Diarrhea
5. Abdominal distention
E. Hematological effects
1. Blood dyscrasia
2. Bone marrow depression
3. Blood coagulation disorders
F. Hepatotoxicity
1. Hepatitis
2. Biliary tract obstruction or spasms
G. Nephrotoxicity: renal insufficiency or failure; kidney stones
H. Drug dependence
1. Physiological: physical need to relieve shaking; pain
2. Psychological: need to relieve feeling of anxiety; stress
I. Teratogenicity: ability of a drug to cause abnormal fetal development

Tolerance and Cross-Tolerance

A. Tolerance: acclimation of the body to a drug over a period of time so larger doses must be given to achieve the same effect
B. Cross-tolerance: tolerance to pharmacologically related drugs

SOURCES OF DRUG INFORMATION

Pharmacology changes rapidly. Nurses need to make use of the multiple resources available to stay current.
A. Resource people
1. Pharmacists
2. Physicians
3. RNs
B. Internet
C. Poison control centers
D. Published sources of information
1. United States Pharmacopeia (USP) and National Formulary (NF)
a. Official references
b. Establish legally binding standards to which drugs must conform
c. Revised every 5 years, with periodic supplements
2. Package insert: Food and Drug Administration (FDA)–approved label for drug products in the United States
3. *Physicians' Desk Reference* (PDR)
a. Published annually, with interim supplements
b. Contains information supplied by manufacturers
c. Is most useful for finding drugs according to brand name
4. American Hospital Formulary Service
a. Contains data on almost every drug available in the United States
b. Kept current by periodic supplements
5. Pharmacology textbooks; drug reference books and cards; online sources often listed from the publisher
6. Nursing journals
7. Online sources, including the American Nurses Association (ANA) and the Centers for Disease Control and Prevention (CDC). Students must consider the site when using online information. There is a great deal of misleading information on the Internet.

NURSING PROCESS

A. Assessment: obtain data on patient regarding problems related to:
1. Route of administration

2. Elimination or metabolism (particular attention paid to persons with renal or hepatic disease)
3. Baseline laboratory values
4. Patient teaching needs
B. Planning
1. Proper timing of administration of ordered dose
2. Ways to improve the effectiveness of the drug
3. Instruction of patient concerning the drug
C. Implementation
1. Proper method of administration
2. Proper timing of administration of ordered dose
3. Instruction of patient concerning the drug
D. Evaluation
1. Effectiveness of drug
a. Subjective: questioning the patient for expected response of the drug (e.g., pain relief, reduction in symptoms)
b. Objective: monitoring physical response by the nurse (e.g., decreased blood pressure [BP], increased cardiac regularity, improvement in signs and symptoms of infection)
c. Documentation of assessment of pain and efforts to relieve it: required by TJC
2. Presence of side effects, adverse reactions
3. Effectiveness of patient teaching
4. If therapy is ineffective, examine possible causes, such as drug interactions, and report to RN or medical doctor (MD).

ADMINISTERING MEDICATIONS

CALCULATION OF DOSAGE

A. Practical nurse responsibility
1. Abide by the guidelines of the health care agency.
2. Check for accuracy in dosage calculation before preparing and administering drug.
3. Check calculations with another knowledgeable person.
4. Measure doses exactly as prescribed by physician.
B. Systems of measurement
1. Household system: measurements commonly used in the home; not as accurate as other systems; examples:
a. 1 teaspoon (tsp or t) = 60 drops (gtt)
b. 3 or 4 tsp = 1 tablespoon (tbsp or T)
2. Apothecary system: an older system, but continues to be used in dosage calculations in several areas of the United States and in several countries outside the United States
a. Common units of measurements
(1) Weight: grain (gr)
(2) Volume
(a) 60 minims = 1 dram (dr or d)
(b) 8 dr = 1 ounce (oz or z)
b. Notations in this system use lowercase Roman numerals; quantities less than 1 are expressed as common factors; exception: one half is written as "ss" in this system only.
3. Metric system: international decimal system
a. Common units of measurement
(1) Weight: unit is expressed in terms of the gram (g).
(a) Prefix *kilo* indicates 1000.
(b) Prefix *milli* indicates 1/1000.
(c) 1 g = 1000 milligrams (mg)

(2) Volume: unit is expressed in terms of the liter (L).
   (a) Prefix *milli* indicates 1/1000.
   (b) 1 L = 1000 milliliters (mL)
   b. Notations in this system use Arabic numbers; fractions are expressed as decimals.
4. Equivalents between systems: a given quantity considered to be of equal value to a quantity expressed in a different system; some common approximate equivalents:
   a. 1 kilogram (kg) = 2.2 pounds (lb)
   b. 1 g = 15 gr
   c. 60 mg = 1 gr
   d. 1 cubic centimeter (cc) = 1 mL
   e. 1000 mL = 1 quart (qt)
   f. 30 mL = 1 oz
   g. 1 mL = 15 or 16 gtt
   h. 1 tsp = 4 or 5 mL
C. Mathematics of conversion within and between systems; ratio and proportion method
   1. Household

   EXAMPLE : 3 tsp = _____ gtt
   teaspoons : drops :: teaspoons : drops
   1 tsp : 60 gtt :: 3 tsp : x gtt
   x = 180
   Answer : 3 tsp = 180 gtt

   2. Apothecary system

   EXAMPLE : 3 oz = _____ dr
   ounces : drams :: ounces : drams
   1 oz : 8 dr :: 3 oz : x dr
   x = 24
   Answer : 3 oz = 24 dr

   3. Metric system

   EXAMPLE : 250 mg = _____ g
   milligram : gram :: milligram : gram
   $1000x = 250 \left(\begin{array}{l} \text{divide } x \text{ into both parts of} \\ \text{the equation to equal } 1x \end{array} \right)$
   x = 0.25
   Answer : 250 mg = 0.25 g

   4. Conversion between systems

   EXAMPLE : gr $\frac{1}{6}$ = _____ mg
   grains : milligrams :: grains : milligrams
   1 : 60 :: $\frac{1}{6}$,: x
   1x = 60 = $\frac{1}{6}$
   x = 10
   Answer : gr $\frac{1}{6}$ = 10 mg

D. Dosage calculations: The dose for oral tablets, capsules, and liquids or solutions for injections can be calculated by use of the following formula:

   Desired dose (D) ÷ Dose on hand (H)
   × Quantity (Q) = Amount to be given

   EXAMPLE : Give 500 mg of tetracycline (Achromycin) using capsules containing 250 mg.
   D ÷ H × Q = 500 mg ÷ 250 mg × 1 capsule =
   Answer : 2 capsules

EXAMPLE : Physician orders digoxin 0.125 mg to be given orally; stock bottle is labeled "digoxin 0.25 mg" scored tablets.
   D ÷ H × Q = 0.125 mg ÷ 0.25 mg × 1 tablet =
   Answer : 0.5 tablet or ½ tablet

EXAMPLE : Erythromycin suspension 750 mg is ordered orally. The bottle is labeled 250 mg/5 mL.
   D ÷ H × Q = 750 mg ÷ 250 mg × 5 mL =
   Answer : 15 mL

EXAMPLE : Morphine sulfate gr $\frac{1}{4}$ is to be given by subcutaneous injection; the vial is labeled "morphine sulfate gr 2/mL."
   D ÷ H × Q = gr $\frac{1}{4}$ ÷ gr 2 × 1 mL =
   Answer : 0.5 mL

EXAMPLE : Penicillin 600,000 units is to be given by intramuscular injection; the vial is labeled "penicillin 300,000 units per mL."
   D ÷ H × Q = 600,000 units ÷ 300,000 units × 1 mL =
   Answer : 2 mL

Note: This formula can be used with any system of measurement. When two systems are involved, converting to the system of measurement of the dose on hand is required.

EXAMPLE : Codeine sulfate gr ss is ordered by mouth; on hand are codeine sulfate tablets labeled "30 mg."
   STEP 1 : CONVERSION BETWEEN SYSTEMS
   grain : milligram :: grain : milligram
   1 : 60 :: ½ : x
   x = 60 × ½
   x = 30
   Answer : codeine gr ss = 30 mg
   STEP 2 : FORMULA
   D ÷ H × Q = 30 mg ÷ 30 mg × 1
   Answer : 1 tablet

CALCULATION OF DRIP RATES FOR INTRAVENOUS INFUSION

A. Information that must be known
   1. Volume of solution to be infused
   2. Length of time over which this volume is to be infused
   3. Number of drops per milliliter delivered by the administration set being used
B. The drip rate may be calculated as follows:
   1. Find the volume of fluid to be administered per hour. Milliliters of fluid to be infused divided by the number of hours for infusion equals milliliters of fluid per hour.
   2. Find the volume of fluid to be administered per minute. Milliliters of fluid per hour divided by 60 min/hr equals milliliters to run per minute.
   3. Multiply the milliliters of fluid to run per minute by the number of drops per milliliter delivered by the infusion set; this gives the number of drops that should fall in the drip chamber per minute.

Milliliters per minute times drops per milliliter equals drops per minute.

$$\frac{\text{Volume (milliliters)}}{\text{Time (minutes)}} \times \text{Drops/milliliter} = \text{Drops/minute}$$

EXAMPLE : Administer 1000 mL of dextrose 5% in water (D5W) over 8 hours using an infusion set that delivers 10 gtt per minute.

$1000 \text{ mL} \div 8 \text{ hr} = 125 \text{ mL/hr}$

$125 \text{ mL/hr} \div 60 \text{ min/hr} = 2.1 \text{ mL/min}$

$2.1 \text{ mL/min} \times 10 \text{ gtt/mL} =$

Answer : 21 gtt/min

EXAMPLE : Administer 250 mL of D5W over 8 hours using a microdrip infusion set that delivers 60 gtt/mL.

$250 \text{ mL} \div 8 \text{ hr} = 31.25 \text{ mL/hr}$

$31.25 \text{ mL/hr} \div 60 \text{ min/hr} = 0.52 \text{ mL/min}$

$0.52 \text{ mL/min} \times 60 \text{ gtt/mL} = 31.2 \text{ gtt/min}$

Answer : 31 gtt/min

C. If the administration rate has been ordered as milliliters per hour, step 1 above is omitted.

D. Alternate formula to calculate drip rate:

Milliliters to administer $\times$ Drops per milliliter
$\div$ (Hours to run $\times$ 60 min/hr) = Drops per milliliter

EXAMPLE : Administer 1000 mL of D5W over 8 hours using an infusion set that delivers 10 gtt/mL.

$1000 \text{ mL} \times 10 \text{ gtt/mL} \div 8 \text{ hr} \times 60 \text{ min/hr} =$

Answer : 21 gtt/min

E. Adjust the flow rate to the number of drops per minute as calculated. Assess the fluid volume at hourly intervals to see that the fluid is being administered at the desired rate. The calculated drip rate is an approximation of the actual flow rate. The type of solution, additives, position of the patient or infusion tubing, height of the reservoir, and volume of fluid in the container can influence the actual drip rate. The LPN/LVN should verify computations with another knowledgeable person before readjusting the drip rate to ensure volume delivery for the prescribed time.

METHODS OF ADMINISTERING MEDICATIONS

A. Nurse's responsibilities
   1. Knowledge of drug
      a. Actions
      b. Ranges of dosage
      c. Methods of administration
      d. Common use
      e. Adverse reactions
      f. Contraindications
      g. Patient education
   2. Assess patient regarding history of allergies or sensitivities to drugs.
   3. Be aware of and follow agency policy regarding procedure for checking the medication order.

4. Know agency system of medication distribution.
   a. Cards (rarely used anymore)
   b. Kardex, Medex, or MAR (medication administration record)
   c. Computer printout sheet
5. Know occasions when and parameters for which drugs may be withheld.
   a. Fasting for diagnostic tests or laboratory work or surgery; illness
   b. Required laboratory blood work before medication administration; certain medications may require therapeutic levels to determine if medication is being maintained in proper range versus nontherapeutic or toxic.
   c. Specific guidelines for certain drugs (e.g., apical pulse rate before cardiotonics; BP readings before antihypertensive agents)
6. Position the patient for proper administration of medications; assist as needed.
7. Observe the six rights of medication administration:
   a. Right patient
   b. Right drug
   c. Right dose
   d. Right route
   e. Right time
   f. Right documentation and right technique— Some sources still refer to the "five rights" of medication; however, more sources have added "right documentation and right technique." Both of these are included in this list of nursing responsibilities.
8. Inform the patient of any anticipated change in normal body functions such as drowsiness, nausea, or change in color of urine.
9. Report patient noncompliance or adverse reactions to other responsible person (i.e., RN, MD).
10. Follow procedure for controlled substances.
11. Remain with patient until medication has been taken.
12. Never leave medications at patient's bedside unless specifically ordered.
13. Ensure accuracy in drug calculation; when in doubt, verify with other responsible person (i.e., RN, pharmacist).
14. Check expiration date on all medication labels and orders.
15. Accurately document medications given and, if omitted or refused, document reason.
16. Document effectiveness of medication.
17. Be aware of and follow agency procedure in event of medication error.
18. Acknowledge and respect patient's request to refuse medication.

B. Safety measures in preparing medications
   1. Environment
      a. Quiet
      b. Free from distractions
      c. Good lighting
   2. Do not leave prepared medications unattended; keep in a locked area.
   3. Do not give medications that someone else has poured.

4. Read each label three times.
   a. When reaching for the container
   b. Immediately before pouring the medication
   c. When replacing or discarding the container
5. Transport drugs for administration by using trays or carts that allow the identifying information and the medication container to be kept together safely.
6. Do not allow tray or cart to be left out of sight during administration.
7. Positively identify patient before administering the medication, preferably by checking his or her identification bracelet, having patient state his or her name, or having second person identify patient; open medication(s) at bedside if possible.
8. Remain with the patient until he or she takes the medication.
9. Document necessary supplemental information (e.g., pulse rate, BP, site of application or injection) according to agency policy.
10. Guidelines for drug safety at home
    a. Keep each drug in original, labeled container.
    b. Be sure that labels are legible.
    c. Discard any outdated medications.
    d. Always finish a prescribed drug unless otherwise instructed.
    e. Dispose of drug(s) as per agency policy.
    f. Do not give one family member a drug prescribed for another family member.
    g. Refrigerate medications if required.
    h. Read labels carefully and follow all instructions.
    i. Use childproof caps when appropriate.
C. Oral administration of medications
   1. General information
      a. Use the simplest and most convenient route.
      b. Liquid preparations
         (1) Pour into a container placed on a flat surface.
         (2) Read at eye level.
         (3) Measure amount by using the bottom of meniscus.
      c. Irritating drugs should be dissolved or diluted and given with food or immediately after a meal.
      d. Distasteful oral medications can be disguised (e.g., by having patient suck on a piece of ice for a few minutes to numb taste buds; storing oily medications in a refrigerator; having patient use a straw; or mixing medication with a small amount of fruit juice, milk, applesauce, or gelatin); always inform patient that a food vehicle contains the medication.
      e. For patients who have difficulty swallowing tablets, some tablets may be crushed to facilitate swallowing; be aware of contraindications for crushing certain medications (e.g., enteric-coated tablets) or for opening capsules containing timed-release medications.
      f. Liquid medications that are harmful to teeth (e.g., liquid iron preparations) should be administered with a straw placed at the back of the tongue.
   2. Specific procedure is described in Table 3-1.

Table 3-1	Administration of Oral Medications
SUGGESTED ACTION	**RATIONALE**
Wash hands before administration, and practice medical asepsis while preparing and administering medication.	Careful handwashing and use of separate medication cups prevent cross-contamination between nurse and patients.
Check the order and read the label three times while preparing the drug.	Frequent checking prevents errors and ensures accuracy.
Pour tablets and capsules into the cap of a stock container and then transfer proper amount into medication cup.	Pouring medications into the nurse's hand contaminates the tablet or capsule.
Pour liquids from the side of the bottle opposite the label.	Liquid that may spill onto the label makes reading the label difficult.
Transport medications to patient's bedside carefully.	Accidental or deliberate disarrangement of medications is prevented.
Keep medications in sight at all times.	This is for safety reasons.
Identify patient carefully. Open medications at the patient's bedside	Illness and different environment can often cause confusion. Safety measure to assure patient receives right medication.
Assist patient to an upright position as necessary.	Proper positioning facilitates swallowing.
Offer sufficient water or other permitted fluids.	Liquids allow for ease in swallowing and help dissolve solid drugs.
Remain with patient until each medication is swallowed.	Patient may discard unwanted medications or accumulate them with intent to harm himself or herself.
Document each medication administered, both promptly and according to agency policy; report or document medications not taken.	The patient's chart is a legal record; prompt documentation avoids the possibility of repeating administration of the same drug.
If patient's intake is being measured, record the amount of fluid taken with the medication.	All fluids taken are to be recorded for determining total intake.

D. Parenteral administration of medications: administration by a route other than through the enteral or GI tract such as intradermal, subcutaneous (SC), intramuscular (IM), or IV routes

Table 3-2 Selection of Syringe and Needle

TYPE OF INJECTION	SYRINGE SIZE	NEEDLE SIZE
Intradermal	1 mL, calibrated in tenths or hundredths of a milliliter or in minims	26 or 27 gauge; ½ or ¾ inch
Subcutaneous	2, 2½, or 3 mL, calibrated in 0.1 mL	25 gauge; ½ or ⅝ inch
Intramuscular	2-5 mL calibrated in 0.2 mL	20 or 22 gauge; 1½ inch
Insulin (subcutaneous)	Insulin syringes in 0.5-1 mL, calibrated in units Insulin syringes also available for patients in premeasured doses	25, 26, or 27 gauge; ½ or ⅝ inch

1. General information: Maintain surgical aseptic technique in preparation and administration. Use of pre-packaged, disposable sterile needles and syringes is preferable.
2. Select syringe and needle. Thick or oily solutions require a large lumen. Short needles are used for children and adults with little adipose tissue; obese individuals may require longer needles to ensure delivery of medications to proper tissue level (Table 3-2).
3. Put the drugs into the syringe.
   a. Manufacturer—prefilled syringes or cartridges: contain the name and dose of the drug and the intended parenteral route; should not be given by any route other than the one specified
   b. Rubber-capped vials: single or multidose container; solution or powder form; dry form of drug dissolved according to label instructions. To remove the drug:
      (1) Remove the soft metal cover on top of the vial.
      (2) Using friction, wipe the rubber cap with a pledget soaked with antiseptic solution.
      (3) Fill syringe with air equal to amount of solution to be withdrawn to increase pressure within the vial and facilitate withdrawal of solution.
      (4) Insert needle into the rubber cap while holding the needle in a slightly lateral position to prevent a piece of the stopper from entering the vial.
      (5) Inject the air and remove prescribed amount of solution while holding the syringe in a vertical position.
   c. Glass ampules: prescored or unscored tops; constricted-neck ampules require that solution be in base of ampule.
      (1) Quickly snap finger on the stem to move the solution into the base of the ampule.
      (2) Hold the ampule in one hand.

   (3) Protecting the fingers of the other hand with a sterile, dry gauze pledget, break off the stem of the ampule; check solution for fragments of glass.
   (4) Insert filter needle into the opened ampule, avoiding needle contamination by not touching the rim of the ampule with the needle.
   (5) Keep needle under solution and withdraw the prescribed amount of the solution.
4. Prepare the skin.
   a. Heavily soiled skin in area of intended injection site should be washed with soap and water.
   b. Antiseptic-soaked gauze or pledget is then used to disinfect injection site and thus prevent injection of harmful organism into body tissue.
      (1) Wipe in a circular motion, starting at point of injection and moving outward to carry debris away from injection site.
      (2) Use firm pressure and friction when wiping to help remove soil.
5. Reduce discomfort.
   a. Use sharp needle.
   b. Use appropriate gauge.
   c. Select site free of irritation or nodules from previous injections.
   d. Numb skin receptors with use of cold compresses or ice cube over injection site.
   e. Hold tissue taut or compress tissue to form a pad, depending on type of injection.
   f. Be sure that no solution is on the needle.
   g. Help patient relax.
   h. Insert needle without hesitation.
   i. Aspirate when appropriate.
   j. Inject solution slowly.
   k. Remove needle quickly. (Heparin should be held for 10 seconds before removal of needle, to decrease bruising.)
   l. Massage area after injection unless contraindicated with certain medications (i.e., insulin) or certain routes (i.e., intradermal, Z-track).
6. Care of equipment after injections: use needle-disposal unit; follow agency policy.
7. Injection sites
   a. Intradermal injection: solutions injected directly under the epidermis into the dermis (10- to 15-degree angle)
      (1) Absorption occurs slowly through the capillaries.
      (2) Common site is inner aspect of the forearm.
      (3) It is a commonly used technique with allergy testing or purified protein derivative testing for TB.
   b. SC injection: solutions injected into the subcutaneous layer of the skin (45- to 90-degree angle)
      (1) Common sites
         (a) Outer aspect of upper arm
         (b) Thigh
         (c) Lower abdomen
         (d) Upper back
      (2) Suggested procedure for SC injection is described in Table 3-3.
   c. IM injection: solutions injected into the muscular layer of tissue (90-degree angle)

Table 3-3 Administration of Subcutaneous Injection

SUGGESTED ACTION	RATIONALE
Verify physician's order, and read medication label three times; check expiration date.	Ensures accuracy and prevents errors.
Obtain and assemble equipment, maintaining sterile technique.	Prevents contamination.
Draw the drug into syringe and protect needle with sterile needle cover.	Prevents needle contamination from exposure to air or contact with moist surface.
Identify patient by identification bracelet and by having patient state name if possible.	Prevents potential medication error.
Select appropriate injection site and cleanse area with antiseptic pledget, using firm, circular motion, moving outward from injection site.	Friction helps clean skin and decreases possibility of introducing bacteria into body.
Grasp the tissue surrounding the injection site and hold it to form a cushion pad.	Ensures placement of medication into subcutaneous tissue and helps prevent deposition of medication into muscle tissue.
Inject the needle quickly at an angle of 45-90 degrees, depending on the quality and amount of tissue and length of needle.	Ensures placement of medication into subcutaneous tissue. Above-average-weight patients require a 90-degree angle. Below-average- or average-weight patients require a 45-degree angle.
After needle is in proper tissue level, release grasp of the tissue.	Reduces discomfort of injection.
Aspirate to determine whether needle is in a blood vessel.	Prevents discomfort and possible serious reaction if medication is injected into vein.
If there is no blood return, inject solution slowly.	Reduces discomfort by reducing pressure in subcutaneous tissue.
Withdraw needle quickly.	Reduces discomfort.
Massage area gently unless contraindicated with certain medications.	Helps to distribute the solution and hasten absorption of the medication.

(1) Common sites
  (a) Dorsogluteal site
  (b) Ventrogluteal site
  (c) Vastus lateralis muscle (most common)
  (d) Deltoid muscle
  (e) Rectus femoris muscle (rarely used)
(2) Suggested procedure for IM injection is described in Table 3-4.

Table 3-4 Administration of Intramuscular Injection

SUGGESTED ACTION	RATIONALE
Verify physician's order and read medication label three times; check expiration date.	Ensures accuracy and prevents errors.
Obtain and assemble equipment, maintaining sterile technique.	Prevents contamination.
Draw the drug into syringe; create small air bubble in the syringe; protect needle with sterile needle cover.	Air bubble forces medication out of needle shaft when injected; exposure to air or contact with moist surfaces contaminates needle.
Identify patient by identification bracelet and by having patient state name if possible.	Prevents potential medication error.
Have the patient assume appropriate position according to site selected.	Helps relax muscles and eases discomfort.
Select appropriate injection site and cleanse area with antiseptic pledget, using firm, circular motion, moving outward from injection site.	Friction helps clean the skin, thus decreasing possibility of introducing bacteria into body tissue.
Press down and hold tissue taut over the injection site.	Ensures that needle reaches muscle layer.
Hold syringe at 90-degree angle and quickly thrust needle into the tissue. Assess patient's body size before injection—a thinner patient may need a smaller angle.	Minimizes discomfort.
Aspirate to determine whether needle is in a blood vessel.	Prevents discomfort and possible serious reaction if medication is injected into vein.
If there is no blood return, inject medication slowly, followed by the air bubble.	Reduces discomfort and allows medication to disperse into the tissue; air bubble clears medication from needle.
Withdraw needle quickly.	Reduces discomfort.
Massage area gently unless contraindicated with certain medications.	Helps distribute the solution and hasten absorption of the medication.

d. Z-track injection: used to prevent damage to and staining of the skin and subcutaneous tissues; common site is the upper outer quadrant of the gluteal region.

e. IV infusion: administration of a large amount of fluid into a vein
   (1) Purposes
      (a) To restore or maintain electrolyte balance and hydration
      (b) To supply drugs for immediate effect
      (c) To replace nutrients and vitamins
      (d) To replace blood loss
   (2) Nurse practice acts and agency policy dictate who may administer IV infusions.
   (3) Nurse's responsibilities for IV infusion
      (a) Verify physician's order.
      (b) Calculate rate of flow.
      (c) Monitor rate of flow.
      (d) Assess patient for adverse reactions
         • Infiltration
         • Circulatory overload
         • Thrombophlebitis

f. Hyperalimentation: total parenteral nutrition (TPN): an IV infusion containing sufficient nutrients to sustain life; provides amino acids, glucose, vitamins, and electrolytes for patients who are unable to ingest nutrients normally for extended periods and for whom standard infusions are inadequate

g. Transfusion: infusion of blood products from a healthy person into a recipient's vein
   (1) Blood is typed and cross-matched before administration to determine compatibility.
   (2) Nurse's responsibilities for blood transfusion (Some states do not allow LPN/LVNs to hang blood.)
      (a) Check and double-check; this is done with a second nurse.
         • Labels
         • Numbers
         • Rh factor
         • Compatibility
      (b) Stay with patient for at least the first 5 minutes (10 to 15 minutes better) after transfusion is started.
      (c) Monitor rate of transfusion.
      (d) Assess patient for signs of adverse reactions.
         • Hemolytic reaction: Stop transfusion immediately, keep vein open with slow-drip normal saline solution, and notify physician. Indications include:
            ○ Headache.
            ○ Sensations of tingling.
            ○ Difficulty in breathing.
            ○ Pain in lumbar region or legs.
         • Allergic reactions: Stop transfusion immediately and notify physician. Indications include:
            ○ Pruritus.
            ○ Hives (urticaria).
            ○ Difficulty in breathing.
         • Febrile reactions resulting from contaminant in the blood: usually occur late in the transfusion or after it is completed. Indications include:
            ○ Flushed skin.
            ○ Elevated temperature.
            ○ Chills, muscular spasms.
            ○ General malaise.
            ○ Signs of systemic infection.
         • Circulatory overload that leads to pulmonary edema. Indications include:
            ○ Increased pulse rate.
            ○ Dyspnea.
            ○ Respiratory distress (crackles on auscultation).
            ○ Moist coughing.
            ○ Expectoration of blood-tinged mucus.
         • Anticoagulant reaction. Indications include:
            ○ Tingling in the fingers.
            ○ Muscular cramping.
            ○ Convulsions.

h. Blood extracts: specific components of whole blood that meet specific needs of the patient
   (1) Packed red blood cells (RBCs)
   (2) Plasma
   (3) Human albumin
   (4) Fibrinogen
   (5) Gamma globulin

PEDIATRIC DRUG ADMINISTRATION

GENERAL RULES

A. The child's age, weight, and level of growth and development should guide pediatric drug therapy.

B. The nurse's approach to the child should convey the impression that he or she expects the child to take the medication.

C. Explanation regarding the medication should be based on the child's level of understanding.

D. The nurse must be honest with the child regarding the procedure.

E. Mixing distasteful medication or crushed tablets with a small amount of honey, applesauce, or gelatin may be necessary.

F. Never threaten a child with an injection if he or she refuses an oral medication.

G. All medications should be kept out of the reach of children, and medications should never be referred to as candy.

CALCULATING THE PEDIATRIC DOSE

Safe dosage ranges of drugs are less well defined for children than they are for adults. Not all drug dosage ranges for children are listed in the literature. Determining the dose of a drug for an infant or child is not the nurse's responsibility; but verifying or calculating a dose as a fraction of the adult dose occasionally may be necessary. The following methods may be used:

A. Body surface area: considered most accurate; requires a nomogram (i.e., a device for rapid estimation of body surface area)

$$\text{Child's dose} = \frac{\text{Body surface area (in square meters)}}{1.73\text{m}^2 \times \text{Adult dose}}$$

B. Clark's rule: based on weight and used for children at least 2 years of age

$$\text{Child's dose} = \frac{\text{Weight (in pounds)}}{150} \times \text{Adult dose}$$

C. Young's rule: based on age and used for children at least 2 years of age

$$\text{Child's dose} = \frac{\text{Age (in years)}}{\text{Age (in years)} + 12} \times \text{Adult dose}$$

D. Fried's rule: used for children younger than 2 years of age

$$\text{Child's dose} = \frac{\text{Age (in months)}}{150} \times \text{Adult dose}$$

IDENTIFYING THE PATIENT

A. Check child's identification bracelet.
B. Ask older child his or her name.
C. Parent or the child's caregiver should be asked to confirm the patient's identity.

ORAL MEDICATION

Verify, calculate, and document all medications.
A. Infants
  1. Draw up liquid medication in a dropper or a syringe without the needle.
  2. Elevate infant's head and shoulders; hold infant in a feeding position.
  3. Depress the chin with the thumb to open infant's mouth.
  4. Using the dropper or syringe, direct the medication toward the inner aspect of the infant's cheek and release the flow of medication slowly.
  5. Release the thumb and allow the infant to swallow.
  6. Liquid medication can also be measured into a nipple; the infant is allowed to suck the medication through the nipple.
  7. Crushed tablets can be mixed with a small amount of honey or applesauce and fed slowly with a teaspoon.
  Note: **Honey should not be given to infants under 1 year of age because of the infant's immature immune system.**
B. Toddlers
  1. Draw up medication in a syringe or measure into a medication cup.
  2. Elevate the child's head and shoulders.
  3. Place the syringe in the child's mouth and slowly release the medication, directing it toward the inner aspect of the cheek, or allow the child to hold the medicine cup and drink it at own pace; offer praise.
C. School-age children
  1. When the child is old enough to take medicine in tablet or capsule form, direct him or her to place the medicine near the back of the tongue and to swallow fluid such as water or juice immediately.
  2. Offer the child praise after he or she has taken medication.

INTRAMUSCULAR INJECTION

A. Infants
  1. Common site: Largest muscle group is the quadriceps femoris, located in the anterolateral thigh. Largest muscle of this group is the vastus lateralis, situated on the anterior surface of the midlateral thigh.
    a. Place infant in supine position.
    b. Compress muscle tissue at upper aspect of thigh, pointing the nurse's fingers toward the infant's feet.
    c. Needle is inserted at a 90-degree angle; maximum length of needle for an infant is 1 inch (2.5 cm).
  2. Alternate site: Rectus femoris muscle, located on the anterolateral surface of the upper thigh. Needle is inserted at a 45-degree angle and is directed toward the knee.
B. Toddlers and school-age children
  1. Dorsogluteal muscle is in the upper outer quadrant; gluteal muscle does not develop until child begins to walk; it should be used for injections only after the child has been walking for 1 year or more.
  2. Ventrogluteal muscle is a dense muscle mass; the disadvantage is that the site is visible to the child.
  3. Deltoid muscle may be used for older, larger children.
  4. Lateral and anterior aspect of thigh is located on upper outer quadrant of thigh.

ADMINISTRATION OF INJECTIONS

A. Infants
  1. Place infant in a secure position to avoid movement of the extremity.
  2. A second person is usually needed to secure the infant.
  3. Hold, cuddle, and comfort the infant after the injection.
B. Toddlers and school-age children
  1. Have syringe and needle completely prepared before contact with the child.
  2. Keep needle outside of child's visual field.
  3. Explain, according to the child's developmental age, the reason for an injection and where it will be given; do not say "it won't hurt."
  4. Inspect injection site before injection for tenderness or undue firmness.
  5. Have a second person available to help secure the child and offer comfort during the procedure.
  6. Allow the child to express fears.
  7. Perform the procedure quickly and gently.
  8. After the injection, praise the child for his or her behavior.

CENTRAL NERVOUS SYSTEM

DEPRESSANTS

A. Characteristics of drug-induced central nervous system (CNS) depression
  1. Mild: disinterest in surroundings, inability to focus on a topic or initiate talking or movement, slowed pulse and respirations
  2. Moderate or progressive: drowsiness or sleep, decreased muscle tone and ability to move, diminished acuity of all senses and sensations—touch, vision, hearing, heat, cold, pain
  3. Severe: unconsciousness or coma, loss of reflexes, respiratory failure, death
B. Analgesics: Nurses have a legal and a moral responsibility to relieve pain. Barriers to effective pain management include:
  1. Fear of developing tolerance.
    a. Tolerance is rarely seen in patients with severe acute or chronic pain.
    b. An increase in pain is usually the result of progression of disease or complications.

2. Fear of addiction.
   a. Risk of addiction in hospitalized patients is minimal.
   b. Psychological dependence is rare in hospitalized patients.
   c. In patients with cancer pain, drug dosage may be titrated to large amounts of opioids to control pain without producing the adverse effects of respiratory depression or excessive sedation.
3. Fear of respiratory depression.
   a. Tolerance develops to the respiratory depression effect but not to the analgesia effect.
   b. Significant respiratory depression is rarely seen because medication has been titrated to meet an individual's requirement.
4. Children. Children are often untreated or inadequately treated for pain.
5. Older adults. Older adults need careful assessment.
   a. Close monitoring to reduce the chances of overtreatment or undertreatment
   b. Greater chance for adverse effects
   c. May have diminished circulatory processes, affecting the absorption of medications
   d. Increased chance for interaction with other medications
C. Analgesics: drugs that relieve pain
   1. Opioid analgesics: act on the CNS; alter the patient's perception of pain; are more often used for severe pain.
      a. Examples include the following: morphine is prototype; natural or synthetic agents that have a morphinelike effect; additional examples in Table 3-5.
      b. Adverse reactions and contraindications
         (1) Depress respiratory and cough centers in the medulla

(2) Cautious use in patients with impaired respiratory function and those with head injury because analgesics obscure CNS evaluation
(3) Inhibit gastric, biliary, and pancreatic secretions; depress GI tract; can cause nausea, vomiting, and constipation. Constipation is seen with increasing doses of opioid medications. A plan to manage this side effect should be in place at the initiation of therapy.
(4) Stimulate release of antidiuretic hormone, resulting in decreased urine volume; can cause urinary retention
(5) Induced hypotension
(6) Decreased heart rate
(7) Pupillary constriction
(8) Pruritus

2. Nonopioid antiinflammatory analgesics: act at the site of the pain; do not alter the patient's perception; used more frequently for mild-to-moderate pain; act by sensitizing peripheral pain receptors; often combined with opioid analgesics to enhance pain control in severe pain; nonsteroidal antiinflammatory drugs (NSAIDs) indicated when an antiinflammatory effect is desired.
   a. Examples can be found in Table 3-6.
   b. Agents
      (1) Acetylsalicylic acid (aspirin)*: effective in managing low-intensity pain
         (a) Adverse reactions
            • Gastric irritation
            • Ulceration and gastric bleeding
            • Intoxication (salicylism): tinnitus, reversible hearing loss, hyperventilation, fever,

Table 3-5 Selected Opioids

GENERIC NAME	TRADE NAME	COMMENTS
OPIOID AGONISTS		
alfentanil	Alfenta	Individualized dosage used in maintenance of anesthesia.
codeine	codeine phosphate, codeine sulfate	Classified as Schedule II drug.
hydrocodone	Hycodan	Respiratory depressant effects are particularly dangerous; have resuscitation equipment nearby.
fentanyl citrate	Sublimaze	Given preoperatively.
hydromorphone	Dilaudid	Potent synthetic compound that maximizes analgesic effects and minimizes some of the common side effects of morphine; hydromorphone has 7-10 times the analgesic action of morphine.
		Adults: Give IM, SC, or PO or as rectal suppository.
levorphanol	Levo-Dromoran	Used to relieve moderate to severe pain; often used preoperatively to reduce apprehension and to prolong analgesia. Relatively longer onset of action than other opioid agonist analgesics.
		May also be given by slow intravenous injection.
meperidine	Demerol	Schedule II drug; synthetic opioid analgesic with less potency than morphine; each dose of syrup should be taken in one-half glass of water, because if undiluted, it can exert a topical anesthetic effect on mucous membranes.
		Give IM, PO, or SC.

Table 3-5	Selected Opioids—Cont'd	

GENERIC NAME	TRADE NAME	COMMENTS
methadone	Dolophine	Schedule II drug; synthetic opioid analgesic used primarily in detoxification, treatment, and maintenance of heroin addicts or for severe pain. When drug is used for severe pain, it is administered IM. Drug is highly addictive. When used for heroin addicts for more than 3 wk, methadone moves from a treatment phase to a maintenance phase.
morphine	Duramorph MS Contin	Schedule II drug; primary opioid analgesic used for relief of severe pain. Morphine is the opioid analgesic against which all others are compared. Also produces sedation and euphoria when pain is present. Traditionally used for preoperative sedation and postoperative analgesia. Morphine is more effective against dull, continuous pain than sharp, spasmodic pain. IV medication should be given slowly over a 4- to 5-min period. Protect drug from light and freezing.
opium combinations	Opium Tincture	Schedule II drug. Opium Tincture is equivalent to 1% morphine. Avoid confusing these two medications.
	Paregoric	Paregoric is equivalent to 0.04% morphine. Paregoric is used for cramps, diarrhea, and teething pain in infants (as a topical application to gums).
oxycodone	OxyContin, Oxycodone	These agents are similar in action and structure but are not identical; they are opium alkaloids and are morphinelike in action.
oxymorphone	Numorphan	Give IV or rectally.
OPIOID ANTAGONISTS		
nalmefene	Revex	Used for postoperative opioid depression or overdose.
naloxone	Narcan	Used for postoperative opioid depression or overdose.
naltrexone	ReVia	Has longer effect than naloxone. Used for alcohol or opioid dependence.
OPIOID AGONIST-ANTAGONISTS		
buprenorphine	Buprenex	Available in subcutaneous, epidural, and rectal forms.
butorphanol	Stadol	Onset of action in 10 min after intramuscular injection and almost immediately after intravenous injection. Respiratory depressant effect is similar to that of morphine, is dose related, and is easily reversed with naloxone. Available in intravenous and intranasal forms. Used for obstetrical analgesia, renal colic, and cancer pain.
nalbuphine	Nubain	Onset in 15 min, duration 3-6 hr. This product tends to be more expensive than other agonist-antagonist products.
		Adults: 10 mg SC, IM, or IV, repeated q3-6h p.r.n.; not to be given more than 20 mg in one dose or more than 160 mg/day.

From Edmunds MW: *Introduction to clinical pharmacology,* ed 7, St Louis, 2013, Mosby.
IM, Intramuscularly; *IV,* intravenously; *PO,* by mouth; *p.r.n., pro re nata* (as needed); *SC,* subcutaneously.

metabolic acidosis, vomiting, hypokalemia, convulsions, coma, death
  (b) Drug interactions with aspirin
    • Anticoagulants: increase likelihood of bleeding
    • Alcohol: increases likelihood of GI irritation and bleeding
  (2) Acetaminophen* (Datril, Tylenol): effective in managing low-intensity pain; does not produce gastric irritation or alter platelet function and bleeding times as does aspirin; does not interact with oral anticoagulants; possible liver and kidney damage from prolonged use or frequent high doses. The recommended maximum daily dose is 4 g. Patients should have their kidney and liver function monitored on a regular basis. The antidote for overdose of acetaminophen is acetylcysteine. Signs of liver toxicity include abdominal pain, nausea, vomiting, and decreased appetite. Renal damage is evidenced by back pain and pedal and/or respiratory edema. It is important for the nurse to know that these signs may take a long time to develop. Any complaint that the patient has should not be ignored. Acetaminophen should not be used in a patient with a history of alcoholism.
  (3) NSAIDs: decrease the inflammatory process; effective in the treatment of osteoarthritis, degenerative joint disease, rheumatic diseases. Agents include:
    • Ibuprofen (Advil).
    • Celecoxib (Celebrex).
There is a potential for bleeding, kidney, and liver damage if NSAIDs are used in high doses or over a prolonged period of time.
  (4) Triptans: selectively used in treating migraines; cause vasoconstriction of cerebral blood vessels

| Table 3-6 | Nonsteroidal Antiinflammatory Drugs (NSAIDs): Pharmacokinetics, Dosage, and Comments |

NSAIDS	ONSET OF ACTION (hr)	HALF-LIFE (hr)	USUAL ADULT DOSAGE (mg/day)	COMMENTS*
ACETIC ACIDS				
Ketorolac IM (Toradol)	10 min (dose dependent)	PO: 4 IM: 6	IM/IV 30 mg, then 10 mg PO every 4-6 h	Should not be given by any route for longer than 5 days. Increased risk of GI bleeding and other severe effects with duration of treatment. Do not give before surgery or intraoperatively if bleeding control is necessary. Severe allergic reactions or anaphylaxis may occur with first dose.
Nabumetone (Relafen)	—	22	500, 750, or 1000 mg daily (hs) or in two divided doses	Prodrug (inactive); converted to active metabolite (6-MNA) in liver. Absorption increased by food and milk. Fewer reports of GI ulceration and bleeding than with other NSAIDs.
COX-2 INHIBITORS				
Celecoxib (Celebrex)			100 to 200 mg PO twice daily	Significant risk for GI bleeding if taken in combination with another NSAID. This group of NSAIDs has considerably less antiplatelet effect and there are fewer bleeding tendencies as a side effect.
PROPIONIC ACIDS				
Ibuprofen (Motrin, Advil)	0.5	2	300-800 mg 3 or 4 times daily	Available in tablet, liquid, and OTC forms. May decrease blood glucose levels. Incidence of GI side effects less than with aspirin.

COX, Cyclooxygenase;
GI, gastrointestinal; *IM*, intramuscular; *PO*, by mouth; *hs*, at bedtime; *IV*, intravenous; *6-MNA*, 6-methoxy-2-naphthylacetic acid; *OTC*, over-the-counter.
* All oral NSAIDs should be taken with 8 oz of water with person remaining upright for at least 15 to 30 min afterward. Newer NSAIDs (e.g., Aleve) are designed to be taken less often.

(a) Agents include:
- Imitrex (sumatriptan).
- Treximet (combination of sumatriptan and naproxen).

(b) NSAIDs and triptans share many common side and adverse effects:
- Heartburn, indigestion
- Nausea, vomiting
- Constipation or diarrhea
- Hypertension
- Dizziness
- Blurred vision
- Skin rash

(c) Serious adverse effects have been seen with triptans and certain NSAIDs, including myocardial infarction (MI) and cerebrovascular accident (CVA) caused by vasoconstrictive effects of these medications. Sudden severe GI bleeding can occur with drugs from both of these classifications.

(d) These medications should be used with caution in any patients with a history of cardiovascular or GI conditions.

(e) Used with caution in older patients, who are prone to upper GI, hepatic, or renal effects.

(f) Administration with anticoagulants may increase risk of GI ulcers or hemorrhage.

(g) Given concurrently may reduce the effectiveness of hypertensive agent.

(h) Used with alcoholic beverages may produce a synergistic effect in causing GI bleeding.

(i) These medications have many adverse side effects, including interactions with other medications. A careful history needs to be taken. Health care providers must be familiar with the details of the individual drug that the patient is taking.

3. Nursing assessment: Determine character, location, onset, contributing factors, duration of pain, time of last dose; presence of head injury; hepatic or renal failure. Ask the patient about pain at least once per shift, and document effectiveness of interventions.

4. Nursing management
   a. Determine the most effective way to manage the pain: drug versus nondrug measure (e.g., positioning, turning). Be creative when trying to relieve a patient's pain; try combinations of drug and nondrug therapies. Documenting the effectiveness of pain relief measures is vital.
   b. Obtain vital signs.
      (1) Be alert to hypotension and hypertension.
      (2) Analyze rate and character of respiration.
      (3) Withhold drug and notify physician in presence of respiratory depression: respiratory rate of 10 or fewer respirations per minute or a decrease of eight or more respirations per minute from baseline data.
   c. Caution patient to remain quiet after drug administration to decrease possible nausea and vomiting.
   d. Implement safety measures: Use side rails and advise patient to remain in bed if changes in mental status, alterations in judgment, or unsteadiness occurs.
   e. Patients need to be instructed to ask for pain medication before the pain becomes severe. The increasing use of patient-controlled analgesia (PCA) pumps has decreased patient anxiety about pain relief.
   f. Initiate intake and output records to determine effectiveness of bladder function.
   g. Determine efficacy of bowel activity. Patients receiving long-term treatment with medications should be on a bowel regimen. Constipation is the one side effect for which patients do not develop a tolerance.
   h. Instruct patient concerning:
      (1) How to take drug.
      (2) Safe storage in the home.
      (3) Avoidance of driving.
      (4) Danger of simultaneous administration of alcohol or other CNS depressant with narcotics.

5. Nursing evaluation
   a. Have patient rate pain before and after administration on a scale of 1 to 10 and document.
   b. Observe for decreased restlessness and anxiety and ability of the patient to function.

D. Narcotic antagonists
1. Action: reverse CNS and respiratory depression caused by overdose of narcotics
2. Agents

Examples	Comment
Levallorphan (Lorfan)	If effects of the narcotic persist, repeat doses may be necessary.
Naloxone (Narcan)	

3. Adverse reactions and contraindications
   a. Arrhythmias
   b. Hypertension
   c. Hypotension
   d. Nausea, vomiting
   e. Return of severe pain
4. Failure to improve indicates need to investigate other causes of CNS and respiratory depression.

E. Dependency: the total psychophysical state of the individual who is addicted to drugs or alcohol and who must receive an increasing amount of the substance to prevent the onset of abstinence symptoms
1. Dependency is rarely seen in hospitalized patients who are taking medication for pain relief, not euphoric effects.
2. Symptoms include runny nose, pilomotor reflex (gooseflesh), tearing, yawning, muscle twitching, abdominal cramping, insomnia, nausea and vomiting, diarrhea.
3. Methadone hydrochloride is used for detoxification and maintenance.
4. With acute toxicity the usual cause of death is respiratory depression; treated with support to respiration and with a narcotic antagonist.

F. Anesthetics: provide a pain-free experience during an operative procedure along with a relaxed state of mind and sense of security
1. General anesthetics: provide loss of pain sensation, loss of consciousness, loss of memory, and loss of voluntary and some involuntary muscle activity
   a. Inhalation agents: The following are examples:
      Cyclopropane
      Ether
      Halothane
      Nitrous oxide
   b. IV agents: The following are examples:
      Droperidol (Inapsine)
      Droperidol and fentanyl (Innovar)
      Ketamine hydrochloride
      Methohexital (Brevital)
2. Regional anesthetics: provide loss of sensation and motor activity in localized areas of the body
   a. Types
      (1) Topical
      (2) Infiltration
      (3) Peripheral nerve blocks
      (4) Spinal
      (5) Epidural
      (6) Caudal

b. Agents: The following are examples:
   Carbocaine
   Novocain
   Nupercaine
   Pontocaine
   Xylocaine
3. Nursing assessment
   a. Preoperative: Obtain health history, including allergies, psychological status, and physiological baseline data. Inform patient about surgical procedure.
   b. Intraoperative: Implement safety measures in presence of explosive or flammable agents.
   c. Postoperative: Determine vital signs and respiratory function.
4. Nursing management
   a. Preoperative: Prepare patient physically and psychologically. Initiate measures to prevent complications: deep-breathing and muscle-strengthening exercises. Administer preoperative medications. Initiate safety measures. Provide quiet environment.
   b. Intraoperative: Maintain quiet during stage 2 anesthesia. Position patient properly and pad pressure points adequately. Transfer patient from operating table in a smooth, coordinated manner to avoid severe hypotension.
   c. Postoperative: Preserve quiet atmosphere. Maintain airway. Assess pain carefully, have patient rate on a scale of 1 to 10, and document. Prevent complications by encouraging deep breathing, coughing, and so on.
5. Nursing evaluation
   a. Preoperative: effects of preoperative medication
   b. Intraoperative: ongoing evaluation of patient's status, usually the responsibility of the anesthesiologist
   c. Postoperative: concerned with pulmonary complications; thrombophlebitis; infection; other complications;, postanesthesia nausea, vomiting, hypotension, tachycardia
G. Anticonvulsants: drugs used to control seizures
   1. Action: not completely understood; thought to depress neuron excitability and modify the ability of brain tissue to respond to stimuli that initiate seizure activity
   2. Agents

Examples	Adverse Reactions
Long-Acting Barbiturates	Sedation, drowsiness, tolerance, nystagmus, ataxia, anemia, congenital malformations in fetus; possible convulsions induced by sudden withdrawal
Phenobarbital (Luminal)*	
Primidone (Mysoline)	
Hydantoins	Nystagmus, ataxia, slurred speech, tremors, nervousness, drowsiness, fatigue, overgrowth of the gums (gingival hyperplasia), occasional folic acid or vitamin D deficiency; congenital malformations in fetus
Mephenytoin (Mesantoin)*	
Phenytoin (Dilantin)*	

Oxazolidinediones	Serious allergic dermatitis, kidney and liver damage, vertigo, photophobia, spontaneous abortion, congenital malformations
Trimethadione (Tridione)	
Benzodiazepines	Drowsiness, ataxia, personality changes
Clonazepam (Klonopin)	
Diazepam (Valium)*	
Clorazepate (Tranxene)	
Lorazepam (Ativan)*	
Miscellaneous	Loss of appetite, drowsiness, confusion, dizziness, ataxia, double vision, GI upset
Acetazolamide (Diamox)*	
Carbamazepine (Tegretol)*	
Lidocaine hydrochloride (Xylocaine)	Depressed heart action
Valproic acid (Depakene)	GI distress, sedation

3. Nursing assessment: Observe course of the seizure. Assist in case finding. Assess baseline data with concentration on areas known to be affected by the drug (e.g., phenytoin {Dilantin}). Assess mouth, teeth, and gums for development of gingival hyperplasia.
4. Nursing management: Instruct patient concerning:
   a. Drug characteristics.
   b. Importance of taking medication even when patient is seizure free; awareness that reaching a therapeutic level may take time.
   c. Impairment of absorption of the anticonvulsant when taken with milk or antacids.
   d. Wearing or carrying identification indicating seizure activity and drugs and dosages being taken.
   e. Reducing gastric irritation by taking drug with meals.
   f. Good gum massage and oral care after each meal.
   g. Gradual dosage reduction that should be designed by health care provider to maintain seizure control.
   h. Contacting patient's physician before taking any OTC medications.
   i. Estrogen-containing birth control pills: use of an alternate form of birth control during treatment.
5. Nursing evaluation: Continue medical follow-up; blood level tests.
H. Skeletal muscle relaxants: drugs used to treat muscle spasticity
   1. Action: inhibit nerve impulse transmission by blocking polysynaptic pathways in the spinal cord
   2. Agents

Examples	Adverse Reactions
Drugs to Treat Spasticity	
Baclofen (Lioresal)	Drowsiness, incoordination, GI upset
Dantrolene sodium (Dantrium)	Liver damage
Diazepam (Valium)	Drowsiness, incoordination

Drugs to Treat Muscle Spasm	Drowsiness, dizziness
Carisoprodol (Rela, Soma)	
Cyclobenzaprine hydrochloride (Flexeril)	
Dantrolene (Dantrium)	
Diazepam (Valium)*	
Methocarbamol (Robaxin)	

3. Nursing assessment: Obtain baseline data, focusing on spasticity, including degree, aggravating factors, associated pain, and interference with activities of daily living. Observe baseline liver function studies.
4. Nursing management: Monitor for drug effectiveness and side effects. Institute safety measures if drowsiness occurs. Teach patient to avoid alcohol and CNS depressants.
5. Nursing evaluation: At regular intervals assess the continuing degree of spasticity.

I. Antiparkinsonian drugs: drugs used in managing Parkinson disease
1. Action: Restore action of the neurotransmitter dopamine to the basal ganglia of the brain or block the effects of excessive action of acetylcholine For further information on the extrapyramidal symptoms, refer to medical/surgical chapter (chapter 5).
2. Agents

Examples	*Adverse Reactions*
Anticholinergics	Dry mouth,
Benztropine mesylate (Cogentin)*	constipation, urinary retention, blurred
Biperiden (Akineton)*	vision; impairment
Cycrimine hydrochloride (Pagitane hydrochloride)	of recent memory, confusion, insomnia,
Ethopropazine hydrochloride (Parsidol)	restlessness
Procyclidine hydrochloride (Kemadrin)	
Trihexyphenidyl hydrochloride (Artane, Pipanol, Tremin)	
Antihistamines	Sedation
Chlorphenoxamine hydrochloride (Phenoxene)	
hydrochloride (Benadryl)*	
Orphenadrine citrate (Disipal)	
Other Drugs	Dry mouth, constipation,
Amantadine hydrochloride (Symmetrel)*	urinary retention, blurred vision
Levodopa (Dopar, Larodopa)	Nausea, vomiting, anorexia, orthostatic hypotension, GI bleeding, cough, hoarseness, dyspnea, blurred vision, increased sex drive
Carbidopa-levodopa (Sinemet)*	Same as levodopa

J. Sedatives, hypnotics, antianxiety drugs
1. Sedatives: small dose to calm an anxious patient
2. Hypnotics: larger dose to induce sleep
3. Antianxiety drugs (minor tranquilizers, anxiolytic): used to treat anxiety
4. Barbiturates: classified according to duration of action—ultrashort acting, short acting, intermediate acting, and long acting
   a. Action: produce CNS depression ranging from sedation to anesthesia
   b. Adverse reactions
      (1) Mild withdrawal symptoms: rebound rapid eye movement (REM) sleep, nightmares, daytime agitation, and a "shaky" feeling—imperative to decrease dosage gradually
      (2) Acute overdose: depression of medullary centers regulating respiration and cardiovascular system—tachycardia, hypotension, loss of reflexes, marked depression of respiration
   c. Agents: The following are examples:
      Amobarbital (Amytal, Tuinal)
      Butabarbital sodium (Butalan, Butisol sodium)
      Pentobarbital (Nembutal)
      Phenobarbital sodium (Luminal)
      Secobarbital (Seconal)
5. Benzodiazepines
   a. Action: produce CNS depression
   b. Adverse reactions: daytime sedation, motor incoordination, dizziness, headaches; Schedule IV substances; decrease of efficacy after 3 to 4 months of use; ineffective in treating psychotic episodes or severe depression; contraindicated in treating patients with glaucoma
   c. Agents: The following are examples:
      Lorazepam (Ativan)*
      Alprazolam (Xanax)*
      Chlordiazepoxide hydrochloride (Librium)
      Clorazepate dipotassium (Tranxene)
      Diazepam (Valium)
      Prazepam (Verstran, Centrax)
      Flurazepam hydrochloride (Dalmane)
      Oxazepam (Serax)
6. Miscellaneous
   a. Action: produce CNS depression; generally short acting. Propofol (Diprivan) is administered IV and used as a short-term hypnotic agent. It is used in the induction and maintenance of general anesthesia.
   b. Agents and adverse effects

Examples	*Adverse Reactions*
Propofol (Diprivan)	Hypotension, transient apnea, pain at infusion site
Zolpidem (Ambien)*	Dizziness, drowsiness, diarrhea, headache, hangover
Hydroxyzine hydrochloride (Vistaril)*	Dry mouth, hypotension, blurred vision

7. Nursing assessment: Give special attention to vital signs, level of consciousness, sleep patterns; can increase toxicity if given with digoxin.

8. Nursing management: Observe for signs of CNS depression; identify nondrug solutions to sleep problems; monitor safety aspects of patient care. The presence of food decreases the effectiveness of zolpidem (Ambien); therefore it should be given immediately before bedtime. Taking for a long period may produce psychological dependence.

9. Nursing evaluation: Review purpose for which drug is given and observe effectiveness; instruct patient concerning self-medication, medical follow-up, and drug-dependence potential.

K. Alcohol
   1. Action: produces CNS depression—sedation, disinhibition, sleep, anesthesia; vasodilation; gastric irritation
   2. Effects of an acute overdose: death, accidents, hangover, upset stomach, thirst, fatigue, headache, depression, anxiety. Long-term toxicity can lead to liver, esophageal, GI, and cardiovascular disorders.
   3. Withdrawal symptoms after long-term use: tremors, anxiety, tachycardia, increased BP, diaphoresis, anorexia, nausea, vomiting, insomnia, hallucinations, seizures, delirium tremens
   4. Withdrawal therapy: one of the benzodiazepines; restoration of normal metabolic functions and administration of vitamins B_1 and B_{12}, and folic acid
   5. Aversion therapy: disulfiram (Antabuse) given to detoxified patient who wishes to avoid drinking again; produces unpleasant reaction 30 minutes to several hours after it is taken in presence of alcohol: flushing, throbbing in head and neck, respiratory difficulty, nausea, copious vomiting, diaphoresis, fainting, dizziness, blurred vision, confusion

PSYCHOTHERAPEUTIC AGENTS

A. Antidepressants: characteristics of drug-induced prevention or relief of depression
   1. Tricyclic antidepressants
      a. Action: primarily used to relieve symptoms of endogenous depression; also used to treat mild exogenous depression. Because of the potential for drug overdose and adverse effects, these agents are more likely to be used only if depression is not responsive to other agents. These drugs are contraindicated in patients with benign prostatic hyperplasia (BPH), diabetes, and narrow-angle glaucoma.
      b. Agents: The following are examples:
         Amitriptyline hydrochloride (Elavil)*
         Doxepin hydrochloride (Adapin, Sinequan)
         Imipramine hydrochloride (Tofranil)
   2. Monoamine oxidase inhibitors (MAOIs)
      a. Action: relieve symptoms of severe reactive or endogenous depression that has not responded to antidepressant therapy with other agents, electroconvulsive therapy, or other modes of psychotherapy
      b. Agents: The following are examples:
         Phenelzine sulfate (Nardil)
         Tranylcypromine sulfate (Parnate)
         These agents are no longer commonly used.

   c. Patients on MAOIs need to be very careful of food containing tyramine (an amino acid in the body). Foods especially high in tyramine include anything that is aged, dried, processed, fermented, salted, smoked, or pickled. Patients should try to avoid processed food as much as possible.
   3. Miscellaneous antidepressants
      a. Action: second-generation antidepressants; inhibit the reuptake of norepinephrine; fewer long-term side effects; individual agents must be considered for advantages and disadvantages
      b. Agents: The following are examples:
         Bupropion (Wellbutrin)*
         Venlafaxine (Effexor)*
   4. Selective serotonin reuptake inhibitors (SSRIs)
      a. Action: treatment for depression
      b. Agents: The following are examples:
         Fluoxetine (Prozac)*
         Paroxetine (Paxil)*
         Sertraline (Zoloft)*
         Escitalopram oxalate (Lexapro)
         Duloxetine (Cymbalta)
   5. Nursing assessment
      a. Obtain complete health history.
      b. Assess for history of insomnia, fatigue, or loss of motivation.
      c. Observe motor movements, facial expression, posture.
      d. Assess for any feelings of suicide; potential for suicide is inherent in any severely depressed patient until a significant remission occurs.
      e. Administer with caution to patients with increased intraocular pressure, prostatic hypertrophy, history of urinary retention, or history of glaucoma because tricyclic antidepressants possess significant anticholinergic properties.
      f. Check medication history carefully for extensive drug interactions.
      g. Use extreme caution in patients with cardiovascular disease because of potential for conduction defects.
      h. Initial dose in adolescent and debilitated patients should be lower and increased gradually.
   6. Nursing management: Administer medication with food to avoid gastric distress.
   7. Nursing evaluation: Observe for adverse effects such as drowsiness.
   8. Patient teaching
      a. Stress compliance with taking medication as ordered.
      b. Instruct patient to avoid using alcohol with sleeping pills and hay fever or cold medications because doing so increases the effects of these medications.
      c. Teach patient to report anticholinergic side effects (blurred vision, altered thought processes, constipation, urinary retention, and eye pain, which may indicate glaucoma).
      d. Food containing tyramine should not be ingested for at least 2 to 3 weeks after discontinuation of therapy; educate patient and family about dietary restrictions. Restrictions on foods containing tyramine refer only to MAOIs; the period during which the patient is on the drug and 2 to 4 weeks after discontinuation should be included.

e. Teach patient that therapeutic effects take 2 to 3 weeks.

f. Instruct patient not to discontinue medication quickly after long-term use; may cause nausea, headache, malaise.

B. Antipsychotic drugs

1. Phenothiazines, thioxanthenes
   a. Action: primarily to reduce or relieve symptoms of acute and chronic psychoses, including schizophrenia, schizoaffective disorders, and involutional psychoses
   b. Agents: The following are examples:
      Chlorpromazine (Thorazine)*
      Haloperidol (Haldol)*
      Promazine hydrochloride (Sparine)
      Thioridazine hydrochloride (Mellaril)
      Trifluoperazine hydrochloride (Stelazine)
      Triflupromazine hydrochloride (Vesprin)

2. Nursing assessment: Obtain complete health history, current use of medications, possibility of pregnancy. Obtain history of emotional unrest, agitation, paranoid ideation, delusions, inability to cope with reality.

3. Nursing management: Administer medication with food or milk to avoid or reduce gastric distress.

4. Nursing evaluation: Observe for adverse effects such as urinary retention, change in vision, sore throat with fever, muscle spasms, trembling or shaking of hands, skin rash, yellow tinge to skin or eyes, uncontrollable movements of the tongue.

C. Antimanic drugs: used to treat manic-depressive psychoses in the acute manic phase and to prevent recurrent episodes of mania in the manic-depressive patient

1. Agent: lithium carbonate (Lithane, Carbolith)

2. Nursing assessment: Obtain complete health history, possibility of pregnancy, medications currently being taken. Observe for restlessness, hyperactivity, aggressiveness.

3. Nursing management: Ensure adequate fluid and electrolyte balance.

4. Nursing evaluation: Monitor serum lithium levels to avoid drug toxicity and reduce side effects. The therapeutic level of lithium is 1 to 1.5 mEq/L.

5. Patient teaching: Stress compliance with taking medication as ordered. Instruct patient to wear medical identification tag.

D. Second-generation antipsychotic medications

1. Action: These are a group of medications used to treat some psychiatric conditions. Examples include: schizophrenia, acute mania, and bipolar disorder.

2. Agents: risperidone (Risperdal), paliperidone (Invega), asenapine (Saphris), clozapine (Clozaril), olanzapine (Zyprexa)

3. To varying degrees these agents cause increased risk of diabetes. Patients should be monitored closely for weight gain and changed lipid profiles. Second-generation antipsychotic medications generally do not cause the same degree of muscle disturbance as drugs in the first generation. Some of these medications to some extent cause cardiovascular-related effects. They must be used with caution in patients with heart conditions.

STIMULANTS

Stimulants are medically accepted only for treatment of narcolepsy, hyperkinetic behavior in children, and obesity. Stimulants are used occasionally for depression in older adults and to reverse respiratory depression from CNS depressants.

A. Amphetamines

1. Action: increase the release and effectiveness of catecholamine neurotransmitters in the brain and peripheral nerves and create increased alertness and sensitivity to stimuli

2. Adverse reactions
   a. GI system: vomiting, diarrhea, abdominal cramps, dry mouth, anorexia
   b. CNS: restless behavior, tremor, irritability, talkativeness, insomnia, mood changes, excessive aggressiveness, confusion, panic, increased libido
   c. Autonomic nervous system: headache, chilliness, palpitation, pallor or facial flushing
   d. Children: growth retardation

3. Agents: The following are examples:
   Amphetamine sulfate
   Dextroamphetamine sulfate (Dexedrine, Ferndex)*
   Methamphetamine hydrochloride (Desoxyn)
   Methylphenidate (Ritalin)*
   Pemoline (Cylert)

4. Nursing assessment: Obtain thorough history of patient's presenting problem. Obtain vital signs, weight, and height in children.

5. Nursing management: Monitor height, weight, vital signs. Inquire about relief of subjective symptoms such as insomnia, agitation, headache, irritability. Begin preparing patient and family for long-term management. Teach patient that last daily dose should be taken at least 6 hours before retiring.

6. Nursing evaluation: Determine success of goals of therapy.
   a. Hyperkinesis: less hyperactivity and a more normal attention span
   b. Narcolepsy: ability to remain awake and alert during specified appropriate time periods

B. Appetite suppressants: used to help control obesity

1. Action: exert an anorectic effect on the appetite-control center in the brain

2. Agents

Examples	Adverse Reactions and Comments
Amphetamine sulfate (Benzedrine)*	See discussion of amphetamines
Benzphetamine (Didrex)	See discussion of amphetamines
Caffeine*	Nervousness, jitteriness, GI bleeding, nausea, vomiting, excessive CNS stimulation, convulsions
Caffeine sodium benzoate injection	Same as for caffeine
Dextroamphetamine sulfate (Dexedrine)	See discussion of amphetamines

Examples	**Adverse Reactions and Comments**
Phenylpropanolamine hydrochloride (Acutrim, Control, Diadax, Dexatrim)	BP increases
Theophylline*	Increased heart rate, nervousness, jitteriness, nausea, vomiting, excessive CNS stimulation, convulsions

3. Nursing assessment: Obtain vital signs and weight. Discuss usual eating habits, and establish reasonable goals for losing weight.
4. Nursing management: Promote weight reduction. Monitor for adverse reactions. Offer support.
5. Nursing evaluation: Instruct patient concerning medication and its potential for drug abuse. Assess achievement of goal—weight loss.

C. Respiratory stimulants (analeptics): used to stimulate respiration when drugs, asphyxiation, or electric shock have depressed it
   1. Action: stimulate CNS medullary centers controlling respiration, vasomotor tone, vagal tone
   2. Agents: see discussion of amphetamines
   3. Nursing assessments: Check respiratory rate and depth of respirations; may measure vital capacity and arterial blood gas levels.
   4. Nursing management: Monitor vital signs with focus on respirations; keep suction machine at bedside.
   5. Nursing evaluation: Observe whether patient is breathing at a rate and depth nearing normal and whether short-term hospitalization is necessary.

AUTONOMIC NERVOUS SYSTEM

CHOLINESTERASE INHIBITORS (CHOLINERGIC AGENTS)

A. Description: drugs that produce a physiological response similar to that of acetylcholine released on nerve stimulation
B. Action
   1. Direct-acting cholinergic stimulants: mimic the action of acetylcholine
   2. Indirect-acting cholinergic stimulants: inhibit the enzyme cholinesterase, which acts to limit acetylcholine action
C. Clinical indications
   1. Postoperative abdominal distention
   2. Urinary retention
   3. Retention of gastric secretions
D. Effects
   1. Vasodilation
   2. Lowered BP
   3. Slowing of heart rate
   4. Salivation
   5. Perspiration
   6. Increased tone and movement in the GI and genitourinary systems
   7. Increased tone and contractility in striated muscles

E. Adverse reactions: heart block, arrhythmias, hypotension, hypertension, nausea, vomiting, cramps, diarrhea, heartburn, muscle weakness, increase in intraocular pressure, urinary retention (bethanechol)
F. Agents
   1. Echothiophate iodide (Phospholine Iodide)
   2. Bethanechol (Urecholine)*
   3. Edrophonium chloride (Tensilon)
   4. Isoflurophate (Floropryl)
   5. Neostigmine bromide (Prostigmin)
   6. Pyridostigmine bromide (Mestinon)*
G. Nursing assessment: Check for history of lung disease, hyperthyroidism, prostate enlargement; patients with obstruction of the intestine or renal disease should not use these products.
H. Nursing management: Monitor vital signs. Insert rectal tube to relieve flatus. Inform patient that drug is not a cure; it only relieves symptoms (myasthenia gravis).
I. Nursing evaluation: Observe for adverse reactions, bowel activity, intake and output records; therapeutic response in treating myasthenia gravis—increased muscle strength and hand grasp, improved muscle gait, absence of labored breathing (if severe).

PARASYMPATHETIC BLOCKING AGENTS (PARASYMPATHOLYTIC OR CHOLINERGIC BLOCKING AGENTS)

A. Action: prevent acetylcholine released by nerve stimulation from exerting its effects
B. Effects
   1. GI system: slow peristalsis
   2. Heart: increase rate
   3. Secretions: depress all body secretions, including perspiration and respiratory, salivary, pancreatic, gastric secretions
   4. Eye: dilate pupils (mydriasis); paralyze ciliary muscles; increase intraocular pressure (see section on eye treatments)
C. Adverse reactions: dry skin, delirium, tachycardia, convulsions, mydriasis, hypertension, dry mouth, urinary retention; not for use in patients with history of glaucoma
D. Agents and clinical indications

Examples	**Clinical Uses**
Atropine sulfate*	Adjunct to anesthesia, antispasmodic, cardiac stimulant
Ropinirole hydrochloride (Requip)	Antiparkinsonian agent, restless leg syndrome
Propantheline bromide (Pro-Banthine)	Antispasmodic
Benztropine mesylate	Antiparkinsonian agent (Cogentin)*

E. Nursing assessment: Monitor vital signs; tachycardia; bowel functions; stimulation or depression of CNS; elevation in temperature; respiratory status; history of urinary difficulty; familial history of glaucoma.
F. Nursing management: Maintain oral hygiene for dry mouth. Initiate methods to prevent abdominal distention and constipation. Initiate safety measures in presence of blurred vision.

G. Nursing evaluation: Establish intake and output records when these drugs are given to older men. Observe for effectiveness of drug: may increase effects of BPH or narrow-angle glaucoma with ropinirole hydrochloride (Requip); falling asleep can occur without warning.

NEUROMUSCULAR BLOCKING AGENTS

A. Action: act at the striated neuromuscular junction to produce paralysis of the voluntary muscles
B. Effects
1. Produce muscular relaxation for insertion of endotracheal tubes during surgical interventions
2. Protect against violent thrashing that occurs with electroconvulsive therapy
3. Alleviate spasms that accompany tetanus
C. Adverse reactions: paralysis of respiration, which may be reversed with neostigmine or edrophonium (Tensilon); hypotension; bronchospasm; tachycardia, cardiac arrhythmias, bradycardia
D. Agents: The following are examples:
1. Decamethonium bromide (Syncurine)
2. Pancuronium bromide (Pavulon)
3. Succinylcholine chloride (Anectine)
4. Tubocurarine chloride (Tubarine)
E. Nursing assessment: Elicit medical history—asthma, myasthenia gravis remission; assess potassium blood levels.
F. Nursing management
1. Cardiopulmonary resuscitation skills are required—have resuscitative equipment available.
2. Monitor vital signs. Continually assess respiratory status, lung sounds, rate and depth of respirations. Have suction and intubation equipment at bedside.
G. Nursing evaluation: Observe for therapeutic effects—sufficient muscle relaxation to allow procedure to be done. Observe for adverse reactions—cough and inability to breathe unassisted and handle secretions.
H. Nursing evaluation: Observe for early signs of flaccid paralysis in muscles of face, neck, eyes.
I. Know that patient may appear to be asleep but can still hear.

SYMPATHOMIMETIC DRUGS: ADRENERGIC STIMULANTS

A. Actions
1. Act directly on adrenergic receptors to produce either excitation or inhibition of a particular effector organ
2. Act indirectly by releasing the stored catecholamines norepinephrine and epinephrine
B. Major effects
1. Excitation of the heart, both its rate and its force of contraction
2. Excitation and constriction of smooth muscles in peripheral blood vessels
3. Inhibition and relaxation of smooth muscles in bronchi, GI tract, and skeletal muscle blood vessels
4. Metabolism: release of fatty acids from adipose tissue and increased gluconeogenesis in muscle and liver
5. Excitation of functions controlled by CNS (e.g., respiration)
6. Suppression of appetite
7. Lessening of fatigue

C. Adverse reactions: anxiety, apprehension, headache, arrhythmias, cerebral hemorrhage, heart failure, pulmonary edema
D. Agents and clinical indications

Examples	*Clinical Indications*
Dopamine hydrochloride (Intropin)*	Hypotension
Ephedrine hydrochloride (Bronkotabs)	Bronchospasms, nasal decongestion, allergy
Epinephrine bitartrate (Medihaler-Epi)	Acute or chronic bronchial asthma, allergic disorders, acute hypersensitivity to drugs
Epinephrine hydrochloride (Adrenalin Chloride)*	Cardiac arrest, heart block, acute asthma, adjunct to local anesthesia, acute hypersensitivity to drugs
	Ophthalmic use: control hemorrhage, decrease intraocular pressure
Isoproterenol hydrochloride (Isuprel)*	Bronchodilation, cardiac stimulant
Isoproterenol sulfate (Medihaler-Iso)	Bronchodilation
Mephentermine sulfate (Wyamine)	Maintain BP during anesthesia
Metaraminol bitartrate (Aramine)	Hypotension
Naphazoline hydrochloride (Privine)	Nasal decongestion
Norepinephrine bitartrate (Levophed, Noradrenalin)*	Shock, cardiac arrest
Nylidrin hydrochloride (Arlidin)	Peripheral vascular disease

E. Nursing assessment: Obtain history of hyperthyroidism, diabetes, hypertension, emotional lability, heart disease.
F. Nursing management: Monitor vital signs. Check infusion rate often. Observe for infusion infiltration. Record bowel and urinary activity. Teach patient to keep fluid intake to at least 2000 mL/day to reduce viscosity of secretions.
G. Nursing evaluation: Monitor effect on BP, pulse rate, regularity of heart rate. Observe for therapeutic and adverse effects.

ADRENERGIC RECEPTOR BLOCKERS AND NEURON BLOCKERS (BETA BLOCKERS)

A. Action: interfere with peripheral adrenergic activity by blocking alpha and beta receptors, depleting peripheral neural stores of norepinephrine, and inhibiting peripheral sympathetic activity through an action on the CNS
B. Adverse reactions: postural hypotension, miosis, inhibition of ejaculation, headache, intense vasoconstriction, diarrhea, nausea, disturbances of vision, insomnia, depression
C. Agents and clinical indications

Examples	Clinical Indications
Guanethidine monosulfate (Ismelin)	Hypertension
Methyldopa (Aldomet)*	Hypertension
Metoprolol tartrate (Lopressor)*	Chronic hypertension, angina prophylaxis
Nadolol (Corgard)*	Chronic hypertension, angina prophylaxis
Phenoxybenzamine hydrochloride (Dibenzyline)	Peripheral vascular disease
Phentolamine mesylate (Regitine)	Hypertension secondary to pheochromocytoma, adrenal tumor surgery
Prazosin hydrochloride (Minipress)	Chronic hypertension
Propranolol hydrochloride (Inderal)*	Chronic hypertension, angina prophylaxis, cardiac arrhythmias, migraine headaches
Reserpine (Serpasil)	Chronic hypertension
Timolol maleate (Timoptic)*	Glaucoma
Tolazoline hydrochloride (Priscoline)	Peripheral vascular disease

D. Nursing assessment: Ascertain if patient has history of ulcer disease, diabetes, ulcerative colitis, emotional depression, renal problems, coronary heart disease, predisposition to asthma, congestive heart failure (CHF).
E. Nursing management: Aim instruction toward patient compliance. Administer medications with meals or milk. Maintain safety measures in presence of postural hypotension. Monitor vital signs.
F. Nursing evaluation: Observe for therapeutic and adverse reactions. Observe for changes in sleep patterns and appetite and depression or suicidal tendencies. Observe for interactions with other arrhythmias or channel blockers; may cause additive effect. Interaction with insulin or hypoglycemic agents can alter insulin requirements and mask signs of hypoglycemia.

GANGLIONIC AGENTS

A. Action: reduce sympathetic tone, particularly in the cardiovascular system
B. Adverse reactions: postural hypotension, pupillary dilation, blurring vision, dry mouth, constipation
C. Agents and clinical indications

Examples	Clinical Indications
Mecamylamine hydrochloride (Inversine)	Hypertensive crisis, chronic hypertension
Trimethaphan camsylate (Arfonad)	Hypertensive crisis

D. Nursing assessment: Obtain baseline vital signs. Assess factors contributing to hypertension such as diet, weight, exercise, lifestyle.
E. Nursing management: Instruction is aimed at patient compliance.
F. Nursing evaluation: Observe for therapeutic effects and adverse reactions.

RESPIRATORY SYSTEM

ANTIHISTAMINES

Antihistamines are found in many OTC medicines and in combination with analgesics, antitussives, and others. Drugs are palliative only and do not protect against allergic reactions.

A. Action: block histamine effects at the receptor site
B. Adverse reactions: sedation, drowsiness, dry mouth, blurred vision, urinary retention, constipation; can also stimulate the nervous system, especially in children, causing insomnia, irritability, nervousness
C. Agents and clinical indications

Examples	Clinical Indications
Brompheniramine maleate (Dimetane)	Colds, allergies
Chlorpheniramine maleate (Chlor-Trimeton, Teldrin, Chlortab)	Colds, allergies
Clemastine fumarate (Tavist)	Allergies
Diphenhydramine hydrochloride (Benadryl)*	Allergic reactions, motion sickness, mild parkinsonism
Fexofenadine hydrochloride (Allegra)*	Allergies
Loratadine (Claritin)*	Allergies
Cetirizine (Zyrtec)*	Allergies
Azelastine (Astral)—nasal spray	Allergies

D. Nursing assessment: Obtain vital signs. Assess respiratory and cardiovascular status. Ascertain if patient has history of allergy and extent and type of rash if present. Obtain drug history. Assess for potential interactions and increased CNS depression.
E. Nursing management: Monitor respiratory response, vital signs, urinary and bowel function. Increase fluid intake to minimize dry mouth. Check specific medication guidelines as to whether they should be administered with meals or on an empty stomach. Older adults may require decreased dosage. Instruct patient to avoid the sun and use sunblock because of increased photosensitivity. Young children are especially susceptible to adverse reactions and may require decreased dosage.
F. Nursing evaluation: Observe for therapeutic effects and adverse reactions; most common adverse reaction is headache. Instruct patient about dangers of operating machinery and about wearing medical identification tag in presence of allergies. Assess therapeutic response—includes absence of allergy symptoms, itching, sneezing.

PROPHYLACTIC ASTHMATIC DRUGS

A. Action: indicated for prevention of bronchospasm and bronchial asthma attacks; inhibit the release of histamines from mast cells
B. Adverse reactions: headache, cough, hoarseness, dry mouth or throat, nasal congestion, sneezing, bad taste in mouth
C. Agents: cromolyn (Intal), montelukast (Singulair)
D. Nursing assessment: Obtain baseline history of the frequency and severity of attacks.
E. Nursing management: Singulair should be administered in the evening for maximum effectiveness. Instruct patient that these medications are taken preventively and not for acute attacks. Advise patient that as long as 4 weeks

may be required before the drug is fully beneficial. Advise patient to avoid OTC products without the physician's permission.

F. Nursing evaluation: Therapeutic effect would be a reduction in the number of attacks, reduced cough, decreased sputum production, a decreased need for other asthma drugs, or any combination.

NASAL DECONGESTANTS

A. Action: sympathomimetic agents (see discussion of drugs for the autonomic nervous system); when applied to nasal mucosa or taken orally, constrict the smooth muscle of arterioles in the nasal mucosa and thus reduce blood flow and edema

B. Adverse reactions: rebound nasal congestion if used too frequently; nervousness, irritability

C. Agents: The following are a few examples of the numerous preparations available:
Afrin*
Neo-Synephrine
Allerest
Privine
Contac
Sine-Off
Coricidin
Sinutab
Dristan
Sudafed

D. Nursing assessment: Obtain history of irritants or environmental conditions contributing to symptoms and objective data such as respiratory rate and vital signs.

E. Nursing management: Instruct patient regarding medication use.

F. Nursing evaluation: Monitor for therapeutic effects and adverse reactions.

EXPECTORANTS, ANTITUSSIVES, MUCOLYTIC DRUGS

A. Definitions
1. Expectorant: increases output of respiratory tract fluid that coats the bronchi and trachea
2. Antitussive: suppresses cough
3. Mucolytic: breaks up viscous mucus to allow for ease in expectoration of drainage

B. Adverse reactions
1. Expectorants—nausea, drowsiness; iodide-based drugs—skin rash, metallic taste, fever, skin eruptions, mucous membrane ulcerations, salivary gland swelling, increased potassium levels
2. Antitussives: nausea, dizziness, constipation
3. Mucolytics: GI upset

C. Agents: The following are examples:
1. Expectorants: Robitussin,* iodinated glycerol (Organidin), potassium iodide
2. Antitussives: codeine, hydrocodone bitartrate, dextromethorphan hydrobromide (Romilar), Benylin, benzonatate (Tessalon)*
3. Mucolytics: acetylcysteine (Mucomyst,* Alevaire)

D. Nursing assessment: Obtain history relevant to cough, vital signs, and objective data relevant only to character and quantity of secretions.

E. Nursing management: Monitor symptoms, vital signs, amount of secretions with mucolytics.

F. Nursing evaluation: Instruct patient regarding drugs—how and when to take them and when they should be discontinued. Encourage patients with persistent coughs to seek follow-up treatment.

BRONCHODILATORS

A. Action: act on bronchial cells to dilate the bronchioles

B. Adverse reactions: CNS stimulation, increased heart rate, muscle tremors, headache, nausea, epigastric pain, bronchospasm

C. Agents: The following are examples:
Aminophylline
Albuterol* (Proventil)
Epinephrine* bitartrate (Asthmahaler, Medihaler-Epi, Primatene Mist)
Isoproterenol* hydrochloride (Iprenol, Isuprel)
Metaproterenol* sulfate (Alupent, Metaprel)
Oxtriphylline (Choledyl)
Salmeterol (Serevent)
Terbutaline (Brethine, Bricanyl)
Theophylline (many preparations)

D. Nursing assessment: Obtain relevant history and vital signs. Note amount and characteristics of secretions. Review medical conditions that may interfere with the administration of individual medications.

E. Nursing management: Monitor vital signs and lung sounds. Closely monitor effects of IV drugs. Teach patient to increase fluid intake to 2000 to 3000 mL/day. These agents are available as inhaled agents and orally; the long-acting preparations are used in treating and preventing asthma attacks. These agents are more effective if given on a fixed schedule. The shorter-acting agents are used for symptom relief during acute attacks and as a preventive measure in exercise-induced asthma; must maintain a therapeutic level with theophylline.

F. Nursing evaluation: Observe for therapeutic effects. Instruct patient regarding drug knowledge and usage.

CARDIOVASCULAR SYSTEM

DRUGS TO IMPROVE CIRCULATION

A. Action: vasoconstriction (direct- and indirect-acting sympathomimetic amines cause release of norepinephrine, which stimulates alpha receptors and thus produces vasoconstriction)

B. Adverse reactions: headache, anxiety, palpitation, nausea, vomiting, insomnia, tremors

C. Agents: The following are examples:
Dobutamine hydrochloride (Dobutrex)
Dopamine hydrochloride (Intropin)
Epinephrine* hydrochloride (Adrenalin Chloride)
Isoproterenol* hydrochloride (Isuprel)
Mephentermine sulfate (Wyamine)
Metaraminol bitartrate (Aramine)
Methoxamine hydrochloride (Vasoxyl)
Norepinephrine bitartrate (Levarterenol Bitartrate; Levophed)
Phenylephrine hydrochloride (Neo-Synephrine Hydrochloride, Isophrin)

D. Principal clinical use: for treating cardiogenic and anaphylactic shock; to maintain BP in life-threatening situations and during anesthesia

E. Nursing assessment: Obtain pulse, respirations, BP. Note level of consciousness.

F. Nursing management: Use infusion-control device to monitor IV administration. Monitor vital signs frequently. Administer through a central IV line.

G. Nursing evaluation: Observe for therapeutic effects.

VASODILATOR DRUGS (ANTIANGINAL DRUGS)

A. Action: dilate arterioles and veins to lower BP, which reduces workload on the heart and decreases the oxygen demand of the heart; increase circulation to cardiac muscle

B. Adverse reactions: hypotension: flushing, headache, dizziness

C. Agents: The following are examples:
Amyl nitrite (Vaporole)
Erythrityl tetranitrate (Cardilate)
Isosorbide dinitrate (Iso-Bid, Isordil, Sorbide, Sorbitrate)
Mannitol hexanitrate (Nitranitol)
Nitroglycerin* (Nitro-Bid)
Nitroglycerin* lingual aerosol (Nitrolingual Spray)
Nitroglycerin* ointment, 2% (Nitrol)

D. Nursing assessment: Obtain vital signs and history relevant to onset and duration of pain.

E. Nursing management: Observe and monitor for additional angina attacks. Instruct patient about prescribed drugs.

F. Nursing evaluation: Observe for therapeutic and adverse effects.

VASODILATOR DRUGS FOR PERIPHERAL VASCULAR DISEASE

A. Action: work directly on vascular smooth muscle to cause relaxation or stimulate beta receptors in blood vessels to produce vasodilation

B. Adverse reactions: GI upset, flushing, hypotension, dizziness, increased heart rate, headache

C. Agents: The following are examples:
Cyclandelate (Cyclospasmol)
Ergoloid mesylates (dihydrogenated ergot alkaloids; Hydergine)
Isoxsuprine hydrochloride (Vasodilan)

D. Nursing assessment: Obtain history of onset and course of vascular disease. Assess BP, pulses, including peripheral pulses, mental status, color and temperature of affected extremities.

E. Nursing management: Monitor presenting signs and symptoms. Instruct patient regarding medications.

F. Nursing evaluation: Observe for therapeutic and adverse effects.

ANTIHYPERTENSIVES

Several drugs used to treat hypertension are also used in the treatment of CHF and MI. Drugs are often used in combinations. The following drugs are used only in the treatment of hypertension.

A. Adrenergic drugs
1. Beta blockers (beta-adrenergic receptor antagonists):
   a. Action: reduce cardiac output; reduce renin release from kidney (blocks response to sympathetic impulses)
   b. Agents:
      Clonidine hydrochloride (Catapres, Catapres-TTS)
      Methyldopa hydrochloride (Aldomet)
2. Alpha$_1$-adrenergic receptor antagonists (alpha blockers)
   a. Action: prevent norepinephrine from constricting blood vessels to increase resistance to blood flow

   b. Agents
      Doxazosin mesylate (Cardura)
      Prazosin hydrochloride (Minipress)
      Terazosin hydrochloride (Hytrin)
Refer to the discussion of the autonomic nervous system for further information on both of the above classifications of drugs.
3. Centrally acting antihypertensive drugs that inhibit the activity of the sympathetic nervous system: decrease sympathetic tone and activate alpha receptors in the medulla that decrease heart rate and cardiac output
4. Vasodilators: relax arteriolar smooth muscle; vasodilators in hypertensive emergencies: rapidly relax smooth muscle
5. Calcium channel blockers: relax the smooth muscles of the peripheral blood vessels, causing a decrease in peripheral resistance
6. Angiotensin-converting enzyme (ACE) inhibitors: decrease peripheral resistance, leading to a reduction in BP

B. Adverse reactions: bradycardia, hypotension, nasal congestion, reflex tachycardia, dry mouth, fluid retention, arthralgia, depression, drowsiness. The most common side effect of ACE inhibitors is a dry hacking cough. Renal dysfunction and hyperkalemia are possible life-threatening effects.

C. Agents: The following are examples:
1. Beta-adrenergic receptor antagonists (beta blockers)
   Metoprolol tartrate* (Lopressor)
   Nadolol* (Corgard)
   Propranolol hydrochloride* (Inderal)
   Atenolol* (Tenormin)
2. Alpha-adrenergic receptor antagonists
   Doxazosin mesylate* (Cardura)
   Terazosin (Hytrin)
   Prazosin hydrochloride (Minipress)
3. Centrally acting antihypertensive drugs
   Clonidine hydrochloride (Catapres)*
   Methyldopa (Aldomet)*
4. Vasodilator
   Hydralazine hydrochloride (Apresoline)*
5. Calcium channel blockers
   Diltiazem (Cardizem)*
   Verapamil (Calan)*
   Nifedipine (Procardia)*
   This group of medications is also used for treating angina.
6. ACE inhibitors
   Captopril (Capoten)*
   Benazepril (Lotensin)*
   Enalapril (Vasotec)*
   Quinapril hydrochloride (Accupril)
   These medications are also used as adjunct therapy in patients with CHF.

D. Nursing assessment: Obtain vital signs and additional baseline data such as weight, diet, serum electrolyte levels for electrolyte imbalances.

E. Nursing management: Monitor vital signs, intake and output, weight, blood studies.

F. Nursing evaluation: Observe for therapeutic effects and adverse reactions.

G. Patient teaching: Stress the importance of knowing acceptable ranges of BP and pulse, taking medication as ordered, preventing orthostatic hypotension, and reporting signs and symptoms of asthma. Instruct patient regarding OTC drugs; to change positions slowly to avoid orthostatic hypotension; that beta blockers mask the signs of hypoglycemia; that hot baths or showers, being outside in heat for prolonged periods, and alcohol intensify hypotension.

H. Nursing considerations
1. Patients who suspect pregnancy should not use ACE inhibitors, the "pril" drugs (e.g., Captopril).
2. Beta blockers, the "olol" drugs (e.g., metoprolol), should not be used by patients with chronic obstructive pulmonary disease (COPD) because these drugs can cause bronchospasm and wheezing.
3. Beta blockers and thiazide diuretics cause the most severe sexual dysfunction.

DIURETICS

A. Action: increase the excretion of sodium ion and thus increase urine flow
B. Agents

Examples	Adverse Reactions
Ethacrynic acid (Edecrin)	Dehydration, thrombosis, emboli, electrolyte imbalance
Furosemide (Lasix)*	Acute dehydration, sodium and potassium depletion, calcium loss, dermatitis, blood dyscrasias
Thiazide Diuretics Chlorothiazide (Diuril) Chlorthalidone (Hygroton) Cyclothiazide (Anhydron) Hydrochlorothiazide (Esidrix, Hydrodiuril) Methyclothiazide (Enduron) Metolazone (Zaroxolyn)	Fluid and electrolyte imbalance, increased calcium serum levels, GI irritation, dizziness, headache, paresthesias, blood dyscrasias, allergy, hypotension
Carbonic Anhydrase Inhibitors Acetazolamide (Diamox)* Ethoxzolamide (Cardrase, Ethamide)	Metabolic abnormalities (acidosis), drowsiness, hematuria, melena
Potassium-Sparing Diuretics Spironolactone (Aldactone) Triamterene (Dyrenium)	Hyperkalemia, fatal cardiac arrhythmias, endocrine alterations, blood dyscrasias

C. Nursing assessment: Perform total patient assessment with emphasis on presenting signs and symptoms, vital signs, laboratory blood studies.
D. Nursing management: Foster drug therapy such as by restricting fluid and monitoring diet. Monitor weight, intake and output, vital signs.

E. Nursing evaluation: Observe for therapeutic effects and adverse reactions. Instruct patient regarding drugs and diet, prevention of orthostatic hypotension.

CARDIOTONIC DRUGS (CARDIAC GLYCOSIDES)

A. Action: act directly on myocardial cells to increase contractility and thus cardiac output; slow heart rate
B. Adverse reactions: anorexia, nausea, vomiting, bradycardia, weakness, fatigue, visual dimming, double vision, altered color vision, mood alterations, hallucinations, arrhythmias
C. Toxic reactions, confusion, heart block, premature ventricular complex
D. Agents: The following is an example:
Digoxin (Lanoxin)*
E. Nursing assessment: Obtain baseline data, weight, vital signs, electrocardiogram.
F. Nursing management: Monitor vital signs (especially pulse), weight, fluid intake and output, serum electrolyte level, especially potassium. Instruct patient regarding drugs, eating foods high in potassium.
G. Nursing evaluation: Observe for therapeutic effects and adverse reactions. Check carefully for signs and symptoms of "digitoxin toxicity" as noted earlier in C.
The apical rate should be monitored before administration of the medication. The dose should be withheld if the pulse is low (60 or below), and the physician notified.
Therapeutic blood levels should be monitored on a scheduled basis.

DRUGS TO CONTROL ARRHYTHMIAS

A. Action: slow conduction through atrioventricular (AV) node; block effects of vagal nerve stimulation; block beta-adrenergic stimulation; suppress automaticity; increase electrical threshold for stimulation
B. Agents

Examples	Adverse Reactions
Atropine	Dry mouth, cycloplegia, mydriasis, fever, urinary retention
Bretylium tosylate (Bretylol)	Angina attacks, bradycardia, hypotension
Disopyramide phosphate (Norpace)	Dry mouth, constipation, urinary retention, blurred vision
Lidocaine (Xylocaine without epinephrine)	Muscle twitching, respiratory depression, coma
Procainamide hydrochloride (Pronestyl)*	Hypotension, decreased cardiac output, GI distress,
Propranolol hydrochloride (Inderal)*	Bradycardia, cardiac arrest, nausea, dizziness, drowsiness

C. Nursing assessment: Obtain baseline data, history of subjective and objective symptoms, vital signs.
D. Nursing management: Monitor vital signs. Instruct patient regarding drugs. Maintain therapeutic blood levels by administering around the clock.
E. Nursing evaluation: Observe for therapeutic effects and adverse reactions.

ANTICOAGULANTS

A. Action: inhibit the aggregation of platelets; interfere with any of the steps leading to the formation of fibrin
B. Adverse reactions: hemorrhage, hematuria, melena, rashes, depression of bone marrow
C. Agents: The following are examples:
   1. Antiplatelet drugs
      Aspirin*
      Dipyridamole (Persantine)*
   2. Heparin* (Liquaemin Sodium, Panheprin, Lipo-Hepin)
   3. Coumarin
      Warfarin sodium (Coumadin, Panwarfin)*
   4. Anisindione (Miradon)
   5. Clopidogrel bisulfate (Plavix)
   6. Aspirin and dipyridamole (Aggrenox)
   7. Enoxaparin sodium (Lovenox)* low molecular weight heparin
D. Drug interactions
   1. Drugs potentiating response: clofibrate (Atromid-S), disulfiram (Antabuse), neomycin sulfate, phenylbutazone (Butazolidin), salicylates, sulfisoxazole (Gantrisin)
   2. Drugs diminishing response: barbiturates, cholestyramine (Questran), ethchlorvynol (Placidyl), glutethimide (Doriden), griseofulvin (Grifulvin V)
E. Antidotes
   1. Heparin: protamine sulfate*
   2. Vitamin K is the antidote for Coumadin overdose. Heparin is not affected by vitamin K.
F. Nursing assessment: Obtain baseline data relevant to general condition of the patient, history of problems with clots, blood coagulation studies—prothrombin time (PT), partial thromboplastin time (PTT), platelet count, clotting times.
G. Nursing management: Monitor blood coagulation study results carefully. Use infusion monitoring device for constant infusions of heparin. Have drug antidotes readily available.
H. Nursing evaluation: Observe for therapeutic effects and adverse reactions.
I. Patient teaching: Stress home safety factors to prevent tissue trauma and bleeding. Advise patient to avoid foods high in vitamin K and avoid aspirin, dextran, dipyridamole, and NSAIDs that increase risk of bleeding. Instruct patient to observe excreta for signs of bleeding. Special care should be taken to observe for internal bleeding that may not be visible; signs and symptoms include abdominal pain, backache, and continuous headache. Instruct patient on obtaining regularly scheduled blood tests to monitor dosage. Plavix may be given with or without food. Children and elderly patients are especially susceptible to side effects and may require lower dose.

THROMBOLYTIC DRUGS

A. Action: promote the digestion of fibrin to dissolve the clot
B. Agents: enzymes urokinase and streptokinase
C. Adverse reaction: hemorrhage. Contraindications to these medications include severe neurotrauma, surgery, bleeding, and severe uncontrolled hypertension.
D. Special considerations: reserved for use with myocardial infarction (MI) (the most common reason this medication is used), acute pulmonary embolism, deep vein thrombosis, CVA, or peripheral arterial occlusion; posttreatment—treated with heparin

E. Nursing assessment: Obtain baseline data relevant to size, location, symptoms of clot. Assess vital signs and peripheral pulses for adequate circulation to extremities.
F. Nursing management: Use only in acute care setting. Monitor laboratory blood studies and for signs of clot dissolution.
G. Nursing evaluation: Observe for therapeutic effects and adverse reactions.

HEMOSTATIC AGENTS

A. Action: inhibit the dissolution of blood clots
B. Adverse reactions: nausea, cramps, dizziness, tinnitus, thrombophlebitis, flushing, vascular collapse
C. Agents and clinical indications

Examples	*Clinical Indications*
Systemic Agents	Used in special surgical situations
Aminocaproic acid (Amicar)	Correction of secondary
Menadiol sodium diphosphate (Synkayvite)	hypoprothrombinemia, correction of severe vitamin K deficiency
Menadione sodium bisulfite (Hykinone)	Oral anticoagulant overdose emergency
Phytonadione; vitamin K (Aquamephyton, Konakion, Mephyton)	
Local Hemostatic Agents	Control bleeding in wound or
Absorbable gelatin sponge (Gelfoam)	at operative site

D. Nursing assessment: Obtain baseline data relevant to type, location, and amount of bleeding, appropriate laboratory blood studies, and general condition of patient.
E. Nursing management: Monitor appropriate laboratory blood studies.
F. Nursing evaluation: Observe for therapeutic effects and adverse reactions.

DRUGS THAT LOWER BLOOD LIPID LEVELS

A. Action: generally lower blood lipid concentrations. Research has shown that lowering cholesterol and low-density lipoprotein (LDL) levels decreases the chances of atherosclerosis and coronary artery disease; these medications are generally ordered when dietary changes and exercise have failed to make changes in the blood level. Ezetimibe (Zetia) works differently by blocking cholesterol that comes from food.
B. Adverse reactions: bloating, fever, dizziness, nausea, constipation, muscle cramps, impotence, flushing, weight loss, insomnia, water retention; contraindicated in patients with liver disease
C. Agents: The following are examples:
   Lovastatin (Mevacor)*
   Atorvastatin (Lipitor)*
   Colestipol hydrochloride (Colestid)
   Niacin; nicotinic acid (Nicobid, Niac, Nicolar)
   Pravastatin (Pravachol)*
   Simvastatin (Zocor)*
   Ezetimibe/simvastatin (Vytorin)
   Ezetimibe (Zetia)
   Rosuvastatin calcium (Crestor)

D. Nursing assessment: Obtain baseline data relevant to weight, serum cholesterol and triglyceride levels, BP, and dietary history. Determine if patient is taking any other medications that may increase lipid levels; examples of these include alcohol and certain cardiac medications. Cholestyramine (Questran) and colestipol (Colestid) should be given with food to increase effectiveness; the others are recommended to be given at night.

E. Nursing management: Observe for any new symptoms. Instruct patient regarding drugs. Restrict intake of fats, cholesterol, alcohol. Instruct patient to stop smoking and follow recommended exercise program. Instruct patient to report unexplained muscle pain, fever, dark brown urine. Monitor liver and renal function test results. These medications are not for anyone who is pregnant, nursing, or planning to become pregnant. Give these medications with food at hour of sleep. Asian subjects show a twofold to fourfold increase in sensitivity to rosuvastatin calcium (Crestor). Monitor for persistent protein in urine; a lower dose may be required.

F. Nursing evaluation: Observe for adverse effects. Monitor blood levels for therapeutic effects.

DRUGS THAT TREAT NUTRITIONAL ANEMIAS

A. Action: supplement or replace essential vitamins and minerals
B. Agents

Examples	*Adverse Reactions*
Iron Salts	
Ferrous sulfate (Feosol, Fer-In-Sol, Fero-Gradumet, Mol-Iron)	Acute toxicity: acute nausea and vomiting, metabolic acidosis, extensive liver and kidney damage
Ferrous gluconate (Fergon, Ferralet Plus, Entron)	Chronic toxicity: bronze coloration of skin, development of diabetes mellitus, heart failure
Ferrocholinate (Chel-Iron, Kelex)	Constipation, cramping
Ferrous fumarate (Ferranol, Feostat)	Abdominal pain
Iron dextran injection (Imferon)	
Vitamin B$_{12}$	
Cyanocobalamin (Betalin 12 Crystalline, Redisol, Rubramin PC, Sytobex)	Virtually free of adverse reactions
Hydroxocobalamin (Alpharedisol)	
Folic Acid for Anemia	
Folic acid (Folvite)	Nontoxic
Leucovorin calcium	

C. Folic acid has been shown to prevent neural tube defects.
D. Nursing assessment: Obtain baseline data for vital signs, weight, dietary history, blood studies, presence of neurological symptoms.
E. Nursing management: Monitor blood study findings (especially complete blood count [CBC]), vital signs.
F. Nursing evaluation: observe for therapeutic effects and adverse reactions. Instruct patient regarding medications.

Use Z-track techniques when injecting iron to avoid staining skin. Use nursing measure to prevent constipation.

G. Patient teaching: Expect dark or black stools and the possibility of GI distress. Maintain nutritionally balanced diet.

GASTROINTESTINAL SYSTEM

Nurses have a responsibility to educate patients in the dangers of self-medication. Many of these drugs are available OTC.

DRUGS THAT INCREASE TONE AND MOTILITY

A. Action: cholinomimetic action to stimulate or restore intestinal tone or urinary bladder tone
B. Adverse reactions: salivation, skin flushing, sweating, diarrhea, abdominal cramps
C. Agents: bethanechol (Urecholine); neostigmine (Prostigmin)
D. Nursing assessment: Obtain baseline data regarding vital signs, bowel sounds, fluid intake and output, bowel activity.
E. Nursing management: Stay with patient at least 15 minutes after administration to observe for adverse reactions. Monitor vital signs, fluid intake and output, bowel activity.
F. Nursing evaluation: Observe for therapeutic effects and adverse reactions.

DRUGS THAT DECREASE TONE AND MOTILITY (ANTICHOLINERGICS)

A. Action: inhibit gastric secretion and depress GI motility
B. Adverse reactions: dry mouth, mydriasis, blurred vision, tachycardia, constipation, acute urinary retention
C. Agents: The following are examples:
Atropine sulfate*
Belladonna extract
Belladonna tincture
D. Nursing assessment: Obtain baseline data for vital signs. Assess frequency and character of stools and presence of occult blood in stools. Assess ability to empty bladder.
E. Nursing management: Monitor vital signs. *Note:* Patients with a history of glaucoma should not receive this medication.
F. Nursing evaluation: Observe for therapeutic effects and adverse reactions. Instruct patient regarding medication.

DRUGS TO TREAT AND PREVENT ULCERS

A. Action
1. Antacids: nonsystemic; neutralize gastric hydrochloric acid; provide soothing effect on lining of GI tract
2. Anticholinergic drugs: see discussion of drugs for the autonomic nervous system
3. Antihistamines: block the histamine receptors and decrease gastric acid production
4. Proton pump inhibitors: act on the parietal cells in the stomach to decrease gastric acid secretion
5. Mucosal protectants: short-term treatment of duodenal ulcers; form a paste that protects stomach wall from hypersecretion; action is local
6. Prostaglandins: a variety of bodily actions, including decreasing hydrochloric acid secretion in the stomach

B. Adverse reactions: constipation, diarrhea; can interfere with absorption of some drugs—tetracycline, digoxin, quinidine. Antihistamines can cause diarrhea, constipation, blurred vision, headaches. Prostaglandins can also cause musculoskeletal pain and renal impairment. Side effects of proton pump inhibitors are relatively low and include GI distress and insomnia.

C. Agents
   1. Agents (antacids): The following are examples:
      Aluminum hydroxide (Amphojel)
      Calcium carbonate (Tums)
      Dihydroxyaluminum sodium carbonate (Rolaids)
      Aluminum hydroxide, magnesium hydroxide (Maalox)
      Aluminum hydroxide gel, magnesium hydroxide, simethicone (Maalox Plus, Mylanta, Gelusil)
      Magaldrate (Riopan)
   2. Agents (H$_2$ histamine receptor antagonists): The following are examples:
      Cimetidine (Tagamet)*
      Nizatidine (Axid)*
      Famotidine (Pepcid)*
      Ranitidine hydrochloride (Zantac)*
   3. Agents (proton pump inhibitors): The following are examples:
      Omeprazole (Prilosec)*
      Lansoprazole (Prevacid)*
   4. Agents (mucosal protectants): The following is an example:
      Sulcrafate (Carafate)
   5. Agents (prokinetic GI agent): The following is an example:
      Metoclopramide (Reglan)

D. Clinical indications: used in treating esophagitis, gastroesophageal reflux disease (GERD), and other hypersecretory disorders. Reglan is indicated in short-term treatment of GERD that fails to respond to traditional treatment. Reglan is also indicated in treating persons with diabetes with gastric stasis.

E. Nursing assessment: Obtain baseline data relevant to vital signs, level of consciousness, character and quality of emesis and stool, appropriate laboratory blood studies, abdominal pain, frank bleeding, and occult bleeding. A careful drug history is needed because many medications interfere with absorption. Calcium and magnesium products increase effect of digoxin and may require dosage adjustment. Fluoroquinolone antibiotics can decrease absorption.

F. Nursing management: monitor vital signs, fluid intake and output, level of consciousness, and character of stools and vomitus. Teach that antacids decrease absorption of many drugs, including iron, tetracyclines. Teach not to take antacids for more than 2 weeks without consulting a physician. H$_2$ blockers need to be administered with meals and at bedtime to enhance effectiveness. Administer antacids at least 2 hours before or 1 hour after any other oral drugs to be certain that these medications are adequately absorbed. Caution should be used in patients with known renal and hepatic impairment. Mucosal protectants should be administered before meals to ensure efficacy. Administer oral Reglan 30 minutes before meals. Monitor for signs and symptoms of hypoglycemia because Reglan causes rapid transit of food through the stomach.

G. Nursing evaluation: Observe for therapeutic effects and adverse reactions.

ANTIEMETICS

A. Action: control nausea and vomiting by reducing stimulation of labyrinthine receptors
B. Adverse reactions: drowsiness, blurred vision, dilated pupils, dry mouth, extrapyramidal symptoms such as shaking
C. Agents: The following are examples:
   1. Phenothiazines
      Prochlorperazine (Compazine)*
      Promethazine (Phenergan)*
   2. Prokinetic GI agent
      Metoclopramide (Reglan)
   3. Serotonin antagonists
      Granisetron (Kytril)
      Ondansetron (Zofran)
   4. Miscellaneous antiemetics
      Dimenhydrinate (Dramamine)
      Diphenhydramine hydrochloride (Benadryl)
      Hydroxyzine pamoate (Vistaril)
      Meclizine hydrochloride (Antivert, Bonine)
      Trimethobenzamide hydrochloride (Tigan)

D. Nursing assessment: Obtain baseline data regarding vital signs. Assess character and quantity of any emesis, presence of bowel sounds. Monitor for constipation, fluid intake and output; dehydrated patients are more likely to experience extrapyramidal symptoms.
E. Nursing management: Monitor vital signs and fluid intake and output.
F. Nursing evaluation: Observe for therapeutic effects and adverse reactions. Advise patient to avoid activities that require mental alertness because of the sedative effect. These drugs are synergistic with other CNS depressants.

ANTIDIARRHEAL AGENTS

A. Action: decrease tone of small and large bowel; depress smooth muscle contraction; decrease release of acetylcholine; absorb toxins
B. Adverse reactions: respiratory depression, constipation, impaction
C. Agents: The following are examples:
   Bismuth subsalicylate (Pepto-Bismol)
   Codeine phosphate
   Codeine sulfate
   Diphenoxylate hydrochloride with atropine sulfate (Diphenatol, Lomotil,* Lofene)
   Loperamide hydrochloride (Imodium)*
D. Nursing assessment: Obtain baseline data relevant to vital signs, fluid and solid intake and output, nature and character of stools, skin turgor, fluid and electrolyte balance.
E. Nursing management: Monitor vital signs, intake and output, frequency and character of stools. Inform patient that diarrhea that lasts for more than 2 days needs to be reported to physician. Bismuth preparations are contraindicated for children recovering from viral infections because they contain salicylates.
F. Nursing evaluation: Observe for therapeutic effects and adverse reactions.

LAXATIVES

A. Action: retain water to keep stools large and soft; stimulate motility in large intestine; inhibit reabsorption of water; attract water by osmosis; soften feces

B. Adverse reactions: loss of bowel tone, dehydration, hypokalemia, hyponatremia, malabsorption of fat-soluble vitamins

C. Agents: The following are examples:
1. Bulk-forming agents
Psyllium hydrocolloid (Effersyllium)
Psyllium hydrophilic mucilloid (Metamucil)*
2. Stimulant cathartics (irritants)
Bisacodyl (Bisco-Lax, Dulcolax)*
Cascara sagrada (Cascara)
Castor oil (Neo-Lid)
Glycerin suppositories
Phenolphthalein (Ex-Lax, Feen-A-Mint, Phenolax)
Senna concentrate (Senokot)*
Senna pod
3. Saline cathartics
Magnesium hydroxide (Milk of Magnesia)
Magnesium sulfate (Epsom Salt)
4. Lubricant
Mineral oil (Agoral Plain, Petrogalar Plain)
5. Fecal softeners
Docusate calcium* (dioctyl calcium sulfosuccinate; Surfak)
Docusate sodium* (dioctyl sodium sulfosuccinate; Colace, Comfolax, D-S-S)
6. Osmotic agents
Glycerin (Glycerol)
Lactulose (Chronulac)

D. Nursing assessment: Obtain baseline data relevant to vital signs, intake and output, presence of bowel sounds, bowel habits, dietary history, medications.

E. Nursing management: Monitor diet and fluid intake. Instruct patient regarding drugs and to increase fiber in diet and fluid intake. Stool softeners are indicated when it is important to avoid straining such as with a cardiac patient. Bulk laxatives need to be given with 8 oz of water to prevent blockage. Mineral oil needs to be used cautiously because it hinders the absorption of fat-soluble vitamins.

F. Nursing evaluation: Observe for therapeutic effects and adverse reactions.

ENDOCRINE SYSTEM

DRUGS AFFECTING THE PITUITARY GLAND

A. Action
1. Antidiuretic hormone: increases permeability of the renal tubule and thus its ability to reabsorb water
2. Oxytocin: promotes uterine contractions during last stages of labor when cervix is fully dilated
3. Growth hormone: anabolic agent that increases cell size and cell numbers and stimulates linear growth
4. Gonadotropic hormone (GTH): regulates maturation and function of male and female sexual organs
5. Adrenocorticotropic hormone (ACTH): stimulates adrenal cortex to release its hormone

B. Adverse reactions: hyponatremia, water retention, glycosuria, vasoconstriction, nausea

C. Agents and clinical indications

Examples	*Clinical Indications*
Desmopressin acetate	Diabetes insipidus
Lypressin (Diapid)	Diabetes insipidus
Posterior pituitary extract (Pituitrin)	Smooth muscle contraction
Vasopressin (Pitressin)	Used in the management of SIADH (syndrome of inappropriate antidiuretic hormone secretion)

D. Nursing assessment: Obtain baseline data relative to excesses or deficiencies of specific hormone.

E. Nursing management: Monitor fluid intake and output, laboratory values. Instruct patient regarding medications.

F. Nursing evaluation: Observe for therapeutic effects and adverse reactions.

DRUGS AFFECTING THE ADRENAL GLANDS

A. Action: replace the normal amount of glucocorticoids in the body; block inflammatory responses; antineoplastic; antagonize autoimmune responses

B. Adverse reactions: impaired glucose tolerance or hyperglycemia; fat deposition; muscle weakness or wasting; peptic ulcer; growth inhibition; mood changes or psychosis; osteoporosis; sodium retention; potassium loss

C. Agents: Dosage is individualized to patient and diagnosis. The following are examples:
Betamethasone valerate (Valisone)
Cortisone acetate (Cortone)
Dexamethasone (Decadron,* Hexadrol)
Hydrocortisone (cortisol; Cortef, Cortril, Hydrocortone)
Hydrocortisone acetate (Cortef)
Methylprednisolone (Medrol, Wyacort)
Methylprednisolone acetate (Depo-Medrol)
Methylprednisolone sodium succinate (Solu-Medrol)
Prednisolone (Delta-Cortef, Paracortol)
Prednisone (Meticorten, Delta-Dome)
Triamcinolone (Aristocort, Kenacort)
Triamcinolone acetonide (Kenalog)

D. Nursing assessment: Obtain baseline data relevant to vital signs, weight, glycosuria.

E. Nursing management: Monitor vital signs, weight, serum electrolyte levels, sugar concentrations in blood and urine, signs of masked infection. Instruct patient regarding medications, additive hypokalemia.

F. Nursing evaluation: Observe for therapeutic effects and adverse reactions.

DRUGS AFFECTING THE THYROID GLAND

A. Hypothyroidism: lack of normal amount of thyroid hormone in the body
1. Action is to replace the normal amount of hormone in the body
a. Signs and symptoms
(1) Hypothyroidism in an adult: gradual slowing of mental and physical functions, puffy hands and feet, thick and leathery skin, hypersensitivity to cold (refer to medical-surgical and pediatric chapters [Chapters 5 and 8] for further information)

b. Agents
   (1) Synthetic thyroid hormones
      Levothyroxine sodium (Eltroxin, Levoid, Synthroid)
      Liothyronine sodium (Cytomel)
      Liotrix (Thyrolar)
   (2) Adenohypophyseal hormones
      Thyroid-stimulating hormone (TSH) (thyrotropin; Thytropar)
      Protirelin (Thypinone)

B. Hyperthyroidism: a condition resulting from an overproduction of thyroid hormone
  1. Action: to decrease the overproduction of thyroid hormone in the body
    a. Signs and symptoms: enlargement of the thyroid gland, protruding eyes, elevation of the basal metabolic rate, nervousness and hyperactivity
    b. Agents:
     (1) Thioamides
       Methimazole (Tapazole)
       Propylthiouracil
     (2) Beta-adrenergic blocker
       Propranolol hydrochloride (Inderal)
     (3) Iodine
       Potassium or sodium iodide (Lugol's Solution)
       Nurses need to question for iodine allergy and increased potassium levels.
     (4) Radioactive iodine (^{131}I)

C. Nursing process related to both hypothyroidism and hyperthyroidism
  1. Nursing assessment: Obtain baseline data relevant to vital signs, weight, level of energy, symptoms of hypofunctioning or hyperfunctioning of gland and serum thyroid levels. Thyroid hormones increase the potency of oral anticoagulants; these drugs also decrease the effectiveness of digoxin.
  2. Nursing management: Monitor vital signs, weight. Instruct patient regarding medications, compliance with therapy.
  3. Nursing evaluation: Observe for therapeutic effects and adverse reactions. Monitor thyroid function study results.

DRUGS AFFECTING THE PARATHYROID GLAND

A. Action: maintain blood calcium levels in the blood
B. Adverse reactions: nausea, local irritation at injection sites, drowsiness, GI complaints, hypertension, facial flushing
C. Agents: The following are examples:
  Calcitonin (Calcimir)
  Calcitriol (Rocaltrol)
  Parathyroid hormone
D. Nursing assessment: Obtain baseline data relevant to vital signs and blood calcium levels.
E. Nursing management: Monitor vital signs, blood calcium levels. Advise to avoid spinach, whole grains, and rhubarb and to maintain adequate intake of calcium and vitamin D.
F. Nursing evaluation: Observe for therapeutic effects (e.g., decreased muscle cramping) and adverse reactions. Instruct patient regarding medications.

FEMALE REPRODUCTIVE SYSTEM

ESTROGENS

A. Action: replace or supplement natural body hormones; alter cell environment in neoplastic processes
B. Adverse reactions: breast tenderness, increased risk of breast and endometrial cancer, nausea, vomiting, anorexia, malaise, depression, salt and water retention
C. Agents: The following are examples:
  Estrogen, conjugated (Premarin)*
  Estradiol (Estraderm)

PROGESTINS

A. Action: suppress endometrial bleeding; tissue sloughing induced by withdrawal of drug
B. Adverse reactions: edema, breast tenderness, depression, midcycle bleeding
C. Agents: The following are examples:
  Medroxyprogesterone acetate (Depo-Provera,* Provera)
  Megestrol acetate (Megace)*
  Norethindrone (Norlutin, Ortho-Novum)

FERTILITY DRUGS

A. Action: stimulate ovulation by pituitary or ovarian mechanisms
B. Adverse reactions: although relatively rare, in some cases abdominal pain
C. Agents: The following are examples:
  Clomiphene citrate (Clomid)*
  Human chorionic gonadotropin (hCG) (Antuitrin S, Follutein)
  Menotropins (Perganol)

CONTRACEPTIVE DRUGS

A. Action: suppress ovulation; induce changes in cervical mucus, making uterine entry by sperm difficult; produce changes in endometrium, making implantation difficult
B. Adverse reactions: thromboembolytic diseases, stroke, hypertension
C. Agents: The following examples contain varying amounts of progesterone and estrogen:
  Brevicon
  Depo-Provera
  Enovid
  Norlestrin
  Ortho-Novum
  Ovrette
  Ovulen
D. Contraceptive effects may be lessened if taken with antibiotics.

OXYTOCIC DRUGS

A. Action: induce contraction of the myometrium
B. Adverse reactions: fetal or maternal cardiac arrhythmias, acute hypertension, nausea, water intoxication, uterine hypertonicity with fetal or maternal injury
C. Agents: The following are examples:
  Ergonovine maleate (Ergotrate)
  Methylergonovine maleate (Methergine)
  Oxytocin (Pitocin, Syntocinon)*

UTERINE RELAXANTS

A. Action: stimulation of beta$_2$-adrenergic receptors produces relaxation of uterine muscle to prevent preterm labor

B. Adverse reactions: heart palpitations, nausea, vomiting, trembling, flushing, headache
C. Agents: ritodrine, terbutaline (Brethine)

NURSING PROCESS

A. Assessment: Obtain baseline data relevant to vital signs, weight, current problem. Elicit history of previous pregnancies and deliveries, fetal heart tones.
B. Management: Inform of possible side effects and benefits. Monitor vital signs, weight. With oxytocics, perform maternal and fetal monitoring. Use infusion monitoring device.
C. Evaluation: Observe for therapeutic effects and adverse reactions. Instruct patient regarding medications.

MALE REPRODUCTIVE SYSTEM

DRUGS USED TO TREAT BENIGN PROSTATIC HYPERPLASIA

A. Action: inhibit the enzyme responsible for prostatic growth and improve urinary flow; also used in treating male pattern baldness
B. Adverse effects: headache, abdominal or back pain, gynecomastia
C. Agent: finasteride (Proscar)*
D. Nursing process: Inform patient that up to 3 months may be required to see relief from symptoms. Monitor urinary patterns for improvement.

MALE HORMONES

Androgens

A. Action: replace or supplement normal body hormone; relieve postpartum breast engorgement; alter cell environment in neoplastic disease in women
B. Adverse reactions: female masculinization; premature closure of epiphyses in children; nausea, vomiting, diarrhea, mood swing
C. Agents: The following are examples:
Danocrine (Danazol)
Fluoxymesterone (Halotestin)
Methyltestosterone (Android)
Testosterone (Delatestryl)
(Testaqua, Oreton)
D. Nursing assessment: Obtain baseline data relevant to vital signs, weight, height (children), current problem.
E. Nursing management: Monitor vital signs, weight, height (children). Review possible effects with patient.
Pregnant women should not handle the crushed tablets or the semen of the patient taking this medication owing to high risk potential to the male fetus.
F. Nursing evaluation: Observe for therapeutic effects and adverse reaction. Instruct patient regarding medications.

Anabolic Steroids

A. Action: increase nitrogen retention and protein formation; stimulate RBC formation and increase bone deposition
B. Adverse reactions: increased libido; priapism (continuous erection), female masculinization, precocious sexual development in children, premature epiphyseal fusion
C. Agents: The following are examples:
Ethylestrenol (Maxibolin)
Methandrostenolone (Dianabol)
Methandriol
Nandrolone phenpropionate (Durabolin)

Oxandrolone (Anavar)
Stanozolol (Winstrol)
D. Nursing assessment: Obtain baseline data relevant to vital signs, weight, height (children), current problem.
E. Nursing management: Monitor vital signs, weight, height (children). Review possible effects with patient.
F. Nursing evaluation: Observe for therapeutic effects and adverse reaction. Instruct patient regarding medications.

EYE

ANTICHOLINERGIC DRUGS

A. Action: cause mydriasis (dilated pupils) and cycloplegia (blurred vision)
B. Adverse reaction: dry mouth and skin, fever, thirst, confusion, hyperactivity
C. Agents: The following are examples:
Atropine sulfate (Atropisol, Isopto Atropine)*
Cyclopentolate hydrochloride (Cyclogyl)
Homatropine hydrobromide (Isopto Homatropine)
Scopolamine hydrobromide (hyoscine hydrobromide; Isopto Hyoscine)
Tropicamide (Mydriacyl)

ADRENERGIC DRUGS

A. Action: cause mydriasis
B. Adverse reactions: rare
C. Agents: phenylephrine (Alconefrin, Mydfrin, Neo-Synephrine)

DRUGS USED TO TREAT GLAUCOMA

A. Action: cause miosis (pupil constriction); reduce resistance to outflow of aqueous humor; decrease production of aqueous humor
B. Adverse reactions: blood vessel congestion causing increased intraocular pressure, ocular pain, headache, tachycardia or bradycardia, hypertension, diaphoresis, anorexia, GI upset, lethargy, depression, diuresis, dehydration
C. Agents: The following are examples:
Acetazolamide (Diamox)* (this drug unlike the others is not eye drops)
Dichlorphenamide (Daranide, Oratrol)
Pilocarpine hydrochloride (Isopto Carpine, Pilocar)
Timolol maleate (Timoptic)*
Urea (Ureaphil, Urevert)
D. Nursing assessment: Obtain history of eye-related symptoms such as difficulty in driving or ambulating. Examine eyes for signs of infection, exudate, tearing, drying. Assess for eye pain.
E. Nursing management: Advise patient about effects of drugs such as blurred vision and photophobia. Instruct patient regarding drugs (e.g., do not skip doses). Teach proper administration of eye medication.
F. Nursing evaluation: Observe for therapeutic effects and adverse reactions.

DRUGS USED TO CONTROL MUSCLE TONE

ACETYLCHOLINESTERASE INHIBITORS (ANTICHOLINERGIC AGENTS)

A. Action: allow the accumulation of acetylcholine at neuromuscular junctions and thus ensure muscle contractility; not used during pregnancy or with patients who have hyperexcitability of muscular symptoms; used to treat conditions such as cystitis, gastritis, and chronic bronchitis

B. Adverse reactions: muscle cramps, fasciculations (rapid, small contractions), weakness; excessive salivation, perspiration, nausea, vomiting

C. Agents: The following are examples:
Ambenonium chloride (Mytelase)
Edrophonium chloride (Tensilon)
Neostigmine bromide (Prostigmin)
Pyridostigmine bromide (Mestinon, Regonol)

D. Nursing assessment: Obtain baseline data relevant to vital signs, ability to swallow, muscle strength, eyelid ptosis, gait, reflexes.

E. Nursing management: Monitor disease symptoms and vital signs; have suction and intubation equipment at bedside.

F. Nursing evaluation: Observe for therapeutic effects and adverse reactions.

DIABETES MELLITUS

INSULIN*

A. Action: restores ability of the cell to use glucose and correct the metabolic changes that occur with diabetes mellitus

B. Adverse reactions: allergic reactions, insulin resistance, injection-site lipoatrophy (Table 3-7)

C. Agents: Table 3-8 lists insulin preparations.

NURSING PROCESS

A. Assessment
1. Obtain baseline data relative to nonfunctioning of the pancreas, vital signs, weight, blood glucose level.
   a. Normal blood glucose level is 70 to 120 mg/dL.
   b. Glycosylated hemoglobin (HgbA$_{1c}$) may be drawn to evaluate treatment effectiveness. The American Diabetes Association (ADA) recommends levels below 7% for good diabetic control; serious action should be taken when levels rise above 8%.
2. Assess for signs and symptoms of hypoglycemia and hyperglycemia (see Table 3-7).

Table 3-8 Insulin Characteristics and Duration of Action

INSULIN	TYPE	ONSET	PEAK	DURATION
RAPID ACTING				
lispro (Humalog)	Clear	5-15 min	30-90 min	3-4 hr
aspart (NovoLog)	Clear	5-15 min	1-3 hr	3-5 hr
glulisine (Apidra)	Clear	5-15 min	30-90 min	3-4 hr
SHORT ACTING				
regular (R)	Clear	30-60 min	2-4 hr	6-8 hr
INTERMEDIATE ACTING				
NPH (N)	Cloudy	2-4 hr	6-10 hr	10-16 hr
LONG ACTING				
glargine (Lantus)	Clear	2 hr	No peak	20-24 hr
detemir (Levemir)	Clear	1 hr	No peak	6-24 hr
MIXTURES				
70/30	Cloudy	15 min	30 min-12 hr	10-16 hr
50/50	Cloudy	30 min	3-5 hr	10-16 hr
Humalog 75/25	Cloudy	15 min	30-90 min	10-16 hr
NovoLog 70/30	Cloudy	5-15 min	1-3 hr	10-16 hr

From Edmunds MW: *Introduction to clinical pharmacology*, ed 7, St Louis, 2013, Mosby.
NPH, Neutral protamine Hagedorn.

Table 3-7 Hyperglycemic and Hypoglycemic Reactions

	HYPERGLYCEMIA: KETOACIDOSIS, DIABETIC COMA, TOO LITTLE INSULIN	HYPOGLYCEMIA: INSULIN REACTION, TOO MUCH INSULIN
Onset	Gradual—days	Minutes to hours
Causes	Neglect of therapy, untreated diabetes, intercurrent disease or infection, increase in emotional or psychological stress	Insulin overdose, omission or delay of meals, excessive exercise before meals
Signs and symptoms	Thirst, headache, excessive urination, nausea, vomiting, abdominal pain, dim vision, coma, flushed face, Kussmaul breathing—rapid, deep, air hunger, dehydration, acetone breath, soft eyeballs, normal reflexes absent	Nervousness, hunger, weakness, cold clammy sweat, nausea, dizziness, double or blurred vision, behavioral changes, stupor, convulsions, pallor, shallow respirations, normal eyeballs, Babinski reflex may be present
Blood glucose	High (>250 mg)	Low (<60 mg)
Blood CO$_2$	Low	Usually normal
Treatment	Insulin, fluid replacement, electrolyte replacement, close observation	Glucose, glucagon, close observation
Response to treatment	Slow	Rapid

B. Interventions
1. Teach patient to follow recommended diabetic diet and use exchange system when planning meals.
2. Teach patient techniques for maintaining serum glucose levels, signs and symptoms of hypoglycemia and hyperglycemia, and actions patient should take; physician should be notified if patient is unable to eat.
3. Teach patient to carry simple sugar and wear identification tag describing medication regimen. A simple sugar should be taken if patient feels signs and symptoms of hypoglycemia. This should be followed by a complex carbohydrate if the next meal is more than 1 hour away.
4. Teach patient the importance of regular exercise, care of feet and nails, self-administration of medications, rotation of injection sites, and how to test blood sugar.
   See Critical Thinking Challenge.

? Critical Thinking Challenge

A nurse is working in an endocrinologist's office and has a patient who has been newly diagnosed with type 1 diabetes. The patient is very apprehensive and asks the nurse for help. What interventions would be appropriate for the nurse to initiate? Keep in mind that it is important that the language used by the nurse needs to be at the appropriate level so the patient can understand all that is being said.

Appropriate interventions for this patient will include instructing the patient of the importance of balancing diet and exercise; understanding the onset, peak, and duration of the specific insulin ordered by the physician; teaching the patient how to administer insulin and monitor blood glucose during certain times during the day; and the importance of follow-up medical care.

It is essential that teaching be reinforced over the course of several sessions which will allow the patient to demonstrate understanding of procedures by verbalizing and performing these procedures under the direct supervision of the nurse.

ORAL HYPOGLYCEMIC AGENTS

Oral hypoglycemic agents are not indicated for patients with type 1 diabetes.

Sulfonylureas

A. Action: stimulate release of insulin from pancreas—effective only as long as pancreas maintains some insulin-producing capacity
B. Adverse reactions: GI distress, muscle weakness, paresthesias, skin reactions, hypoglycemia
C. Agents

Examples	Duration of Action
Tolbutamide (Orinase)*	6-12 hr
Acetohexamide (Dymelor)*	12-24 hr
Tolazamide (Tolinase)*	12-24 hr
Glyburide (Micronase)*	Up to 24 hr
Chlorpropamide (Diabinese)*	24-72 hr
Glipizide (Glucotrol)*	Up to 24 hr
Glimepiride (Amaryl)*	Not available

Biguanides

A. Action: increase the amount of glucose taken up by the muscles and intestinal wall and inhibit hepatic glucose production; raise the body's own sensitivity to insulin
B. Adverse reactions: headache, weakness, GI distress, thrombocytopenia
C. Agents

Examples	Duration of Action
Metformin hydrochloride (Glucophage)*	6-12 hr
Glyburide metformin combination (Glucovance)*	

Alpha-Glucosidase Inhibitors

A. Action: delay the digestion of ingested carbohydrates; result in a smaller rise in blood glucose after meals; do not increase insulin production
B. Adverse reactions: abdominal pain, diarrhea, flatulence
C. Agents

Examples	Duration of Action
Acarbose (Precose)	4-6 hr
Miglitol (Glyset)	4-6 hr

Thiazolidinedione

A. Action: lower blood glucose by improving tissue response to insulin; decrease insulin resistance in the periphery and liver, which results in an increased glucose processing in the body
B. Adverse reactions: palpitations, increased lactate dehydrogenase (LDH), nausea, vomiting, diarrhea, anorexia, nephrotoxicity
C. Agents: The following is an example:
   Pioglitazone (Actos)

Meglitinides

A. Action: improve insulin secretions in response to increased glucose levels; shorter acting and excreted faster than the oral sulfonylurea drugs
B. Adverse effects: similar to oral sulfonylurea drugs with the exception of cardiovascular effects, including hypertension and arrhythmias
C. Agents: The following are examples:
   Nateglinide (Starlix)
   Repaglinide (Prandin)

Incretins

A. Action: work through a glucose-dependent mechanism that decreases glucagon secretion and increases insulin secretion and release
B. Adverse effects: Severe allergic reactions, including shortness of breath, need to be reported immediately. Other effects include headache, sore throat, nausea, stomach pain, and diarrhea.
C. Agents
   Sitagliptin (Januvia)
   Janumet (combination of Metformin and Januvia)

NURSING PROCESS RELATED TO ALL SIX CLASSIFICATIONS OF ORAL HYPOGLYCEMIC AGENTS

A. Assessment
1. Obtain baseline vital signs, weight, blood glucose levels, and other signs and symptoms of the disease.

2. Monitor signs and symptoms of hypoglycemia and hyperglycemia.
B. Management
   1. Monitor vital signs, blood glucose levels, other blood levels.
   2. Instruct patient on medication administration and how to monitor blood glucose levels; teach that stress, fever, trauma, infection, and surgery may increase requirements for medication or necessitate a temporary switch to insulin.
   3. Teach signs and symptoms of hypoglycemia and hyperglycemia and steps to correct them.
   4. Instruct on the avoidance of alcohol to prevent hypoglycemic reactions.
   5. Remind patient to monitor HgbA$_{1c}$ levels for long-term glucose control.
C. Evaluation
   1. Decrease in symptoms associated with diabetes
   2. Blood glucose levels under control

URINARY SYSTEM

URINARY TRACT ANTISPASMODIC ANALGESICS

A. Action: inhibit the effects of smooth muscle on the bladder
B. Adverse effects: headache, dizziness, drowsiness, mental confusion, jaundice, increased intraocular pressure; possible renal failure from prolonged use
C. Agents: The following are examples:
   Flavoxate (Urispas)
   Oxybutynin (Ditropan)*
   Phenazopyridine (Pyridium)
D. Nursing assessment: These medications are contraindicated in patients with glaucoma, GI or genitourinary obstruction, or ileus.
E. Nursing management: Instruct patients to avoid hazardous activity until side effects are known. Teach patients taking Pyridium that urine will be reddish orange in color.
F. Nursing evaluation: Monitor for jaundice, which can be a sign of liver impairment; monitor blood work for any signs of blood dyscrasias.
Note: Diuretics and urinary tract antibiotics are discussed under cardiovascular and immune systems, respectively.

IMMUNE SYSTEM

ANTIBIOTICS USED IN THE TREATMENT AND PREVENTION OF INFECTIONS

Penicillins

A. Action: bactericidal by interfering with the synthesis of the bacterial cell wall
B. Adverse reactions: allergies—rash, anaphylaxis; convulsions with high parenteral doses; GI distress—nausea, vomiting, diarrhea; most common cause of drug allergic reactions
C. Agents: The following are examples:
   Amoxicillin (Amoxil, Larotid, Polymox, Trimox)
   Ampicillin (Amcill, Omnipen, Polycillin, Principen)
   Carbenicillin disodium (Geopen)
   Oxacillin sodium (Bactocill, Prostaphlin)
   Penicillin G potassium (Megacillin)
   Penicillin G procaine (Crysticillin, Duracillin, Wycillin)
   Penicillin V (Pen-Vee K, V-Cillin, Veetids)

D. Clinical indications: useful in treating gram-positive and gram-negative infections, including otitis media, pharyngitis, tonsillitis, pneumonia, syphilis, and gonorrhea; given prophylactically to patients with rheumatic fever
E. Patient teaching
   1. Penicillin should be taken on an empty stomach and with water.
   2. Penicillin is thought to decrease effectiveness of oral contraceptives.

Cephalosporins*

A. Action: interfere with bacterial wall synthesis
B. Adverse effects: symptoms involving GI distress most common. There is a cross-reaction between an allergy to penicillin and an allergy to cephalosporins. Patients and health care providers need to be aware of the possibility of anaphylactic shock.
C. Agents: The following are examples:
   Cefaclor (Ceclor)*
   Cefamandole nafate (Mandol)
   Cefazolin sodium (Ancef, Kefzol)
   Cefoxitin (Mefoxin)
   Cephalexin (Keflex)
   Cefotaxime sodium (Claforan)
   Cefepime (Maxipime)
D. Clinical indications
   1. Wound and skin infections
   2. Respiratory infections, skin infections, urinary tract infections
   3. Each generation is effective against a variety of gram-positive and gram-negative organisms.
E. Patient teaching
   1. Consuming alcohol within 72 hours after discontinuing medication induces disulfiram (Antabuse)-like reaction.
   2. Take with small meal to decrease GI distress.

Erythromycin, Clindamycin (Penicillin Substitutes)

A. Action: bacteriostatic or bactericidal (dosage related) by inhibiting protein synthesis
B. Adverse reactions: abdominal discomfort, cramping, nausea, vomiting, diarrhea, urticaria, anaphylaxis, colitis, liver dysfunction, deafness (vancomycin), permanent kidney damage (systemic bacitracin, vancomycin)
C. Agents: The following are examples:
   1. Erythromycin (E-Mycin, Ilotycin, Robimycin, Rp-Mycin)
   2. Clindamycins, lincomycins
      Clindamycin (Cleocin)
   3. Penicillin substitutes
      Bacitracin
      Novobiocin sodium (Albamycin)
      Spectinomycin hydrochloride (Trobicin)
      Vancomycin hydrochloride (Vancocin)
D. Clinical indications
   1. See clinical indications for penicillins.
   2. Used for patients allergic to penicillin

Macrolides

A. Action: Depending on dosage and organism, macrolides are bacteriostatic or bactericidal.
B. Adverse reactions: relatively few compared with other antibiotics—GI distress, pruritus, reversible hearing loss
C. Agents: The following are examples:
   Erythromycin* (E-Mycin) for ocular infections

Azithromycin* (Zithromax)
Clarithromycin* (Biaxin)
Dirithromycin (Dynabac)
D. Clinical indications: respiratory, skin infections; sexually transmitted diseases

Tetracyclines

A. Action: bacteriostatic by preventing the start of protein synthesis (tetracyclines) or inhibiting protein synthesis (chloramphenicol)
B. Adverse reactions: tetracyclines—nausea, vomiting, stomach pain, diarrhea, superimposed infections, impaired kidney functions, jaundice, delayed blood coagulation, brown discoloration of teeth in children under 8 years of age; known teratogens and should not be given if pregnancy is suspected
C. Agent: The following is an example:
Tetracycline hydrochloride (Achromycin)
D. Clinical indications
1. Gram-negative and gram-positive infections
2. Severe acne vulgaris
3. Used for patients allergic to penicillin
E. Patient teaching: Instruct patient that tetracycline absorption is inhibited with dairy products and many nonsystemic antacids.

Aminoglycosides

A. Action: inhibit early stages of protein synthesis
B. Adverse reactions: eighth cranial nerve damage, renal damage, respiratory paralysis
C. Agents: The following are examples:
Amikacin sulfate (Amikin)
Gentamicin sulfate (Garamycin)
Kanamycin sulfate (Kantrex)
Neomycin sulfate (Mycifradin, Neobiotic)
Streptomycin
Tobramycin sulfate (Nebcin)
D. Clinical indications: Drugs are potentially dangerous and used only in cases of severe infections such as gram-negative bone and joint infections and septicemia. Peak and trough levels need to be drawn to evaluate effectiveness. These medications can be nephrotoxic and ototoxic.

Sulfonamides

A. Action: block bacterial synthesis of folic acid; inhibit bacterial enzymes required for proper metabolism of sugar; interfere directly with deoxyribonucleic acid (DNA) synthesis
B. Adverse reactions: Sulfonamides are not used as frequently as in the past because of the development of drug-resistant bacteria and the development of newer antibiotics. Adverse reactions include allergies, rash, headache, fever, nausea, vomiting, diarrhea, stomatitis, blood dyscrasias, renal calculi, hematuria.
C. Agents: The following are examples:
1. Sulfonamides
Sulfasalazine (Azulfidine, Salazopyrin)
Sulfisoxazole (Gantrisin)
Sulfisoxazole-phenazopyridine hydrochloride (Azo Gantrisin, Sk-Soxazole)
2. Sulfonamides: topical agents and solutions
Mafenide (Sulfamylon)
Silver sulfadiazine (Silvadene)
Sulfisoxazole diolamine (Gantrisin Ophthalmic)

D. Clinical indications
1. Used to treat acute and chronic urinary tract infections
2. Other uses include trachoma, chancroid, toxoplasmosis, acute otitis media, prophylactic therapy in cases of recurrent rheumatic fever
3. Treatment of ulcerative colitis
4. Prophylaxis for patients scheduled for bowel surgery (to prevent renal calculi; teach patient to maintain fluid intake of 2000 to 3000 mL/day)
5. Silver sulfadiazine used topically for burn patients. Apply sparingly to a thickness of ⅙ inch.
E. Patient teaching: adequate fluid intake to prevent crystalluria

Fluoroquinolones*

A. Action: bactericidal against broad spectrum of bacteria
B. Adverse reactions: GI distress, headache, dizziness, superinfections, renal impairment, photosensitivity; not to be given to children under 18 years of age
C. Agents: The following are examples:
Ciprofloxacin hydrochloride* (Cipro)
Levofloxacin* (Levaquin)
Gatifloxacin* (Tequin)
D. Clinical indications: respiratory, urinary, and GI tract infections, sexually transmitted diseases, bone and soft-tissue infections, anthrax
E. Patient teaching: These drugs are synergistic with caffeine, theophylline, warfarin; dosage adjustment may be required; antacids, sucralfate, iron, milk products decrease effectiveness of fluoroquinolones; patients should be taught to wear protective sunscreen and clothing.

Miscellaneous Antibiotics

A. Action: bactericidal
B. Adverse reactions: superinfections, renal toxicity, ototoxicity
C. Agents: The following are examples:
Aztreonam (Azactam)
Clindamycin (Cleocin)
Imipenem (Primaxin)
Vancomycin (Vancocin)
D. Clinical indications
Aztreonam: skin, intraabdominal infections, genitourinary infections, septicemia
Clindamycin: abdominopelvic infections, acne vulgaris
Imipenem: serious respiratory, genitourinary, and pelvic infections, endocarditis, septicemia
Vancomycin*: used to treat life-threatening infections and in the treatment of methicillin-resistant *Staphylococcus aureus* (MRSA) infection. Most common adverse reaction is an allergic reaction to rapid infusion of the medication, characterized by flushing, and erythema of the head and upper body (red man or red neck syndrome). Nephrotoxicity is a major side effect of this medication.
E. Patient teaching
1. Report watery stools to health care providers.
2. These drugs should not be administered to pregnant patients.

NURSING PROCESS FOR ALL ANTIBIOTICS

A. Assessment
1. Obtain baseline data related to signs and symptoms of infection.

2. Monitor blood urea nitrogen (BUN), CBC, liver studies, particularly with IV medications.
3. Antibiotics interact with many medications; an accurate medication history is essential.
4. Antibiotics are effective against bacterial infections; physicians may place high-risk patients with a viral infection on an antibiotic to prevent the development of a secondary bacterial infection.
5. Culture and sensitivity should be performed to determine the appropriate antibiotic.

B. Planning (management)
1. Patients must be taught to take medication for the entire course of therapy to avoid the development of bacterial-resistant strains; they should continue taking medications when symptoms subside.
2. Patients must be instructed on the proper timing and method of administration.
3. Patients need to be taught to report any signs of a superinfection such as vaginal irritation, itching, discharge, black tongue, furry overgrowth, and loose foul-smelling stools.
4. Patients need to be taught to report any rashes and difficulty breathing to health care provider because they may be indications of allergic reaction. Any individual with a history of allergies to other substances is at increased risk for an allergic reaction to antibiotics.
5. Patients need to be taught that overuse of antibiotics or misuse of the medication when they are not certain that it will be beneficial can lead to the development of drug-resistant organisms.
6. Women taking birth control pills should use a barrier method when taking antibiotics. Many antibiotics interfere with the effectiveness of birth control pills, thereby increasing the risk of pregnancy.

C. Implementation
1. Adequate fluid intake should be taken to replace fluids lost with diarrhea and prevent dehydration.
2. Follow appropriate guidelines for each medication; many antibiotics need to be taken at equally spaced intervals around the clock to maintain blood levels.

D. Evaluation: The presenting symptoms of infection are improved.

DRUGS USED TO TREAT TUBERCULOSIS AND LEPROSY

A. Action: alter several metabolic processes in mycobacteria
B. Adverse reactions: peripheral neuropathies, visual disturbances, GI distress, ototoxicity, headache
C. Agents: The following are examples:
1. First-line antituberculin drugs
Isoniazid (INH)
Ethambutol hydrochloride (Myambutol)*
Isoniazid (Isotamine, Niconyl, Nydrazid)*
Para-aminosalicylic acid (PAS) (aminosalicylic acid, Teebacin)*
Rifampin (Rifadin, Rimactane)*
Streptomycin
2. Second-line antituberculin drugs
Capreomycin (Capastat)
Cycloserine (Seromycin)
Ethionamide (Trecator-SC)
Pyrazinamide
3. Antileprosy agents
Clofazimine (Lamprene)

Dapsone (Avlosulfon)
Rifampin (Rifadin, Rimactane)
Sulfoxone sodium (Diasone)

D. Patient teaching: Stress importance of long-term compliance (these medications are often taken for 1 year or longer) and follow-up visits with the physician. Report any adverse reactions promptly. Refrain from consuming alcohol. Refrain from taking other medications without the knowledge and permission of the physician. Wear a medical identification tag indicating medication being taken. Many clinics have adopted directly observed therapy (DOT) to enhance patient compliance.

ANTIFUNGAL DRUGS

A. Action: selectively damage the membranes of fungi
B. Adverse reactions: renal damage, anemia, nausea, diarrhea
C. Agents: The following are examples:
1. Systemic agents
Amphotericin B (Fungizone)
Miconazole (Monistat IV)
Fluconazole (Diflucan)*
Ketoconazole (Nizoral)
2. Topical agents
Amphotericin B (Fungizone)
Clioquinol (Vioform)
Clotrimazole (Gyne-Lotrimin, Lotrimin)*
Griseofulvin (Fulvicin P/G, Grifulvin V, Grisactin)
Miconazole nitrate (Micatin, Monistat)*
Nystatin (Mycostatin, Nilstat)
Tolnaftate (Aftate, Tinactin)
Undecylenic acid—zinc undecylenate (Desenex, Cruex)

D. Clinical indications: Fungal infections can be topical or systemic. Fungal infections are often treated prophylactically in patients who are immunocompromised to prevent secondary infection.
E. Patient teaching: Teach proper administration of vaginal tablets, use of condom by sexual partner to avoid reinfection. Report any signs of liver damage. Instruct patient on "swish and swallow" technique or to hold lozenge in mouth for as long as possible. Patients should refrain from taking alcohol.

DRUGS USED TO TREAT VIRAL DISEASES

A. Action: selective toxicity in various processes of virus reproduction. Most antiviral drugs inhibit the progression of the virus but do not destroy it. A healthy immune system is required to fight off the organism. The development of human immunodeficiency virus (HIV) infection and increasing incidence of herpes have led to the development of medication to decrease the symptoms. These drugs do not cure.
B. Adverse reactions: ataxia, slurred speech, lethargy, local irritation, anorexia, nausea, vomiting, diarrhea, dizziness, headache, anemia and bone marrow suppression (zidovudine), bone marrow depression (ganciclovir), visual haze, irritation, burning of eyes, photophobia (idoxuridine)
C. Agents: The following are examples:
Acyclovir (Zovirax, Cyclovir)*
Valacyclovir (Valtrex)
Amantadine (Symmetrel)
Zidovudine (AZT, Retrovir)
Saquinavir (Invirase)
Nelfinavir (Viracept)
Didanosine (Videx)

D. Clinical indications: Zidovudine (AZT) is used in treatment of acquired immunodeficiency syndrome (AIDS); it prevents replication of HIV, thus delaying disease progression. Acyclovir (Cyclovir) is also useful in treating herpes zoster and other viral infections because the virus changes. The health care provider may vary drug regimen. Drug regimen is most effective before the immune system is compromised. Valacyclovir (Valtrex) is also useful in treating patients with cytomegalovirus (CMV) who are also HIV positive.

  1. Most of the drugs used to treat AIDS are toxic to the liver. Regular blood work should be done, and the patient should refrain from using alcohol.

  2. Complying with exact schedule and dosage is essential to the effectiveness of treatment.

NURSING PROCESS

A. Nursing assessment: Obtain history of allergies. Evaluate baseline data relevant to signs and symptoms of infection; vital signs; pertinent laboratory tests; appearance of wounds, incisions, or lesions; amount and description of drainage; swelling; erythema; subjective symptoms of pain or pressure.

B. Nursing management: Obtain culture for specimens before starting antibiotics. Maintain supportive measures such as rest, comfort, nutrition, fluid and electrolyte balance. Maintain proper administration regarding route, time, dosage. Monitor vital signs and laboratory results.

C. Nursing evaluation. Observe for therapeutic effects and adverse reactions; instruct patient regarding medications to ensure compliance.

NEOPLASTIC DISEASES

SPECIFIC ANTINEOPLASTIC AGENTS

A. Action: selective toxicity during various stages of the cell cycle
B. Agents

Examples	Adverse Reactions
Asparaginase (Elspar)	CNS depression
Chlorambucil (Leukeran)	Bone marrow suppression
Cisplatin (Platinol)	Renal damage, nausea and vomiting, ototoxicity, neurotoxicity, anaphylactic reactions
Cyclophosphamide (Cytoxan)	Hemorrhagic cystitis, bladder fibrosis
Doxorubicin hydrochloride (Adriamycin)	Bone marrow suppression, GI distress, alopecia
Fluorouracil (5-FU, Adrucil)	GI and hematological toxicity
Hydroxyurea (Hydrea)	Bone marrow suppression
Mechlorethamine hydrochloride or nitrogen mustard (Mustargen)	Bone marrow suppression
Medroxyprogesterone (Depo-Provera)	Menstrual irregularities, rashes, thromboembolic diseases
Megestrol acetate (Megace)	Thromboembolic disease
Methotrexate	GI toxicity, bone marrow suppression, immunosuppression
Tamoxifen citrate (Nolvadex)	Hot flashes, nausea, vomiting
Vincristine sulfate (Oncovin)	Alopecia, abdominal pain, peripheral neuropathy

Neoplastic agents are normally administered by a specially trained RN. LPN/LVNs are responsible for monitoring side effects and providing nursing care and comfort measures. LPN/LVNs need to encourage patient compliance with this very difficult course of therapy. Specific effects need to be researched for each agent. Agents affect both healthy cells and tumor cells.

C. Nursing assessment: Obtain baseline data regarding possible adverse reactions of drugs. Evaluate condition of hair, skin, nails; weight; vital signs; and necessary blood laboratory study results (especially white blood cell [WBC], RBC, and platelet counts). Nurses should be familiar with the specific side effects of each of these medications.

These drugs interact with many other medications and herbs. A careful medication history must be taken.

D. Nursing management

  1. Patients need tremendous teaching and emotional support.

  2. Patients are frequently given acetaminophen (Tylenol) and diphenhydramine (Benadryl) after treatment to decrease side effects.

  3. Because of the neutropenia caused by the medication, patients given antineoplastic medications have reduced immunity to infection. They should avoid contact with anyone who has an active infection or is recovering from one. They should also avoid contact with individuals (particularly children) who have received live vaccines. Strict medical asepsis must be maintained when caring for these patients.

  4. Thrombocytopenia is also a side effect of these medications. Protection against injuries needs to be maintained. This includes avoidance of all invasive procedures—for example, not using razors for shaving, using small needles for intramuscular injections, using a soft tooth brush. Patients should be observed carefully for any signs of bleeding, including bruising and nosebleeds.

  5. Good nutrition is a challenge because gastrointestinal side effects are frequent with these medications. Nutritional supplements may be helpful, but they are not a substitute for healthy nutritional choices. Regular inspection of the mouth should be included in care.

E. Nursing evaluation: Observe for therapeutic effects and adverse reactions.

COLONY-STIMULATING FACTORS

A. Action: stimulate proliferation and differentiation of neutrophils; glycoproteins; decrease chances of infection in patients receiving antineoplastics; stimulate RBC production (erythropoietin [Epogen]), restore red bone marrow after transplantation (sargramostim [Leukine])

B. Adverse reactions: fever, nausea, diarrhea, anorexia, alopecia, skeletal pain; elevated BP a possible side effect of erythropoietin

C. Agents: filgrastim (Neupogen),* erythropoietin (Epogen),* sargramostim (Leukine)*

D. Clinical indications: Filgrastim is used to increase the production of neutrophils and decrease the chances of infection in patients who are immunosuppressed. Erythropoietin is used in treating anemia, in patients with AIDS, and in patients with chronic renal failure. Sargramostim is used to restore red bone marrow in patients with transplants.

E. Nursing assessment: Monitor blood study findings. Check vital signs at baseline and during treatment, and assess for bone pain.

F. Evaluation: Infection is absent.

HORMONES

A. Action: one factor controlling rate of RBC production; anemia caused by reduced endogenous erythropoietin production; primarily end-stage renal disease and anemia caused by chemotherapy

B. Adverse reactions: seizures, coldness, sweating, headache, hypertension, bone pain

C. Agent: epoetin alfa (Eprex)

D. Assessment: Assess for CNS symptoms; monitor blood studies.

E. Evaluation: Appetite is increased; RBCs increase in 1 to 2 weeks.

HYPERCALCEMIC AGENTS

A. Action: decrease serum calcium levels to normal or near normal levels; used in treating Paget disease and hypercalcemia associated with malignancy

B. Adverse reactions: contraindicated in patients who are allergic to salmon or fish; facial flushing; nausea

C. Agents: The following are examples:
   Calcitonin-salmon (Calcimar)
   Bisphosphonates-alendronate (Fosamax)*

D. Nursing management: Assess for signs of hypocalcemia with aggressive treatment. Monitor blood work for signs of effectiveness and toxicity. Instruct patient to limit dairy foods, increase intake of fluid to 3000 to 4000 mL/day. Do not administer with other medications or vitamins because of decreased effectiveness.

NUTRIENTS, FLUIDS, AND ELECTROLYTES

Substances required for human nutrition include water, carbohydrates, proteins, fats, vitamins, and minerals necessary to maintain health, prevent illness, and promote recovery from illness.

NUTRITIONAL PRODUCTS: ORAL AND TUBE FEEDINGS

A. Nutritionally complete formulas
   1. Action
      a. Provide U.S. Recommended Dietary Allowance for protein, minerals, and vitamins
      b. Provide 1 calorie per milliliter (Sustagen: 1.84 cal/mL)
   2. Agents: The following are examples:
      Compleat-B
      Ensure
      Isocal
      Osmolite
      Sustacal
      Sustagen

B. Nutritional agents for limited use
   1. Vital H.N.: contains easily digested forms of protein, carbohydrate, fat; used for critically ill patients
   2. Lofenalac: a low-phenylalanine preparation used for infants and children with phenylketonuria (PKU)
   3. Meat-based formula: hypoallergenic infant formula for individuals who are allergic to milk or have galactosemia
   4. Neo-Mull-Soy, ProSobee, Isomil: soybean products used as hypoallergenic, milk-free formulas
   5. Pregestimil: infant formula containing easily digested protein, fat, and carbohydrate; used in infants with diarrhea or malabsorption syndromes

6. Vivonex: nutritionally complete diet containing amino acids as its protein

C. Complete infant formulas
   1. May be used alone for bottle-fed babies or to supplement breast-fed babies; similar to human breast milk; iron deficient
   2. Preparations: Enfamil and Similac are examples.

INTRAVENOUS FLUIDS

A. Dextrose injection: contains 2.5%, 5%, 10%, 20%, 40%, 50%, 60%, and 70% dextrose. The 20% to 50% solutions are used for calories in TPN and administered through a central or subclavian catheter.

B. Dextrose and sodium chloride injection: Most commonly used concentrations are 5% dextrose in 0.25% or 0.45% sodium chloride.

C. Amino acid solution (Aminosyn): Contains essential and nonessential amino acids; most often used with dextrose in TPN.

D. Liposyn, Intralipid: Concentrated calories and essential fatty acids most often used as part of TPN.

VITAMINS

A. General information
   1. Group of substances that act as coenzymes to help in the conversion of carbohydrate and fat into energy and form bones and tissues; necessary for metabolism of fat, carbohydrate, and protein; normally obtained from foods
   2. Subclassified as:
      a. Fat-soluble: A, D, E, K
      b. Water-soluble: B complex, C

B. Agents
   1. Fat-soluble vitamins: The following are examples:
      Vitamin A (Alphalin, Aquasol A)
      Vitamin E (Tocopherol, Aquasol E)
      Vitamin K, menadiol sodium diphosphate (Synkayvite)
      Phytonadione (Mephyton, Aquamephyton)
   2. Water-soluble vitamins: The following are examples:
      B complex
      Calcium pantothenate (B_5) (Pantholin)
      Cyanocobalamin (B_{12}) (Rubramin PC, Betalin 12)
      Folic acid (Folvite)
      Niacin
      Pyridoxine hydrochloride (B_6) (Hexa-Betalin)
      Riboflavin (Riobin-50, B_2)
      Thiamine hydrochloride (B_1) (Betalin S)
   3. Vitamin C: ascorbic acid

MINERALS AND ELECTROLYTES

A. General information: basic constituents of living tissues and components of many enzymes; function to maintain fluid, electrolyte, acid-base balance; maintain muscle and nerve function; assist in transfer of materials across cell membranes and contribute to the growth process

B. Agents: The following are examples:
   Deferoxamine mesylate (Desferal)
   Ferrous gluconate (Fergon)
   Ferrous sulfate (Feosol)
   Iron dextran injection (Imferon)
   Magnesium sulfate
   Potassium bicarbonate–potassium citrate (K-Lyte)
   Potassium chloride (Kay Ciel, K-Lor)
   Potassium gluconate (Kaon)

Sodium bicarbonate
Sodium polystyrene sulfonate (Kayexalate)
Ringer's lactate
Ibandronate sodium (Boniva)

NURSING PROCESS

A. Assessment: Obtain baseline data with emphasis on presenting signs and symptoms, vital signs, laboratory blood studies. With Boniva patient should remain sitting or standing for 60 minutes.

B. Management: Perform nursing actions to foster drug therapy. Monitor diet and laboratory blood studies and electrolyte and renal function. Patient needs adequate intake of calcium and vitamin D. Boniva is indicated to prevent postmenopausal osteoporosis.

C. Evaluation: Observe for therapeutic effects specific to type of nutrient supplement. Instruct patient regarding medications and diet.

Bibliography

Asperheim Favaro MK, Favaro J: *Introduction to pharmacology*, ed 12, St Louis, 2012, Saunders.

Christensen BL, Kockrow EO: *Adult health nursing*, ed 6, St Louis, 2010, Mosby.

Christensen BL, Kockrow EO: *Foundations of nursing*, ed 6, St Louis, 2010, Mosby.

Edmunds MW: *Introduction to clinical pharmacology*, ed 7, St Louis, 2013, Mosby.

Lilley LL, et al: *Pharmacology and the nursing process*, ed 7, St Louis, 2014, Mosby.

Mosby's dictionary of medicine, nursing, and health professions, ed 9, St Louis, 2013, Mosby.

Physicians' desk reference, ed 67, Montvale, NJ, 2013, PDR Network.

Potter PA, et al: *Fundamentals of nursing*, ed 8, St Louis, 2013, Mosby.

Skidmore-Roth L: *Mosby's 2013 nursing drug reference*, St Louis, 2013, Mosby.

Online References

American Nurses Association: www.ana.com.

Centers for Disease Control and Prevention: www.cdc.com.

Diabetes Monitor: www.diabetesmonitor.com.

Drugs.Com: www.drugs.com.

Net Wellness: www. Netwellness.org.

University of Michigan Health System: www.med.umich.edu.

REVIEW QUESTIONS

1. A student nurse questions the nurse about why the patient has 20 mEq of potassium chloride (KCl) in his IV. The nurse explains the purpose and then refers the student to which laboratory test?
   1. Electrolytes
   2. Glucose
   3. Hemoglobin
   4. Arterial blood gases

2. A patient undergoing outpatient anticoagulant therapy asks why he has to have blood drawn every week. The most appropriate answer the nurse should give is:
   1. "The doctor needs to know if the infection is improving."
   2. "The doctor adjusts your dosage to help you maintain a therapeutic level."
   3. "The doctor needs to know if the medication is working."
   4. "We don't want the medicine to become toxic."

3. A patient asks the nurse why he is receiving patches of nitroglycerin instead of just taking it under the tongue when he needs it. The nurse explains that:
   1. "Given in this manner, the medication is absorbed at a slow, steady rate."
   2. "This manner is effective in acute situations."
   3. "This manner allows for more accurate dosage."
   4. "Patches administer a day's to a week's worth of medication."

4. A patient is receiving D5RL at 150 mL/hr. The drip factor for the tubing is 20. The number of drops per minute is:
   Answer: _____ drops/min

5. A patient with cancer has been receiving high doses of morphine for several days. During an assessment, the side effect that the nurse would be likely to see is:
   1. Constipation.
   2. Respiratory depression.
   3. Pain relief.
   4. Diarrhea.

6. The physician has ordered Mycostatin 5 mL, swish and swallow twice daily. The nurse should instruct the patient to:
   1. "Swallow the medication quickly, and follow with 8 oz of water."
   2. "Shake the bottle before administering to help mix the suspension."
   3. "Brush your teeth carefully before each dose."
   4. "Maintain contact with the mucosa as long as possible before swallowing."

7. The nurse will know that the patient understands teaching about self-administration of oral corticosteroids when the patient states that she will take the medication:
   1. Before meals.
   2. With or after meals.
   3. At bedtime.
   4. With orange juice.

8. Which intramuscular site in a child does this picture represent?
   1. Rectus femoris
   2. Vastus lateralis
   3. Ventrogluteal
   4. Deltoid

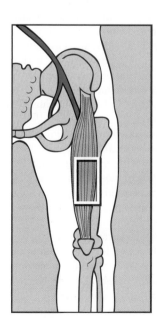

9. After assessment of laboratory work, the physician orders 2 units of packed red blood cells (RBCs) for a patient. The nurse knows that the tests the physician used to assess the need for RBCs were:
   1. Blood glucose
   2. Electrolytes
   3. Hemoglobin and hematocrit
   4. Specific gravity

10. A nurse is making a home visit to care for a patient with chronic obstructive pulmonary disease. When she arrives at the home, she finds that the couple has a big box of medications all mixed together, and some of them are outdated. The first priority should be to:
    1. Examine all the labels to determine which ones are still viable.
    2. Question the couple to see what medications they are taking.
    3. Report the situation to her supervisor so that she can contact the physician.
    4. Contact the social worker to begin placement proceedings for the couple.

11. A physician orders 7.5 mg of iron every day by means of a percutaneous endoscopic gastrostomy tube. The liquid container is labeled 5 mg per 10 mL. How many milliliters are correctly administered?
    Answer: _____ mL

12. An IV infusion is ordered at 60 mL/hr with a drip factor of 60. How many drops per minute should be infusing?
    Answer: _____ drops/min

13. The nurse is going to give a subcutaneous injection to a 42-year-old patient of average weight. The needle length and gauge the nurse will use are:
    1. 19 gauge, 1½ inch
    2. 22 gauge, 1 inch
    3. 24 gauge, 1 inch
    4. 25 gauge, ⅝ inch

14. The order reads 250 mg penicillin IVPB every 6 hours. The dose on hand is 1 g per 10 mL. What is the amount to be given?
    Answer: _____ mL

15. To assess the therapeutic effectiveness of an antiparkinsonian drug, the nurse will observe the patient's:
    1. Increased sleep patterns.
    2. Increased ability to ambulate and speak.
    3. Decreased emotional stability.
    4. Decreased caloric and nutritional intake.

16. A patient is going through withdrawal from alcohol. Which medications would be the treatment of choice to ease delirium tremens?
    1. Diazepam (Valium), vitamins B_1 and B_{12}, folic acid
    2. Aspirin, calcium, Tigan
    3. Vitamin C, aspirin, calcium
    4. Vitamins B_1 and B_2, aspirin

17. A patient with emphysema is taking a bronchodilator. Which instructions or statement would be appropriate for the nurse to give the patient?
    1. "Increase fluids to 2000 to 3000 mL every day."
    2. "Take medication with food."
    3. "Slow-release tablets may be chewed."
    4. "Antibiotics decrease action of these drugs."

18. A patient has been taking phenytoin (Dilantin) for several months, and her seizures are well controlled. Which statement indicates the need for further teaching?
    1. "I understand that I need to continue taking folic acid supplements."
    2. "I cannot wait to stop taking this medication."
    3. "I take my medication with a glass of orange juice every day."
    4. "I always wear my identification tag."

19. A 66-year-old patient with pain associated with angina pectoris is given sublingual nitroglycerin. The nurse knows this medication will:
    1. Dilate blood vessels and increase circulation.
    2. Inhibit the pain sensors in the brainstem.
    3. Increase respirations and cause drowsiness.
    4. Dull nerve endings in the myocardium.

20. Prioritize the following concerns from highest to lowest priority for a nurse visiting a childless couple.
    1. Household cleaners stored under the sink
    2. Insulin syringes on the kitchen cabinet
    3. Husband and wife's medications stored together on the bedside table
    4. Two empty bottles of wine in the trash bin

21. A patient is receiving temazepam (Restoril), 0.015 g orally (PO) at bedtime, for insomnia. The label indicates 15-mg tablets. How many tablets will the nurse give?
    Answer: _____ tablet(s)

22. A nurse is assessing signs of alcohol withdrawal in one of her patients. These assessments would include (select all that apply):
    _____ 1. Tremors.
    _____ 2. Thirst.
    _____ 3. Polyuria.
    _____ 4. Anxiety.
    _____ 5. Increased blood pressure.
    _____ 6. Headache.

23. Identify items that would be appropriate to teach a patient being treated with warfarin (Coumadin). Select all that apply.
    _____ 1. "It is important to avoid eating excessive amounts of broccoli."
    _____ 2. "It is important to avoid foods high in vitamin D."
    _____ 3. "It is important to remember to check your blood sugar twice each day."
    _____ 4. "This medication must be taken early in the morning."
    _____ 5. "It is important to monitor for any signs of bleeding in urine or stool."
    _____ 6. "The physician will regulate your medication according to your blood work."

24. An 89-year-old man is complaining of urinary retention. During the medication history, which assessment would be a priority to report to the physician?
    1. Baclofen (Lioresal)
    2. Diazepam (Valium)
    3. Benztropine (Cogentin)
    4. Cyclobenzaprine hydrochloride (Flexeril)

25. A patient complains to the office nurse that he is experiencing nausea and muscle cramps. He states, "I feel like I always have a virus, but it never develops." The nurse recognizes that these symptoms might be a result of which medication that the patient has just started taking?
    1. Ibuprofen (Motrin)
    2. Diazepam (Valium)

3. Loratadine (Claritin)
4. Atorvastatin (Lipitor)

26. A patient is receiving aminophylline. The nurse knows the medication acts to:
    1. Dilate blood vessels, increasing capillary permeability.
    2. Increase contraction of the bronchi and alveoli.
    3. Decrease contraction of the smooth muscles of the bronchioles.
    4. Decrease the amount of mucus secretion from the bronchi.

27. An adverse reaction to atropine sulfate that may be serious for patients with underlying heart disease is:
    1. Delirium.
    2. Tachycardia.
    3. Constipation.
    4. Dry mouth.

28. When a nurse is giving dietary instructions appropriate to a person taking ibandronate sodium (Boniva), it would be especially important to include which of the following:
    1. "Maintain adequate intake of calcium and vitamin D."
    2. "Increase fiber, whole grains, and rhubarb."
    3. "Increase intake of vitamin C."
    4. "Maintain appropriate calories to avoid gaining weight."

29. An athlete asks the school nurse why using steroids to increase athletic ability is so dangerous. The nurse explains that the drugs:
    1. Stimulate red blood cell formation.
    2. Are difficult to withdraw from, and a tolerance may develop.
    3. Are illegal if given without a prescription.
    4. Are a risk for many adverse side effects, including cardiac failure.

30. A patient in the intensive care unit goes into life-threatening cardiogenic shock. The primary effect that the nurse would look for after a norepinephrine bitartrate (Levophed) drip is initiated on an infusion pump is:
    1. Decreasing hyperventilation.
    2. Decreasing polyuria.
    3. Increasing blood pressure.
    4. Increasing orientation.

31. The nurse in a physician's office interviews a patient being treated for asthma. The patient is jittery and complains of nausea. A statement that might indicate a cause for the jitteriness would be:
    1. "I have been taking diazepam (Valium) for my nerves."
    2. "I am overdue to have a theophylline level drawn."
    3. "I am taking cimetidine (Tagamet) for my epigastric pain."
    4. "I take a laxative when I am constipated."

32. A patient who has been taking phenytoin (Dilantin) for 1 week is very upset and states, "I don't understand why I am still having seizures." The nurse explains:
    1. "We may need to speak with the physician about changing your medication."
    2. "Therapeutic effectiveness may take several weeks."
    3. "Maybe we need to add an additional medication."
    4. "Improvement will be gradual."

33. A patient who has been taking Claritin for allergy relief for several weeks complains to the nurse that the medication is no longer working. The nurse suspects that the patient may have developed a(n):
    1. Tolerance.
    2. Cumulation.

3. Synergistic reaction.
4. Antagonistic effect.

34. A child is being treated with Ritalin. How would the therapeutic effectiveness be evaluated?
    1. Decreased hyperactivity and a more normal attention span
    2. Decreased irritability and a more normal sleep pattern
    3. Decreased headache pain and a more normal appetite
    4. Decreased nausea and vomiting

35. Indicate in which order of priority the nurse should administer the medications to these patients (from highest priority to lowest priority).
    1. A cardiac patient receiving a daily dose of digoxin (Lanoxin)
    2. An asthmatic patient receiving a daily dose of montelukast (Singulair)
    3. A patient receiving an antibiotic four times per day for a wound infection
    4. A patient with diabetes receiving a daily dose of insulin

36. A nurse is obtaining the medication history of a newly admitted patient. The patient has been taking escitalopram oxalate (Lexapro) for 14 days. Which effect would be observed if the drug is therapeutic?
    1. Absence of diarrhea
    2. Decreased nausea and vomiting
    3. Decreased depression
    4. Decreased insomnia

37. During an admission interview, the nurse learns that a patient has been taking dipyridamole (Persantine) for several months. This assessment is an indication for:
    1. Assessing respirations after activity.
    2. Monitoring blood pressure sitting, standing, and lying.
    3. Assessing temperature every 4 hours.
    4. Monitoring white blood cells (WBCs) to check for infection.

38. Patients who are receiving vancomycin (Vancocin) by IV infusion should be assessed before and during the administration for:
    1. Blurred vision.
    2. Constipation.
    3. Hearing damage.
    4. Muscle cramps.

39. A nurse assesses that a patient with diabetes is reporting increased episodes of hypoglycemia. What is the likely explanation?
    1. Decreasing usual exercise patterns without changing insulin
    2. Increasing caloric intake without changing insulin
    3. Increased exercise patterns with a decreased insulin dosage
    4. Decreased caloric intake and increased exercise pattern

40. A nurse is interviewing a patient about her medication history. The patient denies taking any over-the-counter (OTC) medicines. The nurse then asks about dietary habits. The patient removes a bottle of Pepto-Bismol from her purse and states that she has been taking this "food" for years for her stomach pain. She also has a bottle of vitamin pills, which she takes for her eyes. The first priority for the nurse at this point is to:
    1. Assess the "stomach pain."
    2. Ask the patient what foods irritate her stomach.

3. Investigate what might be wrong with her eyes.

4. Explain to the patient that these are considered medications and investigate further.

41. The nurse is taking an admission history for a person being seen by a physician for an initial visit. Which statement most indicates the need for further investigation?

1. "Once in a while when I get constipated, I take a laxative."

2. "I have been taking spironolactone (Aldactone) for many years."

3. "I am a fanatic about taking a vitamin every day."

4. "I have been taking famotidine (Pepcid) almost every day for a month."

42. A patient is being started on isoniazid (INH) therapy for the treatment of tuberculosis. Identify all items that should be included in his discharge instructions. Select all that apply.

_____ 1. Take the medication with meals.

_____ 2. Avoid smoked fish, tuna, and milk products.

_____ 3. Monitor blood glucose levels regularly.

_____ 4. Do not drink alcohol.

_____ 5. Maintain follow-up contact with physician.

_____ 6. Limit contact with others during the course of therapy.

43. Identify diagnoses that are appropriate indications for antihistamine therapy. Select all that apply.

_____ 1. Upper respiratory tract infections

_____ 2. Asthmatic attacks

_____ 3. Lower respiratory tract infections

_____ 4. Narrow-angle glaucoma

_____ 5. Benign prostatic hyperplasia

_____ 6. Anaphylactic reactions

44. Which assessment concerning an IV infusion would be a priority to report to the charge nurse?

1. The drops are falling too slowly.

2. A small, reddened area is near the insertion site.

3. The infusion slows when the patient bends his arm.

4. The piggyback infusion is complete.

45. A nurse is admitting a patient diagnosed with deep vein thrombosis. He is starting treatment with IV anticoagulation therapy. Which assessment is most important to report to the physician?

1. The patient takes psyllium (Metamucil) occasionally for constipation.

2. The patient uses ibuprofen (Motrin) for treating osteoarthritis.

3. The patient takes loratadine (Claritin) for treating allergies.

4. The patient takes nifedipine (Procardia) for treating hypertension.

46. A physician orders an IV infusion of 3000 mL of Ringer's lactate with 5% dextrose (D5RL) for his patient over the next 24 hours. The drip factor for the tubing is 10. How many drops per minute will deliver the correct amount of fluid?

Answer: _____ drops/min

47. A nurse is administering an antibiotic to a patient at midnight. The patient refuses to take the medication, stating, "I already received my pills before I went to sleep." The most appropriate action for the nurse to take is:

1. Verify that the medication order is current and correct.

2. Explain to the patient that the physician has ordered the medication to cure his infection.

3. Explain to the patient that he received his sleeping pill before going to sleep.

4. Check previous documentation to be certain that the time of administration was not changed during the previous shift.

48. A clinic nurse is concerned when a patient diagnosed with active tuberculosis (TB) returns to the clinic after 2 weeks of treatment and reports a worsening cough and recurring night sweats. These findings most likely indicate:

1. Noncompliance with medication regimen.

2. Additional exposure to infected individuals.

3. The need for additional medication.

4. The need for follow-up care for family members.

49. A patient who is being administered dialysis is placed on a 1200-mL fluid restriction in 24 hours. The best allocation for the fluid would be:

1. 600 mL on the 7:00 to 3:00 shift, 400 mL on the 3:00 to 11:00 shift, and 200 mL on the 11:00 to 7:00 shift

2. 500 mL on the 7:00 to 3:00 shift, 500 mL on the 3:00 to 11:00 shift, and 200 mL on the 11:00 to 7:00 shift

3. Liquids only at mealtimes

4. As long as 100 mL is left for medications, the patient should regulate his or her own fluids.

50. A patient is taking Gantrisin. Which statement would indicate that the patient understands the purpose of this medication?

1. "I have had urinary frequency and burning for the last 2 days."

2. "I am allergic to penicillin."

3. "I have had a runny nose for 3 days."

4. "I have loose, foul-smelling diarrhea."

51. The nurse will do a daily assessment of the integrity of the oral mucosa when the patient is receiving:

1. Antibiotics.

2. Cancer drugs.

3. Antiparkinsonian drugs.

4. Vitamins.

52. Identify the site most commonly used for intravenous insertions (A, B, or C).

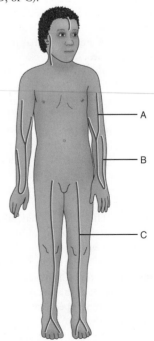

53. The nurse knows that an 80-year-old patient taking medication would be prone to:
    1. Developing a tolerance to medication
    2. Metabolizing medications more rapidly
    3. Developing more frequent adverse reactions
    4. Experiencing more cumulative effects

54. Many drugs have anticholinergic side effects. Examples of these effects would include:
    1. Dryness of the mouth and constipation.
    2. Increased salivation and diarrhea.
    3. Polyuria and thirst.
    4. Tachycardia and diarrhea.

55. A patient is being treated with pyridostigmine (Mestinon) for myasthenia gravis. How would the nurse evaluate the therapeutic effectiveness of this medication?
    1. Decreased arrhythmias
    2. Decreased nausea and vomiting
    3. Increased perspiration
    4. Increased muscle strength

56. A 3-year-old patient has been receiving high doses of metoclopramide (Reglan) for side effects associated with chemotherapy. The nurse is reinforcing home care instructions related to adverse medication effects. Which symptoms should be reported to the health care provider immediately?
    1. Mild sedation and fatigue
    2. Rigidity and tremors
    3. Constipation and dry mouth
    4. Headache and insomnia

57. A nurse is administering amoxicillin PO to a 3-year-old child diagnosed with an ear infection. The most appropriate approach with the child would be to:
    1. Give a detailed explanation to the child about why he needs this medicine.
    2. Explain that it is time to take your "pink medicine."
    3. Have the parent hold the child in his or her arms, and inject it quickly into the child's mouth.
    4. Administer the medication in 240 mL of apple juice.

58. The patient is to receive an IV infusion of lactated Ringer's at 75 mL/hr. The drop factor is 20 gtt/mL. The nurse will run the IV at how many gtt per minute?
    Answer: _____ gtt/min

59. A postoperative patient receives 5000 units of heparin (Heparin Sodium) subcutaneously (SC) bid. The dosage available is 10,000 units per milliliter. The correct amount of medication to be administered is:
    Answer: _____ mL

60. Atropine, 1/150 grain, is ordered as a preoperative medication. On hand is 0.4 mg/mL. The appropriate amount of fluid to be administered is:
    Answer: _____ mL

61. A nurse is assisting at a clinic where a 3-month-old infant is required to have an IM injection. The most appropriate site for this injection is the:
    1. Vastus lateralis.
    2. Dorsogluteal.
    3. Deltoid.
    4. Ventrogluteal.

62. A nurse is assigned to administer morning medications to four patients. Place the patients in order of priority from highest to lowest for those medications.

    1. Ascorbic acid (vitamin C), Os-Cal, furosemide (Lasix)
    2. Metformin (metformin) digoxin (Lanoxin)
    3. Escitalopram (Lexapro), multivitamin, ascorbic acid
    4. Metoprolol, multivitamins, aspirin

63. The nurse has been monitoring a patient in his home. Two weeks ago he was diagnosed with active tuberculosis (TB). Which of these statements would most indicate that he understands his treatment?
    1. "I'm so glad that the treatment is over so that I can go back to work."
    2. "I will need support and assistance to take this medication for such a long time."
    3. "I have to learn to eat healthier foods."
    4. "I can't believe I am going to be contagious for a year."

64. A statement that would most indicate that an adolescent is beginning to understand his diagnosis of type 1 (insulin-dependent) diabetes mellitus would be:
    1. "I am going to hang out with my friends like I always did."
    2. "Swimming is an important part of my life."
    3. "I will need to make sure that I eat healthy snacks between meals."
    4. "I hate being different from my friends."

65. The nurse will administer thyroid drugs:
    1. In a single dose, usually before breakfast.
    2. In divided doses before meals.
    3. In divided doses after meals.
    4. As the patient's energy level decreases.

66. The physician's order reads to administer 3 L of 5% dextrose, 0.45% normal saline IV over 24 hours. The drip factor is 10 gtt/mL. The nurse will regulate the IV at:
    Answer: _____ gtt/min

67. A patient with asthma has been placed on a metered-dose inhaler. Which statement indicates the need for further teaching?
    1. "I need to press down on the inhaler to release one puff while inhaling slowly."
    2. "The inhalers can be used on a multidose basis."
    3. "I should inhale both puffs in quick succession."
    4. "After each puff I should hold my breath for approximately 10 seconds."

68. The patient is to receive an IV of 5% dextrose, 0.33 normal saline at 1000 mL/8 hr. The drip factor is 10 gtt/mL. The nurse will run the IV at:
    1. 7 gtt/min.
    2. 14 gtt/min.
    3. 20 gtt/min.
    4. 28 gtt/min.

69. Fluoxetine (Prozac) has been ordered for a 49-year-old man with depression. In teaching him about his new medicine, the nurse will tell him that:
    1. It should be taken at bedtime.
    2. A feeling of euphoria will occur within 24 hours.
    3. Two to 3 weeks will be required before the effects of the drug will be felt.
    4. It should be taken with meals.

70. A 20-year-old male patient is taking ciprofloxacin (Cipro) for a urinary tract infection. He also takes theophylline

for asthma. In teaching him about his medication, the nurse knows that:
1. Fluids should be restricted while taking ciprofloxacin.
2. The patient should not be started on ciprofloxacin until culture results have been obtained.
3. Theophylline levels may be elevated and can become toxic.
4. The two medications should be given at alternate times.

71. A 64-year-old patient with congestive heart failure takes a digitalis preparation every day. Before administering the medication, the nurse will:
1. Weigh the patient.
2. Check the patient's apical pulse.
3. Take the patient's blood pressure.
4. Monitor the patient's clotting time.

72. The patient will be taught to take his iron preparation:
1. At bedtime.
2. Before breakfast.
3. With meals.
4. Between meals.

73. The nurse gives the 59-year-old patient atropine sulfate as a preoperative medication. The nurse tells the patient that he will not be allowed out of bed because:
1. The central nervous system is depressed.
2. Vertigo might occur because of dilation of the pupils.
3. An adverse effect of the drug is orthostatic hypotension.
4. Diaphoresis may predispose to a chill.

74. Identify substance interactions that are antagonistic to one another. Select all that apply.
_____ 1. Antacids and bran
_____ 2. Erythromycin and citrus foods
_____ 3. Calcium and vitamin D
_____ 4. Warfarin and vitamin K

75. A patient diagnosed with cancer is taking erythropoietin (Epogen). The blood test that should be checked to indicate the effectiveness of this medication would be:
1. Blood glucose level.
2. Blood urea nitrogen and creatinine
3. Hemoglobin and hematocrit.
4. White blood cell (WBC) count.

76. While taking a medication history on a preoperative patient, the nurse is concerned when she discovers that the patient is being treated with acetazolamide (Diamox) for narrow-angle glaucoma. She knows that this is important to communicate to the physician because the patient should not receive which medication?
1. Meperidine (Demerol)
2. Atropine sulfate (Isopto Atropine)
3. Pentazocine (Talwin)
4. Naloxone hydrochloride (Narcan)

77. A patient is admitted for the treatment of gastroesophageal reflux disease. His treatment has not responded to first-line medications, so the physician is planning to place him on a regimen of metoclopramide (Reglan) for a short period. The nurse should instruct the patient on all items except:
1. Advise the patient to avoid alcohol and other central nervous system (CNS) depressants.
2. Monitor carefully for signs of hyperglycemia because the food is more efficiently absorbed into the bloodstream.

3. Avoid tasks that require concentration.
4. Administer the oral dose 30 minutes before meals and at bedtime.

78. A patient arrives at a clinic with complaints of dysuria, pain frequency, and incontinence. A complete history is taken. The patient has a list of medications. Which medication is used to treat dysuria?
1. Furosemide (Lasix)
2. Metolazone (Zaroxolyn)
3. Oxybutynin (Ditropan)
4. Spironolactone (Aldactone)

79. Protease inhibitors should be taken:
1. With meals to improve absorption.
2. 1 hour before or 2 hours after meals.
3. With only a small sip of water.
4. With the scheduled vitamins.

80. Zidovudine (Retrovir) is commonly prescribed for patients with human immunodeficiency virus. The nurse knows that the ideal time for beginning treatment is:
1. When symptoms of immune deficiency first begin to appear.
2. After other antiviral medicines have been tried.
3. Before symptoms of immunodeficiency appear.
4. At the end stage of the disease.

81. A nurse is teaching a woman newly diagnosed with diabetes and her daughter how to administer insulin when they return home. Which statement indicates the need for further teaching?
1. "Rotating the sites is important to prevent complications."
2. "Checking blood glucose is important after the insulin has been administered."
3. "Eating is important after the insulin has been administered."
4. "My daughter will be able to help me if I am sick."

82. A vancomycin level is ordered for your patient. The nurse knows that it is important to check blood levels because a therapeutic blood level:
1. Means that an adequate amount of medication is present to combat infection.
2. Shows that the antibiotic is being excreted adequately.
3. Needs to be reached gradually to avoid toxicity.
4. Will show that the bacterial infection is sensitive to the medication.

83. A student nurse is worried that a patient with a terminal illness is receiving too high a dose of morphine in her continuous morphine drip. The oncology nurse explains that:
1. "The high dose is needed to relieve pain, and the excessive sedation is a side effect."
2. "Pain relief is important; the high dose is why we have to monitor her carefully for respiratory depression."
3. "Patients with cancer pain can be administered gradually increasing doses without side effects of respiratory depression and sedation."
4. "Increasing pain must be treated because of the progression of the disease."

84. A postoperative patient is reluctant to take pain medication, even though he is rating his pain as an 8 on a scale of 1 to 10. The nurse assesses the patient's feelings and concludes that he has a fear of addiction. She explains to him that:
1. He is wise to limit his pain medication because psychological dependence is a potential complication.

2. He should continue to wait as long as possible for his pain medication to increase effectiveness.

3. Addiction is minimal in hospitalized patients.

4. Fear of tolerance developing is warranted with post-operative patients.

85. Patients should be taught to take all of their antibiotics as prescribed because:

1. They increase their risk for dehydration if they do not finish.

2. They increase their risk for developing bacterial-resistant strains.

3. They increase their risk for abdominal distress.

4. It is not cost-effective if another prescription is required.

86. The nurse in an outpatient clinic is concerned because a patient comes to the clinic complaining of heartburn that she has been experiencing for the last 2 weeks. She has been self-medicating with sodium bicarbonate. The nurse anticipates that the physician will order which blood test?

1. Complete blood count

2. Blood urea nitrogen

3. Electrolytes

4. Blood glucose levels

87. A patient asks the nurse why his aluminum hydroxide (Amphojel) is always given 1 hour before meals. The nurse replies:

1. "The presence of food decreases the absorption of aluminum hydroxide."

2. "An empty stomach allows the medication to decrease hydrochloric acid secretion more effectively."

3. "This medication is less likely to cause diarrhea if given on an empty stomach."

4. "Rebound acidity is less likely to occur if the medication is given on this schedule."

88. A nurse is taking a medication history of a patient diagnosed with a urinary tract infection. The physician has prescribed ciprofloxacin (Cipro) to treat the infection. Which medication taken by the patient would be of most concern to the nurse?

1. Mylanta

2. Aspirin

3. Ibuprofen

4. Birth control pills

89. A patient at a walk-in clinic has been on an extended overseas trip. He is complaining of diarrhea. The physician prescribes polycarbophil (FiberCon). The nurse also instructs the patient to:

1. Limit fluid intake because fluid retention may be a problem.

2. Take this medication with his other oral drugs because this will help him remember.

3. Take aspirin as needed for any fever that may develop.

4. Report back to the physician if diarrhea persists more than 2 days.

90. A student nurse asks her instructor why sucralfate (Carafate) has to be given 1 hour before meals and 2 hours after other medications. The instructor explains that:

1. Sucralfate is better able to protect the lining of the stomach if it is able to come in contact with it.

2. Spicy foods might interfere with the effectiveness of sucralfate.

3. Sucralfate is less likely to cause diarrhea on an empty stomach.

4. Sucralfate is synergistic with many other medications and may increase their effect.

91. A patient is being discharged home taking levothyroxine (Synthroid). Which statement indicates the need for further teaching?

1. "I may feel very sleepy at first when I am on this medication."

2. "I should let my physician know if I feel my heart is beating fast."

3. "I will have to be certain to eat healthier food."

4. "I will take this with my other medications so I remember."

92. A preoperative patient is being treated with heparin before surgery. The purpose of this medication is to:

1. Minimize blood loss during surgery.

2. Decrease the risk of deep vein thrombosis.

3. Improve red blood cell (RBC) production.

4. Minimize the chance of a potential infection.

93. A patient is being discharged on warfarin sodium (Coumadin). Which of these instructions is appropriate for the nurse to give him?

1. The visiting nurse will administer the medication subcutaneously on a daily basis.

2. Checking carefully for any signs of infection is important.

3. Report any signs of bleeding to your health care provider.

4. Your blood levels need to be checked in 3 months before your next visit with your physician.

94. Which is inappropriate when giving instructions to a patient who is being treated with nitroglycerin for acute attacks of angina?

1. The patient should use a plastic wrap over his patch to avoid stains on his clothing.

2. Allow the tablet to dissolve under the tongue.

3. The dose may be repeated twice at 5-minute intervals.

4. Sustained-release nitroglycerin should be swallowed whole.

95. A patient is admitted for the treatment of congestive heart failure. He is started on digoxin (Lanoxin) and furosemide (Lasix). A loading dose of digoxin is given for the purpose of:

1. Gradually bringing the patient into the therapeutic range.

2. Eliminating fluid from the lungs.

3. Giving the patient an adequate blood level.

4. Decreasing the possibility of toxicity.

96. Identify all of the pairs of substances listed below that are potentially antagonistic to each other.

_____ 1. Vitamin B_{12} (cyanocobalamin) and fish

_____ 2. Calcium carbonate and bran

_____ 3. Salicylates and ascorbic acid

_____ 4. Warfarin (Coumadin) and green leafy vegetables

97. A patient is being started on celecoxib (Celebrex) for treating osteoarthritis. Which statement indicates that the patient understands the nurse's teaching?

1. "I need to take this medication three times each day with meals."

2. "I need to take this when I feel the soreness starting."

3. "I should take this medication once each day."
4. "If I take this with breakfast, I will not have any nausea."

98. A patient has been given gabapentin (Neurontin) over the last year after having had a craniotomy for a subdural hematoma. The directions given him at this time would be:
    1. "The physician will monitor liver function test results and complete blood counts to ensure that the medications are not toxic."
    2. "This medication needs to be discontinued on a gradual schedule initiated by the physician."
    3. "Avoid driving or operating any hazardous machinery while you are taking this medication."
    4. "Use sunscreen and protective clothing to avoid photosensitivity reaction while taking this medication."

99. A patient has been treated with sertraline (Zoloft) for 1 week. She tells her nurse that she is discouraged because she is not feeling any better. The nurse replies:
    1. "You must not drink alcohol while you are on this therapy."
    2. "Speak with your physician about changing medications."
    3. "It may take a few weeks for a change to be noticed."
    4. "Tell me more about what you are feeling."

100. A student nurse asks why a patient is taking insulin when no history of diabetes is in her chart. The nurse explains that one of the medications she is taking sometimes causes hyperglycemia. This medication would be:
    1. Dexamethasone (Decadron).
    2. Rosiglitazone (Avandia).
    3. Digoxin (Lanoxin).
    4. Glucophage (Metformin).

101. Which medicine has priority when giving scheduled medications at 8:00 am before breakfast?
    1. Digoxin (Lanoxin)
    2. Glipizide (Glucotrol)
    3. Donepezil hydrochloride (Aricept)
    4. Atorvastatin (Lipitor)

102. The order reads Ceclor 0.5 g. On hand is Ceclor 250 mg/tablet. How many tablets will the nurse give?
    Answer: _____tablet(s)

103. A child is being treated with methylphenidate (Ritalin) for attention-deficit hyperkinetic disorder. The parent should be instructed to schedule the medication:
    1. At bedtime.
    2. Before dinnertime
    3. After meals.
    4. In the early morning.

104. A postpartum patient complains of dysuria. The physician prescribes which of these medications to ease symptoms?
    1. Phenazopyridine (Pyridium)
    2. Furosemide (Lasix)
    3. Loperamide (Imodium)
    4. Sulfisoxazole (Gantrisin)

105. An adverse side effect of oxybutynin (Ditropan) that needs to be reported immediately is:
    1. Jaundice.
    2. Restlessness.
    3. Bradycardia.
    4. Fatigue.

106. Which terms describe the pharmacokinetics of medication in the body?
    1. Digestion, excretion, metabolism, catabolism
    2. Absorption, catabolism, metabolism, excretion
    3. Absorption, distribution, metabolism, excretion
    4. Anabolism, distribution, metabolism, excretion

107. A patient has just been started on furosemide (Lasix). What is the most important nursing intervention at this time?
    1. Monitoring potassium levels
    2. Checking the patient's weight and vital signs
    3. Reporting severe diarrhea
    4. Assessing lung and bowel sounds

108. A patient is being discharged taking bisphosphonates—alendronate (Fosamax). Which instructions are not appropriate?
    1. "Drinking 3000 to 4000 mL of fluid will help your kidneys excrete the medication."
    2. "Increasing your intake of dairy products will help this medication to work better."
    3. "Remember to take your other vitamins at least 30 minutes after this pill."
    4. "Laboratory work needs to be scheduled to make sure this medication is working."

109. One of the most common side effects of enalapril (Vasotec) is:
    1. Dry hacking cough.
    2. Hypertension.
    3. Constipation.
    4. Irritability.

110. A patient is receiving bisphosphonates—alendronate (Fosamax). The proper time to schedule this medication is:
    1. With meals.
    2. With other medications early in the day.
    3. 30 minutes before other medications.
    4. 30 minutes before uncomfortable procedures.

111. Which is a sign of salicylate toxicity?
    1. Tinnitus
    2. Headache
    3. Dizziness
    4. Irritability

112. Which dietary pattern would be contraindicated for the administration of enoxaparin (Lovenox)?
    1. Hyperalimentation
    2. A kosher diet
    3. A vegetarian diet
    4. A low-sodium diet

113. Identify all of the instructions listed below that are necessary for a patient starting antibiotic therapy.
    _____ 1. The doctor will prescribe medicine based on the results of the culture and sensitivity.
    _____ 2. Avoid dairy products.
    _____ 3. Always monitor renal and liver functions for any long-term use.
    _____ 4. Avoid excessive exposure to the sun.
    _____ 5. Always take with meals.
    _____ 6. Monitor for signs of superinfection.

114. Which classification would be used to facilitate the examination of the eyes?
    1. Cholinergic agents
    2. Mydriatic agents

3. Ceruminolytic
4. Ocular decongestant

115. A postoperative patient is rating his operative pain as an 8 on a scale of 1 to 10. He is refusing pain medication. The most appropriate action for the nurse at this time would be to:
    1. Document his report and the refusal of pain medication.
    2. Assess the location, duration, and radiation of his pain.
    3. Investigate why he is not receptive to medication.
    4. Report the situation to the charge nurse.

116. Identify the landmarks listed for the deltoid site pictured below:
    _____ Brachial artery
    _____ Radial nerve
    _____ Clavicle
    _____ Humerus
    _____ Deltoid muscle
    _____ Acromion process

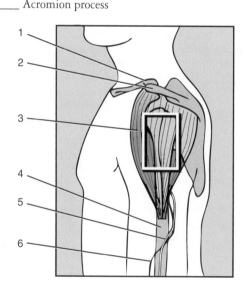

117. A patient has been taking loratadine (Claritin) for 2 weeks. The nurse would know the drug is effective if the patient reports:
    1. Increased ability to sleep through the night.
    2. Decreased sneezing and runny nose.
    3. Decreased nausea and vomiting.
    4. Decreased number of migraines.

118. A patient with type 2 diabetes is hospitalized for surgery. He has been maintaining glycemic control using an oral hypoglycemic agent. He is concerned that his blood sugar has been elevated and that he has been needing to receive insulin. The best response for the nurse at this time would be:
    1. "Don't worry about that now. Ask your doctor after you have recovered."
    2. "As you get older, very often the resistance of your cells to insulin increases."
    3. "Stress often temporarily increases blood glucose levels in your body."
    4. "We are carefully monitoring your blood glucose levels."

119. Using the sliding scale below, indicate the amount of regular insulin an individual with a blood glucose of 260 would receive.
    Answer: _____units
    <200 mg/dL: No insulin

201-250 mg/dL: 2 units regular insulin
251-300 mg/dL: 4 units regular insulin
301-350 mg/dL: 6 units regular insulin
351-400 mg/dL: 8 units regular insulin
>400 mg/dL: Call doctor for insulin order

120. Identify the parts of the intravenous apparatus shown below in their proper order from top to bottom.
    1. Volume control center, macrodrip chamber, secondary port, plastic bag, roller clamp
    2. Major port, volume control center, macrodrip chamber, roller clamp
    3. Plastic bag, roller clamp, volume control chamber, macrodrip chamber, secondary port
    4. Plastic bag, volume control center, roller clamp, secondary port insertion site

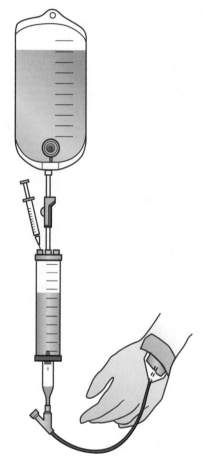

121. A patient is brought into the emergency room after having taken an overdose of secobarbital (Seconal). Which of these is the priority for the nurse?
    1. Maintain patient's safety (e.g., elevate side rails) to prevent injuries because of agitation upon awakening.
    2. Prepare for the initiation of dialysis.
    3. Prepare to draw blood work to determine if level is toxic.
    4. Prepare for the intravenous administration of phenytoin (Dilantin).

122. A patient receiving clonazepam (Klonopin) should be taught (select all that apply):
    _____ 1. Make sure seizures are controlled before driving.

_____ 2. Monitor for decreased effectiveness.

_____ 3. Monitor blood pressure for signs of hypertension.

_____ 4. Use caution when operating machinery.

_____ 5. Check carefully for the development of secondary infections.

123. A patient with a diagnosis of congestive heart failure (CHF) is admitted to the emergency room. The doctor orders digoxin and the nurse knows that important considerations for this drug include (select all that apply):

_____ 1. Checking for signs of toxicity

_____ 2. Checking blood pressure for therapeutic levels

_____ 3. Monitoring for a steady decrease in the rate and an increase in the strength of the heartbeat

_____ 4. Monitoring for visual disturbance

_____ 5. Checking the pulse rate before administration

_____ 6. Monitoring for a decrease in fever

124. A 30-year-old female patient with a diagnosis of varicose veins visits the doctor's office. She said that surgery for her varicose veins is scheduled at the time of her vacation (in 6 months). She wants a prescription for birth control pills. The most effective thing for the nurse to say is:

1. "Varicose veins can be aggravated during pregnancy, so it is a good thing that you are planning ahead."

2. "An alternative form of birth control would be safer because of the potential side effects of birth control pills."

3. "We can only give you a 3-month supply of birth control pills."

4. "An IUD (intrauterine device) would be the preferred choice of birth control right now for you."

125. A student nurse is accompanying a visiting nurse on a home visit. A 70-year-old woman is complaining of what she calls "indigestion." She says she has been experiencing this symptom for about 2 weeks. Her husband says she has been "popping" Prevacid (lansoprazole) three or four times a day. In addition to assessing symptoms and encouraging medical care, the nurse should be concerned with which medication(s)? Select all that apply.

_____ 1. Digoxin

_____ 2. Coumadin

_____ 3. Dilantin

_____ 4. Ibuprofen

126. A postoperative patient is refusing any medication for pain. Which intervention would be a priority for the nurse?

1. Assess the severity of the patient's pain on a scale of 1 to 10.

2. Praise the patience for his tolerance of pain.

3. Try nursing measures (e.g., repositioning, back rub) to relieve pain.

4. Determine what information the patient understands concerning his medications.

127. A patient is experiencing seizures. The physician has prescribed the anticonvulsant carbamazepine (Tegretol). The nurse understands that this drug can be used to treat all except:

1. The treatment of trigeminal nerve pain

2. Grand mal seizures

3. Petit mal seizures

4. Pain caused by neuritis

128. A patient enters a clinic. The student nurse is assigned to assist the nurse with a physical assessment and history taking. The patient complains of decreased energy levels,

inability to concentrate, and increased sensitivity to cold. The student nurse might expect to see which physical signs? Select all that apply.

_____ 1. Puffy hands and feet

_____ 2. High or increased blood pressure

_____ 3. Bruises

_____ 4. Protruding eyes

_____ 5. Dry or leathery skin

129. After the physician has made a diagnosis of hypothyroidism in the previous scenario, the student nurse asks the physician about the patient's prognosis. The physician's response would be:

1. After surgery, she has a 50% chance of recovery.

2. With surgery and radiation treatment, the prognosis is good.

3. With the administration of thyroid hormones, the prognosis is good.

4. Methimazole (Tapazole) inhibits synthesis of the thyroid hormones.

130. A patient is halfway through a 10-day course of Bactrim (co-trimoxazole). She is complaining of itching on her extremities. Which questions should be included in the assessment interview? Select all that apply.

_____ 1. Have you been exposed to any individuals with a respiratory infection in the past 7 days?

_____ 2. What other medications have you taken in the week?

_____ 3. Are there any other symptoms that you have noticed recently?

_____ 4. Have you obtained relief from this medication?

131. A patient is 7 days postoperative after abdominal surgery. He arrives in the ER with a temperature of 104°. Place the following physician orders in priority of action from highest to lowest priority.

1. Administer antipyretic.

2. Obtain blood work for culture and sensitivity.

3. Administer intravenous antibiotic.

4. Perform irrigation and dressing change.

5. Perform cool sponge baths.

132. A mother accompanies her 7-year-old child to the physician's office. The child has been recently diagnosed with type 1 diabetes. Which statement indicates that the mother is beginning to understand the treatment regimen?

1. "Once my child loses weight, he can switch to the pills I heard about on TV."

2. "When he gets cold and clammy in the afternoon, I will give him a snack."

3. "He is learning to exercise on a regular basis."

4. "He knows to report to me how he is feeling."

133. A 56-year-old patient is referred to an ENT (ear, nose, and throat) specialist for complaints of decreased hearing. Which medication in the patient's history would be of the most concern to the physician?

1. The patient was treated 2 years ago with kanamycin sulfate (Kantrex) for a prolonged respiratory infection.

2. The patient has been treated with sumatriptan succinate (Imitrex) for migraine headaches.

3. The patient is taking pregabalin (Lyrica) for the treatment of fibromyalgia.

4. The patient has been treated with clindamycin (Cleocin) for recurring pneumonia.

8. Application, implementation, physiological integrity, (a).
   1. ***The rectus femoris muscle lies medial to the vastus lateralis muscle but does not cross the midline of the anterior thigh.***
   2. The vastus lateralis muscle is located on the anterior lateral thigh away from blood vessels and nerves.
   3. The ventrogluteal muscle is a large muscle mass free of major nerves and adipose tissue.
   4. The deltoid muscle is located in the arm.
9. Comprehension, assessment, physiological integrity, (a).
   3. ***These tests measure the levels of hemoglobin (the oxygen-carrying component of the RBC) in the blood and the hematocrit (the number of packed RBCs found in 100 mL of blood) and provide an index to the severity of possible anemia.***
   1. A fasting blood sugar measures the amount of glucose in the bloodstream during a period of fasting; coagulation studies (PT and PPT) are used to monitor anticoagulant therapy.
   2. Electrolytes measure the amount of elements essential to bodily function (potassium, sodium, calcium); an elevated WBC indicates the presence of inflammation or infection.
   4. A change from the normal specific gravity indicates dehydration or inadequate kidney function; a routine urinalysis provides information about renal function and systemic health.
10. Analysis, implementation, health promotion and maintenance, (b).
    3. ***The physician needs to know to verify any needed prescriptions.***
    1, 2. These are subsequent steps but not first priorities.
    4. This is very premature. The couple may need education and support.
11. Comprehension, implementation, physiological integrity, (a).
    Answer: 15 mL
    $5 mg / 10 mL \times 7.5 mg / x$
    $5x = 75$
    $x = 15 mL$
12. Knowledge, implementation, physiological integrity, (a).
    Answer: 60 drops/min
    Drip factor of 60 mL/hr = 60 drops/min
13. Application, planning, physiological integrity, (a).
    4. ***This is the correct size needle to reach subcutaneous tissue.***
    1, 2, 3. These needles are too long; they could pass through subcutaneous tissue to underlying muscle and possibly bone.
14. Application, planning, physiological integrity, (b).
    Answer: 2.5 mL
    $1 g = 1000 mg$
    $2500 = 1000x$
    $x = 2.5 mL$
15. Application, evaluation, physiological integrity, (a).
    2. ***This is the therapeutic effect that is desired for the patient.***
    1. Sleep patterns are not affected by antiparkinsonian drugs.
    3. Emotional stability is not affected by antiparkinsonian drugs.
    4. Diet and nutrition are not affected by antiparkinsonian drugs.

16. Comprehension, planning, physiological integrity, (b).
    1. ***A tranquilizer will ease tremors, and vitamins will improve metabolism.***
    2. Aspirin would be appropriate to relieve a headache from an overdose, and Tigan might be appropriate for complaints of nausea. Calcium is prescribed for potential or actual bone loss, not for withdrawal.
    3. Vitamin C is prescribed for wound healing, aspirin for a headache, and calcium to promote healthy bones.
    4. Vitamins B_1 and B_2 might be prescribed for long-term increased use of nutrients; however, aspirin is most helpful for headaches.
17. Analysis, implementation, physiological integrity, (b).
    1. ***Fluids help thin secretions and help prevent dehydration. Dehydration is particularly common in the elderly and in children.***
    2. Medication should be taken with water. Food affects absorption.
    3. Chewing speeds up absorption.
    4. Certain antibiotics (particularly erythromycin) increase action of theophylline.
18. Analysis, evaluation health promotion and maintenance, (c).
    2. ***Discontinuing this medication may or may not be possible, depending on the cause of the seizure. If it is discontinued, it must be done gradually under the direction of a physician.***
    1. Folic acid deficiency is an adverse reaction to this medication and should be documented by the physician.
    3. This is fine; the stomach should not be empty.
    4. This practice is safe.
19. Application, evaluation, physiological integrity, (b).
    1. ***This is an action of the drug.***
    2. Nitroglycerin has no effect on the brainstem.
    3. Nitroglycerin does not affect respiration or alertness.
    4. Nitroglycerin acts on the myocardial blood vessels, not nerve endings.
20. Application, planning, safe and effective care environment, (a).
    Correct order: 3124.
    3. ***The potential for medication errors increases tremendously when two individuals' medicines are stored in the same place.***
    1. ***This item would be of more concern in a household with young children.***
    2. ***This item would be of more concern in a household with young children.***
    4. ***There is no indication of excessive drinking. They may have had a dinner party. Further investigation is needed.***
21. Comprehension, planning, physiological integrity, (b).
    Answer: 1 tablet
    To change grams to milligrams, multiply grams by 1000.
    $0.015 g \times 1000 = 15 mg = 1$ tablet
22. Comprehension, assessment, physiological integrity, (a).
    __X__ 1. ***Tremors are a sign of alcohol withdrawal, along with tachycardia, diaphoresis, anorexia, nausea, vomiting, insomnia, hallucinations, and seizures.***
    _____ 2. Thirst is a sign of diabetes.
    _____ 3. Polyuria is a sign of diabetes.
    __X__ 4. ***Anxiety is a sign of alcohol withdrawal.***

___X___ 5. *Increased blood pressure is a sign of alcohol withdrawal.*

_____ 6. Headache is a sign of overdose.

23. Analysis, implementation, health promotion and maintenance (b).

___X___ 1. *Broccoli contains large amounts of vitamin K, which is synergistic with Coumadin.*

_____ 2. Foods high in vitamin D do not need to be avoided with this medication.

_____ 3. The level of blood sugar is not affected by warfarin.

_____ 4. This medication should be administered in the afternoon.

___X___ 5. *Bleeding may occur if the dosage is not regulated properly.*

___X___ 6. *The dosage is managed by monitoring the therapeutic level.*

24. Analysis, implementation, physiological integrity, (b).

3. *This is a cholinergic-blocking agent. Urinary retention is an adverse side effect.*

1, 4. These are skeletal muscle relaxants; a side effect is urinary frequency.

2. This is an antianxiety agent. Urinary retention is not a side effect.

25. Analysis, implementation, physiological integrity, (b).

4. *These are side effects of this cholesterol-lowering medication.*

1. This is a nonsteroidal antiinflammatory drug; nausea may be a side effect at times, but the drug is generally given to relieve muscle cramps.

2. This is a skeletal muscle relaxant; these are not common side effects of this medication.

3. This is an antihistamine given to relieve allergy symptoms; these are not common side effects of this medication.

26. Comprehension, evaluation, physiological integrity, (c).

2. *This is the correct action.*

1. This is an action of histamine.

3. This is an action of a beta antagonist.

4. This is the action of a decongestant.

27. Comprehension, evaluation, physiological integrity, (b).

2. *Heart rate can increase.*

1. This is a serious symptom not related to an adverse reaction to atropine.

3. This is caused by lack of bulk in the diet.

4. This is an expected reaction of atropine; it would have no effect on heart disease.

28. Application, planning, physiological integrity, (c).

1. *Patients being treated with Boniva require calcium supplements to maintain blood levels.*

2. Fiber promotes calcium excretion.

3. Calcitonin does not affect vitamin C.

4. This is true for everyone.

29. Application, planning, physiological integrity, (b).

4. *Other effects include diabetes, impotence, amenorrhea, and acromegalic syndrome.*

1, 3. These are true; however, they do not answer the question.

2. This is true; however, it is not the best answer.

30. Comprehension, evaluation, physiological integrity, (b).

3. *The purpose is to maintain and improve blood pressure.*

1. Respiration needs to slow down and be more effective. Respiratory depression needs to be avoided.

2. Urinary output is decreased in shock. It needs to be maintained to keep circulation adequate.

4. This would not be the first sign. Increasing orientation is a sign of improvement.

31. Comprehension, assessment, physiological integrity, (b).

2. *Theophylline can cause these effects; a level is necessary to determine if the medication is in the therapeutic range.*

1. Valium may be used in an emergency asthmatic situation. It is not used on a routine basis.

3. Tagamet does not cause jitteriness, and it is given to decrease nausea.

4. These are not side effects of laxatives.

32. Application, evaluation, physiological integrity, (b).

2. *This is the truth, and patients need encouragement to comply.*

1. There is no indication of the need to change medication.

3. It is not within the scope of practice for the nurse to add a medication, nor is there any indication that the physician should do so.

4. This is true; however, it does not answer the question.

33. Comprehension, assessment, physiological integrity, (a).

1. *This is the correct definition.*

2. Cumulation is the inability of one drug to be completely excreted before another dose is administered; this may lead to toxicity.

3. The synergistic effect occurs when the effects of two drugs are greater when given together than when given separately. An example would be central nervous system depressants and alcohol.

4. An antagonistic effect occurs when the effect of two drugs is less when given together than when given separately. An example would be vitamin K and warfarin (Coumadin).

34. Comprehension, evaluation, physiological integrity, (b).

1. *These are the therapeutic effects desired in children with hyperactivity.*

2. Irritability is an adverse reaction to the medication. Drug should be given at least 6 hours before bedtime to avoid insomnia.

3. Headache is an adverse reaction, as is anorexia.

4. These are adverse reactions.

35. Comprehension, planning, physiological integrity, (b). **Correct order: 4321.**

4. *Insulin is time sensitive and must be administered a certain number of minutes before a meal*

3. *Antibiotics need to be given at scheduled intervals to maintain a therapeutic level*

2. *Montelukast (Singular) is given to prevent attacks and is not used during acute situations.*

1. *Digoxin (Lanoxin) is a daily dose and is not time sensitive.*

36. Comprehension, assessment, physiological integrity, (b)

3. *This is the therapeutic effect; it takes 2 to 3 weeks to reach a therapeutic level.*

1, 2, 4. Diarrhea, nausea, vomiting, and insomnia are adverse reactions to the drug.

37. Comprehension, assessment, physiological integrity, (b).

2. *This medicine is used to treat transient ischemic attacks; orthostatic hypotension is a common side effect.*
   1. This is not a necessary parameter to monitor.
   3. This does not affect temperature.
   4. This does not affect WBCs and may increase risk of bleeding.
38. Comprehension, assessment, physiological integrity, (b).
   3. *Vancomycin is both ototoxic and nephrotoxic.*
   1, 2. Blurred vision and constipation would be characteristic side effects of cholinergic-blocking agents such as atropine.
   4. Muscle cramps would be characteristic of an anticholesterol agent, such as Zocor.
39. Application, assessment, physiological integrity, (b).
   4. *Less food and more exercise are most likely to cause decreased blood sugar.*
   1. Decreasing exercise is more likely to cause hyperglycemia.
   2. This is more likely to cause hyperglycemia.
   3. Exercise decreases the need for insulin. Increasing calories is another option.
40. Application, assessment, physiological integrity, (c).
   4. *A cultural influence may cause her to believe that these medicines are food; however, a knowledge deficit definitely exists.*
   1. This is definitely a necessary assessment, but further information about the entire pattern of OTC medicines is needed.
   2. This is a necessary assessment, but it is not a priority.
   3. Documentation of any subjective or objective items concerning her eyes is definitely needed. It is not a priority at the moment.
41. Application, assessment, physiological integrity, (c).
   4. *Patients should be advised about the danger of taking over-the-counter medicines for more than 2 weeks without consulting a physician. The location and characteristics of the pain need to be investigated.*
   1. Occasional use of a laxative is not dangerous, but further dietary teaching may be indicated.
   2. Assessment of blood pressure is called for; but if it is stable, this is considered ongoing care.
   3. Taking a vitamin every day is fine as long as it is not used as a substitute for good nutrition.
42. Comprehension, planning, physiological integrity, (b).
   ____ 1. The medications should be taken on an empty stomach.
   __X__ 2. *These products contain ingredients that are antagonistic to the prescribed medications.*
   ____ 3. Blood glucose levels do not need to be monitored.
   __X__ 4. *Alcohol and these medications can cause a toxic reaction.*
   __X__ 5. *Follow-up care with the physician is essential, because if these medications are not taken properly for the prescribed period of time, the bacillus that causes tuberculosis can recur.*
   ____ 6. It is not necessary to restrict contact with others during the course of treatment.

43. Comprehension, planning, physiological integrity, (b).
   __X__ 1. *These drugs block histamines at their receptor sites, thereby decreasing the symptoms of these conditions.*
   ____ 2. These drugs affect the cholinergic nervous system, which would make the symptoms of these conditions worse.
   ____ 3. These drugs affect the cholinergic nervous system, which would make the symptoms of these conditions worse.
   ____ 4. These drugs affect the cholinergic nervous system, which would make the symptoms of these conditions worse.
   ____ 5. These drugs affect the cholinergic nervous system, which would make the symptoms of these conditions worse.
   __X__ 6. *These drugs block histamines at their receptor sites, thereby decreasing the symptoms of these conditions.*
44. Comprehension, assessment, physiological integrity, (b).
   2. *This may indicate infiltration.*
   1. This can be corrected (if the insertion site is still patent) by repositioning and making certain that the dial is set correctly.
   3. This can be corrected with positioning.
   4. This is important; however, the primary infusion normally begins when the "piggyback" is completed.
45. Comprehension, assessment, physiological integrity, (b).
   2. *Concurrent use of heparin and nonsteroidal antiinflammatory drugs may predispose the patient to hemorrhage.*
   1. Psyllium is not contraindicated with heparin. It should not be given at the same time as aspirin or digoxin; absorption may be inhibited.
   3. This is a central nervous system depressant and is synergistic with other groups in this classification.
   4. The need here would be to monitor the cumulative effects of other hypertensive agents.
46. Comprehension, implementation, physiological integrity, (a).
   Answer: 21 gtt/min
   The formula is:
   milliliters/hour × gtt factor/60
   = 125 mL/hr × 10/60
47. Comprehension, implementation, physiological integrity, (b).
   4. *It is possible that the evening shift obtained permission to give the medication early so the patient would not be awakened.*
   1. This should be done before administration.
   2. This is true; however, it does not answer the question.
   3. This may also be true, but it does not answer the question.
48. Application, implementation, safe and effective care environment, (b).
   1. *TB medications must be taken over an extended period (6 months to 2 years) to ensure effective treatment.*
   2. There is no indication of this, and continued exposure would not be a factor if the medication regimen were being followed.
   3. There may be a need for additional medication in the future, but it would have to be determined if multidrug-resistant TB has developed.
   4. Family members should have already received follow-up medical care.

49. Comprehension, implementation, physiological integrity, (a).
    1. **This allocation allows for two meals on the 7:00 to 3:00 shift, one meal on the 3:00 to 11:00 shift, and fluids for medications on the 11:00 to 7:00 shift.**
    2. There are two meals on the 7:00 to 3:00 shift; most patients prefer fluids with meals.
    3. Fluids must be allowed for medication.
    4. Patients need to be encouraged to save fluids during the day to increase comfort.
50. Comprehension, assessment, physiological integrity, (a).
    1. **This is the most common antibiotic used to treat urinary tract infections.**
    2. A penicillin substitute such as erythromycin would be used if the symptoms warranted.
    3. This may or may not call for an antibiotic; it may be viral in nature. If an antibiotic were called for, it would probably be penicillin or a substitute.
    4. This may be an indication of a superinfection.
51. Comprehension, assessment, physiological integrity, (b).
    2. **Cancer drugs can affect the integrity of the oral mucosa.**
    1. Antibiotics do not affect the oral mucosa.
    3. Antiparkinsonian drugs do not affect the oral mucosa.
    4. Vitamins do not affect the oral mucosa.
52. Knowledge, planning, physiological integrity, (c).
    The most common site for intravenous insertions is the basilic vein (B). A is the cephalic vein, and C is the femoral vein.
53. Comprehension, assessment, physiological integrity, (c).
    4. **Elderly persons metabolize drugs more slowly because of declining body function, thus prolonging the half-life of the drug, resulting in drug accumulation.**
    1. Age does not make a difference in tolerance.
    2. Older adults metabolize drugs at a decreased rate.
    3. Age does not cause more frequent adverse effects.
54. Knowledge, evaluation, physiological integrity, (a).
    1. **These medications decrease the effects of the parasympathetic nervous system.**
    2. These are opposites of what the side effects would be.
    3. Thirst is a side effect, but polyuria is not.
    4. Tachycardia may occur, but not diarrhea.
55. Comprehension, evaluation, physiological integrity, (b).
    4. **Increased muscle strength would indicate an improvement in the symptoms.**
    1. Slowing of the heart rate is an effect. It is not given to treat arrhythmias.
    2. This is a side effect; however, it is not a therapeutic effect.
    3. This is a side effect; however, it is not a therapeutic effect.
56. Application, evaluation, physiological integrity, (c).
    2. **Children taking high doses of Reglan are particularly prone to the extrapyramidal effects of the drug. Presence of these effects should be reported to the health care provider immediately so the dose can be adjusted or a new drug prescribed.**
    1, 3, 4. These are common side effects and need not be reported.
57. Application, planning, physiological integrity, (b).
    2. **Explanations should be geared to the child's ability to understand.**

    1. Long explanations to a child under 5 years of age only increase anxiety.
    3. Of course, the parent can hold the child; however, injecting it quickly can cause aspiration.
    4. Administering some medication in juice may be appropriate; however, the nurse must be certain that the child will drink all of the juice to receive a correct dose.
58. Knowledge, implementation, physiological integrity, (a).
    Answer: 25 gtt/min
    Calculation:
    milliliters/hour × gtt factor/60
    75/1 × 20/60=1500/60=25 gtt/min
59. Knowledge, implementation, physiological integrity, (a).
    Answer: ½ mL
    Calculation:
    1 mL/10,000 = ½ mL/5000 units
60. Knowledge, implementation, physiological integrity, (a).
    Answer: 1 mL
    Calculation:
    0.4 mg = ¹/₁₅₀ grain
61. Comprehension, implementation, physiological integrity, (a).
    1. **This is the preferred site for children under age 3 years because it is well developed at birth.**
    2. This site should not be used for injections at all until the child has been walking for at least 1 year.
    3. This site can be used with older, larger children.
    4. This site can be used for children older than 3 years who have been walking for 1 or 2 years; however, it has a disadvantage of being visible to the child.
62. Comprehension, planning, physiological integrity, (b).
    Correct order: 2143 or 2134 (see rationale below).
    2. Metformin (metformin), digoxin (Lanoxin)
    1. Ascorbic acid (Vitamin C), Os-Cal, furosemide (Lasix)
    4. Metoprolol, multivitamins, aspirin
    3. Escitalopram (Lexapro), multivitamin, ascorbic acid Metformin (metformin) is an oral hypoglycemic agent that should be given before breakfast. Furosemide (Lasix) should be given early in the morning. The remaining medications are not time sensitive.
63. Comprehension, planning, physiological integrity, (b).
    2. **Follow-up care by health professionals and support of family and friends are vital because patients may need to take medications for as long as 2 years.**
    1. The treatment may need to continue for 6 months to as long as 12 months.
    3. This is necessary to assist in maintaining the immune system. However, it does not answer the question.
    4. Patients are contagious in the initial stages of TB. Good health habits should always be maintained to prevent exposure to others.
64. Comprehension, evaluation, health promotion and maintenance, (b).
    3. **It may be a "drag," but at least he acknowledges that it has to be done.**
    1. This is fine. There is no problem with him hanging out with his friends.
    2. Exercise is fine as long as it is balanced with diet and medication.
    4. Peers are important to adolescents. This statement does not indicate understanding that he has measures necessary to manage his diabetes, but his activities are not restricted.

65. Application, implementation, physiological integrity, (b).
    1. **This allows peak drug activity (better absorption) during daytime hours.**
    2, 3, 4. Thyroid medicine is most effective when given in a single dose before breakfast. This allows the patient to have the maximum benefit during daylight hours.

66. Knowledge, implementation, physiological integrity, (b). **Answer: 21 gtt/min**

$$\frac{\text{Volume}\,(\text{mL})}{\text{Time}} \times \text{Drops/mL} = \text{Drops/min}$$

300 mL ÷ 24 hr = 125 mL/hr
125 mL/hr ÷ 60 min/hr = 2.1 mL/min
2.1 mL/min × 10 gtt/mL = 21 gtt/min

67. Application, evaluation, physiological integrity, (b).
    3. **One minute should be allowed between puffs.**
    1. This is the correct procedure; it allows for maximal absorption.
    2. This is true.
    4. This is true; it aids in absorption.

68. Knowledge, implementation, physiological integrity, (b).
    3. **This is the correct calculation.**
    1, 2, 4. These are incorrect calculations.

69. Application, implementation, physiological integrity, (b).
    3. **The action of the drug takes 2 to 3 weeks while blood levels are building.**
    1. It should be taken in the morning so the effects of the drug are the strongest during waking hours.
    2. The action of the drug does not occur in 24 hours; 2 to 3 weeks are required while blood levels are building.
    4. This is not necessary.

70. Application, implementation, physiological integrity, (c).
    3. **Ciprofloxacin (Cipro) can increase theophylline levels.**
    1. Fluids should be forced.
    2. Ciprofloxacin should be started while results are pending.
    4. The two medications can be given together.

71. Application, implementation, physiological integrity, (b).
    2. **Check the apical pulse 1 full minute and hold medication if it is less than 60.**
    1. The patient should be weighed every week.
    3. Pulse is more significant.
    4. Digitalis level, not clotting time, is monitored.

72. Comprehension, implementation, physiological integrity, (a).
    3. **Drug is irritating to the gastrointestinal tract; taking the drug with meals decreases irritation.**
    1. Taking the drug at bedtime can irritate the GI tract.
    2. Taking the drug before breakfast can irritate the GI tract.
    4. Taking the drug between meals can irritate the GI tract.

73. Comprehension, implementation, physiological integrity, (a).
    3. **This can cause patient injury.**
    1. This is not an action of atropine.
    2. Dilation of pupils does not cause vertigo.
    4. This medication decreases diaphoresis.

74. Knowledge, planning, physiological integrity, (a).
    X 1. **Bran interferes with the ability of the antacid to coat and protect the stomach.**

    X 2. **Citrus foods are antagonistic to erythromycin and therefore decrease its effectiveness.**
    _____ 3. Calcium and vitamin D actually work together in many functions in the body, including the formation of healthy bones and teeth.
    X 4. **Vitamin K is the antidote to warfarin (Coumadin). Warfarin is given as an anticoagulant, and vitamin K functions inside the body in the formation of clots.**

75. Knowledge, evaluation, physiological integrity, (b).
    3. **Epoetin (Epogen) is indicated for treating low hemoglobin and hematocrit in anemia.**
    1. This test would be used in the management of diabetes.
    2. This test would manage the healthiness of the renal system.
    4. An elevated WBC count would indicate the presence of infection; a depressed WBC count would indicate neutropenia.

76. Comprehension, assessment, physiological integrity, (c).
    2. **Atropine is a cholinergic-blocking agent that increases pupil dilation.**
    1. Meperidine (Demerol) would be contraindicated for patients with head injury, seizures, asthma, and other similar conditions. It is not recommended for patients with glaucoma.
    3. Pentazocine (Talwin) is an analgesic and would be contraindicated for a patient with a head injury.
    4. This is used to reverse the effects of respiratory depression of opioid analgesia.

77. Application, planning, physiological integrity, (c).
    2. **Metoclopramide (Reglan) is more likely to cause hypoglycemia because the food moves more rapidly through the gastrointestinal tract.**
    1. Reglan is synergistic with other CNS depressants.
    3. A side effect of metoclopramide is CNS depression.
    4. Administering it at this time increases effectiveness because it can act on the food that is present.

78. Comprehension, planning, physiological integrity, (c).
    3. **Oxybutynin (Ditropan) is an antispasmodic agent useful in treating these symptoms and neurogenic bladder.**
    1. This is a diuretic used in treating edema.
    2. This is an antihypertensive medication.
    4. This is a potassium-sparing diuretic used in treating hypertension.

79. Application, implementation, physiological integrity, (c).
    2. **These medications are better absorbed on an empty stomach.**
    1. These medications are better absorbed on an empty stomach.
    3. Patients should be instructed to drink at least 1.5 L of fluid to prevent nephrolithiasis.
    4. Vitamins should be taken; however, they do not affect the time of administration.

80. Comprehension, planning, physiological integrity, (c).
    3. **The aim of this therapy is to reduce the viral load as much as possible for as long as possible.**
    1. The medication has decreased effectiveness with an increased viral load.
    2. Other antiviral medications in combinations are often used as treatment.

4. These medications are not effective at the end stage; resistant strains may have developed, and an increased viral load is present.

81. Application, evaluation, physiological integrity, (b).
    2. Blood glucose should be tested before insulin is administered, to prevent hypoglycemia.
    1. This is true; failing to rotate sites can cause tissue damage.
    3. Food is necessary to prevent hypoglycemia.
    4. This is the purpose of having a family member involved in the education.

82. Comprehension, evaluation, physiological integrity, (b).
    1. A therapeutic level must be achieved and maintained to combat infection. In addition, a level should not be toxic.
    2. A therapeutic level shows adequacy and not toxicity.
    3. A therapeutic level needs to be reached as quickly as possible.
    4. Culture and sensitivity would show whether a medication is effective against an organism.

83. Comprehension, evaluation, physiological integrity, (c).
    3. Patients develop a tolerance to all side effects except constipation.
    1. Excessive sedation does not develop when doses are gradually titrated.
    2. Pain relief is vital. The patient develops a tolerance to respiratory depression.
    4. This is true; however, it does not answer the question.

84. Analysis, evaluation, physiological integrity, (c).
    3. Risk of addiction is minimal in patients who are taking medication to relieve pain and not for psychological reasons.
    1. This is rare in hospitalized patients.
    2. Pain medication should be administered before the pain becomes severe, to increase effectiveness.
    4. Tolerance is rare in severe acute or chronic pain.

85. Comprehension, implementation, physiological integrity, (b).
    2. Bacteria can mutate and become resistant if the entire course of antibiotics is not taken.
    1. Adequate fluids can prevent the risk of dehydration present with some groups of antibiotics.
    3. Following proper administration directions (e.g., taking with a small snack) is required.
    4. Certain antibiotics can be expensive; however, it is not the primary concern.

86. Comprehension, planning, physiological integrity, (b).
    3. Older patients on long-term use of alkalizing agents are especially susceptible to electrolyte disorders.
    1. This test would be ordered for suspected bleeding disorders.
    2. This test would be ordered for suspected renal disease.
    4. This test is ordered if diabetes is suspected.

87. Application, planning, physiological integrity, (b).
    2. It has a protective effect and is better able to work if it can come in contact with the lining of the stomach.
    1. Aluminum hydroxide (Amphojel) is not absorbed systemically.
    3. Aluminum preparations are more likely to cause constipation. The schedule of administration does not affect the occurrence of diarrhea.

4. Rebound acidity occurs with prolonged use and is not related to schedule of administration.

88. Analysis, assessment, physiological integrity, (b).
    1. Mylanta binds with ciprofloxacin and may decrease effectiveness.
    2, 3. Aspirin and ibuprofen are not known to interfere with absorption.
    4. Penicillin and tetracycline antibiotics have been shown to interfere with the effectiveness of birth control pills.

89. Application, implementation, physiological integrity, (c).
    4. The cause of the diarrhea needs to be investigated if it persists beyond 2 days.
    1. Fluid intake needs to be increased to prevent dehydration.
    2. This medication needs to be taken at least 2 hours before or after other medications because the other medications will interfere with absorption.
    3. A fever is a sign that an infection may be present, and it needs to be reported. This medication also decreases absorption of salicylates.

90. Comprehension, implementation, physiological integrity, (c).
    1. The action of sucralfate (Carafate) is to line and protect the stomach; it is better able to do so if the medication can come in contact with the stomach.
    2. Patients taking this medication are usually being treated for ulcers. They should avoid spicy foods; however, any food would interfere with the action of this medication.
    3. Constipation is the most common complication of this medication.
    4. Sucralfate interferes with the absorption and decreases the effectiveness of many medications.

91. Application, evaluation, physiological integrity, (b).
    1. A side effect of this medication is sleeplessness.
    2. A side effect that should be reported is tachycardia.
    3. This is fine; however, it does not answer the question.
    4. Levothyroxine (Synthroid) can be taken with other medications. It is antagonistic to digoxin and synergistic with oral anticoagulants.

92. Comprehension, planning, physiological integrity, (a).
    2. Heparin is an anticoagulant; it is given to decrease the risk of thrombosis and deep vein thrombosis (DVT).
    1. The risk of blood loss is actually increased slightly.
    3. Epoetin (Epogen) is given to improve RBC production.
    4. Heparin is not an antibiotic.

93. Analysis, implementation, health promotion and maintenance, (b).
    3. It is critical that patients taking warfarin (Coumadin) report any signs of bleeding, including any blood observed in excreta.
    1. Warfarin is usually taken orally, not subcutaneously.
    2. This should be routine in every patient teaching situation.
    4. Blood levels are checked more frequently than every 3 months, especially during the initiation phase of treatment.

94. Analysis, planning, physiological integrity, (c).
    1. This is true; however, topical nitroglycerin is used preventively, and its absorption is unpredictable.
    2. This is the proper method for sublingual nitroglycerin.

3. This is true; however, if pain persists after three tablets, the person should report to the physician.

4. This is true; however, this method is not used in acute attacks.

95. Application, planning, physiological integrity, (b).

 3. To achieve therapeutic relief as quickly as possible, patients are given a loading dose. A maintenance dose is given to maintain the therapeutic stage.

1. Patients need relief and cannot wait to be brought into the therapeutic range.

2. Furosemide (Lasix) will help decrease edema in the body.

4. All patients need to be monitored for signs of toxicity.

96. Knowledge, planning, physiological integrity, (a).

 _____ **1. Fish is a major source of vitamin B$_{12}$.**

 __X__ **2. Bran prevents the absorption of calcium.**

 __X__ **3. Ascorbic acid increases the effect of salicylates.**

 __X__ **4. Green leafy vegetables contain large amounts of vitamin K, which is the antihemorrhagic vitamin and is used as an antidote for warfarin (Coumadin).**

97. Comprehension, evaluation, physiological integrity, (c).

 3. Celecoxib (Celebrex) is taken once per day to decrease prostaglandin synthesis.

1. Celecoxib can be taken without regard to meals.

2. Celecoxib is taken preventively to maintain a certain level of effectiveness that cannot be attained if taken p.r.n.

4. Nausea is a possible side effect; food may decrease effectiveness.

98. Application, implementation, health promotion and maintenance, (b).

 2. This medication should not be discontinued abruptly, to protect against possible seizures after the surgery.

1. These tests are done on a regular basis during therapy, not just at this point in time.

3. This is an ongoing direction until the effect of the medication can be judged.

4. This is an ongoing direction.

99. Analysis, implementation, physiological integrity, (b).

 3. Teach patient the importance of complying with therapy; effectiveness may take a few weeks.

1. This is true; however, it does not answer the patient's concerns.

2. This is not indicated at this point.

4. This is fine; however, it does not answer the concern of the patient.

100. Analysis, implementation, health promotion and maintenance, (b).

 1. Steroids cause hyperglycemia as an adverse effect.

2, 4. These are oral hypoglycemics.

3. This is a cardiac medication that does not cause hyperglycemia.

101. Analysis, implementation, health promotion and maintenance, (b).

 2. This is an oral hypoglycemic that is more effective when given at this time.

1. This is a cardiac medication that does not need to be given before breakfast.

3. This does not need to be given with food.

4. This should be given at bedtime to increase effectiveness.

102. Application, implementation, safe and effective care environment, (a).

 Answer: 2 tablets

 $250\,mg \times 2 = 500\,mg$ or $0.5\,g = 2$ tablets

103. Application implementation, physiological integrity, (b).

 3. This time would minimize impact on nutrition and growth and development.

1. Increased activity is not desirable at bedtime.

2. The appetite in growing children should not be suppressed.

4. The appetite before breakfast should not be suppressed.

104. Analysis, planning, physiological integrity, (b).

 1. Phenazopyridine (Pyridium) is a urinary tract analgesic that is prescribed for these symptoms.

2. This is a diuretic.

3. This is used to treat diarrhea.

4. This is an antibiotic used to treat urinary tract infections.

105. Comprehension, planning, physiological integrity, (b).

 1. This may indicate liver damage.

2. Restlessness is not an expected side effect.

3. Tachycardia is a more likely side effect.

4. Fatigue is an expected side effect.

106. Knowledge, assessment, physiological integrity, (b).

 3. These are the correct terms for the processes that all medications go through in the body.

1. Oral medications need to be digested as part of absorption; other routes do not require digestion. *Catabolism* means breaking down from complex to simple.

2. These are not the correct terms.

4. *Anabolism* means building up from simple to complex.

107. Analysis, implementation, health promotion and maintenance, (b).

 2. Weight and vital signs must be determined to establish a baseline to determine effectiveness of therapy.

1. For long-term therapy potassium levels should be monitored.

3. This is a side effect of long-term therapy and should be reported.

4. These assessments should be done on all patients on a routine basis.

108. Application, implementation, physiological integrity, (c).

 2. Patients should limit intake of dairy products because of their high calcium content.

1. Fluids help these medications to be excreted effectively.

3. This medication is more effective if taken without other medications.

4. Laboratory work needs to be checked to make sure that the medication is therapeutic.

109. Assessment, evaluation, physiological integrity, (b).

 1. A cough is commonly associated with angiotensin-converting enzyme inhibitors, resulting from increased sensitivity of cough reflex.

2. Hypotension is a therapeutic effect.

3. Diarrhea, nausea, and vomiting are common side effects.

4. This is not a documented side effect.

110. Comprehension, planning, physiological integrity, (a).

 3. This medication is more effective if given by itself.

1. This medication is less effective if given with food.

2. Medication is not effective when given with other medications.

4. This would be appropriate for analgesics.

111. Knowledge, evaluation, physiological integrity, (a).
    1. This is one of the earliest signs of toxicity.
    2. Aspirin is given to relieve headaches.
    3, 4. These may be signs of a blood sugar or a blood pressure that is too low.

112. Comprehensive, planning, physiological integrity, (b).
    2. This product is partially made from pork.
    1. A patient on hyperalimentation is usually unable to take anything by mouth and therefore requires a supplement either enterally or intravenously. This is not a contraindication for receiving an anticoagulant.
    3, 4. Patients on either of these diets are not restricted from receiving this medication.

113. Application, implementation, physiological integrity, (b).
    __X__ **1. This is important with all antibiotics.**
    _____ 2. This would be significant with erythromycin and penicillin.
    __X__ **3. This is important with all antibiotics.**
    _____ 4. This would be a consideration with tetracycline.
    _____ 5. This would also depend on the individual medication. Many of the newer antibiotics such as ciprofloxacin (Cipro) need to be taken only once each day.
    __X__ **6. This is important with all antibiotics.**

114. Knowledge, planning, physiological integrity, (b).
    2. Drugs of this classification block the effects of the parasympathetic system and are used to dilate the pupil for examination.
    1. Cholinergic agents are used to treat certain kinds of glaucoma and decrease intraocular pressure.
    3. These are used to remove cerumen from the ear.
    4. This is used for short-term treatment of ocular congestion.

115. Analysis, implementation, health promotion and maintenance, (b).
    3. He may be afraid of addiction or respiratory depression.
    1. This is not sufficient; a patient needs relief for a successful recovery.
    2. This should have been done before offering medication.
    4. This is appropriate but not before completing No. 3.

116. Knowledge, implementation, physiological integrity, (a).
    __5__ **Brachial artery**
    __6__ **Radial nerve**
    __1__ **Clavicle**
    __4__ **Humerus**
    __3__ **Deltoid muscle**
    __2__ **Acromion process**

117. Analysis, evaluation, health promotion and maintenance, (b).
    2. This is an antihistamine used to treat symptoms of allergic rhinitis.
    1. This may be a side effect, but it is not the reason the drug is given.
    3, 4. These are not reasons the drug is given.

118. Analysis, implementation, physiological integrity, (c).
    3. This is true and is the least anxiety-producing effect for the patient.
    1. This denies the patient's feelings and closes communication.
    2. This is true; however, it does not answer the question.
    4. This is a given; however, it does not answer the question.

119. Comprehension, implementation, physiological integrity, (a).
    Answer: 4 units. This patient would receive 4 units of regular insulin. Patients with diabetes are frequently given rapid-acting insulin based on the results of their Chemstrips.

120. Knowledge, implementation, physiological integrity,
    3. The correct order is plastic bag, roller clamp, volume control chamber, macrodrip chamber, secondary port insertion site.

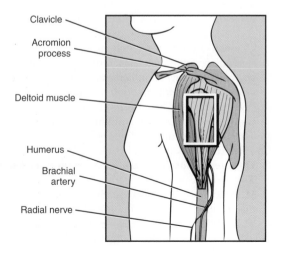

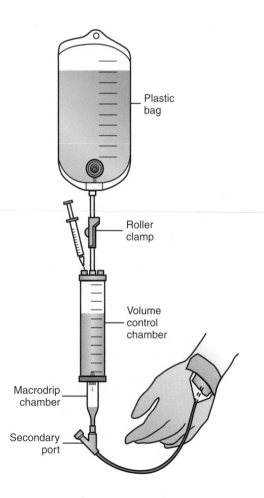

121. Comprehension, implementation, physiological integrity, (b).
    2. Barbiturate poisoning is treated with dialysis to cleanse the blood.
    1. Maintaining the patient's safety should be done with all patients. This patient will be sedated, not agitated.
    3. Blood work should also be done but dialysis is a priority.
    4. Phenytoin (Dilantin) may be used to control seizures but it is a CNS depressant.

122. Comprehension, implementation, physiological integrity, (b).
    X   1. Drowsiness is a side effect of clonazepam.
    X   2. Clonazepam is used to treat absence or partial seizure tolerance may develop decreasing effectiveness.
    _____ 3. Hypertension is not a documented side effect of clonazepam.
    X   4. Seizures should be controlled before driving or operation machinery.
    _____ 5. Secondary infections may develop with the administration of certain antibiotics.

123. Comprehension, implementation, physiological integrity, (b).
    X   1. The most important action of digoxin is to slow and strengthen the heartbeat. These actions improve the circulation. Therapeutic blood levels need to be drawn on a periodic basis.
    _____ 2. Monitoring blood pressure is not an indication of therapeutic level. This is always appropriate for cardiac patients.
    X   3. An overdose can lead to a heart rate that is lower than the desired rate of 60 to 80 beats/min.
    X   4. Green-yellow vision or other disturbances are early signs of digoxin toxicity.
    X   5. The pulse should always be checked before administration.
    _____ 6. An elevated temperature is not a side effect of digoxin. It may be an indication of a secondary infection.

124. Comprehension, implementation, physiological integrity (b).
    2. Birth control pills should not be used with a patient who has a history of circulatory conditions.
    1. It is true that varicose veins can be aggravated during pregnancy but this does that answer the question.
    3. This may or may not be true but it does not rule out the birth control pills as an alternative.
    4. An IUD may be a choice but it is not the only alternative.

125. Comprehension, assessment, safe and effective care environment, (c).
    X   1. The effect of this medication is enhanced because it interferes with the body's metabolism of the medication. Therefore the medication is available in the body longer. Patients should undergo regular digoxin level and INR measurements to assess for therapeutic levels.
    X   2. See the rationale for digoxin.
    X   3. See the rationale for digoxin.

    _____ 4. Although both are nephrotoxic, ibuprofen and Prevacid do not interfere with the effectiveness of each other.

126. Application, assessment, physiological integrity, (b).
    4. The patient may believe that she will become addicted if she takes the pain medicine. Reassure her that this is not true for the overwhelming majority of patients who take medications on a short-term basis.
    1. It is always important to assess a patient's pain. However, assessment alone does nothing to relieve pain.
    2. Patients should not be encouraged to endure pain. This is judgmental on the nurse's part.
    3. Nursing measures should always be used, but not in the place of medication.

127. Knowledge, assessment, physiological integrity, (b).
    3. This medication is ineffective in the treatment of petit mal seizures.
    1, 4. Carbamazepine can be used carefully for controlling certain types of pain. Side effects are dangerous and include aplastic anemia, liver failure, and congestive heart failure (CHF). This drug should not be used if the patient responds to other medications.
    2. Carbamazepine is used to control grand mal seizures.

128. Knowledge, assessment, physiological integrity, (a).
    X   1. This symptom is commonly associated with hypothyroidism. Thyroid hormones promote metabolism, growth, and development.
    _____ 2. This is characteristic of hyperthyroidism.
    _____ 3. This is characteristic of hyperthyroidism.
    _____ 4. This is characteristic of hyperthyroidism.
    X   5. This symptom is commonly associated with hypothyroidism. Thyroid hormones promote metabolism, growth, and development.

129. Knowledge, planning, physiological integrity, (a).
    3. The treatment of adults with hypothyroidism involves this medication. It is generally successful because unlike with children, growth and development are complete.
    1, 2. These are not indicated for this condition.
    4. This medication inhibits synthesis of the thyroid hormone, which is contraindicated in hypothyroidism.

130. Application, evaluation, physiological integrity, (b).
    _____ 1. Respiratory infections are not generally responsible for itching (pruritus) reactions.
    X   2. There are many medications that interfere with sulfa drugs.
    X   3. It is always important to assess for additional symptoms.
    X   4. It is always important to assess for relief.

131. Comprehension, implementation, health promotion and safety, (c).
    Correct order: 12345.
    1. The priority is to lower the dangerous fever as soon as possible.
    2. Obtaining blood work should be done as soon as possible to determine potential causes.
    3. A broad spectrum antibiotic may be ordered—blood cultures will narrow the choice.

4. *The wound should be assessed for signs and symptoms of infection.*

5. *Giving a tepid (cool) sponge bath may feel good to the patient, but does little to lower a high fever in a short period of time.*

132. Evaluation, implementation, safe and effective care environment, (b).

   4. *All diabetic patients including children need to learn sensitivity to what their body is telling them.*

   1. Oral pills require that the pancreas has some remaining capacity to produce insulin. Oral pills are not appropriate for type 1 diabetes.

   2. This is true. However, if the child is getting cold and clammy on a regular basis, he may need an adjustment in insulin to prevent hypoglycemia.

   3. Exercise is important. It needs to be balanced with meals and snacks.

133. Evaluation, assessment, health promotion and safety, (b).

   1. *This medication has an adverse effect of ototoxicity.*

   2. These medications are not generally ototoxic.

   3, 4. These side effects are not common with these medications.

134. Knowledge, assessment, health promotion and maintenance, (a).

   4. *Antihistamines must be used with caution in elderly adults because they do cause CNS depression. A smaller dose may be required.*

   1. Lisinopril is used to treat hypertension and congestive heart failure (CHF). Confusion is not an expected side effect.

   2. This is not an expected side effect of Vitamin D.

   3. This is a diuretic, and confusion is not an expected side effect.

135. Comprehension, implementation, physiological integrity, (b).

   3. *There are many reasons for a patient's noncompliance, as far ranging as unpleasant side effects and the inability to open a childproof cap.*

   1. This is incorrect because lack of financial resources is not the only reason for noncompliance. The nurse is making an assumption here.

   2. If the patient persists in not taking her medication despite nursing intervention, the physician will need to be notified.

   4. This is of course appropriate, but it does not solve the problem.

136. Comprehension, implementation, health promotion and safety, (b).

   _____ 1. Hypocalcemia should be corrected before the initiation of medication therapy. Calcium supplements should be taken as prescribed by the MD. These medications inhibit the reabsorption of calcium from bone to the bloodstream.

   __X__ **2. *An empty stomach promotes quicker absorption and decreases GI upsets, which are common side effects.***

   _____ 3. Food in the stomach will decrease the absorption rate.

   _____ 4. Exercise facilitates absorption.

   __X__ **5. *Osteomyelitis of the jaw is a common adverse effect.***

137. Knowledge, implementation, physiological integrity, (a).

   1. *The medication helps promote calcium entering and remaining in the bones.*

   2, 3, 4. These are all true statements, but they do not answer the question.

138. Knowledge, assessment, physiological integrity, (a).

   4. *Imitrex is used to treat migraine headaches. It causes vasoconstriction and blocks nerve fibers that transmit pain impulses.*

   1. Phenytoin (Dilantin) is one of several agents used to treat epilepsy.

   2. There are many medications used to treat depression, including bupropion (Wellbutrin) and escitalopram (Lexapro).

   3. Parkinson disease is treated with levodopa and carbidopa (Sinemet).

139. Comprehension, implementation, physiological integrity, (b).

   2. *Diuretics should be taken early in the morning to avoid enuresis.*

   1. Hypotension is a side effect of diuretics. This is caused by electrolyte disturbance.

   3. This is true because hypokalemia is a side effect of diuretics.

   4. These foods are high in potassium.

140. Comprehension, assessment, health promotion and maintenance, (b).

   1. *Sulfa drugs increase the sensitivity of the skin to the sun. The face and arms are exposed during golf.*

   2. An allergic reaction to a kitten would be respiratory.

   3. An allergic reaction to a chemical in the pool would be more widespread on the body.

   4. Mexican food may cause allergies but the symptoms would be more extensive. They would include possible intestinal and respiratory symptoms.

141. Comprehension, assessment, physiological integrity, (a).

   4. *Because of a slower metabolism, elderly patients have increased susceptibility to the CNS effects of many types of medications. This also includes the possible interactions of over-the-counter medicines, prescription medications, and herbal remedies.*

   1. This is important but it does not answer the immediate concern.

   2. This is also important and may be a contributing or causal factor of the confusion experienced by the patient. It does not help with the immediate concern.

   3. This is important and may help determine a cause.

142. Comprehension, implementation, health promotion and maintenance, (b).

   3. *Mineral oil is no longer recommended to treat constipation because it interferes with the absorption of soluble vitamins. There is also a danger of pneumonia if mineral oil is aspirated.*

   1. This is true. However, it does not help with the patient's immediate concern.

   2. This is also true. However, it does not inform the patient of concerns over the use of mineral oil.

   4. Prune juice does not help prevent constipation, but it also does not answer the immediate concern.

143. Knowledge, implementation, physiological integrity, (a).
    __X__ **1. *These are central nervous system depressants. The first drug in the combination relieves pain. The second drug has sedating and/or tranquilizing effects.***
    __X__ **2. *These are central nervous system depressants. The first drug in the combination relieves pain. The second drug has sedating and/or tranquilizing effects.***
    __X__ **3. *These are central nervous system depressants. The first drug in the combination relieves pain. The second drug has sedating and/or tranquilizing effects.***
    _____ 4. Xylocaine is used for local anesthetic purposes.
    _____ 5. Codeine is given by mouth. This is not possible if the preoperative patient is NPO.

144. Comprehension, implementation, physiological integrity, (c).
    3. *This behavior frequently resolves when the pain is adequately assessed and treated.*
    1. Drug-seeking behaviors may occur when the patient's pain is undertreated. Many patients with acute pain are anxious when the pain is not relieved.
    2. Nursing interventions are always appropriate. They should not be used in the place of medications.
    4. This may be possible, but the physician should order adequate oral medications to equal intramuscular.

145. Knowledge, intervention, health promotion and maintenance, (b).
    1. *Albuterol is a short-acting agent used for acute asthma attacks.*
    2. Tiotropium bromide is intended for a long-term once-daily maintenance dose.
    3. This drug is intended for the prevention of asthma.
    4. Cromolyn sodium (Intal) is ineffective in the treatment of acute asthma. It is used for the prevention of asthma attacks.

146. Knowledge, assessment, health promotion and maintenance, (a).
    1. *Constipation is a side effect that the patient does not develop a tolerance to, unlike respiratory depression.*
    2. Urinary retention is not a common side effect
    3. The patient may or may not be on a vitamin supplement. It is not as crucial as a laxative.

4. An anxiolytic may be appropriate to decrease anxiety, but it is not standard.

147. Comprehension, implementation, safe and effective care environment, (b).
    3. *This is the procedure recommended by pharmacists. Nurses should follow their organization policies.*
    1. It is no longer recommended that medications be disposed of in the toilet. This practice has been found to cause environmental contamination.
    2. Many pharmacies will not accept discarded medications.
    4. This practice may lead to confusion and medication errors.

148. Knowledge, implementation, safe and effective care environment, (b).
    2. *This medication is applied topically to treat acne. This is not a steroid.*
    1. This is a low-potency topical corticosteroid that would be used to treat more severe acne. Corticosteroids have antiinflammatory side effects. They may also have adverse systemic effects. Steroids should always be continued as ordered.
    3. This medication is a high-potency topical steroid and not used to treat severe acne.
    4. This is an immunosuppressant drug when applied topically. It is used to treat atopic dermatitis (eczema).

149. Knowledge, assessment, physiological integrity, (a).
    2. *Prolonged use of Celebrex (a COX-2 inhibitor) is a significant risk factor for gastrointestinal bleeding.*
    1, 3. These are not common side effects of this medication.
    4. Celebrex can be used to replace chronic pain although it is not usually used to treat headaches.

150. Application, implementation, safe and effective care environment, (b).
    3. *Older patients are especially sensitive to the effects of central nervous system depression. Benadryl and oxycodone have a synergistic effect on the CNS.*
    1. Assessment is important in identifying the potential cause, but it does not deal with the immediate concern for safety.
    2. This is important for any patient at high risk of falling.
    4. This would be advisable for any patient experiencing insomnia.

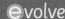
Objectives

After studying this chapter, the student should be able to:

1. Identify five principles of nutrition as presented in this chapter.
2. Describe the functions of nutrients found in the foods people eat.
3. Explain the strategies of the Dietary Guidelines for Americans 2010.
4. Review importance of economic considerations in meal planning.
5. Describe nutrition throughout the life cycle.
6. Demonstrate a beginning understanding of both standard hospital diets and diets ordered for specific conditions.

Nutrition is the combination of processes by which the body uses food for growth, energy, and maintenance. It is also the study of food and its relationship to health and disease. Increasing emphasis is being placed on the role of balanced nutrition in preventing many chronic illnesses. The body works to maintain balance in its chemical processes through homeostasis. The nurse plays an especially important role in the nutritional aspects of patient care. Because of close and continual contact with the patient, the nurse is able to evaluate and monitor the patient's nutritional status and inform the dietician or appropriate dietary person about the patient's nutritional needs and acceptance of the nutritional plan of care. Good nutrition is essential to good health throughout the life cycle, and the nurse is in an excellent position to encourage sound nutritional practice for each patient and the patient's family.

HEALTH PROMOTION

A. Goal: to increase the level of health of individuals, families, groups, and communities; requires a lifestyle change that will lead to new positive health behaviors
B. In 1990 the U.S. Department of Health and Human Services (USDHHS) issued a national report, *Healthy People 2000*, which outlined national health promotion and disease prevention objectives for people in the United States to be achieved by the year 2000. Nutrition was the key to these goals. This study was updated as *Healthy People 2010*. *Healthy People 2010* challenged everyone—individuals, communities, and professionals—to take specific steps to ensure that good health and long life are enjoyed by all. In December 2010, USDHHS launched *Healthy People 2020*, which has four overarching goals:
    1. Attain high-quality, longer lives free of preventable disease, disability, injury, and premature death
    2. Achieve health equity, eliminate disparities, and improve the health of people in all groups
    3. Create social and physical environments that promote good health for all
    4. Promote quality of life, healthy development, and healthy behaviors across all life stages

DEFINITIONS COMMONLY USED IN NUTRITION

Absorption: the process by which end products of digestion are absorbed from the small intestine into circulation to be distributed to the cells

Anabolism: the process by which food molecules are built up into more complex chemical compounds

Basal metabolism: the energy required for the body to sustain life while in a resting state

Calorie: standard unit for measuring energy needed to raise the temperature of water by $1\,^{\circ}C$ as the standard temperature

Catabolism: the breakdown of food molecules into carbon dioxide and water, which releases energy

Cellulose: a polysaccharide that makes up a framework of plants

Chemical digestion: action of enzymes that breaks large food molecules into smaller molecules

Cholesterol: a complex fat-related compound

Complementary proteins: foods that, when eaten together, supply the amino acid that is missing or in short supply in other food

Complete proteins: foods that contain all nine of the essential amino acids

Condensed: water removed and sugar added so carbohydrate content is increased

Conditionally indispensable amino acids: amino acids that the body can manufacture from other amino acids and that must be consumed in the diet under certain physiological conditions

Dietary fiber: the total amount of naturally occurring material in foods, mostly plants, that is not digested by the human digestive system and therefore is not absorbed

Digestion: the process of changing foods so they can be absorbed and used by cells

Disaccharides: double sugars

Dispensable amino acids: five amino acids that the body can manufacture from other amino acids

Enriched: the addition of nutrients to a food

Evaporated: heated above the boiling point so more than half of the water evaporates

Extracellular: all body fluids outside cells

Fortified: the replacement in food of nutrients lost during processing

Homeostasis: a condition in which the biological or physical body is not lacking any nutrients

Homogenized: fat particles evenly dispersed so cream does not separate

Hydrogenation: the process of adding hydrogen to a liquid or polyunsaturated fat and changing it to a solid or semisolid state

Hypervitaminosis: the excess of one or more vitamins

Hypoglycemia: low blood sugar

Incomplete proteins: foods that lack one or more of the essential amino acids

Indispensable amino acids: five amino acids that the body cannot manufacture from other amino acids

Intracellular: fluid within cells

Invisible fats: fats in which the fat is less obvious

Kilocalorie: the unit most often used in nutritional guidelines, equal to 1000 calories

Mechanical digestion: chewing, swallowing, peristalsis; breaks food into small pieces, mixes it with digestive juices, and moves it along the digestive tract

Monosaccharides: single sugars

Nutrients: chemical substances that are present in food and needed by the body to function

Nutrition: process by which the body uses food for growth, energy, and maintenance

Pasteurized: heated to a specific temperature to destroy pathogenic bacteria

Polysaccharides: complex carbohydrates

Precursor: substance that precedes and can be changed into an active vitamin

Saturated fats: organic compounds that are completely filled with all the hydrogen they can hold

Synthetic: manufactured vitamins

Unsaturated fats: hydrogen can be added to one or more places in a chemical structure

Visible fats: fats that are readily seen

Vitamins: organic compounds needed in small amounts for growth and maintenance of life

ABBREVIATIONS

AI: adequate intake

DRI: dietary reference intake

EAR: estimated average requirement

HDL: high-density lipoprotein (good cholesterol)

LDL: low-density lipoprotein (bad cholesterol)

RDA: recommended dietary allowance

TC: total cholesterol

TFAs: trans fatty acids

TPN: total parenteral nutrition

Type 1 diabetes mellitus (formerly called *IDDM*): insulin-dependent diabetes mellitus

Type 2 diabetes mellitus (formerly called *NIDDM*): non–insulin-dependent diabetes mellitus

UL: upper intake level

WIC: women, infants, and children

PRINCIPLES OF NUTRITION

A. Functions of food
   1. Provides energy
   2. Builds and repairs body tissues

   3. Regulates and controls the chemical processes in the body, which are essential for providing energy and building tissues
B. Evidence of good nutrition (Table 4-1)
   Individuals who receive less than desired amounts of nutrients have a greater risk of physical illness, are limited in physical work and mental capacity, and have lower immune system function than do people receiving adequate nutrients.
C. Primary causes of nutritional deficiency
   1. Dietary lack of specific essential nutrients caused by:
      a. Anorexia (resulting from a variety of causes).
      b. Alcoholism (and the resulting lack of proper nutrition).
      c. Poor food habits or eating nutritionally deficient foods.
      d. Anorexia nervosa or bulimia.
   2. Inability of the body to use a specific nutrient properly as a result of:
      a. Diseases of the digestive tract such as ulcerative colitis.
      b. Faulty absorption in digestive tract: malabsorption syndrome or excessive use of mineral oil.
      c. Metabolic disorders such as diabetes.
      d. Drug interactions or toxicity or both.
D. Classification of nutrients
   1. Nutrients are chemical substances that are present in food and needed by the body to function.
   2. Six prime nutrients
      a. Carbohydrates
      b. Fats
      c. Proteins
      d. Vitamins
      e. Minerals
      f. Water
   3. Individual nutrients have many specific metabolic functions. No nutrient ever works alone. In addition, the lack of one nutrient may inhibit the absorption or use of another nutrient.
E. Culture and nutrition
   1. Food habits are among the oldest and most deeply rooted aspects of many cultures. They are established early in childhood and can be difficult to change.
   2. In many cultures foods take on significance in life events, including serious illness.
   3. If possible, cultural preferences should be considered when any dietary modifications are planned.
   4. In many instances religion will greatly influence nutritional practice (Table 4-2).

ASSIMILATION OF NUTRIENTS
Digestion and Absorption

A. Digestion: the process of changing foods to be absorbed and used by cells; mechanical and chemical digestion occur simultaneously.
   1. Mechanical digestion (chewing, swallowing, peristalsis) breaks food into small pieces, mixes it with digestive juices, and moves it along the digestive tract.
   2. Chemical digestion occurs through the action of enzymes, which break large food molecules into smaller molecules.

Table 4-1 Clinical Signs of Nutritional Status

FEATURES	GOOD	POOR
General appearance	Alert, responsive	Listless, apathetic; cachectic
Hair	Shiny, lustrous; healthy scalp	Stringy, dull, brittle, dry, depigmented
Neck glands	No enlargement	Thyroid enlarged
Skin, face, and neck	Smooth, slightly moist, good color, reddish-pink mucous membranes	Greasy, discolored, scaly
Eyes	Bright, clear; no fatigue circles	Dryness, signs of infection, increased vascularity, glassiness, thickened conjunctivae
Lips	Good color, moist	Dry, scaly, swollen, angular lesions (stomatitis), cheilosis
Tongue	Good pink color; surface papillae present; no lesions	Papillary atrophy, smooth appearance; swollen, red, beefy (glossitis)
Gums	Good pink color; no swelling or bleeding; firm	Marginal redness or swelling; receding, spongy
Teeth	Straight, no crowding; well-shaped jaw; clean, no discoloration	Unfilled cavities, absent teeth, worn surfaces; mottled, malpositioned
Skin, general	Smooth, slightly moist; good color; good turgor	Rough, dry, scaly, pale, pigmented, irritated; petechiae, bruises
Abdomen	Flat	Swollen
Legs, feet	No tenderness, weakness, swelling; good color	Edema, tender calf; tingling, weakness
Skeleton	No malformations	Bowlegs, knock-knees, chest deformity at diaphragm, beaded ribs, prominent scapulae
Weight	Normal for height, age, body build	Overweight or underweight
Posture	Erect, arms and legs straight, abdomen in, chest out	Sagging shoulders, sunken chest, humped back
Muscles	Well developed, firm	Flaccid, poor tone; undeveloped, tender
Nervous control	Good attention span for age; does not cry easily; not irritable or restless	Inattentive, irritable
GI function	Good appetite and digestion; normal, regular elimination	Anorexia, indigestion, constipation or diarrhea
General vitality	Endurance; energetic; sleeps well at night; vigorous	Easily fatigued; no energy; falls asleep in school; looks tired, apathetic

Modified from Schlenker E, Long SL: *Williams' essentials of nutrition and diet therapy,* ed 10, St Louis, 2011, Mosby.
GI, Gastrointestinal.

a. Carbohydrate digestion begins in the mouth and occurs primarily in the small intestine; carbohydrates are reduced to simple sugars (monosaccharides) such as glucose for absorption. Sorbitol, a naturally occurring sugar that is not absorbed, may cause diarrhea in children.

b. Protein digestion begins in the stomach and is completed in the small intestine; proteins are broken down into amino acids for absorption.

c. Fat digestion begins in the stomach but occurs primarily in the small intestine; fats are reduced to fatty acids and glycerol for absorption.

B. Absorption: the process by which end products of digestion (fatty acids, glycerol, amino acids, glucose) are absorbed from the small intestine into circulation (blood and lymph) to be distributed to the cells. Vitamins may require proper pH to be absorbed. Patients with achlorhydria may develop vitamin B_{12} deficiency. Certain foods or beverages such as grapefruit juice can alter the metabolism or absorption of medications.

Metabolism

A. Use of food by the body cells for producing energy and building complex chemical compounds

B. Consists of two processes
1. Catabolism: the breakdown of food molecules into carbon dioxide and water, which releases energy; carbohydrates are primarily catabolized for energy.
2. Anabolism: the process by which food molecules are built up into more complex chemical compounds; proteins are primarily anabolized (used for building).

Energy

A. Energy is required for the metabolic processes of catabolism and anabolism; energy needs of the body are based on three factors.
1. Physical activity: the type of activity and how long it is performed
2. Basal metabolism: the energy required for the body to sustain life while in a resting state (1 calorie per kilogram of body weight per hour)

Table 4-2	Effects of Culture and Religion on Nutrition
GROUP	**COMMON DIETARY PRACTICES**
CULTURAL	
African Americans	Foods associated with the southern United States; milk and dairy foods may be lacking in the diet because of lactose intolerance prevalent in the group
Mexican Americans	Liberally seasoned food; many corn products used
Chinese Americans	Include staples of rice, wheat, and soy
Japanese Americans	Include rice, wheat, and seafood
Korean Americans	Include rice, wheat, highly seasoned foods such as cabbage
Italian Americans	Include pasta, breads, sauces, and cheese
Greek Americans	Include lamb, goat milk products, and cheese products
RELIGIOUS	
Jewish—orthodox	No pork products; meat must be slaughtered and prepared according to ritual; no mixing of meat and milk; only fish with fins and scales permitted
Muslim	Pork and alcohol strictly prohibited; 1-month period of daylight fasting observed during Ramadan; children, pregnant women, and ill individuals exempt from the fasting period
Hindu	Primarily vegetarians; beef not eaten
Roman Catholic	Restrictions on eating meat on Fridays (voluntary); special observance from Ash Wednesday through Easter voluntarily observed by some members of group

3. Thermal effects of food: energy required for the digestion, absorption, and metabolism of foods

B. Measurement of energy
   1. The calorie is the unit used to measure the energy value of food.
   2. Fuel values of basic nutrients
      a. Carbohydrate: 4 calories/g
      b. Fat: 9 calories/g
      c. Protein: 4 calories/g
   3. Total number of calories needed per day
      a. Moderately active man: 20.5 calories per pound (0.45 kg) of ideal weight
      b. Moderately active woman: 18 calories per pound (0.45 kg) of ideal weight

Drugs and Nutrition

A. Drugs affect taste, appetite, intestinal motility, absorption, metabolism, and excretion of nutrients and cause nausea and vomiting. Many of these interactions may compromise nutritional status and health.

B. If a nutrient binds with a medication, decreased solubility of both the nutrient and the drug can result. Interactions between certain foods and certain medications may alter the amount of drug that is available to the body. Foods or beverages containing alcohol can trigger a reaction in a patient taking disulfiram (Antabuse), a treatment for alcoholism.

C. People at greatest risk of undesirable drug-nutrient interaction are those taking medication for long periods, those taking two or more medications, and those not eating well. Elderly people fall into the high-risk category.

D. Certain medications may cause weight gain through retained fluid or increased appetite.

NUTRIENTS

Carbohydrates

A. Classification
   1. Monosaccharides: single sugars, which require no digestion and are easily absorbed into the bloodstream (e.g., glucose, fructose, galactose)
   2. Disaccharides: double sugars, which must be broken down before absorption (e.g., sucrose [table sugar], lactose, maltose)
   3. Polysaccharides: complex carbohydrates composed of many sugar units (e.g., starches, glycogen, dietary fiber)

B. Functions
   1. Provide energy (glucose is the only form of energy that can be used by the central nervous system)
   2. Protein-sparing effect (allows protein to be used for tissue building rather than energy production)
   3. Essential for complete metabolism of fats (incomplete fat metabolism leads to buildup of ketones and acidosis)

C. Sources
   1. Polysaccharides (complex carbohydrates): bread, cereal, pasta, rice, corn, baked goods
   2. Disaccharides (double sugars): table sugar, sugar cane, molasses
   3. Monosaccharides (simple carbohydrates): fruit, honey, milk

D. Digestion and metabolism
   1. Carbohydrate digestion occurs primarily in the small intestine and is acted on by three enzymes: sucrase, lactase, and maltase. Gas in the intestinal tract is largely a result of incomplete digestion of carbohydrates.
   2. Carbohydrates must be broken down into monosaccharides before being absorbed.
   3. Monosaccharides are carried to the liver, where glucose is released to the cells.

4. Excess glucose is stored as glycogen to be used when needed or converted to fat and stored as fat tissue.
5. Insulin regulates the use of glucose for use by the cells, thereby lowering blood sugar.
6. The hormone glucagon regulates the conversion of glycogen back to glucose, causing an increase in blood glucose.
7. The speed with which food raises the blood glucose is the glycemic index.
8. Hypoglycemia in people who do not have diabetes can be managed with small feedings approximately every 3 hours from a diet that is low in sugar and high in fiber.

E. Excess carbohydrates in diet may lead to:
1. Obesity.
2. Tooth decay and gum disease.
3. Malnutrition (if empty-calorie foods such as candy and soft drinks are consumed extensively).

F. Dietary considerations
1. The greater portion of carbohydrates should come from starches, and the least from simple sugars (which provide empty calories).
2. Encourage the intake of whole-grain bread and cereal products; if refined cereal products are used, they should be enriched.

G. Dietary fiber
1. Definition: the total amount of naturally occurring material in foods, mostly plants, that is not digested by the human digestive system and therefore is not absorbed. Adequate amounts are needed to facilitate proper bowel movements and reduce serum cholesterol and blood glucose levels and the risk of cancer.
2. There are two categories of dietary fiber: soluble and insoluble, based on the solubility in water.

Protein

A. Composed of amino acids
1. Essential amino acids: amino acids that the body cannot manufacture in sufficient quantity, or at all, and that therefore must be supplied in the diet. There are nine (essential) amino acids.
2. Nonessential amino acids: amino acids that the body can manufacture from other amino acids; therefore they are not necessary in the diet.
3. Conditional amino acids: amino acids that are usually not essential, except in times of illness and stress.

B. Functions
1. Build and repair body tissue (primary function)
2. Furnish energy if carbohydrate or fat is insufficient for this purpose
3. Maintain normal circulation of tissue and blood vessel fluids through the action of plasma protein
4. Aid metabolic functions by combining with iron to form hemoglobin; used to manufacture enzymes and hormones
5. Aid body defenses by manufacturing lymphocytes and antibodies

C. Digestion and metabolism
1. Digestion of protein begins in the stomach, where it is acted on by the enzyme pepsin. Digestion is completed in the small intestine by three enzymes: trypsin, chymotrypsin, and carboxypeptidase.
2. Protein must be broken down into amino acids to be absorbed and distributed to the cells. Accumulation of uric acid, a byproduct of purine catabolism, can cause gout. High intake of animal protein is associated with kidney stones.
3. End products of protein metabolism are hydrogen, oxygen, nitrogen, water, uric acid, and urea.
4. Dietary deficiencies of B-complex vitamins may cause elevated levels of homocysteine, an amino acid product linked to vascular disease in coronary and renal blood vessels.

D. Types and sources
1. Complete proteins: foods that contain all nine essential amino acids in amounts capable of meeting human requirements (mainly animal sources such as meats, fish, poultry, eggs, milk, cheese)
2. Incomplete proteins: foods that lack one or more of the essential amino acids (mainly plant sources such as cereal grains, nuts, legumes, lentils)
3. Complementary proteins: foods that, when eaten together, supply the amino acid that is missing or in short supply in the other food (e.g., peanut butter with bread, beans with rice, baked beans with brown bread). A rule of thumb is that a grain and a legume eaten together supply all the essential amino acids.

E. Dietary considerations
1. To build a healthier plate, dietary guidelines recommend varying one's protein food choices.
2. Dietary proteins are not stored in the body as amino acids. Proteins are the main components needed to build and repair body tissues. If the right amount and types are not available, the nitrogen is broken off, and the remainder of the protein is used for energy or stored as fat. The need for cell building and maintenance is continuous. For a supply of proteins to be available on a regular basis, a source of complete proteins should be eaten at every meal.
3. Increased protein is necessary during periods of growth, illness, injury, or stress; after surgery; and when bed rest is prescribed (especially for older adults). Protein supplements such as creatine may not enhance growth or endurance, despite marketers' claims.
4. Kwashiorkor, a protein-deficiency disease, is seen in many underdeveloped countries.
5. Marasmus is overt starvation caused by a deficiency of calories from any source.
6. Leptin and other hormones secreted by adipose tissue act on the brain to control appetite.

Fats (Lipids)

A. Functions
1. Supply energy for body activities when carbohydrates are not available. All body tissues except brain and nervous cells can use fat for energy. Most concentrated form of energy yields 9 calories/g.
2. Act as insulation to maintain body temperature and protect organs from mechanical injury
3. Carry fat-soluble vitamins A, D, E, and K and aid in their absorption
4. Provide a feeling of fullness and satisfaction after eating because of their slow rate of digestion

5. Furnish the essential fatty acid linoleic acid, which is found primarily in vegetable oils; called *essential* because they cannot be synthesized in the body and are vital to body functioning

6. Omega-3 fatty acids (polyunsaturated fat), which are found in fatty fish, may contribute to lower risks of heart disease.

B. Types

1. Saturated fats: The chemical structure is completely filled with all the hydrogen it can hold. They are usually from animal sources and solid at room temperature (e.g., fats in meat, dairy products, eggs; coconut oil, palm oil, and chocolate are also highly saturated). Trans fatty acids (TFAs) tend to raise low-density lipoprotein (LDL) ("bad") cholesterol and lower high-density lipoprotein (HDL) ("good") cholesterol when used instead of fatty acids or natural oils.

2. Unsaturated fats: The chemical structure has one or more places where hydrogen can be added. They are less dense, are usually liquid at room temperature (with the exception of margarine), and are chiefly from plant sources (e.g., vegetable oils such as cottonseed, soybean, corn oil).

   a. Monounsaturated fats have one place for hydrogen to be added.

   b. Polyunsaturated fats have two or more places for hydrogen to be added.

   c. Hydrogenation is the process of adding hydrogen to a liquid or polyunsaturated fat and changing it to a solid or semisolid state (however, hydrogenation reduces the polyunsaturated fat content and therefore possibly reduces its health value).

   d. Triglycerides are fats eaten in foods or made in the body from other sources such as carbohydrates. Excess calories consumed in a meal are converted and transported to fat cells for storage.

C. Digestion and metabolism

1. Digestion of fat begins in the stomach, where gastric lipase acts on emulsified fats.

2. Major portions of fat digestion occur in the small intestine, where bile emulsifies fats (breaks it into small droplets); pancreatic lipase changes the emulsified fats into fatty acids and glycerol, the end products of fat digestion.

3. Fats are carried as lipoproteins to body cells, where they are either broken down for use as energy or stored as adipose tissue.

D. Sources

1. Visible fats: those readily seen (e.g., butter and margarine, salad oils, shortening, fat in meats)

2. Invisible fats: those in which the fat is less obvious (e.g., milk, avocado, cheese, lean meat)

E. Cholesterol: a complex fat-related compound

1. A normal component of blood and of all body cells, especially brain and nerve tissue

2. Necessary for normal body functioning as structural material in cells, in the production of vitamin D, and in the production of a large number of hormones

3. Supplied by food (mainly animal sources). Some are synthesized within the body, mainly in the intestinal walls and liver, in response to need. Excess calories consumed are converted into triglycerides for storage as fat.

4. A variety of factors, including diet, heredity, emotional stress, and exercise, affect blood cholesterol levels. Saturated fats tend to raise blood cholesterol, whereas polyunsaturated fats are recommended for lowering cholesterol levels.

5. Cholesterol is carried to and from body cells by special carriers called *lipoproteins*.

   a. HDL, or "good" cholesterol, carries cholesterol away from the arteries and back to the liver for removal from the body.

   b. LDL, or "bad" cholesterol, tends to circulate in the bloodstream and form plaque on the inner walls of arteries.

6. Risk is classified according to total cholesterol level as follows:

   a. Desirable: less than 200 mg/dL

   b. Borderline high risk: 200 to 239 mg/dL

   c. High risk: 240 mg/dL and over

7. If the total cholesterol level is borderline high or high, the levels and ratio of LDL and HDL should be evaluated.

8. High cholesterol levels predispose individuals to atherosclerosis, the underlying pathological factor of coronary heart disease, and other serious health problems.

9. Foods high in cholesterol are organ meats, animal fat, egg yolk, and shellfish.

F. Dietary considerations

1. The Dietary Guidelines for Americans 2010 ChooseMyPlate illustrates the five food groups that are the building blocks for a healthy diet through use of a familiar image—a place setting for a meal. Before you eat, think about what goes on your plate or in your cup or bowl. Further recommendations are to eat fewer foods that are high in solid fats.

2. To decrease dietary fat:

   a. Use leaner cuts of meat and more poultry; trim fats from all meats.

   b. Use egg substitute products or fewer eggs.

   c. Use low-fat milk products.

   d. Limit use of fat in cooking as much as possible.

   e. Decrease consumption of red meat.

G. Effects of excess fat intake

1. Obesity

2. Predisposition to serious conditions such as heart disease, diabetes, and stroke

3. Increased surgical risk

Vitamins

See Table 4-3.

A. Definitions

1. Vitamins: organic compounds needed in small amounts for growth and maintenance of life

2. Precursor (or provitamin): substance that precedes and can be changed into an active vitamin (e.g., carotene is the precursor of vitamin A)

3. Hypervitaminosis: the excess of one or more vitamins

4. Synthetic: manufactured vitamins

5. Enriched: the addition of nutrients to a food, often in amounts larger than might be found naturally in that food

6. Fortified: the replacement in food of nutrients lost during processing

Table 4-3	Vitamins		
VITAMIN	**SOURCES**	**FUNCTIONS**	**DEFICIENCY SYMPTOMS**
FAT-SOLUBLE VITAMINS			
A (retinol); precursor: carotene	Fish liver oils Liver Green leafy vegetables Yellow vegetables (corn, carrots, potatoes) Yellow fruits (apricots, peaches) Egg yolk Whole milk	Regenerates visual purple (necessary for good vision) Formation of bones and teeth Maintains skin and mucous membranes	Night blindness Retardation of skeletal growth Dry, scaly skin Dry mucous membranes Susceptibility to epithelial infection Xerophthalmia (corneal cells become opaque, slough off, can lead to blindness)
D (calciferol)	Sunshine Fish liver oils Fortified milk	Regulates calcium and phosphorus absorption and metabolism Essential for normal formation of bones and teeth	Lowered levels of calcium and phosphorus in blood Soft bones Rickets Malformed teeth
E (tocopherol)	Wheat germ Vegetable oils Dark green leafy vegetables	Inconclusive at present Preserves integrity of RBCs Antioxidant (protects materials that oxidize easily) Protects structure and function of muscle	Increased hemolysis (breakdown) of RBCs Anemia Breakdown of vitamin A and essential fatty acids
K (menadione sodium bisulfate; Aquamephyton)	Synthesis by intestinal bacteria Green leafy vegetables Pork liver	Formation of prothrombin (necessary in blood clotting)	Prolonged clotting time (bleeding tendencies) Hemorrhagic diseases
WATER-SOLUBLE VITAMINS			
C (ascorbic acid)	Citrus fruits Tomatoes Broccoli Strawberries Green peppers Cantaloupes Potatoes	Formation and maintenance of capillary walls and collagen formation Aids in absorption of iron	Scurvy (deficiency disease) Sore gums Tendency to bruise easily Poor wound healing Anemia
B_1 (thiamine)	Wheat germ Whole or enriched grains Legumes Pork and organ meats	Maintains carbohydrate metabolism Maintains muscle and nerve functioning	Beriberi (deficiency disease) Anorexia, fatigue, nerve disorders, irritability
B_2 (riboflavin)	Milk Organ meats Green leafy vegetables Enriched bread and cereals	Maintains appetite Maintains healthy eyes Maintains color and structure of lips Metabolism of nutrients	Sensitivity to light, dim vision Inflammation of lips and tongue, cheilosis Loss of appetite and weight
B_6 (pyridoxine hydrochloride)	Red meats (especially organ meats) Whole-grain cereals Pork, lamb, veal	Synthesis and metabolism of proteins Hemoglobin synthesis Maintenance of muscles and nerves	Nausea, vomiting, anorexia, anemia, irritability, CNS dysfunction, kidney stones, dermatitis INH can cause deficiency
B_{12} (cobalamin)	Found only in animal products Organ and muscle meats Dairy products	Protein metabolism Production of RBCs Nervous system function	Pernicious anemia (resulting from lack of intrinsic factor needed for vitamin B_{12} absorption)
Niacin (nicotinic acid); precursor: tryptophan	Meats (especially organ meats) Poultry and fish Peanut butter	Essential for normal functioning of digestive and nervous systems Essential for growth and metabolism	Pellagra (deficiency disease) Nervous disorders Diarrhea and nausea Dermatitis
Folic acid (folacin)	Citrus fruits Eggs Green leafy vegetables Milk products Organ meat Seafood Whole grains	Essential in formation of all body cells, especially RBCs Protein metabolism Prevents neural tube deficiency in newborn	Anemia (macrocytic) GI disturbances Glossitis Stomatitis

CNS, Central nervous system; *GI,* gastrointestinal; *INH,* isonicotinic acid hydrazide; *RBC,* red blood cell.

B. Characteristics
   1. Contain no calories
   2. Essential to life because they generally cannot be synthesized by the body and are necessary for cell metabolism
   3. Functions include tissue building and regulation of body functions.
   4. Needed in minute amounts (milligrams [mg] or micrograms [mcg]); the safety of taking megadoses is debatable.
   5. Well-balanced diet should provide adequate vitamins to fulfill body requirements.
C. Classified on basis of solubility
   1. Fat-soluble vitamins: A, D, E, K
      a. Sufficient fats needed in diet to carry fat-soluble vitamins
      b. Stored in body so deficiencies are slow to appear
      c. Absorbed in the same manner as are fats. Thus anything that interferes with absorption of fats interferes with absorption of fat-soluble vitamins (e.g., mineral oil, an indigestible substance, carries fat-soluble vitamins with it out of the body).
      d. Fairly stable in cooking and storage
   2. Water-soluble vitamins: C and B complex
      a. Not stored in body; possible deficiency if vitamins are not consumed in the daily diet.
      b. Easily destroyed by air and in cooking

Special Vitamin Considerations
A. Current research indicates that the effects of megadoses of vitamin C on the common cold are minimal.
B. Effects of vitamin C on cancer still require further study.
C. Claims list vitamin E as a "cure-all," especially in prolonging virility in men, preventing miscarriages, and curing muscular weakness.
D. Current research has not established the validity of these claims; however, the amounts usually taken in supplements have caused no damage.

Minerals
A. Definition: inorganic elements essential for growth and normal functioning (Table 4-4)
B. Types
   1. Major minerals, or macrominerals, are found in the largest amounts in the body and are needed in large amounts (100 mg or more per day); they are calcium, phosphorus, potassium, sodium, chlorine, magnesium, and sulfur.
   2. Microminerals, or trace elements, are needed in small amounts; examples include iron, zinc, copper, iodine.
C. Characteristics
   1. Found in all body tissues and fluids
   2. Occur naturally in foods (especially unrefined foods)
   3. Do not furnish energy but regulate body processes that furnish energy
   4. Remain stable in food preparation
D. Functions
   1. Constitute bones and teeth (calcium, phosphorus)
   2. Transmit nerve impulses and aid in muscle contraction
   3. Control water balance (sodium, potassium)
   4. Maintain acid-base balance
   5. Synthesize essential body compounds (e.g., iodine for thyroxine)
   6. Act as catalysts for tissue reactions (e.g., calcium needed for blood clotting)

Water
A. Water makes up 50% to 65% of the weight of an average adult.
   1. Intracellular: fluid within cells composed of water plus concentrations of potassium and phosphates; contains minerals, potassium, magnesium, and phosphorus
   2. Extracellular: all body fluids outside cells, including interstitial fluid, plasma, and watery components of body organs and substances; contains minerals and sodium chloride
B. Functions
   1. Essential component of all tissues and fluids
   2. Transportation of nutrients from the digestive tract to the bloodstream and from cell to cell; removal of waste products from cells to outside the body
   3. Lubrication of joints
   4. Maintenance of stable body temperature (as temperature increases, sweating occurs, evaporates, and cools the body)
   5. Solvent for all chemical processes in the body
C. Overall water balance in the body
   1. Intake: Under ordinary conditions adults need 2 to 3 L of liquid per day—five or six glasses of which should be water.
      a. Ingested fluids such as water, soups, and beverages
      b. Water in foods that are eaten
      c. Water formed from cell oxidation (when nutrients are burned)
   2. Output: averages 2600 mL daily
      a. Normal routes of excretion are primarily the kidneys but also the skin, lungs, and feces.
      b. Abnormal and extensive losses can occur from vomiting and diarrhea, open or draining wounds, fever, extensive burns, hemorrhage, and anything that causes excessive perspiration.
D. Additional fluids are required:
   1. By infants.
   2. During fever or disease process (especially kidney stones).
   3. In warm weather.
   4. During heavy work or extensive physical activity.

Cellulose
A. Definition: a polysaccharide that makes up the framework of plants; provides bulk (fiber or roughage) for the diet; cannot be broken down by the human digestive system and therefore is not absorbed
B. Function: to absorb water, provide bulk, and stimulate peristalsis
C. Found in the stalks and leaves of plants, the skins of fruit and vegetables, and the outer covering of seeds and cereals (refined cereals have most of the fiber removed and provide little bulk)

NUTRITIONAL GUIDELINES

DIETARY REFERENCE INTAKES
A. Developed by the Food and Nutrition Board of the National Academy of Sciences, this revised the recommended dietary allowances (RDAs)
B. Four types of Dietary Reference Intake (DRI) reference values
   1. The estimated average requirement (EAR)
   2. The RDA

Table 4-4 **Major Minerals and Microminerals (Trace Elements)**

MINERAL	SOURCES	FUNCTIONS	DEFICIENCY SYMPTOMS
MAJOR MINERALS			
Calcium (Ca): absorption aided by vitamin D	Milk and milk products Cheese Some green leafy vegetables (turnips, collards, kale, broccoli)	Bone and tooth formation Blood clotting Muscle (including heart muscle) contraction Nerve transmission Cell wall permeability	Poor bone and tooth formation Rickets (deficiency disease) Stunted growth Osteoporosis Poor blood clotting Tetany
Phosphorus (P): absorption with Ca aided by vitamin D	Milk and cheese Meat Egg yolk Whole grains (diet adequate in protein and Ca should be adequate in P)	Functions as calcium phosphate in calcification of bones and teeth Energy metabolism Regulation of acid-base balance Cell structure and enzyme activity	Poor bone and tooth formation Rickets (deficiency disease) Retarded growth Weakness Anorexia
Sodium (Na)	Salt Baking powder and soda Dairy products Meat, fish, and poultry Range of 500-2400 mg daily	Regulation of acid-base balance Fluid balance Nerve transmission and muscle contraction	Nausea and vomiting Apathy Exhaustion Abdominal and muscle cramps Glucose absorption
Potassium (K)	Meat, fish, and poultry Whole-grain breads and cereals Fruits (oranges, bananas) Green leafy vegetables	Regulates nerve conduction and muscle contraction Necessary for regular heart rhythm Fluid and acid-base balance Cell metabolism	Abnormal heartbeat Muscle weakness Nausea and vomiting Deficiency results from dieresis
Chlorine (Cl)	Table salt (NaCl)	Formation of hydrochloric acid and maintenance of gastric acidity Maintenance of acid-base balance, osmotic pressure, and water balance	Deficiency results from fluid loss through vomiting, diarrhea, and heavy sweating
Magnesium (Mg)	Green leafy vegetables Legumes Milk Whole grains	Component of bones and teeth Enzymes essential in general Metabolism Conduction of nerve impulses Muscle contraction	Tremors leading to convulsive seizures
Sulfur (S)	Protein foods Meat Milk Eggs Cheese Nuts and legumes	Component of all body cells; important in building connective tissue Component in several B vitamins and several amino acids Energy metabolism	None documented
MICROMINERALS			
Iron (Fe): absorption enhanced by vitamin C, decreased by ASA (acetylsalicylic acid)	Organ meats (especially liver) Egg yolk Green leafy vegetables Lean red meats Dried fruits (apricots, raisins)	Synthesis of hemoglobin General metabolic activities	Anemia
Iodine (I)	Iodized salt Saltwater fish	Normal functioning of thyroid gland	Goiter
Zinc (Zn)	Oysters Liver High-protein foods	Component of enzymes Assists in regulation of cell growth Protein synthesis	Impaired wound healing Poor taste sensitivity Retarded sexual and physical development
Copper (Cu)	Liver Cocoa Nuts Raisins	Aids in absorption of iron Component of hemoglobin Component of enzymes	Unknown at present, although secondary conditions may develop

3. The adequate intake (AI)
4. The tolerable upper intake level (UL)
C. Primary goals are to prevent nutrient deficiencies and reduce the risk of chronic diseases such as osteoporosis, cancer, and cardiovascular disease.

U.S. DIETARY GOALS OR DIETARY GUIDELINES

A. Developed by the U.S. Department of Agriculture and USDHHS
B. Established in 1980 and updated every 5 years; the current Nutrition and Your Health: Dietary Guidelines for Americans 2010 was released January 2011. These guidelines emphasize three major goals for Americans. They are:
   1. Balance calories with physical activity to manage weight.
   2. Consume more of certain foods and nutrients such as fruits, vegetables, whole grains, fat-free and low-fat dairy products, and seafood.
   3. Consume fewer foods with sodium (salt), saturated fats, trans fats, cholesterol, added sugars, and refined grains.
C. The 2010 Dietary Guidelines for Americans include 23 key recommendations for the general population and six additional key recommendations for specific population groups, such as pregnant women. The recommendations are intended to help people choose an overall healthy diet.

Nutritional Labeling and Education Act of 1990

A. This regulation has increased consumer access to safe products and knowledge of what nutrients are in food.
B. The nutrition facts panel must include the serving size, calories (and calories from fat), and nutrients (i.e., how much of each nutrient and the percent daily value [%DV]).
C. Ingredients labeled GRAS are "generally recognized as safe" for ingestion by anyone. See www.fda.gov/Food/FoodIngredientsPackaging/GenerallyRecognizedasSafeGRAS/ default.htm for listing.

Nutritional Assessment

A. Two phases: screening and assessment. The purpose is to screen for nutritional risks and apply specific assessment techniques to determine an action plan.
B. Components of nutritional assessment: anthropometric measurements (e.g., body mass index), biochemical tests, clinical observations, dietary and personal histories. Techniques such as hair analysis have not been demonstrated to provide useful information about nutritional status. All components work together to allow determination of the best action plan for the individual in the healthy and sick populations within the context of the individual's personal, social, and economic background. Techniques such as the "energy panel" can be used to determine if nutritional status is adequate to support an active immune system.

ChooseMyPlate

Originally identified in the Child Obesity Task Force report, which noted that simple, actionable advice for consumers is needed, MyPlate replaces the MyPyramid image as the government's primary food group symbol as an easy-to-understand visual cue to help consumers adopt healthy eating habits consistent with the 2010 Dietary Guidelines for Americans. MyPyramid will remain available to interested health pro-

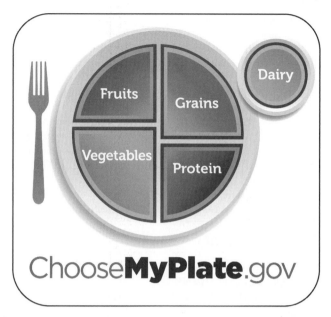

FIGURE 4-1 ChooseMyPlate. (Courtesy U.S. Department of Agriculture, 2010, Washington, DC.)

fessionals and nutrition educators in a special section of the new website (www.choosemyplate.gov). See Figure 4-1. *Note:* ChooseMyPlate illustrates the five food groups that are the building blocks for a healthy diet using a familiar image—a place setting for a meal. Before you eat, think about what goes on your plate or in your cup or bowl. The following are the guideline messages:

A. Balancing calories
   1. Enjoy your food but eat less.
   2. Avoid oversized portions.
B. Foods to increase
   1. Make half your plate fruits and vegetables.
   2. Make at least half your grains whole grains.
   3. Switch to fat-free or low-fat (1%) milk.
C. Foods to reduce
   1. Compare sodium in foods like soup, bread, and frozen meals—and choose foods with lower numbers.
   2. Drink water instead of sugary drinks.
D. ChooseMyPlate provides a list of 10 tips for a great plate.
   1. Balance calories—Find out how many calories *you* need for a day as a first step in managing your weight.
   2. Enjoy your food but eat less—Eating elsewhere may lead to eating too many calories. Pay attention to hunger and fullness cues before, during, and after meals. Use them to recognize when to eat and when you've had enough.
   3. Avoid oversized portions—Use a smaller plate, bowl, and glass.
   4. Food to eat more often—Eat more vegetables, fruits, whole grains, and fat-free or 1% milk and dairy products.
   5. Make half your plate fruits and vegetables—Choose red, orange, and dark-green vegetables like tomatoes, sweet potatoes, and broccoli, along with other vegetables for your meals. Add fruit to meals as part of main or side dishes or as dessert.
   6. Switch to fat-free or low-fat milk—They have the same amount of calcium and other essential nutrients as whole milk, but fewer calories and less saturated fat.

7. Make half your grains whole grains—To eat more whole grains, substitute a whole-grain product for a refined product, such as eating whole wheat bread instead of white bread or trying brown rice instead of white rice.

8. Foods to eat less often—Cut back on foods high in solid fats, added sugars, and salt.

9. Compare sodium in foods—Use the Nutrition Facts label to choose lower-sodium versions of foods like soup, bread, and frozen meals. Select canned foods labeled "low sodium," "reduced sodium," or "no salt added."

10. Drink water instead of sugary drinks—Cut calories by drinking water or unsweetened beverages.

FOOD MANAGEMENT

FOOD FADS AND FACTS: MEAT EATERS VERSUS VEGETARIANS

A. Problems occur when too large a portion of the diet consists of meat.
   1. Excess calories tend to be consumed. Meat (and the fat therein) is high in calories. Because of the taste, the tendency is to eat more than is required.
   2. When a large portion of the meal is meat, a smaller portion of fruits and vegetables is consumed; therefore less fiber and fewer of the nutrients in fruits and vegetables are consumed.
B. Vegetarians also can have nutritional deficiencies.
   1. Calories may be insufficient despite consumption of large amounts of foods.
   2. Protein can be lacking; incomplete protein must be supplemented with complementary proteins.
   3. Strict vegetarians may need supplements of cobalamin (vitamin B_{12}) because it is found only in animal proteins.
C. The ideal diet combines both types of diet with a variety of foods.
   1. Meat eaters should eat smaller servings of leaner meats with more fruits, vegetables, and cereals.
   2. Vegetarians should improve the quality of their diet by adding dairy products such as eggs and milk. (If no dairy products are taken, complementary proteins should be selected carefully.)

ECONOMIC CONSIDERATIONS IN MENU PLANNING

A. Plan menus in advance.
   1. Take advantage of specials and sales to plan balanced meals.
   2. Shop from a list to avoid impulse buying.
   3. Supplemental food may be available from programs such as the Women, Infants, and Children (WIC) program or Meals on Wheels.
B. Choose foods wisely.
   1. Buy foods in season and in good supply.
   2. Buy in quantity if adequate storage is available (larger quantities may cost less per unit).
   3. Buy sale items only if they can be used.
   4. Use unit pricing to find the best buys among brands.
   5. Know grades and brands of foods. Grading of canned goods has no bearing on nutritive value. Generic labeling can save up to 25% of name-brand items.
   6. Purchase staple and canned goods when on sale.

7. Remember that cost per serving rather than per pound is important, especially in buying meat.
8. Compare labels for weights and ingredients.
9. Buy less expensive forms of food (margarine is less expensive than butter).
10. Limit purchase of empty-calorie foods.
11. Decrease the cost of protein in the diet by using small amounts of meats, fish, and poultry and lower grades and less expensive cuts of meat; legumes, peanut butter, eggs, and cheese are good sources of less expensive protein.
12. Try to avoid convenience foods (any food bought partially prepared and ready to eat with little home preparation); they are usually more expensive than foods prepared entirely at home and less nutritionally balanced, containing high proportions of fat, calories, and sodium.
C. Care for foods after purchase.
   1. Store foods properly to avoid spoilage and loss of nutrients.
   2. Consume leftover foods quickly.

STORAGE AND PREPARATION OF BASIC FOODS

A. Milk
   1. Store milk refrigerated in covered container; powdered milk should be stored in a cool, dry place; refrigerate powdered milk after reconstituting.
   2. Cook over low heat; avoid scorching.
B. Cheese
   1. Refrigerate well, wrapped or in tight containers.
   2. It is most palatable if served at room temperature; cook at low temperatures for a short time.
C. Eggs
   1. Refrigerate promptly; avoid purchase of eggs that are already cracked (eggs that are cracked later should be used only in foods that will be well cooked).
   2. Cook at lower temperatures to prevent discoloration, curdling, or toughness.
D. Cereals and breads
   1. Store in cool, dry place; bread retains freshness best at room temperature but molds faster; it freezes well.
   2. Cook cereals according to directions; overcooking reduces vitamin content.
E. Meat, fish, and poultry
   1. Store in refrigerator for a short time or freeze for longer storage.
   2. Less expensive meats, although nutritionally equivalent to more expensive ones, require longer cooking at lower temperatures.
F. Fruits and vegetables
   1. Store ripe fruits and vegetables in the refrigerator (fruits ripen best at room temperature).
   2. Cook only until tender (steaming), using as little water as possible (cooking liquids contain valuable nutrients and should be used if possible); raw fruits and vegetables are especially nutritious.

TYPES OF MILK

A. Skim: fat and vitamin A removed (may have vitamins A and D added); contains all other nutrients of whole milk
B. Homogenized: fat particles evenly dispersed so cream does not separate

C. Pasteurized: heated to a specific temperature to destroy pathogenic bacteria (but nutrients are not affected)

D. Condensed: water removed and sugar added so carbohydrate content is increased; low in calcium and vitamins and high in sugar compared with whole milk

E. Evaporated: heated above the boiling point so more than one half of the water evaporates

F. Low fat: contains 0.5% to 2% fat; lower in calories than whole milk but comparable in nutrient value

G. Powdered or dry: water removed; least expensive form of milk on the market; when reconstituted has the same nutrient value as the milk from which it was made.

COMMON TYPES OF FOOD POISONING

STAPHYLOCOCCAL FOOD POISONING

A. Caused by *Staphylococcus aureus* bacteria; resistant to heat

B. Involves foods such as custard; potato, macaroni, egg, and chicken salads; cheese; ham; and salami

C. Exhibited by symptoms such as abdominal cramps, diarrhea, and vomiting; lasts 1 to 2 days; usually mild and attributed to other causes

D. Prevented by keeping foods above 140°F (60°C) or below 40°F (4°C); toxin is destroyed by boiling for several hours or heating in a pressure cooker at 240°F (138.5°C) for 30 minutes.

CLOSTRIDIAL FOOD POISONING

A. Perfringens poisoning – the most common causative agent of gas gangrene
  1. Caused by *Clostridium perfringens,* spore-forming bacteria that grow in the absence of oxygen
  2. Involves foods such as stews, soups, and gravies made from poultry and red meat
  3. Exhibited by symptoms such as nausea without vomiting, diarrhea, and acute inflammation of the stomach and intestine; usually lasts 1 day
  4. Prevented by storing foods properly and keeping foods above 140°F (60°C) or below 40°F (4°C)

B. Botulism
  1. Caused by *Clostridium botulinum,* spore-forming bacteria that grow and produce toxins in absence of oxygen (anaerobic)
  2. Involves canned low-acid foods, especially home-canned foods such as meats, corn, peas, green beans, asparagus, and mushrooms
  3. Exhibited by symptoms such as inability to swallow, double vision, and progressive respiratory paralysis; fatality rate high if condition is untreated.
  4. Prevented by pressure cooking canned foods for specified length of time; any can or jar with a bulging top should be discarded.

SALMONELLOSIS

A. Caused by salmonellae, bacteria widespread in nature that live in the intestinal tracts of humans and animals; transmitted by eating infected food or by contact with people who are infected or are carriers of the disease; also transmitted by insects or rodents

B. Involves poultry, red meats, dairy products, and eggs

C. Exhibited by symptoms such as severe headache, vomiting, diarrhea, abdominal cramps, and fever; usually last 2 to 7 days

D. Prevented by heating foods at 140°F (60°C) for 10 minutes or at higher temperatures for less time

ESCHERICHIA COLI INFECTION

A. Caused by pathogenic *E. coli;* some types are normally found in human intestinal system

B. Pathogenic *E. coli* found in raw ground beef

C. Bacterium attacks intestinal wall and spreads to body.

D. Exhibited by symptoms such as bloody diarrhea, cramps, fever, chills, dehydration, kidney problems; can be fatal

E. Prevented by using well-cooked meats and sanitary food handling

NUTRITION THROUGHOUT THE LIFE CYCLE

INFANT NUTRITION

A. Infants require more protein and calories per pound of body weight than adults do because infants have more body surface in proportion to weight and because of their growth and activity.

B. Breast-feeding is the recommended method of feeding, if possible. More vitamin C is provided, and protein and sugar are more easily digested than those in cow's milk. The infant is also provided with antibodies against disease, and breast-feeding assists in establishing the mother-child bond. In addition, breastfed babies have fewer allergies and intolerances and easier digestion.

C. Bottle-feeding is an acceptable alternative if close mother-child contact is maintained. Most mothers use a commercially prepared formula such as Enfamil; a soy-based product such as Isomil can be used if the infant is allergic to milk products. At no time during the first year of life should an infant be fed regular whole cow's milk. Concentration of cow's milk may cause gastrointestinal (GI) bleeding or renal discomfort. Skim milk or low-fat milk provides infants with too little energy and linoleic acid.

D. The American Academy of Pediatrics recommends breast milk supplemented by vitamin D and fluoride from birth and iron supplements after 4 months of age.

E. Introduction of solid foods varies among pediatricians, with most favoring a delay until the infant is at least 6 months of age.
  1. Infant cereal is usually given first (often with added iron to supplement a possible lack in the infant's diet; prenatal iron reserves last 5 to 6 months). Rice cereal is given first because it is easy to digest and provokes few allergies.
  2. Fruits, vegetables, and egg yolk are frequently given next. (Because of possible allergic reactions, egg white is delayed until late in the first year.)
  3. Solid foods should be introduced one at a time and at 4- to 5-day intervals to observe for any allergic reactions.
  4. Adding sugar or salt to an infant's food is undesirable.
  5. Infants can choke on small foods such as berries, corn, popcorn, hot dogs, or candy.
  6. Infants should not eat honey because it contains botulism spores, which can harm the infant (even though quantities are too low to harm older children and adults).

PRESCHOOL CHILDREN

A. Growth rate is slower and more erratic, and food intake varies accordingly.

B. A variety of foods should be offered.
  1. Finger foods such as carrot sticks are enjoyed.

2. Serve small amounts because too large a serving can discourage a child from eating.
3. Avoid refined sweets.
4. Do not coax a child to eat; if a food is refused, offer it at a later time.
5. Nutritious snacks are a viable alternative for a child who is a poor eater.

C. Teach healthy eating habits; avoid rewarding good behavior with food.

SCHOOL CHILDREN (5 TO 10 YEARS OF AGE)

A. Growth increase is gradual at this age (approximately equal for boys and girls).
B. Proper nutrition is important for proper mental and physical development; an adequate breakfast is important for alertness during class.
C. Children are usually good eaters at this age and should be encouraged by the examples set at home and at school. Promote healthy eating.

ADOLESCENTS

A. Tremendous growth spurt occurs at puberty (age of sexual maturity).
   1. For girls, usually between 10 and 13 years of age
   2. For boys, between 13 and 16 years of age
B. Diets are influenced by peers, with many empty-calorie foods being consumed. Adolescents tend to skip lunch. Eating disorders such as anorexia or bulimia may develop with impaired self-esteem issues.
C. Boys gain mostly lean muscle tissue; they consume large amounts of food to meet energy requirements.
D. Girls gain more fat tissue; their diets may be more influenced by a desire to remain thin; girls frequently require iron supplements to meet their needs; adequate nutrition during adolescence helps avoid complications during pregnancy. Promote healthy eating along with exercise.

ADULTS

A. Adequate nutrition throughout the life span is important for avoiding many serious illnesses.
B. Proper nutrition is based on guidelines set by U.S. government agencies (e.g., ChooseMyPlate).
C. Persons who consume a balanced diet usually do not need vitamin supplements.
D. If a woman of childbearing age is a smoker and has poor dietary intake, a vitamin C supplement of 100 mg/day is recommended.

OLDER ADULTS

A. Physiological changes affect nutrition of older adults.
   1. Aging slows the basal metabolic rate (BMR); combined with decreased activity, the result is decreased energy requirements and decreased number of calories needed.
   2. Taste may be adversely affected by gradual diminishing of the senses of smell, sight, and taste.
   3. Loss of teeth may affect proper chewing, food intake, or enjoyment. Older adults, children, and psychiatric patients may "pouch" or "cheek" foods or medications and should be checked to make sure that intake is indeed swallowed.
   4. Reduced saliva makes swallowing more difficult and digestion less efficient.
   5. Decreased movement of wastes through intestines contributes to constipation.
   6. Marginal deficiencies of ascorbic acid, thiamine, and riboflavin have occurred in some elderly patients.
   7. Decrease in absorption and use of nutrients results from decreased digestive juices and gastric motility reduction.

B. Economic and social considerations
   1. Decrease in income among older adults, combined with an increase in the amount spent for medical care, leaves less for adequate nutrition; the tendency is to eat less protein (which is expensive) and more carbohydrates (which are cheaper and easier to prepare).
   2. Loss of spouse, friends, or mobility results in isolation, depression, and often a decreased will to obtain adequate nutrition.

C. Planning diets
   1. Diet should be well balanced in protein, vitamins, and minerals (especially calcium and iron) to allow for diminished absorption.
   2. Calories should be sufficient to maintain energy and activity (reduced from those previously required).
   3. Soft bulk should be added to diet to prevent constipation (cooked fruits and vegetables).
   4. Increased fluid intake is required to eliminate metabolic wastes.
   5. Meals should be light and easily digested (i.e., contain only a small amount of fats); frequent small meals may be easier to digest than three large meals.
   6. Individual preferences should be respected, and the diet built around them; make changes slowly.
   7. Meals eaten with others are often more appetizing than those eaten alone.

PREGNANCY

A. A well-balanced diet with increased amounts of essential nutrients is important to the well-being of the mother and baby.
   1. A protein increase of 50% or 25 g/day over the normal diet is recommended to allow for growth of the baby, placenta, and maternal tissues and increased circulating blood volume, amniotic fluid, and storage.
   2. An increase in calories meets increased energy demands and allows protein to be used for tissue building. Calorie needs are approximately an extra 300 calories per day, which can be gained by adding a serving of dairy foods.
   3. The following are needed: increased amounts of calcium, phosphorus, and vitamin D for the mother and for the bones and teeth of the baby; iron for hemoglobin and prenatal storage for the baby; iodine for thyroxin for the mother's increased BMR; and vitamins A, B complex, and C.
   4. Weight should not be severely restricted; a gain of 25 to 35 pounds is considered healthy.
   5. Severe restriction of salt is unfounded.

B. Vomiting (morning sickness)
   1. Lower fat intake with more high-carbohydrate foods
   2. Fluids between instead of with meals
   3. Dry toast or crackers on awakening
   4. Avoidance of cooking odors

LACTATION

A. A baby requires 2 to 8 ounces of breast milk per feeding up to 6 months of age; the maternal need for all nutrients is increased during lactation.

B. Diet of a lactating mother should be high in protein and calories (approximately 500 extra calories per day).

C. Increased fluids are also required; at least 6 cups (1.5 L) of fluid in some form is recommended but preferably 3 L/day.

DIET THERAPY

NURSING RESPONSIBILITIES

A. Nutritional assessment: Assess physical characteristics of patient. Individualize care to allow for patient differences.

B. Evaluate the patient's tolerance to diet, and provide feedback to other health team members.

C. Assist patient in learning about required dietary changes; reinforce information and answer questions.

D. If possible, incorporate patient preferences to increase compliance with the nutritional care plan.

E. Prepare the patient for mealtime; assist as necessary.

F. See that each person receives the correct tray unless foods are being withheld.

G. Serve and remove tray promptly.

H. Teach patients the value of proper nutrition, and urge compliance with the nutritional care plan.

PURPOSES OF DIET THERAPY

A. To increase or decrease weight

B. To allow a particular organ or system to rest (e.g., a low-fat diet in gallbladder disease)

C. To regulate the diet to correspond with the ability of the body to metabolize a specific nutrient (e.g., diabetes)

D. To correct conditions caused by deficiencies

E. To eliminate harmful substances from the diet (e.g., caffeine, cholesterol, alcohol)

F. To nourish the body

DIET MODIFICATIONS

A. Calories may be increased or decreased.

B. Nutrients may be adjusted (high or low protein, low fat, low sodium).

C. Certain foods may be omitted (gluten, phenylalanine, or tyramine; those that might contain allergens) or added.

D. Texture may be modified (e.g., consistency—soft diet).

E. Meals are more frequent than the standard three.

F. Enteral feedings (tube feedings based on individual needs) or parenteral feedings for patients with compromised GI function may be used.

STANDARD HOSPITAL DIETS (MODIFICATIONS IN CONSISTENCY)

A. Clear liquid (surgical liquid)

1. Temporary diet of clear liquids—nonresidue, nonirritating, non–gas-forming; protein, vitamins, minerals, and calories inadequate; oral intake restricted in the absence of bowel sounds

2. Used after surgery to replace fluids, before certain tests, and to lessen amount of fecal matter in colon

3. Includes water, coffee, tea, fat-free broth, pulp-free fruit juices (apple), gelatin, and ginger ale

B. Full liquid diet

1. Foods that are liquid at room or body temperatures; may be adequate if carefully planned, although frequently deficient in iron

2. Used after surgery as a transition between clear and soft diet, in infections and acute gastritis; in febrile conditions, and for patients who are unable to chew or swallow or have an intolerance to food for other reasons

3. Includes all clear liquids; milk; creamed soups; ice creams; sherbets; plain puddings; and thin, strained cereal

C. Soft diet

1. Normal diet modified in consistency to have limited fiber; easily digested; nutritionally adequate

2. Used between full liquid and regular, for chewing difficulties, and in GI disorders

3. Includes tender meats and tender, well-cooked vegetables (those with a great deal of fiber should be pureed or omitted); fruits (no fiber) and plain cakes allowed; no spicy or coarse foods allowed.

D. Regular (general or house) diet

1. Adequate, well-balanced diet designed to appeal to most people

2. Used for individuals who do not require a modified or therapeutic diet

3. Includes all foods from ChooseMyPlate

ADDITIONAL MODIFIED (OR THERAPEUTIC) DIETS

Table 4-5 lists diets, foods allowed and omitted, and the purpose of the diets.

DIETS FOR SPECIFIC CONDITIONS

DIABETES MELLITUS

A. Classification

1. Type 1: onset is usually before 20 years of age. It is difficult to manage and requires dietary restrictions, insulin injections, and exercise.

2. Type 2: maturity onset. It usually develops after age 35 years. It is frequently controlled by diet alone; insulin or oral hypoglycemics or both may also be needed. Medications should be taken as prescribed under the direction of a physician. An alarming increase in the incidence of type 2 diabetes has occurred in children, adolescents, and young adults.

B. Diet is determined by age, gender, body build, weight, and activity. Maintenance requirements are the same as for a patient without diabetes. Blood glucose levels are monitored with fasting or postprandial specimens and hemoglobin A_{1c} (HgbA$_{1c}$) (done approximately every 3 months).

1. Calories should be sufficient to maintain ideal body weight (approximately 30 calories/kg ideal weight).

2. Protein as outlined in the DRIs.

3. Carbohydrates should be obtained with the greatest portion from complex carbohydrates such as starches and the least from simple sugars. Readily digestible sugars may be needed to counteract hypoglycemic episodes. Hypoglycemic symptoms associated with premenstrual syndrome do not respond to dietary modifications.

4. Fats should be moderately controlled, with less than 7% from saturated fat.

5. High-fiber foods, which decrease postprandial blood glucose levels, are encouraged.

C. Exchange system is used for planning the diabetic diet.

1. It is based on a simple grouping of common foods according to equivalent nutritional values.

Table 4-5   **Modified or Therapeutic Diets**

DIET	CONDITION	FOODS ALLOWED	PURPOSE OF DIET

High-calorie	Underweight (10% or more)
	Anorexia nervosa
	Hyperthyroidism
		Emphasis on increase in calories
		Easily digested foods
		    (carbohydrates) recommended
		Full meals with high-calorie snacks
			Meet the increased metabolic
			    needs of the body or provide
			    increased calories for weight
			    gain

Low-calorie	Overweight	Fruits and vegetables especially
		    recommended
			Reduce the caloric intake below
			    body requirements so weight
			    loss will occur

High-protein	Children who need additional
	    protein for growth
	After surgery
	Pregnancy and lactation
	Conditions that cause protein loss
	Extensive burns
		Added amounts of poultry, meat,
		    fish, milk, cheese, and eggs
		Nonfat dry milk added to soups
		    and baked goods
			Increase the intake of high-
			    protein foods for maintaining
			    and rebuilding tissues and
			    correcting protein loss

Low-protein	Liver disease
	Kidney diseases leading to renal
	    failure
		Fruits and vegetables
		Severely limited in amounts
		    of meats, fish, poultry, eggs,
		    and dairy products
			Limit the end products of protein
			    metabolism to avoid disturbing
			    the fluid, electrolyte, and acid-
			    base balances

High-residue	Constipation (atonic) Diverticulitis (when inflammation has ceased)	Increased whole-grain cereals Increased fruits and raw vegetables Fibrous meats	Mechanically stimulate the GI tract

Low-residue	Before and after bowel surgery
	Ulcerative colitis
	Diverticulitis (during inflammatory
	    stage)
	Diarrhea
		Soft cheeses
		Tender meats
		Refined cereals and breads
		Pureed fruits and vegetables
		Plain puddings
			Soothe and be nonirritating to
			    GI tract

Low-fat	Gallbladder disease
	Obesity
	Cardiovascular disease
		Vegetables and fruits
		Skim milk
		Sherbet
		Increased carbohydrates and
		    proteins
			Lower fat content in diet (may be
			    deficient in fat-soluble vitamins)

Low-cholesterol	Cardiovascular disease	Lean meats and fish
		Poultry without the skin
		Liquid vegetable oils
		Skim milk
			Decrease the blood cholesterol
			    levels or maintain them at
			    acceptable levels

High-iron	Anemias	Regular diet with high-iron foods Liver and organ meats Red meats Dried fruits Egg yolks	Correct an iron deficiency

Sodium-restricted	Kidney disease
	Cardiovascular disease
	Hypertension
		Natural foods without salt
		Milk and meat in limited quantities
			Control or correct the retention of
			    sodium and water in the body
			    by controlling sodium intake

High-carbohydrate	Preparation for surgery
	Liver disease
	Kidney disease
		Emphasis on carbohydrate foods
		Full meals with high-carbohydrate
		    snacks
			Provide increased energy and
			    spare protein for tissue building

Low-carbohydrate	Dumping syndrome
	Hyperinsulinism
	Diabetes mellitus (although severe
	    restriction of carbohydrates is
	    currently considered unwarranted)
		Proteins
		Only enough carbohydrate to
		    maintain health and perform
		    activities
			Decrease the amounts of glucose
			    in the bloodstream (increased
			    blood glucose causes increased
			    amounts of insulin to be
			    produced by the body)

Lactose-restricted	Lactose intolerance	Avoid foods containing lactose
		    such as milk, cheese,
		    and ice cream
			Eliminate or cut down on
			    lactose—a substance certain
			    individuals cannot metabolize

GI, Gastrointestinal.

2. There are six basic food groups or food exchanges; each food within the group contains approximately the same food value as other foods within the same group.
   a. Milk: equal to 1 cup (240 mL) whole milk
   b. Vegetables: variety of low-carbohydrate vegetables
   c. Fruit: fresh or canned without sugar
   d. Bread: starchy items (breads, pasta, cereals, and vegetables equal to 1 slice bread)
   e. Meat: protein food equal to 1 oz (28 g) lean meat
   f. Fat equal to 1 tsp (5 mL) margarine
3. Total exchanges per day are determined by individual nutritional needs based on nutritional standards. (Table 4-6 shows a sample diet based on the exchange system.)
4. Advantages of exchange system
   a. Easy to understand
   b. Allows patients with diabetes more freedom to choose foods they like
   c. Allows choice of foods that fit into their economic status
   d. Can be used for other types of diets
   e. Does not require dietetic or specialized diabetic foods

? Critical Thinking Challenge

A 13-year-old patient has type I diabetes. Because he is starting puberty and is active with extra-curricular activities, these considerations have to be taken into account when planning his carbohydrate intake for each meal. The patient prefers to do self-injection prior to each meal. Below is a typical lunch for this patient who is on a 2200-kcal diet.

Lunch—Vegetable soup	(1 g CHO)
Tuna sandwich on whole-wheat bread	(16 g CHO)
Tuna ½ cup, drained	
Reduced fat mayonnaise (2 tsp.)	
Chopped dill pickle	
Chopped celery	
1 fresh pear	(15 g CHO)

Given the above lunch for this type I diabetic patient, calculate the amount of regular insulin this patient should inject prior to this meal.

The rule of thumb is to give 1 unit of insulin for every 15 g of CHO. Add the number of CHOs given (1+16+15=32 g of CHO. Then set up the problem in a ratio proportion.

15 g: 1 unit = 32 g: x units
15x = 32
32 divided by 15 = 2.1
x = 2.1 units

SURGERY

A. Surgery increases the nutritional demands on the body.
   1. Protein is increased for tissue repair, to prevent tissue breakdown, and to help replace blood and fluid losses.
   2. Carbohydrates are increased to meet body demands for energy and to spare protein for tissue building.
   3. Vitamins are especially important in wound healing; vitamin C cements cells and builds connective tissue and capillaries.
   4. Minerals, especially zinc, are also essential to wound healing.

Table 4-6 1800-Calorie Diet with Food Exchanges*

EXCHANGE GROUP	TOTAL EXCHANGES FOR THE DAY
Milk	2
Vegetables	2
Fruit	5
Bread	9
Meat	8
Fat	7

SAMPLE DIET	EXCHANGE LIST
BREAKFAST	
Black coffee	Free
2 eggs	2 meat
2 pieces toast	2 bread
with butter	2 fat
Cereal	1 bread
with milk	1 milk
and plain blueberries	1 fruit
LUNCH	
Turkey sandwich (3 oz [84 g])	2 breads, 3 meat
with mayonnaise (2 tsp [10 mL])	2 fat
with tomatoes	1 vegetable
Sponge cake	1 bread
with strawberries	1 fruit
and whipped cream	2 fat
EVENING MEAL	
Roast beef (3 oz [84 g])	3 meat
Mashed potatoes	3 bread
with butter	1 fat
Carrots	1 vegetable
and butter	1 fat
Applesauce	1 fruit
Small apple	1 fruit
Snack	
Raspberries (1 cup [224 g])	1 fruit
in light cream (2 tbsp [30 mL])	1 fat
Milk (8 oz [240 mL])	1 milk

* Rule of thumb for people with type 1 diabetes—1 unit of insulin for every 15 g of carbohydrates.

B. Types of feeding available after surgery
   1. Intravenous feeding is immediately administered to supply essential water, electrolytes, and vitamins and is intended only as a short-term fluid and electrolyte supplement.
   2. Parenteral hyperalimentation (total parenteral nutrition [TPN]) is administered through a larger central vein such as the superior vena cava because the TPN solution is hypertonic (high osmolarity) and must enter the body in a

region of high blood flow so the solution is rapidly diluted. It provides a higher percentage of water, glucose, amino acids, fats, vitamins, minerals, and electrolytes. It requires surgical insertion, careful monitoring, and special care. It may also be indicated before surgery or for debilitated patients whose intake does not meet body requirements.

3. Oral feedings: Most patients should begin oral feedings as soon as bowel sounds return. Oral feedings provide nutrients essential to recovery; they should progress from clear liquid onward.

BURNS

A. Rate of tissue breakdown and loss of other body nutrients are greater with serious burns compared with any other disease process.
B. Increase of fluids and nutrients is required.
1. Increased energy requires 2000 to 6000 calories.
2. Protein increase must be more than 50% above normal.
3. Vitamin C requirements are greatly increased for wound healing.
4. B vitamins are increased for higher metabolic rate.
5. Fluids must be increased to replace lost body fluids and help eliminate waste products.
C. Intravenous dextrose, electrolytes, and plasma are given initially; a high-protein, high-calorie diet is given when oral foods can be taken.
D. Victims of extensive burns may require parenteral hyperalimentation to meet their extensive nutritional requirements.

CANCER

A. The National Cancer Institute and the American Cancer Society have issued the following guidelines for cancer prevention:
1. Eat a variety of healthful foods, with an emphasis on plant sources.
2. Maintain a healthy weight.
3. Eat a variety of both fruits and vegetables every day.
4. Eat more high-fiber foods such as whole-grain breads and cereals, legumes, vegetables, and fruits.
5. Limit consumption of red meats, especially processed meats and those high in fat.
6. Limit consumption of alcoholic beverages.
B. Diet for the patient with cancer must supply enough protein, fats, carbohydrates, vitamins, minerals, and fluids to meet increased energy demands, prevent weight loss, and rebuild body tissues during treatment. Energy and protein needs may increase up to 20%. Dietary supplements may be given to supply all necessary nutrients. Foods at room temperature may be more palatable for the patient with stomatitis.
C. The wasting away that can occur as a result of the disease itself or from radiation and chemotherapy is termed *cancer cachexia* and can decrease the life of the individual if not prevented or treated early.
D. When the GI tract cannot be used, nutritional support may be given by TPN.
E. Nutritional factors most likely are involved in the development of some cancers. Both excesses and deficiencies have been implicated. Further evaluation is needed.
F. No one food causes cancer, and no one food can prevent it. Diet is considered to be one of the most important environmental and lifestyle factors in the cause and prevention of cancer in the United States.

ACQUIRED IMMUNODEFICIENCY SYNDROME

A. Nutritional support is vital to the survival of all individuals with acquired immunodeficiency syndrome (AIDS). Weight loss is a major symptom in human immunodeficiency virus (HIV) infection. Malnutrition itself contributes to the suppression of immune function.
B. Good nutritional care is essential to preserve lean body mass, maintain weight and strength, and improve the response of the body to medication.
C. Nutritional status of individuals with AIDS can be compromised by decreased oral intake, anorexia, nausea, vomiting, dyspnea, fatigue, neurological disease, and disorders of mouth and esophagus.
D. Techniques to help with food intake include small meals; readily available snacks; adequate hydration; a high-caloric, high-protein diet; and nutritional supplements. Administer medications after meals.
E. General goals of nutrition intervention are to:
1. Preserve optimal somatic and visceral protein status.
2. Prevent nutrient deficiencies or excesses known to compromise immune function.
3. Minimize nutrition-related complications that interfere with either intake or absorption of nutrients.
4. Enhance the quality of life.
5. Educate individuals about the importance of consuming a well-balanced diet.

CARDIOVASCULAR DISEASE

A. Cardiovascular diseases are the primary causes of death in the United States. Research has shown that diet may be a risk factor in determining whether a person develops heart disease. Lifestyle modifications will probably need to continue after desired goals are achieved.
B. Objectives in dietary treatment of heart disease
1. Provide an adequate diet.
2. Prevent gas- and bulk-forming foods from distending stomach and exerting pressure against the heart.
3. Maintain patient's weight as near to ideal as possible to reduce workload of heart.
4. Prevent edema by lowering sodium intake.
5. Reduce the risk of atherosclerosis by reducing circulating blood lipids (low–saturated fat, low-cholesterol diet).
6. Reduce the workload on the damaged heart after a myocardial infarction.
C. Sodium restriction
1. Sodium restriction is a component of many diets for cardiovascular diseases.
2. It helps reduce excess edema and is thought to reduce the risk of hypertension.
3. Sources of sodium
a. It is naturally present in foods, especially animal products such as meat, poultry, fish, milk, and eggs. Fruits have little sodium.
b. Sodium is added to foods in the form of table salt and preservatives in processed foods. Most canned, packaged, and frozen foods have either monosodium glutamate or sodium added.
c. Water supplies may have high sodium content; water softeners add a significant amount of sodium to a diet.
d. Nonprescription medicines and home remedies such as baking soda, alkalizers for indigestion, cough medicines, and laxatives may contain large amounts of sodium.

4. Sodium-restricted diets limit the intake of sodium to a level prescribed by the physician.
   a. A mild sodium-restricted diet (2 to 3 g) contains approximately one half of the salt previously used; additional salting of processed foods is not permitted; no salty foods are allowed.
   b. A 1000-mg sodium diet is considered moderate.
   c. A 500-mg sodium diet is considered strict.
   d. A 250-mg sodium diet is considered severe.

PEPTIC ULCER DISEASE

A. Current advances in drug therapy to decrease acid secretion and promote healing have decreased the need for a highly restrictive, bland diet.
B. These bland diets have been shown to be ineffective and lacking in nutrients to support the healing process. Therapy is based on an individual's response to food choices; avoiding foods that cause gastric stimulation (e.g., caffeine) is recommended.

CHRONIC RENAL FAILURE

A. Patients with chronic renal failure require strict monitoring of protein, water, and electrolyte balance. Specific nutritional therapy varies greatly, depending on the patient's age and the stage of the disease. Enough protein should be supplied to repair and maintain tissues and avoid the use of protein for energy.
B. The blood urea nitrogen (BUN) level and creatinine clearance levels are monitored to assist in regulating protein levels.
C. Homocysteine levels may be associated with vascular damage; dietary sources of this amino acid should be limited in renal patients.

Bibliography

Christensen BL, Kockrow EO: Adult health nursing, ed 6, St Louis, 2010a, Mosby.

Christensen BL, Kockrow EO: Foundations of nursing, ed 6, St Louis, 2010b, Mosby.

Food and Nutrition Information Center: Dietary Guidance, 2013, United States Department of Agriculture. Available at http://fnic.nal.usda.gov/dietary-guidance.

Grodner M, Roth SL, Walkingshaw BC: Nutritional foundations and clinical applications: a nursing approach, ed 5, St Louis, 2012, Mosby.

Leifer G: Maternity nursing: an introductory text, ed 11, St Louis, 2012, Mosby.

Mahan LK, Escott-Stump S, Raymond JL: Krause's food and the nutrition care process, ed 13, Philadelphia, 2012, Saunders.

Nix S: Williams' basic nutrition and diet therapy, ed 14, St Louis, 2013, Mosby.

Peckenpaugh NJ, Poleman CM: Nutrition: essentials and diet therapy, ed 11, Philadelphia, 2010, Saunders.

Physicians' desk reference, ed 67, Montvale, 2013, PDR Network.

Schlenker E, Long SL: Williams' essentials of nutrition and diet therapy, ed 10, St Louis, 2011, Mosby.

U.S. Food and Drug Administration: How to understand and use the nutrition facts label, Silver Spring, Md, 2012, U.S. Food and Drug Administration under the auspices of the U.S. Department of Health and Human Services.

Venes D: Taber's cyclopedic medical dictionary, ed 21, Philadelphia, 2010, FA Davis.

Wold GH: Basic geriatric nursing, ed 5, St Louis, 2012, Mosby.

Online References

American Cancer Society: Diet and Physical Activity: "What's the Cancer Connection? www.cancer.org/cancer/cancercauses/dietandphysicalactivity/diet-and-physical-activity.

Dietary Guidelines for Americans: health.gov/dietaryguidelines.

Dietary Reference Intakes: http://fnic.nal.usda.gov/dietary-guidance/dietary-reference-intakes.

Food and Nutrition Information Center: http://fnic.nal.usda.gov/.

Guide to Nutrition Labeling and Education Act (NELA) Requirements: www.fda.gov/ICECI/Inspections/InspectionGuides/ucm114100.htm.

Healthy People 2020: http://www.healthypeople.gov/2020/.

Produce for Better Health Foundation: http://www.fruitsandveggies-morematters.org.

Amino Acids (Medline Plus): www.nlm.nih.gov/medlineplus/ency/article/002222.htm.

USDA Choose My Plate.gov: www.choosemyplate.gov/food-groups/.

U.S. Food and Drug Administration: Food. www.fda.gov/Food/default.htm.

REVIEW QUESTIONS

1. A third-grade student asks a nurse who is working in a school why the salt on the table has iodine in it. The nurse responds that iodine is essential to health because it:
   1. Strengthens bone and teeth.
   2. Is necessary for blood clotting.
   3. Assists in the ability of the body cells to grow.
   4. Allows oxygen to travel safely to cells.

2. A nurse is explaining a discharge plan to an individual who has had surgery. In planning an adequate diet to promote tissue healing, the nurse advises the patient to increase his intake of the vitamins:
   1. A and D.
   2. A and C.
   3. B_6 and C.
   4. B_{12} and D.

3. A patient hospitalized with peptic ulcer disease is distressed to find that he has no coffee on his meal tray. Which statement by the nurse conveys the reason for a caffeine-restricted diet in patients with peptic ulcer disease?
   1. "Caffeine hydrates the body."
   2. "Caffeine increases gastric emptying."
   3. "Caffeine neutralizes stomach acidity."
   4. "Caffeine stimulates gastric acid secretions."

4. A pregnant patient asks how much weight she should expect to gain if she follows a balanced diet and exercise program. The nurse explains:
   1. "Weight gain should not exceed 10 pounds."
   2. "Your physician will be concerned if you gain more than 20 pounds."
   3. "Acceptable weight gain now averages around 30 pounds."
   4. "You may gain as much as 40 pounds."

5. The nurse correctly advises the pregnant patient to increase the number of calories in her daily diet by:
   1. 340.
   2. 500.
   3. 750.
   4. 1000.

6. Which dietary modification provides an athlete with maximum endurance during a marathon run?
   1. High fat
   2. High carbohydrate
   3. Increased consumption of all nutrients
   4. High protein

7. Which resource is most appropriate in assisting the consumer to better follow a sodium-restricted diet?
   1. Handbooks from the local pharmacist
   2. Package labels
   3. The butcher at the grocery store
   4. Websites on nutrition

8. The nurse is preparing to give an injection of vitamin B$_{12}$ to a nursing home resident. The nurse is giving the injection to prevent the disorder:
   1. Scurvy.
   2. Pellagra.
   3. Marasmus.
   4. Pernicious anemia.

9. A patient who is receiving chemotherapy is concerned because she is unable to eat well because of stomatitis. Which intervention should the nurse recommend?
   1. Eat as much as possible when able.
   2. Drink as much fluid as possible along with food at meals.
   3. Eat small, frequent meals consisting of foods at room temperature.
   4. Eat protein-rich foods when able.

10. A dietary modification that shows evidence of reducing the risk of cancer is:
    1. Increasing intake of saturated fats.
    2. Decreasing intake of saturated fats.
    3. Decreasing intake of raw fruits and vegetables.
    4. Increasing intake of smoked and salt-cured meats.

11. Which statement by a patient indicates to the nurse that the patient is following a diet for the management of gout?
    1. "I eat a high-calorie diet."
    2. "I don't eat foods high in purine."
    3. "I drink a glass of wine each night."
    4. "I restrict my fluid intake to 1000 mL/day."

12. In teaching a patient who has recently been started on angiotensin-converting enzyme (ACE) inhibitors to control his hypertension, the nurse advises him to avoid:
    1. Vigorous exercise and physical exertion.
    2. Salt substitutes containing potassium chloride.
    3. Prolonged exposure to the sun.
    4. Packaged lunchmeats containing nitrites.

13. A patient of Middle Eastern descent refuses to eat during the day and then asks for a double serving during the evening. The patient is newly diagnosed with type I diabetes mellitus. What is the best response by the nurse?
    1. "I know that this is Ramadan, but you have to eat during the day."
    2. "We will need to hold your insulin during the day and then double it at night."
    3. "I think I should talk with your physician. It is very difficult to manage your diabetes."
    4. "We need to find a way for you to observe your religion and also manage your diabetes."

14. The consumption of substances usually considered inedible and without nutrient value such as cornstarch, red clay, or ice cubes describes which term?
    1. Effleurage
    2. Lightening
    3. Pica
    4. Rugae

15. Which of the following should the nurse include when teaching a patient about magnesium deficiency?
    1. The major food sources are red meats and grains.
    2. The major role of magnesium is in tissue growth and repair.
    3. Magnesium deficiency is a relatively uncommon occurrence.
    4. Frequent urination may produce magnesium deficiency.

16. A nurse's aide is passing out evening snacks to a group of residents. Which snack should the nurse recommend for the resident with type 1 diabetes mellitus?
    1. Ice cream
    2. Cookies and milk
    3. Cheese and crackers
    4. Slice of chocolate cake

17. In teaching a patient on a weight loss diet, the nurse includes what information about the hormone leptin?
    1. The hormone is secreted by the pancreas.
    2. The lipogenic activity of insulin is increased by this hormone.
    3. It is believed to be involved with body weight regulation and may promote satiety.
    4. Studies suggest that obese individuals have an excess of leptin.

18. Cheilosis, a common condition in older patients, is the result of a deficiency of which vitamin?
    1. Cobalamin (vitamin B$_{12}$)
    2. Niacin (vitamin B$_3$)
    3. Riboflavin (vitamin B$_2$)
    4. Thiamine (vitamin B$_1$)

19. A postoperative patient has been on intravenous (IV) fluids for several days. What remark made by the patient indicates that she is probably ready to be started on oral feedings?
    1. "I can't wait to see some real food rather than this IV bottle!"
    2. "I'm so glad I don't have any more nausea—what a nuisance that was!"
    3. "My stomach is really rumbling. I don't know why—there's nothing in it!"
    4. "My stomach is feeling a little bloated because I haven't had anything in it for so long."

20. An 80-year-old woman complains to the nurse that she is "burping acid" on a daily basis. What recommendations from the nurse would be most likely to reduce the patient's discomfort?
    1. Eat one large meal per day to allow the stomach to empty thoroughly.
    2. Be sure to have a high-carbohydrate snack before bedtime.
    3. Avoid fatty foods, alcohol, caffeine, and nicotine.
    4. Try a glass of wine before meals and at bedtime.

21. Apple juice can cause diarrhea and abdominal discomfort in young children because of:
    1. Ascorbic acid
    2. Pectin
    3. Sorbitol
    4. Potassium

22. A patient states that she manages her hypoglycemia with a very low–carbohydrate diet but that she is having increased episodes of nervousness, headaches, and hunger a couple hours after eating. The nurse should suggest what to the patient?
    1. Increasing simple carbohydrates to maintain blood glucose levels

2. Limiting dietary fiber
3. Increasing protein intake
4. Eating a diet rich in complex carbohydrates and dietary fiber

23. Which foods should the nurse recommend to a patient to reduce triglycerides?
    1. Red meats, coconut oil, and shrimp
    2. Poultry, eggs, and whole milk
    3. Soybeans, green vegetables, and olive oil
    4. Lamb, lobster, and yogurt

24. Place an X beside all the assessment data that indicate the patient is experiencing problems while on enteral nutrition. Select all that apply.
    _____ 1. Bowel sounds in four (4) quadrants
    _____ 2. Able to change position in bed without assistance
    _____ 3. Bone pain
    _____ 4. Oral dryness
    _____ 5. Thirst

25. A patient who is newly diagnosed with human immunodeficiency virus (HIV) is angry and withdrawn. He verbalizes to the nurse that he does not understand why she is even bothering to tell him about nutrition when he is going to die anyway. What should the nurse say at this point?
    1. "When you are ready to listen, we will talk again."
    2. "I will leave written material here for you to read."
    3. "I know you feel you have lost control over your life."
    4. "Eating well is a way you can maintain your immune system."

26. Place an X beside the factors that contribute to overweight children and adolescents. (Select all that apply).
    _____ 1. Behavior
    _____ 2. Environment
    _____ 3. Genetics
    _____ 4. Overseasoning
    _____ 5. Psychosocial

27. Determine the first step in following the DASH (Dietary Approach to Stop Hypertension) diet.
    1. Appropriate amount of activity.
    2. Appropriate energy level.
    3. Appropriate number of servings per day.
    4. Appropriate serving sizes.

28. Which statement by the nurse explains to the patient the reason why her physician has prescribed vitamin E?
    1. "It helps the liver make blood-clotting factors and helps reduce the risk of hip fracture."
    2. "It promotes normal bone growth, helps control cell reproduction, and may help treat skin disorders such as psoriasis."
    3. "It helps your eyes adapt to light and to dark, and it prevents skin conditions such as follicular hyperkeratosis."
    4. "It helps promote your immune system, reduces the risk of heart disease and stroke, and seems to help prevent some age-related dementias."

29. Select from the list below the 4 Ds that characterize the disease pellagra.
    _____ 1. Death
    _____ 2. Dementia
    _____ 3. Dermatitis
    _____ 4. Diarrhea
    _____ 5. Disorientation
    _____ 6. Dizziness

30. Which prenatal patient is most at risk for nutritional complications?
    1. A patient in her third trimester who has gained 39 pounds
    2. A woman in her third trimester with complaints of heartburn
    3. An underweight adolescent who confesses to eating erratically
    4. A 36-year-old primigravida in her second trimester who is slightly anemic

31. What occurs in the body of a severely burned patient during the immediate shock period? Select all that apply.
    _____ 1. Blood pressure drops
    _____ 2. Loss of water, electrolytes, and protein
    _____ 3. Respiratory rate increases
    _____ 4. Serum potassium levels fall
    _____ 5. Urine output increases

32. What has been linked with hypertension in the general population? Select all that apply.
    _____ 1. African-American women
    _____ 2. Acute stress
    _____ 3. Obesity
    _____ 4. Physical activity
    _____ 5. Sodium intake

33. A patient who is taking isonicotinic acid hydrazide (INH) for treatment of tuberculosis asks the nurse if any special attention should be paid to her dietary intake while she is on the medication. The nurse's reply should be:
    1. "You will need to take more vitamin C than usual."
    2. "You need to make sure that you get enough vitamin B_6."
    3. "You must make sure that you don't get too much calcium."
    4. "You should avoid milk products."

34. Which foods rich in tyramine should a patient be instructed to avoid while taking a monoamine oxidase inhibitor (MAOI) medication?
    1. Whole grain
    2. Chicken liver
    3. Green, leafy vegetables
    4. Citrus fruits

35. Which common food allergen elicits the most severe reaction?
    1. Eggs
    2. Peanuts
    3. Shellfish
    4. Wheat

36. Which strategy is the focus of diet therapy for a patient with phenylketonuria (PKU)?
    1. Allowing unlimited aspartame intake
    2. Using as many milk-based foods as possible
    3. Including high levels of phenylalanine on a daily basis
    4. Individualizing diet plans containing some aspartame, with careful monitoring of phenylalanine levels

37. Trans fatty acids (TFAs) should be limited in the diet because of their tendency to:
    1. Inhibit the absorption of fat-soluble vitamins.
    2. Add calories to the daily intake.
    3. Increase blood levels of low-density lipoproteins (LDLs).
    4. Reduce the amount of high-density lipoprotein (HDL) in the blood.

38. Which action should a patient with diabetes mellitus take when general illness occurs?
    1. Contact the physician only as a last resort.

2. Do not omit insulin.
3. Monitor blood glucose levels a little less frequently.
4. Skip a meal if needed.

39. Which dinner selection would be best suited for a patient admitted with chronic renal failure?
    1. Ground round steak, asparagus, bread and butter, fruit cup, and milk
    2. Hamburger with tomato on a bun, potato chips, and a glass of chocolate milk
    3. Liver, cottage cheese with peach half, deviled eggs, and coffee with cream and sugar
    4. Apple juice, 1 oz roasted chicken, asparagus, sliced tomatoes, fruit cup, and tea with sugar

40. A patient who was admitted for treatment of peptic ulcer disease asks the nurse if eating too many spicy foods caused the disease. The nurse should explain to him that:
    1. Smoking and alcohol use are the causes of ulcers.
    2. Spicy foods and alcohol cause ulcers.
    3. The cause is an organism named *Helicobacter pylori.*
    4. Stress and worry are the primary causes of ulcers.

41. A patient is admitted with a diagnosis of suspected myocardial infarction. He complains about his soft diet order. The nurse explains to the patient that the purpose of this diet is to:
    1. Reduce the workload on the heart.
    2. Decrease irritation to the digestive tract.
    3. Reduce the number of calories in his diet.
    4. Decrease peristalsis within the digestive tract.

42. To reduce the risk of developing hypertension, sodium intake should be limited to how many grams per day?
    1. 1.5 g/day
    2. 2.4 g/day
    3. 3.4 g/day
    4. 4.4 g/day

43. A patient who has been experiencing severe pain from gallstones is scheduled for surgery in 2 weeks. To minimize discomfort until then, the nurse should instruct the patient to modify her diet in which ways?
    1. Limit fat intake as much as possible.
    2. Reduce the total number of calories.
    3. Increase the amount of dairy products.
    4. Limit carbohydrate foods.

44. A patient receiving medical nutritional therapy for coronary heart disease asks the nurse why the physician recommended an increase in the amount of fiber in his diet. The nurse should explain that:
    1. Fiber slows glucose absorption.
    2. The time that food takes to pass through the intestine increases when additional fiber is added to the diet.
    3. Fiber helps increase low-density lipoprotein (LDL) cholesterol in the colon.
    4. The stomach empties faster when fiber is present in the diet.

45. What should the nurse take into consideration when planning meals for patients with chronic renal disease?
    1. Maintain normal serum blood levels of magnesium and bicarbonates.
    2. Reduce the levels of chloride and sulfates in the blood.
    3. Maintain adequate protein and calorie intake.
    4. Restrict fluids to avoid edema.

46. The wife of a patient with cancer asks for suggestions to work around his lack of interest in eating resulting from fatigue and a sore mouth. What recommendations might the nurse suggest?
    1. "Limit the amount of gravy, sauces, or butter added to foods."
    2. "Offer salty, spicy, or acidic foods to stimulate his appetite through taste."
    3. "Avoid snacking; it will spoil his appetite."
    4. "Try shakes made from frozen liquid supplements or milk shakes with protein powders added."

47. What problems might an adolescent with bulimia experience other than intake and absorption?
    1. Dental erosion
    2. Gastroesophageal reflux
    3. Constipation
    4. Hyperglycemia

48. Which bacterial poisoning might a patient contract from eating raw eggs?
    1. *Escherichia coli*
    2. *Salmonella*
    3. *Clostridium botulinum*
    4. *Staphylococcus*

49. How many protein calories would a patient consume from an 18-g soy burger?
    Answer: _____ calories

50. A middle-aged woman is concerned because her mother has just been diagnosed with osteoporosis. She asks what she can do to limit her chances for getting osteoporosis. What should the nurse recommend?
    1. "Increase the potassium in your diet."
    2. "Try to increase dairy products in your diet."
    3. "You should limit the amount of salt you eat."
    4. "Increase the amount of protein you consume each day."

51. Which dietary source of potassium might a patient consider in addition to bananas?
    1. Whole grains
    2. Green, leafy vegetables
    3. Red meats
    4. Dairy products

52. Trace elements in the body are defined as:
    1. Minerals that are not essential to health.
    2. Essential nutrients that are found in very small amounts.
    3. Only minerals that are found in the blood.
    4. Minerals that are undetectable by blood studies.

53. What are recommended supplements for patients with end-stage renal disease with high levels of homocysteine in the blood?
    1. Saturated fats and cholesterol
    2. Ascorbic acid and choline
    3. Folic acid and vitamin B$_{12}$
    4. Potassium and sodium

54. What is likely to have the greatest impact on the eating habits of adolescents?
    1. Nutrition knowledge
    2. Availability of nutritious foods
    3. Instructions from parents and health care professionals
    4. Personal beliefs about nutrition

55. Which diet strongly predisposes humans to the development of colon cancer?
    1. High in fiber and vegetables, low in fats and calories

2. Low in fats and calories, high in fruits and fibers
3. High in fats and calories, low in fruits and fibers
4. Low in calories and vegetables, high in fruits and fats

56. After 30 years of age, as lean body mass declines, a gradual but accelerated decrease occurs in:
    1. Body mass index.
    2. Basal metabolic rate.
    3. Bone mineral density.
    4. Blood glucose metabolism.

57. The mother of a 16-year-old girl reports to the nurse that her daughter has been eating large amounts of food sometimes and throwing up afterward. In addition, the girl is exercising much more than she did in the past. Which condition should the nurse explore?
    1. Anorexia nervosa
    2. Bulimia nervosa
    3. Binge-eating disorder
    4. Compulsive-eating disorder

58. It has been shown that a direct relationship exists between excess body weight and:
    1. Renal disease and type 2 diabetes
    2. Gallbladder disease and hypertension
    3. Hypertension and type 2 diabetes
    4. Hypertension and degenerative joint disease

59. Guidelines for nutrition during lactation include:
    1. Decreasing the amount of calories consumed during pregnancy to prevent additional weight gain.
    2. Limiting fluids to four to six glasses per day to prevent fluid overload.
    3. Increasing the energy intake by approximately 500 kilocalories more than the usual adult allowance.
    4. Increasing the amount of fat in the diet to ensure ample absorption of fat-soluble vitamins by the baby.

60. A patient who does not like to drink water asks the nurse if it is okay to drink six to eight glasses of tea each day instead. The nurse should tell her:
    1. "Tea is a good substitute, especially if you like the taste. Be sure to add enough sugar to make it flavorful too."
    2. "Tea is a diuretic and increases your need for fluids. You might try sparkling water or water flavored with fruit flavors."
    3. "Drinking tea with meals helps absorb iron from the foods."
    4. "Tea is better than coffee because it does not contain caffeine."

61. The macronutrients with the greatest sources of energy in the diet are:
    1. Protein and carbohydrates.
    2. Carbohydrates and fats.
    3. Fats and proteins.
    4. Carbohydrates and vitamins.

62. A patient who was admitted for treatment of food poisoning mentions to the nurse that he saw a bandage on the hand of the person at the fast-food restaurant where he bought his chicken dinner. The nurse explains to the patient that he most likely has been infected with:
    1. *Clostridium perfringens.*
    2. *Salmonella typhi.*
    3. *Escherichia coli.*
    4. *Staphylococcus aureus.*

63. A female patient says that during premenstrual syndrome she has symptoms of hypoglycemia that do not respond to eating food. What should the nurse tell the patient about this phenomenon?
    1. "You are probably eating the wrong foods. You should include high-calorie carbohydrates such as candy or fruit juice."
    2. "Although the symptoms are similar, this is probably not hypoglycemia and will not respond to the same treatment."
    3. "Have you tried taking crackers and milk for the symptoms?"
    4. "The next time this happens, be sure to get a blood sugar done so we can prescribe a proper diet for you."

64. On a 2000 calories/day diet, what is the lowest number of calories that should come from fat?
    Answer: _____ calories

65. On the low end of a 2000 calories/day diet, how many calories should come from carbohydrates?
    Answer: _____ calories

66. Which action describes the term *pouching?*
    1. Development of enlarged villi in the small intestine that are known as *diverticula*
    2. Development of adipose deposits around the middle of the body that give the appearance of an abdominal pouch
    3. Retaining pieces of food or medications between the cheeks and gums
    4. Carrying a small bag with emergency food and medications in case of a diabetic reaction away from home

67. The Women, Infants, and Children (WIC) program is designed to meet which of the following needs? Select all that apply.
    _____ 1. Nutrition education
    _____ 2. Vouchers for prescribed supplemental foods
    _____ 3. Meals on Wheels for homebound older patients
    _____ 4. Community meals for any low-income adult
    _____ 5. Dietary counseling for patients with eating disorders

68. The designation *GRAS* means that food additives are:
    1. Derived from plant origins.
    2. Unsafe for use by small children and pregnant women.
    3. Added to genetically modified foods to retain freshness.
    4. Generally recognized as safe.

69. Why are food additives such as alginate, lecithin, agar, and carrageenan used?
    1. To improve nutritive value
    2. To impart and maintain desired consistency
    3. To enhance flavor
    4. To maintain appearance, palatability, and wholesomeness

70. A patient who has been taking a tricyclic antidepressant for several weeks complains to the nurse that she is gaining weight and cannot seem to lose it. The most appropriate response by the nurse should be:
    1. "This is an alarming occurrence, and you should make an appointment with your psychiatrist immediately."
    2. "Have you been eating more junk food and snacks? That can put on the pounds pretty quickly."
    3. "This is a common side effect of tricyclic antidepressants. Let's take a look at your food diary and see if there is a way we can help control this while you continue to take the medication."
    4. "You should stop taking the medication right away and see if you can lose the weight."

71. A patient who has been taking disulfiram (Antabuse) reports to the nurse that at a banquet last night he had a flushing reaction and had to leave the dinner. He is very embarrassed and wants to know how to prevent this from happening again. Which statement by the nurse is the most appropriate in response to the patient's concern?
    1. "In addition to alcoholic beverages, a reaction can be triggered from eating foods with alcohol in them such as sauces that may not have been cooked thoroughly and may still have an alcoholic content."
    2. "That was probably just a freak accident. I'm sure it won't take place again."
    3. "As long as you never eat the same foods again, you should be okay."
    4. "Are you sure you didn't use too much aftershave or cologne before you left the house?"

72. A patient with diabetes calls and reports to the nurse that she is nauseated and coughing a lot. She is not able to manage solid foods and wants to know if she should skip her diabetes medication until she feels better. The nurse should explain to her:
    1. "Yes, because otherwise you will have a hypoglycemic reaction."
    2. "Even though you can't take solid foods, you will need the medication to cover soft and liquid foods that you may have consumed."
    3. "Don't take the medication again until you can tolerate a full diet of solid foods."
    4. "It's okay to stop the medication, but you should start taking it again if you have any symptoms of a reaction."

73. The foods that are the most likely to raise serum cholesterol levels are foods that:
    1. Have no trans fatty acids.
    2. Are high in unsaturated fats.
    3. Are fat free.
    4. Are high in saturated fats.

74. Which is a common side effect of narcotic analgesics?
    1. Anxiety
    2. Constipation
    3. Diarrhea
    4. Tachypnea

75. Which type of dietary fiber is noncarbohydrate?
    1. Cellulose
    2. Lignin
    3. Mucilages
    4. Pectin

76. Sugar alcohols are often used as sugar replacements. An upside of using sugar alcohols is that they do not promote:
    1. Constipation.
    2. Diarrhea.
    3. Indigestion.
    4. Tooth decay.

77. What is the fuel factor for carbohydrates per gram?
    Answer: _____

78. Which food would be used more frequently in a low–saturated fat diet to lower the risk of heart disease?
    1. Bacon
    2. Eggs
    3. Palm oil
    4. Olive oil

79. Which person has the lowest energy needs per unit of body weight?
    1. 6-month-old girl
    2. 31-year-old mother
    3. 37-year-old father
    4. 78-year-old grandmother

80. A 3-oz piece of chicken breast contains 16 g protein, 2 g fat, and 0 carbohydrates. What is its kilocalorie value?
    Answer: _____ kilocalories

81. Which food source supplies the greatest amount of vitamin E?
    1. Chicken liver
    2. Safflower oil
    3. Whole-grain cereal
    4. Whole milk

82. Which foods should the nurse teach the patient to choose to increase intake of vitamin C?
    1. Bread and rice
    2. Eggs and milk
    3. Safflower oil
    4. Tomatoes and kiwi

83. What percentage of the calcium in the body is found in bones and teeth?
    Answer: _____ %

84. Which mineral, if it becomes deficient or toxic in the body, can cause cardiac problems?
    1. Calcium
    2. Chloride
    3. Potassium
    4. Sulfa

85. Which suggestions should make child-feeding easier? Select all that apply.
    _____ 1. Be patient.
    _____ 2. Offer a variety of foods.
    _____ 3. Overseason.
    _____ 4. Serve dessert first.
    _____ 5. Serve small portions.

86. For prevention of bacterial food infection, four steps for food safety should be followed. Place the following steps in order:
    1. Chill
    2. Clean
    3. Cook
    4. Separate

87. Food fads appeal to which vulnerable groups? Select all that apply.
    _____ 1. Teenagers
    _____ 2. Older individuals
    _____ 3. Religious persons
    _____ 4. Athletes
    _____ 5. Obese individuals
    _____ 6. Movie stars

88. Which nutritional components of a regular diet can be modified? Select all that apply.
    _____ 1. Energy
    _____ 2. Condiments
    _____ 3. Nutrients
    _____ 4. Texture

89. Individual differences in energy needs, along with social pressures, have led many overweight persons to use extreme measures to lose weight. Pictured are several such extreme measures. Choose the procedure named *gastric banding*.

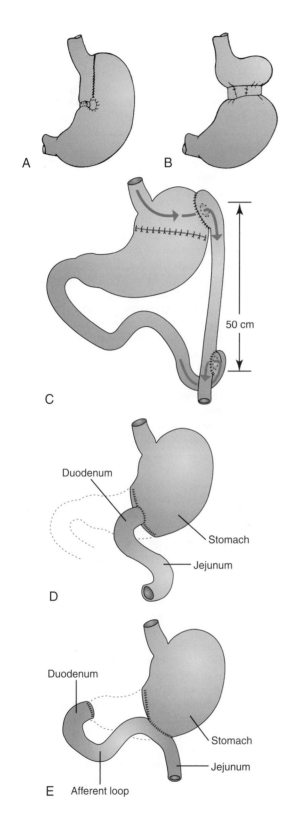

A   B

C

50 cm

Duodenum

Stomach

Jejunum

D

Duodenum

Stomach

Jejunum

E   Afferent loop

____ 3. Note if the patient avoids food.

____ 4. Observe tooth enamel.

____ 5. Describe the patient's self-esteem.

92. A patient is concerned with her intake of calories that come from foods containing fat. There are 11 g of fat in 1 tablespoon of butter. The nurse needs to caution the patient that _____ calories will be consumed every time she eats that amount of butter.

93. All of the following processes occur with digestion in the mouth and esophagus. In which order should they occur?
    1. Gravity aids the movement of food down the esophagus.
    2. The mixed mass of food particles is swallowed.
    3. Biting and chewing begin the breakdown.
    4. Muscles at the base of the tongue facilitate swallowing.
    5. Gastroesophageal sphincter relaxes to allow swallowing and entrance into the stomach.

94. Which assessment finding does the nurse recognize as indicative of potassium depletion?
    1. Decrease in the number of RBCs
    2. Edema of the extremities
    3. Muscle weakness
    4. Reduced bone mass

95. Which assessment finding(s) does the nurse recognize as indicative of beta carotene excess in a patient's diet?
    1. Burning, tingling and itching
    2. Malformation of bones
    3. Orange skin tint
    4. Poor blood clotting

96. Which diet choices of a diabetic patient would the nurse assess to be in compliance?
    1. Breakfast—1 poached egg, black coffee, 1 medium fresh peach
    2. Lunch—tuna sandwich on whole-wheat bread, chips, 1 cookie
    3. Dinner—broiled pork chop, 1 cup white rice, 1 cup green beans, 1 cup applesauce
    4. Snack—1 cup buttered popcorn, 1 can diet soda, 1 large apple

97. In what anatomic area should the nurse assessing bowel sounds expect to locate the area in which most of the water is absorbed in the large intestines?

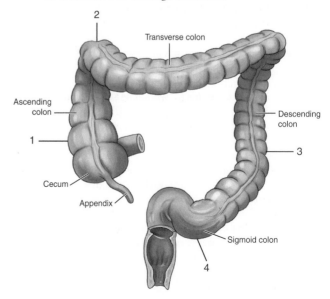

2

Transverse colon

Ascending colon

Descending colon

1

3

Cecum

Appendix

Sigmoid colon

4

90. Which food is allowed on a clear liquid diet?
    1. Bouillon
    2. Grits
    3. Milk
    4. Yogurt

91. Which nursing actions will the nurse take to assess a patient for bulimia nervosa? Select all that apply.
    ____ 1. Assess oral mucous membranes.
    ____ 2. Comment on the length of the fingernails.

1. 1
2. 2
3. 3
4. 4

98. A nurse is reviewing objective data from the physical examination of a newly diagnosed diabetic patient. Which assessment finding does the nurse recognize as abnormal?

Tab 1 **Examination of the Eyes**	Tab 2 **Examination of Lab TestResults**	Tab 3 **Examination of the Skin**
Pupils are equal and react to light	Blood glucose 105 mg/dL	Skin clear with quick elastic return
Vision blurred	Triglycerides <150 mg/dL	Skin warm to touch

1. Blood glucose 105 mg/dL
2. Skin warm to touch
3. Triglycerides <150 mg/dL
4. Vision blurred

99. Which assessment finding does the nurse recognize as indicative of a drug interaction of calcium channel blockers with grapefruit juice?
1. Bradycardia
2. Diaphoresis
3. Elevated blood sugar
4. Weight loss

100. Which exchange choice made by the patient is an appropriate choice for a diabetic diet?
1. Fruit—1 cup applesauce
2. Milk—1 cup whole milk
3. Cereals—¾ cup bran
4. Vegetables—½ cup sweet potato

ANSWERS AND RATIONALES

1. Application, implementation, physiological integrity, (b).
   3. This explanation is short, geared to the child's knowledge level, and accurately condenses what the purpose of iodine is in the body.
   1. This correctly explains why calcium and phosphorus are necessary for the body.
   2. Calcium and vitamin K are essential for blood clotting.
   4. This explains the role iron plays in hemoglobin.
2. Application, planning, physiological integrity, (b).
   2. Vitamins essential for wound healing include A and C.
   1. Vitamins A and D can be readily found in fortified milk and assist in healing fractures.
   3. Vitamins B_6 and C, although important in an adequate diet, are not specific for tissue healing.
   4. These vitamins are also not specific for tissue healing, although they are important in the diet.
3. Comprehension, implementation, physiological integrity, (b).
   4. Caffeine stimulates gastric acid secretions, potentially aggravating peptic ulcer disease.
   1. Caffeine dehydrates the body.
   2. Fluids increase gastric emptying.

3. Caffeine does not neutralize stomach acidity.
4. Comprehension, implementation, health promotion and maintenance, (b).
   3. This is the truest statement. In the past weight was restricted, but the focus is now on gaining enough weight to safeguard the baby's health.
   1. This is not true for the majority of pregnant women.
   2. This does not provide information to the patient and blocks communication.
   4. Although true in the past, this weight gain is probably too much for most pregnant women.
5. Application, implementation, health promotion and maintenance, (b).
   1. The caloric needs of the pregnant woman increase by 340 kcal/day in the second trimester and 450 kcal/day in the third trimester.
   2. The lactating mother needs to increase her calories to 330 kcal/day + 170 kcal/day from maternal stores, yielding a total of 500 kcal/day.
   3. Unless the pregnant woman is severely malnourished, 750 calories is generally too many additional calories.
   4. Unless the pregnant woman is instructed by a physician, 1000 calories is too much of an increase.
6. Comprehension, planning, health promotion and maintenance, (b).
   2. A high-carbohydrate diet (80% of calories) consumed for several days before an event can greatly improve endurance time and performance.
   1. A high-fat diet (90% of calories) increases endurance approximately one half as much as does a high-carbohydrate diet.
   3. Increasing all nutrients probably will not decrease endurance and performance.
   4. Protein is not one of the nutrients that fuel activity.
7. Analysis, evaluation, health promotion and maintenance, (b).
   2. The labels right on the package are the best sources for food information giving information like calories, fats, proteins, sodium, and calcium content.
   1 & 3. The local pharmacists and butchers will also refer the consumer to these labels.
   4. All websites are not accurate, so be careful of where information is obtained.
8. Application, implementation, physiological integrity, (b).
   4. Vitamin B_{12} injections are given to elderly patients because of the decrease of intrinsic factor in their stomach acid. Vitamin B_{12} cannot be absorbed without intrinsic factor and must be supplemented to prevent pernicious anemia from developing.
   1. Vitamin C prevents scurvy.
   2. Pellagra is caused by a deficiency in niacin.
   3. *Marasmus* is a term for general starvation.
9. Comprehension, planning, physiological integrity, (c).
   3. Many individuals with stomatitis are able to eat foods that are neither hot nor cold and may find eating more comfortable if the food is served at room temperature.
   1. This is a dietary recommendation for anorexia.
   2. Swallowing fluids may be uncomfortable for the patient because taking in solids with large amounts of fluids fills the stomach at the expense of nutrients.
   4. This may not be possible, and protein-rich foods do not help the problem of stomatitis.

10. Knowledge, planning, health promotion and maintenance, (b).
    2. The Dietary Guidelines for people in the United States recommend that individuals decrease their intake of saturated fats.
    1. This is likely to increase the risk of cancer.
    3. Studies have shown that raw fruits and vegetables can alleviate some types of cancer.
    4. The preservatives in smoked and salt-cured meats have been linked to some types of cancer.
11. Application, evaluation, physiological integrity, (a).
    2. Although diet therapy is not as effective in managing gout as are medications, the general acceptance is that a diet low in purine diminishes uric acid in the body.
    1. Weight loss is usually indicated and would require a low-calorie diet. Fatty foods precipitate attacks.
    3. Alcohol precipitates exacerbations and should be avoided.
    4. A liberal fluid intake is encouraged to flush the minerals from the body.
12. Application, assessment, physiological integrity, (c).
    2. One side effect of ACE inhibitor antihypertensive medication is retention of potassium.
    1. Aerobic exercise may be helpful in weight reduction and blood pressure management.
    3. Photosensitivity is not a side effect of ACE inhibitors.
    4. The negative effects of nitrites are related to their correlation with cancer.
13. Application, implementation, physiological integrity, (c).
    4. This is the only response that preserves the patient's need for religious influence while recognizing that a solution to this problem must be found.
    1. This response is condescending to the patient and will likely be met with resistance.
    2. This is not conducive to the management of diabetes mellitus.
    3. This response places the patient in a dependent, passive role.
14. Knowledge, evaluation, physiological integrity, (a).
    3. Pica is the consumption of substances usually considered inedible and without nutritional value.
    1. Effleurage is a technique of gentle abdominal massage often taught in childbirth classes.
    2. Lightening is what happens when the fetus begins to settle in the maternal pelvis and descend toward the pelvic outlet.
    4. Rugae are folds in the vagina that allow it to stretch considerably during childbirth.
15. Comprehension, planning, physiological integrity, (a).
    4. In addition to conditions such as diabetes, low levels of magnesium in the blood can be caused by alcoholism, malabsorption, hyperthyroidism, use of steroids, and massive blood transfusions.
    1. The major food sources of magnesium are those containing chlorophyll, such as dark green, leafy vegetables.
    2. Magnesium plays a role in metabolic processes at a cellular level and in muscle contractions.
    3. This is a relatively common mineral deficiency in the general population.
16. Application, implementation, safe and effective care environment, (b).

3. **The cheese and crackers provide the patient with type 1 diabetes with complex carbohydrates, which are used to stabilize blood glucose levels.**
    1. Ice cream would provide too many calories and not enough complex carbohydrates.
    2. Cookies have too much refined sugar and would raise the person's blood glucose level too high.
    4. Although it would depend on the ingredients in the cake, generally chocolate cake has too much refined sugar.
17. Comprehension, planning, physiological integrity, (b).
    3. Leptin alters the levels of neuropeptides and affects weight regulation and feeling satisfied after eating.
    1. Leptin acts within the hypothalamus.
    2. Leptin decreases the lipogenic activity of insulin.
    4. Obese individuals may be resistant to leptin at a cellular level.
18. Knowledge, planning, physiological integrity, (b).
    3. Riboflavin deficiency often results in cheilosis and general dermatitis, especially among older adults.
    1. Cobalamin deficiency is associated with pernicious anemia.
    2. Niacin deficiency is associated with pellagra.
    4. Thiamine deficiency is associated with neuropathy.
19. Application, assessment, physiological integrity, (b).
    3. Stomach rumbling indicates return of bowel sounds; peristalsis has started, and oral feedings may be indicated.
    1. Hunger is not an accurate predictor of return of bowel function.
    2. Although she may be able to tolerate foods, this does not mean peristalsis has returned.
    4. Distention can indicate lack of peristalsis.
20. Comprehension, application, physiological integrity, (b).
    3. Avoiding these helps the esophageal sphincter to function better, thereby helping prevent reflux.
    1. Frequent small meals help to reduce pressure on the stomach.
    2. Reflux is more likely when the patient lies down with a full stomach.
    4. Alcohol makes it harder for the esophageal sphincter to work properly, increasing the likelihood of reflux.
21. Knowledge, assessment, physiological integrity, (b).
    3. Sorbitol, a naturally occurring sugar that is not absorbed, is found in high amounts in apple juice.
    1. Citrus juices have a higher content of vitamin C than does apple juice and are more likely to cause diarrhea from that vitamin.
    2. Pectin is found in apples, but it is more likely to prevent or cure diarrhea than cause it.
    4. An average apple provides about 60 mg of magnesium, which is beneficial in the treatment of diarrhea as an electrolyte replacement.
22. Comprehension, planning, physiological integrity, (c).
    4. Current research indicates that frequent small meals of complex carbohydrates and fibers maintain a more stable blood glucose level.
    1. Reactive hypoglycemia may result from the intake of simple sugars.
    2. Fiber slows gastric emptying and carbohydrate absorption, thus supporting a consistent release of glucose into the bloodstream.

3. A high-protein, low-carbohydrate diet restricts the ability of the body to obtain sufficient amounts of glucose to achieve and maintain normal blood glucose levels.

23. Comprehension, planning, physiological integrity, (b).

   3. These are plant foods that have no saturated fats.
   1. These are foods that are high in saturated fats.
   2, 4. These animal foods are high in saturated fats.

24. Analysis, evaluation, physiological integrity, (b).

   _____ 1. Bowel sound in four (4) quadrants is a normal finding.
   _____ 2. The patient changing positions in bed by himself or herself is a good sign that he or she can alleviate pressure so that skin will not become a problem.
   __X__ **3. Bone pain indicates a problem with malabsorption.**
   __X__ **4. Oral dryness is a problem when the patient cannot drink.**
   __X__ **5. Thirst is a problem when the patient cannot drink.**

25. Application, implementation, psychosocial integrity, (b).

   4. Malnutrition contributes to a compromised immune system. Participating in his meal planning and preparation is one way for him to have control over his health.
   1. This closes communication; the patient may never be "ready" to communicate if no supportive intervention takes place.
   2. Written material is more appropriate after a discussion, as a way of reinforcing the information given.
   3. This sets up a barrier to communication because the nurse has no way of knowing if this is true or not.

26. Analysis, evaluation, health promotion and maintenance, (b).

   __X__ **1. Behavior**
   __X__ **2. Environment**
   __X__ **3. Genetics**
   _____ 4. Overseasoning
   _____ 5. Psychosocial

   Overweight _is defined as a body mass index of greater than the 95th percentile on the CDC 2000 growth charts. Prevalence of overweight among U.S. children and adolescents (ages 2 to 19 years) according to the National Health and Nutrition Examination Surveys indicates the contributing factors to be genetics, behavioral factors, and environmental factors._

27. Analysis, evaluation, health promotion and maintenance, (b).

   2. The first step in following the DASH diet is to determine the appropriate energy level based on desired weight and activity level.
   1, 3, 4. Are also included in the DASH plan; they are just not the first step.

28. Application, planning, physiological integrity, (b).

   4. Vitamin E is a powerful antioxidant that has effects on cell membranes and stimulates immune function in elderly people.
   1. This is true of vitamin K.
   2. This is true of vitamin D.
   3. This is true of vitamin A.

29. Analysis, evaluation, physiological integrity, (b).

   __X__ **1. Death**
   __X__ **2. Dementia**
   __X__ **3. Dermatitis**
   __X__ **4. Diarrhea**

   _____ 5. Disorientation
   _____ 6. Dizziness

   1, 2, 3, and 4 are the 4 Ds that characterize pellagra; 5 and 6 do not.

30. Application, assessment, health promotion and maintenance, (b).

   3. Irregular eating habits and age are two factors that would cause the nurse concern.
   1. This pattern of weight gain is not excessive and should meet the nutrition demands of the baby.
   2. This is typical of this time of pregnancy, caused by the uterus pressing on the diaphragm.
   4. Physiological anemia in pregnancy is often caused by increased blood volume. True anemia is diagnosed by blood studies and treated by a physician.

31. Analysis, assessment, physiological integrity, (b).

   __X__ **1. Blood pressure drops**
   __X__ **2. Loss of water, electrolytes, and protein**
   __X__ **3. Respiratory rate increases**
   _____ 4. Serum potassium levels fall
   _____ 5. Urine output increases

   Events that occur within the body of a severely burned patient.

   Blood pressure drops; there is considerable loss of water, electrolytes, and protein; and respiratory efforts increase due to obstruction of upper airway passages from swelling.

   Serum potassium levels rise; they do not fall. Urine output decreases; it does not increase.

32. Analysis, assessment, physiological integrity, (b).

   __X__ **1. African-American women**
   _____ 2. Acute stress
   __X__ **3. Obesity**
   _____ 4. Physical activity
   __X__ **5. Sodium intake**

   African-American women, obesity, and sodium intake are all links to hypertension in the general population.

   Inactivity, not physical activity, is linked to hypertension. Chronic stress is linked to hypertension, not acute stress.

33. Knowledge, planning, physiological integrity, (b).

   2. INH blocks the conversion of vitamin B$_6$ to an active form in the body and can lead to deficiency of this vitamin.
   1. INH does not affect vitamin C.
   3. INH does not affect calcium.
   4. INH does not affect nutrients found in milk.

34. Application, planning, physiological integrity, (b).

   2. Other foods rich in tyramine include certain cheeses, red wines, and fava beans.
   1, 3, 4. These foods are not rich in tyramine.

35. Analysis, evaluation, health promotion and maintenance, (b).

   2. Peanuts elicit the most severe reaction.
   1, 3, 4. These are common food allergens, but their reaction is not as severe.

36. Knowledge, planning, health promotion and maintenance, (b).

   4. Because aspartame is an essential amino acid and therefore necessary for growth, it must be included in the diet; but careful monitoring of blood levels must be followed.
   1. Aspartame is 50% phenylalanine.
   2. Milk is high in phenylalanine. Dietary management would include using a milk substitute.

3. This would lead to central nervous system damage in the patient.

37. Application, planning, physiological integrity, (a).
    3. TFAs raise the level of LDL cholesterol even more than do saturated fats.
    1. TFAs do not affect vitamin absorption.
    2. All types of fats increase calorie consumption.
    4. TFAs do not reduce the level of HDL in the blood.

38. Analysis, implementation, physiological integrity, (b).
    2. Do not omit insulin; follow an adjusted dosage if needed.
    1. Contact a physician if the illness lasts more than a few days, not only as a last resort.
    3. Blood glucose levels should be monitored more frequently during illness.
    4. Maintain food intake every day; do not skip meals.

39. Application, planning, physiological integrity, (b).
    4. The low protein provided on this diet limits end products of protein metabolism—an important consideration in kidney disease.
    1. Steak and milk provide more protein than is desirable for this patient.
    2. Hamburger and milk provide protein not desirable in this situation.
    3. Liver, cottage cheese, eggs, and cream provide a high-protein diet.

40. Knowledge, application, physiological integrity, (b).
    3. Although spicy foods can aggravate peptic ulcer disease, the causative agent is the bacterium H. pylori.
    1. Although smoking and alcohol use contribute to ulcer development, they are not the primary cause.
    2. Although these aggravate the disease, they are not the causes.
    4. Adequate rest and relaxation enhance the natural healing process of the body, but stress is not the primary cause of ulcers, although it may contribute to peptic ulcer disease.

41. Knowledge, implementation, physiological integrity, (b).
    1. Soft diets are easier to digest, thereby reducing the workload of the heart.
    2. Decreasing irritation to the digestive tract is not important in the diet therapy for cardiovascular disease.
    3. Unless the patient is overweight, no specific reason exists to reduce calories.
    4. This is not the primary reason for the soft diet in this situation.

42. Knowledge, planning, health promotion and maintenance, (b).
    2. 2.4 g/day is the recommended limit.
    1. This is below the recommended limit.
    3, 4. Both are well over the recommended limit.

43. Comprehension, planning, physiological integrity, (b).
    1. Fat is the principal cause of contraction of the diseased gallbladder.
    2. The patient still needs to consume adequate intake for energy and metabolism.
    3. Dairy products tend to be high in fat and may aggravate the pain of gallbladder disease.
    4. Carbohydrates should be the primary source of energy, especially during the acute phase of gallbladder disease.

44. Application, planning, physiological integrity, (b).
    1. Inclusion of high-fiber foods in menu planning facilitates lowered blood glucose and blood cholesterol.
    2. Fiber slows intestinal transit time.
    3. Fiber helps clear LDL cholesterol in the colon.
    4. Fiber delays gastric emptying time.

45. Knowledge, planning, physiological integrity, (b).
    3. Because of anorexia, many patients with chronic renal disease do not have adequate intake of calories or protein.
    1. Patients with chronic renal disease need to maintain normal serum potassium and sodium blood levels.
    2. Patients with chronic renal disease need to maintain acceptable levels of phosphate and calcium.
    4. Fluid balance is needed to prevent dehydration or fluid overload.

46. Application, implementation, physiological integrity, (b).
    4. This option provides soothing texture and temperature along with essential nutrients.
    1. Fatty sauces such as gravy are easier to swallow and add taste appeal to food items.
    2. These foods might irritate his mouth and make him less likely to want to eat.
    3. Snacks and frequent small meals are a good way to provide nutrition with less energy expenditure on the part of the patient.

47. Comprehension, assessment, physiological integrity, (b).
    1. Purging after eating can cause irreversible damage to the enamel of teeth because of increased acid content of the mouth.
    2, 3. These are not commonly associated with bulimia.
    3. The person with bulimia is more likely to experience hypoglycemia because of inadequate intake or retention of food.

48. Knowledge, assessment, physiological integrity, (a).
    2. Raw eggs can be contaminated with Salmonella, and vulnerable groups such as older adults, persons who are ill, babies, and pregnant women should avoid them.
    1. *E. coli* infections are associated with undercooked beef or raw milk.
    3. Botulism is associated with inadequately processed or preserved foods.
    4. *Staphylococcus* infections are associated with skin contaminants.

49. Application, implementation, physiological integrity, (b).
    Answer: 72 calories: 4 kcal/g × 18 g = 72

50. Comprehension, planning, health promotion and maintenance, (b).
    2. Increasing dairy products will increase the woman's calcium intake, which can prevent the development of osteoporosis.
    1. This is not significant in preventing osteoporosis.
    3. This does not affect the development of osteoporosis.
    4. Protein does not prevent osteoporosis, but increasing calcium-rich protein foods does.

51. Application, planning, physiological integrity, (b).
    2. Based on kilocalories and carbohydrates, green leafy vegetables contain more potassium than bananas and orange juice.
    1, 3, 4. These foods are not good food sources of potassium.

52. Comprehension, assessment, physiological integrity, (b).
    2. *This accurately describes the role of trace elements in the body.*
    1. Trace elements are essential to health.
    3. This is not accurate.
    4. Most of the minerals can be detected in bodily fluids.

53. Comprehension, planning, physiological integrity, (b).
    3. *These vitamins reduce the levels of homocysteine, but the low-protein, low-potassium diet for patients with end-stage renal disease reduces the food sources of these.*
    1, 2, 4. These would not help reduce the levels of homocysteine.

54. Comprehension, planning, health promotion and maintenance, (b).
    4. *These beliefs shape the choices teens make in selecting foods to eat.*
    1, 2. Studies show that these do not influence adolescents' eating habits.
    3. This may not influence adolescents' eating habits.

55. Comprehension, planning, health promotion and maintenance, (b).
    3. *A diet high in fat and energy and low in fruits, vegetables, and dietary fiber strongly predisposes humans and animals to the development of colon cancer.*
    1, 2. These diets are likely to help prevent colon cancer.
    4. This diet is not likely to help prevent or promote colon cancer.

56. Knowledge, assessment, physiological integrity, (b).
    2. *As lean body mass declines after 30 years of age, a gradual, but accelerating, decrease occurs in the basal metabolic rate.*
    1, 3, 4. These do not necessarily decrease with age.

57. Knowledge, assessment, physiological integrity, (b).
    2. *This disorder is characterized by recurrent episodes of bingeing, purging, fasting, and excessive exercise.*
    1. This disorder does not feature episodes of overeating.
    3, 4. These disorders are characterized by overeating without the compensatory purging behaviors.

58. Comprehension, assessment, physiological integrity, (b).
    3. *Hypertension and type 2 diabetes are the two conditions in which research has shown that a direct relation to excessive weight exists.*
    1. Obese individuals could be at risk for renal disease.
    2. Obese individuals could be at risk for gallbladder disease.
    4. Obese individuals are also at risk for degenerative joint disease.

59. Comprehension, planning, physiological integrity, (b).
    3. *This brings the total to approximately 2500 to 2700 calories/day.*
    1. Additional energy is needed for both producing milk and ensuring adequate calorie content of the fluid.
    2. Ample fluid intake, in the range of 8 to 10 glasses daily, is needed before and during lactation.
    4. This does not contribute to the health of the mother or the baby.

60. Application, implementation, physiological integrity, (b).
    2. *Tea causes diuresis and increases the need of the body for water.*
    1. Tea is not a good substitute, and adding sugar to the diet is not a healthy choice.

3. Tea can reduce the amount of iron that the body absorbs.
4. Tea contains nearly as much caffeine as coffee and is considered a stimulant.

61. Knowledge, planning, health promotion and maintenance, (b).
    2. *Carbohydrates and fat are the primary fuels that the body uses to maintain energy reserves.*
    1, 3. Protein has only a small role as a fuel substrate in energy production; it may be used only when fuel supply from carbohydrates and fats is insufficient.
    4. See rationale for Nos. 1 and 3; vitamins are not macronutrients.

62. Comprehension, implementation, safe and effective care environment, (b).
    4. *The source of contamination for most S. aureus food poisonings is from an infection on the hand of a worker preparing food.*
    1. *Clostridium* infections are usually caused by inadequately prepared or preserved foods.
    2. *Salmonella* poisonings usually result from eating contaminated raw eggs.
    3. *E. coli* infections are usually the result of improperly cooked, contaminated beef.

63. Comprehension, assessment, physiological integrity, (b).
    2. *Although eating balanced meals at regular times is a prudent approach, nutrition has no known effect on premenstrual syndrome.*
    1, 3, 4. Nutrition has no known effect on premenstrual syndrome.

64. Knowledge, planning, physiological integrity, (b).
    Answer: 400 calories
    The lowest amount of calories from fat in the diet is 20%, which translates to 400 calories.

65. Knowledge, planning, physiological integrity, (b).
    Answer: 900 calories
    The lowest amount of calories from carbohydrates in a 2000-calorie diet is 45%, which translates to 900 calories.

66. Comprehension, assessment, safe and effective care environment, (b).
    3. *This can be unsafe because of the possibility of infection or fermentation of retained substances and because the patient is deprived of the benefit of the nutrition or therapeutic effect of medication. It is common in children, psychiatric patients, and confused patients.*
    1. This process is known as *diverticulosis*.
    2. This is associated with increased morbidity and mortality related to obesity.
    4. Although this is a prudent practice, it is not known as pouching.

67. Knowledge, implementation, health promotion and maintenance, (b).
    __X__ 1. *The WIC program is designed to provide nutritional education.*
    __X__ 2. *WIC provides vouchers for prescribed supplemental foods and is aimed at promoting the growth of the young child.*
    _____ 3. Meals on Wheels are delivered to homebound elderly patients.
    _____ 4. Community meals for any low-income adult would come under the Nutrition Services Incentive Program, not WIC.

_____ 5. Dietary counseling for patients with eating disorders is a psychological aspect, and patients would require treatment on an individual basis.

68. Comprehension, planning, physiological integrity, (b).
   4. Substances on the list meet strict guidelines for inclusion.
   1. Food additives come from many different sources.
   2. Substances on the list are determined to be generally safe for consumption.
   3. Some of the food additives designed to retain freshness may not be on the GRAS list.

69. Application, planning, physiological integrity, (b).
   2. These agents emulsify tiny particles of one liquid in another to improve texture and consistency.
   1. Typical additives in this category are vitamins, minerals, milk, and iodized salt.
   3. Typical additives in this category are spices, citrus oils, and amyl acetate.
   4. Typical additives in this category are butylated hydroxytoluene, benzoates, and propionic acid.

70. Application, assessment, physiological integrity, (b).
   3. Most antipsychotic drugs have this effect, caused in part by increased appetite.
   1. This is a false statement and would frighten the patient.
   2. This does not address the issue of the side effect of the medication.
   4. This is not a prudent comment for the nurse to make under the circumstances, and it does not address the issue of the side effect of the medication.

71. Application, planning, physiological integrity, (b).
   1. In many instances desserts such as trifle have a liqueur poured over them; tiramisu may have a coffee liqueur incorporated into it. Patients must be educated to avoid all sources of alcohol, not just alcoholic beverages.
   2, 3, 4. These statements address neither the patient's concerns nor the real risk of ingesting alcohol that is not obvious.

72. Application, implementation, physiological integrity, (b).
   2. Stopping diabetes medication, whether oral hypoglycemic agents or insulin, is best done only with a physician's supervision.
   1, 3. Advising the patient not to take her medication can lead to a hyperglycemic reaction if the patient has soft or liquid foods without medication.
   4. This is not a prudent comment for the nurse to make. Stopping diabetes medication, whether oral hypoglycemic agents or insulin, is best done only with a physician's supervision.

73. Comprehension, planning, physiological integrity, (b).
   4. Saturated fatty acids raise blood cholesterol, which raises the risk of coronary heart disease and stroke.
   1. Trans fatty acids, or hydrogenated fats, tend to raise total blood cholesterol levels and low-density lipoprotein ("bad") cholesterol and to lower high-density lipoprotein ("good") cholesterol.
   2. Monounsaturated fatty acids seem to lower blood cholesterol when substituted for saturated fats.

   3. These foods do not contribute to raising the serum cholesterol.

74. Knowledge, assessment, physiological integrity (a)
   2. Constipation is a common side effect of narcotic analgesics.
   1, 3, 4. These are not side effects of narcotic analgesics.

75. Knowledge, assessment, physiological integrity (b),
   2. Lignin is the only noncarbohydrate type of dietary fiber.
   1, 3, 4. These are types of dietary fiber, but lignin is the only noncarbohydrate.

76. Comprehension, assessment, physiological integrity (b),
   4. Sugar alcohols are sugar substitutes; therefore they do not contribute to tooth decay.
   1. Constipation does not result because of the slowing of digestion but could be a downside.
   2. Diarrhea may result from sugar alcohols, which would be a downside.
   3. Indigestion does not result.

77. Knowledge, assessment, physiological integrity, (b).
   Answer: 4
   To meet energy needs of the body, carbohydrates burn at the rate of 4 kcal/g, which makes the fuel factor for carbohydrates 4.

78. Analysis, assessment, health promotion and maintenance, (c).
   4. Olive oil is a monounsaturated fat, meaning it has one unfilled spot; therefore it is not saturated. A patient wishing to lower his risk of heart disease needs to avoid saturated fats.
   1, 2, 3. Bacon, eggs, and palm oil are saturated fats.

79. Analysis, evaluation, physiological integrity, (c).
   4. The 78-year-old grandmother would have the lowest energy need per unit of body weight because in the aging process the gradual decline in basal metabolic rate and physical activity decreases the total energy requirement.
   1. The 6-month-old girl has the highest energy needs.
   2, 3. The 31-year-old mother and 37-year-old father have achieved full adult growth, and their energy needs have leveled off.

80. Comprehension, evaluation, physiological integrity, (b).
   Answer: 82 kilocalories
   16 g (protein) × 4 kcal/g = 64 kcal
   2 g (fat) × 9 kcal/g = 18 kcal
   64 kcal + 18 kcal = 82 kcal

81. Analysis, evaluation, physiological integrity (b)
   2. The richest sources of vitamin E are vegetable oils such as safflower oil.
   1. The meat and poultry group is not an important source of vitamin E.
   3. The bread and cereal group is not an important source of vitamin E.
   4. The dairy group is not an important source of vitamin E.

82. Application, implementation, health promotion and maintenance, (b).
   4. The vegetable and fruit group is an excellent source of vitamin C.
   1. The bread and cereal group is not an important source of vitamin C.
   2. The dairy group is not an important source of vitamin C.

3. The fats and oil group is not an important source of vitamin C.

83. Comprehension, assessment, physiological integrity, (b).
    Answer: 99%

    Most of the calcium supply in the body, more than 99%, is found in teeth and bones, whereas an approximate 1% to 2% of normal adult body weight is attributed to calcium.

84. Comprehension, assessment, physiological integrity, (b).
    3. The heart is very sensitive to potassium levels because these contribute to nerve impulse transmission to stimulate muscle action.

    1. Calcium is responsible for bone and tooth formation, blood clotting, metabolic reactions, and muscle and nerve action, but calcium is not as sensitive as potassium.
    2. Chloride is a key element in hydrochloric acid and therefore is involved with digestion; chloride ions also assist red blood cells to transport large amounts of CO_2 to the lungs for release in breathing.
    4. Functions of sulfa deal with hair, skin, nails, general metabolic functions, vitamin structure, and collagen structure.

85. Application, implementation, health promotion and maintenance, (b).
    X   1. Be patient; toddlers are just learning to pick up a fork, and they take longer to eat.
    X   2. Offering a variety of foods helps to develop broad taste.
    _____ 3. Avoid overseasoning; let tastes develop gradually.
    _____ 4. Keep the main meal on the table before serving dessert; often if they are still hungry they will eat more food.
    X   5. It is best to serve small portions and then let them ask for seconds if they are still hungry.

86. Analysis, application, safe and effective care environment, (c).
    Correct order: 2431.
    2. Clean.
    4. Separate
    3. Cook.
    1. Chill
    Based on campaign (Fight BAC) to prevent foodborne illness developed by the Partnership for Food Safety Education.

87. Comprehension, assessment, health promotion and maintenance, (b).
    X   1. Teenagers (young persons) are often figure conscious and concerned about how they might appear to people of the opposite sex, which often results in their resorting to crash diets or other fads to attain a "perfect" body.
    X   2. Older persons, especially those with chronic illness, may also turn to food fads that promise a "cure."
    _____ 3. Persons following food mandates of their religion are not considered vulnerable based solely on those mandates.
    X   4. Athletes and their coaches are prime candidates for miracle supplements so they can gain a competitive edge.
    X   5. Obese persons face a multitude of diets and supplements that promise easy and fast weight loss.

X   6. Movie stars must maintain a certain appearance to maintain their careers.

88. Analysis, implementation, health promotion and maintenance, (c).
    X   1. Energy
    _____ 2. Condiments are not components of diets
    X   3. Nutrients
    X   4. Texture
    1, 3, 4. These are all components of a regular diet that can be modified.

89. Analysis, assessment, physiological integrity, (c).
    Answer: B

    A demonstrates a vertical banded gastroplasty. C is a roux-en-Y procedure, D is a Billroth I gastroduodenostomy, and E is a Billroth II gastrojejunostomy.

90. Knowledge, planning, physiological integrity, (a).
    1. Bouillon is a broth that is allowed on a clear liquid diet.
    2, 3, 4. These are allowed only on a full liquid diet; they are not clear.

91. Application, assessment, health promotion and maintenance, (b).
    X   1. The purging behavior may involve oral mucosal irritation.
    _____ 2. The length of the fingernails is not a direct effect of this condition.
    _____ 3. These patients have episodes of binge eating, not avoiding food.
    X   4. Tooth enamel erosion comes from the purging behavior.
    X   5. Individuals with bulimia nervosa often have low self-esteem and are depressed.

92. Application, implementation, physiological integrity, (b).
    Answer: 99 calories
    1 g of fat=9 kcal; 11×9=99 kcal

93. Analysis, planning, physiological integrity, (a).
    Correct order: 32415.
    3. Biting and chewing begins the breakdown.
    2. The mixed mass of food particles is swallowed.
    4. Muscles at the base of the tongue facilitate swallowing.
    1. Gravity aids the movement of food down the esophagus.
    5. The gastroesophageal sphincter relaxes to allow swallowing and entrance into the stomach.
    The first process that occurs in the mouth is mastication (biting and chewing), by which food is broken down into smaller particles. After the food has been chewed, the mixed mass of food particles is swallowed; the muscles at the base of the tongue aid in swallowing. Gravity then aids the movement of food down the esophagus. Then the gastroesophageal sphincter relaxes to allow the food to enter into the stomach.

94. Analysis, assessment, physiological integrity, (c).
    3. Characteristic findings of potassium depletion include heart muscle, respiratory, and intestinal muscle weaknesses.

    1. A decrease in the number of RBCs is indicative of poor iron intake in the diet or some other underlying clinical manifestation.
    2. Edema of the extremities could indicate poor compliance with the drug regimen or increased intake of sodium.
    4. Reduced bone mass is seen in osteoporosis.

95. Analysis, assessment, physiological integrity, (c).

3. Excess intake of beta carotene will result in an orange skin tint.

1 Burning, tingling, and itching can result from excessive amounts of niacin.

2. Malformation of bones can result from a deficiency of vitamin D.

4. Poor blood clotting can be caused by lack of vitamin K.

96. Analysis, assessment, physiological integrity, (c).

1. Breakfast—1 poached egg, coffee, and 1 medium fresh peach are the correct choices for a diabetic patient because the poached egg is rich in protein and a good meat substitute, black coffee has no carbohydrates, and 1 medium fresh peach has 15g carbohydrates, no fat, and no protein for added carbohydrates.

2. The lunch choice adds chips and a cookie, which are high in carbohydrates and fats.

3. Dinner should include ½ cup of brown rice, ½ cup applesauce, and ½ cup of green beans; the choices as presented provide too many carbohydrates.

4. The snack choice with the buttered popcorn adds too many carbohydrates with the extra butter. The diet soda is fine. If an apple is added, it should be a small one not a large one, for fewer carbohydrates.

97. Analysis, assessment, health promotion and maintenance, (b).

2. Most water in the chyme entering the large intestine is absorbed in the first half of the colon; the ascending and transverse colon can accomplish this task.

1. The cecum area is not large enough to accomplish this task.

3, 4. The descending colon and sigmoid colon help to form and eliminate the feces.

98. Analysis, assessment, physiological integrity, (c).

4. Blurred vision can be one of the first signs of diabetes.

1, 2, 3. All other assessment findings are within normal limits.

99. Analysis, assessment, physiological integrity, (c).

1. Bradycardia is an assessment finding indicative of an interaction between a calcium channel blocker and grapefruit juice.

2, 3, 4. All other options (diaphoresis, elevated blood sugar, and weight loss) are not indicative of a drug-food interaction between a calcium channel blocker and grapefruit juice.

100. Analysis, assessment, health promotion and maintenance, (b).

4. One-half cup of sweet potato is an appropriate exchange or choice for a diabetic diet according to the exchange list.

1. A better choice for fruit would be the plain fruit itself, such as a medium or small apple.

2. A better milk choice is fat-free or low-fat milk, which provides fewer carbohydrates.

3. A cereal choice of bran is a good choice, but only ½ cup, not ¾ cup, which provides fewer carbohydrates.

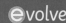
Medical-Surgical Nursing

Objectives

After studying this chapter, the student should be able to:

1. Describe the nursing care responsibilities surrounding diagnostic tests.
2. Identify signs and symptoms of common medical diagnoses.
3. Plan nursing interventions for individuals with nursing diagnoses.

4. Evaluate the effectiveness of nursing interventions for individuals with select nursing diagnoses.
5. Describe the responsibilities of the nurse regarding the patient who is undergoing surgery.

This chapter presents the nursing assessment of medical-surgical patients and is organized according to the body systems affected. Following the nursing process, frequent patient problems and recommended nursing care are identified and discussed. A selected group of major diagnoses, medical management, and nursing care plans is included. Although assessment of the functioning and problems of each system is isolated, the student must remember that total patient assessment is necessary each time a patient is given care. The chapter begins with a brief overview of anatomy and physiology before moving on to the anatomy and physiology of the individual body systems.

ANATOMY AND PHYSIOLOGY: AN OVERVIEW

A. Anatomy: the study of the structure of the body, its many parts, and their relationship to one another
B. Physiology: the study of how the body and its many parts function
C. Homeostasis: a state of constancy or dynamic equilibrium within the body
D. Anatomical terminology
   1. Anatomical position: the body is erect, with arms at sides and palms turned forward
   2. Anterior: toward the front of the body
   3. Posterior: toward the back of the body
   4. Cranial: near the head
   5. Superior: toward the head
   6. Inferior: toward the lower aspect
   7. Medial: toward the midline
   8. Lateral: toward the side
   9. Proximal: nearest the origin of a structure (elbows are proximal to the fingers, shoulder is proximal to the elbow)
   10. Distal: farthest from the origin of a structure
E. Body cavities
   1. Dorsal: pertaining to the back; has two subdivisions that are continuous with each other
      a. Cranial: the space inside the skull; contains the brain
      b. Spinal: extends from the cranial cavity nearly to the end of the vertebral column; contains the spinal cord

   2. Ventral: pertaining to the front; contains structures of the chest and abdomen; has two subdivisions
      a. Thoracic: chest cavity; contains the heart, lungs, and large blood vessels; separated from the lower cavity by the diaphragm
      b. Abdominopelvic: one large cavity with no separation
         (1) Abdominal: upper portion; contains stomach, liver, gallbladder, pancreas, spleen, kidneys, and most of the intestines
         (2) Pelvic: lower portion; contains urinary bladder, lower part of intestines, and internal reproductive organs

STRUCTURAL UNITS

Cell

A. Definition: basic unit of structure and function of all living things; made of protoplasm (meaning "original substance"), which is composed of oxygen, hydrogen, nitrogen, carbon, sulfur, and phosphorus; varies in size and shape
B. Structure and function
   1. Structural parts
      a. Cytoplasmic membrane: keeps cell whole and intact; allows certain substances to pass through and prevents others from entering (semipermeable membrane)
      b. Cytoplasm: area in which most cellular activity occurs; the working and storage area
      c. Nucleus: the control center; directs cell activity and is necessary for reproduction; the site of the genetic material, deoxyribonucleic acid (DNA)
   2. Characteristics of cells
      a. Irritability: respond to stimuli
      b. Growth and reproduction: get larger in size and are able to increase in number
      c. Metabolism: chemical reaction consisting of:
         (1) Anabolism: forming new substances to build new cell material; constructive
         (2) Catabolism: breaking down of substances into simpler substances and disposing of waste; destructive
      d. Contractility: the ability to shorten and thicken in response to a stimulus

e. Conductivity: ability to transfer an electrical charge or impulse
3. Functions
   a. Movement of substances through cell membranes
      (1) Diffusion: movement of dissolved particles through a semipermeable membrane from an area of high concentration of particles to an area of low concentration of particles. Diffusion continues until the particles are evenly distributed.
      (2) Osmosis: movement of water through a semipermeable membrane from an area in which a large amount of water (dilute solution) exists to an area of a low concentration of water (a concentrated solution). Osmosis occurs until the water is evenly distributed.
      (3) Filtration: movement of water and particles through a membrane because of a greater pushing force on one side of the membrane (hydrostatic pressure)
   b. Reproduction mitosis: process of cell division; distributes identical chromosomes (DNA molecules) to each cell formed; enables cells to reproduce their own kind

Tissues
A. Definition: groups of similar cells having like functions
B. Classifications and functions
   1. Epithelial: cells are packed closely together; contain no blood vessels; three main types:
      a. Simple squamous: single layer of cells through which substances can pass; function is absorption; lines air sacs of lungs, lines blood vessels, and covers membranes that line body cavity
      b. Stratified squamous: several layers of closely packed cells; protect the body against invasion of microorganisms; outer layer of skin, epidermis
      c. Simple columnar: single layer of cells; lines the stomach, intestines, and respiratory tract; specializes in secreting mucus and absorption
   2. Connective: cells are separated by intercellular material; located in all parts of the body; various types include areolar, adipose, bone, and cartilage; function to support and protect
   3. Muscle: three types of muscle tissue
      a. Skeletal or striated (voluntary): cells have striations; attach to bones; contractions are controlled voluntarily; cause movement.
      b. Cardiac or striated (involuntary): cells have cross-striations; cardiac muscle cells have the inherent power of rhythmical contraction.
      c. Visceral or nonstriated (smooth involuntary): cells appear smooth; help form walls of blood vessels and intestines; contractions cannot be controlled; cause movement.
   4. Nerve: composed of cells called *neurons;* all neurons receive and conduct electrochemical impulses; important in control of the entire body.

Membranes
A. Definition: thin, soft sheets of tissue that cover, line, lubricate, and anchor body parts
B. Classification and functions
   1. Epithelial: lubricate and protect the body against infection; two types
      a. Mucous: line body cavities that open to the exterior (mouth, nose, intestinal tract, urinary tract, vaginal canal); secrete mucus, which protects against bacterial invasion
      b. Serous: line cavities that do not open to the exterior; cover the lungs, stomach, and heart; secrete thin fluid that prevents friction
   2. Connective: cover bone or hold body parts in place
      a. Skeletal: cover bones and cartilage; support the bony structure
      b. Synovial: line joint cavities and secrete synovial fluid, which lubricates
      c. Fascial or fibrous: hold organs in place; superficial—connect the skin to underlying structures; deep—support the internal organs (the viscera)

Organs
Organs are structures composed of several tissues grouped together. They perform a more complex function than does a single tissue. The composition and structure depend on their function.

Systems
A. Definition: groups of organs that contribute to the function of the whole; they perform a more complex function than does a single organ. No system can function independently of another system.
B. Body systems and functions
   1. Integumentary (skin): covers and protects the body; aids in fluid balance
   2. Musculoskeletal: supports and allows movement; framework of the body
   3. Circulatory: transports food, water, oxygen, and waste
   4. Digestive: processes food and eliminates waste
   5. Respiratory: supplies oxygen and eliminates carbon dioxide
   6. Urinary: excretes waste
   7. Nervous: controls and coordinates body activities
   8. Endocrine: regulates body activities
   9. Reproductive: increases the number of the species

MUSCULOSKELETAL SYSTEM

ANATOMY AND PHYSIOLOGY OF THE SKELETAL SYSTEM (FIGURE 5-1)
A. Functions
   1. Support: forms framework for body structures and provides shape
   2. Protection: protects the internal organs
   3. Movement: supplies levers that are activated by the contraction of an attached muscle
   4. Mineral storage: stores calcium and minerals used by the body when needed
   5. Produces blood cells: forms erythrocytes and thrombocytes and red marrow of bone
B. Bone composition
   1. Composed of 33% organic material and 67% inorganic mineral salts
   2. Collagen: organic part derived from a protein; fibrous material with a jellylike substance between the fibers; gives bone flexibility

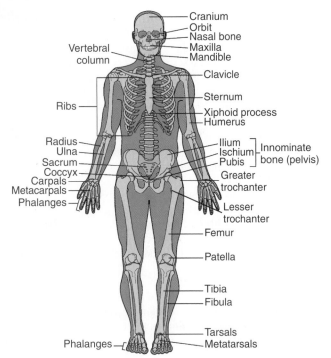

Cranium
Orbit
Nasal bone
Maxilla
Mandible
Vertebral column
Clavicle
Sternum
Ribs
Xiphoid process
Humerus
Radius
Ulna
Sacrum
Coccyx
Carpals
Metacarpals
Phalanges
Ilium
Ischium — Innominate
Pubis — bone (pelvis)
Greater trochanter
Lesser trochanter
Femur
Patella
Tibia
Fibula
Tarsals
Phalanges
Metatarsals

FIGURE 5-1 Bones of the body. (From Sorrentino SA, Remmert LN: *Mosby's textbook for nursing assistants,* ed 8, St Louis, 2012, Mosby.)

3. Inorganic substance consists of large amount of mineral salts: calcium phosphate, calcium carbonate, calcium fluoride, magnesium phosphate, sodium oxide, and sodium chloride, which give bone its hardness and durability

C. Classification of bones
1. Long bone: consists of diaphysis, epiphysis, and medullary cavity (e.g., femur)
2. Short bone: contains more spongy bone than compact; generally cube shaped (e.g., wrist bone)
3. Flat bone: thin and flat; two thin layers of compact bone with a spongy bone between them; red blood cells (RBCs) manufactured here (e.g., sternum)
4. Irregular: do not fall into preceding categories; are not symmetrical (e.g., vertebrae)

D. Structure of long bones
1. Long bones are similar to other bones in the body in structure, development, and function.
2. They are longer than wide and have a shaft with heads at both ends. Bones of extremities are long bones.
3. Diaphysis or shaft: hollow cylinder of hard, compact bone; contains medullary canal, which is filled with yellow bone marrow. In the adult it is primarily a storage area for adipose tissue.
4. Epiphysis: ends of the diaphysis composed of spongy bone covered by a thin layer of compact bone; contains red marrow where some RBCs are manufactured during childhood and adolescence. Erythropoietic activity in the adult occurs mainly in flat bones and vertebrae.
5. Periosteum: strong fibrous membrane that covers the bone and contains blood vessels; lymph vessels; nerves; and bone cells necessary for growth, repair, and nutrition.

6. Epiphyseal disk (flat plate made up of hyaline cartilage): allows for lengthwise growth of long bones. At puberty when growth stops, it calcifies and becomes the epiphyseal line.
7. Haversian canals: run lengthwise through bone matrix, carrying blood vessels and nerves to all areas of the bone. They nourish the osteocytes, or bone cells.

E. Processes: bony prominences that serve as landmarks
1. Acromion: highest point of the shoulder
2. Olecranon: upper end of the ulna; forms the point of the elbow
3. Iliac crest: curved rim along the upper border of the ilium
4. Ischial spine: lies at the back of the pelvic outlet
5. Acetabulum: deep socket in the hip bone
6. Greater trochanter: large protuberance located at the top of the shaft of the femur

F. Factors that affect bone growth and maintenance
1. Heredity: Each person has a genetic potential for height, with genes inherited from both parents
2. Nutrition: Nutrients such as calcium, phosphorus, and proteins are raw materials of which bones are made; without nutrients, bones cannot grow properly.
3. Hormones: Produced by endocrine glands, they help regulate cell division, protein synthesis, calcium metabolism, and energy production.
4. Exercise: bearing weight such as walking. Without exercise, bones become weak and fragile because of the loss of calcium.

G. Joints: points at which bones meet; classification determined by the extent of movement
1. Synarthroses: Fibrous connective tissue holds joining bones close together with no movement (e.g., sutures in skull).
2. Amphiarthroses: There is slight movement (e.g., joints between the vertebrae).
3. Diarthroses: Free movement; all have a joint capsule, a joint cavity, and a layer of cartilage.
   a. Ball-and-socket joint: Ball-shaped head of one bone fits into a concave socket of another bone (e.g., hip joint).
   b. Hinge joint: It allows movement in only two directions, flexion and extension (e.g., knee).
   c. Pivot joint: A small projection of one bone pivots in an arch of another bone (e.g., vertebrae of the neck).
   d. Saddle joint: It exists only between the metacarpal bone and a carpal bone of the wrist (e.g., thumb and wrist).
   e. Gliding joint: Bone surfaces slide over one another (e.g., wrist, ankle).

H. Ligaments: connective tissue bands that hold bones together
I. Tendons: connective tissue bands that attach bones to muscles
J. Bursa: a sac or cavity filled with fluid (synovia or synovial fluid) that reduces friction at joints

ANATOMY AND PHYSIOLOGY OF THE MUSCULAR SYSTEM (FIGURE 5-2)

A. Functions
1. Produces movement by contraction (Table 5-1)
2. Maintains posture
3. Produces heat and energy

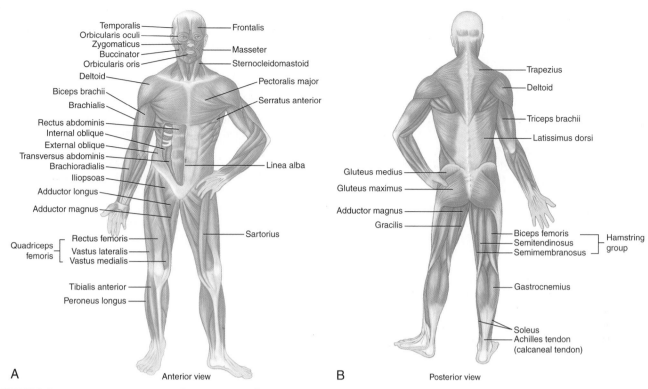

FIGURE 5-2 Major muscles of the body. **A**, Anterior view. **B**, Posterior view. (From Herlihy B: *The human body in health and illness,* ed 4, St Louis, 2011, Saunders.)

Table 5-1 **The Skeletal Muscles**

MUSCLE	LOCATION	FUNCTION
Sternocleidomastoid	Neck	Flexion and rotation of head
Trapezius	Upper back	Helps hold head erect; also assists in moving head sideways
Latissimus dorsi	Lower back	Extension and adduction of upper arm
Pectoralis major	Chest	Flexion and abduction of upper arm
Deltoid	Shoulder	Adduction of upper arm
Biceps brachii	Anterior upper arm	Flexion of arm and forearm
Triceps brachii	Posterior upper arm	Extension of arm and forearm
Gluteus maximus	Fleshy part of hips and buttocks	Extension of thigh
Gluteus medius	Lateral part of hips and buttocks	Abduction of thigh when limb is extended
Hamstring group	Posterior thigh	Flexion of lower leg and extension of thigh
Quadriceps femoris	Anterior thigh	Flexion of thigh and extension of lower leg
Gastrocnemius	Calf of leg	Helps in extension of foot and flexion of leg

B. Structure and types
  1. Striated: skeletal, voluntary muscle; attached to bones and accounts for body movement; controlled consciously
  2. Smooth: visceral, nonstriated, involuntary muscle; found in the walls of internal organs and blood vessels; works automatically
  3. Cardiac: found only in the heart; striated, branched, and involuntary
C. Characteristics
  1. Excitability: capacity to respond to stimulus

  2. Contractility: ability to shorten and thicken in response to a stimulus
  3. Extensibility: ability to stretch
  4. Elasticity: ability to regain original size and shape
  5. Tonicity: ability to maintain steady contraction
D. Contraction and movement
  1. Muscles move bones by pulling on them; as muscle contracts, it pulls insertion bone toward its original bone.
    a. Origin: attached to fixed structure of bone
    b. Insertion: attached to movable part

2. Several muscles contract at the same time to produce movement.
   a. Agonist: prime mover; responsible mainly for producing movement
   b. Antagonists: responsible for relaxing when the prime mover is contracting
   c. Synergists: aid the prime mover in producing movement
3. To contract, muscle must first be stimulated by nerve impulses.
   a. Subminimal stimulus: does not cause contraction
   b. Minimal stimulus: does cause contraction
   c. Maximal stimulus: causes all muscle fibers in muscle to contract
   d. Supramaximal stimulus: strength of stimulus above maximal; no effect on strength of contraction
4. Types of contractions
   a. Isometric: increase the tension without causing movement
   b. Isotonic: produce movement
   c. Tonic: do not produce movement but increase firmness of muscles that maintain posture
   d. Twitch: a quick, jerky contraction
   e. Tetanic (tetanus): sustained contraction
5. Types of movement
   a. Flexion: makes angle at joint smaller
   b. Extension: makes angle at joint larger
   c. Abduction: moves part away from midline
   d. Adduction: moves part toward midline

MUSCULOSKELETAL CONDITIONS AND DISORDERS

Musculoskeletal disorders may be acute or chronic. Acute problems are usually related to simple injuries. Chronic disorders may be more distressing to the patient because of loss of mobility and changes in self-image. The nurse needs to possess excellent observational skills, provide safe positioning of the patient, and exercise care in use of equipment. The nurse is probably the most important preventive health care provider associated with complications of immobility.

NURSING ASSESSMENT

A. Observation (objective data)
   1. General appearance
      a. Age
      b. Weight loss or weight gain
      c. Height changes: loss
      d. Abnormal gait
      e. Absence of extremity
      f. Deformity
      g. Crepitus
      h. Malalignment
      i. Use of assistive devices
      j. Spinal curvature (kyphosis, scoliosis, lordosis)
   2. Respirations
      a. Rate
      b. Depth
      c. Character: any difficulty (wheezing, shortness of breath, crackles)
   3. Pulse
      a. Presence of pulse above and below injured part or part in a cast
      b. Rate, quality, character

   4. Neurovascular status
      a. Assessment of skin color and temperature
      b. Pulses, presence of
      c. Intact sensation (with numbness noted)
      d. Motor function
      e. Sensation and capillary refill
   5. Motor function
      a. Comparison of affected and unaffected sides
      b. Limited ability or loss of ability to move body part
      c. Diminished muscle strength to passive resistance
      d. Limited range of motion (ROM)
      e. Degree of ability to perform activities of daily living (ADLs)
   6. Pain and swelling
      a. Location, character, intensity, frequency, duration, alleviating or aggravating factors
      b. Bony enlargements or soft-tissue swelling
B. Patient description (subjective data)
   1. Pain
      a. Patient's account of location, character, frequency, duration, onset
      b. May use the PQRST method of assessment
         P: provoking incident: What initially caused the pain?
         Q: quality of pain: Is the pain throbbing, stabbing, or burning?
         R: region: Where is the pain? Does the pain radiate? What measures relieve the pain?
         S: severity of the pain: Is the pain mild, moderate, or severe?
         T: timing of pain: When is the pain worse?
   2. Stamina
      a. Weakness, fatigue
      b. Changes in ability to perform ADLs
   3. Report of recent injury
      a. Description
      b. Evaluation and treatment
   4. Motor function
      a. Pain with movement
      b. Limited movement; difficult gait
   5. General
      a. Maintenance of weight
      b. Changes in appetite
      c. Tolerance of ADLs

DIAGNOSTIC TESTS AND METHODS

A. Serum laboratory studies
   1. Complete blood count (CBC): an aid in determining anemia or the presence of infection
   2. Erythrocyte sedimentation rate (ESR): if elevated, evidence of an inflammatory process
   3. Rheumatoid factor: protein found in the blood of most people with rheumatoid arthritis
   4. Uric acid: high concentration found in persons who have gout
   5. Lupus erythematosus (LE) cell
      a. A cell identified in persons with LE
      b. Normally no LE cells in the blood
B. Procedures
   1. Roentgenogram (x-ray): film to determine the presence of a deformity, fracture, or tumor of the skeletal system
   2. Aspiration: withdrawal of fluid from a joint to obtain a specimen for diagnostic purposes

3. Bone biopsy: removal and examination of bone tissue
4. Bone scan: isotope imaging of the skeleton
5. Computed tomography (CT): use of roentgen rays to obtain accurate images of thin cross-sections of the body
   a. Nursing care for CT
      (1) An informed consent must be obtained.
      (2) Ascertain allergies to iodine or seafood.
      (3) Most CT scans require NPO (nothing by mouth) status.
6. Magnetic resonance imaging (MRI): aids in diagnosing musculoskeletal conditions through the clear differentiation of various types of tissue such as bones, fat, and muscle; nursing care includes removal of metal jewelry and assessing for metal implants
7. Arthroscopy: endoscopic examination that allows for direct visualization of a joint
8. Electromyography (EMG): used to evaluate nerve conduction in skeletal muscle
9. Positron emission tomography (PET): using an isotope, scans the brain for evaluation of structure function
10. Myelogram: x-ray examination of the spinal cord after injection with radiopaque dye (important to inquire about any known allergies to dyes)

C. Nursing interventions after a myelogram
1. After procedure, patient must remain flat in bed for 8 to 12 hours before resumption of usual activities.
2. Encourage fluids to 2000 to 3000 mL every 24 hours.
3. Observe for alterations in normal motor and sensory states.
4. Observe for nausea and vomiting.
5. Administer medication as ordered by physician should patient complain of headache after the procedure.

FREQUENT PATIENT PROBLEMS AND NURSING CARE

A. Disturbed body image related to immobility
1. Provide atmosphere of acceptance; be an active listener
2. Express empathy, warmth, and friendliness.
3. Encourage acceptance of self-limitations.
4. Encourage self-performance.

B. Impaired skin integrity: potential breakdown related to immobility and assistive devices
1. Change patient's position frequently (usually every 2 hours).
2. Keep the skin clean, dry, and lubricated.
3. Massage bony prominences.
4. Provide sheepskin, polyurethane foam padding, or alternating pressure mattress when appropriate.

C. Risk for injury: joint contracture related to incorrect body alignment
1. Place hands, feet, and knees in the natural position of function.
2. Provide devices to protect against poor alignment of body part.
3. Assist in performing active and passive ROM exercises.
4. Provide trapeze over patient's bed.
5. Avoid pillows under knee or any prolonged pressure on popliteal space.

D. Ineffective airway clearance related to increased secretions resulting from immobility
1. Change patient's position frequently (usually every 2 hours).

2. Encourage coughing and deep breathing and use of incentive spirometer if provided.
3. Observe for coughing, fever, and green-yellow sputum.
4. Increase fluids unless contraindicated.

E. Ineffective tissue perfusion: potential for thrombi and emboli related to impaired physical mobility or edema
1. Inquire about history of deep vein thrombosis (DVT), other varicosities.
2. Encourage patient to move lower extremities.
3. Encourage adequate hydration.
4. Avoid use of pillows under knee.
5. To avoid release of emboli, never rub legs.
6. Encourage use of antiembolism stockings.
7. Take daily calf measurements.

F. Acute pain related to bone fracture or disease
1. Inspect and palpate the painful site, looking for inflammation, edema, bruising, tenderness, and skin warmth; do not rub site, to avoid causing emboli.
2. Support the affected body part.
3. Apply warm, moist compress to affected body part where prescribed. Use ice for injuries within the first 24 to 48 hours.
4. Give prescribed analgesic.
5. Evaluate effectiveness of pain relief measures.
6. Patient teaching for early recognition and reporting of discomfort or pain.

G. Impaired physical mobility related to cast or traction confinement, joint pain, stiffness, or inflammation
1. Explain the reason for and intended effect of ROM exercises.
2. Have patient maintain body alignment.
3. Provide total exercising of muscles and joints unless severe pain or inflammation is present. Movement is contraindicated if recent surgery was performed on or near the joint.

H. Acute pain related to cast
1. Massage the area around the cast except for leg casts.
2. Pad rough edges.
3. Elevate extremity to reduce swelling.
4. Inspect the skin for irritation.
5. Observe for cyanosis and assess capillary refill times of the extremity in a cast.
6. Observe for complaints of numbness and tingling of the extremity in a cast.
7. Observe cast for indentations.

I. Self-care deficits (feeding, bathing, hygiene) related to impaired physical mobility
1. Assist with ADLs.
2. Provide self-care aids or devices.
3. Teach self-care activities.

MAJOR MEDICAL DIAGNOSES
Rheumatoid Arthritis

A. Definition: chronic, systemic disease in which inflammatory changes occur throughout the connective tissue in the body, destroying joints internally. Joints most involved are hands, wrists, elbows, knees, and ankles.
B. Pathology: cause is unknown. Related theories include autoimmune causes, microorganisms, viruses, and genetic predisposition.

C. Signs and symptoms
1. Subjective
   a. Sore, achy joint or joints
   b. Fatigue
   c. Weakness
   d. Malaise
   e. Loss of appetite
   f. Morning stiffness
   g. Joint pain
2. Objective
   a. Low-grade fever
   b. Weakened grip
   c. Anemia
   d. Weight loss
   e. Subcutaneous nodes
   f. Enlarged lymph nodes
   g. Joint deformity
   h. Muscle atrophy
   i. Limited ROM
   j. Edema and tenderness of joint
   k. Extraarticular symptoms: lung, heart, blood vessels, muscle, eye, and skin
D. Diagnostic tests and methods
1. Elevated ESR
2. Slightly elevated white blood cell (WBC) count
3. Presence of serum rheumatoid factors
4. Synovial fluid aspiration
5. X-ray film to reveal joint deformity
6. Low hemoglobin (Hgb) and hematocrit (Hct)
E. Treatment
1. Antiinflammatory agents, analgesics, corticosteroids, gold salts, antineoplastics (methotrexate), immunosuppressive drugs
2. Heat applications such as paraffin dip, hot packs, and warm tub baths or showers for analgesia or muscle relaxation
3. Surgical intervention to prevent deformities or remove damaged joints
4. Physical therapy to maintain optimal function
F. Nursing interventions
1. Provide undisturbed periods of rest—should receive 8 to 10 hours of sleep per night with frequent naps during the day.
2. Use firm mattress, footboards, splints, and sandbags to maintain proper body alignment.
3. Encourage self-performance activities such as combing hair, feeding self, and brushing teeth. Provide assistive devices for improving hand grasp and participation in ADLs as per occupational therapy.
4. Assist with ROM exercises within limits of pain tolerance.

Osteoarthritis (Degenerative Joint Disease)
A. Definition: local joint disorder affecting weight-bearing joints (hips, knees); results in disintegration of the cartilage covering the ends of bones
B. Pathology: cause is unknown; predisposing factors include aging, joint trauma, and obesity
C. Signs and symptoms
1. Subjective
   a. Pain after exercise; relieved by rest
   b. Morning stiffness

   c. Muscle spasms
   d. Reduced strength
2. Objective
   a. Limited ROM
   b. Crepitant joint
   c. Prominent bony enlargement—Bouchard nodes are present at the interphalangeal joints of the fingers; Heberden nodes are present at the distal joints of the fingers.
D. Diagnostic tests: X-ray studies reveal joint abnormalities.
E. Treatment
1. Weight reduction to relieve strain
2. Heat and massage for aching and stiffness
3. Physical therapy to maintain optimum level of functioning
4. Drugs to relieve symptoms
   a. Analgesics
   b. Antiinflammatory agents
   c. Steroids
5. Surgical intervention to prevent deformity, relieve inflammation, delay progression, or replace affected joint
6. Alternative therapies
   a. Massage
   b. Imagery
   c. Nutritional supplements—glucosamine and chondroitin sulfate
F. Nursing interventions
1. Encourage patient to express feelings concerning disorder.
2. If ordered, provide moist heat, massage, and prescribed exercise, to relax muscle and relieve stiffness or discomfort.

Gouty Arthritis (Gout)
A. Definition: disorder in which excessive amounts of uric acid are retained in the blood
B. Pathology
1. Cause is related to a disorder of purine metabolism.
2. Uric acid crystals are deposited in the joints and cartilage and form calculi (tophi).
3. Deposits cause local irritation and an inflammatory response; big toe most common site.
4. Men older than 30 years of age are most commonly affected.
C. Signs and symptoms
1. Subjective
   a. Acute pain, swelling, and inflammation of great toe (most affected joint)
   b. Headache
   c. Malaise
   d. Anorexia
   e. Pruritus (local)
2. Objective
   a. Skin over joint swollen, warm, and red
   b. Limited ROM
   c. Tophi located in cartilage of ears, hands, and feet
D. Diagnostic tests and methods
1. Elevated serum uric acid level
2. Elevated ESR and WBC count
E. Treatment
1. Dietary restriction of foods high in purine such as organ meats

2. Uricosuric drugs to increase uric acid excretion; allopurinol to inhibit uric acid formation
3. Weight loss and periodic blood glucose screening because a relationship may exist between gouty arthritis and insulin resistance
4. Colchicine to reduce pain and relieve swelling
5. Alkaline ash diet to increase urinary pH (includes foods that reduce to an alkaline ash such as milk, cheese, cream)

F. Nursing interventions
1. Instruct patient to avoid foods high in purine content.
2. Encourage physical activity to promote optimal muscular and skeletal function.
3. Use bed cradle (or tent sheets over side rails) to prevent pressure of linen on feet and legs.
4. Encourage fluid intake of 2000 to 3000 mL daily to avoid renal calculi unless contraindicated.
5. Instruct patient to limit alcohol intake, which may precipitate an acute attack.
6. Instruct patient to avoid salicylates because of antagonistic actions of uricosuric drugs.

Systemic Lupus Erythematosus
A. Definition: chronic multisystem inflammatory disorder involving the connective tissues such as the muscles, kidneys, heart, and serous membranes; may affect the skin, lungs, and nervous system
B. Pathology
1. Cause is unknown; it is believed to be an autoimmune disorder.
2. Inflammation produces fibroid deposits and structural changes in connective tissue of organs and blood vessels.
3. It results in problems with mobility, oxygenation, and elimination.
C. Signs and symptoms
1. Subjective
   a. Abdominal, joint, and muscle pain
   b. Weakness; fatigue
   c. Depression
   d. Anorexia, (loss of appetite)
2. Objective
   a. Low-grade fever
   b. Weight loss
   c. Butterfly skin rash over bridge of nose and cheeks, which increases with exposure to the sun
   d. Anemia
   e. Alopecia
D. Diagnostic tests
1. Positive LE test
2. Elevated ESR
3. Increased gamma globulin levels
4. Positive antinuclear antibody titer
5. High anti-DNA test
E. Treatment
1. Corticosteroids, analgesics, and medications for anemia
2. Hydroxychloroquine (antimalarial drug) and chemotherapy drugs indicated in some individuals
3. Avoidance of exposure to sunlight
F. Nursing interventions
1. Provide emotional support to patient and family in coping with poor prognosis.
2. Encourage alternative activities and planned rest periods.

3. Instruct to avoid persons with infections, undue exposure to sunlight, and emotional stress, which can cause exacerbations.
4. Encourage intake of foods high in iron: liver, shellfish, leafy vegetables, and enriched breads and cereals.
5. Encourage patient to seek medical attention before conceiving.

Scleroderma (Progressive Systemic Sclerosis)
A. Definition: fiberlike changes in the connective tissue throughout the body caused by collagen deposits and subsequent fibrosis
B. Pathology
1. An insidious, chronic, progressive disorder; scleroderma usually begins in the skin.
2. Skin becomes thick and hard; fingers and toes become fixed in a position.
3. Other disorders that occur are difficulty in swallowing, impaired gastrointestinal (GI) mobility, cardiac and renal problems, and osteoporosis.
C. Signs and symptoms
1. Subjective
   a. Sweating of hands and feet
   b. Stiffness of hands
   c. Muscle weakness
   d. Joint pain
   e. Dysphagia
2. Objective
   a. Increased pigmentation or dyspigmentation
   b. Dilated capillaries of lips, fingers, face, and tongue
D. Diagnostic tests and methods
1. Positive LE cell test result
2. False-positive syphilis test result
E. Treatment
1. Skin care to prevent formation of decubitus ulcers
2. Physical therapy
3. Analgesics for joint pain
4. Corticosteroids
F. Nursing interventions
1. Provide emotional support to patient and family in addressing physical and psychological needs.
2. Encourage moderate exercise to promote muscular and joint function.
3. Force fluids; encourage fluid intake of at least 1500 to 2500 mL/day unless contraindicated by patient's condition.
4. Advise to avoid cold temperatures; use gloves to remove items from freezer.
5. Plan rest periods.
6. Provide assistive devices to help with ADLs (eating, grooming).

Osteomyelitis
A. Definition: bone inflammation caused by direct or indirect invasion of an organism
B. Pathology: bacteria enter bloodstream through an open fracture or wound or by secondary invasion from bloodborne infection from a distant site such as bone or infected tonsils
C. Signs and symptoms
1. Subjective
   a. Tenderness over the bones
   b. Painful movement; limited mobility
   c. Malaise

2. Objective
   a. Fever
   b. Chills
   c. Heat, swelling, and redness of the skin over the bone
   d. Signs of sepsis
   e. Wound drainage
D. Diagnostic tests and methods
   1. Positive blood cultures
   2. Elevated ESR
   3. Elevated WBC count
   4. X-ray film may not reveal abnormalities for 5 to 10 days from onset.
E. Treatment
   1. Long-term intravenous (IV) antibiotic therapy
   2. Drainage from abscess with continuous irrigation of wound
   3. Surgical removal of necrotic bone
F. Nursing interventions
   1. Use strict aseptic technique when changing dressings.
   2. Keep affected limb in proper alignment with pillows and sandbags.
   3. Maintain drainage and secretion precautions for disposal of dressings.
   4. Provide a high-calorie, high-protein diet and adequate hydration.
   5. Provide undisturbed rest periods.
   6. Move affected body part gently because of severe pain.

Osteoporosis

A. Definition: metabolic bone disorder in which bone mass is decreased. Bones become weak and brittle. Prevention is crucial; adequate calcium intake must be maintained throughout life.
B. Pathology
   1. Common in postmenopausal women, especially Caucasian and Asian individuals
   2. May be caused by deficit of estrogen and androgens, prolonged immobilization, insufficient calcium intake or absorption, vitamin D deficiency, or endocrine disorder
   3. Sites usually affected are vertebrae, pelvis, hip, wrist, and femur
C. Signs and symptoms
   1. Subjective: backache that worsens with sitting, standing, coughing, and sneezing
   2. Objective
      a. Kyphosis (abnormal condition of the thoracic spine)
      b. Loss of height
      c. Pathological fractures
D. Diagnostic test: X-ray film reveals bone demineralization and compression of vertebrae.
E. Treatment
   1. Physical activity and exercise to prevent atrophy
   2. Estrogen replacement to provide calcium balance
   3. Diet high in protein and calcium
   4. Vitamin D supplements
   5. Support of spine with brace or corset
   6. The medications alendronate (Fosamax), risedronate (Actonel), and ibandronate (Boniva) are bone resorption inhibitors and are used to help alleviate bone loss.
F. Nursing interventions
   1. Encourage patient to use a walker or cane to stabilize balance when ambulating.

2. Encourage fluid intake of 2000 to 3000 mL daily, unless contraindicated, to avoid formation of renal calculi.
3. Give instruction on foods that are high in protein and calcium content.
4. Emphasize need to follow prescribed daily activity and exercise.
5. If confined to bed, give passive ROM exercises and assist with active ROM exercises.
6. Teach safety measures to protect from fractures.
7. Teach patient about relationship between sun exposure and vitamin D.

Osteogenic Sarcoma

A. Definition: tumor located in the bone and composed of cells derived from connective tissue
B. Pathology
   1. Highly malignant tumor that may metastasize to the lungs
   2. Affects children, adolescents, and young adults
   3. Usually occurs in shaft of long bones, especially affecting the femur
C. Signs and symptoms
   1. Subjective: pain
   2. Objective
      a. Restricted ROM
      b. Swelling
      c. Weight loss
      d. Anemia
D. Diagnostic tests and methods
   1. X-ray examination to reveal lesion in the extremity and chest; CT scan
   2. Biopsy examination to evaluate cells
   3. Frozen section for rapid diagnosis of possible malignant lesion
E. Treatment
   1. Chemotherapeutic agents to reduce and retard growth
   2. Radiation therapy to destroy malignant tissue
   3. Amputation of affected limb or resection of tumor
   4. Use of cadaver bone to preserve function after bone removal
F. Nursing interventions
   1. Provide emotional support to patient and family to reduce fear and anxiety.
   2. Provide diet high in protein and caloric content.
   3. If patient undergoes amputation procedure, follow special nursing actions. (Refer to discussion of amputation.)
   4. If patient is receiving radiotherapy:
      a. Provide noninfectious environment.
      b. Avoid ointments, lotions, powders, and washing of port (treated) areas.
      c. Do not remove markings on skin.
      d. Observe site for redness, swelling, itching, and drying.
   5. If patient is receiving chemotherapy:
      a. Administer antiemetic agents as ordered.
      b. Provide small frequent feedings, supplements, frequent oral care; encourage intake of fluids.
      c. Monitor for dyspnea, edema; encourage turning, coughing, and deep breathing.
      d. Assess sensation.

Fibromyalgia Syndrome

A. Definition: musculoskeletal–chronic pain syndrome
B. Pathology
  1. Unknown cause
  2. Causes pain in muscles, bones, or joints at certain trigger points
C. Signs and symptoms
  1. Subjective
    a. Pain in neck and lower back
    b. Early-morning muscle stiffness
    c. Poor sleep
    d. Headache
    e. Forgetfulness
  2. Objective: periodic limb movement, restless legs
D. Diagnostic tests and methods
  1. No definitive diagnostic tests to confirm diagnosis
  2. Clinical manifestations
E. Treatment
  1. Patient education concerning aggravating factors
    a. Cold or humid weather
    b. Physical and mental fatigue
    c. Anxiety and stress
    d. Irritable bowel syndrome
  2. Use of tricyclic antidepressants and muscle relaxants has been helpful in some patients.
F. Nursing interventions
  1. Identify functional goals.
  2. Teach stretching exercises and promote an exercise program.

Osteitis Deformans (Paget Disease of Bone)

A. Definition: inflammatory condition in which certain bones become soft, thick, and deformed
B. Pathology
  1. Unknown cause; occurs mainly in men of middle age or older
  2. Disturbs new bone tissue, with bones becoming enlarged and coarse in texture
C. Signs and symptoms
  1. Subjective
    a. Bone pain; worsens at night
    b. Tenderness on pressure of the bones
    c. Back pain
    d. Headache from enlarged skull
    e. Deafness or blindness caused by pressure from overgrowth of bone
  2. Objective
    a. Pathological fractures
    b. Decrease in height
    c. Bowing of femur and tibia
    d. Enlarged skull
D. Diagnostic tests and methods
  1. Skeletal x-ray film to reveal bone enlargement and denseness
  2. Elevated serum alkaline phosphate value
  3. Urinary excretion of hydroxyproline increased
E. Treatment
  1. Androgen therapy for men; estrogen therapy for women to reverse hypercalciuria, if present
  2. Salicylates for pain
F. Nursing interventions
  1. Observe for stress fractures; signs and symptoms include tenderness, pain at site, and limited movement.

  2. Emphasize need for maintenance of normal weight.
  3. If fracture occurs and patient becomes immobilized:
    a. Limit calcium intake to avoid renal calculi.
    b. Provide high fluid intake to avoid hypercalcemia.
  4. Explain safety measures to prevent fractures; include making sure of a clear pathway, reducing clutter, rolling if individual does fall, and limiting high-risk activities.

Herniated Nucleus Pulposus
(Slipped Disk or Rupture of Intervertebral Disk)

A. Definition: protrusion of the nucleus pulposus, which compresses the nerve roots of the spinal cord
B. Pathology
  1. Site usually affected is between L4 and L5, L5 and sacrum, C5 and C6, or C6 and C7.
  2. Causes may be straining the spine in an unnatural position (poor body mechanics), degenerative changes, heavy lifting when bending from the waist, and accidents.
C. Signs and symptoms
  1. Subjective
    a. Cervical disk
      (1) Stiff neck
      (2) Shoulder pain descending down the arm into the hand
      (3) Numbness of arm and hand
    b. Lumbosacral disk: low-back pain radiating down the posterior thigh
  2. Objective
    a. Cervical disk
      (1) Sensory disturbances of the hand
      (2) Atrophy of biceps and triceps
      (3) Muscle strength diminished
    b. Lumbosacral disk
      (1) Difficulty in ambulating
      (2) Lasègue sign: pain in back and leg while raising heel with knee straight; numbness of leg and foot
      (3) Footdrop
D. Diagnostic tests and methods
  1. X-ray examination to reveal narrowing disk space
  2. Myelogram to localize site
  3. EMG
  4. CT scan of the spine
  5. MRI of the spine
E. Treatment
  1. Cervical traction (cervical disk); traction to lower extremities (lumbosacral disk)
  2. Bed rest, heat application, and analgesics
  3. Surgical interventions
    a. Laminectomy: removal of a portion of the vertebra and excision of the ruptured portion of the nucleus pulposus
    b. Spinal fusion: permanent binding of the vertebrae
    c. Chemonucleolysis: dissolving of the affected disk through the injection of chymopapain
F. Nursing interventions
  1. Encourage patient to verbalize feelings related to immobility, fears, and future impairment.
  2. Observations of traction:
    a. Check that it is hanging free and has not fallen or become caught in bed grooves.
    b. Observe for frayed cords and loosened knots.

3. Give back care to promote circulation and relax muscles.
4. Have patient maintain proper body alignment.
5. Provide diet high in fiber, with adequate hydration to avoid constipation and straining.
6. Instruct patient on principles of body mechanics.
7. Assess for muscle spasms, which may indicate weights are too heavy
8. If patient undergoes EMG:
   a. Position flat for period prescribed by physician.
   b. Encourage adequate hydration.
9. If patient undergoes surgical intervention, follow general postoperative nursing actions.
   a. Observe for leakage of cerebrospinal fluid on surgical dressing; reinforce dressing until inspected by physician.
   b. Change position by logrolling to prevent motion of spinal column.
   c. Provide straight-backed chair in which patient can sit; feet must be on floor.
   d. Discharge instructions
      (1) Avoid heavy lifting and climbing stairs.
      (2) Avoid riding in car.
      (3) Avoid forward flexion of head (cervical laminectomy).

Fractures

A. Definition: break in the continuity of bone that may be accompanied by injury of surrounding soft tissue, producing swelling and discoloration
B. Pathology
   1. Most fractures are a result of trauma; pathological fractures result from disorders such as osteoporosis, malnutrition, bone tumors, and Cushing syndrome.
   2. Types of fractures
      a. Closed (simple): Skin is intact over the site.
      b. Open (compound): Break in skin is present over the fracture site; the ends of the bone may or may not be visible.
      c. Complete: Fracture line extends completely through the bone.
      d. Incomplete (partial): Fracture line extends partially through the bone; one side breaks while the opposite side bends.
      e. Comminuted: More than one fracture is present, with bone fragments either crushed or splintered into several pieces.
      f. Greenstick: One side of a bone splinters (most often seen in children because of soft bone structure).
      g. Impacted: One bone fragment is driven into another bone fragment.
C. Signs and symptoms
   1. Subjective
      a. Pain on movement of body part
      b. Tenderness
      c. Loss of function
      d. Muscle spasms
   2. Objective
      a. Deformity
      b. Edema
      c. Bruising
      d. Crepitus
D. Diagnostic test: x-ray examination to confirm location and direction of fracture line

E. Treatment
   1. Reduction of the fracture consists of pulling the broken bone ends to correct alignment and regain continuity. A cast is usually applied, or the part may be placed in a traction device.
      a. Closed reduction: manual manipulation to bring ends into contact
      b. Open reduction: surgical intervention to cleanse the area and attach devices to hold the bones in position
   2. Cast application to immobilize, support, and protect the part during the healing process
   3. Traction to apply a pulling force in two directions to realign the bones
      a. Skin traction applied temporarily: light weights that are attached to the skin with strips of adhesive tape
         (1) Buck extension: exerts a straight pull on the limb; used for fractures of upper and lower leg, hip dislocation, and pelvic injuries
         (2) Bryant traction: vertical extension of lower extremities, hip flexed 90 degrees, knees extended, and buttocks clear of the bed for reduction of femur or hip dislocation in very young children
         (3) Russell traction: sling placed behind the knee to create an upward pull of the knee; at the same time horizontal force exerted on the tibia and fibula; used for fractures of femurs
      b. Skeletal traction provides continuous reduction by the attachment of a device to the bone.
         (1) Kirschner wires or Steinmann pins are surgically inserted through the skin and bone; a traction bow or stirrup is attached to the wire or pin to exert a longitudinal pull and control rotation.
         (2) Crutchfield tongs are inserted into parietal areas of the skull to achieve hyperextension; used for spinal fractures.
         (3) Halo traction–halo loop for alignment of cervical area. Loop is attached to a halo vest or cast.
         (4) Skeletal pins (external fixators): devices to stabilize a fracture. They consist of pins that enter the skin and are affixed to a metal framework.
F. Nursing interventions
   1. Provide emergency nursing care of fractures (see Chapter 10).
   2. Provide nursing care for patient with a cast.
      a. Observe for neurovascular impairment of limb (Box 5-1).
      b. Elevate extremity (use palms of hands) in cast on pillow to reduce edema. (Avoid plastic pillow until cast is dry.)
      c. Promote drying of cast by exposing it to air.

Box **5-1**	Signs of Neurovascular Impairment

Compare extremity with cast with other extremities when assessing the following:
- Cyanosis
- Slow capillary refill times (more than 3 seconds)
- Poor pulse
- Lack of sensation
- Complaints of numbness and tingling

d. Inspect for skin irritation under edges of cast: apply lotion, pad edges, and apply tape to edge of cast.

e. If drainage is present on the cast, measure and note.

f. Observe for possible infection: increased temperature, foul odor from cast, edema, and "hot spots" over the cast.

g. Ice may be applied for first 24 hours to reduce edema.

h. Observe for complications.

(1) Pulmonary emboli: If embolus lodges in the lungs, patient may experience dyspnea, anxiety, restlessness, chest pain, cough, hemoptysis, and increase in temperature.

(2) Fat emboli: These are similar to pulmonary emboli, except that the emboli are fat globules, probably arising from central area of the fractured bone (patients with fat emboli are more likely to experience petechiae).

(3) Compartment syndrome occurs when circulation to the muscles is compromised; look for changes in neurocirculatory status.

i. Educate patient on home cast care.

3. Provide nursing care for patient in traction.

a. Inspect and maintain ropes, knots, and pulleys; taut rope rides easily over pulleys; knots should not slip and should be unobstructed.

b. Inspect and maintain weights: hang freely off the floor and free of bedding.

c. Observe for skin traction.

(1) Inspect skin condition at distal ends of bandages (wrist and heel) for possible skin breakdown.

(2) Ensure that tapes do not encircle a limb, are applied smoothly, and are applied on skin that is free of irritation.

(3) Assess neurovascular status: color, pulses, warmth, and sensation.

d. Observe for skeletal traction complications.

(1) Inspect insertion points daily for signs and symptoms of infection.

(2) Provide dressing change or wound care aseptically to prevent infection.

(3) Inspect pins, wires, and skeletal apparatus for sharp ends that may catch on bed linen.

(4) Cleanse pin sites to prevent pin site infections.

(5) Assess neurovascular status.

e. Examine and give skin care to all pressure points on which patient rests.

f. Provide foot support to prevent footdrop, especially for patients with Russell traction or Buck extension.

g. Observe for thrombophlebitis, especially in patient with Russell traction because of pressure to the popliteal space.

h. Encourage diet high in protein and vitamins to promote healing.

i. Encourage 2000- to 3000-mL fluid intake daily to prevent complications such as constipation, renal calculi, and urinary tract infections.

j. Encourage patient to perform ROM and isometric exercises.

k. Have patient maintain proper position and good alignment.

l. Assess for pain, and medicate as needed.

Fractured Hip

A. Definition: fracture of the hip joint

B. Pathology

1. Site of fracture

a. Inside the joint (intracapsular or neck of the femur)

b. Outside the joint (extracapsular or base of the neck of the femur)

2. Elderly women experience high incidence because of osteoporosis.

C. Signs and symptoms

1. Subjective: pain

2. Objective

a. Leg appears shorter than unaffected extremity.

b. Foot points upward and outward on affected side (external rotation).

c. Edema

d. Discoloration

D. Diagnostic test: x-ray study to confirm discontinuity of the bone

E. Treatment

1. Russell traction or Buck extension: before open reduction to prevent muscle spasms if surgery is not contraindicated

2. Closed reduction with application of hip spica cast if fracture occurred in intertrochanteric site

3. Open reduction and implantation of a prosthesis to replace head and neck of femur or fixation device to secure fragments of the fracture

a. Austin Moore prosthesis

b. Thompson prosthesis

c. Neufeld nail and screws

d. Smith-Petersen nail

e. Zickel nail

F. Nursing interventions

1. Provide nursing care of patient in traction as outlined previously in the section on fractures; assess level of pain and provide medications as ordered.

2. Be aware of coexisting problems such as diabetes or cardiac, vascular, or neurological disorders.

3. Considerations for the older patient

a. Complications of immobility

b. Reduced tolerance to drugs

c. Delayed healing because of nutritional problems related to the aging process

4. Keep side rail up and provide trapeze to facilitate movement.

5. Encourage patient to participate in ADLs: eating, bathing, and combing hair.

6. Provide postoperative care.

a. Inspect dressings and linen for drainage and bleeding.

b. Provide trochanter roll to prevent external rotation of legs.

c. Provide and maintain proper alignment. Use an abductor pillow to prevent adduction. Adduction, external rotation, or acute flexion can dislocate hip before it is healed.

d. Encourage quadriceps-setting exercises.

e. Assist patient in learning to use walker and ambulating with a non–weight-bearing technique.

f. Instruct on the use of an elevated toilet seat to prevent hip flexion.

Arthroplasty

A. Definition: replacement of a joint, which may be necessary to restore function, relieve pain, and correct deformity

B. Pathology: arthritic changes damage the joint, resulting in impaired mobility, pain, and deformity. Hip, knee, fingers, elbow, and shoulder commonly are affected.

C. Signs and symptoms
 1. Subjective
   a. Pain
   b. Limited ROM
   c. Limited weight-bearing ability
 2. Objective
   a. Limited ROM
   b. Edema and skin character changes around affected joint

D. Diagnostic tests and methods
 1. X-ray studies to confirm joint changes and damage
 2. Arthroscopy to provide direct visualization and inspection of joint changes

E. Treatment: a prosthetic device used to replace the articulating joint surfaces (hip, knee, shoulder, elbow, fingers)

F. Nursing interventions
 1. Maintain proper positioning after surgery (e.g., if hip is replaced, maintain affected leg in abduction).
 2. Wound care: Monitor drains, note blood loss, and monitor dressing status.
 3. Monitor continuous passive ROM machine, if used for knee replacement.
 4. Assist with prescribed activity and encourage prescribed exercise.
 5. Monitor pain; provide pain control.
 6. Assess neuromuscular function.
 7. Monitor skin integrity.

Amputation

A. Definition: surgical removal of part or all of an extremity

B. Pathology
 1. Most amputations result from blood vessel disorders, causing inadequate oxygen supply to the tissue.
 2. Other indications for amputation are gas gangrene, malignant tumors, septic wounds, severe trauma, and burns.
 3. A skin flap is usually constructed for prosthetic equipment.

C. Signs and symptoms of conditions that may necessitate this intervention
 1. Subjective
   a. Gas gangrene and septic wounds: pain
   b. Peripheral vascular diseases
    (1) Pain
    (2) Tingling
    (3) Cold or cool extremity
    (4) Change in color
 2. Objective
   a. Gas gangrene and septic wounds
    (1) Fever
    (2) Edema
    (3) Foul odor
    (4) Bronze or blackened wound caused by necrosis
   b. Peripheral vascular diseases
    (1) Edema
    (2) Pallor
    (3) Shiny, hairless skin
    (4) Hyperpigmentation
    (5) Ulcer formation

   c. Arterial diseases
    (1) Pallor
    (2) Cyanosis
    (3) Diminished pulses
    (4) Pain on pressure

D. Diagnostic tests and methods
 1. Oscillometry
 2. Arteriography
 3. Skin temperature studies
 4. X-ray examination
 5. Doppler flow studies

E. Treatment
 1. Psychological preparation
 2. Rehabilitation preparation
 3. Nutritional status buildup
 4. Prosthetic device

F. Nursing interventions
 1. Provide preoperative care.
   a. Encourage expression of feelings by providing honesty concerning loss of limb.
   b. Explain to patient the possibility of experiencing pain in the amputated limb (phantom limb pain).
   c. Explain to patient that he or she will undergo a program of exercises that includes strengthening of upper extremities, transferring from bed to chair, and ambulating with a walker or crutches.
 2. Provide postoperative care.
   a. Provide routine postoperative care.
   b. Monitor for hemorrhage; if it occurs, apply manual pressure and notify physician.
   c. Apply elastic (Ace) bandages in a crisscross or figure-of-eight pattern only.
   d. Elevate the residual limb 8 to 12 hours on a pillow; remove after 12 hours to prevent hip contracture; place in prone position 1 hour out of every 4 hours to prevent hip contracture.
   e. Prevent outward rotation by placing trochanter roll along the outer side of the residual limb.
   f. Instruct patient not to hang the residual limb over the edge of the bed, wheelchair, chair, or handrail of his or her crutches to avoid residual limb contracture.
   g. When conditioning of the residual limb is ordered, begin by having patient push the residual limb against a pillow and progress to pushing against a firmer surface.
   h. Teach patient to massage the residual limb to soften the scar and improve vascularity.
   i. Teach use of transcutaneous electrical nerve stimulation (TENS) unit for relief of phantom limb pain.
   j. Medicate as prescribed for phantom limb pain.
   k. Encourage progressive ambulation and physical therapy.

RESPIRATORY SYSTEM

ANATOMY AND PHYSIOLOGY

A. Respiration: the taking in of oxygen, its use in the tissues, and the giving off of carbon dioxide; has two stages
 1. External: exchange of oxygen and carbon dioxide between body and outside environment; consists of inhalation and exhalation; also known as *ventilation*

2. Internal: exchange of carbon dioxide and oxygen between the cells and the interstitial fluid surrounding the cells; also known as *perfusion*

B. Organs (Figures 5-3 and 5-4)

1. Nose
   a. Divides into two cavities separated by nasal septum
   b. Ciliated mucosa lines the cavities and traps inhaled foreign particles.
   c. Filters, warms, and moistens air
   d. Serves as organ of smell
      (1) Receptors are located in olfactory epithelium of upper part of nasal cavity.
      (2) It stimulates appetite and flow of digestive juices.
      (3) Senses of smell and taste work together to give flavor to food.
   e. Paranasal sinuses: lighten skull, act as resonance chamber in speech

2. Pharynx: passageway for food and air; divided into three parts
   a. Nasopharynx (behind nose): contains adenoids; eustachian tube, which drains the middle ear, opens into the nasopharynx
   b. Oropharynx (mouth): contains tonsils, which are lymphatic tissue
   c. Laryngopharynx: opens into larynx toward front and into esophagus toward back

3. Larynx (voice box)
   a. Formed by nine cartilages in boxlike formation
   b. Thyroid cartilage, which forms the Adam's apple
   c. Epiglottis: flap of elastic cartilage that closes off the larynx when food is swallowed

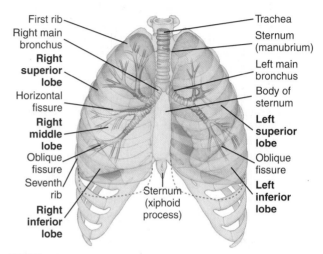

FIGURE 5-4 Projection of the lungs and trachea in relation to the rib cage and clavicles. (From Thibodeau GA, Patton KT: *Structure and function of the body,* ed 12, St Louis, 2004, Mosby.)

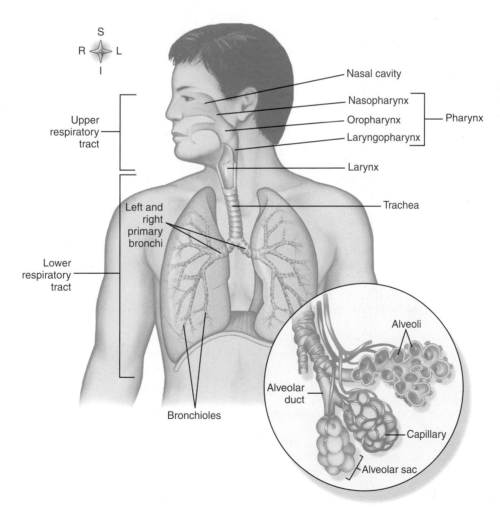

FIGURE 5-3 Structural plan of the respiratory organs. (From Thibodeau GA, Patton KT: *Structure and function of the body,* ed 12, St Louis, 2004, Mosby.)

d. Produces sound; vibration of vocal cords with expelled air

e. Passageway for air to the trachea

4. Trachea (windpipe): tube reinforced by C-shaped rings. Open ends of rings face posteriorly toward the esophagus and allow it to expand when food is swallowed; solid portion keeps the trachea open for the passage of air.

5. Bronchi
   a. They are formed by the division of the trachea into two branches; distribute air to the interior of the lungs; called *bronchial tree.*
   b. Right main bronchus is larger and more vertical; aspiration is more common by this route.
   c. Bronchi divide into smaller branches called *bronchioles.*
   d. Bronchioles divide into smaller tubes and terminate in the alveoli.
   e. Alveoli: microscopic air sacs that resemble bunches of grapes; composed of a single, thin layer of squamous epithelium; external surface surrounded by spider-web pulmonary capillaries; here gas exchanges occur, oxygen passes from the alveoli into the capillary blood, and carbon dioxide leaves the blood to enter the alveoli.

6. Lungs
   a. Cone shaped: Upper part is the apex; broad lower part is the base. Base is concave and rests on diaphragm. Right side has three lobes, and left side has two lobes.
   b. Tissue is porous and spongy.
   c. Pleura: thin, moist, slippery membrane covering lungs. It prevents friction during breathing movement.

C. Physiology
   1. Two phases of breathing: inspiration and expiration
   2. Respiration is controlled by respiratory center in medulla oblongata.
   3. Carbon dioxide stimulates respiration.
   4. Muscles of respiration
      a. Diaphragm: dome shaped; separates thoracic and abdominal cavities; contracts and relaxes
      b. Intercostals: between the ribs; elevate the ribs and enlarge the thorax during inspiration
   5. Mechanism of inspiration
      a. Contraction of diaphragm causes the thorax to expand.
      b. The lungs cling to the thoracic wall as a result of the attachment of the pleural membranes.
      c. Intrathoracic pressure decreases.
      d. The volume within the lungs (intrapulmonary) increases, and gases in the lungs spread out to fill the space.
      e. Result is a decrease in gas pressure, and a partial vacuum sucks air into the lungs. Air continues to move into the lungs until intrapulmonary pressure equals atmospheric pressure.
   6. Mechanism of expiration
      a. Respiratory muscles relax, and thorax decreases in size.
      b. Intrathoracic and intrapulmonary volumes decrease.
      c. As volume decreases, gases are forced closer together, and intrapulmonary pressure rises higher than atmospheric pressure.
      d. Gases flow out of lungs and equalize pressure inside and outside the lung.

7. Volumes of air exchanges
   a. Total lung capacity (TLC): total volume of air present in the lungs after maximum inspiration
   b. Vital capacity (VC): volume of air that can be expelled after maximum inspiration
   c. Tidal volume (TV): volume of air exhaled after normal inspiration
   d. Residual volume (RV): amount of air remaining in lung after maximum expiration

RESPIRATORY CONDITIONS AND DISORDERS

All cells of the body depend on adequate oxygenation and removal of carbon dioxide for health. The respiratory system depends on central nervous system (CNS) regulation and on the cardiovascular system for blood supply. Respiratory distress or dysfunction may be secondary to disease in another system. Many pulmonary diseases are chronic. Therefore the nurse must make a complete respiratory assessment of all patients and include this in nursing care planning, even when the primary diagnosis is unrelated to the respiratory system.

The following terms are used to describe respirations:

- Bradypnea: slow respirations
- Cheyne-Stokes: periods of apnea alternating with rapid respirations
- Dyspnea: difficulty breathing; may be subjective or objective
- Dyspnea on exertion (DOE)
- Kussmaul's breathing: fast, deep, and labored respirations
- Orthopnea: difficulty breathing in a supine position; relieved by sitting up
- Paroxysmal nocturnal dyspnea: transient episodes of acute dyspnea that occur a few hours after falling asleep
- Shortness of breath
- Tachypnea: rapid respirations
- Wheeze: sound as air moves out through bronchi and bronchioles that have been narrowed by spasm, swelling, and secretions

NURSING ASSESSMENT

A. Observations (objective data)
   1. Respirations
      a. Rate
      b. Depth
      c. Characteristics (wheezing); any difficulty breathing; DOE
   2. Oxygen deprivation (note any)
      a. Restlessness
      b. Yawning
      c. Anxiety
      d. Drowsiness
      e. Confusion
      f. Disorientation
      g. Flaring nostrils
      h. Retractions
   3. Cough
      a. Frequency
      b. Relationship to activity and precipitating factors
      c. Production of sputum
      d. Complete description (e.g., dry, productive, nonproductive, hoarse, barking, moist, or hacking)

4. Lung sounds (adventitious)
   a. Crackles: caused by fluid, mucus, or pus in the small airways and alveoli
   b. Wheezes: sound created by narrowed bronchioles
   c. Friction rub: coarse sound caused by inflammation and pleurisy
   d. Stridor: whooping sound created by a severely narrowed airway
   e. Rhonchi: created by secretions trapped in the trachea or large bronchi
5. Sputum; note the following:
   a. Consistency (e.g., thick, tenacious, watery, frothy)
   b. Amount (e.g., scant, moderate, copious)
   c. Color (e.g., white, yellow, pink, rust, blood-tinged, green)
   d. Odor
6. Skin color
   a. Pallor, ashen, or ruddy
   b. Cyanosis (bluish discoloration): observe lips, nail beds, and mucous membranes
7. Skin
   a. Temperature
   b. Diaphoresis
8. Vital signs
   a. Pulse: note rate, quality, and characteristics
   b. Blood pressure
   c. Temperature (rectal, tympanic, temporomandibular)
   d. Pulse oximetry
9. Nasal discharge
10. Voice: huskiness

B. Patient description (subjective data)
   1. Cough
   2. Pain
   3. Difficulty breathing, shortness of breath
   4. Fatigue or weakness, dizziness or fainting
   5. Sputum, congestion
C. Patient history
   1. History of orthopnea—use of extra pillows needed to sleep
   2. Respiratory illness or difficulty
   3. Injuries
   4. Use of medications or respiratory aids
   5. Smoking
   6. Seasonal exacerbations
   7. Exposure to environmental irritants
   8. Known allergies
   9. Coexisting chronic illness (e.g., human immunodeficiency virus [HIV], diabetes, immunocompromised conditions, therapies)

DIAGNOSTIC TESTS AND METHODS

A. Chest x-ray examination: a visualization of lung tissue from different angles. Based on a knowledge of normal anatomy and usual changes in disease, diagnosis of many conditions can be made (e.g., tumors, pneumonia). No preparation and no special care or observations are required after x-ray examination.
B. Bronchoscopy
   1. Direct inspection of the trachea and bronchi through a scope passed via the nose or mouth. With this procedure, specimens are obtained for biopsy and culture; foreign bodies (e.g., fish bones) can be removed.
   2. Nursing responsibilities: provide general preparation as for a surgical procedure (see Chapter 2); after the procedure monitor vital signs, provide oral hygiene, and observe for cough and blood-streaked sputum; do not allow patient to eat or drink until gag reflex returns.
C. Bronchogram
   1. Visualization of bronchial tree through x-ray examination after introduction of radiopaque dye; patient is given sedative and antispasmodic.
   2. Nursing responsibilities: Provide postural drainage to aid in removal of dye (usually done by a respiratory therapist). Encourage deep breathing and coughing. Do not allow patient to eat or drink until gag reflex returns.
D. CT scan: produces clear, anatomical images of the chest cavity
E. Ultrasound: image of area created by high-frequency sound; used for specific data relative to lung capacities
F. MRI: scan created by magnetic resonance imaging, a non-invasive procedure
G. Thoracentesis
   1. Needle aspiration of fluid from pleural cavity (space). Local anesthesia is used.
   2. Nursing responsibilities: Maintain proper positioning. Support and reassure patient during the procedure. Monitor vital signs during and after the procedure.
H. CBC: WBC count changes (increase or elevation in WBC count) from normal values may indicate infection.
I. Arterial blood gas analysis
   1. Measurement of the partial pressure of oxygen and carbon dioxide in the blood. Arterial puncture is performed.
   2. Nursing care: Once the blood sample has been obtained, apply constant pressure to the site for 5 minutes. Apply pressure dressing. Inspect site frequently for hematoma and pain, distally for skin temperature and color.
J. Culture and sensitivity
   1. Throat or nasopharynx
   2. Sputum
      a. Identifies organisms and specific medication to which patient will respond
      b. Nursing responsibilities: obtain before starting antibiotics. First sputum in the morning usually has the most organisms.
K. Sputum analysis
   1. Acid-fast bacillus (AFB): determines presence of *Mycobacterium tuberculosis*
   2. Cytology: assists in the diagnosis of lung carcinoma
L. Pulmonary function test: determines extent of respiratory difficulty and evaluates function of respiratory system. No special preparation or nursing care is required after testing. A spirometer is used to diagram air movement, lung volumes, and air flow. The computer determines the actual value, predicted value, and percentage of the predicted value. Examples of these tests include:
   1. Volumes: TV, expiratory reserve volume, RV, and inspiratory reserve volume
   2. Capacities: TLC, functional residual capacity, VC, inspiratory capacity
M. Lung scan, PET: Radioisotopes are inhaled or administered intravenously. A scanning device records the pattern of radioactivity. These scans are used in diagnosing vascular diseases (e.g., pulmonary embolism). No special preparation or nursing care is required.

N. Biopsy examination
1. Removal of a small amount of tissue to identify disease; biopsy may be of a lymph node to determine if the disease has spread into the lymphatic system.
2. Nursing care: provide general preoperative and postoperative care (see Chapter 2)

FREQUENT PATIENT PROBLEMS AND NURSING CARE

A. Activity intolerance related to fatigue caused by body cell demand for oxygen not being met; patient tires easily and becomes short of breath.
1. Protect from exertion; provide care; space activities appropriately.
2. Plan care to include rest periods.
3. Leave call bell and all personal belongings within easy reach.
4. Provide oxygen with humidity as ordered.
5. Limit conversation.
B. Risk for injury related to dizziness caused by diminished oxygen to the brain cells
1. Provide all care as in preceding list.
2. Maintain safety; use side rails.
3. Perform neurological assessment every 4 hours.
4. Assist when patient is out of bed.
C. Impaired oral mucous membrane related to mouth breathing
1. Encourage fluids if allowed.
2. Provide oral hygiene every 2 hours.
3. Lubricate lips with non–petroleum-based product.
D. Ineffective breathing pattern related to orthopnea
1. Place a pillow longitudinally under back.
2. Provide table with pillow for headrest in extreme difficulty.
3. Use footboard to prevent slipping down in bed.
4. Use semi-Fowler to high Fowler position.
E. Ineffective tissue perfusion (cardiopulmonary); impaired gas exchange related to dyspnea and coughing
1. Oxygen therapy: Maintain safety of equipment and proper care and observations.
2. Organize care and work efficiently to conserve patient's energy.
3. Plan rest periods.
4. Position in semi-Fowler to high-Fowler position; use two pillows.
5. Provide soft diet and small, frequent feedings.
6. Avoid gas-forming foods.
7. Prevent constipation and straining.
8. Use rectal thermometer; take tympanic temperature.
9. Make accurate observations about cough and sputum.
10. Obtain specimens as needed.
11. Provide tissues and bag for disposal within easy reach for infection control.
12. Provide sputum cup if specimen needed; instruct patient on correct technique.
13. Change position every 2 hours.
14. Encourage deep breathing.
15. Encourage fluids every 2 hours.
16. Provide oral hygiene every 2 hours.
17. Provide postural drainage if ordered (see Chapter 2).
18. Give expectorants as ordered (see Chapters 2 and 3).
19. Suction as necessary (*pro re nata* [p.r.n.]).

F. Anxiety related to dyspnea, fatigue, and weakness
1. Maintain quiet environment.
2. Help patient remain calm.
3. Explain everything slowly and carefully.
4. Provide physical and mental rest.
5. Answer call lights promptly.
6. Provide frequent contacts.
7. Offer realistic encouragement.
8. Provide restful diversion (e.g., music).
9. Encourage patient to express feelings and concerns.
G. Imbalanced nutrition: less than body requirements, related to dry mouth from mouth breathing, foul taste and odor from sputum, and fatigue; may affect desire for food
1. Make mealtime pleasant.
2. Provide oral hygiene before each meal.
3. Remove used tissues and sputum cups.
4. Request food preferences.
5. Give small, frequent, attractively served meals. Change to nasal cannula if permitted.

MAJOR MEDICAL DIAGNOSES
Sinusitis

A. Definition: inflammation of one or more of the sinuses of the frontal, ethmoid, sphenoid, or maxillary bones; secretions become infected; is acute but becomes chronic if not treated or leads to complications: septicemia, meningitis, brain abscess
B. Cause: results from the spread of organisms from the nose or trapped secretions interfering with drainage (e.g., nasal polyps, edema from allergy)
C. Signs and symptoms
1. Subjective: pain and headache
2. Objective
a. Nasal secretions, possibly purulent and blood tinged
b. Elevation of temperature; mild leukopenia
c. Pain or tenderness to palpation or percussion
D. Diagnostic tests and methods
1. Patient history and physical assessment
2. X-ray examination, transillumination
3. Culture and sensitivity
E. Treatment
1. Irrigation and inhalation of steam
2. Antibiotics and decongestants (see Chapter 3)
3. Surgery (e.g., Caldwell-Luc procedure [infected maxillary sinus is removed through an incision under the upper lip] or ethmoidectomy)
F. Nursing interventions
1. Administer nonnarcotic analgesics or nasal constrictors (see Chapter 3).
2. Provide moist steam; a hot, dry environment increases congestion; a vaporizer may thin secretions and soothe passages.
3. Provide hot wet pack; may relieve pain and congestion of overinvolved sinus.
4. Give general preoperative and postoperative care (see Chapter 2). Note specific orders for care or observations.

Epistaxis (Nosebleed)

A. Definition: bleeding from the nose
B. Cause: may be spontaneous, related to direct trauma or a result of systemic diseases (e.g., hypertension, blood dyscrasias); may be caused by local irritation from chronic infections or low-humidity environment
C. Sign: bleeding; shock if profuse

D. Diagnostic tests and methods
1. Patient history and physical examination
2. Platelet, Hct, and Hgb if profuse
E. Treatment (only if bleeding cannot be stopped)
1. Nasal packing
2. Cauterization of site with 10% silver nitrate stick
3. Epinephrine spray
4. Treatment of systemic disease
5. Hemostatic agents
F. Nursing interventions
1. Maintain patent airway (direct patient to breathe through mouth); have suction available.
2. Control bleeding: pinch nose firmly with fingers on soft part of nose. Place patient in high Fowler position with head forward.
3. Instruct patient to expectorate blood (swallowing will cause vomiting).
4. Apply ice or cold compresses to nasal area or back of neck to constrict blood vessels.
5. Monitor vital signs.
6. Avoid hot liquids.
7. Provide oral hygiene.
8. Reassure patient and family.

Deviated Septum

A. Definition: airway obstruction caused by deflection of bone and cartilage in the nasal septum
B. Causes
1. Trauma
2. Congenital
C. Diagnostic tests and methods
1. Patient history
2. Physical assessment
3. X-ray examination
D. Treatment: surgery—submucous resection (SMR), performed through the mucous membrane within the nares. Bone and cartilage are removed.
E. Nursing interventions
1. Provide general preoperative and postoperative care (see Chapter 2).
2. Before surgery, inform patient that nasal packing will be in place 24 to 48 hours; nasal breathing will not be possible; a temporary loss of smell will occur; sneezing must be avoided; and pain, discoloration, and swelling around the eyes will be present.
3. Maintain airway. Place patient on side or in semi-Fowler position. Monitor respirations.
4. Provide oral hygiene every 1 to 2 hours.
5. Provide ice compresses. Note bleeding on dressing; inspect back of throat for trickle of blood.
6. Use rectal or tympanic thermometer.
7. Provide liquid diet when tolerated. Encourage fluids. Prevent constipation.
8. Discourage forceful coughing.

Polyps

A. Definition: grapelike swellings of tissue. Nasal polyps obstruct breathing and block sinus drainage (see discussion of sinusitis).
B. Treatment: surgical removal
C. Nursing interventions
1. Surgical preparation
2. Close check on postoperative bleeding

Laryngitis

A. Definition: inflammation and swelling of the mucous membrane lining of the larynx
B. Cause: local irritation (e.g., smoking, spread of infection from elsewhere in the upper respiratory tract, abuse of vocal cords)
C. Signs and symptoms
1. Subjective: pain
2. Objective
a. Hoarseness
b. Loss of voice
c. Cough
D. Diagnostic tests and methods
1. Physical assessment
2. Patient history
3. Indirect laryngoscopy
E. Treatment and nursing interventions
1. Rest voice; provide alternate means of communication. Even whispering increases strain.
2. Remove the cause.
3. Provide steam inhalations.
4. Administer astringent or antiseptic spray (see Chapter 3).

Carcinoma of the Larynx

A. Description: Squamous cell carcinoma grows, spreads, and metastasizes. The rate of growth is determined by location of the lesion in the larynx.
B. Causes: related to heavy smoking, chronic laryngitis and vocal abuse, and alcohol consumption
C. Signs and symptoms
1. Subjective: anxiety (i.e., concerning surgery, confirmation of diagnosis, disfigurement)
2. Objective
a. Hoarseness
b. Signs of metastasis: pain; lump in throat; difficulty swallowing; dyspnea; and enlarged, painful lymph nodes
D. Diagnostic tests and methods
1. Patient history
2. Visual examination (laryngoscopy)
3. Biopsy examination
4. Laryngeal tomography
E. Treatment: surgery
1. Removal of larynx (laryngectomy) (partial or complete)
2. Radical neck dissection: wide excision, including lymph nodes, epiglottis, thyroid cartilage, and muscle tissue. A permanent tracheostomy is performed.
3. Radiotherapy with surgery
F. Nursing interventions
1. Provide general preoperative and postoperative care (see Chapter 2).
2. Provide immediate postoperative care.
a. Maintain patent airway. Patient may have a permanent tracheostomy (see Chapter 2). There will be a shorter tube (laryngectomy tube). Place patient in semi-Fowler position. Provide frequent mouth care.
b. Examine dressing every hour. Connect wound drains to suction as ordered. Prevent movement of head.
3. Provide continued postoperative care.
a. Provide method of communication (e.g., magic slate). Leave call bell close to hand, and answer promptly in person.

b. Assist and be supportive as alternate methods of speech are learned (e.g., esophageal speech, use of mechanical voice box).

c. Provide high-calorie, high-protein diet (tube feedings may be required at first).

d. Arrange for a visit from someone who has had a similar operation and satisfactory rehabilitation.

e. Investigate lifestyle changes (e.g., smoking, alcohol consumption) to decrease further risk of complications.

Pneumonia

A. Definition: inflammation (infection) of the lungs or part of the lung (e.g., left lower lobe pneumonia). Secretions fill the alveolar sacs and are a good medium for bacterial growth. The inflammation spreads to adjacent sacs. Spaces of the lung consolidate with thick exudate. Irritation may cause bleeding, and sputum has a characteristic rusty color; exchange of air is difficult and in advanced conditions not possible.

B. Causes: bacterial infections and viruses that are spread by respiratory secretions (droplets); chemical irritation; fungi and other organisms; aspirations. Patients with poor health and low natural resistance to infection are more susceptible (e.g., older adults, persons with chronic illness, and immunocompromised individuals should consider receiving Pneumovax vaccine as a preventive measure for the most common type of bacterial pneumonia).

C. Signs and symptoms
1. Subjective
   a. Dyspnea, shortness of breath
   b. Pain on inspiration
   c. Shallow breathing, signs of air hunger, orthopnea, and oxygen deprivation
2. Objective
   a. Marked elevation in temperature
   b. Cough: painful and dry at first, then productive with copious amounts of thick sputum (color according to organism)
   c. X-ray results
   d. Wheezes, crackles, or rhonchi heard in the lungs

D. Diagnostic tests and methods
1. Patient history
2. Physical assessment with auscultation of chest
3. Chest x-ray examination
4. Sputum culture and sensitivity
5. CBC

E. Treatment
1. Specific and broad-spectrum antibiotics (see Chapter 3)
2. Antipyretics, analgesics (codeine), expectorants, and bronchodilators (see Chapter 3)
3. IV fluids; encourage oral fluids.
4. Oxygen with humidity; incentive spirometer

F. Nursing interventions
1. Provide optimum rest: Provide care, help patient conserve energy, schedule rest periods, limit conversation, and keep personal items and call bell within easy reach. Alleviate anxiety.
2. Maintain oxygen with humidity.
3. Isolate as indicated, especially patients with oral and nasal secretions; provide for proper disposal (see Chapter 2).

4. Liquefy secretions: Encourage fluids (3000 mL daily or more. Observe and document production of sputum; suction as necessary.
5. Provide oral hygiene every 2 hours.
6. Monitor vital signs every 4 hours; use rectal thermometer. Monitor lung sounds.
7. Assist with loosening secretions: Have patient turn, cough, and deep breathe every 2 hours (splint chest if painful). Observe and document cough. Patient may need aerosol treatment.
8. Maintain adequate nutrition: Provide liquid-to-soft diet high in protein and calories.
9. Maintain IV fluids and medication schedule to ensure continued blood levels.
10. Position for comfort (high Fowler position or lying on affected side).

Pleurisy and Pleural Effusion

A. Definition: inflammation of the pleural membranes (local or diffuse); may or may not have fluid exudate. When fluid is present, the condition is pleural effusion; when purulent, the condition is empyema.

B. Cause: infections (e.g., pneumonia, lung abscess, trauma, fungus, tuberculosis, lung cancer, congestive heart failure [CHF], ascites)

C. Signs and symptoms
1. Subjective
   a. Sharp pain on inspiration (referred to shoulder, abdomen, or affected side)
   b. Dyspnea
   c. Anxiety
2. Objective
   a. Cough
   b. Elevation of temperature
   c. Decreased breath sounds (shallow respirations)
   d. Pleural rub

D. Diagnostic tests and methods
1. Chest x-ray examination
2. Patient history
3. Physical assessment, including auscultation of chest
4. Examination of pleural fluid obtained via thoracentesis and laboratory analysis

E. Treatment (according to cause)
1. Analgesics and antibiotics
2. Drainage of fluid: thoracentesis, then chest tubes to underwater-seal drainage with suction
3. Oxygen if dyspnea is severe; alleviation of pain by turning patient to affected side

F. Nursing interventions
1. See plan for patient with chest tubes (Box 5-2).
2. Provide diet high in protein, calories, minerals, and vitamins.
3. Alleviate anxiety.

Pneumothorax, Hemothorax, and Empyema

A. Definition
1. Pneumothorax: air in pleural space allowing for partial or complete collapse of the lung
2. Hemothorax: blood in the pleural space
3. Empyema: exudates in the pleural space

B. Causes
1. May be spontaneous
2. Trauma (e.g., knife wound, fractured rib that punctures lung)

Box 5-2   Patient with Chest Tubes

DESCRIPTION

Drainage tubes are inserted between the ribs into the pleural cavity to allow for drainage of secretions, blood, or air; the tube or tubes are attached to an underwater-seal system to allow for expansion of the lung and to prevent air from entering the pleural cavity; the drainage system may or may not be attached to suction.

INDICATIONS

- Chest surgery
- Stab wounds to the chest
- Pleural effusion
- Spontaneous pneumothorax

NURSING INTERVENTIONS

- Do complete assessment of the respiratory system q2h. Place patient in semi-Fowler position; provide oxygen with humidity.
- Prevent complications of immobility. Have patient turn, deep breathe, and cough q2h. Encourage patient to ambulate as ordered and as condition allows. Splint chest to cough.
- Encourage fluids to liquefy secretions. Provide tissues and bag for proper disposal. Provide sputum cup.
- Provide oral hygiene q2h.
- Anticipate pain; medicate as needed. Observe respirations 30 minutes after administration of sedative or analgesic.
- Observe underwater-seal system every hour:
  - Drainage color and amount
  - Rise and fall of water in bottle (or suction) going to patient
  - Bubbling (if connected to suction)
- Alleviate anxiety.
- Pace activities to allow for periods of rest.
- Monitor chest tube drainage.

3. Postoperative (e.g., when the thoracic cavity has been entered)
4. Diagnostic (e.g., central venous pressure [CVP] line, thoracentesis, pleural biopsy)

C. Signs and symptoms
  1. Subjective
    a. Sudden, sharp chest pain (when spontaneous)
    b. Vertigo
  2. Objective
    a. Diaphoresis, rapid pulse, and rapid respirations
    b. Decreased blood pressure
    c. Decreased or absent breath sounds
    d. Dyspnea

D. Diagnostic tests and methods
  1. Patient history and physical assessment
  2. Chest x-ray examination
  3. Auscultation
  4. Observation

E. Treatment
  1. Closure of wound with airtight dressing
  2. Aspiration of fluids and air; water-seal drainage
  3. Analgesics
  4. Thoracentesis

F. Nursing interventions
  1. Provide nursing care and observations as necessary for primary diagnosis.

2. Place patient in high-Fowler position.
3. Monitor vital signs.
4. Administer oxygen.
5. Provide nursing care for a patient with chest tubes as described in Box 5-2.
6. Provide instructions on tube or dressing care if discharged with chest tube in place.

Influenza

A. Definition: acute disease that may occur as an epidemic. Recovery is usually complete. No permanent immunity results. Complications and death may occur in patients with chronic or debilitating conditions, especially cardiac or pulmonary conditions.

B. Cause: virus

C. Preventive: Flu vaccine is indicated for elderly and at-risk individuals each year.

D. Signs and symptoms
  1. Subjective
    a. Headache, chest pain, and muscle ache
    b. Dry throat
  2. Objective
    a. Neck stiffness
    b. Elevated temperature
    c. Coughing, sneezing, nasal discharge, and herpetic lesions
  3. GI symptoms; nausea, vomiting, and anorexia
  4. Weakness

E. Diagnostic tests and methods: patient history and physical assessment

F. Treatment
  1. Prevention with vaccines; influenza vaccine recommended on annual basis
  2. Relief of symptoms
  3. Antiviral therapy: amantadine hydrochloride for the prophylaxis and treatment of influenza A virus

G. Nursing interventions
  1. Provide rest, assist with care, provide quiet environment and dim lighting.
  2. Encourage fluids.
  3. Relieve symptoms: Provide antipyretics, analgesics.

Pulmonary Tuberculosis

A. Definition: chronic, progressive infection. Alveoli are inflamed, and small nodules called *primary tubercles* are produced. The tubercle bacillus is at the center of the nodule (these become fibrosed); the area becomes calcified and can be identified on x-ray film. The person who has been infected harbors the bacillus for life; it is dormant unless it becomes active during physical or emotional stress.

B. Cause: *M. tuberculosis,* Koch bacillus, an AFB spread by droplets from an infected person

C. Signs and symptoms
  1. Subjective
    a. Malaise; patient is easily fatigued
    b. Chest pain
    c. Anorexia and weight loss
    d. Anxiety (e.g., fear of chronic disease, fear of public rejection)
  2. Objective
    a. Cough and hemoptysis (coughing up blood from the respiratory tract)
    b. Elevation of temperature and night sweats

D. Diagnostic tests and methods
1. Patient history and physical assessment, coexisting chronic illness
2. Chest x-ray examination
3. Sputum specimen for AFB; aspiration of gastric fluid for AFB if unable to obtain specimen
4. Tuberculin skin testing (e.g., Mantoux test)
E. Treatment
1. Combination of two or three antituberculin drugs for 6 to 9 months and sometimes longer for extrapulmonary disease (see Chapter 3)
2. Rest (physical and emotional)
3. Diet high in carbohydrates, proteins, and vitamins (especially vitamin B_6)
4. Surgical resection of affected lung tissue or involved lobe (only when necessary)
F. Nursing interventions
1. Provide rest. Assist with or provide care. Plan rest periods. Limit conversation. Leave personal items in easy reach.
2. Prevent transmission: Ensure proper isolation (AFB, tuberculosis); provide tissues and bag for disposal; encourage proper use of tissues; insist that patient cover mouth and nose when coughing or sneezing; provide mask for patient if necessary. Room must be equipped with special means of ventilation.
3. Provide frequent, small meals and nutritious snacks. Provide mouth care after meals.
4. Help patient avoid chills. Keep patient's skin dry and clean. Protect from drafts, especially at night.
5. Allay fears of patient and family about transmission: Encourage proper adherence to drug maintenance. Explain how organism is carried, transmitted, and destroyed (nurse must be aware that a tuberculin test is recommended for all contacts with a person with tuberculosis). A positive test result does not mean that the disease has developed but indicates that the organism has entered the body and the body has produced antibodies at some point. Explain need for multiple, long-term drug therapy.

Chronic Obstructive Pulmonary Disease

Chronic obstructive pulmonary disease (COPD) includes chronic and frequently progressive pulmonary disorders that affect expiratory air flow; asthma, chronic bronchitis, and pulmonary emphysema may occur independently or together.

Asthma

A. Definition: spasms of the bronchial muscle. Edema and swelling of the mucosa produce thick secretions. Air flow is obstructed; air enters and is trapped. A characteristic wheeze accompanies attempts to exhale through narrowed bronchi. Breathing is labored. Patient attempts to cough but fails to expectorate satisfactory amounts. Patient experiences great anxiety. The attacks last 30 to 60 minutes, often with normal breathing between attacks. An attack that is difficult to control and is resistant to all forms of treatment is called *status asthmaticus*.
B. Causes
1. Recurrent respiratory infection
2. Allergic reaction
3. Physical or emotional stress may provoke attack in a person with asthma.

C. Signs and symptoms
1. Subjective: anxiety or feeling of suffocation, dyspnea
2. Objective
a. Shortness of breath, expiratory wheeze, labored respirations, diaphoresis, use of accessory muscles, and flaring nostrils
b. Thick, tenacious sputum (after acute attack)
D. Diagnostic tests and methods
1. Patient history and physical examination
2. Arterial blood gas analysis, allergy testing, pulmonary function
3. Peak flow meter
E. Treatment
1. Removal of cause (source of allergy) or desensitization
2. Low-flow, humidified oxygen
3. Bronchodilators, mast cell inhibitors, corticosteroids, or sedatives (see Chapter 3); metered-dose inhalers
F. Nursing interventions
1. Reduce anxiety: Provide time to listen; do not leave patient alone during attack.
2. Remove cause: Keep environment free from dust and other allergens.
3. Provide continuous humidity as ordered.
4. Encourage fluids; maintain IV line as ordered.
5. Position for maximal comfort and breathing: Have patient sit in high-Fowler position with arms supported by an over-bed table.
6. Prevent secondary infections: Avoid staff and visitors with upper respiratory infections.
7. Teach abdominal breathing.
8. Do not allow smoking; refer patient for help in quitting.
9. Have patient avoid exposure to cold, wet weather.
10. Instruct on preventive treatment for exertional asthma.
11. Instruct on medications, use of inhalers, peak flow meter.

Chronic Bronchitis

A. Definition: chronic, progressive infection accompanied by hypersecretion of mucus by the bronchioles. Without treatment and prevention of acute attacks, the alveolar sacs and capillaries will extend and be destroyed.
B. Causes
1. Asthma
2. Acute respiratory tract infections (e.g., pneumonia, influenza, smoking, and air pollution contribute to incidence)
3. Familial tendency
C. Signs and symptoms
1. Subjective
a. Worsening dyspnea
b. Exertional dyspnea
2. Objective
a. Results of diagnostic tests
b. Cough productive with thick, white sputum; sputum is blood tinged as disease progresses (cough is greatest on arising).
c. May progress to wheezing, prolonged expiratory time, use of accessory muscles
D. Diagnostic tests and methods
1. Patient history
2. Pulmonary testing to rule out other disease (e.g., tuberculosis, malignancy)
3. Chest x-ray analysis

E. Treatment
1. Prevent irritation of bronchial mucosa: Encourage patient to discontinue smoking and change aggravating conditions in occupation or home environment.
2. Prevent upper respiratory tract infection: Maintain optimum health, adequate rest, and high-protein, high-vitamin diet.
3. Provide bronchodilators, antibiotics, corticosteroids, and influenza vaccine during epidemics (see Chapter 3).
F. Nursing interventions
1. Provide care to relieve patient problems. (See discussion of frequent patient problems and nursing care earlier in this chapter.)
2. Loosen, liquefy, and remove secretions: Provide postural drainage and chest percussion as ordered; encourage fluids.
3. Involve patient and family in care and care planning.
4. Do not allow smoking; refer patient for help in quitting.

Emphysema

A. Definition: chronic, progressive condition in which the alveolar sacs distend, rupture, and destroy the capillary beds; the alveoli lose elasticity, and inspired air is trapped. Inspiration is difficult, and expiration is prolonged. The lung tissue becomes fibrotic. Exchange of gases is impaired. Anxiety increases. Signs of oxygen deprivation are evident.
B. Cause (see discussion of chronic bronchitis)
C. Signs and symptoms
1. Subjective
a. DOE (later, dyspnea on slightest exertion and orthopnea)
b. Anorexia, weakness, feels isolated owing to chronic cough
2. Objective
a. Results of diagnostic tests
b. Wheezing, prolonged expiratory time
c. Chronic cough; productive, purulent sputum in copious amounts
d. Speaks in short, jerky sentences
e. Cerebral anoxia: is drowsy and confused; may become unconscious and go into coma
f. Barrel chest
g. Weight loss
D. Diagnostic tests and methods
1. Patient history and physical examination
2. Chest x-ray examination
3. Pulmonary function tests
4. Arterial blood gas analysis, CBC
5. Sputum analysis
E. Treatment (see chronic bronchitis)
F. Nursing interventions
1. Loosen, liquefy, and remove secretions: Provide postural drainage and chest percussion as ordered; encourage fluids; administer expectorants as needed.
2. Promote respiratory function: breathing exercises and coughing.
3. Administer oxygen; oxygen is administered in low concentrations only (1 to 2L). A high carbon dioxide level in the blood can be dangerous. The respiratory center of the brain becomes accustomed to the low blood oxygen level; if oxygen increases, respiratory rate slows significantly.
4. Prevent and control infections: Administer antibiotics; avoid contact with people with upper respiratory tract infections. Avoid smoking.

5. Provide rest: Limit exertion of any type; provide care; minimize conversation; assist with all movements (e.g., turning, getting into chair).
6. Include family in care and care plan; be understanding that this condition is chronic.
7. Teach pursed-lip and abdominal breathing.
8. Teach prolonged expiration and breathing.
9. Encourage small, frequent meals.
10. Encourage activities to alleviate loneliness or feelings of isolation.

Cancer of the Lung

A. Definition: primary or secondary (from metastasis [e.g., from prostate]) malignant tumor. Bronchogenic carcinoma is the most common primary tumor. Usually symptoms are absent until late stages, when metastasis has occurred to brain, spinal cord, or esophagus. Treatment is difficult in late stages and is based on symptoms. Prognosis is poor unless the cancer is detected and treated early.
B. Cause: strongly related to smoking, air pollution, and chemical irritants
C. Signs and symptoms (occur in late stages)
1. Subjective
a. Dyspnea and chest pain
b. Fatigue, anorexia
2. Objective
a. Results of diagnostic tests
b. Productive cough with blood-streaked sputum
c. Weight loss
D. Diagnostic tests and methods
1. CT scan, MRI
2. Examination of sputum for cells (cytology)
3. Bronchial biopsy examination
E. Treatment
1. Surgery: Procedure depends on size and location of tumor (lobectomy, pneumonectomy, or laparoscopic thoracotomy).
2. Radiation
3. Chemotherapy
4. Photodynamic therapy with laser
F. Nursing interventions
1. Provide nursing care for symptoms. (See discussion of frequent patient problems and nursing care earlier in the chapter.)
2. Provide preoperative and postoperative nursing care (see Chapter 2).
a. Maintain patent airway; administer oxygen; have patient turn, cough, and deep breathe every 2 hours. A patient with a pneumonectomy must not cough. Do not turn on operative side until physician orders (prevent mediastinal shift).
b. Provide special care for a patient with chest tubes (rarely used but still a possibility).
c. Provide care to radiation sites.
d. Monitor for side effects of chemotherapy.

Obstructive Sleep Apnea

A. Definition: complete or partial upper airway obstruction during sleep, causing apnea and hypopnea. Stroke, arrhythmias, and hypertension may occur.
B. Cause: obstruction from the tongue or soft palate
1. Occurs more frequently in older, obese men

2. Nasal allergies and a receding chin may be precipitating factors.

C. Signs and symptoms
1. Subjective
    a. Frequent awakening at night
    b. Insomnia
    c. Excessive daytime sleepiness
    d. Morning headaches
    e. Personality changes
    f. Irritability
2. Objective
    a. Witnessed apneic episodes
    b. Snoring

D. Diagnostic tests and methods: Sleep study—polysomnography results show multiple episodes of apnea.

E. Medical treatment
1. Weight loss
2. Oral appliances to enlarge airway space
3. Nasal continuous positive airway pressure (CPAP)
4. Bilevel positive airway pressure (BiPAP)
5. Surgical removal of tissue causing obstruction

F. Nursing interventions
1. Educate patient regarding avoidance of sedatives and alcoholic beverages before sleep.
2. Educate regarding use of the CPAP or BiPAP devices.

Severe Acute Respiratory Syndrome (SARS)

A. Definition: acutely infectious respiratory condition in which 10% to 20% of those affected develop severe breathing difficulties

B. Cause
1. Caused by a coronavirus that is spread by close physical contact
2. Virus may be found within 10 days of traveling to one of the SARS regions (Toronto, Taiwan, Singapore, Hong Kong, Vietnam).

C. Signs and symptoms
1. Subjective—develop within 2 to 7 days of exposure
    a. Fever
    b. Headache
    c. Malaise
    d. Muscle aches
2. Objective
    a. Dry cough
    b. Shortness of breath

D. Diagnostic tests and methods
1. Chest x-ray examination: Results initially may be normal, later show patchy infiltrated lung tissue
2. Serum antibodies
3. Positive tissue cultures
4. Elevated WBCs late in disease
5. Elevated creatine phosphokinase (CPK)

E. Treatment: Begin treatment before diagnosis is confirmed.
1. Respiratory isolation, including particulate filters
2. Antiviral medication: ribavirin
3. Antibiotic: may not be beneficial but could treat secondary infections
4. Corticosteroids

F. Nursing interventions
1. Notify local public health department.
2. Educate on disease and need for Isolation Precautions.
3. Instruct that patient may be discharged 10 days after fever has resolved.

CARDIOVASCULAR, PERIPHERAL, AND HEMATOLOGICAL SYSTEMS

ANATOMY AND PHYSIOLOGY OF THE CIRCULATORY SYSTEM

A. Functions
1. Major function: transports oxygen, carbon dioxide, cell wastes, nutrients, enzymes, and antibodies throughout the body
2. Secondary function: contributes to bodily metabolic functions and maintenance of homeostasis

B. Heart (Figure 5-5)
1. Hollow, cone-shaped muscular organ the size of a man's fist; functions as a pump
2. Positioned in thoracic cavity between the sternum and thoracic vertebrae
3. Apex extends slightly to the left and rests on the diaphragm, approximately at the level of the fifth rib; point at which apical pulse is assessed
4. Layers
    a. Pericardium: outer covering; consists of two layers of serous membrane that is lubricated and prevents friction when the heart beats
    b. Myocardium: dense, fibrous connective tissue; the heart wall
    c. Endocardium: thin, serous lining that helps the blood flow smoothly through the heart; lines the heart chamber
5. Chambers
    a. Atria: upper chambers—primarily receiving chambers; do not exert the major pumping force of the heart
        (1) Right atrium: receives deoxygenated blood from the coronary sinus and the superior and inferior venae cavae
        (2) Left atrium: receives oxygenated blood from the lungs by way of the four pulmonary veins
    b. Ventricles: lower chambers—the pumping chambers; have the major responsibility of forcing blood out into large arteries
        (1) Right ventricle: receives blood from right atrium and pumps blood to lungs by way of the pulmonary artery
        (2) Left ventricle: does the major work of the heart; has the thickest muscular wall; pumps blood to all parts of the body by way of the aorta
        (3) Interventricular or interatrial septum: divides the heart longitudinally

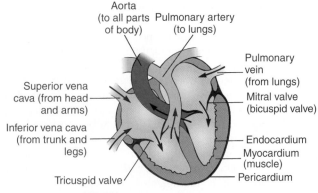

FIGURE 5-5 Structures of the heart.

6. Valves: permit flow of blood in only one direction
   a. Atrioventricular (AV) valves
      (1) Tricuspid: allows blood to flow from right atrium into right ventricle
      (2) Mitral or bicuspid: allows blood to flow from left atrium to left ventricle
   b. Semilunar valves
      (1) Pulmonary semilunar: allows blood to flow out of right ventricle into pulmonary artery
      (2) Aortic semilunar: allows blood to flow out of left ventricle into aorta
7. Physiology
   a. Cardiac cycle: refers to one complete heartbeat, consisting of contraction or systole and relaxation or diastole of the atria and ventricles
   b. Auscultatory sounds: heard through a stethoscope. The first sound, systolic, is longer and louder because of the closure of the cuspid valves; the second sound, diastole, is shorter and softer because of the closure of the semilunar valves.
   c. Conduction system
      (1) Functions: initiates heartbeat; conducts electrical impulses around heart; coordinates heartbeat
      (2) Components
         (a) Sinoatrial (SA) node: pacemaker of the heart; sets and regulates the beat by sending electrical impulses to the atria and the AV node
         (b) AV node: receives impulses from SA node; transmits electrical impulses by way of bundle of His to the ventricles
         (c) Bundle of His: fibers that begin at AV node and follow the interventricular septum; divide into Purkinje fibers
         (d) Purkinje fibers: conducting fibers; stimulate ventricles to contract
   d. Heart rate: controlled by internal and external factors
      (1) Bradycardia: slower than normal rate, less than 60 beats/min
      (2) Tachycardia: faster than normal rate, more than 100 beats/min
      (3) Extrasystole: premature beat
      (4) Sinus arrhythmia: deviation from the normal pattern of the heartbeat resulting from changes in the rate and depth of breathing or other benign causes

C. Blood vessels
   1. Arteries: elastic, muscular conducting tubes; carry blood away from the heart and to the capillaries. All arteries (except pulmonary) carry oxygenated blood.
      a. Aorta: the largest artery, from which all other arteries branch out and become smaller and smaller
      b. Arterioles: extremely small arteries; branch into the capillaries
   2. Veins: thin-walled tubes that have one-way valves to prevent backflow of blood; transport blood back to the heart. All veins (except pulmonary) carry deoxygenated blood.
      a. Venae cavae: largest veins; enter the right atrium
         (1) Superior vena cava: returns blood from the head, arms, and thoracic region
         (2) Inferior vena cava: returns blood from body regions below the diaphragm
      b. Venules: extremely small veins; collect blood from the capillaries

   3. Capillaries: microscopic vessels; carry blood from arterioles to venules. Exchange of nutrients and waste products occurs in capillaries.
D. Types of circulation
   1. Systemic: Blood flows from the left ventricle into the aorta, through the body, and back to the right atrium; provides oxygen-rich, nutrient-laden blood to body organs.
   2. Pulmonary: Blood flows from the right ventricle into the pulmonary artery, to the lungs, and then back to the left atrium through the pulmonary vein. Its function is to carry blood to the lungs for gas exchange and return it to the heart.
   3. Portal: Detour of venous blood from the stomach, pancreas, intestines, and spleen through the liver, where it is processed and returned by way of the inferior vena cava. Excess glucose is removed and stored in the liver as glycogen; poisonous substances are removed and detoxified.
E. Blood
   1. Functions
      a. Transports oxygen and carbon dioxide to and from lungs
      b. Transports nutrients, hormones, and waste products
      c. Helps maintain acid-base, electrolyte, and fluid balance
      d. Carries substances that help fight infection
      e. Acts to maintain homeostasis
   2. Composition
      a. Plasma: liquid, straw-colored portion of blood
         (1) Approximately 90% water
         (2) Contains blood proteins (fibrinogen, prothrombin, albumin, gamma globulin)
         (3) Contains mineral salts (electrolytes), hormones, nutrients, oxygen, carbon dioxide, and waste products (urea, lactic acid, uric acid)
      b. Formed elements
         (1) Erythrocytes: RBCs
            (a) Contain Hgb, which carries oxygen to cells and carbon dioxide from cells
            (b) Originate in red bone marrow
            (c) Life span: 100 to 120 days
            (d) Destroyed by the spleen, liver, and bone marrow
            (e) Normal range: male, 4.5 to 6.2 million per cubic millimeter (mm^3); female, 4 to 5.5 million/mm^3
         (2) Leukocytes: WBCs
            (a) Principal function: to fight infection
            (b) Able to multiply rapidly
            (c) Classified according to whether they contain visible granules in their cytoplasm
               • Granulocytes: include neutrophils, eosinophils, and basophils
               • Agranulocytes: include lymphocytes and monocytes
            (d) Form in red bone marrow and by lymphatic tissue in lymph nodes, thymus, and spleen
            (e) Normal range: 5000 to 10,000/mm^3
         (3) Thrombocytes: platelets
            (a) Aid in clotting process
            (b) Originate in bone marrow
            (c) Normal range: 200,000 to 400,000/mm3

3. Blood types
   a. Every person belongs to one of the four groups (type A, B, AB, or O) and is classified as either Rh positive or Rh negative.
   b. Type A blood: type A antigens in RBCs, anti-B antibodies in plasma
   c. Type B blood: type B antigens in RBCs, anti-A antibodies in plasma
   d. Type AB blood: type A and type B antigens in RBCs; no anti-A or anti-B antibodies in plasma; a person with type AB is called a *universal recipient*.
   e. Type O blood: no type A or type B antigens in RBCs; both anti-A and anti-B antibodies in plasma; a person with type O is called a *universal donor*.
   f. Rh-positive blood: Rh-factor antigen in RBCs
   g. Rh-negative blood: no Rh factor in RBCs; no anti-Rh antibodies in plasma
   h. Harmful effects can result from a blood transfusion if donor's RBCs become agglutinated by antibodies in the recipient's plasma.
F. Lymphatic system: represents an accessory route for return of fluid from interstitial spaces to cardiovascular system; consists of lymphatic vessels, lymph nodes or glands, and spleen
   1. Lymph: transparent fluid in surrounding spaces between tissue cells; made of water and end products of cell metabolism; referred to as *intercellular* or *interstitial fluid*
   2. Function of system
      a. Lymphatic vessels: return fluid and proteins to blood
      b. Lymph nodes: filter injurious particles such as microorganisms and cancer cells
      c. Tonsils: filter and remove bacteria or pathogens entering the throat
      d. Thymus: most active during early life (childhood); regulates immune system response through puberty; atrophies at adulthood
   3. Spleen: consists of lymphoid tissue
      a. Forms lymphocytes and monocytes
      b. Destroys old RBCs
      c. Stores blood until needed and then releases it into circulation
G. Immunity: the body's defense system against diseases and substances interpreted as "nonself"; mediated by T and B lymphocytes of the circulatory system. Functions of lymphocytes in immunity by cell type are:
   1. T lymphocytes: originate from stem cells in thymus; responsible for cellular immunity (a slow response) to an antigen; act against most bacteria, viruses, tumor cells, and foreign organs or grafts; clone into types of regulatory cells—helpers and suppressors
      a. Helper T cells: interact directly with B cells by stimulating activity of B cells on killer T cells
      b. Killer T cells: directly attack virus-infected cells; promote lysis
      c. Suppressor T cells: terminate normal immune response
   2. B lymphocytes: originate mainly in fetal liver and lymphoid tissue during first few months of life; responsible for humoral immunity (a rapid response) to an antigen
      a. Clone antibody-producing plasma cells
      b. Protect against toxins

3. Naturally acquired immunity
   a. Active: acquired through contact with disease
   b. Passive: acquired from antibodies obtained through placenta and mother's milk
4. Artificially acquired immunity
   a. Active: immunization with vaccines
   b. Passive: administration of immune serum

CARDIOVASCULAR CONDITIONS AND DISORDERS

Diseases related to the cardiovascular system are the leading cause of death in the United States. Cardiovascular health problems occur along the age continuum. To reduce death and disability, three major objectives are early detection of the disease; appropriate treatment to control the disease progression; and reduction of predisposing factors by promoting screening, education, and patient care of cardiovascular health.

NURSING ASSESSMENT
A. Observations
   1. Vital signs
      a. Temperature
      b. Pulse: character, rate, rhythm, and any irregularities
      c. Respiration: character, rate; note abnormalities
      d. Blood pressure: hypotension or hypertension
      e. Pulse oximetry: measures the amount of dissolved oxygen in capillary blood
      f. Pain: character, source, radiation, location, severity
   2. General appearance
      a. Skin temperature, character, and color (jaundice, cyanosis, pallor); note clamminess
      b. Distended neck veins
      c. DOE
      d. Limited or reduced ability to perform ADLs
      e. Clubbing of fingers
      f. Presence of edema; pedal, pulmonary, ascites, or sacral (if supine)
   3. Heart sounds
      a. Note bruits (whooshing sounds caused by turbulent blood flow) in carotids
      b. Abnormal heart sounds: arrhythmias, murmurs
      c. Precordial movements, thrills
B. Patient description (subjective data)
   1. Chest pain
      a. Onset, location, frequency, duration, radiation
      b. Alleviating or aggravating factors
      c. May occur during periods of physical and emotional stress (emotions, eating, exercise, environment); may radiate to arm or jaw or may occur at rest
   2. Easily fatigued
      a. Can no longer perform usual activities without frequent rest periods
      b. Intolerance of exercise or exertion
   3. Palpitations
   4. Dizziness and feelings of fatigue, especially when arising or standing
   5. Cough
      a. Frothy or blood tinged (hemoptysis)
      b. Nocturnal cough
   6. Family history of heart disease and hypertension
   7. DOE

DIAGNOSTIC TESTS AND METHODS

A. Electrocardiogram (ECG); also known as EKG
   1. Tracing of the electrical activity of the heart
   2. Used to identify abnormal cardiac rhythms (arrhythmias) and coronary atherosclerotic heart disease
   3. Reassure patient that the ECG is recording the electrical impulses of the heart and not delivering any electrical impulses to the body.
   4. May be done on ambulatory patients through the use of telemetry units; signals from a box that patient carries are conveyed to a monitor at a nurses' station.
B. Stress test
   1. A procedure designed to detect cardiac ischemia that develops during exercise or exertion
   2. A heart tracing (ECG) is recorded and monitored while a patient performs an activity such as stair climbing, pedaling a stationary bicycle, or walking on a treadmill.
   3. May be pharmacologically induced
C. Blood tests
   1. CBC: analyzes components of the blood
      a. Low Hgb and Hct indicate anemia.
      b. Elevated WBC count indicates inflammation, infection.
   2. ESR: may indicate inflammation
   3. Blood urea nitrogen (BUN) and creatinine: detect the effects of heart disease on the kidneys
   4. Serum enzymes and isoenzymes (serum glutamic oxaloacetic transaminase [SGOT], CPK, lactate dehydrogenase [LDH]): Troponin is elevated in a myocardial infarction.
   5. Serum lipids: Elevated blood lipids have been associated with coronary disease.
   6. Blood cultures: performed if bacterial endocarditis is suspected
   7. Coagulation studies: prothrombin time (PT) and partial thromboplastin time (PTT); useful in monitoring anticoagulant therapy
   8. Serum electrolytes: detect imbalances in sodium, potassium, and calcium
   9. Arterial blood gas analysis: monitors oxygenation and acid-base balance
D. Urinalysis: to determine the effects of heart disease on the kidney
E. Holter monitoring
   1. Portable monitor designed and equipped to record patient's heartbeat during a 24-hour period; a written record of patient's activity kept simultaneously; helpful in determining arrhythmias
   2. Assists patient in the recording of activity
F. Coronary angiography
   1. A roentgenogram of the coronary circulation facilitated by introducing contrast medium into the artery to outline the vessel and determine the extent of the disease process
   2. After the study patient must be observed for bleeding from the puncture site and undergo a cardiovascular status check of the involved area (pulses and skin temperature).
G. Chest x-ray examination: A standard chest roentgenogram is used to determine heart size and shape.
H. Echocardiography (ultrasound cardiography)
   1. Echoes from sound waves are used to study the movements and dimensions of cardiac structures; determines abnormalities.
   2. Information derived includes size of cardiac structures.

I. Radionuclide studies
   1. Tracing material is injected intravenously, and the radioactivity concentration over a body part is recorded.
   2. Size, shape, and filling of the heart chambers can be recorded; heart damage and cardiac circulation can also be evaluated.
J. Cardiac catheterization
   1. A cardiac catheter is introduced through a vein or artery and advanced through the system; pressures of the heart chambers and pulmonary arteries are recorded, and blood is analyzed; a contrast dye can be injected for visualization of certain structures to detect defects.
   2. Patient may feel a warm flushing sensation on injection of the dye; some patients experience chest pain.
   3. Patient observations after examination: monitor bleeding at the insertion site, check pulses and skin warmth in the involved area and check heart rate and rhythm.
K. Oscillometry: a noninvasive test that measures the amplitude of pulsations over an artery

FREQUENT PATIENT PROBLEMS AND NURSING CARE

A. Acute or chronic pain related to decreased cardiac output; overactivity
   1. Evaluate and record onset, duration, and intensity.
   2. Note any associated symptoms (nausea, vomiting, dyspnea).
   3. Monitor vital signs and record.
   4. Give vasodilators as prescribed; monitor for effectiveness and observe for side effects.
   5. If pain is unrelieved in 15 minutes by drugs or rest, notify physician.
   6. Reinforce patient teaching regarding diet, drugs, planned exercise, and stress management.
   7. Administer oxygen as prescribed.
   8. Record reactions to treatment and nursing care.
B. Ineffective breathing pattern related to dyspnea
   1. Monitor vital signs and record.
   2. Note character and rate of respirations.
   3. Elevate the head of the bed at least 30 degrees.
   4. Help patient assume an orthopneic position when necessary.
   5. Auscultate chest and note the presence of abnormal lung and heart sounds.
   6. Monitor oxygen therapy.
   7. Monitor intake and output.
   8. Record reactions to treatment and nursing care.
   9. Give diuretics, cardiotonics, and bronchodilators as prescribed, and monitor for side effects.
   10. Note color, character, and amount of sputum.
C. Decreased cardiac output related to arrhythmias
   1. Monitor vital signs and record.
   2. Note and report any changes in the vital signs.
   3. Auscultate chest, noting any abnormal heart sounds, and report abnormalities.
   4. Give antiarrhythmic drugs as prescribed, and monitor for side effects.
   5. Monitor for and report any associated symptoms.
D. Risk for peripheral neurovascular dysfunction related to edema
   1. Note and record location and degree of edema.
   2. Elevate legs.

3. Change positions when patient is in bed.
4. Note degree of pitting.
5. Note "weeping" of skin areas.
6. Monitor for skin breakdown.
7. Give prescribed diuretics and cardiotonics.
8. Note the presence of tenderness in the upper quadrant of the abdomen.
9. Note the presence of ascites.
10. Note daily weight.
11. Record intake and output.
12. Limit fluid intake as prescribed.
13. Reinforce teaching for reduction of dependent edema.

E. Activity intolerance related to reduced cardiac reserve
1. Encourage progressive ambulation.
2. Encourage progressive resuming of ADLs.
3. Provide for planned activity and rest periods.
4. Monitor for signs of fatigue.
5. Stop activity at the first sign of intolerance.
6. Encourage ROM exercises.
7. Provide prescribed diet.
8. Reinforce patient instruction of planned exercise.

F. Ineffective tissue perfusion related to decreased cardiac output
1. Observe for presence of postural hypotension—orthostatic vital signs. (Note if blood pressure drops when patient is standing.)
2. Assist patient to dangle legs over the side of the bed before standing, to reduce dizziness.
3. Instruct patient to get up slowly.
4. Assess patient's pulse when he or she is standing.

G. Excess fluid volume related to decreased cardiac output
1. Daily weight; report weight changes.
2. Record intake and output.
3. Monitor serum electrolytes.
4. Limit fluids as indicated.
5. Provide salt-restricted diet if ordered.
6. Give diuretic medication as prescribed.
7. Reinforce instructions regarding diet, drugs, and weight control.

H. Ineffective tissue perfusion related to hypertension
1. Monitor vital signs and report changes.
2. Provide sodium-restricted diet as prescribed.
3. Provide cholesterol-controlled diet if prescribed, and monitor for side effects.
4. Instruct in the avoidance of risk factors (smoking, stress, obesity).
5. Reinforce teaching in the areas of diet, weight control, avoidance of risk factors, and home monitoring of blood pressure.

MAJOR MEDICAL DIAGNOSES
Arteriosclerosis and Atherosclerosis
A. Definition
1. Arteriosclerosis: a process in which the arterial walls harden, thicken, and lose their elasticity, resulting in restricted blood flow
2. Atherosclerosis: one form of arteriosclerosis; fatty plaques that form on the intima (inner layer) of the arteries

B. Pathology
1. The underlying mechanism is the formation of fatty plaque deposits in the arteries.
2. The plaque increases in size and ultimately obstructs blood flow to vital areas.

C. Arteriosclerosis is associated with the following health problems:
1. Coronary artery disease
2. Angina pectoris
3. Myocardial infarction
4. Hypertension
5. Peripheral vascular disease
6. Cerebrovascular accidents (CVAs) (strokes)

D. Signs and symptoms vary, depending on the arteries affected by the sclerosing process.
1. Extremity involvement
a. Cramping pain (intermittent claudication)
b. Numbness and tingling
c. Reduced circulation, causing ulceration or pain
d. Outward changes: skin pallor, cool skin, reduced or absent pulses, loss of leg hair, and skin ulceration
2. Coronary involvement
a. Chest pain
b. Dyspnea
c. Palpitations
d. Fainting (syncope)
e. Fatigue

E. Diagnostic tests and methods
1. Patient history and physical examination
2. Arteriograms
3. ECG
4. Oscillometry

F. Treatment
1. Dietary restriction of fat and cholesterol, sodium
2. Vasodilator drugs
3. Cholesterol-lowering drugs
4. Elimination or reduction of risk factors (Box 5-3)
5. Weight management
6. Planned exercise
7. Prevention of pressure in extremities
8. Use of special devices such as bed cradles
9. Bypass surgery or removal of plaques may be considered.

G. Nursing interventions
1. Assess and document signs and symptoms.
2. Protect the extremity from trauma.
3. Monitor protective devices (e.g., bed cradles, pads).
4. Provide skin care to ulcerated areas or areas affected by reduced circulation.
5. Monitor pulses and skin character of involved extremities.
6. Report changes in the involved extremities.
a. Absence of pulse
b. Cyanosis
c. Increased pain
d. Temperature change (coldness)
7. Monitor for signs and symptoms of infection in ulcerated areas.
8. Provide slow, progressive physical activity as prescribed.
9. Administer prescribed diet.

Box 5-3	Risk Factors in the Development of Atherosclerosis

- Obesity
- Sedentary lifestyle
- Smoking
- Stress
- High-fat diet

10. Administer prescribed drugs.
11. Relieve pain from ischemia.
12. Avoid cold and provide adequate warmth to prevent vasoconstriction.
13. Avoid constrictive clothing.
14. Educate patient and family regarding avoidance of risk factors, management of diet, medication, and activity.

Angina Pectoris

A. Definition: episodes of acute chest pain resulting from insufficient oxygenation of myocardial tissue, which in turn is caused by decreased blood flow to the area (ischemia)
  1. Episodes occur most frequently during periods of physical or emotional exertion.
     a. Exercise
     b. Eating a heavy meal
     c. Environmental temperature extremes
  2. Episodes seldom last more than 15 minutes.
B. Causes
  1. The major cause is atherosclerosis.
  2. Narrowed coronary arteries obstruct blood flow; thus oxygen carried by the blood cannot sufficiently meet tissue demands, particularly during periods of exertion.
C. Signs and symptoms
  1. Substernal chest pain, usually brought on by exertion
  2. Radiation of pain to the jaw or an extremity
  3. Dyspnea
  4. Anxiety or feeling of impending doom
  5. Tachycardia
  6. Diaphoresis
  7. Sensation of heaviness, choking, or suffocation
  8. Indigestion
D. Diagnostic tests and methods
  1. Patient history and physical examination
  2. ECG
  3. Holter monitoring
  4. Coronary angiography
  5. Stress testing
  6. Chest x-ray examination
  7. Serum lipid and enzyme values
E. Treatment
  1. Relieving chest pain by using vasodilator drugs (e.g., nitrates, beta blockers, calcium channel blockers), sedatives, and analgesics
  2. Dietary restriction of fat and cholesterol
  3. Planned exercise
  4. Weight management
  5. Stress management
  6. If conservative measures are unsuccessful, coronary bypass surgery or an angioplasty may be considered.
F. Nursing interventions
  1. Assess and document signs and symptoms and reactions to treatment.
  2. Administer vasodilator medication, and monitor for side effects.
  3. Instruct patient to inform the nursing staff at the onset of an anginal attack.
  4. Provide emotional support and assurance.
  5. Provide prompt relief of pain.
  6. Monitor vital signs, particularly during an attack.
  7. Educate patient and family regarding diet, activity, drug therapy, and avoidance of risk factors.

Hypertension (High Blood Pressure)

A. Definition: characterized by persistent elevation of blood pressure (see Box 5-4 for current classification system)
  1. Primary hypertension (essential): a persistent elevation of blood pressure without an apparent cause
     a. Actual cause is unknown; known as the "silent killer" because patient frequently does not experience symptoms until organ damage has occurred.
     b. Primarily small blood vessels are affected; peripheral resistance increases, and blood pressure rises.
     c. Constricted blood vessels eventually cause damage to organs that rely on a blood supply from these vessels.
  2. Secondary hypertension: a persistent elevation of blood pressure associated with another disease state
     a. Renal disease
     b. Toxemia
     c. Adrenal dysfunction
     d. Atherosclerosis
     e. Coarctation of the aorta
B. Predisposing factors
  1. Smoking
  2. Obesity
  3. Heavy salt and cholesterol intake
  4. Heredity
  5. Aggressive, hyperactive personality
  6. Age: develops between 30 and 50 years of age
  7. Gender: primarily men older than 35 years of age and women older than 45 years of age
  8. Race: African Americans have twice the incidence of Caucasians
  9. Birth-control pills and estrogens
C. The heart, brain, kidneys, and eyes can be damaged if the hypertensive state continues without correction.
D. Signs and symptoms may be insidious and vague; a person can have the disorder and not know it.
  1. Tinnitus
  2. Light-headedness
  3. Blurred vision
  4. Irritability
  5. Fatigue
  6. Tachycardia and palpitations
  7. Occipital, morning headaches
  8. Nosebleeds (epistaxis)
  9. DOE
E. Diagnostic tests and methods
  1. Patient history and physical examination
  2. Series of resting blood pressure readings

Box **5-4**   How to Classify Hypertension

Take two or more blood pressure readings, and average the results. Use this average and averages from other blood pressure readings to classify the patient's risk for hypertension.

Category	Systolic Reading (mm Hg)	Diastolic Reading (mm Hg)
Normal	<120 and	<80
Prehypertension	120-139 or	80-89
Stage I	140-159 or	90-99
Stage II	≥160 or	≥100

Data from American Heart Association, 2009.

3. Routine urinalysis, BUN, and serum creatinine to screen for renal involvement
4. Serum electrolytes to screen for adrenal involvement
5. Blood sugar levels to screen for endocrine involvement
6. Lipid profile
7. Chest x-ray examination
8. ECG
9. Holter monitoring
10. Funduscopic eye examination

F. Treatment
1. Lifestyle modifications such as exercise, smoking cessation, heart-healthy diet
2. Lowering blood pressure by using diuretics and antihypertensive drugs
3. Sodium-restricted diet
4. Cholesterol-controlled diet
5. Weight management
6. Stress management
7. Reduction or elimination of smoking
8. Planned exercise

G. Nursing interventions
1. Assess and document signs and symptoms and reactions to treatments.
2. Administer prescribed medication.
3. Observe for and report drug-related side effects.
4. Monitor weight every day to evaluate initial diuretic therapy.
5. Monitor intake and output to evaluate initial diuretic therapy.
6. Monitor vital signs, particularly blood pressure, under the same conditions every day.
7. Provide planned activity and rest periods.
8. Provide prescribed diet.
   a. Calorie-controlled
   b. Sodium-restricted
   c. Cholesterol-controlled
9. Educate patient and family.
   a. Drug therapy and side effects
   b. Dietary restrictions; weight management
   c. Elimination of risk factors such as smoking
   d. Activity
   e. Blood pressure monitoring
   f. Need for participation in and compliance with the prescribed regimen

Myocardial Infarction (Heart Attack)

A. Definition: obstruction of a coronary artery or one of its branches
1. The obstruction results in the death of the myocardial tissue supplied by that vessel.
2. The myocardial tissue dies because of oxygen deprivation (infarction or necrosis).
3. The ability of the heart to regain or maintain its function depends on the location and size of the area of infarction.

B. A myocardial infarction can occur whenever a coronary artery or branch of the artery becomes occluded by a thrombus, emboli, or the atherosclerotic process.

C. Signs and symptoms
1. "Crushing" chest pain lasting longer than 15 minutes and unrelieved by rest or drugs; this pain may radiate to the arms (usually left), jaw, head, or shoulder.
2. Shortness of breath

3. Nausea and vomiting
4. Tachycardia
5. Diaphoresis and pallor
6. Temperature rise after 48 hours
7. Elevation of the cardiac enzymes
8. Arrhythmias
9. Anxiety
10. Females may have atypical pain in back of neck, occipital region.

D. Diagnostic tests and methods
1. Patient history and physical examination
2. ECG
3. Cardiac enzyme studies (troponin, SGOT, LDH, CPK-MB)
4. Chest x-ray examination

E. Treatment
1. Analgesic drugs to relieve pain
2. Oxygen to relieve respiratory distress
3. Vasopressor drugs to prevent circulatory collapse (cardiogenic shock)
4. Cardiac monitoring to detect arrhythmias
5. Hemodynamic monitoring: internal monitoring of blood pressure and pulmonary artery pressure
6. Bed rest with progressive activity to allow the damaged myocardium to heal
7. IV fluids to provide for IV drug administration
8. Cardiopulmonary resuscitation in the event of cardiac standstill (arrest)
9. Pacemaker insertion
10. Anticoagulant therapy
11. Thrombolytic therapy to dissolve blood clot and restore blood flow
12. Nitrates

F. Nursing interventions
1. Provide pain relief.
2. Provide ongoing assessment and documentation of symptoms and reactions to treatment.
3. Administer and monitor oxygen.
4. Record vital signs hourly during the acute period.
5. Record intake and output hourly during the acute period.
6. Provide bed rest during the acute period and progressive activity as prescribed.
   a. Apply antiembolism stockings.
   b. Allow patient out of bed to use bedside commode (less taxing to the cardiovascular system).
   c. Monitor pulse during periods of activity.
7. Avoid activities that produce straining (Valsalva maneuver) to avoid stimulation of the vagus nerve, which induces bradycardia.
   a. Administer stool softeners as prescribed.
   b. Caution patient against straining when attempting a bowel movement.
8. Provide diet as prescribed.
   a. Patient may begin on liquids and then progress.
   b. Sodium and cholesterol may be restricted.
   c. Caffeine may be restricted.
9. Give prescribed antiarrhythmics, and monitor for side effects.
10. Give prescribed cardiotonics and diuretics, and monitor for side effects.
11. Monitor for complications.

a. Cardiogenic shock: circulatory collapse caused by decreased cardiac output. The vital organs are not being perfused.

(1) Monitor vital signs every 15 minutes.

(2) Record intake and output hourly.

(3) Report changes in rate, rhythm, and conductivity.

(4) Observe and report signs and symptoms: restlessness, diaphoresis, pallor, low blood pressure, and tachycardia.

(5) Administer and monitor prescribed vasopressors and antiarrhythmics.

(6) Administer oxygen as prescribed.

(7) Provide cardiac and hemodynamic monitoring. (*Hemodynamic monitoring* refers to the internal monitoring of blood pressure and pulmonary artery pressure.)

b. Pulmonary edema: left ventricle failure (pumping mechanism) caused by strain on a diseased heart. Cardiac output (the amount of blood pumped out by the heart to the body per minute) is reduced, resulting in lung congestion.

(1) Observe and report symptoms: anxiety; dyspnea; orthopnea; frothy, pink-tinged sputum; crackles in the lungs; decreased urine output; and dependent edema.

(2) Record vital signs every 15 minutes.

(3) Record intake and output hourly.

(4) Place bed in high-Fowler position.

(5) Administer cardiotonics and diuretics as prescribed, and monitor for side effects.

(6) Administer and monitor oxygen therapy.

(7) Be prepared to administer analgesics to allay anxiety and reduce respiratory rate.

(8) Provide emotional support to patient and family.

Heart Failure

A. Definition: failure of the pumping mechanism of the heart, resulting in an insufficient blood supply to meet bodily needs

B. Causes

1. The underlying mechanism in heart failure (HF) involves the failure of the pumping mechanism of the heart to respond to the metabolic changes of the body.

2. The result is a heart that cannot supply a sufficient amount of blood in relation to bodily needs and to the amount of blood returning to the heart (venous return); pressure builds up in the vascular beds on the affected side of the heart.

C. HF is described in terms of left-sided or right-sided failure, depending on which ventricle is affected.

D. Signs and symptoms are divided into left-sided and right-sided failure, although both sides may be affected.

1. Left-sided failure leads to pulmonary congestion.

a. Dyspnea

b. Orthopnea

c. Nonproductive cough that worsens at night

d. Frothy, blood-tinged sputum noted (pulmonary edema) as severity of failure increases

e. Anxiety and restlessness

f. Fatigue

2. Right-sided failure may follow left-sided failure and results in systemic venous congestion.

a. Weight gain caused by fluid accumulation in the tissues

b. Dependent edema in the form of ankle edema or sacral edema

c. Ascites caused by the collection of fluid in the abdominal cavity; may also hinder respiration

d. Fatigue

e. GI symptoms such as nausea, vomiting, and anorexia

f. Decreased urine output

g. Distended neck veins

E. Diagnostic test and methods

1. Patient history and physical examination, including the findings of edema, abnormal heart sounds, and the presence of crackles with dyspnea

2. Chest x-ray examination

3. ECG

4. Arterial blood gas studies

5. Liver function studies

6. Renal function studies

F. Treatment

1. Drug therapy: digitalization, diuretics, and sedatives

2. Recording of weight daily

3. Monitoring of intake and output

4. Oxygen therapy

5. Hemodynamic monitoring

6. Restriction of fluids

7. Restriction of dietary sodium

8. Bed rest with progressive activity

9. Elevation of the head of the bed on blocks

10. Monitoring of vital signs

G. Nursing interventions

1. Provide ongoing assessment and documentation of signs, symptoms, and reactions to treatment.

2. Monitor oxygen therapy.

3. Record vital signs every 15 minutes to 2 hours during the acute phase.

4. Record intake and output hourly during the acute phase.

5. Weigh patient daily.

6. Administer and monitor prescribed cardiotonics, diuretics, and sedatives; observe for side effects.

7. Determine the amount of activity that produces the least discomfort to patient.

8. Monitor for dependent edema.

a. Ankle edema when sitting upright

b. Sacral edema when in supine position

9. Raise the head of the bed as prescribed.

10. Observe for complications of bed rest.

a. Have patient turn, cough, and take deep breaths.

b. Apply antiembolism stockings.

11. Provide emotional support to patient and family.

12. Provide a diet low in sodium if prescribed.

13. Educate patient and family concerning dietary management, drug therapy, and activity.

14. Restrict fluids as ordered.

Valvular Conditions

A. Valvular dysfunction results in either stenosis or insufficiency of the heart valves.

1. Valvular stenosis results from cardiac infections; the valve leaflets (cusps) become fibrotic and thicken and may even fuse together, thus hindering blood flow.

2. Valvular insufficiency occurs in much the same way as does valvular stenosis; after repeated infections the valve leaflets (cusps) become inflamed and scarred and can no longer close completely; the incomplete closure allows blood to leak from the left ventricle into the left atrium during systole.

B. Blood flow through the heart is altered, resulting in decreased cardiac output, systemic and pulmonary congestion, and dilation of the heart chambers.

C. Causes
   1. Rheumatic heart disease is the primary cause of valvular dysfunction.
   2. Other causes include syphilis, bacterial endocarditis, and congenital malformations.

D. Signs and symptoms
   1. Mitral stenosis
      a. DOE
      b. Orthopnea
      c. Pink-tinged sputum
      d. Fatigue
      e. Palpitations
      f. Heart murmur
   2. Mitral insufficiency
      a. Fatigue
      b. DOE
      c. Heart murmur
      d. Orthopnea
      e. Pulmonary congestion
   3. Aortic stenosis
      a. Fatigue
      b. Angina
      c. Syncope
      d. Heart murmur
      e. HF
   4. Aortic insufficiency
      a. Palpitations
      b. Dyspnea
      c. Fatigue
      d. Orthopnea
      e. Anginal pain occurring even at rest

E. Diagnostic tests and methods
   1. Patient history and physical examination; murmur a common finding of the examination
   2. ECG
   3. Chest x-ray examination to determine heart size
   4. Cardiac catheterization to reveal possible pressure changes
   5. Echocardiogram: provides information concerning structure and function of valves
   6. Laboratory studies

F. Treatment
   1. Mitral stenosis
      a. Antibiotics administered as prophylaxis to prevent recurrences of causative agents, especially before invasive procedures (dental visit or podiatric visit)
      b. Drug therapy: diuretics, cardiotonics, and antiarrhythmics
      c. Restricted sodium diet
      d. Planned activity and avoidance of symptom-producing activity
      e. Surgical correction of the defect
         (1) Mitral commissurotomy: fused valve leaflets are separated, and the mitral opening may be dilated.
         (2) Valve replacement: diseased valve is replaced with a prosthetic valve.
   2. Mitral insufficiency
      a. Planned exercise and avoidance of symptom-producing activity
      b. Sodium-restricted diet
      c. Drug therapy: diuretics, cardiotonics, antiarrhythmics, and vasodilators
      d. Surgical correction
         (1) Valvuloplasty: repair of the existing valve
         (2) Valve replacement
   3. Aortic stenosis
      a. Prevention of infective endocarditis
      b. Treatment of symptoms
      c. Drug therapy: diuretics, nitrates, and cardiotonics
      d. Sodium-restricted diet
      e. Valve replacement

G. Nursing interventions
   1. Assess and document signs and symptoms and reaction to treatments.
   2. Administer prescribed medication and observe patient for side effects.
   3. Provide a calm, quiet environment.
   4. Allow patient and family to verbalize their anxieties and fears.
   5. Monitor vital signs and report changes.
   6. Weigh patient daily.
   7. Provide the prescribed diet.
      a. Nutritionally well balanced
      b. Sodium restricted to prevent fluid retention
   8. Encourage progressive activity as prescribed.
      a. Consider patient's limitations.
      b. Provide rest periods.
   9. Monitor intake and output if diuretics are used.
   10. Educate patient and family concerning diet, drugs, activity, and need for compliance.
   11. Vocational counseling may be needed if patient has a demanding job.

Inflammatory Disorders of the Heart

A. Definition: diseases resulting from acute or chronic inflammation of the lining of the heart and valves caused by bacteria or viruses, trauma, or other factors
   1. Pericarditis: an inflammation of the pericardium
      a. The result is a loss of elasticity or fluid accumulation within the pericardial sac.
      b. HF and cardiac tamponade (compression of heart as a result of blood or fluid in pericardial sac) may result.
   2. Myocarditis: an inflammation of the myocardium
      a. The result is impairment of contractility.
      b. Myocardial ischemia and necrosis may result.
   3. Endocarditis: an inflammation of the inner lining of the heart and valves associated with a streptococcal infection
   4. Rheumatic heart disease
      a. It is usually associated with rheumatic fever.
      b. Rheumatic fever is an inflammatory process that can affect all the layers of the heart.
      c. Cardiac impairment results from swelling and scarring of valve leaflets, leading to valvular changes (mitral insufficiency, aortic insufficiency, pericarditis).

B. Signs and symptoms
   1. Chest pain
   2. Dyspnea
   3. Chills and intermittent fever

4. Weakness and fatigue
5. Diaphoresis
6. Anorexia
7. Arrhythmias
8. Elevated cardiac enzymes
9. Friction rubs (auscultatory sound created by the rubbing together of two serous surfaces)
10. Presence of Aschoff bodies (collection of cells and leukocytes in the interstitial layers of the heart)
11. New heart murmur or an abnormal heart sound
12. Existing streptococcal infection
13. Cardiac enlargement
14. Joint involvement

C. Diagnostic tests and methods
1. Patient history and physical examination
   a. History of recent infections
   b. History of heart disease
2. ECG
3. Chest x-ray examination
4. Cardiac enzyme studies
5. Blood cultures
6. Echocardiogram to assess valvular disease and vegetation (growth of scar tissue)
7. Laboratory studies: CBC, electrolytes, ESR
8. Radionuclide studies to assess heart structure and heart damage

D. Treatment
1. Identification and elimination of the infecting agent
2. Drug therapy: antibiotics, cardiotonics, antiinflammatory agents, analgesics, and corticosteroids
3. Blood cultures
4. Oxygen
5. Rest and planned activity
6. Well-balanced diet
7. Prevention of exposure to other infectious agents

E. Nursing interventions
1. Assess and document signs and symptoms and reactions to treatment.
2. Maintain a calm, quiet environment.
3. Administer prescribed drugs, and monitor for side effects.
4. Evaluate patient's understanding of the disease process and the need for compliance.
5. Alleviate pain.
6. Allay patient's and family's fears and anxieties.
7. Monitor vital signs and report changes.
8. Observe for signs and symptoms of complications (tachycardia, dyspnea, orthopnea).
9. Educate patient concerning the illness, diet, drugs, activity, avoidance of infections, dental care, vocational counseling, and compliance with the regimen.

PERIPHERAL VASCULAR CONDITIONS AND DISORDERS

Peripheral vascular disease refers to vascular disorders exclusive of those affecting the heart. The underlying factor in peripheral vascular disease is the arteriosclerotic process. Blood flow is slowed because of vessels that are narrowed or obstructed. The lack of normal blood flow causes tissue changes (see discussion of arteriosclerosis and atherosclerosis). Vascular disease related to the lower extremities is discussed in this section.

NURSING ASSESSMENT
A. Observations
1. Skin of the lower extremities
   a. Redness (hyperemia) of the leg when in a dependent position
   b. Cold or blue feet
   c. Varicose veins
   d. Sparse hair distribution
   e. Lesions or stasis ulcers
   f. Edema
   g. Dermatitis or brown pigmentation of the skin
2. Delayed capillary filling
3. Diminished or absent pulses
   a. Rigidity (hardness) of the vessels
   b. Palpable vibration of the vessels (thrill)
4. Assessing major arteries for bruits (an auscultatory sound taking the form of a whooshing, buzzing, or humming sound caused by turbulent blood flow)
5. Differences in leg circumference
6. Thickening of nail beds

B. Patient description (subjective data)
1. Leg cramps
2. Aching calves
3. Leg numbness
4. Leg pain occurring during exercise (claudication)
5. Loss of sensation in one or both legs
6. Past or present history
   a. Alcohol excess
   b. Diabetes mellitus
   c. Hypertension
   d. Thrombophlebitis

DIAGNOSTIC TESTS AND METHODS
A. Chest x-ray examination for abnormalities
B. Oscillometry: noninvasive test that measures the amplitude of pulsations over an artery
C. Doppler ultrasonography: device that emits sound waves that can be used to measure the amount of blood flow through a vessel
D. Arteriography: used to determine the location and extent of the disease process
E. Venography: radiographic study used to determine the location and size of a blood clot, vessel distention, and development of collateral circulation
F. Trendelenburg test
1. Used to determine valvular competency
2. The leg is elevated to 90 degrees, and a tourniquet is placed around the thigh.
3. Patient stands, and the vein-filling pattern is observed.
4. Normally the veins fill slowly from below in 20 to 30 seconds; the rate of filling should not greatly accelerate when the tourniquet is removed.
G. Lung scan
1. It is used to assess the presence of pulmonary embolism and lung damage.
2. An IV radiographic isotope is injected into the patient.
3. Pulmonary circulation is assessed with a scanning device.
4. The patient also inhales a radioactive gas and is scanned to determine lung distribution of this gas.
H. Arterial blood gas analysis: used to assess the adequacy of ventilation

I. X-ray examination of the abdomen: may show evidence of an aneurysm
J. Blood tests
   1. CBC: for routine evaluation
   2. ESR to determine the presence of an inflammatory process
   3. Coagulation studies (platelet count, bleeding time, PT, PTT) to determine the existence of blood disorders

FREQUENT PATIENT PROBLEMS AND NURSING CARE

A. Pain related to intermittent claudication
   1. Evaluate and record onset, duration, and intensity.
   2. Provide rest during the episode.
   3. Determine the amount of exercise patient can tolerate before claudication occurs.
   4. Assess for and report claudication occurring without activity.
   5. Educate patient on avoiding exposure to cold and maintaining warmth.
B. Excess fluid volume as evidenced by edema of the lower extremities or decreased cardiac output or both
   1. Note and record location and degree.
   2. Instruct patient to avoid activity that places the legs in a dependent position for prolonged periods.
   3. Instruct patient to avoid wearing constricting clothing around the legs.
   4. Monitor for skin breakdown.
   5. Elevate legs.
C. Impaired skin integrity related to stasis ulcers
   1. Note location and character of ulceration.
   2. Maintain bed rest with leg elevation.
   3. Perform prescribed wound care.
   4. Instruct patient to avoid trauma to the legs.
   5. Instruct patient in proper skin care measures. Refer to Chapter 2 for skin care measures.
   6. Reinforce patient teaching in the area of drugs, diet, activity, and skin care.

MAJOR MEDICAL DIAGNOSES

Arteriosclerosis Obliterans

A. Definition: chronic arterio-occlusive disease
   1. Progression is slow and insidious.
   2. The medial and intimal layers of arteries become inflamed and thrombosed.
   3. Vessels lose elasticity, and plaques obstruct blood flow.
   4. Vessels primarily affected are the femoral and carotid arteries.
B. Causes
   1. It is associated with atherosclerotic process.
   2. Predisposing factors include hypertension, smoking, hyperlipidemia, obesity, and a positive family history.
C. Signs and symptoms
   1. Intermittent claudication
   2. Pain in the legs at rest
   3. Impotence
   4. Paresthesia
   5. Pallor or blanching on elevation of leg
   6. Hyperemia (redness) or dusky appearance of the leg or legs when dependent
   7. Loss of hair on extremities
   8. Absent or diminished pulses

D. Diagnostic tests and methods
   1. Patient history and physical examination
   2. Oscillometry
   3. Doppler ultrasonography
   4. Arteriography
   5. Laboratory studies
E. Treatment
   1. Protection of extremity from injury
   2. Prevention and control of infection
   3. Drug therapy: vasodilators, analgesics, and antibiotics
   4. Weight-reduction diet if patient is obese
   5. Bed rest
   6. Avoidance of smoking
   7. Surgical management: endarterectomy (removing the obstructing plaque) or a bypass graft
F. Nursing interventions
   1. Assist patient in obtaining body warmth and warmth to the extremity.
      a. Warm room
      b. Warm bath
      c. Warm clothes such as socks
   2. Avoid applying direct heat to the affected part.
   3. Protect the affected part from trauma and pressure.
      a. Use bed cradle.
      b. Assess skin lesions, and monitor for signs of infection.
      c. Caution patient against wearing anything that constricts.
   4. Give prescribed drugs, and monitor for side effects.
   5. Assess the affected part daily.
      a. Assess skin color, temperature, and circulation.
      b. Monitor for pain.
   6. Provide emotional support.
   7. Educate patient and family regarding:
      a. Hygiene and avoidance of infection.
      b. Rest and planned exercise.
      c. Protection from injury.
      d. Diet.
      e. Drugs.
      f. Improvement of circulation.

Buerger Disease (Thromboangiitis Obliterans)

A. Definition: inflammatory process affecting primarily arteries that causes occlusion, thrombosis, and ultimately ischemia
   1. Medium-size distal arteries of the legs are primarily affected.
   2. Veins can also be affected.
B. Causes
   1. Exact cause unknown
   2. Associated with smoking
   3. Men in the 25- to 40-year age-group who smoke at risk
   4. Familial tendency
C. Signs and symptoms
   1. Coldness of the extremities
   2. Diminished or absent pulses
   3. Numbness and tingling
   4. Cramping pain (intermittent claudication)
   5. Pain at rest, not associated with activity
   6. Skin ulceration
   7. Aggravation of symptoms by exposure to cold environment
   8. Change in appearance of extremities

9. Muscle atrophy
10. Slow-healing cuts
11. Gangrene
12. Sensitivity to cold

D. Diagnostic tests and methods
  1. Patient history and physical examination
  2. Oscillometry
  3. Doppler ultrasonography
  4. Arteriography
  5. Laboratory studies
  6. ECG
  7. Chest x-ray examination

E. Treatment
  1. Restriction of smoking
  2. Drug therapy: vasodilator drugs, analgesics, and anticoagulants
  3. Moderate exercise
  4. Avoidance and treatment of infection
  5. Protection from trauma
  6. Sympathectomy (disruption of nerve impulses to a particular area)
  7. Nerve blocks (drug injections to block nerve impulses)
  8. Amputation as a last resort

F. Nursing interventions
  1. Support patient in his or her effort to stop smoking.
  2. Give prescribed vasodilators, analgesics, and anticoagulants; monitor for side effects.
  3. Document location and character of pain.
  4. Assist patient in maintaining warmth.
  5. Educate patient and family concerning drug therapy, activity, and avoidance of smoking, exposure to cold, constricting clothing, and trauma.

Raynaud Disease

A. Definition: peripheral vascular disease affecting digital arteries
  1. Disease occurs primarily in women.
  2. Exposure to environmental cold, emotional stress, or tobacco use produces spasms of the arteries.
  3. Hands and arms are usually affected.

B. Cause
  1. Exact cause unknown
  2. Associated with collagen diseases in women

C. Contributing factors
  1. Pressure to the fingertips such as that encountered by typists and pianists
  2. Using handheld vibrating equipment on a regular basis

D. Signs and symptoms
  1. Numbness and tingling
  2. Blanching of digits and cyanosis
  3. Hyperemia
  4. Coldness
  5. Dryness and atrophy of the nails
  6. Pain
  7. Punctate (small hole) lesions of the fingertips
  8. Eventual gangrene of the fingertips

E. Diagnostic tests and methods
  1. Patient history and physical examination
  2. Doppler ultrasonography
  3. Arteriography
  4. ECG
  5. Chest x-ray examination

F. Treatment
  1. Drug therapy with vasodilators
  2. Sympathectomy in advanced cases
  3. Elimination of smoking
  4. Avoidance of stressful situations
  5. Avoidance of exposure to cold

G. Nursing interventions
  1. Document location and characteristics of pain.
  2. Observe affected areas daily.
  3. Administer prescribed vasodilators and analgesics; monitor for side effects.
  4. Instruct patient to avoid activities that precipitate spasms.
  5. Instruct patient to avoid exposing hands to the cold without proper protection.
  6. Support patient's effort to give up smoking.
  7. Offer emotional support and allay anxiety.
  8. Educate patient and family concerning drug therapy, avoidance of cold, protection from trauma and infection, and prevention of spasms.

Aneurysms

A. Definition: enlargement or ballooning of an artery, usually caused by trauma, congenital weakness, arteriosclerosis, or infection. The aorta is the most frequently affected artery.

B. Causes
  1. Causes are varied, but the prime culprit is arteriosclerosis. Plaque formation causes degenerative changes, leading to loss of vessel elasticity, weakness, and dilation.
  2. Syphilis
  3. Infections
  4. Congenital disorder
  5. Trauma
  6. Risk factors: obesity, smoking, hypertension, stress, high blood cholesterol levels

C. Signs and symptoms
  1. Abdominal
    a. Increased blood pressure
    b. Visible or palpable pulsating mass
    c. Pain or tenderness in the abdominal area
  2. Thoracic
    a. Dyspnea
    b. Dysphagia
    c. Hoarseness or cough
    d. Severe chest pain
  3. Ruptured aneurysm
    a. Anxiety
    b. Restlessness
    c. Pain
    d. Diminished pulses
    e. Hypotension and shock

D. Diagnostic tests and methods
  1. Patient history and physical examination
  2. Chest x-ray examination
  3. Abdominal x-ray examination
  4. Ultrasonography
  5. Angiography, arteriography
  6. Routine ECG
  7. Laboratory studies

E. Treatment
  1. Conservative measures
    a. Drug therapy: antihypertensives, pain relievers, and negative inotropic agents

b. Correction of hydration and electrolyte imbalances

c. Decreased activity

2. Surgical repair

a. Resection and replacement with a prosthesis of Teflon or Dacron

b. Resection and replacement with a graft

F. Nursing interventions

1. Provide immediate postoperative care.

a. Assess vital signs and peripheral pulses every 15 minutes, then decrease frequency as ordered.

b. Record intake and output hourly.

c. Compare extremities for warmth and color.

d. Administer IV fluids at prescribed rate.

e. Relieve pain with prescribed analgesic.

f. Monitor oxygen therapy.

g. Give prescribed prophylactic antibiotics as ordered.

h. Assess level of consciousness (LOC) every 1 to 2 hours.

i. Auscultate lung sounds and bowel sounds at least every 4 hours.

j. Monitor for arrhythmias.

k. Have patient turn, cough, and deep breathe at least every 2 hours.

2. Other postoperative considerations

a. Provide antiembolism stockings.

b. Provide emotional support and allay anxiety.

c. Encourage early ambulation as prescribed.

d. Instruct patient to observe for changes in the extremities such as color and warmth.

e. Instruct patient about assessment of peripheral pulses.

Phlebitis and Thrombophlebitis

A. Definition: inflammatory disorders of the veins

1. Phlebitis: inflammation of a vein

2. Thrombophlebitis: inflammation of a vein with clot formation

B. Causes

1. The inflammation and clot formation are associated with venous stasis, vessel damage, and enhanced blood coagulability.

2. Situations that produce venous stasis include decreased mobility, prolonged periods of sitting and standing, wearing of confining clothing, and increased abdominal pressure.

C. Signs and symptoms

1. Redness and pain along vein path

2. Elevation of temperature

3. Swelling

4. Positive Homans sign (pain on dorsiflexion of the foot)

5. Area sensitive to the touch

D. Diagnostic tests and methods

1. Patient history and physical examination

2. Doppler ultrasonography

3. Venography

4. Laboratory studies: CBC, ESR, and coagulation studies

5. Lung scan to rule out pulmonary embolism

E. Treatment

1. Bed rest

2. Anticoagulant therapy (see Chapter 3)

3. Thrombolytic therapy (see Chapter 3)

4. Vasodilators (see Chapter 3)

5. Warm, moist packs to the affected leg (some physicians prefer ice packs to the area)

6. Antiembolism stockings

7. Elevation of affected extremity

8. Surgical intervention required in only a small percentage of patients

F. Nursing interventions

1. Assess and document signs and symptoms.

2. Administer analgesics as ordered, and monitor for side effects.

3. Elevate leg as ordered. Avoid using a knee gatch or pillow under the affected knee. Avoid crossing legs.

4. Apply warm, moist heat as ordered.

5. Assess thigh and calf measurements daily.

6. Monitor vital signs every 4 hours.

7. Maintain bed rest as ordered.

8. Apply antiembolism stockings on unaffected leg.

9. Avoid massaging calf of affected leg.

10. Avoid constrictive clothing.

11. Monitor anticoagulant therapy.

12. Monitor for bleeding tendencies.

a. Bleeding gums

b. Epistaxis

c. Easy bruising

d. Melena

e. Petechiae

13. Monitor Hgb and Hct levels.

14. Educate patient and family concerning drug therapy, avoidance of activities that aggravate the existing state, and monitoring for signs and symptoms of complications.

15. Monitor patient for complications such as an embolism.

Embolism

A. Definition: blood clot circulating in the blood

B. Causes

1. The clot may be a fragment of an arteriosclerotic plaque, or it may have originated in the heart.

2. If large, an embolism may lodge in a vessel bifurcation and obstruct the flow of blood to vital organs or tissues.

3. Most emboli arise from deep-vein thrombi; the embolus travels in the bloodstream until it lodges in a narrowed area, usually the lungs.

C. Signs and symptoms: depend on the area involved

1. Pain at the site

2. Shock (refer to Chapter 10 for signs and symptoms of shock)

3. Areas supplied by the involved vessel: pallor, coldness, numbness, tingling, and cyanosis

4. Sudden onset of dyspnea

5. Cough and hemoptysis

6. Chest pain

7. Tachycardia

8. Tachypnea

D. Diagnostic tests and methods

1. Patient history and physical examination

2. Lung scan

3. Chest x-ray examination

4. Arterial blood gas analysis

E. Treatment

1. Oxygen therapy

2. IV fluids

    3. IV anticoagulants
    4. Analgesics
    5. Thrombolytic agents
F. Nursing interventions
    1. Assess and document signs and symptoms and reactions to treatments.
    2. Monitor vital signs.
    3. Monitor arterial blood gas reports.
    4. Administer prescribed analgesic, and monitor for side effects.
    5. Administer anticoagulants as prescribed, and monitor for bleeding tendencies.
    6. Monitor oxygen therapy.
    7. Give ROM exercises.
    8. Provide antiembolism stockings.
    9. Educate patient and family concerning drug therapy, monitoring for bleeding tendencies, and restricting activities.

Varicose Veins

A. Definition: dilated, tortuous leg veins resulting from blood backflow caused by incomplete valve closure, which leads to congestion and further enlargement
B. Causes
    1. Basic cause of varicosities unknown
    2. Predisposing factors: heredity, pregnancy, obesity, and aging
C. Signs and symptoms
    1. Leg fatigue and aching
    2. Leg cramping and pain
    3. Heaviness in the legs
    4. Dilated veins
    5. Ankle edema
D. Diagnostic tests and methods
    1. Patient history and physical examination
    2. Venography
    3. Trendelenburg test
E. Treatment
    1. Rest with elevation of legs
    2. Exercise
    3. Support stockings
    4. Avoidance of prolonged standing, sitting, and crossing the legs
    5. Weight management
    6. Surgical vein stripping, ligation; vein sclerosing
    7. Laser
F. Nursing interventions
    1. After surgery, check legs for color, movement, temperature, and sensation.
    2. Provide leg exercises as prescribed.
    3. Reinforce the importance of weight management.
    4. Instruct patient to avoid prolonged sitting and standing.
    5. Avoid constrictive clothing.

HEMATOLOGICAL CONDITIONS AND DISORDERS

Disorders of hematopoiesis are problems of the blood-forming tissues such as the blood cells, bone marrow, spleen, and lymph system. This discussion includes descriptions of the anemias, leukemia, and acquired immunodeficiency syndrome (AIDS).

NURSING ASSESSMENT

A. Observations
    1. Pulse
        a. Character, rate, rhythm
        b. Note tachycardia or periods of palpitations
    2. Respirations
        a. Character, rate, rhythm
        b. Tachypnea
        c. DOE (dyspnea on exertion)
        d. Shortness of breath
    3. Blood pressure: hypotension, perhaps orthostatic
    4. Temperature: unexplained occurrences of elevation, sometimes accompanied by chills and sweating
    5. Skin
        a. Color: pallor, cyanosis
        b. Pruritus
        c. Bruising
        d. Slow to heal cuts
        e. Bleeding from nose or mouth
    6. Oral mucosal changes
        a. Mouth ulcerations
        b. Bleeding gums
        c. Smooth tongue
    7. Motor
        a. Lack of coordination
        b. Loss of usual stamina
        c. Changes in ability to perform activities
        d. Intolerance to exertion (climbing stairs, usual housework, walking)
B. Patient description (subjective)
    1. Changes in ability to perform ADLs
    2. Self-reported increase in weakness and fatigue
    3. DOE
    4. Changes in appetite
        a. Weight loss
        b. Anorexia
        c. Nausea and vomiting
    5. Skin
        a. Easy bruising
        b. Bleeding from gums, nose
    6. Mood changes: irritable
    7. Progressive symptoms
        a. Onset of headaches
        b. Onset of fatigue
        c. Numbness, tingling, burning feet
        d. Intermittent swollen, tender lymph nodes

DIAGNOSTIC TESTS AND METHODS

A. RBC count
    1. The blood study is used in routine screenings and provides information about the hematological system.
    2. Circulating RBC counts rise in conditions such as anemia and hypoxia.
B. Erythrocyte indexes (mean cell volume, mean cell Hgb concentration, mean cell Hgb)
    1. Aid in describing the anemias
    2. Provide a relationship among the number, size, and Hgb content of the RBCs
C. Hgb and Hct levels
    1. Levels provide an index to the severity of the anemia.
    2. Hct is the number of packed RBCs found in 100 mL of blood.

3. Hgb is the oxygen-carrying component of the RBC and is more reliable in determining the severity of the anemia.

D. Reticulocyte count: number of newly formed RBCs
   1. Provides information concerning the cause of the anemia
   2. Indicates whether the anemia is a result of diminished production or excessive loss or destruction of RBCs

E. ESR
   1. Not specific to anemias
   2. If elevated, suggests the presence of an underlying disease process; further studies possibly indicated

F. Serum iron
   1. Helpful in classifying the anemia
   2. Useful in differentiating an acute from a chronic disorder

G. Total iron-binding capacity (TIBC): helpful in classifying the anemia and differentiating between an acute and a chronic disorder

H. Serum bilirubin
   1. Useful in evaluating the degree of RBC hemolysis
   2. Bilirubin is formed from the Hgb of destroyed RBCs.
   3. Elevations may indicate the increased destruction of RBCs caused by a particular disease process.

I. Schilling test
   1. Used in classifying anemias, particularly a vitamin B_{12} disorder
   2. Helps differentiate between an intrinsic factor deficiency and an intestinal absorption disorder
   3. Patient preparation
      a. Patient may be instructed to be NPO before the test.
      b. Oral radioactive vitamin B_{12} is administered.
      c. Nonradioactive parenteral dose is given 2 hours later.
      d. Urine collection follows.
      e. One third of the vitamin appears in the urine. Little or no radioactivity in the urine suggests a GI malabsorption problem.
      f. Procedure may be repeated with the addition of intrinsic factor to the oral vitamin B_{12}.
      g. Nonabsorption of vitamin B_{12} without intrinsic factor but absorption with intrinsic factor suggests pernicious anemia.
   4. Nursing interventions
      a. Explain the basic procedure to patient.
      b. Maintain NPO status.
      c. Collect the urine at the specified time.

J. Vitamin B_{12} level
   1. Used to help identify pernicious anemia
   2. Provides an index for determining the adequacy of vitamin B_{12} levels and the need for further evaluation
   3. Vitamin B_{12} is important for normal hematopoiesis.

K. Serum folate level
   1. Folic acid is another important factor in hematopoiesis.
   2. Level of serum folate is useful in folic acid–deficiency anemia.

L. Gastric analysis
   1. Nasogastric tube is inserted, and histamine (H_2) is injected to stimulate gastric secretions.
   2. Gastric contents are aspirated and analyzed.
   3. Achlorhydria (absence of hydrochloric acid) is a feature of pernicious anemia because of a lack of intrinsic factor in the stomach.

M. Sickle cell preparation
   1. The reaction of the blood specimen in hypoxia is observed.

2. Sickling of cells in hypoxia suggests sickle cell trait or sickle cell anemia.

N. Hgb electrophoresis
   1. An electric field separates the specimen into the various types of Hgb present.
   2. Hgb S and A suggest sickle cell anemia or trait.
   3. Hgb F suggests thalassemia.

O. Bone marrow biopsy
   1. Bone marrow aspiration provides information about blood cell production.
   2. Test may be used in patients suspected of having leukemia, aplastic anemia, and other hematological disorders.
   3. Sample of marrow may be obtained from the sternum, iliac crest, vertebrae, or vertebral body.
   4. Procedure
      a. The skin over the designated area is prepared and anesthetized.
      b. The needle is inserted into the center of the bone, and a small amount of marrow is aspirated.
   5. Nursing interventions
      a. Allay patient's anxiety before the examination.
      b. Assist with the marrow as instructed.
      c. Place patient in a comfortable position after the procedure.
      d. Monitor pain status (soreness remains for several days).
      e. Monitor puncture site for bleeding.

P. WBC count and differential
   1. Determines the total number of leukocytes
   2. Differential: helps analyze each type of WBC and determine if the amount present is in proper proportion
   3. Aids in diagnosing infection and blood disorders such as leukemia

Q. Platelet count
   1. Evaluates adequacy of platelet levels
   2. If platelet levels drop below a certain level, spontaneous hemorrhage is possible.

R. Serum for HIV: determines the presence of the HIV antibodies

S. Lymphangiography: radiological examination used to detect lymph node involvement

FREQUENT PATIENT PROBLEMS AND NURSING CARE

A. Activity intolerance related to weakness and fatigue
   1. Provide planned activity and rest periods.
   2. Monitor for signs of fatigue.
   3. Reinforce patient teaching of planned activity and exercise.
   4. Assist patient with ADLs.
   5. Assess vital signs as ordered.

B. Ineffective tissue perfusion related to hypotension
   1. Observe for evidence of postural hypotension.
   2. Assist patient in dangling legs over the side of the bed before standing.
   3. Instruct patient to get up slowly.
   4. Assess patient's pulse when he or she is standing.

C. Ineffective breathing pattern related to DOE
   1. Note degree or kind of activity that causes dyspnea.
   2. Note character and rate of respirations during the episodes.
   3. Instruct patient to stop the activity and relax when dyspnea is experienced.

4. Assist patient in planning activities so dyspnea does not occur.

5. Reinforce patient teaching regarding planned exercise and rest periods.

D. Impaired oral mucous membranes caused by ulcerations of the mouth and tongue
   1. Assess ulcerated areas daily.
   2. Provide mouth care with a soft-bristle brush or cotton swab.
   3. Offer soothing mouthwashes every 2 to 4 hours.
   4. Instruct patient to avoid ingesting food or drink that may aggravate the ulcers.

E. Deficient fluid volume related to hemorrhage
   1. Assess for signs of bleeding.
      a. Tarry stools
      b. Hematuria
      c. Bleeding gums
      d. Bleeding tendency
      e. Petechiae
      f. Epistaxis
   2. Protect from trauma and injury.
   3. Avoid parenteral injections.
   4. Have patient use soft-bristle brush for mouth care.
   5. Monitor vital signs at least every 4 hours.
   6. Monitor Hgb and Hct values.
   7. Encourage intake of fluids and the prescribed diet.

F. Risk for infection related to interference with the immune system
   1. Prevent exposure to others with infection.
   2. Monitor for signs and symptoms of infection.
   3. Give prescribed drugs, and monitor for side effects.
   4. Place in Protective Isolation (may be known as Neutropenic Precautions) if ordered.

G. Pain related to sickling and dehydration (sickle cell anemia covered in Chapter 8)

MAJOR MEDICAL DIAGNOSES
Anemia Caused by Decreased Red Blood Cell Production

A. A balance normally exists between RBC production and RBC destruction; however, alterations occur that significantly affect RBC production.
   1. Iron-deficiency anemia
      a. Results from insufficient dietary intake of iron, which is needed for the formation of Hgb and RBCs
      b. Other causes: malabsorption, blood loss, and hemolysis
   2. Pernicious anemia
      a. Caused by a lack of intrinsic factor in the GI tract
      b. Intrinsic factor is needed for the absorption of vitamin B_{12}.
      c. Anemia usually results from a loss of the mucosal surface of the GI tract, which secretes intrinsic factor.
      d. Patients undergoing total gastrectomy and small-bowel resection are at risk.
   3. Folic acid–deficiency anemia
      a. Folic acid is required in the synthesis of DNA, which in turn is necessary for the production of RBCs.
      b. Common causes: poor diet (lacking in green leafy vegetables, citrus fruits, liver, grains, and dried beans), malabsorption, and drugs that interfere with the absorption of folic acid

   4. Thalassemia
      a. Unlike the other three anemias, thalassemia is a genetic disorder resulting in abnormal Hgb synthesis.
      b. The main problem is an inadequate production of normal Hgb; hemolysis is a secondary problem.
      c. People of Mediterranean ancestry are at risk.
      d. Mild forms of this anemia (thalassemia minor) may be asymptomatic.
      e. Patients with a more severe hemolytic form (thalassemia major) may experience hepatomegaly, splenomegaly, jaundice, and bone marrow hypertrophy.

B. Signs and symptoms
   1. Skin changes
      a. Pallor
      b. Jaundice
      c. Pruritus
      d. Dermatitis
   2. Eye and visual disturbances
      a. Blurred vision
      b. Scleral icterus
   3. Mouth
      a. Glossitis
      b. Smooth tongue
      c. Ulcerations of the mucosa
   4. Cardiovascular
      a. Tachycardia
      b. Murmurs
      c. Angina
      d. CHF
      e. Hypotension
   5. Respiratory
      a. Tachypnea
      b. DOE
      c. Orthopnea
   6. Neurological
      a. Dizziness
      b. Headaches
      c. Irritability
      d. Depression
      e. Incoordination
      f. Impaired thought processes
   7. GI
      a. Nausea and vomiting
      b. Anorexia
      c. Hepatomegaly
      d. Splenomegaly
   8. General
      a. Weight loss
      b. Weakness and fatigue
      c. Bone pain
      d. Numbness, tingling, and burning of the feet

C. Diagnostic tests and methods
   1. Patient history and physical examination
   2. Routine chest x-ray examination
   3. Routine ECG
   4. Schilling test
   5. Gastric analysis
   6. CBC and RBC indexes
   7. Bone marrow aspiration or biopsy
   8. Serum iron level

D. Treatment
   1. Iron therapy

2. Increased dietary iron intake
3. Vitamin B$_{12}$ replacement (pernicious anemia)
4. Folic acid replacement
5. Hematinics
6. Blood transfusions (thalassemia)

E. Nursing interventions
1. Assess and document signs and symptoms and reactions to treatments.
2. Provide planned activity alternated with rest periods.
3. Assist patient with ADLs to avoid fatigue.
4. Monitor supplemental oxygen therapy in use.
5. Administer prescribed drugs, and monitor for side effects.
6. Monitor blood transfusions.
7. Provide oral hygiene, particularly if mouth ulcers are present.
8. Provide the prescribed diet.
9. Instruct patient to get up from bed or chair slowly to avoid dizziness.
10. Educate patient about avoiding and preventing exposure to infection.
11. Support patient and allay anxiety.
12. Educate patient and family concerning drugs, diet therapy, and planned activity.

Anemia Caused by Red Blood Cell Destruction

A. Definition: process in which RBCs are destroyed faster than they are produced
B. Known causes of RBC destruction
1. Snake venom
2. Infections
3. Drugs or chemicals
4. Heavy metals or organic compounds
5. Antigen-antibody reaction
6. Splenic dysfunction
7. Congenital causes
   a. Thalassemia: a group of hereditary hemolytic anemias characterized by a defect or defects in one or more of the Hgb polypeptide chains
   b. Sickle cell anemia (see Chapter 8)
   c. Spherocytosis: a hemolytic anemia characterized by spherocytes (small, globular erythrocytes without the characteristic central pallor) in the blood. The spleen destroys abnormal cells.
   d. Glucose-6-phosphate dehydrogenase (G6PD) deficiency: a hemolytic disorder brought on by stressors such as infection, certain drugs, acidosis, and toxic substances. Individuals with this genetic disorder are relatively symptom free until they experience the stressor that initiates the hemolytic process.
C. Signs and symptoms
1. Anemia
2. Jaundice
3. Splenomegaly
4. Hepatomegaly
5. Weakness and fatigue
6. Skin pallor
7. Anorexia
8. Weight loss
9. Dyspnea
10. Tachycardia
11. Tachypnea
12. Hypotension
13. Cholelithiasis (gallstones): caused by excessive bilirubin

D. Diagnostic tests and methods
1. Patient history and physical examination
2. Laboratory studies
3. Routine chest x-ray examination
4. Routine ECG
5. Bone marrow biopsy
6. Renal studies to monitor kidney status
E. Treatment
1. Identification and treatment of the causative agent
2. Blood or blood product replacement
3. Supportive care
4. Genetic counseling
5. Splenectomy to halt the destruction of abnormal RBCs by the spleen
6. Maintenance of renal function
7. Maintenance of fluid and electrolyte balance
F. Nursing interventions
1. Assess and document signs and symptoms and reactions to treatment.
2. Monitor vital signs as ordered, and report abnormalities.
3. Allay fears and anxieties.
4. Provide planned exercise and rest periods.
5. Caution patient to get up slowly from the bed or chair to avoid postural hypotension.
6. Assist patient with ADLs.
7. Monitor intake and output.
8. Monitor laboratory study results.
9. Encourage intake of fluids.
10. Provide prescribed diet.
11. Administer prescribed drugs, and monitor for side effects.
12. Educate patient and family concerning drugs, diet, activity, and compliance with the prescribed regimen.

Aplastic Anemia (Hypoplastic)

A. Definition: failure of the bone marrow to produce adequate amounts of erythrocytes, leukocytes, and platelets
B. Exact cause is unclear (idiopathic).
1. May be congenital
2. Related to radiation exposure
3. Results from a disorder that suppresses bone marrow (cancer)
4. Exposure to toxic substances possibly a contributing factor
C. Signs and symptoms
1. General symptoms of anemia; refer to the preceding outlines in this section.
2. Susceptibility to infection
3. Fever
4. Bleeding tendencies
D. Diagnostic tests and methods
1. Patient history and physical examination
2. Laboratory studies, particularly WBC count and platelet count; a reduced WBC count predisposes patient to infection; a low platelet count predisposes patient to a bleeding disorder.
3. Bone marrow biopsy examination to evaluate blood cell production
4. Routine chest x-ray examination
5. Routine ECG

E. Treatment
 1. Identification of the causative agent
 2. Supportive care
 3. Administration of blood or blood products
 4. Hydration with IV fluids
 5. Protection from injury and infections
 6. Prevention of hemorrhage
 7. Splenectomy
 8. Bone marrow transplant
F. Nursing interventions
 1. Assess and document signs and symptoms and reactions to treatment.
 2. Monitor vital signs at least every 4 hours.
 3. Monitor for and report signs of bleeding.
 4. Give prescribed medication, and monitor for side effects.
 5. Avoid fatiguing patient; provide planned exercise and rest periods.
 6. Prevent injury and exposure to infection.
 7. Neutropenic Precautions may be necessary.
 8. Monitor supplemental oxygen if ordered.
 9. Provide and encourage the prescribed diet.
 10. Allay fears and anxiety.
 11. Provide oral hygiene, avoiding aggravation of bleeding gums.
 12. Provide skin care using protective devices and frequent repositioning.
 13. Educate patient and family concerning drug therapy, diet, planned activity, avoidance of injury and infection, monitoring for bleeding tendencies, and compliance with the regimen.

Leukemia

A. Definition: disorder of the hematopoietic system characterized by an overproduction of immature WBCs
 1. As the disease progresses, fewer normal WBCs are produced.
 2. The abnormal cells continue to multiply and eventually infiltrate and damage the bone marrow, spleen, lymph nodes, and other organs.
B. Classification of leukemias
 1. Two major categories: acute and chronic
  a. Acute leukemia has a rapid onset; cells in this phase are young, undifferentiated, and immature.
  b. Chronic leukemia has a gradual onset; cells are mature and differentiated.
 2. Further classification: identifying the type of WBC involved
  a. Acute granulocytic leukemia (nonlymphocytic): the myeloblasts proliferate; myeloblasts are the precursors of granulocytes.
  b. Acute lymphoblastic leukemia: immature lymphocytes proliferate in the bone marrow.
  c. Chronic granulocytic leukemia (nonlymphocytic): excessive neoplastic granulocytes are found in the bone marrow.
  d. Chronic lymphocytic leukemia: inactive, mature-appearing lymphocytes characterize it.
C. Leukemia is considered a neoplastic process; cause is unknown.
D. Predisposing factors
 1. Familial tendency

 2. Viral origin
 3. Exposure to chemicals
 4. Exposure to radiation
E. Once leukemia has been diagnosed, the aim of therapy is to prolong survival by attaining a state of remission.
 1. Management of acute leukemia is aggressive.
 2. Management of chronic leukemia aims to control the disorder and maintain remission.
 3. All forms of leukemia are fatal if untreated.
F. Signs and symptoms
 1. General symptoms of anemia
 2. Decreased resistance to infection
 3. Fever
 4. Bleeding tendencies
 5. Enlarged lymph nodes
 6. Splenomegaly
 7. Hepatomegaly
 8. Elevated WBC count
 9. Low platelet count and low Hgb and Hct levels
 10. Poor appetite
 11. Mouth ulcers
 12. Diarrhea
G. Diagnostic tests and methods
 1. Patient history and physical examination
 2. Laboratory studies to evaluate peripheral blood
 3. Bone marrow biopsy
 4. Routine chest x-ray examination
 5. Routine ECG
 6. Lymph node biopsy examination
H. Treatment
 1. Drug therapy: chemotherapeutic agents, analgesics, sedatives, and antibiotics
 2. Radiation therapy (prophylactic measure)
 3. Bone marrow transplants—still under investigation
 4. Hydration with IV fluids
 5. Replacement of blood and blood products
 6. Monitoring renal status
 7. Protection against infection (Neutropenic Precautions if needed)
 8. Prevention of hemorrhage
I. Nursing interventions
 1. Assess and document signs and symptoms and reactions to treatment.
 2. Prevent patient from being exposed to infection.
  a. Screen visitors.
  b. Monitor WBC counts.
  c. Practice good handwashing.
  d. Neutropenic Precautions may be required.
 3. Avoid fatigue.
  a. Provide planned exercises and rest periods.
  b. Assist patient with ADLs.
 4. Monitor for bleeding tendencies.
 5. Administer blood or blood components as ordered, and monitor for side effects.
 6. Monitor intake and output.
 7. Encourage intake of fluids.
  a. Keep fluids at the bedside.
  b. Provide patient with favorite fluids.
 8. Administer prescribed medication as ordered, and monitor for side effects.
  a. Analgesics and sedatives
  b. Antiemetics

9. Monitor IV fluids.
   a. Monitor the IV site for infiltration.
   b. Monitor rate.
10. Allay anxieties and fears.
11. Monitor vital signs at least every 4 hours, and report abnormalities. (An elevated temperature may be the only sign of infection in an immunocompromised patient.)
12. Monitor supplemental oxygen if ordered.
13. Provide and encourage the prescribed diet.
14. Provide oral hygiene, which protects against aggravation of bleeding and drying of the mouth; carefully monitor oral status.
15. Provide skin care to include the use of protective devices and frequent repositioning.
16. Educate patient and family concerning drug therapy, diet, activity, monitoring for bleeding tendencies, avoidance of injury and infection, and compliance with the regimen.

Acquired Immunodeficiency Syndrome

A. Definition: viral disorder that disrupts the balance of T lymphocytes and ultimately destroys them, rendering the body incapable of defending itself against infection; course is progressive and fatal.
B. Cause: infection with HIV
   1. The virus is spread by sexual contact (primarily through anal intercourse), sharing of infected needles, and contact with infected blood and blood products.
   2. Infected mothers can pass the virus to the unborn baby during the gestational period, the birth process, or breastfeeding.
   3. The virus may also enter the body when contaminated blood or body fluids come in contact with broken skin surfaces.
C. Signs and symptoms (vary with each patient; may harbor the virus but be asymptomatic for months or years)
   1. Swollen lymph glands
   2. Recurrent fever, night sweats
   3. Weight loss, diminished appetite
   4. Chronic diarrhea
   5. Fatigue
   6. White patches or lesions in the mouth
   7. Presence of opportunistic infections such as *Pneumocystis jiroveci* (not pneumonia) and Kaposi sarcoma (purplish skin lesions)
   8. Dry cough, shortness of breath
   9. Centers for Disease Control and Prevention clinical categories (Table 5-2)
      a. Category A: Categories B and C have not occurred; asymptomatic HIV infection; persistent, generalized lymphadenopathy; acute HIV infection.
      b. Category B: Category C has not occurred; presence of conditions commonly associated with HIV.
      c. Category C: Once in this category, person remains in it; all clinical conditions listed as associated with advanced HIV disease or AIDS.
   10. Symptoms may occur as early as 2 to 6 weeks after exposure, or individual may be asymptomatic for months

Table 5-2	1993 Revised Classification System for HIV Infection and Expanded AIDS Surveillance Case Definition for Adolescents and Adults		
	CLINICAL CATEGORIES*		
CD4 CELL CATEGORIES	**(A) ASYMPTOMATIC OR PGL**	**(B) SYMPTOMATIC, NOT (A) OR (C) CONDITIONS**	**(C) AIDS-INDICATOR CONDITIONS**
>500/mm³	A1	B1	C1
200-499/mm³	A2	B2	C2
<200/mm³ AIDS-indicator cell count	A3	B3	C3

Modified from Harkness G, Dincher JR: *Medical-surgical nursing: total patient care*, ed 9, St Louis, 1996, Mosby; Centers for Disease Control and Prevention: Impact of the expanded AIDS surveillance case definition on AIDS case reporting—U.S. first quarter, 1993, *MMWR Morb Mortal Wkly Rep* 42:308-310, 1993.
AIDS, Acquired immunodeficiency syndrome; *HIV,* human immunodeficiency virus; *PGL,* persistent generalized lymphadenopathy.
* Description of clinical categories:
A: One or more of the conditions listed below with documented HIV infection. Conditions listed in categories B and C must not have occurred.
  • Asymptomatic HIV infection
  • PGL
  • Acute (primary) HIV infection with accompanying illness or history of acute infection
B: Symptomatic conditions that meet at least one of the following criteria: (a) the conditions are attributed to HIV infection and/or are indicative of a defect in cell-mediated immunity; or (b) the conditions are considered by physicians to have a clinical course or management that is complicated by HIV infection. Examples of conditions in clinical category B include, but are not limited to, the following:
  • Bacterial endocarditis, meningitis, pneumonia, or sepsis
  • Candidiasis, vulvovaginal, that is persistent (greater than 1-month duration) or poorly responsive to therapy
  • Candidiasis, oropharyngeal (thrush)
  • Cervical dysplasia, severe; or carcinoma
  • Constitutional symptoms, such as fever (38.4° C) or diarrhea lasting more than 1 month
  • Hairy leukoplakia, oral
  • Herpes zoster (shingles), involving at least two distinct episodes or more than one dermatome
  • Idiopathic thrombocytopenic purpura
  • Listeriosis
  • Mycobacterium tuberculosis, pulmonary
  • Nocardiosis
  • Pelvic inflammatory disease
  • Peripheral neuropathy
C: Any condition listed in the 1993 surveillance case definition for AIDS. The conditions in clinical category C are strongly associated with severe immunodeficiency, occur frequently in HIV-infected individuals, and cause serious morbidity or mortality.

or years; seroconversion (when the blood work changes from negative to positive for HIV antibodies) may not occur for 8 to 12 weeks or longer. Retesting is advisable 6 months after exposure, then at 1 year; further testing is left up to the health care provider.

D. Diagnostic tests and methods
  1. Patient history and physical examination
  2. Serum for HIV antibodies
  3. Presence of opportunistic infections
    a. *P. jiroveci* pneumonia
    b. Kaposi sarcoma
  4. Bronchial biopsy (tests for presence of opportunistic infections)
  5. Lumbar puncture (tests for neurological evidence of infections)
  6. CT scan
  7. Enzyme-linked immunosorbent assay (ELISA): detects antibodies for HIV; possible false positives
  8. Western blot test to confirm the results of a positive ELISA test: detects HIV antibodies
  9. CD4 cell counts: if lower than 200, the risk for opportunistic infections increases (see Table 5-2).

E. Treatment
  1. Treatment instituted according to symptoms
  2. Protection of patient from opportunistic infections
  3. Zidovudine (azidothymidine [AZT], Retrovir)
  4. Didanosine
  5. Zalcitabine
  6. Nutritional support
  7. Treatment of opportunistic infections

F. Nursing care
  1. Assess and document signs and symptoms and reactions to treatment.
  2. Monitor vital signs.
  3. Monitor arterial blood gas, CBC, and platelet count.
  4. Administer prescribed medication, and monitor for side effects.
  5. Use Blood and Body Fluid Precautions. (*Note:* This practice should be followed when caring for all patients.)
    a. Wear protective clothing (e.g., gloves, masks, goggles, gowns) as needed for the procedure.
    b. Wash hands thoroughly.
    c. Label specimens appropriately.
    d. Dispose of contaminated articles properly.
  6. Plan activity followed by rest periods.
  7. Encourage physical independence.
  8. Monitor oxygen therapy.
  9. Monitor pain status and provide analgesia and comfort measures.
  10. Offer support to patient and allay anxiety.
  11. Educate patient and family concerning mode of spread, protective measures, and home care.

Lymphoma

A. Definition: group of malignancies originating in the stem cell of the bone marrow
B. Causes: unknown, possibly linked to viruses, genetics, environmental exposures; possible autoimmune links
C. Two main types
  1. Hodgkin disease
  2. Non-Hodgkin lymphoma

D. Signs and symptoms
  1. Swollen, painless lymph nodes; may be unilateral
  2. Fever, chills
  3. Weight loss
  4. Night sweats
  5. Fatigue
  6. Loss of usual stamina; changes in ability to perform ADLs

E. Diagnostic tests and methods
  1. History and physical examination
  2. CBC and RBC indexes
  3. Blood chemistry: alkaline phosphatase, gamma globulin
  4. Serum protein electrophoresis
  5. Urine electrophoresis
  6. Lymph node biopsy
  7. Bone marrow biopsy

F. Treatment
  1. Staging laparotomy with splenectomy (to improve response to chemotherapy)
  2. Chemotherapy
  3. Radiation therapy

G. Nursing care
  1. Assess and document signs and symptoms and reactions to treatment.
  2. Monitor vital signs.
  3. Monitor laboratory studies.
  4. Assist in preventing infection and recognizing early signs.
  5. Assist in planning activity; provide rest periods.
  6. Monitor oxygen therapy if ordered.
  7. Monitor pain status and provide comfort measures.
  8. Give support and allay anxiety.
  9. Maintain hydration.

GASTROINTESTINAL SYSTEM

ANATOMY AND PHYSIOLOGY

A. Organs (Figure 5-6)
  1. Mouth (buccal cavity)
    a. Receives food; aids in digestion; aids in speaking
    b. Consists of hard and soft palate, teeth, tongue, and salivary glands
      (1) Teeth
        (a) Deciduous: baby teeth
        (b) Permanent: appear at approximately 6 years of age
        (c) Incisors: cut food
        (d) Canines: tear food
        (e) Molars: grind food
      (2) Salivary glands (parotid, submandibular, sublingual): manufacture saliva, which contains ptyalin to begin the chemical breakdown of starches
      (3) Tongue: also organ of taste
        (a) Receptors (taste buds, located in tongue): stimulated only if substance is in solution
        (b) Four kinds: sweet (tip of tongue); sour (side of tongue); salty (tip of tongue); bitter (back part of tongue)
        (c) Stimulates appetite and flow of digestive juices
    c. Functions
      (1) Ingestion of food
      (2) Mastication of food
      (3) Lubrication of food
      (4) Digestion of starch with salivary amylase

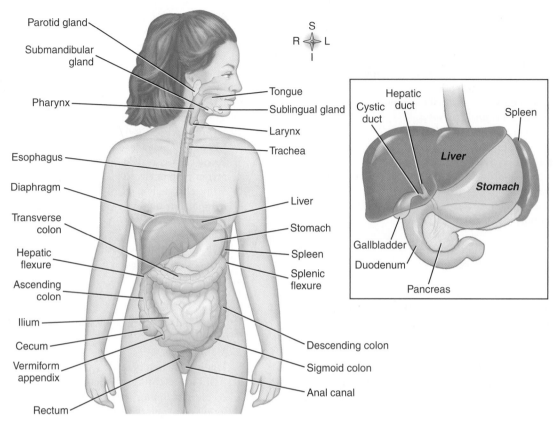

FIGURE 5-6 Location of digestive organs. (From Thibodeau GA, Patton KT: *Structure and function of the body,* ed 14, St Louis, 2012, Mosby.)

2. Pharynx: transports food
3. Esophagus: muscular tube; uses peristalsis to conduct food from pharynx to stomach
4. Stomach
   a. J-shaped pouch; varies in size, depending on contents; stores food and changes it into chyme
   b. Three divisions
      (1) Fundus: upper portion; the cardiac sphincter between the esophagus and fundus. The fundus controls the entrance of food.
      (2) Body: the largest, central portion
      (3) Pylorus: lower portion above the small intestine. The pyloric sphincter controls the passage of food into the duodenum.
   c. Special cells in the stomach secrete gastric juices and enzymes (including hydrochloric acid). The chemical breakdown of protein begins in the stomach.
      (1) Pepsin: begins digestion of protein
      (2) Lipase: acts on emulsified fat
      (3) Renin: acts on casein (a protein) in milk
      (4) Gastrin (hormone): related to the control of gastric secretions; not an enzyme
      (5) Hydrochloric acid: makes stomach content acid and activates enzymes
   d. Chyme: the semiliquid contents of the stomach, consisting of partially digested food and gastric enzymes
   e. Functions
      (1) Storage of food
      (2) Breakdown of food by churning
      (3) Liquefying of food with hydrochloric acid
      (4) Digestion of protein with enzyme (pepsin)

5. Small intestine: extends from the pyloric sphincter to the ileocecal valve, which prevents backflow of material and regulates forward flow
   a. Size: approximately 20 ft (600 cm) long and 1 inch (2.5 cm) in diameter
   b. Three major divisions
      (1) Duodenum: approximately 10 inches (25 cm) long; curves around head of the pancreas. Pancreatic duct and common bile duct enter below pyloric sphincter.
      (2) Jejunum: approximately 8 ft (240 cm) long
      (3) Ileum: approximately 12 ft (360 cm) long; terminal part
   c. Functions
      (1) Digestion of food
      (2) Absorption of food
   d. Intestinal glands, pancreas, liver, and gallbladder secrete digestive enzymes that complete the chemical breakdown of food.
      (1) Bile (formed in the liver and stored in the gallbladder): not an enzyme; emulsifies fat
      (2) Trypsin (pancreas): digests proteins into amino acids
      (3) Amylase (pancreas): digests starches into sugars
      (4) Lipase (pancreas): digests fat into simplest forms (fatty acids and glycerol)
      (5) Erepsin (intestine): digests proteins into amino acids
      (6) Lactase, maltase, sucrase (secretions of the small intestine): digest sugar into simplest forms (glucose, fructose, galactose)

6. Large intestine
   a. Size: approximately 5 to 6 ft (150 to 180 cm) long and 2.5 inches (6 cm) in diameter
   b. Divisions
      (1) Cecum: a blind pouch approximately 3 inches (7.5 cm) long; appendix attaches to distal end; located in right lower quadrant
      (2) Colon: ascending, continues up right side; transverse, extends across to the left; descending, descends on left side of pelvis
      (3) Sigmoid: S-shaped portion; extends to rectum
      (4) Rectum: approximately 8 inches (20 cm) long
      (5) Anus: terminal opening, guarded by internal and external sphincters
   c. Functions
      (1) Reabsorption of fluids and sodium
      (2) Temporary storage of fecal matter; defecation
B. Accessory organs (see Figure 5-6)
   1. Liver: largest organ in body; lies below diaphragm in upper right quadrant of abdominal cavity
      a. Metabolizes carbohydrates, fats, and proteins
      b. Detoxifies harmful substances
      c. Produces and stores heparin and fibrinogen
      d. Stores glycogen and vitamins A, B, B$_{12}$, K, D, E
      e. Manufactures bile. Hepatic duct drains bile into gallbladder.
   2. Gallbladder: small sac embedded in the interior surface of the liver
      a. Concentrates and stores bile
      b. Releases bile through the common bile duct into the duodenum when fat enters the small intestine
   3. Pancreas: long, triangular gland; lies behind the stomach; produces enzymes that break down food particles; secretes enzymes into the duodenum; has two functions
      a. Exocrine gland: secretes digestive enzymes that neutralize chyme
      b. Endocrine gland: islets of Langerhans; secretes insulin for use of glucose; secretes glucagons to regulate blood sugar level
C. Functions
   1. Digestion: two processes
      a. Mechanical: chewing, swallowing, and peristalsis of food; ends with elimination
      b. Chemical: breakdown of food into simpler compounds by the action of enzymes
   2. Absorption
      a. Occurs in small intestine
      b. Most water absorbed in large intestine.
   3. Metabolism: the sum of all bodily functions to convert simple compounds into living tissue
      a. Catabolism: process by which substances are broken down into simpler substances, resulting in the release of heat and energy
      b. Anabolism: the building phase in which simpler substances are combined to form more complex substances (conversion of food into living tissues)
      c. Basal metabolism: the amount of energy (calories) used by the body when at rest

GASTROINTESTINAL CONDITIONS AND DISORDERS

The GI system provides a means by which food and fluids enter the body and are converted into elements that help maintain the human organism. It is important to note that other systems of the body influence this system. The endocrine system, CNS, and autonomic nervous system all serve as regulators of the GI system.

NURSING ASSESSMENT
A. Observations (objective data)
   1. Vital signs
   2. Skin and mucous membrane character and color
      a. Gingivitis
      b. Stomatitis
      c. Jaundice
   3. Hematemesis: Emesis resembles coffee grounds in appearance, signifying digested blood.
   4. Stool changes
      a. Melena (tarry stool)
      b. Clay-colored (lack of bile pigment)
      c. Frothy, foamy, foul-smelling (seen in pancreatitis)
      d. Constipation
      e. Diarrhea
      f. Changes in size or shape or both (may indicate colon lesion)
   5. Urine color: dark urine (tea-colored)
   6. Hemorrhoids
   7. Abdominal distention
   8. Edema
   9. Bowel sounds
B. Patient description (subjective data)
   1. General
      a. History of GI-related problems
      b. Family history of GI-related problems
   2. Weight
      a. Loss or gain
      b. Appetite changes: increase or decrease
   3. Dietary and eating changes
      a. Presence of nausea and vomiting
      b. Difficulty chewing
      c. Dysphagia
      d. Occurrence of indigestion or dyspepsia
      e. Intolerance to certain foods
      f. Presence of pain: relationship to meals and eating
   4. Changes in bowel habits
      a. Diarrhea
      b. Constipation
      c. Alternating diarrhea and constipation
      d. Gas formation
   5. Easy bruising

DIAGNOSTIC TESTS AND METHODS
A. Patient history and physical examination
B. Examination of stool
   1. Examination of stool for occult (hidden) blood
   2. Fecal analysis: analysis of stool for mucus, pus, blood, parasites, and fat content
   3. Stool for ova and parasites must be taken to the laboratory while it is still warm.
   4. Nursing interventions

a. Instruct patient in the proper collection of the specimen.

b. Take specimen to the laboratory promptly.

C. Radiographic examination

1. Upper GI series
   a. Patient ingests contrast medium (barium).
   b. Movement of the medium through the esophagus and into the stomach is observed by fluoroscopy; x-ray films are also taken.
      (1) Aids in identification of esophageal and stomach pathology
      (2) Nursing interventions
         (a) Explain procedures to patient.
         (b) Patient is usually on NPO status before the examination.
         (c) Enemas or cathartics may be given before and after the examination.
         (d) Allay patient's anxiety.

2. Lower GI series (barium enema)
   a. The filling of the colon with barium is observed by fluoroscopy; x-ray films of the colon are also taken.
   b. Aids in the detection of abnormalities or defects in the colon such as lesions, polyps, tumors, and diverticula
   c. Nursing interventions
      (1) Explain procedures to patient.
      (2) Patient is usually on NPO status before the examination.
      (3) Enemas or cathartics may be given before and after the examination.
      (4) Allay patient's anxiety.

3. Gallbladder series (oral cholecystography)
   a. Patient is given an oral radiographic dye to ingest the evening before the examination.
   b. The gallbladder is visualized to detect gallstones and obstruction of the biliary tract.
   c. Nursing interventions
      (1) Explain procedures to patient.
      (2) Administer the radiographic dye as prescribed.
      (3) Maintain NPO status after the dye has been given.
      (4) Allay patient's anxiety.

4. Ultrasound of the gallbladder

5. Cholangiography
   a. Aids in the visualization of the biliary duct system
   b. Three methods
      (1) IV cholangiography (IVC): A radiographic dye is administered intravenously, and x-ray films are taken.
      (2) Percutaneous transhepatic cholangiography: With fluoroscopy a cannula is inserted into the liver and bile duct. A radiographic dye is injected into the duct, and filling is observed.
      (3) Operative or T-tube cholangiography: Contrast medium is instilled into the common bile duct, cystic duct, or gallbladder with use of a fine needle or catheter during surgery or via an existing T tube after surgery.
   c. Nursing interventions
      (1) Explain procedures to patient.
      (2) Maintain NPO as ordered.
      (3) Monitor patient for bleeding or bile leakage if the percutaneous approach was used.

6. Barium swallow: barium contrast study used to detect esophageal abnormalities and reasons for dysphagia

D. Endoscopy

1. Endoscopy of the upper GI tract (esophagoscopy, gastroscopy, gastroduodenoscopy, esophagogastroduodenoscopy)
   a. Visualization of the esophagus, stomach, or duodenum with a lighted scope
   b. Useful in detecting inflammation, ulceration, tumors, and other lesions
   c. Nursing interventions
      (1) Explain procedures to patient.
      (2) Obtain signed consent.
      (3) Maintain NPO status as ordered.
      (4) Administer preoperative medication as ordered.
      (5) After the examination, maintain NPO status until the gag reflex returns.

2. Colonoscopy, sigmoidoscopy
   a. Visualization of the internal structures of the colon with a fiberoptic scope
   b. Lesions, tumors, and polyps may be visualized, and a biopsy may be performed.
   c. Nursing interventions
      (1) Explain procedures to patient.
      (2) Prepare patient with enemas and cathartics as ordered.
      (3) After the examination, observe for rectal bleeding and signs of perforation (malaise, distention, tenesmus).

E. Ultrasonography

1. Noninvasive test that uses echoes from sound waves to visualize deep structures of the body
2. Requires no special preparation
3. Useful for procedures such as detecting masses, fluid accumulation, cysts, and tumors

F. Scans (liver, pancreas)

1. Assessment of size, shape, and position of the organ
2. Radionuclide is injected intravenously, and a scanning device picks up the radioactive emissions, which are recorded on paper.
3. Nursing interventions
   a. No preparation is required for liver scanning.
   b. Fasting and dietary preparation may be ordered for pancreatic scanning.
   c. Explain procedures to patient.
   d. Allay patient's anxiety.

G. CT scan

1. Noninvasive, radiological imaging technique that takes exposures of the body or body part at different depths
2. Requires no special preparation

H. Liver biopsy

1. Invasive procedure in which a needle is inserted into the liver through a small incision in the skin and a sample of liver tissue is obtained
2. The incision is usually made on the right side at the sixth, seventh, eighth, or ninth intercostal space.
3. Nursing interventions
   a. Obtain signed consent.
   b. Explain procedure to patient.
   c. Take baseline vital signs.
   d. Provide assistance during the procedure.
   e. After the procedure, monitor the vital signs every 15 to 60 minutes. Carry out prescription for bed rest (position flat or on the right side), assess the site, and monitor for complications.

I. Laboratory studies
1. Serum amylase
   a. Measures the secretion of amylase by the pancreas
   b. Useful in diagnosing pancreatitis
2. Serum lipase
   a. Measures the secretion of lipase by the pancreas
   b. Useful in diagnosing pancreatitis
3. Serum bilirubin and spot urine amylase: indicate the ability of the liver to conjugate and excrete bilirubin
4. Coagulation studies (PT, PTT): useful in analyzing hemostatic functions
5. Liver enzyme studies (SGOT, serum glutamic-pyruvic transaminase [SGPT], LDH): elevations usually indicate liver damage.
6. Hepatitis-associated antigen (HAA): presence suggests hepatitis.
7. Ammonia levels: elevated in advanced liver disease
8. Urine amylase: elevated amylase levels indicate pancreatic dysfunction.

J. Gastric analysis
1. Gastric contents are analyzed primarily for hydrochloric acid content.
2. Acidity (pH), volume, and cytology may also be determined.

K. D-Xylose tolerance test
1. This study evaluates absorption.
2. Xylose in water is given orally.
3. A urine collection of several hours follows; the amount of D-xylose in the urine is measured.
4. Abnormal amounts of D-xylose in the urine indicate a malabsorption problem.
5. Nursing interventions
   a. Explain procedure to patient.
   b. Maintain NPO status before the examination.
   c. Give patient instructions for collecting the urine.

FREQUENT PATIENT PROBLEMS AND NURSING CARE

A. Pain related to impaired oral mucous membranes
1. Give soft, bland foods.
2. Encourage intake of fluids that do not aggravate the condition.
3. Encourage use of soothing mouth rinses.
4. Administer topical medication as prescribed.

B. Impaired swallowing related to gingivitis
1. Give mouth irrigations as prescribed.
2. Offer soft, bland foods and liquids.
3. Instruct patient in the benefit of good oral hygiene and professional dental cleaning.

C. Deficient fluid volume related to nausea and vomiting
1. Observe character and quantity of emesis.
2. Observe for associated symptoms.
3. Observe for precipitating factors.
4. Administer antiemetics as prescribed.
5. Offer ice chips.
6. Maintain cool environment.
7. Apply a cool compress to the neck and forehead for comfort.
8. Offer sips of clear liquids such as 7-Up or ginger ale.
9. Reduce environmental stimuli such as noise, unpleasant odors, and unpleasant sights.
10. Encourage rest and deep breathing.
11. Serve patient's favorite foods.
12. Limit food servings.
13. Provide mouth care after episodes of emesis.

D. Risk for aspiration related to dysphagia
1. Provide patient with favorite foods arranged attractively.
2. Provide soft, bland foods that can be chewed easily.
3. Provide small, frequent feedings.
4. Avoid irritating food and fluid.
5. Monitor intake.
6. Administer topical medication as ordered.
7. Follow Aspiration Precautions; use high-Fowler position for eating, avoid distractions, and position chin down for swallowing.

E. Impaired nutrition, less than body requirements, related to anorexia
1. Assess status of the anorexia.
2. Monitor intake of food and fluid.
3. Determine patient's food likes and dislikes.
4. Prepare patient for meals.
   a. Relieve pain.
   b. Provide mouth care.
   c. Assist patient to a comfortable position.
   d. Use patient screen for privacy.
   e. Remove unpleasant stimuli from patient's view.
5. Prepare food tray.
   a. Serve food at proper temperature.
   b. Make the tray attractive.
   c. Serve appropriate quantities. (Large quantities may reduce the appetite.)

F. Deficient fluid volume related to diarrhea
1. Document character, consistency, number, and appearance of stools.
2. Assess for associated symptoms.
3. Monitor intake and output.
4. Administer antidiarrheals as prescribed, and monitor for side effects.
5. Avoid milk and milk products.
6. Increase fluid intake to at least 3000 mL daily.
7. Monitor vital signs at least every 4 hours.
8. Identify symptoms of electrolyte imbalance.
9. Monitor laboratory reports for electrolyte values.

G. Constipation related to decreased peristalsis or activity
1. Administer enemas, stool softeners, and cathartics as ordered.
2. Encourage fluids to at least 3000 mL daily.
3. Provide hot drinks to stimulate peristalsis.
4. Encourage a diet high in fiber.
5. Check for an impaction.
6. Encourage exercises.
7. Instruct patient concerning proper diet, increased fluid intake, exercise, and avoidance of laxative abuse.

MAJOR MEDICAL DIAGNOSES
Esophagitis

A. Definition: inflammation of the esophagus; more common in middle age
B. Causes
1. Inflammation of the esophagus may be brought on by irritants (food, tobacco), bacteria, or trauma (also see discussion of hiatal hernia).
2. Fungal: *Candida*
3. Gastroesophageal reflux disease (GERD): term for reflux esophagitis. An incompetent lower esophageal sphincter allows a reflux of gastric contents into the esophagus.

4. Malignancy
5. Prolonged nasogastric intubation
6. Repeated vomiting
C. Signs and symptoms
1. Heartburn (epigastric distress)
2. Pain with eructation or regurgitations
3. Dysphagia
4. Pain associated with ingestion of citrus liquids, alcohol, or hot or cold fluid
5. Symptoms aggravated by lying down after meals
6. Bleeding
D. Diagnostic tests and methods
1. Patient history and physical examination
2. Barium swallow
3. Esophagoscopy and biopsy
4. Routine chest x-ray examination
E. Treatments
1. Avoid food and fluids that aggravate the symptoms.
2. Administer antacids, analgesics, and sedatives.
3. Elevate head of bed on shock blocks.
4. Maintain bland diet.
5. Medications are used to decrease the amount of gastric acid produced (Pepcid, Zantac, Axid, among others).
6. Surgery may be necessary if conservative measures fail.
   a. Fundoplication: plication (making tucks) in the fundus of the stomach around the lower end of the esophagus
   b. Vagotomy and pyloroplasty: interruption of the impulses carried by the vagus nerve to reduce gastric secretions. The pylorus is also surgically manipulated to provide a larger conduit between the stomach and the duodenum.
F. Nursing interventions
1. Assess signs and symptoms and reactions to treatments.
2. Provide small, frequent feedings of bland, low-roughage foods.
3. Discourage intake of food close to bedtime.
4. Administer medication as prescribed, and monitor for side effects.
5. Place patient in semi-Fowler position.

Esophageal Varices

A. Definition: dilated vessels that occur at the lower end of the esophagus
B. Causes
1. Dilation of these vessels is usually a complication arising from cirrhosis of the liver.
2. Veins in the lower esophagus become distended as a result of increased portal pressure. The varices may rupture, causing hemorrhage and subsequent shock.
C. Signs and symptoms
1. Usually none until the varices become ulcerated
2. Hematemesis and coffee-ground emesis
3. Melena
4. Tachycardia
5. Hypotension
6. Low Hgb and Hct levels
D. Diagnostic tests and methods
1. Patient history and physical examination: history of alcoholism may be present.
2. Fiberoptic endoscopy
3. Laboratory studies: Hgb, Hct, and liver function studies

4. Angiography
5. Barium swallow
6. CT scan
7. Ultrasound
E. Treatment
1. Blood and blood product replacement
2. Control of bleeding through balloon tamponade and vitamin K therapy
3. Laboratory studies to monitor bleeding status and effectiveness of treatments
4. Hydration with IV fluids
5. Monitoring intake and output
6. Surgery if needed to control bleeding
7. Injection of bleeding varices with a sclerosing agent to control the bleeding
F. Nursing interventions
1. Provide ongoing assessment of signs and symptoms and reactions to treatment.
2. Monitor vital signs at least every 4 hours and every 30 minutes if bleeding is occurring.
3. Record intake and output hourly if varices are bleeding.
4. Monitor fluids: assess the site and monitor flow rate.
5. Give prescribed medication as ordered, and monitor for side effects.
6. Allay patient's anxieties and fears.
7. Assess all emesis and stool for the presence of blood.
8. Monitor laboratory studies and inform physician of incoming laboratory test values.
9. Keep head of bed elevated.
10. Monitor the Sengstaken-Blakemore tube if in use. Keep scissors taped to head of bed in case of emergency.
11. Note the character of respirations.

Hiatal Hernia

A. Definition: protrusion of the proximal area of the stomach through a weakened area of the diaphragm into the thoracic cavity (Figure 5-7)
B. Causes
1. Congenital weakness
2. Increased abdominal pressure
3. Trauma
4. Relaxation of the musculature
5. Gastric reflux may flow into the esophagus, causing inflammation and ulceration.
C. Signs and symptoms
1. Heartburn (pyrosis)
2. Sternal pain after a heavy meal
3. Regurgitation
4. Feeling of fullness
5. Dysphagia
6. Dyspnea
D. Diagnosis tests and methods
1. Patient history and physical examination
2. Upper GI series (barium swallow)
3. Esophagoscopy
4. Routine chest x-ray examination
E. Treatment
1. Conservative
   a. Elevation of the head of the bed on shock blocks
   b. Bland diet with frequent small feedings
   c. Avoidance of caffeine, alcohol, and chocolate

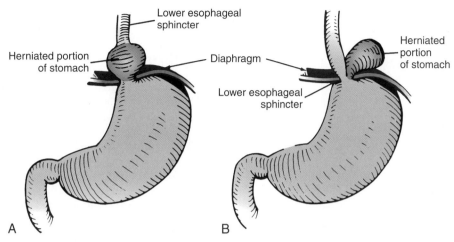

FIGURE 5-7 Hiatal hernia. **A,** Sliding hernia. **B,** Paraesophageal hernia. (From Monahan FD et al: *Phipps' medical-surgical nursing: health and illness perspectives,* ed 8, St Louis, 2007, Mosby.)

d. Drug therapy with anticholinergics, H_2 blockers, and antacids

e. Weight management

f. Avoidance of activities that increase intraabdominal pressure

2. When conservative measures fail, surgery indicated: fundoplication—"wrapping" the upper part of the stomach around the esophageal sphincter to prevent reflux

a. Nasogastric tube

b. IV therapy

c. Drug therapy with analgesics and antiemetics

d. Monitoring of vital signs

e. Monitoring of intake and output

F. Nursing interventions

1. Assess and document signs and symptoms and reactions to treatments.

2. Administer prescribed drugs, and monitor for side effects.

3. Monitor vital signs at least every shift and more often if surgery was performed.

4. Monitor intake and output if surgery was performed.

5. Provide prescribed diet.

6. Inform physician if patient reports gastric reflux after surgery.

7. Educate patient and family concerning drug therapy, diet, activities to avoid, and the need for compliance.

Gastritis

A. Definition: inflammation in the mucosal lining of the stomach; may be acute or chronic

B. May be caused by bacteria, alcohol, drugs, or toxins that cause the lining of the stomach to become inflamed and edematous

C. Signs and symptoms

1. Nausea and vomiting

2. Anorexia

3. Epigastric tenderness

4. Feeling of fullness

5. Cramping

6. Diarrhea

7. Fever

D. Diagnostic tests and methods

1. Patient history and physical examination

2. Identification of a causative agent

3. Laboratory studies

4. Stool culture

5. Endoscopy with biopsy

6. Gastric analysis

E. Treatment

1. Supportive care

2. Bed rest

3. Continued NPO status if nausea or vomiting is severe

4. Hydration with IV fluids

5. In severe cases, insertion of a nasogastric tube

6. Drug therapy: antiemetics, antacids, and H_2-receptor antagonists

7. Progressive diet when acute symptoms subside

8. Restriction of smoking

F. Nursing interventions

1. Assess and document signs and symptoms and reactions to treatments.

2. Monitor vital signs at least every 4 hours.

3. Monitor intake and output.

4. Provide the prescribed diet.

5. Administer medication as prescribed, and monitor for side effects.

6. Note amount and character of emesis and diarrhea.

7. Monitor IV fluids.

8. Educate patient and family concerning drug therapy, diet, activities, and any restrictions.

Cancer of the Stomach

A. Can develop anywhere in the stomach

B. Causes

1. Exact cause unknown

2. Familial tendency suspected

3. Predisposing conditions: chronic gastric ulcers and gastritis

C. Signs and symptoms

1. Loss of appetite, early satiety

2. Weight loss

3. Weakness, fatigue

4. Pain

5. Melena

6. Anemia
7. Hematemesis
8. Dizziness
9. Indigestion or dysphagia
10. Constipation
D. Diagnostic tests and methods
1. Patient history and physical examination
2. Laboratory studies
3. Stool analysis
4. Gastric analysis
5. Barium studies
6. Gastroscopy
E. Treatment
1. Preoperative therapy
a. Correction of nutritional deficiencies
b. Treatment of anemias
c. Blood replacement
d. Gastric decompression with a nasogastric tube
2. Surgery: removal of the cancerous lesion or tumor along with a margin of normal tissue
3. Radiation therapy and chemotherapy, whether or not patient is having surgery
a. Combination therapy has a better response rate.
b. Single-agent therapy has proved to be of little value.
F. Nursing interventions
1. Preoperative care
a. Offer support to patient and family.
b. Assess and document signs and symptoms and reactions to treatments.
c. Provide and encourage the prescribed diet.
d. Monitor vital signs at least every 8 hours.
e. Monitor blood and fluid replacement therapy.
f. Provide preoperative teaching.
2. Postoperative care (immediate)
a. Have patient turn, cough, and breathe deeply.
b. Monitor nasogastric suctioning and tube patency.
c. Monitor vital signs as ordered.
d. Record intake and output.
e. Administer prescribed medication, and monitor for side effects.
f. Assess dressing.
g. Assess for bowel sounds.
h. Encourage early ambulation and ROM exercises to prevent thrombosis.
i. Provide antiembolism stockings.
j. Relieve pain with drugs and supportive measures.
3. Postoperative period
a. Provide six to eight small feedings.
b. Weigh patient daily while in hospital to monitor weight loss.
c. Reduce fluids taken with meals if not tolerated.
d. Educate patient and family concerning drug therapy, dietary restrictions, activity, wound care, and compliance with the regimen.

Peptic Ulcers

A. Definition: ulcerations in the mucosal lining of the distal esophagus, stomach, or small intestine (duodenum or jejunum); duodenal ulcers more common than gastric ulcers, and men more prone to ulcers than women
B. Cause: exact causes unknown; recurrent or refractory ulcers linked to *Helicobacter pylori* infections

C. Predisposing factors
1. Stress
2. Smoking
3. Heavy caffeine ingestion
4. Ingestion of certain drugs (acetylsalicylic acid [ASA], steroids, nonsteroidal antiinflammatory drugs [NSAIDs])
5. Infection of the mucosa by *H. pylori*
D. Signs and symptoms
1. Loss of appetite
2. Weight loss or gain
3. Pain (gnawing, burning)
4. Melena
5. Anemia
6. Hematemesis; coffee-ground emesis
7. Occasional nausea or vomiting
8. Dark, tarry stools
E. Diagnostic tests and methods
1. Patient history and physical examination
2. Gastroscopy and duodenoscopy
3. Barium studies
4. Gastric analysis
5. Laboratory studies
F. Treatment
1. Conservative
a. Rest
b. Drug therapy: antacids, anticholinergics, proton pump inhibitors, H_2 receptor antagonists, sedatives, analgesics, and in some cases antibiotics
c. Elimination of smoking and caffeine
d. Reduction of stress
e. Bland diet with small, frequent feedings
f. In acute situations, patient may be on NPO status and have nasogastric tube inserted.
2. Surgical interventions
a. Closure if perforation has occurred
b. Pyloroplasty and vagotomy if the gastric outlet is obstructed
c. Total or partial resection of the stomach to remove the ulcerated areas
G. Nursing interventions
1. Conduct ongoing assessment of signs and symptoms and reactions to treatments.
2. Monitor vital signs at least every 4 hours.
3. Administer the prescribed medication, and monitor for side effects.
4. Provide the prescribed diet.
5. Provide physical and emotional rest.
6. Monitor for signs and symptoms of complications (perforation, hemorrhage, obstruction).
7. Instruct patient regarding eliminating smoking, avoiding certain foods, and reducing stress.
8. Educate patient and family concerning drug therapy, diet and dietary restrictions, avoidance of stress, and the need for compliance with the prescribed regimen.

Obstruction

A. Definition: mechanical or neurological abnormality inhibiting the normal flow of gastric or intestinal contents
B. Obstructions may result from scar tissue formation, cancer, or strangulated hernias; all are mechanical barriers to the normal flow of gastric or intestinal contents.

C. A neurological obstruction in the form of a paralytic ileus causes interference with innervation, thus hindering normal peristaltic activity.

D. Signs and symptoms
1. Abnormal pain and distention
2. Projectile vomiting
3. Nausea
4. Possible absence of bowel sounds or increase in bowel sounds
5. Cramping
6. Abdomen may be tense (distended)
7. Obstipation (chronic constipation)

E. Diagnostic tests and methods
1. Patient history and physical examination
2. Flat plate of the abdomen
3. Laboratory studies

F. Treatment
1. Surgery for treating mechanical obstructions
2. Gastric or intestinal decompression to decrease nausea and vomiting
3. Hydration with IV therapy
4. Prophylactic antibiotics
5. Monitoring intake and output
6. Supportive care

G. Nursing interventions
1. Assess and document signs and symptoms and reactions to treatments.
2. Monitor vital signs at least every 4 hours.
3. Record intake and output.
4. Monitor the decompression tube and assess quantity and character of drainage.
5. Provide mouth care while patient is intubated.
6. Administer prescribed medication, and monitor for side effects.
7. Maintain NPO status.
8. Monitor the states of distention and hydration.
9. Provide routine postoperative care if patient undergoes surgery.

Crohn Disease (Regional Enteritis)

A. Definition: inflammatory disease affecting primarily the small bowel and also possibly the large bowel; the intestinal lining ulcerates, and scar tissue forms; bowel becomes thick and narrow.

B. Cause is unknown. Stricture, obstruction, and perforation can occur as a result of this disorder. Malabsorption of fluid and nutrients is also associated with this disorder.

C. Signs and symptoms (aggravated by illness or stress)
1. Abdominal pain and cramping
2. Diarrhea
3. Weight loss
4. Fever
5. Anemia
6. Weakness and fatigue
7. Anorexia
8. Abdominal tenderness

D. Diagnostic tests and methods
1. Patient history and physical examination
2. Laboratory studies: CBC, electrolytes, clotting studies
3. Stool examination
4. Endoscopy
5. Proctosigmoidoscopy and biopsy examination
6. Barium studies

E. Treatment
1. Drug therapy: sedatives, antidiarrheals, antibiotics, steroids, hematinics, anticholinergics, and analgesics
2. Hydration with IV therapy
3. Correction of nutritional deficiencies
4. Provision of symptomatic relief
5. In severe cases patient may be on NPO status, have a nasogastric tube, and require blood transfusions.
6. High-calorie, high-protein, low-residue diet
7. Surgery is indicated if fistula formation, bleeding, perforation, or obstruction is present.

F. Nursing interventions
1. Assess and document signs and symptoms and reactions to treatments.
2. Monitor vital signs every 4 hours.
3. Record intake and output.
4. Provide and encourage the prescribed diet.
5. Assist with ADLs.
6. Monitor the number, amount, and character of stools.
7. Monitor hydration status.
8. Assess for abdominal distention.
9. Maintain skin integrity, and monitor for anal excoriation.
10. Provide support to patient.
11. Administer prescribed medication, and monitor for side effects.
12. Educate patient and family concerning drug therapy, dietary restrictions, and compliance. Provide information on ostomy care if applicable.

Ulcerative Colitis

A. Definition: inflammatory disorder of the large bowel; The inflammatory process begins in the distal segments of the colon and ascends.
1. The mucosa ulcerates, bleeds, and becomes edematous and thickens.
2. Perforations and abscesses can occur.
3. The colon eventually loses its elasticity, and its absorptive ability is reduced.

B. Cause is unknown, although the condition has been associated with stress, autoimmune factors, and food allergies.

C. Signs and symptoms
1. Abdominal cramping pain with diarrhea
2. Nausea
3. Dehydration
4. Cachexia
5. Weight loss
6. Anorexia
7. Bloody diarrhea
8. Anemia

D. Diagnostic tests and methods
1. Patient history and physical examination
2. Laboratory studies to reveal anemia and electrolyte imbalance: CBC, electrolytes
3. Stool examination
4. Proctosigmoidoscopy
5. Barium studies

E. Treatment
1. Drug therapy: sedatives, antidiarrheals, antibiotics, steroids, hematinics, anticholinergics, and analgesics
2. Correction of malnutrition
3. Hydration with IV therapy
4. Colectomy with ileostomy if other medical treatment fails

5. Provision of symptomatic relief
6. Monitoring of weight
7. Monitoring of intake and output
8. Parenteral hyperalimentation if necessary
9. Psychotherapy

F. Nursing interventions
1. Assess and document signs and symptoms and reactions to treatments.
2. Provide emotional and physical rest.
3. Monitor number, amount, and characteristics of stools.
4. Provide skin care measures to avoid anal excoriation.
5. Monitor intake and output.
6. Monitor vital signs every 4 hours.
7. Weigh patient daily.
8. Increase intake of fluids.
9. Provide the prescribed diet.
10. Administer prescribed medication, and monitor for side effects.
11. Assess bowel sounds every 4 hours.
12. Assist with ADLs.
13. Provide emotional support.
14. Educate patient and family concerning drug therapy, dietary restrictions, avoidance of stress, and compliance with the prescribed regimen.

Diverticulosis and Diverticulitis

A. Definition: diverticulum—an outpouching of the mucosa of the colon
1. Diverticulosis: the existence of diverticula in the large intestine
2. Diverticulitis: an inflammation of the diverticulum
B. Cause of diverticulosis is unknown. Theories include a congenital weakness of the colon, colon distention, constipation, and inadequate dietary fiber.
C. Signs and symptoms
1. Abdominal cramps
2. Lower-quadrant tenderness
3. Constipation or constipation alternating with diarrhea
4. Fever
5. Occult bleeding
6. Elevated WBC count
D. Diagnostic tests and methods
1. Patient history and physical examination
2. Laboratory studies
3. Stool examination for occult blood
4. Sigmoidoscopy
5. Colonoscopy
6. Barium studies
E. Treatment
1. High-residue diet
2. Drug therapy: bulk laxatives, antibiotics, stool softeners, and anticholinergics
3. In more severe cases patient may be on NPO status and require IV therapy.
4. Surgery: colon resection for obstruction and hemorrhage
F. Nursing interventions
1. Assess and document signs and symptoms and reactions to treatments.
2. Provide increased fiber in the diet.
3. Increase intake of fluids.
4. Administer prescribed medication, and monitor for side effects.

5. Instruct patient to avoid activity that increases intraabdominal pressure (straining at stool, lifting, bending, wearing restrictive clothing).
6. Educate patient and family concerning drug therapy, dietary restrictions, and avoidance of constipation and activity that increases intraabdominal pressure.

Colon and Rectal Cancer and Polyps

A. Definition: Cancerous process can invade the large intestine. Cancer of the colon and rectum may take the form of a well-defined tumor or cancerous polyp: a polyp is a pouchlike structure projecting from the wall of the bowel; polyps may be cancerous or benign.
B. Cause of colon cancer is unknown. Persons with colon polyps, lesions, diverticula, or ulcerative colitis are monitored closely for malignant changes in the bowel.
C. Signs and symptoms
1. Changes in bowel pattern
2. Rectal bleeding
3. Changes in the shape of stool
4. Weakness and fatigue
5. Weight loss
6. Rectal pain
7. Abdominal pain
8. Anemia
D. Diagnostic tests and methods
1. Patient history and physical examination
2. Laboratory studies
3. Barium studies
4. Proctosigmoidoscopic examination
E. Treatment
1. Surgical resection of the affected area; creation of a colostomy if necessary
2. Chemotherapy
3. Radiation therapy
4. Supportive therapy
F. Nursing interventions (also see nursing interventions for cancer of the stomach)
1. Assess and document signs and symptoms and reactions to treatments.
2. Monitor vital signs at least every 4 hours and more often during the postoperative periods.
3. Record intake and output.
4. Monitor dressings and wound drainage.
5. Relieve pain.
6. Administer prescribed medication, and monitor for side effects.
7. Provide psychological support.
8. Monitor colostomy site.
9. Monitor perineal area if drain or packing has been inserted.
10. Assist patient with sitz baths if ordered.
11. Assist patient with ADLs as needed.
12. Monitor hydration status.
13. Encourage increased fluid intake.
14. Educate patient and family concerning drug therapy, diet, activities, colostomy care, and adaptation to everyday activity.

Hemorrhoids

A. Definition: varicosities or dilated vessels in the rectal and anal area
B. Cause: Hemorrhoids result from increased abdominal pressure such as that during pregnancy and from prolonged

periods of sitting and standing. Constipation and obesity are also predisposing factors.

C. Signs and symptoms vary from no symptoms at all to pain, itching, and bleeding.

D. Diagnostic tests and methods
  1. Patient history and physical examination
  2. Digital examination
  3. Proctoscopy

E. Treatment
  1. Symptomatic relief in mild cases
    a. Topical medication to shrink the mucous membrane
    b. Stool softeners and laxatives to keep stool soft and avoid straining
    c. Sitz baths to relieve pain
    d. High-fiber diet to keep stools soft
  2. Rubber-band ligation of internal hemorrhoids: the constriction impairs circulation; the tissues become necrotic and slough off.
  3. Hemorrhoidectomy: the surgical excision of hemorrhoids
    a. Removal may be by clamp, excision, or cautery.
    b. Postoperative treatments are similar to those identified previously for symptomatic relief.

F. Nursing interventions
  1. Assess and document signs and symptoms and reactions to treatments.
  2. Alleviate pain with analgesics, positioning, and sitz baths.
  3. Administer prescribed medication, and monitor for side effects.
  4. Monitor vital signs at least every 4 hours.
  5. Monitor dressings for drainage.
  6. Monitor voiding after surgery.
  7. Assist with gradual return to activity.
  8. Encourage increased fluid intake.
  9. Provide patient with rationale for avoiding constipation and prolonged sitting and standing.
  10. Educate patient and family concerning drug therapy, high-fiber diet, activity, and avoidance of constipation.

Cholelithiasis and Cholecystitis

A. Definition
  1. Cholelithiasis: the presence of gallstones in the gallbladder or biliary tree
  2. Cholecystitis: an inflammation of the gallbladder usually associated with the presence of gallstones

B. Causes
  1. Cholelithiasis is believed to be precipitated by chemical changes in bile.
    a. Bile stasis, infections of the gallbladder, and metabolic changes can precipitate stone formation.
    b. Stones may lodge in the biliary tree, causing obstruction and biliary colic (Figure 5-8).
  2. Cholecystitis may be brought on by cholelithiasis or the presence of an organism in the gallbladder.

C. Signs and symptoms
  1. Indigestion after a meal high in fat
  2. Nausea and vomiting
  3. Flatulence
  4. Belching
  5. Right upper-quadrant pain radiating to the back or shoulder
  6. Fever
  7. Jaundice
  8. Clay-colored stools

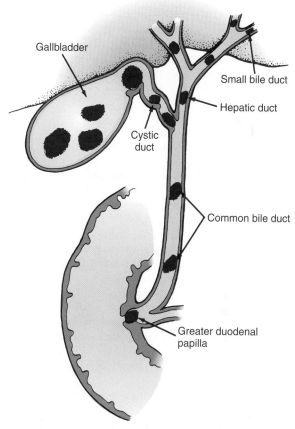

FIGURE 5-8 Common sites of gallstones. (From Monahan FD et al: *Phipps' medical-surgical nursing: health and illness perspectives,* ed 8, St Louis, 2007, Mosby.)

  9. Dark-colored urine
  10. Elevated WBC count

D. Diagnostic tests and methods
  1. Patient history and physical examination
  2. Laboratory studies
  3. Oral cholecystography
  4. IVC
  5. Ultrasound examination of gallbladder

E. Treatment
  1. Hydration with IV fluids
  2. Drug therapy: analgesics, antibiotics, and antispasmodics
  3. Drug therapy to dissolve stones has been effective in certain patients.
  4. Low-fat diet
  5. Lithotripsy (use of shock waves to disintegrate gallstones) has been attempted in patients having few stones.
  6. Surgical removal of the gallbladder (cholecystectomy) or gallstones (cholecystostomy)
  7. Laparoscopic cholecystectomy (removal through an endoscope inserted through the abdominal wall)

F. Nursing interventions
  1. Assess and document signs and symptoms and reactions to treatments.
  2. Administer prescribed medication, and monitor for side effects.
  3. Alleviate pain and promote comfort.
  4. Monitor IV therapy.
  5. Provide the prescribed diet.
  6. Monitor the state of hydration.

7. Assess vital signs at least every 4 hours.
8. Provide postoperative care: monitor dressing, nasogastric tube, and T tube (tube is inserted into the common bile duct during surgery if the common bile duct is explored) (Figure 5-9).
9. Educate patient and family concerning drug therapy, dietary restrictions, and wound care if surgery was performed.

Hepatitis

A. Definition: inflammation of the liver
B. Causes
   1. Drugs or chemicals (toxic hepatitis)
   2. Viral origin
   3. Multiple blood transfusions
   4. Hepatitis A
      a. Transmitted by the fecal-oral route
      b. Incubation period approximately 2 to 7 weeks
      c. May be spread by contaminated food, water, milk, and shellfish
   5. Hepatitis B
      a. Associated with contaminated needles and syringes
      b. Transmitted through blood or blood products and pricking of the skin with contaminated equipment
      c. May also be spread through feces, urine, saliva, and semen
      d. Patients are prone to exacerbations and complications (cirrhosis) from the disease.
      e. Incubation period is approximately 6 to 26 weeks.
      f. Immunization is available: it is given to newborn, then again at 2 and 6 months of age.

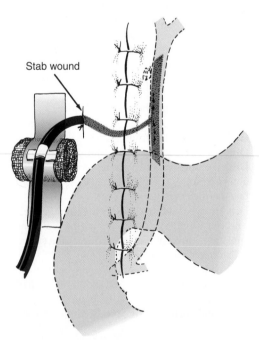

Stab wound

FIGURE 5-9 Section of T tube emerging from stab wound may be placed over roll of gauze anchored to skin with adhesive tape to prevent its lumen from being occluded by pressure. (From Monahan FD et al: *Phipps' medical-surgical nursing: health and illness perspectives*, ed 8, St Louis, 2007, Mosby.)

6. Hepatitis C virus (HCV; formerly known as non-HAV, non-HBV) and hepatitis E
   a. Name given to forms of hepatitis caused by a virus genetically different from hepatitis A or B
   b. Associated with blood transfusions, particularly from paid donors; previous IV drug use
   c. No specific antigen associated with the form
   d. Similar to hepatitis B in characteristics but insidious course in the beginning
   e. All blood donors now tested for HCV
C. Signs and symptoms (early symptoms of hepatitis A may be more severe)
   1. Fever and chills
   2. Headache
   3. Respiratory symptoms
   4. Anorexia
   5. Nausea and vomiting
   6. Liver tenderness
   7. Jaundice and itching
   8. Elevated liver enzymes
   9. Elevated PT values
   10. Elevated bilirubin levels
   11. Presence of hepatitis virus in feces and serum
   12. Presence of the hepatitis surface antigen (HBsAg)
   13. Clay-colored stools and dark-colored urine
D. Diagnostic tests and methods
   1. Patient history and physical examination
   2. Laboratory studies: HAA, liver profile
   3. Stool examination
   4. Urinary bilirubin and urobilinogen
   5. Liver biopsy
   6. Serum ammonia levels: protein restricted if ammonia levels are elevated
E. Treatment
   1. Monitoring of liver function study results
   2. Bed rest with bathroom privileges
   3. High-calorie, high-carbohydrate, high-protein, moderate-fat diet
   4. Topical lotions to alleviate dry, itchy skin
   5. Hydration with IV therapy
   6. Administration of vitamin K preparations
   7. Monitoring for bleeding tendencies and progression of the illness
   8. Blood and Body Fluid Precautions
   9. Passive immunity
F. Nursing interventions
   1. Assess and document signs and symptoms and reactions to treatments.
   2. Monitor skin, stool, and urine color.
   3. Promote balanced activity and rest periods.
   4. Maintain Blood and Body Fluid Precautions.
   5. Monitor IV therapy.
   6. Assess intake and output.
   7. Monitor vital signs at least every 4 hours.
   8. Provide and encourage the prescribed diet.
   9. Offer support to patient and family.
   10. Administer prescribed medication, and monitor for side effects.
   11. Monitor for bleeding tendencies.
   12. Educate patient and family concerning drug therapy, the prescribed diet, activity level, and monitoring for complications.

Cirrhosis

A. Definition: cell degeneration occurring in the liver wherever scar tissue replaces normally functioning tissue

B. A complication of alcoholism, hepatitis, biliary disease, and certain metabolic disorders.

C. Whatever the cause of the liver destruction, the course of cirrhosis is the same.
1. Liver parenchyma die and regenerate, and fibrous tissue (scarring) occurs.
2. This alteration in structure progresses in the liver, causing problems in hepatic blood flow and normal liver function. In time the liver fails.

D. Major complications of cirrhosis
1. Portal hypertension: hypertension resulting from the obstruction of normal blood flow through the portal system, which in turn is caused by changes in the liver from the cirrhotic process.
2. Esophageal varices (see discussion of esophageal varices)
3. Ascites: accumulation of fluid in the peritoneal or abdominal cavity, which is a later symptom in cirrhosis
4. Hepatic coma (encephalopathy): a condition of advanced liver disease; the entrance of blood into the general circulation without being properly detoxified by the liver

E. Signs and symptoms
1. Headache
2. Nausea and vomiting
3. Weight loss
4. Anorexia
5. Jaundice
6. Abdominal pain
7. Fatigue and weakness
8. Liver enlargement and fibrosis
9. Bleeding disorders caused by disruption in the manufacture of vitamin K–dependent factors
10. Edema
11. Telangiectasis (blood vessels develop a spiderlike appearance)
12. Ascites
13. Esophageal varices
14. Hepatic coma

F. Diagnostic tests and methods
1. Patient history and physical examination
2. Laboratory studies to assess liver function
3. Liver scan
4. Liver biopsy; monitoring for bleeding at site

G. Treatment
1. Rest with activity as tolerated
2. Nutritious diet with protein level determined by liver functioning
3. If ascites is present, restriction of fluid and sodium, monitoring of weight, and abdominal girth measurement daily
4. Monitoring for complications such as ascites, esophageal varices, and hepatic coma
5. Drug therapy to reduce ammonia levels, prevent bleeding, reduce edema, and provide comfort

H. Nursing interventions
1. Assess and document signs and symptoms and reactions to treatments.
2. Administer prescribed medication, and monitor for side effects.
3. Provide and encourage prescribed diet.
4. Promote comfort.
5. Monitor vital signs at least every 4 hours, and report abnormalities.
6. Monitor status of ascites.
   a. Record weight.
   b. Assess measurements of extremities and abnormal girth.
   c. Monitor intake and output.
7. Provide planned exercise and rest periods.
8. Assist patient with ADLs.
9. Monitor skin status and take measures to prevent skin breakdown.
10. Protect against infection.
11. Provide diversional activity.
12. Offer emotional support.
13. Provide ongoing assessment for evidence of hepatic encephalopathy.
    a. Monitor for symptoms of lethargy, confusion, twitching, tremors, sweetish breath odor, fever, and increasing somnolence.
    b. Eliminate dietary protein to decrease serum ammonia levels that contribute to the encephalopathy.
    c. Administer prescribed drugs and enemas to reduce ammonia levels.
    d. Monitor IV fluids.
    e. Give narcotics and sedatives cautiously.
14. See care of patient with esophageal varices (see discussion on esophageal varices).
15. Educate patient and family concerning homebound care.

Pancreatitis

A. Definition: acute or chronic inflammation of the pancreas

B. Associated with biliary disease, infections, drug toxicity, nutritional deficiencies, and ingestion of alcohol; some cases possibly idiopathic

C. The digestive enzymes of the pancreas are released into the pancreatic tissue, causing inflammation.
1. As the condition progresses, ischemia, duct obstruction, and necrosis may occur.
2. Bleeding occurs if tissue necrosis affects vessels.
3. Pancreatic abscesses may occur if bacteria invade the necrotic tissue.
4. In chronic pancreatitis the tissue becomes fibrotic, and normal function is compromised.

D. Signs and symptoms
1. Acute pancreatitis
   a. Severe epigastric pain that radiates to the back
   b. Pain aggravated by eating
   c. Patient assuming a side-lying position with knees bent for comfort.
   d. Nausea and vomiting
   e. Low-grade fever
   f. Hypotension
   g. Tachycardia
   h. Jaundice
   i. Elevated WBC count
   j. Shock: if blood vessel or tissue erosion is present
2. Chronic pancreatitis
   a. Abdominal pain
   b. Weight loss
   c. Steatorrhea (foul-smelling, foamy stool)
   d. Diabetes mellitus if beta cell function is affected

E. Diagnostic tests and methods
   1. Patient history and physical examination
   2. Laboratory tests, particularly electrolytes, amylase, lipase, and liver enzymes
   3. Pancreatic scan and sonography
   4. Visualization of the pancreatic duct (endoscopy)
   5. X-ray studies
F. Treatment
   1. Control of pain
   2. Hydration with IV fluids
   3. Correction of any bleeding
   4. Nasogastric tube and NPO status to reduce pancreatic secretions
   5. Drug therapy: analgesics, antibiotics, steroids, vitamins, and pancreatic extracts
   6. Diet that does not stimulate pancreatic secretions
   7. Control of blood glucose levels if beta cells are affected
G. Nursing interventions
   1. Assess and document signs and symptoms and reactions to treatments.
   2. Administer prescribed medication, and monitor for side effects.
   3. Provide prescribed diet.
   4. Explain dietary restrictions to patient.
   5. Monitor vital signs at least every 4 hours.
   6. Monitor IV therapy.
   7. Promote comfort and relieve pain.
   8. Provide emotional support.
   9. Assess intake and output.
   10. Relieve nausea and vomiting if present.
   11. Note color, character, and amount of urine and stool.
   12. Monitor jaundice if present.
   13. Monitor the nasogastric tube and secretions.
   14. Educate patient and family concerning drug therapy, diet and dietary restrictions, avoidance of alcohol, monitoring of steatorrhea, monitoring of blood glucose (glucometer), and compliance with the regimen.

Cancer of the Pancreas

A. Cancer of the pancreas can affect any portion of the pancreas, including the beta cells. Metastasis readily occurs to adjacent structures.
B. Cancerous tissue impairs normal pancreatic function, primarily by causing obstruction and hindering the flow of pancreatic secretions.
C. Signs and symptoms
   1. Early symptoms may be vague.
      a. Nausea and vomiting
      b. Anorexia
      c. Weight loss
      d. Weakness and fatigue
   2. Later symptoms
      a. Pain
      b. Jaundice
      c. Diabetes mellitus
D. Diagnostic tests and methods
   1. Patient history and physical examination
   2. Laboratory studies
   3. Pancreatic scan and sonography
   4. X-ray studies
   5. Visualization of the pancreatic duct

E. Treatment
   1. Supportive therapy
   2. Surgical excision: Whipple procedure—removal of the head of the pancreas, lower portion of the common bile duct, distal portion of the stomach, and the duodenum
   3. Palliative surgery to restore bile and pancreatic output
   4. Chemotherapy
F. Nursing interventions: see discussion of cancer of the stomach

Appendicitis

A. Definition: inflammation of the appendix
B. Signs and symptoms
   1. Right lower-quadrant pain with possible rebound tenderness
   2. Periumbilical pain
   3. Nausea and vomiting
   4. Anorexia
   5. Fever
   6. Elevated WBC count
C. Diagnostic tests and methods
   1. Patient history and physical examination
   2. Laboratory tests, particularly WBC count
D. Treatment
   1. Supportive therapy
   2. Immediate surgical removal (appendectomy)
E. Nursing interventions
   1. Assess and document signs and symptoms and reactions to treatments.
   2. Monitor IV fluids.
   3. Provide comfort measures such as an ice pack to the abdomen and analgesia.
   4. Administer prescribed drugs, and monitor for side effects.
   5. Monitor vital signs as ordered.
   6. Encourage progressive ambulation after surgery.
   7. Monitor the dressing and operative site after surgery.
   8. Educate patient and family concerning drug therapy, activity restrictions, and care of the operative site.

Peritonitis

A. Definition: infection and subsequent inflammation of the peritoneal membrane by trauma or bacterial invasion (see Critical Thinking Challenge box)

? Critical Thinking Challenge

Peritonitis

A patient is 1 day postoperative after a small bowel resection. The patient has been restless most of the night and is running a low-grade fever of 99.9° F. All other vital signs are stable. The patient's NG tube is draining a greenish brownish substance. The Foley catheter is draining clear yellow urine. The morning labs are drawn, with the following abnormal results:

   WBC 23.7

   The patient may likely be developing peritonitis because the WBC has increased from 11.2 (yesterday morning) to 23.7 this morning. The nurse would alert her supervisor to the increased WBC count, and the physician will need to be notified of the result. An abdominal CT scan will most likely be ordered, as well as additional antibiotics.

CT, Computed tomography; *NG,* nasogastric; *WBC,* white blood cell.

B. The inflammation may be localized or widespread and may affect the organs of the abdominal cavity. Adhesions, abscesses, and obstructions may occur.
C. Signs and symptoms
1. Nausea and vomiting
2. Abdominal pain
3. Abdominal rigidity and distention
4. Fever
5. Paralytic ileus
6. Fluid and electrolyte imbalance
7. Elevated WBC count
8. Constipation, diarrhea
D. Diagnostic tests and methods
1. Patient history and physical examination
2. Laboratory tests, including a WBC count, electrolytes, and blood cultures
E. Treatment
1. Identification of the causative agent
2. Intestinal decompression
3. Hydration with IV therapy
4. Control of pain
5. Drug therapy: analgesics and antibiotics
6. Monitoring of vital signs
7. Monitoring of intake and output
8. Control of the spread of infection
F. Nursing interventions
1. Assess and document signs and symptoms and reactions to treatment.
2. Assess vital signs every 1 to 2 hours during the acute period.
3. Monitor intake and output.
4. Administer prescribed medication, and monitor for side effects.
5. Provide comfort and relief of pain.
6. Assess bowel sounds.
7. Maintain NPO status during the acute period.
8. Maintain nasogastric tube, and monitor output during the acute period.
9. Offer support to patient and allay anxieties.
10. Place patient in semi-Fowler position.
11. Have patient turn, cough, and deep breathe at least every 2 hours.

Hernia

A. Definition: protrusion of an organ or structure through the muscle wall of the containing cavity
B. May occur around the umbilical area, inguinal area, diaphragm, and femoral ring and at the site of an incision
C. Hernias are categorized as:
1. Reducible: can be returned to the normal position
2. Irreducible: cannot be returned to the normal position
3. Incarcerated: obstruction of intestinal flow
4. Strangulated: blood supply cut off (occluded)—surgical emergency
D. Causes
1. Congenital weakness in the containing wall
2. Weakness in containing wall related to straining and the aging process
3. Trauma
4. Increased intraabdominal pressure (obesity or pregnancy)

E. Signs and symptoms
1. Protrusion of a structure without symptoms
2. Appearance of a protrusion when straining or lifting
3. Pain in certain instances
4. If intestine is obstructed, possible distention, pain, nausea, and vomiting
F. Diagnostic methods: patient history and physical examination
G. Treatment
1. Surgery is the treatment of choice.
   a. Herniorrhaphy: surgical repair of the hernia
   b. Hernioplasty: the surgical reinforcement of the weakened area
2. Use of a truss (a support worn over the hernia to keep it in place)
H. Nursing interventions
1. Assess and document signs and symptoms and reactions to treatments.
2. Assess vital signs every shift before surgery.
3. Report any symptoms of coughing, sneezing, or upper respiratory tract infection noted before surgery because this will weaken the surgical repair.
4. Apply ice packs as ordered to control pain and swelling.
5. Monitor voidings after inguinal hernia repair.
6. Educate patient and family concerning care of the operative site, activity restrictions, and avoidance of constipation.

NEUROLOGICAL SYSTEM

ANATOMY AND PHYSIOLOGY

The nervous system acts as a coordinated unit, both structurally and functionally.
A. Functions
1. Regulates system; responsible for coordinating bodily functions and responding to changes in or stimuli from the internal and external environment
2. Controls communication among body parts
3. Coordinates activities of body system
B. Divisions
1. CNS: brain and spinal cord; interprets incoming sensory information and sends out instruction based on past experiences
2. Peripheral nervous system (PNS): cranial and spinal nerves extending out from brain and spinal cord; carry impulses to and from brain and spinal cord
3. Autonomic nervous system: functional classification of the PNS; regulates involuntary activities
4. Somatic nervous system: functional classification of the PNS; allows conscious or voluntary control of skeletal muscles
C. Structure and physiology
1. Neurons or nerve cells: respond to a stimulus, connect into a nerve impulse (irritability), and transmit the impulse to neurons, muscle, or glands (conductivity); consist of three main parts:
   a. Cell body: contains nucleus and one or more fibers or processes extending from cell body
   b. Dendrites: conduct impulses toward cell body. A neuron has many dendrites.
   c. Axons: conduct impulses away from cell body. A neuron has one axon.

2. Types of neurons
   a. Motor (efferent) neurons: conduct impulses from CNS to muscle and glands
   b. Sensory (afferent) neurons: conduct impulses toward CNS
   c. Connecting (internuncial) neurons: conduct impulses from sensory to motor neurons
3. Synapse: chemical transmission of impulses from axon to dendrites
4. Myelin sheath: protects and insulates the axon fibers; increases the rate of transmission of nerve impulses
5. Neurilemma: sheath covering the myelin; found in PNS; function is regeneration of nerve fiber
6. Neuroglia: connective or supporting tissue; important in reaction of nervous system to injury or infection
7. Ganglia: clusters of nerve cells outside the CNS
8. White matter: bundles of myelinated nerve fibers; conducts impulses along fibers
9. Gray matter: clusters of neuron cell bodies; fibers not covered with myelin; distributes impulses across selected synapses

D. CNS
   1. Brain (Figure 5-10)
      a. Cerebrum: largest part of brain; outer layer called *cerebral cortex;* cortex composed of dendrites and cell bodies; controls mental processes; highest level of functioning (Table 5-3)
      b. Cerebellum: controls muscle tone coordination and maintains equilibrium
      c. Diencephalon: consists of two major structures located between the cerebrum and midbrain
         (1) Hypothalamus regulates the autonomic nervous system; controls blood pressure; helps maintain normal body temperature and appetite; controls water balance and sleep.
         (2) Thalamus acts as a relay station for incoming and outgoing nerve impulses. It produces emotions of pleasantness and unpleasantness associated with sensations.
      d. Brainstem: connects the cerebrum with the spinal cord
         (1) Midbrain: relay center for eye and ear reflexes

Table 5-3	Specific Functions of Cerebral Cortices
Frontal cortex	Conceptualization
	Abstraction
	Judgment formation
	Motor ability
	Ability to write words
	Higher level centers for autonomic functions
Parietal cortex	Highest integrative and coordinating center for perception and interpretation of sensory information
	Ability to recognize body parts
	Left versus right
	Motor movement
Temporal cortex	Memory storage
	Auditory integration
	Hearing
Occipital cortex	Visual center
	Understanding of written material

Adapted from Monahan FD et al: *Phipps' medical-surgical nursing: health and illness perspectives,* ed 8, St Louis, 2007, Mosby.

   (2) Pons: connecting link between cerebellum and rest of nervous system
   (3) Medulla oblongata: contains center for respiration, heart rate, and vasomotor activity
   2. Spinal cord
      a. Inner column composed of gray matter, H-shaped, composed of dendrites and cell bodies; outer part composed of white matter, composed of bundles of axons called *tracts*
      b. Function: Sensory tract conducts impulses to brain; motor tract conducts impulses from brain; center for all spinal cord reflexes.
   3. Protection for CNS
      a. Bone: Vertebrae surround cord; skull surrounds brain.
      b. Meninges: three connective tissue membranes that cover brain and spinal cord
         (1) Dura mater: white fibrous tissue; outer layer
         (2) Arachnoid: delicate membrane, middle layer; contains subarachnoid fluid
         (3) Pia mater: inner layer; contains blood vessels
      c. Spaces
         (1) Epidural space: between dura mater and the vertebrae
         (2) Subdural space: between dura mater and arachnoid
         (3) Subarachnoid space: between arachnoid and pia mater; contains cerebrospinal fluid
      d. Cerebrospinal fluid: acts as a shock absorber; aids in exchange of nutrients and waste materials

E. PNS
   1. Carries voluntary and involuntary impulses
   2. Cranial nerves (Table 5-4)
   3. Spinal nerves: 31 pairs; conduct impulses necessary for sensation and voluntary movement; each group named for the corresponding part of the spinal column

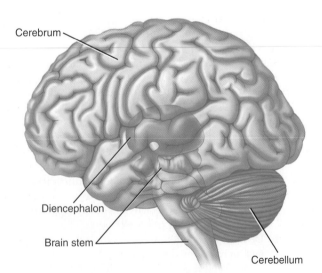

FIGURE 5-10 Areas of the brain. (From Herlihy B: *The human body in health and illness,* ed 4, St Louis, 2011, Saunders.)

Cerebrum

Diencephalon

Brain stem

Cerebellum

Table 5-4   Cranial Nerves

	CRANIAL NERVES	CONDUCT IMPULSES	FUNCTION
I	Olfactory	From nose to brain	Sense of smell
II	Optic	From eye to brain	Vision
III	Oculomotor	From brain to eye and eye muscles	Contraction of upper eyelid; maintains position of eyelid; papillary reflexes
IV	Trochlear	From brain to external eye muscles	Eye movements
V	Trigeminal	From skin and mucous membranes of head and teeth to chewing muscles	Sensations of head and teeth; chewing muscles
VI	Abducens	From brain to external eye muscles	Eye movements
VII	Facial	From taste buds of the tongue and facial muscles to muscles of facial expression	Taste, facial expression
VIII	Acoustic	From organ of Corti to brain	Hearing
	Vestibular branch	From semicircular canals to brain	Balance
IX	Glossopharyngeal	From pharynx and posterior third of tongue to brain; also from brain to throat muscles and salivary glands	Sensations of tastes, sensations of pharynx; swallowing; secretion of saliva
X	Vagus	From throat and organs in thoracic and abdominal cavities to brain; to muscles of throat and abdominal cavities	Important in swallowing, speaking, peristalsis, and production of gastric juices
XI	Accessory	From brain to shoulder and neck muscles	Rotation of head and raising shoulders
XII	Hypoglossal	From brain to muscles of tongue	Tongue movement

F. Autonomic nervous system
  1. Part of PNS; controls smooth muscle, cardiac muscle, and glands
  2. Two divisions
    a. Sympathetic: "fight or flight" response; increases heart rate and blood pressure; dilates pupils
    b. Parasympathetic: dominates control under normal conditions; maintains homeostasis

NEUROLOGICAL CONDITIONS AND DISORDERS

Pathological conditions of the CNS arise from injuries, new growths, vascular insufficiency, and infections and as complications secondary to other diseases. Patient problems are related to interference with normal functioning of the affected tissue.

The following terms are used in describing patients with a neurological impairment:
- Anesthesia: complete loss of sensation
- Aphasia: loss of ability to use language
  - Auditory or receptive aphasia: loss of ability to understand
  - Expressive aphasia: loss of ability to use spoken or written word
- Ataxia: uncoordinated movements
- Coma: state of profound unconsciousness
- Convulsion: involuntary contractions and relaxation of muscle
- Delirium: mental state characterized by restlessness and disorientation
- Diplopia: double vision
- Dyskinesia: difficulty in voluntary movement
- Flaccid: without tone, limp

- Neuralgia: intermittent, intense pain along the course of a nerve
- Neuritis: inflammation of a nerve or nerves
- Nuchal rigidity: stiff neck
- Nystagmus: involuntary, rapid movements of the eyeball
- Papilledema: swelling of optic nerve head
- Paresthesia: abnormal sensation without obvious cause and with numbness and tingling
- Spastic: convulsive muscular contraction
- Stupor: state of impaired consciousness with brief response only to vigorous and repeated stimulation
- Tic: spasmodic, involuntary twitching of a muscle
- Vertigo: dizziness

NURSING ASSESSMENT

A. Observations
  1. Mental status: drowsiness or lethargy, ability to follow commands
  2. LOC: ability to be aroused in response to verbal and physical stimuli; ranges from awake and alert to coma. Glasgow Coma Scale (Table 5-5) is the usual guide for assessing and describing the degree of conscious impairment, based on three determinants:
    a. Eye opening
    b. Motor response
    c. Verbal response
  3. Orientation
    a. Time: knows month or year
    b. Place: has general knowledge of where he or she is (e.g., hospital)
    c. Person: knows own name; is able to name relative or friend

Table 5-5 **Glasgow Coma Scale**

	STIMULI	SCORE
Eyes open	Spontaneously	4
	To speech	3
	To pain	2
	None	1
Best verbal response	Oriented	5
	Confused	4
	Inappropriate words	3
	Incomprehensible	2
	None	1
Best motor response	Obeys commands	5
	Localizes to pain	4
	Flexes to pain	3
	Extends arm to pain	2
	None	1

Adapted from Monahan FD et al: *Phipps' medical-surgical nursing: health and illness perspectives,* ed 8, St Louis, 2007, Mosby.

4. Behavior: Is it appropriate for the situation?
5. Emotional response: Is it appropriate for the situation?
6. Memory: capability for early and recent recall; remote, recent, and new learning ability
7. Speech: presence of aphasia, appropriate speech, words distinct or slurred, quality, rate, loudness, and fluency
8. Vital signs: temperature, pulse, respirations, and blood pressure; pulse pressure
9. Ability to follow simple directions
10. Eyes
    a. Pupillary reaction to light: The pupils are periodically assessed with a flashlight to evaluate and compare size, configuration, and reaction; differences between the eyes and from previous assessments are compared for similarities and differences.
    b. Movement of lids and pupils
11. Motor function: coordination, gait, balance, posture, strength, functioning, and muscle tone
12. Bladder and bowel control
13. Ears for drainage (may indicate cerebrospinal fluid leak)
14. Facial expression for symmetry
15. Sensation for:
    a. Pain
    b. Light touch, pressure
    c. Smell
16. Rancho Los Amigos scale: a scale of cognitive functioning that was developed to aid in assessment and treatment after traumatic brain injury (TBI)
    a. No response: completely unresponsive to any stimuli
    b. Generalized response: reacts inconsistently and without purpose to stimuli

c. Localized response: reacts specifically yet inconsistently to stimuli
d. Confused-agitated: is in agitated state yet has decreased ability to process information
e. Confused-inappropriate: appears alert; is able to respond to simple commands fairly consistently
f. Confused-appropriate: has goal-directed behaviors; needs cues
g. Automatic-appropriate: oriented; does daily routine; has shallow recall of actions
h. Purpose-appropriate: aware and oriented; is able to recall and integrate past and recent events
17. Grooming, personal hygiene
18. Thoughts, perceptions, attention span
B. Patient description (subjective data)
   1. History of head injury, loss of consciousness, vertigo, weakness, headache, sleep problems, paralysis, seizures, or diplopia
   2. Complaints of pain, numbness, problems with elimination, memory loss, difficulty concentrating, drowsiness, or visual problems
   3. Medications taken
C. History from family
   1. Medical
   2. ADLs
   3. Behavior

DIAGNOSTIC TESTS AND METHODS

A. CT (CAT) scan: computer analysis of tissues as x-rays pass through them; has replaced many of the usual tests; no special preparation or care after test
B. Lumbar puncture (spinal tap)
   1. Description: With patient under local anesthesia, a puncture is made at the junction of the third and fourth lumbar vertebrae to obtain a specimen of cerebrospinal fluid; cerebrospinal fluid pressure can be measured. This procedure is also used to inject medications (e.g., spinal anesthesia) and in diagnostic x-ray examination to inject air or dye (e.g., myelogram).
   2. Nursing interventions
      a. Monitor vital signs.
      b. Keep patient supine 4 to 8 hours.
      c. Observe for headache and nuchal rigidity.
      d. Monitor site for leakage.
C. Cerebral angiography
   1. Description: intraarterial injection of radiopaque dye to obtain an x-ray film of cerebrovascular circulation
   2. Nursing interventions after procedure
      a. Related to dye: Observe for allergic reaction—urticaria, decreased urinary output, respiratory distress, and difficulty swallowing. Have tracheostomy set available.
      b. Related to injection site
         (1) Provide ice pack and bed rest.
         (2) Monitor vital signs.
         (3) Observe for pain, tenderness, bleeding, temperature, and color.
D. Electroencephalography (EEG)
   1. Description: Electrodes are placed on unshaven scalp with tiny needles and electrode jelly.
   2. Nursing interventions
      a. Anticipate patient's fears about electrocution; do not give stimulants or depressants before test.

b. No smoking or caffeinated beverages. Patient needs to eat a full meal before the test; fasting may cause hypoglycemia and alter brain waves.

c. If ordered, withhold antiseizure medications or tranquilizers.

d. Stress need for restful sleep before test; sleep deprivation may cause abnormal brain waves.

e. Wash hair and scalp after procedure, to remove jelly.

f. Patient may resume all previous activities.

E. Brain scan

1. Description: After an IV injection of a radioisotope, abnormal brain tissue absorbs more rapidly than normal tissue; this can be detected with a Geiger counter to diagnose brain tumors.

2. Nursing interventions

a. No observations are necessary.

b. Patient may resume all previous activities.

F. MRI

1. Description: MRI uses a combination of radio waves and a strong magnetic field to view soft tissue (does not use x-rays or dyes); produces a computerized picture that depicts soft tissues in high-contrast color.

2. Nursing interventions

a. Before the procedure instruct patient to remain perfectly still in the narrow cylinder-shaped machine.

b. Inform patient that no pain or discomfort will occur but there must be no movement during the MRI.

c. No specific care or observations are necessary after the procedure.

G. Myelography (MEG)

1. Description: injection of a radiopaque dye into the subarachnoid space via a lumbar puncture; performed to locate lesions of the spinal column or ruptured vertebral disk

2. Types of agents used: metrizamide and iophendylate (Pantopaque). If metrizamide is used, patient should not take phenothiazines, tricyclic antidepressants, CNS stimulants, or amphetamines for 24 to 48 hours before test. After the procedure is completed, Pantopaque dye is removed; leaving it in would cause meningeal irritation. Metrizamide is water soluble and does not need to be removed.

3. After procedure with Pantopaque, patient lies flat in bed for 6 to 8 hours; after procedure with metrizamide, patient's head must be elevated 30 to 50 degrees for 6 to 8 hours. Fluids are encouraged. Common side effects include nausea, vomiting, and possibly seizures. Check with physician regarding when medications withheld before test may be given. With both types of agents, observe site for leakage of cerebrospinal fluid; assess strength and sensation in lower extremities; encourage fluids; maintain bed rest; monitor vital signs; observe for headache, pain, and dizziness.

H. PET scan

1. Patient inhales or is injected with a radioactive substance.

2. The computer can diagnose and determine level of functioning of an organ.

3. Exposure to radiation is minimal, and no special care is indicated.

I. Skull x-ray examination: no preparation. No nursing care or observations are indicated afterward.

FREQUENT PATIENT PROBLEMS AND NURSING CARE

A. Impaired physical mobility related to progression of primary disease

1. Give specific care and perform assessment as required (see Chapter 2).

2. Perform neurological assessment every 2 to 4 hours.

3. Initiate nursing care measures to prevent complications of immobility.

4. Use assistive devices.

B. Risk for injury or infection related to "fixed eyes" (no blinking)

1. Protect with eye shields.

2. If necessary, remove dried exudate with warm saline solution and mineral oil.

3. Have patient close eyes.

4. Inspect for inflammation.

C. Ineffective breathing pattern related to neuromuscular impairment

1. Maintain patent airway, suction as needed, and elevate head 20 to 30 degrees.

2. Have tracheostomy set available.

3. Provide oxygen with humidity.

4. Monitor vital signs every 2 hours.

5. Provide oral hygiene every 2 hours.

6. Lubricate patient's lips.

D. Risk for hyperthermia, hypothermia related to neuromuscular impairment

1. Assess rectal temperature every 2 hours.

2. Use external heating and cooling (e.g., hypothermia or hyperthermia machine).

E. Risk for aspiration related to neuromuscular impairment

1. Maintain NPO status.

2. Position patient on side; turn every 2 hours.

3. Provide nasogastric tube feedings.

4. Monitor IV fluids.

F. Risk for injury related to restlessness, involuntary motions, or seizures

1. Maintain safety (e.g., padded side rails, bed in low position).

2. Follow precautions, care, and observations for a patient with seizures (see discussion of convulsive disorders)

G. Risk for impaired urinary elimination related to neuromuscular impairment

1. Urinary retention

a. Provide indwelling catheter care.

b. Monitor intake and output hourly.

2. Incontinence

a. Wash, dry, and inspect skin as needed.

b. Implement measures to prevent skin breakdown.

c. Implement bladder training.

H. Bowel incontinence, constipation related to neuromuscular impairment

1. Incontinence

a. Wash, dry, and inspect skin as needed.

b. Implement measures to prevent skin breakdown.

c. Implement bowel training.

2. Constipation

a. Record bowel movements.

b. Provide stool softeners, laxatives, and enemas as ordered.

   c. Check for impaction; perform disimpaction as needed.

   d. Encourage fluids as tolerated.

   e. Encourage activity as tolerated.

   f. Increase fiber in the diet.

I. Fear and anxiety related to pain; complications; surgery; possible disfigurement, disability, or dependency; fatal prognosis

   1. Explain nursing actions thoroughly.

   2. Encourage patient to express feelings.

   3. Report to health team.

   4. Involve family or significant others in care.

J. Other possible patient problems include:

   1. Self-care deficit: perform own ADLs related to sensory-motor impairments

   2. Imbalanced nutrition; less than body requirements related to dysphagia and fatigue

   3. Grieving related to actual or perceived loss or uncertain future or both

   4. Impaired swallowing related to chewing difficulties, muscle paralysis

   5. Activity intolerance related to fatigue and difficulty in performing ADLs

   6. Fatigue related to weakness, spasticity, fear of injury, and stressors

   7. Risk for social isolation related to spasticity, change in body image

   8. Risk for injury related to visual field, motor, or perception deficits

   9. Interrupted family processes related to physiological deficits, role disturbances, uncertain future

   10. Disturbed sensory perception specifically related to hypoxia secondary to trauma, progression of disease process

   11. Impaired verbal communication related to dysarthria or aphasia secondary to physiological changes

   12. Risk for deficient fluid volume related to vomiting secondary to increased intracranial pressure (IICP)

Special Situations

A. Patient in a coma

   1. Unconscious state in which patient is unresponsive to verbal or painful stimuli; occurs with many primary diseases. Patient depends on the nurse for maintenance of all basic human needs: nourishment, bathing, elimination, respiration, prevention of complications, and assessment and provision of care for problems (see the preceding section).

   2. Nursing interventions

     a. Include family in nursing care and care planning as much as possible.

     b. Note LOC (see discussion of nursing assessment for neurological conditions and disorders) every 15 minutes if LOC decreases; assess every 1, 2, or 4 hours as LOC improves.

     c. Demonstrate respect in patient's presence.

     d. Provide a quiet, restful environment.

     e. Speak to patient; use proper name; introduce self, and explain all care before starting.

     f. Provide privacy.

B. Patient with paralysis

   1. Paraplegia: paralysis of the lower extremities from sudden injury (e.g., automobile accident) or progressive degenerative disease (e.g., multiple sclerosis) to the spi-

nal cord. No motion or sensory function or reflexes may be evident. Uncontrollable muscle spasms may occur. Perspiration ceases and then becomes profuse. A loss of bladder and bowel control occurs. Sexual dysfunction, anxiety, fear, depression, anger, and embarrassment are major patient problems. Patient may be totally dependent.

   2. Quadriplegia (tetraplegia): paralysis of all four extremities from sudden injury (e.g., diving accident) or progressive degenerative disease (e.g., amyotrophic lateral sclerosis [ALS]). Symptoms and patient problems include autonomic dysreflexia and those encountered with paraplegia.

   3. Nursing interventions

     a. Take measures to prevent complications of immobility.

     b. Provide bowel and bladder training.

     c. Prevent deformity; maintain joint mobility and correct alignment.

     d. Encourage fluid intake.

     e. Provide high-protein diet.

     f. Encourage independence according to ability.

     g. Communicate and work closely with the physiatrist, physical therapist, occupational therapist, and other members of the rehabilitation team.

     h. Include family in nursing care and planning.

MAJOR MEDICAL DIAGNOSES

Increased Intracranial Pressure

A. Description: Fluid accumulation or a lesion takes up space in the cranial cavity, producing IICP. The brain is gradually compressed, or life-sustaining functions cease. Onset may be sudden, or condition may progress slowly.

B. Causes: tumors, hematoma, edema from trauma or stroke, and abscesses from infections

C. Signs and symptoms: related to primary diagnosis

   1. Headache, restlessness, and anxiety

   2. Vomiting: recurrent, projectile, and not related to nausea or meals

   3. Change in pupil response to light

   4. Seizures

   5. Respiratory difficulty: irregular, Cheyne-Stokes, or Kussmaul breathing

   6. Elevated blood pressure, with wide pulse pressure

   7. Increases in pulse at first, then slowing to 40 to 60 beats/min, regular and strong

   8. Altered LOC: becomes lethargic, speech slows, becomes confused, and shows decreased level of response

   9. Visual disturbances: diplopia and blurred vision

   10. Progressive weakness or paralysis

   11. Loss of consciousness, coma, and death

D. Diagnostic tests and methods: neurological assessment by physician and nurse

E. Treatment: depends on cause

   1. Surgical intervention (craniotomy)

   2. Steroids, anticonvulsants, mannitol, dexamethasone (Decadron), or urea to decrease edema

F. Nursing interventions

   1. Elevate head to semi-Fowler position; never place in Trendelenburg position.

   2. Monitor vital signs every 15 minutes.

   3. Prevent aspiration; place patient on side.

4. Maintain airway; provide oxygen therapy as necessary.
5. Observe pupillary response (usually unequal and may not react to light).
6. Report any change in LOC immediately.
7. Provide special care and observation when a patient has a seizure.
8. Provide care and safety for an unconscious patient.
9. Monitor IV fluids closely to prevent overhydration.

Convulsive Disorders

A. Description: Frequently a convulsion or seizure is not a disease but a symptom of a neurological disorder. Epilepsy is a disease characterized by a disposition for seizures. The following are types of seizures:
   1. Tonic-clonic (formerly *grand mal*): A premonition or sign (aura) may occur. The individual cries out, loses consciousness, and enters a tonic phase (the body is rigid, and the jaw is clenched); then a clonic phase occurs, with jerking movements of muscles, cessation of respirations, and fecal and urinary incontinence. Seizure lasts 1 to 2 minutes, followed by a short period of unresponsiveness.
   2. Absence (formerly *petit mal*): loss of consciousness that lasts 5 to 30 seconds, during which time normal activities may or may not cease. Amnesia concerning this time may occur.
B. International Classification of Epileptic Seizures (Box 5-5)
C. Causes
   1. May be secondary to another condition: CVA, head injury, brain tumor, markedly elevated temperature, toxins, or electrolyte imbalance
   2. Epilepsy may have no known cause; onset is usually in childhood or before 30 years of age.
D. Patient problems
   1. Related to primary disease
   2. Fear of injury
   3. Anxiety related to a chronic disease
   4. Embarrassment
   5. Fear of public rejection
   6. Side effects of drug therapy
E. Diagnostic tests and methods
   1. Specific tests to identify lesions
   2. EEG, CT scan, MRI, and brain mapping
   3. Serum chemistries
F. Treatment
   1. Treatment and removal of cause, if known
   2. Anticonvulsant drugs (see Chapter 3)
   3. Surgery: stereotactic (electrical stimulation to locate and resect [destroy] epileptogenic focus)

Box 5-5   International Classification of Epileptic Seizures

- **Partial (focal) seizures (consciousness may not be impaired):** with motor symptoms, with special sensory symptoms, with autonomic symptoms, with psychic symptoms; may become complex partial seizures; may evolve to generalized seizures
- **Generalized seizures (involve the entire brain; consciousness is lost):** may last from several seconds to minutes; types: absence seizures, tonic-clonic seizures, atonic seizures
- **Unclassified seizures:** unable to classify because of incomplete or inadequate data

---

G. Nursing interventions
   1. Provide accurate observation and documentation, including the following: aura, time of onset, whether seizure is generalized or focal, specific parts of body involved, progression of seizure, duration of seizure, eye movement, loss of consciousness, loss of bowel and bladder control, condition after seizure, memory loss, weakness, and any injury caused by seizure.
   2. Encourage patient to wear medical identification tag.
   3. Have suction available.
   4. Secure airway for easy accessibility.
   5. During generalized (grand mal) seizure:
      a. Maintain airway.
      b. Prevent head injury.
      c. Place patient on side if possible.
      d. Protect extremities from injury by guiding movements.
      e. Do not restrain.
      f. Loosen clothing.
      g. Remove pillows.
      h. Maintain safety until patient is fully conscious.

Transient Ischemic Attack (TIA)

A. Definition: altered cerebral tissue perfusion related to a temporary neurological disturbance
   1. Exhibited by sudden loss of motor or sensory function
   2. Lasts for a few minutes to a few hours
   3. Caused by a temporarily diminished blood supply to an area of the brain
   4. Patient is at high risk for developing a stroke.
B. Medical management is indicated (control of hypertension, low-sodium diet, possible anticoagulant therapy, smoking cessation).
C. Nursing care would include close observation and assessment; specific care is based on treatment.

Cerebrovascular Accident (Stroke, Brain Attack) and Cerebrovascular Disruptions

A. Description: decreased blood supply to a part of the brain caused by rupture, occlusion, or stenosis of the blood vessels. Onset may be sudden or gradual; symptoms and patient problems depend on location and size of area of brain with reduced or absent blood supply (left CVA results in right-sided involvement often associated with speech problems; right CVA results in left-sided involvement often associated with safety and judgment problems).
B. Causes: increased incidence with aging
   1. Atherosclerosis
   2. Embolism
   3. Thrombosis
   4. Hemorrhage from a ruptured cerebral aneurysm
   5. Hypertension
C. Signs and symptoms
   1. Subjective
      a. Change in mental status: decreased attention span, decreased ability to think and reason, difficulty following simple directions
      b. Headaches
   2. Objective
      a. Altered LOC
      b. Communication: motor or sensory aphasia: difficulty reading, writing, speaking, or understanding

c. Bowel or bladder dysfunction: retention, impaction, or incontinence

d. Seizures

e. Limited motor function: paralysis, dysphagia, weakness, hemiplegia, loss of function, or contractures

f. Loss of sensation or perception

g. Loss of temperature regulation and elevated temperature, pulse, and blood pressure

h. Absent gag reflex (aspiration)

i. Unusual emotional responses: depression, anxiety, anger, verbal outbursts, and crying; emotional lability

j. Problems related to immobility (see Chapter 2)

D. Diagnostic tests and methods

1. Physical assessment and patient or family history

2. EEG, CT scan, lumbar puncture, cerebral angiography or carotid ultrasonography, Doppler flow studies

E. Treatment

1. Removal of cause, prevention of complications, and maintenance of function; rehabilitation to restore function

2. Antihypertensives, anticoagulants, antiplatelet aggregation, antifibrinolytics, and stool softeners (see Chapter 3)

3. Surgical removal of clot, repair of aneurysm, carotid endarterectomy, balloon angioplasty, stents

F. Nursing interventions

1. Maintain bed rest. Provide complete care. Use turning sheet, footboard, firm mattress, pillows; use trochanter rolls to maintain proper body alignment. Anticipate needs, and leave things within reach (e.g., call bell).

2. Reposition patient every 2 hours. Provide passive and active ROM exercises. Place patient in chair as soon as allowed. Use flotation mattress or sheepskin.

3. Provide bath, inspect skin, and provide nursing measures to prevent decubitus ulcers.

4. Provide oxygen with humidity. Have patient cough and take deep breaths every 2 hours if possible. Maintain airway; suction as needed; prevent aspiration; keep head turned to side. Place in semi-Fowler position.

5. Ensure adequate nutrition and fluid and electrolyte balance. Provide nasogastric or gastrostomy tube feeding. Maintain IV fluids. Provide soft diet when tolerated. Use total parenteral nutrition (TPN). Follow Aspiration Precautions.

6. Establish means of communication: call bell, pad and pencil, and nonverbal gestures. Use simple commands, speak slowly, explain all care, provide speech therapy.

7. Be nonjudgmental about personality changes. Encourage family participation. Provide diversional activities. Praise accomplishments realistically.

8. Assess LOC. Maintain safety in environment, use side rails, restrain only as necessary.

9. Observe for IICP.

10. Monitor vital signs every 4 hours.

11. Ensure elimination: check bowel sounds, monitor bowel movements, monitor intake and output, provide indwelling catheter care, then conduct bowel and bladder training.

12. Provide care, safety, and precautions for a patient with seizures.

13. Provide support for family.

14. Schedule physical and occupational therapy as soon as possible.

15. Provide nursing measures to prevent complications of immobility (see Chapter 2).

16. Encourage self-care.

Brain Tumor

A. Definition: benign or malignant growth that grows and exerts pressure on vital centers of the brain, depressing function and causing increased pressure

B. Cause: unknown

C. Signs and symptoms: individual, depending on location and size

1. Personality changes, fear, and anxiety

2. Headaches, dizziness, and visual disturbance (e.g., double vision)

3. Seizures

4. Pituitary dysfunction

5. Signs of IICP

6. Local paresthesia or anesthesia

7. Aphasia

8. Problems with coordination, gait

D. Diagnostic tests and methods

1. Patient history and physical examination

2. Neurological assessment, including EEG, CT scan, angiography, MRI, PET scan

E. Treatment: surgical removal if possible (craniotomy), frequently combined with radiotherapy and chemotherapy

F. Nursing interventions

1. Perform timely neurological assessment and documentation.

2. Provide safety and assist with care as needed.

3. Be nonjudgmental about personality changes; encourage patient to express feelings.

4. Provide postoperative care.

a. Anticipate and provide care as needed to maintain airway.

b. Provide safety and observation during a seizure.

c. Regulate body temperature.

d. Position on unoperated side.

e. Elevate head only under medical order.

f. Inspect dressing every 30 minutes for hemorrhage or drainage (leakage of cerebrospinal fluid).

g. Make neurological assessment hourly until patient is stable and then every 4 hours; observe for IICP.

h. Provide care for patient in coma as indicated earlier in this section.

Head Injuries

A. Definition: trauma to scalp, skull, or brain. A fracture to the skull may result in either a simple break in the bone or bone fragmentation that penetrates the brain tissue; hemorrhage, concussion, or contusion can also result.

1. Cerebral concussion: injury to the head. Patient may be dazed or unconscious for a few minutes. Some functions (e.g., memory) may be impaired for as long as several weeks.

2. Cerebral contusion: head injury causing bruising of brain tissue. Person experiences stupor, confusion, or loss of consciousness. If the contusion is severe, the person may go into coma.

3. Cerebral laceration: a break in continuity of brain tissue

B. Cause: blow to the head (e.g., from a fall or automobile accident)

C. Signs and symptoms: individual, according to location and extent of blow
  1. Nausea and vomiting, dizziness, vertigo
  2. Lethargy: increasing loss of consciousness to impending coma
  3. Disorientation
  4. Drainage of cerebrospinal fluid from ear or nose (Battle sign)
  5. Convulsions
  6. Problems related to IICP

D. Diagnostic tests and methods
  1. Patient history and physical and neurological assessment
  2. X-ray examination
  3. Angiography, Doppler studies
  4. CT scan, MRI
  5. PET scan

E. Treatment
  1. Anticonvulsants, corticosteroids, mannitol (if cerebral edema)
  2. Maintenance of fluid balance
  3. Surgery

F. Nursing interventions
  1. Provide care as discussed for a patient with IICP (see discussion of IICP).
  2. Perform neurological assessment hourly.
  3. Maintain airway.
  4. Give care as required for the unconscious patient if necessary.
  5. Take precautions for a patient with seizures.
  6. Observe for serous or bloody discharge from ears or nose.

Multiple Sclerosis

A. Description: a chronic, progressive disease of the brain and spinal cord. Lesions cause degeneration of the myelin sheath and interfere with conduction of motor nerve impulses. Periods of remissions and exacerbations occur. Onset occurs in young adults; progression is unpredictable.

B. Cause: unknown; exacerbated with stress

C. Signs and symptoms vary with individual.
  1. Ataxia
  2. Paresthesia, numbness, tingling
  3. Weakness and loss of muscle tone, fatigue
  4. Loss of sense of position
  5. Vertigo
  6. Blurred vision, diplopia, nystagmus, patchy blindness that may progress to total blindness
  7. Inappropriate emotions: euphoria, apathy, depression
  8. Dysphagia
  9. Slurred speech
  10. Bladder and bowel dysfunction: incontinence or retention
  11. Sexual dysfunction: impotence, diminished sensation
  12. Spasticity as disease progresses

D. Diagnostic tests and methods
  1. Patient history and physical and neurological assessment
  2. CT scan
  3. MRI
  4. Examination of cerebrospinal fluid
  5. PET scan
  6. Evoked responses

E. Treatment: symptomatic; corticosteroids during acute exacerbations

F. Nursing interventions
  1. Provide care to prevent complications of immobility (see Chapter 2).
  2. Encourage patient to maintain independence.
  3. Encourage patient to participate in care plan.
  4. Encourage high-caloric, high-vitamin, high-protein diet. Provide nutrition that can be swallowed easily.
  5. Provide bowel and bladder training (may have indwelling catheter).
  6. Provide diversional activities.
  7. Provide safety measures.
  8. Allow time for patients to express concerns about disabilities and dependencies: be supportive.
  9. Avoid precipitating factors that cause exacerbations (fatigue, cold, heat, infections, stress).
  10. Provide patient and family education.

Parkinson Disease

A. Definition: progressive, degenerative disease that causes destruction of nerve cells in the basal ganglia of the brain as a result of a deficiency of dopamine. Limbs become rigid, fingers have characteristic pill-rolling movement, and head has to-and-fro movement. Patient has a bent position and walks in short, shuffling steps. Facial expression becomes blank, with wide eyes and infrequent blinking (Parkinson mask); intelligence is not affected.

B. Cause: unknown

C. Signs and symptoms
  1. Tremor
  2. Voluntary movement is slow and difficult; coordination is poor (ataxia).
  3. Impaired chewing and eating; excessive salivation and drooling occur.
  4. Speech is slow, and patient is soft-spoken; written communication is difficult.
  5. Sweating is excessive.
  6. Emotional changes include depression, paranoia, and eventually confusion.
  7. Dependency
  8. Results of diagnostic tests
  9. Side effects of drugs
  10. Autonomic manifestations such as urinary incontinence, constipation, hypotension

D. Diagnostic tests and methods
  1. Patient history and physical assessment
  2. Neurological assessment, examination of cerebrospinal fluid, and CT scan

E. Treatment: Many patients respond to drug therapy, and the disease is controlled with medication for the remainder of their lives. Others have no response, and the disease progresses to a state of invalidism and immobility (usually treated with a combination of drugs) (see Chapter 3); surgeries (stereotaxic, fetal dopamine transplant, adrenal medullary transplant) may be performed.

F. Nursing interventions
  1. Encourage patient to maintain independence as much as possible in hygiene and dressing. Include patient in planning all aspects of care as much as possible.
  2. Encourage participation in previous work and social and diversional activities (avoid social withdrawal).

3. Help patient avoid embarrassment while eating; use straws, wipe drooling saliva, use bib, and keep clothing clean. Use utensils with large handles for easy grip.
4. Recommend a soft diet or one of a consistency that patient is able to chew.
5. Provide diversion (activity therapy).
6. Encourage daily exercises as tolerated, especially walking. Take safety measures (avoid rubber-soled shoes; these increase risk of falls because the rubber grips the floor, and patients fall forward).
7. Encourage patient to avoid fatigue.
8. Help patient to avoid frustration; emphasize capabilities rather than limitations.
9. Reinforce speech, physical, and occupational therapy treatment protocols.
10. Administer stool softeners to avoid constipation.
11. Provide bowel and bladder training.
12. Be patient when patient is slow or clumsy.
13. Establish a means of communication.
14. Enhance cognitive skills (reorient frequently).
15. Prevent pneumonia; force fluids; turn patient when in bed, and encourage patient to be out of bed as much as possible.
16. Provide mouth care every 4 hours.
17. Encourage family participation in all aspects of rehabilitation.

Amyotrophic Lateral Sclerosis

A. Definition: Also known as *Lou Gehrig disease,* ALS is a degenerative disease that affects the upper or lower motor neurons of the brain, the spinal cord, or both.
B. Cause: unknown; a genetic link or a slow-moving viral infection is suspected.
C. Signs and symptoms
  1. Fatigue, weight loss
  2. Difficulty doing fine motor tasks (buttoning a shirt)
  3. Progressive muscle weakness, muscle wasting, atrophy
  4. Dysphagia (difficulty swallowing)
  5. Dysarthria (difficult speech)
  6. Tongue fasciculation (twitching)
  7. Jaw clonus (involuntary tightening and relaxing of muscles)
  8. Spasticity of flexor muscles
  9. Respiratory difficulty
  10. Involvement of upper or lower extremities; one side of body affected more than other (late in disease process)
  11. No sensory loss; patient remains alert.
  12. Death usually occurs 5 to 10 years from onset; caused by respiratory or bulbar paralysis.
D. Diagnostic tests and methods: No specific test is available to diagnose ALS; EMG may be done initially to rule out other neuromuscular diseases.
E. Treatment: symptomatic relief as disease progresses. Surgery may be necessary to insert a gastrostomy tube during the later stages of the disease.
F. Nursing interventions
  1. Provide care to prevent complications of immobility.
  2. Promote adequate nutrition; implement safety measures.
  3. Provide adequate rest periods; instruct to avoid hot baths or traveling in hot weather.

4. Provide alternative means of communication.
5. Prevent bowel and bladder problems with adequate diet. Provide medications to prevent urinary tract infections and constipation. Bowel and bladder training programs may be necessary.
6. Promote skin integrity.
7. Assist in maintaining ADLs.
8. Assist in maintaining a clear airway. Encourage use of a tucked chin position when eating or drinking. Encourage use of a suction machine. Ventilator may be used for respiratory assistance during later stages of disease.
9. Provide patient and family education.
10. Facilitate coping and adjustment. Be supportive and allow patient and family to express their concerns. Refer to local support group.

SPINAL CORD IMPAIRMENT

The vertebral column houses the spinal cord. A small cartilage disk acts as a cushion between vertebrae. All sensory and motor nerves to the neck, trunk, and extremities branch out from the spinal cord. The degree of disability and patient problems is related to the part of the body controlled by the injured or diseased nerves. For herniated intervertebral disks, see the discussion of musculoskeletal conditions and disorders.

Spinal Cord Lesion

A. Definition: growth compressing the spinal cord; may be benign or malignant; interferes with nerve function
B. Cause: unknown
C. Signs and symptoms: individual, according to area involved
D. Diagnostic tests and methods
  1. Patient history
  2. MEG, CT, MRI
  3. Neurological assessment
E. Treatment: surgical removal
F. Nursing intervention: See care of a patient with a laminectomy (p. 179).

Spinal Cord Injuries

A. Description: Trauma to spinal cord may cause complete or partial severing of the spinal cord. If severing is complete, permanent paralysis of body parts below site of injury occurs; when partial damage occurs, edema may cause a temporary paralysis.
B. Cause: accident (e.g., automobile, shooting, diving)
C. Signs and symptoms: individual, according to level of spinal cord involved (signs of spinal shock)
  1. Respiratory distress
  2. Paralysis
D. Diagnostic tests and methods: physical examination
E. Treatment
  1. Immobilization: Crutchfield tongs, halo traction, back brace, or body cast
  2. Surgery, corticosteroids, mannitol
F. Nursing interventions
  1. See care of a patient with paralysis (p. 230); observe for complications of spinal shock.
  2. Maintain airway and respiratory function.
  3. See emergency care of a patient with a spinal cord injury, Chapter 10.

ENDOCRINE SYSTEM

ANATOMY AND PHYSIOLOGY

A. Classification and secretions
1. Exocrine glands: have ducts (tubes). Secretions are carried to an external or internal surface of the body by ducts (e.g., lacrimal gland).
2. Endocrine glands: ductless. Secretions by glands (hormones) are carried to body tissue by blood and lymph.
B. Endocrine glands and hormones (Figure 5-11 and Table 5-6)
1. Pituitary: located at base of the brain in a saddlelike depression of the sphenoid bone at the base of brain; called the *master gland,* approximately the size of a grape; composed of two parts
   a. Anterior lobe: secretes many hormones
   b. Posterior lobe: secretes two hormones
2. Thyroid: located in the neck inferior to the Adam's apple; easily palpated; the largest of the endocrine glands; consists of two lobes joined by a narrow band (isthmus)

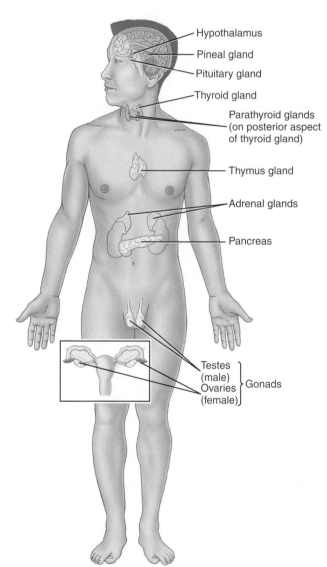

3. Parathyroid (four glands): located on posterior surface of the thyroid; regulates calcium level in the blood
4. Adrenal
   a. Two small glands; curve over the top of the kidneys
   b. Each gland has two separate parts: inner area (medulla) and outer area (cortex); produce different hormones.
   c. Medulla: mimics the action of the sympathetic nervous system
   d. Cortex: outer part of the adrenals: produces three major groups of steroid hormones
5. Gonads (sex glands)
   a. Ovaries in woman: located in pelvic cavity; produce ova and two hormones, estrogen and progesterone; do not function until puberty
   b. Testes in man: suspended in a sac called the *scrotum* outside the pelvic cavity; produce sperm and sex hormone, testosterone
6. Islets of Langerhans: located within the pancreas; consist of alpha and beta cells
   a. Alpha cells: produce glucagon
   b. Beta cells: secrete hormone insulin
7. Pineal: lies just above midbrain; secretes melatonin, which inhibits gonadotropic hormone secretion; exact function in humans is unclear.
C. Functions: regulators of body functions
1. Growth and development
2. Reproduction
3. Metabolism
4. Fluid and electrolyte balance

ENDOCRINE SYSTEM CONDITIONS AND DISORDERS

The endocrine system is composed of numerous glands and hormones. These hormones are chemical messengers for other target glands or cells. A disturbance in one of the secreting glands may affect regulation of another gland; therefore the patient may experience multiple problems and have varying needs. Some of the hormonal disturbances may affect patient appearance, personality, and stamina. Part of the nursing intervention is aimed at providing support and education for the patient and family. Some patients must undergo lifelong hormonal therapy as a result of their endocrine disorder.

NURSING ASSESSMENT

A. Observations
1. General appearance
2. Vital signs
3. Weight
4. Skin
   a. Color
      (1) Pallor
      (2) Flushed
      (3) Yellow pigmentation
      (4) Bronze pigmentation
      (5) Purple striae over obese areas
   b. Temperature
   c. Dry
   d. Moist
   e. Excess diaphoresis
   f. Poor wound healing

FIGURE 5-11 Major endocrine glands of the body. (From Herlihy B: *The human body in health and illness,* ed 4, St Louis, 2011, Saunders.)

Table 5-6   Endocrine Glands, Hormones, and Actions

ENDOCRINE GLANDS AND HORMONES	ACTIONS OF HORMONES
ANTERIOR PITUITARY	
Corticotropin (adrenocorticotropic hormone [ACTH])	Stimulates the adrenal cortex to produce and secrete glucocorticoid hormones
Somatotropic hormone (STH)	Stimulates growth of body cells
Thyroid-stimulating hormone (TSH)	Stimulates the thyroid gland to produce and release thyroid hormone
Gonadotropic hormones (GTHs)	Affect growth, maturity, and function of primary and secondary sex organs
Luteinizing hormone (LH)	
Lactogenic hormone (prolactin)	
Follicle-stimulating hormone (FSH)	
POSTERIOR PITUITARY	
Antidiuretic hormone (ADH)	Promotes sodium and water retention in the kidney; increases blood pressure
Oxytocin	Initiates and maintains labor; influences the breasts to release milk
THYROID	
Thyroxine	Regulates the metabolic rate of all body cells
PANCREAS	
Insulin	Promotes glucose use by the cell and decreases blood sugar level
Glucagon	Promotes glucose release from the liver and increases blood sugar level
ADRENAL CORTEX	
Glucocorticoids (include cortisol and cortisone)	Help the body respond to stress; concerned with carbohydrate, fat, protein metabolism; reduce inflammation
Mineralocorticoids (include aldosterone)	Promote sodium and water retention in the kidney and potassium excretion
Sex hormones (androgens, estrogen, progesterone)	Mainly affect development of secondary sex characteristics
ADRENAL MEDULLA	
Epinephrine (adrenaline) and norepinephrine (noradrenaline)	Constrict blood vessels and channel the blood to vital internal organs to prepare the body for emergency situations
OVARIES	
Estrogen	Promotes development of female sex characteristics, growth of female sex organs, and development of the uterine wall for implantation of the fertilized ovum; regulates menstruation
Progesterone	Prepares the uterine wall for implantation of the fertilized ovum; maintains the placenta and pregnancy; regulates menstruation
TESTES	
Androgens (includes testosterone)	Stimulates development of the secondary male sex characteristics; essential for normal functioning of male sex organs

5. Hair
   a. Dry
   b. Brittle
   c. Thin
6. Nails
   a. Dry
   b. Thin
   c. Thick
7. Musculoskeletal
   a. Muscle mass distribution
   b. Fat distribution
   c. Change in height

d. Changes in body proportions: enlarged ears, nose, jaws, hands, and feet
e. Diminished muscle strength
8. CNS
   a. Personality changes
   b. Alterations in consciousness
      (1) Listlessness
      (2) Slowed cognitive ability
      (3) Stupor
      (4) Seizures
      (5) Confusion
      (6) Coma

    c. Slowed, hoarse speech

    d. Reflexes

      (1) Trousseau sign

      (2) Chvostek sign

  9. Eyes

    a. Periorbital edema

    b. Protruding eyeball (exophthalmos)

    c. Drooping eyelids (ptosis)

  10. GI system

    a. Anorexia

    b. Polyphagia

    c. Polydipsia

    d. Constipation

    e. Diarrhea

    f. Nausea and vomiting

  11. Cardiovascular system

    a. Hypertension

    b. Hypotension

    c. Tachycardia

    d. Bradycardia

  12. Respiratory system

    a. Tachypnea

    b. Acetone breath

    c. Kussmaul respirations

  13. Renal system

    a. Polyuria

    b. Oliguria

  14. Reproductive system

    a. Menstrual disturbances

    b. Libido disturbances

    c. Galactorrhea (excess mammary gland secretion in women)

    d. Gynecomastia (increased breast tissue in men)

B. Patient description (subjective data)

  1. Pain

    a. Headache

    b. Skeletal pain

    c. Back pain

    d. Muscle spasms

  2. Appetite

    a. Anorexia

    b. Polyphagia

  3. Weakness

  4. Numbness

  5. Tingling

  6. Mood swings

  7. Nausea

  8. Intolerance to heat or cold

  9. Polydipsia

  10. Polyuria, nocturia, and dysuria

  11. Decreased libido and impotence

  12. Frequent infections

DIAGNOSTIC TESTS AND METHODS

A. Serum laboratory studies

  1. Protein-bound iodine (PBI)

    a. The thyroid hormone thyroxine (T_4) contains iodine that binds itself to blood proteins; therefore the function of the thyroid gland is evaluated by measuring the amount of this iodine.

    b. Factors that may alter test findings

      (1) Ingestion of drugs or administration of dyes containing iodine

      (2) Mercurial diuretics or estrogen

      (3) Pregnancy

  2. Radioactive iodine thyroid uptake (iodine-131 uptake)

    a. Measures the amount of radioactive iodine that has concentrated in the thyroid gland after ingestion of the iodine preparation

    b. Test findings may be altered by recent ingestion of iodides or use of radiographic dyes.

    c. A normal thyroid gland removes 15% to 50% of iodine from the bloodstream.

  3. Basal metabolic rate (BMR): measures the amount of oxygen consumed by the body while patient is in a state of complete mental and physical rest

  4. Triiodothyronine (T_3): measures thyroid function indirectly by evaluating whether radioactive T_3 binds to a serum specimen

  5. T_4: measures the amount of T_4 in the circulation

  6. Thyroid-stimulating hormone (TSH) radioimmunoassay: indicator of TSH production based on pituitary function; measures TSH levels

  7. Fasting blood sugar (FBS)

    a. Measures the amount of glucose in the bloodstream during a fasting period

    b. No food is permitted for 12 hours before the test.

    c. Normal value: 60 to 99 mg/dL

  8. Postprandial blood sugar

    a. Evaluates patient's ability to dispose of blood glucose after a meal

    b. Normal value: under 140 mg/dL serum

  9. Glucose tolerance test (GTT)

    a. Determines patient response to a measured dose of glucose

    b. Normal value: Blood glucose climbs to a peak of 140 mg/dL serum in the first hour and returns to normal by the second or third hour.

  10. Glycosylated Hgb

    a. Determines patient's control of blood glucose over a 3-month period

    b. Normal value for a person without diabetes is 4% to 6%; patients with diabetes mellitus have ranges from 7% to 9% or more.

  11. Serum potassium

    a. Measures the amount of potassium in the bloodstream

    b. Normal range: 3.5 to 5.5 mEq/L

  12. Serum sodium

    a. Measures the amount of sodium in the bloodstream

    b. Normal range: 135 to 145 mEq/L

  13. Total serum calcium

    a. Measures the amount of calcium in the bloodstream

    b. Normal range: 4.8 to 5.2 mEq/L (9 to 11 mg/dL)

  14. Serum ketones: determine the amount of ketones produced by the metabolism of fat

  15. Blood pH

    a. Measures the acid-base status of the blood

    b. Normal arterial blood findings: pH 7.35 to 7.45

    c. Normal venous blood findings: pH 7.31 to 7.41

  16. Serum phosphorus: measures the amount of serum phosphorus in the bloodstream

  17. Adrenocorticotropic hormone (ACTH) stimulating test (or glucocorticoid-stimulating test)

    a. Evaluates the changes in adrenocortical function produced by the administration of ACTH

b. ACTH is administered intramuscularly or intravenously.
c. For the intramuscular (IM) method a blood specimen is obtained 1 hour after administration of ACTH.
d. For the IV method a 24-hour urine specimen is collected and analyzed.
18. Cortisone suppression test: used to differentiate between Cushing syndrome and Cushing disease
19. Plasma cortisol
    a. Hormonal study of the adrenal cortex
    b. Low levels are seen in Addison disease.
    c. Elevated levels indicate Cushing syndrome.
20. Plasma cortisol response to ACTH
    a. Hormonal study of the adrenal cortex
    b. Patient's blood specimen is drawn in a fasting state and examined for plasma cortisol levels.
    c. Next, ACTH is administered intramuscularly, and a second blood sample is withdrawn.
    d. Rise in the plasma cortisol level in the second specimen is normal.
21. Urine 17-ketogenic steroids
    a. Measure adrenocortical function
    b. Urine specimen is collected for a 24-hour period and should be kept cold.
B. Urine laboratory studies
    1. 24-hour quantitative sugar specimen
        a. Evaluation of patient's glucose loss over a 24-hour period
        b. Urine normally free of sugar
        c. Nursing interventions
            (1) Have patient void and discard the specimen at the beginning of the 24-hour period.
            (2) Save all urine voided in a container provided by the laboratory.
            (3) At the end of the 24 hours have patient void again and save the specimen in the container.
    2. Urine pH
        a. Measures the acid-base balance of the urine
        b. Normal range: pH 4.8 to 7.5
    3. Quantitative urinary calcium: measures the amount of calcium in a 24-hour urine specimen after a period of calcium deprivation
    4. Vanillylmandelic acid (VMA) test
        a. Determines the amount of urinary excretion of the end product of catecholamine metabolism
        b. Factors that may alter test findings
            (1) Ingestion of coffee, tea, chocolate, bananas, vanilla-containing food, or aspirin
            (2) Stress
C. Scans
    1. Thyroid scan: radionuclide study of the thyroid to determine function
    2. CT scan: used to visualize cross-sections of tissue

FREQUENT PATIENT PROBLEMS AND NURSING CARE

A. Risk for situational low self-esteem related to changes in appearance from fluctuating hormones
    1. Observe patient for loss of appetite, insomnia, disinterest in self, and unwillingness to discuss alteration in body image.
    2. Encourage patient to express feelings.
    3. Encourage communication with significant other.

B. Imbalanced nutrition, less than body requirements, related to noncompliance with therapeutic diet
    1. Observe patient for diet intolerance such as refusal to eat, complaints about foods, and eating foods that are contraindicated.
    2. Explain to patient and family the reason for and intended effect of therapeutic diet and necessity of maintaining it until discontinued by physician.
    3. Instruct patient and family about prescribed food selection.
C. Deficient knowledge related to prescribed medication
    1. Explain to patient and family the dosage and method of administering prescribed drugs.
    2. Provide information about the purpose of the drug and potential side effects.
    3. Describe symptoms that should be reported to the physician.
    4. Explain where therapeutic supplies may be obtained.
    5. Evaluate patient's response to teaching.
D. High risk for injury related to toxic effects of iodine preparations; discontinue iodides if evidence of the following exists:
    1. Swelling of buccal mucosa
    2. Excessive salivation
    3. Swelling of neck glands
    4. Skin eruptions
E. High risk for injury related to hypoglycemia (see Critical Thinking Challenge box)

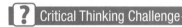 **? Critical Thinking Challenge**

Diabetes Mellitus

The nurse is passing 9 PM medications. She obtains a glucometer reading of 104 from a patient who is to receive 96 units of Levemir if the glucometer reading is greater than 100. The patient has met that parameter and the nurse administers the insulin.

At 3 AM the nurse finds the patient cold, sweaty, and confused. The nurse checks a glucometer reading and finds the blood glucose to be 56. She immediately alerts the RN and administers 15 g of carbohydrates to the individual (via orange juice). Fifteen minutes later the patient is more alert with a glucometer reading of 81.

The nurse did not know that the patient had been ill the night before. After administering the Levemir (for which the patient had just barely met the parameter for administration), the nurse was called to another floor to help out. During that time the patient had an emesis and refused the evening snack ordered for him. The combination of lack of food intake and insulin administration resulted in the patient having a dangerously low blood sugar level.

1. Observe for complaints of headache, nervousness, hunger, dizziness, pallor, and sweating (diaphoresis).
2. Assess vital signs.
3. Give quick-acting carbohydrate:
    a. Orange juice
    b. Cola
    c. Granulated sugar
    d. Crackers
    e. Hard candy
4. If patient is unconscious: Give instant glucose (buccally); glucagon (subcutaneously); IV glucose.

5. Have laboratory draw serum specimen for glucose assessment.
6. Assess reason for reaction after situation has been controlled.
   a. Length of time since last meal
   b. Correct amount of food eaten or meal omitted
   c. Correct dosage of insulin
   d. Kinds of activities or situation before reaction
F. High risk for injury (seizures) related to hypocalcemia
   1. Observe for complaints of numbness, tingling, cramping, or spastic movements of extremities.
   2. Emergency treatment requires administration of IV calcium.
   3. Prevent airway obstruction.
      a. Keep airway at bedside.
      b. Provide suction machine at bedside.
      c. Provide tracheostomy set at bedside.
   4. Prevent injury by putting padding along side rails, easing patient to floor, or removing constrictive clothes.
   5. Monitor and record vital signs.
   6. Note frequency, time, LOC, and length of seizure.

MAJOR MEDICAL DIAGNOSES

Hyperpituitarism

A. Definition: overproduction of growth hormone by the anterior pituitary gland
B. Pathology
   1. Increased activity of the gland usually results from a secreting pituitary tumor.
   2. Two major disorders arise from hypersecretion.
      a. Gigantism: develops in children; hypersecretion before the growth plate closes, results in bone and tissue growth
      b. Acromegaly: disorder in adults caused by hypersecretion after closure of the epiphyses of the long bones
C. Signs and symptoms
   1. Subjective
      a. Headache
      b. Visual disturbances
      c. Weakness
   2. Objective
      a. Coarse facial features: enlarged ears, nose, lips, tongue, and jaws
      b. Broad hands, fingers, and feet
      c. Palpable, enlarged visceral organs
      d. Disturbances in carbohydrate metabolism, menstruation, and libido
      e. Gynecomastia in men; galactorrhea in women
      f. Symmetrical bone overgrowth (gigantism)
      g. Increased heights; 8 to 9 ft (gigantism)
D. Diagnostic tests and methods
   1. X-ray studies of jaws, sinuses, hands, and feet
   2. Changes in physical appearance
   3. CT scan to identify tumor
   4. Cerebral arteriography to identify tumor
   5. Growth hormone assay
E. Treatment
   1. Surgical intervention: hypophysectomy (excision of the pituitary gland); excision of tumor with laser
   2. Irradiation of the pituitary gland
   3. Medication to treat symptoms related to other hormonal disturbances as a result of hypersecretion

F. Nursing interventions
   1. Assist patient to accept altered body image, emphasizing person's value as an individual.
   2. Explain basis for altered sexual functioning.
   3. Emphasize need for lifelong medical follow-up.
   4. If patient has undergone hypophysectomy:
      a. Perform nursing care as for patient who has undergone intracranial surgery.
      b. Observe for potential postoperative complications.
         (1) Adrenal insufficiency
         (2) Hypothyroidism
         (3) Diabetes insipidus

Hypopituitarism (Simmonds Disease)

A. Definition: total absence of all pituitary secretions
B. Pathology: occurs after destruction of the pituitary gland by surgery, infection, injury, hemorrhage, or tumor
C. Signs and symptoms
   1. Subjective
      a. Lethargy
      b. Loss of muscle strength
      c. Weakness
      d. Menstrual irregularities
   2. Objective
      a. Emaciation
      b. Pallor
      c. Dry, yellow skin
      d. Diminished axillary and pubic hair
      e. Decreased muscle size
      f. Increased susceptibility to infection
D. Diagnostic tests and methods
   1. T_3 and T_4
   2. Urine 17-ketogenic steroids
E. Treatment
   1. Replacement hormones
   2. Surgical ablation if tumor is present in pituitary gland
F. Nursing interventions
   1. Emphasize need for lifelong medical follow-up.
   2. Teach patient self-administration of drug: purpose, proper dosage, and potential side effects.
   3. Perform nursing care as for patient who has undergone intracranial surgery.

Hyperthyroidism (Graves Disease and Thyrotoxicosis)

A. Definition: overactivity of the thyroid gland with hypersecretion of T4
B. Pathology
   1. Metabolic rate is increased, resulting in a high amount of energy and oxygen expenditure.
   2. May be caused by decreased production of TSH by malfunctioning pituitary gland, which results in high T_4 serum concentration.
   3. May be attributed to enlarged thyroid gland caused by decreased iodine intake.
C. Signs and symptoms
   1. Subjective
      a. Polyphagia
      b. Hyperexcitability, personality changes
      c. Heat intolerance
      d. Insomnia
      e. Amenorrhea
      f. Diarrhea, constipation

g. Increased appetite

h. Fatigue, weakness

2. Objective

    a. Weight loss

    b. Exophthalmos

    c. Excessive sweating

    d. Increased pulse rate

    e. Fine hand tremors

    f. Warm, flushed skin

    g. Elevated blood pressure

    h. Bruit over thyroid

D. Diagnostic tests: increased laboratory values of T_3, T_4, iodine-131 uptake, PBI, and BMR to confirm hyperthyroidism; thyroid scan

E. Treatment

1. Medication to inhibit T_4 production

2. Radioactive iodine to destroy thyroid gland cells to decrease T_4 secretion

3. Drugs to control tachycardia and hyperexcitability

4. Subtotal or total thyroidectomy

F. Nursing interventions

1. Teach patient and family signs and symptoms of hypothyroidism when patient is receiving thyroid-inhibiting drugs.

    a. Increased body weight

    b. Sensitivity to cold

    c. Fatigue

    d. Dry skin, hair, and nails

    e. Slow, hoarse speech

    f. Constipation

2. Encourage adequate nutrition for increased energy expenditure.

    a. High-calorie, high-vitamin, and high-carbohydrate intake

    b. Between-meal snacks

    c. Increased fluid intake

    d. Avoidance of caffeine

3. Plan undisturbed rest periods to restore energy; provide cool, quiet, nonstressful environment.

4. Advise patient to elevate the head of bed while recumbent to improve eye drainage.

5. If patient has undergone surgery:

    a. Place him or her on back in low-Fowler or semi-Fowler position to avoid strain on sutures.

    b. Observe dressing for hemorrhage or constriction of the throat; examine back of neck for pooling of blood.

    c. Keep tracheostomy set at bedside in event of respiratory obstruction caused by hemorrhage, edema of glottis, laryngeal nerve damage, or tetany.

    d. Encourage him or her to cough and expectorate secretions from throat and bronchi.

    e. Observe for signs of thyroid storm (may occur as a result of gland manipulation during surgery): fever, tachycardia, and restlessness.

    f. Observe for signs of tetany (may occur if parathyroids are accidentally removed): numbness and tingling around mouth, carpopedal spasms, and convulsions.

Hypothyroidism

A. Definition: absence or decreased production of T_4 by the thyroid gland

B. Pathology

1. The disorder causes a depression of metabolic activity, resulting in physical and mental sluggishness.

2. Three classifications of hypothyroidism

    a. Cretinism: total absence of T4 from birth

    b. Hypothyroidism without myxedema: mild thyroid failure in older children and adults

    c. Hypothyroidism with myxedema: a severe form of gland failure in adults

C. Signs and symptoms

1. Subjective

    a. Lethargy

    b. Fatigues easily

    c. Cold intolerance

    d. Constipation

2. Objective

    a. Increased body weight with loss of appetite

    b. Coarse facial features

    c. Slow, hoarse speech

    d. Dry skin, hair, and nails

    e. Bradycardia

    f. Impaired memory

    g. Slowed thought process

    h. Personality changes

D. Diagnostic tests: decreased laboratory values of T_3, T_4, iodine-131 uptake, PBI, and BMR to confirm hypothyroidism; thyroid scan

E. Treatment: thyroid-replacement drugs

F. Nursing interventions

1. Educate patient on self-administration of drug: purpose, proper dosage, and potential side effects.

2. Emphasize need for lifelong medical follow-up.

3. Teach patient and family signs and symptoms of hyperthyroidism when receiving thyroid-replacement drugs: chest pain, tachycardia, nervousness, headache, excessive sweating, heat intolerance, and weight loss.

4. Encourage decreased caloric intake to avoid weight gain.

5. Encourage application of emollients to soothe dry skin.

Hyperparathyroidism

A. Definition: oversecretion of parathormone by one or more parathyroid glands

B. Pathology

1. Results in calcium loss from the bones and increased secretion of calcium and phosphorus by the kidneys

2. Usually the result of a parathyroid tumor

C. Signs and symptoms

1. Subjective

    a. Fatigue

    b. Thirst; poor appetite

    c. Nausea

    d. Back pain

    e. Skeletal pain

    f. Pain on weight bearing

    g. Constipation

    h. Visual disturbances

2. Objective

    a. Pathological fractures

    b. Vomiting

    c. Kidney stones composed of calcium phosphate

D. Diagnostic tests

1. Quantitative urinary calcium

2. Total serum calcium

3. Serum phosphorus

4. X-ray film to reveal skeletal changes

E. Treatment: surgical resection of parathyroid gland

F. Nursing interventions

   1. Observe for postoperative conditions (refer to postoperative nursing interventions for hyperthyroidism [Graves disease and thyrotoxicosis]).

   2. Observe for tetany: tingling of hands and feet, facial muscle spasms, and muscle twitching.

   3. Protect from accidents: position carefully, keep bed low, keep side rails up, and assist to ambulate.

   4. Explain rationale for low-calcium, low-phosphorus diet.

   5. Encourage adequate hydration and dietary fiber to avoid constipation.

Hypoparathyroidism

A. Definition: undersecretion of parathormone by the parathyroid glands

B. Pathology

   1. Insufficiency of parathormone causes a decrease of the serum calcium level and slows bone resorption.

   2. Increased serum phosphorus value

   3. Increased neuromuscular irritability that results in tetany

C. Signs and symptoms

   1. Subjective

     a. Lethargy

     b. Painful muscle spasms

     c. Tingling of hands and feet

     d. Visual disturbances

   2. Objective

     a. Dry skin, hair, and nails

     b. Respiratory distress caused by laryngeal spasms

     c. Convulsions

D. Diagnostic tests and methods

   1. Quantitative urinary calcium

   2. Total serum calcium

   3. Positive Trousseau sign (spasms of fingers and hands after application of blood pressure cuff to arm)

   4. Presence of Chvostek sign (hyperactivity of facial muscle in response to tapping near the angle of the jaw)

   5. X-ray studies reveal increased bone density.

E. Treatment

   1. Calcium replacement in chronic cases

   2. Calcium gluconate intravenously for emergency treatment

   3. Diet high in calcium and low in phosphorus

   4. Vitamin D preparation

F. Nursing interventions

   1. Keep endotracheal tube and tracheostomy set at bedside at all times when caring for patients with acute tetany.

   2. Promote rest with a quiet, calm, and dimly lit environment.

   3. Explain need for diet high in calcium but low in phosphorus: encourage avoidance of milk, cheese, and egg yolks.

   4. Emphasize importance of lifelong medical follow-up; serum calcium level should be assessed at least three times each year.

Diabetes Mellitus

A. Definition: insufficiency or absence of insulin production by pancreatic islets, creating a disturbance in carbohydrate metabolism and a deficiency in protein and fat conversion

B. Pathology

   1. Develops when a persistent deficiency of insulin occurs

   2. May be caused by trauma, infection, or tumor of the pancreas or increased insulin requirements attributable to obesity, pregnancy, infection, or stress

   3. Persons at risk: women older than 40 years and individuals who are obese or who have a familial tendency to diabetes

   4. Two classifications

     a. Type 1: insulin-dependent diabetes mellitus (IDDM) (formerly juvenile diabetes): rapid onset, with no production of insulin; affects children and adolescents; is controlled with insulin

     b. Type 2: non–insulin-dependent diabetes mellitus (NIDDM) (formerly adult onset): gradual onset; may be controlled by diet, oral hypoglycemic drugs, or insulin injection

   5. Lack of insulin disrupts transportation of glucose into cells, and cells become energy exhausted; cells must use proteins and fats as a compensatory mechanism.

   6. Blood sugar level becomes elevated because of lack of insulin in the cells.

   7. Cellular dehydration occurs because blood sugar pulls water from the cells into the bloodstream.

   8. Glucose builds up in urine, creating osmotic pull; kidneys cannot reabsorb water.

C. Signs and symptoms

   1. Subjective

     a. Polyuria and nocturia

     b. Polydipsia

     c. Polyphagia

     d. Weakness

     e. Blurred vision

   2. Objective

     a. Hyperglycemia

     b. Glycosuria

     c. Polyuria

     d. Ketosis

     e. Weight loss

     f. Retarded wound healing

D. Diagnostic tests and methods

   1. Presence of polyuria, polydipsia, and polyphagia

   2. Family and medical history

   3. Laboratory studies: FBS, postprandial blood sugar, GTT, and glycosylated Hgb

   4. 24-hour urine quantitative sugar specimen

E. Treatment

   1. Drug therapy for hyperglycemia; refer to Chapter 3 for indicated nursing actions.

   2. Therapeutic diet with controlled calories to correct and avoid obesity

     a. American Diabetes Association (ADA) food exchange list; widely prescribed by physicians

     b. Identifies calorie intake of protein (15% to 20%), carbohydrates (50% to 60%), fats (no more than 30%)

F. Nursing interventions

   1. Assist patient in adjusting to condition. Allow verbalization of feelings, offer reassurance, and give support at patient's own pace.

   2. Emphasize need to comply with diet and eat meals at prescribed times.

3. Instruct patient and family on signs of impending hypoglycemia: diaphoresis; pale, cold, and clammy skin; nervousness; hunger; mental confusion. Give orange juice, sugar, or hard candy.
4. Encourage prompt treatment of minor injuries to or irritation of skin.
5. Emphasize importance of continued medical follow-up, regular vision examinations, and foot care.
6. Patient teaching should include:
   a. Self–blood-glucose-level monitoring.
   b. Self-injection of insulin: selection of equipment, sites of injection, rationale for rotation, accurate withdrawal of insulin, injection technique, and peak action time of insulin.
   c. How to use food substitution if using the ADA meal plans.
   d. How to count carbohydrates and administer insulin accordingly if using carbohydrate-counting method for insulin administration.
   e. Instructions on foot care: hygiene, proper trimming of toenails, proper fit of shoes and stockings, and treatment of minor abrasions.
   f. Relationship between exercise and blood glucose.
7. Instruct patient and family about signs and symptoms of impending ketoacidosis: hot, dry, flushed skin; polydipsia; fruity odor of breath; nausea; and abdominal pain.
8. Administer insulin by way of pump.
   a. Method of needle insertion and filling of syringe
   b. Instruction on site rotation and needle change every 4 to 8 hours
   c. Removal of pump and covering of needle and tubing for bathing

Diabetic Coma (Ketoacidosis)

A. Definition: excess glucose and acid (ketones) in the bloodstream
B. Pathology
   1. A response to insufficient insulin levels primarily seen in type 1 diabetes mellitus (IDDM)
   2. Fats are mobilized for energy; fatty acids are rejected by muscles, resulting in buildup of acids in the bloodstream.
   3. Body's buffer system becomes exhausted.
C. Signs and symptoms
   1. Subjective
      a. Weakness
      b. Polydipsia
      c. Abdominal pain
      d. Nausea
      e. Headache
      f. Polyphagia
   2. Objective
      a. Hot, dry, flushed skin
      b. Listlessness and drowsiness
      c. Kussmaul respirations
      d. Sweet or acetone breath
      e. Hypotension
      f. Confusion
      g. Polyuria
      h. Nausea and vomiting
      i. Coma

D. Diagnostic tests
   1. Elevated serum glucose level
   2. Elevated serum and urinary ketones
   3. Lowered blood pH
E. Treatment
   1. Insulin replacement
   2. Correction of electrolyte and pH imbalance
   3. Fluid replacement
F. Nursing interventions
   1. Give insulin as ordered; have another person check to prevent error.
   2. Monitor and record vital signs and intake and output.
   3. Test for glucose and acetone levels; record on diabetic flow sheet.
   4. Position patient with head of bed elevated 30 degrees.
   5. Maintain patent airway.
   6. Give oral care every 4 hours and p.r.n.; keep lips and mouth moist.
   7. Assess LOC.
   8. Observe patient for signs of hypoglycemia: pale, cool, clammy skin; lethargy; and hypotension.
   9. Instruct patient and family on factors and signs of impending ketoacidosis.
   10. Explain importance of balance among diet, exercise, and insulin.
   11. Before discharge, provide diabetic alert band or chain.

Hyperglycemic Hyperosmolar Nonketotic Coma (HHNC)

A. Definition: similar to ketoacidosis but occurs primarily in type 2 diabetes mellitus (NIDDM). Ketosis does not develop.
B. Pathology: high serum glucose levels increase osmotic pressure, leading to polyuria. Dehydration occurs at the cellular level.
C. Signs and symptoms
   1. Subjective
      a. Polyuria
      b. Polydipsia
      c. Drowsiness
      d. Confusion
   2. Objective
      a. Dry, hot skin
      b. Flushed skin
      c. Hyperglycemia
      d. Glycosuria
      e. Hypotension
D. Diagnostic tests (see section on diabetic coma [ketoacidosis])
E. Treatment (see section on diabetic coma [ketoacidosis])
F. Nursing interventions (see section on diabetic coma [ketoacidosis])

Hypoglycemia (Insulin Shock)

A. Definition: abnormally low level of glucose in the bloodstream
B. Pathology
   1. Accelerated glucose removed from the serum
   2. May be caused by overproduction or overdosage of insulin
   3. Omission of a meal or too little food eaten by a patient receiving insulin
   4. Too much exercise without extra food; rapid onset

C. Signs and symptoms
1. Subjective
   a. Hunger
   b. Weakness
   c. Visual disturbances
   d. Tingling lips and tongue
   e. Nervousness
2. Objective
   a. Pale, moist skin
   b. Tremors
   c. Tachycardia
   d. Hypotension
   e. Muscle weakness
   f. Disorientation
   g. Coma
D. Diagnostic test: lowered serum glucose level
E. Treatment
1. Sweetened fluids or sugar given orally; oral glucose preparations
2. Glucagon subcutaneously or intramuscularly
3. Glucose intravenously
F. Nursing interventions
1. Give medications as ordered.
2. Monitor and record vital signs and intake and output.
3. Patient teaching should include the following:
   a. Always carry and ingest quick-acting carbohydrate when initial signs appear: fruit juices, sweetened sodas, granulated sugar, or hard candy.
   b. Prevent medication error by having another person check dosage.
   c. Record each administration of medication to avoid duplication.
   d. Always wear medical identification tag.
   e. To prevent a rebound effect, remember to eat a regular meal after raising glucose level.

Diabetes Insipidus

A. Definition: water metabolism disorder related to hyposecretion of antidiuretic hormone (ADH) by the posterior pituitary lobe
B. Pathology
1. Renal tubules are unable to reabsorb water, resulting in elimination of large amounts of water.
2. Hyposecretion may occur in conjunction with lung cancer, head injuries, pituitary tumor, myxedema, or encephalitis.
3. Other causes may result from malfunctioning, surgical removal of, or atrophy of the pituitary gland.
C. Signs and symptoms
1. Subjective
   a. Polydipsia
   b. Polyuria
2. Objective
   a. Signs of dehydration (loss of skin turgor, dry skin and mucous membranes, cracked lips)
   b. Low specific gravity (sp gr) (1.001 to 1.006)
   c. Increased fluid intake (5 to 40 L/24 hr)
   d. Increased urine output (5 to 25 L/24 hr)
   e. Electrolyte imbalance
D. Diagnostic method: restriction of fluid intake to observe changes in urine volume and concentration
E. Treatment: vasopressin replacement

F. Nursing interventions
1. Monitor and record intake and output.
2. Monitor specific gravity.
3. Weigh patient daily.

Primary Hyperaldosteronism (Conn Syndrome)

A. Definition: hypersecretion of aldosterone by the adrenal cortex
B. Pathology
1. Usually caused by a tumor or tumors, which results in renal retention of sodium and excretion of potassium
2. Leads to inability of kidneys to concentrate urine (acidify)
C. Signs and symptoms
1. Subjective
   a. Headache
   b. Polyuria and polydipsia
   c. Paresthesia
2. Objective
   a. Hypertension with postural hypotension
   b. Signs of kidney damage: flank pain, chills, fever, and increased frequency of voiding
   c. Low specific gravity
D. Diagnostic tests
1. Low serum potassium level
2. Elevated serum sodium value
3. Elevated urinary aldosterone level
4. Increased urine pH
5. X-ray study reveals cardiac hypertrophy caused by chronic hypertension.
E. Treatment: surgical removal of adrenal tumor
F. Nursing interventions
1. Monitor and record blood pressure, specific gravity, and intake and output.
2. Identify and explain diet high in potassium and low in sodium.
3. Provide fluids to meet excessive thirst.
4. If patient has undergone adrenalectomy:
   a. Protect from exposure to infections.
   b. Follow general postoperative nursing actions.
5. Once patient is convalescent, teach self-administration of drugs: purpose, proper dosage, and potential side effects.
6. Before discharge obtain medical identification tag.

Cushing Syndrome

A. Definition: hyperactivity of the adrenal cortex
B. Pathology
1. Excessive cortisol is secreted.
2. Disorder results from abnormal growth of cortices or tumor to one of the glands.
3. May occur because of pituitary gland dysfunction, causing excessive production of ACTH
C. Signs and symptoms
1. Subjective
   a. Weakness
   b. Easy bruising
   c. Amenorrhea
   d. Decreased libido
   e. Changes in secondary sex characteristics
2. Objective
   a. Fat deposits to face, back of neck, and abdomen
   b. Decreased muscle mass on limbs
   c. Unusual growth of body hair
   d. Purple striae over obese areas

    e. Impaired wound healing

    f. Hypertension

    g. Mood lability

D. Diagnostic tests

   1. Increased plasma cortisol levels

   2. ACTH stimulating test

   3. Cortisone suppression test

E. Treatment

   1. Drugs to inhibit cortisol production

   2. Bilateral adrenalectomy

   3. Resection of pituitary gland

   4. Potassium supplements

   5. Diet with sodium restriction

F. Nursing interventions

   1. Assist patient in adjusting to altered body image.

   2. Place in noninfectious environment.

   3. Maintain diet low in calories, carbohydrates, and sodium and high in potassium.

   4. Weigh patient daily.

   5. Monitor glucose and acetone levels.

   6. Follow general postoperative nursing actions if patient undergoes adrenalectomy.

   7. Once patient is convalescent, instruct on self-administration of replacement hormones and drugs: proper dosage, purpose, and potential side effects.

Addison Disease (Adrenocortical Insufficiency)

A. Definition: hypofunction of adrenal cortex

B. Pathology

   1. As a result of dysfunction, adrenal cortex shrinks and atrophies.

   2. Disorder usually originates within the adrenal cortex (gland unable to secrete sufficient hormones) or may result from destruction of the adrenal cortex.

   3. Results in disturbances of sodium and potassium

C. Signs and symptoms

   1. Subjective

    a. Weakness and fatigue

    b. Anorexia and nausea

    c. Depression

    d. Diarrhea

    e. Abdominal pain

   2. Objective

    a. Weight loss

    b. Hypotension

    c. Hypoglycemia

    d. Bronze or tan skin pigmentation

    e. Susceptibility to infection

    f. Arrhythmias

D. Diagnostic tests

   1. 8-hour IV ACTH test

   2. Plasma cortisol response to ACTH

   3. Low serum sodium level

   4. High serum potassium level

E. Treatment

   1. Replacement of adrenal cortex hormones

   2. Restoration of sodium and potassium balance

   3. Diet high in sodium and low in potassium, with adequate fluids

F. Nursing interventions

   1. Monitor and record vital signs and intake and output.

   2. Weigh patient daily.

   3. Observe for sodium imbalance: increased body weight, pitting edema, puffy eyelids, coughing, and diaphoresis.

   4. Observe for potassium imbalance: lethargy, flaccid muscles, anorexia, hypotension, and arrhythmias.

   5. Provide small, frequent feedings.

   6. Observe for hypoglycemia: weakness, clammy skin, tremors, and mental confusion.

   7. Before discharge, obtain medical identification tag.

   8. Emphasize need for compliance with diet and medication regimen.

   9. Observe for addisonian crisis (causes: stress, surgery, trauma, infection, withdrawal of medication): hypotension, asthenia, abdominal pain, confusion, shock, and vascular collapse.

  10. Teach patient to avoid infections and stressful situations.

Pheochromocytoma

A. Definition: hyperactivity of the adrenal medulla

B. Pathology: caused by tumor in adrenal medulla, resulting in increased secretion of epinephrine and norepinephrine

C. Signs and symptoms

   1. Subjective

    a. Headache

    b. Visual disturbances

    c. Nervousness

    d. Heat intolerance

   2. Objective

    a. Hypertension (blood pressure may be as high as 220/140 mm Hg)

    b. Orthostatic hypotension

    c. Tachycardia

    d. Hyperglycemia

    e. Blanching of skin

    f. Weight loss

    g. Arrhythmias

    h. Diaphoresis

D. Diagnostic tests

   1. Chemical and pharmacological drug tests to differentiate from hypertension or hyperthyroidism

   2. X-ray studies to reveal adrenal medullary tumor

   3. 24-hour urine collection for VMA and metanephrines

   4. Arteriography

   5. CT scan

   6. IV pyelogram (IVP)

E. Treatment

   1. Surgical excision of tumor

   2. Drugs to control hypertension and arrhythmias

F. Nursing interventions

   1. Monitor blood pressure every 4 hours and record.

   2. Plan undisturbed rest periods: cool, quiet, nonstressful environment.

   3. Encourage adequate hydration; record intake and output.

   4. If patient undergoes adrenalectomy, follow general postoperative nursing actions: observe for adrenal crisis—falling blood pressure, tachycardia, elevated temperature, restlessness, convulsions, and coma.

   5. Patient teaching should include:

    a. Self-administration of medications: purpose, proper dosage, and potential side effects.

    b. Signs of impending adrenal crisis.

c. Avoidance of exposure to infection; reporting of symptoms of infections to physician.

d. Avoidance of stressful situations.

e. Emphasis on need for adequate rest and good nutrition.

6. Provide medical identification tag.

RENAL (URINARY) SYSTEM

ANATOMY AND PHYSIOLOGY

A. Organs (Figure 5-12)

1. Kidneys: bean shaped and reddish brown; lie against posterior abdominal wall; right kidney is slightly lower than left.

a. External structure

(1) Hilus: concave notch. Blood vessels, nerves, lymphatic vessels, and ureters enter the kidneys at this point.

(2) Renal capsule; protective fibrous tissue surrounding kidneys

b. Internal structure

(1) Cortex: outer portion. The greater portion of the nephron is located here.

(2) Medulla: inner portion; consists of 12 cone-shaped structures (pyramids). Tip of pyramid points toward renal pelvis and drains waste and excess water into pelvis.

(3) Pelvis: funnel shaped; forms upper end of ureter and receives waste and water

c. Nephron: basic unit of function; microscopic structure composed of capillaries; approximately 1 million per kidney; controls the processes of filtration, reabsorption, and secretion (Figure 5-13)

(1) Glomerulus: filtering unit. Process of urine formation begins here.

(2) Renal tubules: Reabsorption occurs in the proximal convoluted tubules, through Henle loops, and the distal convoluted tubules. The collecting tubules then pass the final urine product into the pelvis.

2. Ureters: two long, narrow tubes; transport urine from kidney to bladder by peristalsis

3. Bladder: elastic, muscular organ, capable of expansion; stores urine; assists in voiding (micturition: the release of urine or voiding)

4. Urethra: narrow, short tube from bladder to exterior; exterior opening called the *meatus*

a. In women: approximately 1¼ to 2 inches (3 to 5 cm) long; transports urine

b. In men: approximately 8 inches (20 cm) long; transports urine and is a passageway for semen

B. Functions

1. Excretion: Nitrogen-containing waste (urea, uric acid, creatinine) is excreted. Normal daily output is 1200 to

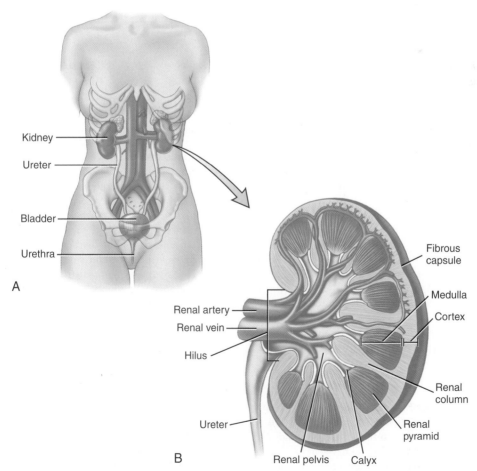

FIGURE 5-12 **A,** Organs of the urinary system. **B,** Internal structure of a kidney. (From Herlihy B: *The human body in health and illness,* ed 4, St Louis, 2011, Saunders.)

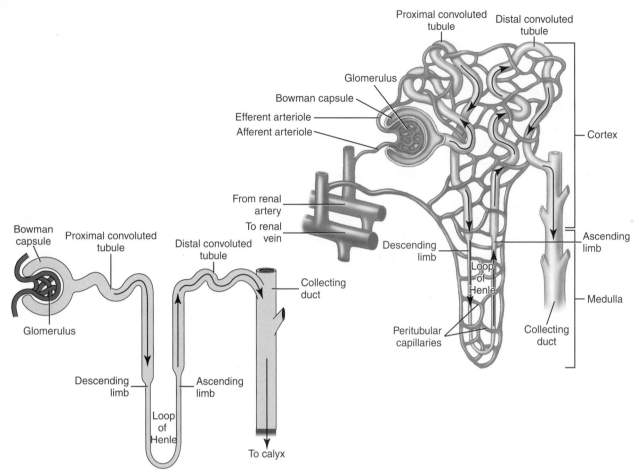

FIGURE 5-13 The nephron unit. (From Herlihy B: *The human body in health and illness,* ed 4, St Louis, 2011, Saunders.)

1500 mL. Primary function is to regulate the volume and composition of extracellular fluid.

2. Maintenance of water balance: absorbs more or less water, depending on intake. Normally intake is approximately equal to output.
3. Other major functions include renin secretion and blood pressure control, erythropoietin production, vitamin D activation, and acid-base balance.

C. Urine composition
1. Clear, yellowish, slightly aromatic, and slightly acid
2. Contains 95% water and 5% solids, which include urea, uric acid, creatinine, ammonia, sodium, and potassium; specific gravity indicates amount of the dissolved solids; normal range: 1.003 to 1.035.
3. Abnormal substances: glucose, blood protein, RBCs, bile, and bacteria

RENAL (URINARY) SYSTEM CONDITIONS AND DISORDERS

The urinary system regulates the composition and volume of the blood. It excretes metabolic wastes and fluids and maintains fluid, electrolyte, and acid-base balance. Malfunction of this system has generalized effects on the normal physiology of the body. Frequently patients are older and have chronic medical problems (e.g., cardiac conditions); these problems must be considered when nursing care is planned (e.g., many diagnoses and procedures require additional fluids as a natural irrigation;

increased fluids might be contraindicated in the patient with a cardiac condition). Problems of the male reproductive system are discussed in this section.

The following terms are used to describe urine output:
- Anuria: absence of urine output
- Bacteriuria: bacteria in the urine
- Costovertebral angle tenderness: Examiner strikes one or more light blows to the area where the lower ribs meet the vertebrae (flank); tenderness in this area may indicate renal disorders.
- Dribbling: voiding without stream, in small amounts, frequently or constantly
- Dysuria: painful or difficult urination
- Enuresis: involuntary voiding while asleep
- Frequency: voiding often and in small amounts
- Hematuria: blood in the urine
- Hesitancy: inability to immediately empty the full bladder when the desire is present
- Hydronephrosis: dilation of the pelvis and calices of one or both kidneys resulting from obstruction of the flow of urine
- Incontinence: partial or complete inability to control urine output
- Micturition: voiding, urination
- Nocturia: awakening to void
- Overflow incontinence: leakage of urine in small amounts while bladder remains full and distended
- Polyuria: excessive production and excretion of urine

- Residual urine: urine remaining in the bladder after voiding
- Retention: inability to excrete urine from bladder
- Urgency: an intense stimulus to void (may cause incontinence)
- Voiding: micturition, elimination of urine

NURSING ASSESSMENT

A. Observations
1. Observe bladder for distention: lower abdominal area is rigid, tense, swollen, and sensitive to the touch.
2. Assess urine: amount, color, odor, opacity (clear or cloudy), and presence of sediment, mucus, or clots.
3. Check catheter (if indwelling) for drainage and meatus for irritation or secretions.
4. Check genitalia (scrotum, labia, anal area) for irritation, rashes, and lesions.
5. Monitor fluid and electrolyte balance.
6. Check eyes, extremities, presacral area, and scrotum for edema.
7. Monitor vital signs; note elevation of temperature and blood pressure.
8. Note problems related to aging (e.g., urgency, stress incontinence).

B. Patient description (subjective data)
1. Change in voiding habits
2. Problems with elimination or changes in patterns of urination
   a. Frequency
   b. Nocturia
   c. Hesitancy of stream
   d. Urgency
   e. Retention
   f. Incontinence
   g. Enuresis
   h. Dribbling
3. Urethral discharge
4. Burning on voiding
5. Pain: suprapubic or flank

C. Obtain patient history regarding:
1. Normal urinary and bowel elimination habits.
2. Medical problems with the urinary system (e.g., stones, sexually transmitted diseases [STDs]).
3. Medical problems with other body systems (e.g., cardiac conditions), trauma.
4. Medications.
5. Diet.
6. Food or medication allergies.
7. Decreased urinary stream.
8. Pain or spasms: what precipitated this, and what relieved it?
9. Discharge.
10. Edema.

DIAGNOSTIC TESTS AND METHODS

A. Blood studies
1. BUN: Normal level is 10 to 20 mg/dL. Urea is an end product of protein metabolism and is excreted by the kidneys in urine; an increase indicates impaired renal function.
2. Creatinine: Normal level is 0.5 to 1.3 mg/dL; elevation indicates decreased renal function.
3. Acid and alkaline phosphatase: Normal value varies with laboratory; increase may indicate metastasis to bone or liver from the kidney. Nurse must assess for bone fracture or pathological conditions of the liver.
4. Albumin/globulin ratio is usually 2:1. A change indicates damage to nephron and loss of albumin in the urine; patient retains fluid and has edema.

B. Urine studies
1. Routine urinalysis: a single voided specimen to observe and compare with known normal specimens. Results give information about renal function and systemic health.
2. Specific gravity: normal value 1.003 to 1.035; change indicates dehydration or inadequate kidney function. A single voided specimen is required.
3. Urine culture and sensitivity (see Chapter 2)
4. Creatine: 24-hour urine collection to measure creatinine excreted. Oral fluids are encouraged (see Chapter 2).

C. X-ray procedures, radiographic studies
1. Kidneys, ureter, bladder (KUB): an abdominal x-ray study that gives baseline information about size, shape, and placement of organs; flatus and stones are visualized; no preparation or care after procedure is required.
2. IVP: an IV injection of a radiopaque dye that is rapidly excreted by the kidney. This tests renal function; x-ray films outline renal pelvis, ureters, bladder, and urethra. Nursing responsibilities: Maintain NPO status before procedure; after procedure observe for allergic reaction to dye; note voiding.
3. Retrograde pyelogram: visualization of upper genitourinary (GU) tract by injection of radiopaque dye through ureteral catheters to locate obstruction (e.g., stone, tumor). Nursing responsibilities: Preparation is the same as preoperative preparation (see Chapter 2). After procedure monitor vital signs, anticipate pain, and administer analgesics; note voiding and observe urine.
4. Cystoscopy: a direct visualization of the bladder and urethral orifices. A cystoscope is inserted through the urethra into the bladder; the bladder is distended with sterile solution. Stones, tumors, and polyps can be diagnosed; urine can be observed entering the bladder from each ureter to evaluate renal function. Instruments may be passed through the cystoscope to crush stones, take biopsy specimens, or pass catheters into ureters. Nursing responsibilities: Provide general preoperative and postoperative care (see Chapter 2). After procedure determine what was done during procedure; assess urinary function, observe urine; provide care and observation of a patient with indwelling catheter (see Chapter 2).
5. Renogram: also called *renal angiogram;* for before and after procedure see discussion of retrograde pyelogram.
6. CT scan

D. Other procedures
1. MRI
2. Urodynamic studies

FREQUENT PATIENT PROBLEMS AND NURSING CARE

A. Incontinence (types: urge, total, stress, reflex, functional) related to catheter use, infection, tissue damage, immobility
1. Minimize embarrassment; provide privacy.

2. Wash, dry, and inspect skin; take measures to prevent decubitus ulcers (pressure sores).

3. Provide bladder training.

B. Impaired skin integrity related to retention of metabolic wastes and resulting toxicity (uremia)

1. Urea is excreted through the skin, causing odor and pruritus. Provide frequent and thorough skin care; wash and pat dry.

2. Confusion and disorientation; may progress to state of unconsciousness and coma. Provide all care; maintain safety (see nursing care of a patient in a coma in section on special situations, p. 230)

3. Nausea and vomiting: Provide mouth care every 2 hours.

4. Renal failure: See nursing interventions for chronic renal failure (end-stage renal disease) later in this chapter.

C. Pain related to bladder spasms: Bladder spasms caused by catheter irritation are intermittent in the suprapubic area, radiating to the urethra.

1. Assess type, location, and severity of pain.

2. Check catheter for obstruction; irrigate as ordered.

3. Administer medication as ordered (see discussion of urinary tract antispasmodic analgesics, Chapter 3).

4. Reassure patient that spasms are not abnormal.

D. Deficient fluid volume related to dehydration

1. Use hydration methods (encourage fluids).

2. Monitor intake and output.

E. Risk for infection or injury (hematuria) related to surgery or pathogens

1. Monitor signs and symptoms, vital signs.

2. Administer medication as ordered.

3. Note characteristics of urine at each voiding.

4. Encourage fluids if not contraindicated.

5. Report and document clots noted in urine.

6. Maintain patency and gravity drainage of catheters.

7. Assess for signs of anemia (weakness and fatigue).

8. Provide nursing care and safety as indicated.

9. Reassure patient that blood-tinged urine is not unusual after instrumentation or surgery.

F. Urinary retention related to surgery

1. Perform nursing measures to assist patient with voiding (see Chapter 2).

2. Monitor intake and output.

3. Encourage fluids if not contraindicated.

G. Anxiety related to sexual dysfunction, impending surgery, or possible change in body image or function

1. Provide time to listen to patient express feelings.

2. Explain all care and procedures; reassure often.

3. Be honest, provide privacy, avoid embarrassing situations.

4. Praise patient's progress toward discharge goals.

H. Risk for excess fluid volume related to inability to filter urine

1. Assess deep skin (e.g., sacral, feet).

2. Monitor lung sounds.

MAJOR MEDICAL DIAGNOSES

Cystitis

A. Definition: inflammation of the bladder mucosa; difficult to cure; recurs and may be chronic

B. Pathology: usually from a bacterial infection

1. May be secondary to infection elsewhere in urinary system (e.g., urethritis)

2. Contamination during catheterization or instrumentation

3. An obstruction causing urinary stasis in the bladder (e.g., enlarged prostate, urethral stricture)

C. Signs and symptoms

1. Subjective

a. Burning, dysuria, urgency, frequency, nocturia, hematuria, and pyuria

b. Low-back pain and bladder spasms

2. Objective: elevation of temperature

D. Diagnostic tests and methods

1. Patient history and assessment

2. Urine culture, IVP, voiding cystoureterogram

E. Treatment: systemic medications, urinary antiseptics, antibiotics, sulfonamides, and antispasmodics (see Chapter 3)

F. Nursing interventions

1. Encourage fluids: 3000 mL daily over that of dietary intake unless contraindicated.

2. Provide and supervise proper perineal care.

3. Provide diet that acidifies urine (e.g., cranberry juice).

4. Monitor temperature and administer antipyretics as ordered.

5. Provide sitz baths.

6. Teach preventive measures.

a. Taking full course of antibiotic therapy as prescribed

b. Emptying bladder completely

c. Maintaining a consistent fluid intake of 2 L per day

d. Voiding after sexual intercourse

Urethritis

A. Definition: inflammation of the urethra; may result in formation of scar tissue and stricture, causing obstruction, cystitis, and nephritis

B. Pathology

1. Prostatitis; injury during instrumentation or catheterization

2. Gonococcus infection; chlamydial infection

C. Signs and symptoms

1. Subjective

a. Urgency

b. Frequency

c. Dysuria

d. Burning on urination

2. Objective

a. Purulent discharge

b. Results of urine culture

D. Diagnostic tests and methods

1. Patient history and physical examination

2. Culture of discharge

E. Treatment

1. Antibiotics

2. Dilation for stricture

F. Nursing interventions

1. Provide sitz baths.

2. Demonstrate and supervise thorough handwashing.

3. Teach monitoring and care of Foley catheter.

4. Avoid unnecessary catheterization and instrumentation.

Pyelonephritis

A. Definition: infection of the kidney; may be acute or become chronic. Kidney becomes edematous, mucosa is inflamed, and multiple abscesses may form. Kidney becomes fibrotic, and uremia may develop.

B. Pathology
  1. Ascending infection from an infection lower in the GU tract
  2. Staphylococcal or streptococcal infection carried in the blood
C. Signs and symptoms
  1. Subjective
     a. Nausea
     b. Chills
     c. Dysuria, burning, frequency
     d. Costovertebral angle tenderness
  2. Objective
     a. Markedly elevated temperature (102° to 105° F)
     b. Vomiting
     c. Pyuria, hematuria
     d. Increased WBC count
     e. Results of urine cultures and IVP
D. Diagnostic tests and methods
  1. Urine culture and sensitivity
  2. Patient history and physical examination
  3. IVP
E. Treatment: urinary antiseptics and specific antibiotics (see Chapter 3); follow-up care for at least 1 year
F. Nursing interventions
  1. Prevent dehydration; encourage fluids and maintain IV therapy.
  2. Provide rest and conserve energy.
  3. Prevent chill; keep skin dry and clean.
  4. Provide mouth care every 2 hours.
  5. Provide soft diet.
  6. Provide and assist with perineal care. Demonstrate proper technique and handwashing.
  7. Anticipate pain; administer analgesics and local heat.
  8. Administer antiemetic as needed.
  9. Control temperature; administer antipyretics.

Calculi (Lithiasis)
A. Definition: formation of stones in the urinary tract caused by deposits of crystalline substance that normally remains in solution and is excreted in the urine; may be found in the kidney, ureters, or bladder; vary in size from renal calculi that can be as large as an orange or as small as grains of sand; can obstruct urine flow, causing chronic infection, backflow, hydronephrosis, and gradual destruction of kidney. Many small stones pass spontaneously.
B. Cause
  1. Infection
  2. Urinary stasis
  3. Dehydration and concentration of urine
  4. Metabolic diseases (e.g., gout, hyperparathyroidism)
  5. Immobility (see dangers of immobility, Chapter 2)
  6. Familial tendency
  7. Elevated uric acid
  8. Excessive calcium intake
C. Signs and symptoms
  1. Subjective
     a. Pain (can be extreme) radiating down flank to pubic area
     b. Frequency and urgency
  2. Objective
     a. Hematuria and pyuria
     b. Diaphoresis, nausea, vomiting, pallor (related to pain)
     c. Results of diagnostic tests

D. Diagnostic tests and methods: x-ray studies (KUB, IVP), urine studies (ultrasonography, cystoscopy, serial blood calcium and phosphorus levels)
E. Treatment: depends on location—removal of stones, restoration of normal urine production and elimination, prevention of recurrence
  1. Cystoscopy and crushing of stones (lithotripsy)
  2. Dislodgement of ureteral stone by passage of ureteral catheter; laser lithotripsy
  3. Surgery to remove ureteral or kidney stone
     a. Pyelolithotomy: removal of stones from renal pelvis
     b. Nephrolithotomy: incision through kidney and removal of stone
     c. Ureterolithotomy: removal of ureteral calculus
     d. Transcutaneous shock wave lithotripsy: ultrasonic waves used to disintegrate renal calculi
     e. Percutaneous stone dissolution: chemical agents injected into a nephrostomy tube to dissolve the stone
F. Nursing interventions
  1. Provide general preoperative and postoperative nursing care (see Chapter 2).
  2. Supervise and explain diet restrictions as ordered according to type of stone.
  3. Provide analgesics as ordered.
  4. Observe, describe, and strain all urine.
  5. Maintain gravity drainage; never clamp ureteral or nephrostomy catheters.
  6. Observe patency of catheters; in most cases never irrigate renal or ureteral catheters.
  7. Record output from each catheter separately; immediately report scanty output from one tube.
  8. Encourage fluids (but keep NPO if nausea, vomiting, or abdominal distention occurs).

Hydronephrosis
A. Definition: accumulation of fluid in the renal pelvis; distention of the renal tubules, calyces, and pelvis present; renal tissues destroyed from pressure; leads to uremia (azotemia)
B. Pathology
  1. Congenital defective drainage; blockage from stones or scar tissues
  2. Reflux (backup) from obstructed bladder neck in benign prostatic hypertrophy
C. Signs and symptoms
  1. Subjective
     a. Related to cause; in some patients no symptoms or mild pain
     b. Severe colicky renal pain
     c. Flank pain radiating to groin
     d. Dysuria
     e. Oliguria to anuria
     f. Nausea
     g. Abdominal fullness
     h. Dribbling, hesitancy
  2. Objective
     a. Hematuria, pyuria
     b. Results of diagnostic tests
D. Diagnostic tests and methods
  1. Patient history and physical examination
  2. Blood serum tests (urea, creatinine)
  3. IVP, ultrasonography

E. Treatment
1. Removal of the cause
2. Provision of adequate urinary drainage (e.g., bladder catheter, nephrostomy tube)
3. Antibiotics
F. Nursing interventions
1. Provide rest.
2. Provide medication and care as needed for symptoms (e.g., elevation of temperature, pain).
3. Assess for and provide care as indicated for patient with uremia.

Bladder Tumors

A. Definition: benign or malignant lesions that ulcerate into the mucous membrane; bladder capacity decreased. Benign tumors tend to recur and become malignant.
B. Pathology
1. Related to cigarette smoking and exposure to dyes (environmental: nitrates, benzene, rubber, petroleum)
2. Chronic bladder irritation (e.g., stones, infection)
3. Related to aging
C. Signs and symptoms
1. Subjective: signs of bladder infection: dysuria, frequency, urgency, chills
2. Objective
a. Painless, gross hematuria
b. Anemia
D. Diagnostic tests and methods
1. Patient history and physical examination
2. X-ray studies: IVP, KUB, and retrograde pyelogram
3. Cystoscopy and biopsy examination
4. Renoscan, ultrasonography, CT, and MRI
E. Treatment
1. Removal of tumor through cystoscopy if benign
2. Administration of antineoplastic agents into bladder through urinary catheter
3. Surgery
a. Partial cystectomy
b. Cystectomy: total removal of bladder and provision for urinary diversion
c. Radiation, intravesical, external
d. Chemotherapy, intravesical
e. Fulguration (coagulation)
f. Experimental therapy (photodynamic therapy: use of photosensitivity agent and laser destruction of tumor cells)
g. Interferon (Roferon-A)
F. Nursing interventions: perform according to method of treatment (see specific sections).
1. Be supportive of patient concerns expressed.
2. Provide general preoperative and postoperative care (see Chapter 2).

Urinary Diversion

A. Definition: surgical intervention to allow for urinary elimination. The bladder is removed; the procedure is permanent.
1. Ileal conduit (ileal passageway): A small segment of ileum is separated from the intestine, and the distal end is brought out of the abdomen to form a stoma. The ureters are implanted into this ileal pouch; urine flows continuously from the renal pelvis through the ureters into the ileal pouch and into a collecting bag.
2. Ureterointestinal implant: Ureters are anastomosed into the sigmoid colon or rectum; urine is mixed with feces, and evacuation is controlled from the anal sphincter.
3. Cutaneous ureterostomies: Ureters are implanted on the abdomen, forming one or two stomas that drain urine continuously into drainage bags.
4. Continent ileal urinary reservoir (Koch pouch): Ureters are anastomosed to an isolated segment of ileum, which has a one-way valve; urine is drained by periodic insertion of a catheter.
5. Nephrostomy (may be long term): Tubes are inserted in the pelvis of each kidney, brought through the skin, and connected to a closed-drainage system.
B. Indication: cancer of the bladder
C. Patient problems (depends on procedure)
1. Susceptibility to infection
2. Anxiety or depression about diagnosis and change in body image
3. Inability to control elimination
4. Embarrassment
5. Odor if urine leaks onto skin; risk for impaired skin integrity
6. Impaired skin integrity resulting from the incision and ostomy
7. Pain from surgical incision or urinary obstruction or both
D. Nursing interventions (vary with procedures)
1. Provide general preoperative and postoperative care (see Chapter 2).
2. Provide time to listen to patient fears and anxieties.
3. Assess for fluid and electrolyte imbalance.
4. Maintain skin integrity: clean, inspect, and change drainage bag as needed.
5. Monitor temperature.
6. Monitor urine output from each catheter or tube; maintain separate output records for each. If nephrostomy tubes are used, contact physician if tube fails to drain urine, urine is grossly bloody, or patient complains of sudden severe flank pain.
7. Provide stoma care; stoma may need to be dilated in postoperative period.
8. Monitor fluid and electrolyte balance.
9. Prevent infection: maintain asepsis; encourage fluids. Patient must know when to seek medical attention for pain or elevation of temperature.
10. Do not give patient laxatives or enemas.
11. Arrange a visit from a person who has undergone a similar procedure (with permission of physician and patient).
12. Provide elimination of odor in drainage bags; use weak solution of vinegar or a liquid appliance deodorant.
13. Empty or change pouch when one-third to one-half full.
14. Instruct patient to avoid odor-producing foods such as onions, fish, eggs, and cheese and to drink cranberry juice.

Kidney Tumor

A. Definition: Most tumors of the kidney are malignant; no early symptoms occur.
B. Cause: unknown
C. Signs and symptoms (only in late stages)
1. Hematuria with no pain
2. Low-grade temperature
3. Weight loss

    4. Anemia

    5. Symptoms related to metastasis (e.g., bone pain)

D. Diagnostic tests and methods
    1. Renal arteriogram: IVP, KUB
    2. Renal biopsy examination

E. Treatment
    1. Surgery: radical nephrectomy
    2. Radiation
    3. Chemotherapy
    4. Biological response modifiers (interferon)

F. Nursing interventions
    1. Provide nursing care for individual symptoms.
    2. Provide general nursing care: before and after surgery, during radiation (see Chapter 2), and for a patient undergoing chemotherapy (see Chapter 3).

Acute Renal Failure

A. Definition: sudden damage to the kidneys, causing cessation of function and retention of toxins, fluids, and end products of metabolism. Patient may recover, or disease may become chronic or be fatal; may be prerenal, intrarenal, or postrenal.

B. Causes: blood transfusion reaction, shock, toxins, burns, renal ischemia, nephrotoxins, trauma, reaction to chemotherapy

C. Signs and symptoms
    1. Subjective
        a. Nausea, weakness
        b. Metallic taste in mouth
    2. Subjective
        a. Lethargy, headache, drowsiness; convulsion; may go into coma
        b. Vomiting and diarrhea
        c. Sudden oliguria or anuria
        d. Increased bleeding time
        e. Electrolyte imbalance
        f. Abnormal BUN and creatinine levels
        g. Paresthesia
        h. Hypotension

D. Diagnostic tests and methods
    1. Patient history and physical examination
    2. Blood serum tests, especially potassium
    3. Renal scan, renal biopsy, KUB
    4. Nephrotomography
    5. Retrograde pyelogram
    6. Ultrasonography, CT, MRI
    7. Urinalysis, CBC

E. Treatment
    1. Removal of cause
    2. Peritoneal dialysis
    3. Hemodialysis

F. Nursing interventions
    1. Provide nursing observations and care as indicated for primary problem.
    2. Provide care and observations as indicated for patient with chronic renal failure (see section on chronic renal failure [end-stage renal disease]).
    3. Provide nursing care as indicated for patient receiving peritoneal dialysis (see section on peritoneal dialysis).
    4. Provide nursing care as indicated for patient receiving hemodialysis (see section on hemodialysis).
    5. Offer emotional support.

Chronic Renal Failure (End-Stage Renal Disease)

A. Definition: progressive kidney damage; the nephron deteriorates; the kidneys stop functioning. This is the final stage of many chronic diseases (e.g., hypertension).

B. Causes
    1. Glomerulonephritis, pyelonephritis, polycystic kidney, urinary tract obstruction, diabetes
    2. Essential hypertension
    3. Lupus erythematosus
    4. Toxic agents
    5. Vascular disorders

C. Signs and symptoms (Figure 5-14)
    1. Subjective
        a. Malaise
        b. Nausea
        c. Headaches and visual disturbances
    2. Objective
        a. Anemia
        b. Oliguria
        c. Hyperkalemia
        d. Twitching (from low serum calcium and increased phosphorus levels); pathological fracture
        e. Hypertension (from fluid retention)
        f. Very susceptible to infection: delayed wound healing and ulcers in the mouth
        g. Bleeding tendency
        h. Uremic frost: Urea is excreted in perspiration onto the skin, and small crystals can be seen; this causes severe pruritus.
        i. Vomiting
        j. Decreased erythropoietin
        k. Disorientation, convulsions, coma
        l. Results of diagnostic tests

D. Diagnostic tests and methods
    1. Patient history and physical examination
    2. Serum blood tests
    3. Kidney function tests: BUN, creatinine level
    4. X-ray studies
    5. Renal arteriograms, renal ultrasound
    6. Nephrotomograms
    7. Kidney biopsy

E. Treatment
    1. Removal (treatment) of cause
    2. Hemodialysis
    3. Peritoneal dialysis
    4. Kidney transplant

F. Nursing interventions
    1. Monitor fluid balance: Weigh patient daily; record intake and output.
    2. Maintain asepsis: Provide catheter care, prevent infections, and encourage frequent handwashing. Do not expose patient to staff or visitors with upper respiratory tract infections.
    3. Instruct patient to conserve energy. Provide care; maintain rest periods.
    4. Provide safety (see nursing care of patient in a coma in the section on special situations, p. 230).
    5. Relieve pruritus: Wash patient frequently with tepid water, do not use soap, handle skin gently, use skin lotion, cut nails, apply calamine lotion.
    6. Assist with administration of transfusion; biological response modifiers; epoetin alfa (erythropoietin).

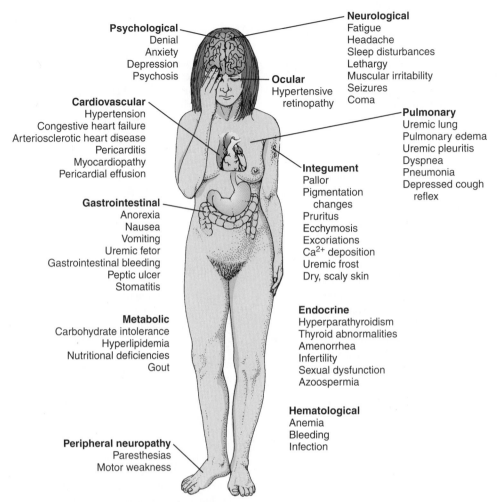

Psychological
Denial
Anxiety
Depression
Psychosis

Neurological
Fatigue
Headache
Sleep disturbances
Lethargy
Muscular irritability
Seizures
Coma

Ocular
Hypertensive
retinopathy

Cardiovascular
Hypertension
Congestive heart failure
Arteriosclerotic heart disease
Pericarditis
Myocardiopathy
Pericardial effusion

Pulmonary
Uremic lung
Pulmonary edema
Uremic pleuritis
Dyspnea
Pneumonia
Depressed cough
    reflex

Integument
Pallor
Pigmentation
    changes
Pruritus
Ecchymosis
Excoriations
Ca^{2+} deposition
Uremic frost
Dry, scaly skin

Gastrointestinal
Anorexia
Nausea
Vomiting
Uremic fetor
Gastrointestinal bleeding
Peptic ulcer
Stomatitis

Endocrine
Hyperparathyroidism
Thyroid abnormalities
Amenorrhea
Infertility
Sexual dysfunction
Azoospermia

Metabolic
Carbohydrate intolerance
Hyperlipidemia
Nutritional deficiencies
Gout

Hematological
Anemia
Bleeding
Infection

Peripheral neuropathy
Paresthesias
Motor weakness

FIGURE 5-14 Clinical manifestations of chronic uremia. (Modified from Lewis SM et al: *Medical-surgical nursing: assessment and management of clinical problems,* ed 7, St Louis, 2007, Mosby.)

7. Provide oral hygiene every 1 to 2 hours. Use cotton swabs and soft toothbrush. Hard candy and mouthwash minimize bad taste in mouth and alleviate thirst.
8. Provide soft, high-carbohydrate, low-potassium, low-sodium, low-protein diet in small feedings.
9. Restrict fluids as ordered.
10. Anticipate cardiac arrest; monitor vital signs.
11. Assess LOC; orient as necessary.
12. Provide nursing care and precautions as indicated for a patient with seizures (see section on convulsive disorders).
13. Provide nursing measures to prevent dangers of immobility (see Chapter 2).
14. Anticipate and prevent bleeding.
    a. Observe stool, urine, sputum, and vomitus.
    b. Monitor vital signs, laboratory values.
    c. Use soft swab for mouth care.
    d. Avoid injections if possible.
15. Reinforce instructions for kind of drug therapy (i.e., erythropoietin, iron, minerals, antihypertensives, phosphate binders, ion-exchange resins).

Peritoneal Dialysis (Figure 5-15)
A. Description: Toxins, end products of metabolism, and fluids are removed from the blood through the peritoneal membrane; a catheter is passed into the peritoneal cavity; dialyzing fluid, which is similar to plasma, is instilled by gravity into the abdominal cavity, and the catheter is clamped. Toxins and electrolytes, which are in greater concentration in the blood vessels of the peritoneal membrane, pass into the dialyzing fluid. After a specified dwell time the catheter is unclamped, and the fluid drains out by gravity.
B. Types
    1. Intermittent peritoneal dialysis (IPD)
    2. Continuous ambulatory peritoneal dialysis (CAPD)

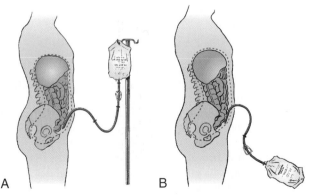

A   B

FIGURE 5-15 Peritoneal dialysis. A, Inflow. B, Outflow. (From Thompson JM et al: *Mosby's clinical nursing,* ed 5, St Louis, 2002, Mosby.)

3. Continuous cycling peritoneal dialysis (CCPD)
4. Access devices may be temporary or permanent.
C. Patient problems
   1. Risk for infection related to dialysis procedure
   2. Self-care deficit related to discomfort and immobility
   3. Deficient or excess fluid volume
   4. Disturbed body image
D. Nursing interventions
   1. Record baseline vital signs; complete assessment; carefully measure fluid instilled or drained.
   2. Maintain surgical asepsis; prevent peritonitis.
   3. Assist patient with self-care activities.
   4. Observe for complications (hypotension, pain, respiratory distress, hypovolemia, peritonitis, atelectasis).

Hemodialysis

A. Description: Blood leaves patient through an arterial cannula and travels through coils placed in a solution. Dialysis takes place, and the detoxified blood returns to patient's venous circulation. A surgically created arteriovenous fistula (AVF) (connection) is necessary for repeated dialysis.
B. Patient problems
   1. Situational low self-esteem related to threatened self-image
   2. Powerlessness related to dependency on machine
   3. Risk for infection related to the hemodialysis procedure
   4. Anxiety related to lifelong, life-threatening disease
   5. Excess fluid volume related to fluid accumulation, inadequate dialysis
   6. Deficient fluid volume related to rapid removal of body fluid during treatment
C. Nursing interventions
   1. Maintain surgical asepsis.
   2. Assess AVF fistula, graft, or shunt for patency. Normally a thrill can be felt by palpating the area of anastomosis, and a bruit can be heard with a stethoscope; the bruit and thrill are created by arterial blood rushing into the vein.
   3. Provide emotional support; alleviate anxiety.
   4. Provide patient teaching.

Kidney Transplant

A. Removal of the diseased kidney and transplantation of a normal kidney are sometimes performed for patients with advanced renal failure; restores normal function; less expensive than dialysis after first year.
B. Patient problems
   1. Risk for infection related to altered immune system secondary to medications
   2. Anxiety related to possibility of organ rejection
   3. Fear of pain, rejection
   4. Disturbed body image
   5. Deficient knowledge (surgery, drug therapies, nutrition, activities, follow-up care)

MALE REPRODUCTIVE SYSTEM

ANATOMY AND PHYSIOLOGY (FIGURE 5-16)

A. External genitalia
   1. Scrotum: skin-covered pouch; lies outside of pelvic cavity; contains testes, epididymis, and lower part of vas

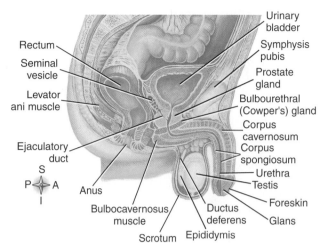

FIGURE 5-16 Male reproductive organs. (From Thibodeau GA, Patton KT: *Anatomy and physiology,* ed 6, St Louis, 2007, Mosby.)

deferens. Lower body temperature here is necessary for reproduction.
   2. Penis: erectile tissue; organ of coitus (sexual intercourse); serves as passageway for urine and semen
B. Testes: small oval glands in scrotum; produce spermatozoa; secrete testosterone
C. Ducts
   1. Seminiferous tubules: formation of sperm
   2. Epididymis: narrow, tightly coiled tubes; provides temporary storage space for immature sperm
   3. Vas deferens: continuation of epididymis; lies near surface of scrotum; called the *spermatic cord*
   4. Ejaculatory: pass through prostate; ejaculate semen into urethra
D. Accessory glands
   1. Seminal vesicles: located on each side of the prostate; empty secretion into the prostatic ampulla
   2. Prostate: encircles the upper area of the urethra; secretes alkaline fluid; increases sperm motility
   3. Cowper gland: located below prostate; produces an alkaline secretion that is primarily a lubricant during sexual intercourse
E. Semen: alkaline fluid (pH 7.5). The major bulk (60%) is secreted by the seminal vesicles; the remaining 40% is secreted by other accessory organs.
F. Function
   1. Reproduction
   2. Production of testosterone

MALE GENITOURINARY SYSTEM CONDITIONS AND DISORDERS

The male reproductive and urinary systems are so closely related that disorders that occur in one system greatly influence the other. Aging changes in the male reproductive system predispose these systems to many disorders. Collecting information about these body systems is often difficult because the patient is embarrassed to discuss such matters. The nurse should project an open, nonjudgmental attitude during data collection.

NURSING ASSESSMENT

A. Observations (objective data)
1. General appearance
2. Vital signs
3. Weight
4. External genitalia: penis
   a. Lesions
   b. Drainage
   c. Tenderness
5. Scrotum
   a. Enlargement
   b. Presence of testes in scrotum
6. Urine
   a. Color, clarity, amount
   b. Incontinence
B. Patient description—subjective data
1. Pain
2. Change in urinary stream, urgency
3. Impotence
4. Swelling

FREQUENT PATIENT PROBLEMS AND NURSING CARE

A. Anxiety related to modesty
1. Keep patient's body covered at all times.
2. Provide privacy.
3. Speak with patient during the examination or procedure.
B. Deficient knowledge related to diagnostic examinations
1. Provide factual information related to the examination process.
2. Teach testicular self-examination.
   a. Should be done on a monthly basis
   b. More comfortable if done in shower
   c. Check each scrotal sac for any abnormalities in size and shape.
3. Risk for sexual dysfunction
   a. Allow patient to express emotions, fears.
   b. Provide literature on aids or medications to assist in achieving satisfactory sexual experiences.

MAJOR MEDICAL DIAGNOSES

Benign Prostatic Hypertrophy or Hyperplasia (BPH)

A. Description: The prostate gland slowly enlarges (hypertrophies) and extends upward into the bladder. Outflow of urine is obstructed; the urinary stream is smaller, and voiding is difficult. A pouch is formed in the bladder as the gland continues to enlarge. Stasis of urine occurs; obstruction causes gradual dilation of ureters and kidneys; may cause hydronephrosis. When obstruction is complete, acute urinary retention occurs.
B. Cause: unknown; increased incidence with age, usually older than 50 years; related to smoking
C. Signs and symptoms
1. Subjective
   a. Dysuria, frequency, nocturia, urgency, retention, hesitancy
   b. Burning on urination, decreased force of stream, end-stream dribbling
2. Objective
   a. Urinary tract infection
   b. Acute urinary retention

c. Hematuria
d. Enlarged prostate gland
e. Results of diagnostic tests
D. Diagnostic tests and methods
1. Patient history and assessment; palpation through rectal examination
2. IVP, cystoscopy, retrograde pyelography
3. Urine culture
4. BUN, CBC
5. Serum creatinine
6. Transrectal ultrasonography
E. Treatment
1. Immediate
   a. Bladder drainage with indwelling catheter
   b. Decompression
   c. Antibiotics as indicated
   d. Suprapubic cystotomy and insertion of catheter for long-term drainage
2. Surgery: Type depends on patient's age and size of enlargement (open approaches).
   a. Transurethral resection of the prostate (TURP): An instrument is passed through the urethra to the prostate. Under direct visualization small pieces of the obstructing gland are removed with electric wire; bleeding points are cauterized. No incision is required; bleeding is a common postoperative problem.
   b. Suprapubic (transvesical) prostatectomy: A low incision is made over the bladder. The bladder is opened, and the prostatic tissue is removed through an incision into the urethral mucosa. Two drainage tubes are inserted (a cystotomy tube and a Foley catheter); these tubes are connected to a continuous bladder irrigation setup.
   c. Retropubic prostatectomy: A low abdominal incision is made; the bladder is not entered.
   d. Perineal prostatectomy: The gland is removed through an incision in the perineum; the entire gland and capsule are removed.
   e. Bilateral vasectomy may be performed with a prostatectomy to reduce risk of epididymitis.
3. Other treatment methods
   a. Finasteride (Proscar), an androgen hormone inhibitor, can be used to decrease symptoms; may arrest prostate enlargement.
   b. Transcystoscopic urethroplasty: balloon dilation of prostatic urethra
   c. Transurethral incision of the prostate (TUIP) at bladder neck
   d. Treatment of short-term effects involving microwaves
   e. Implantation of intraurethral prostatic stent
F. Nursing interventions
1. On admission complete assessment related to:
   a. Aging.
   b. Possible infection.
   c. Anxiety.
   d. Medical problems associated with aging: examples are diabetes, cardiovascular, hearing, sight, GI problems.
2. Encourage fluids if not contraindicated; monitor intake and output.
3. Maintain gravity drainage of indwelling catheter.
4. Provide general preoperative and postoperative care (see Chapter 2).

5. Provide specific postoperative care, depending on procedure performed.
   a. Continue to maintain gravity drainage of indwelling catheter.
   b. Keep irrigation flowing (note clots). Maintain a closed, continuous irrigation. Ensure that drainage is not obstructed.
   c. Maintain asepsis. Change dressing when it becomes wet (may need physician's order). Fecal incontinence may be present if a perineal prostatectomy was performed.
   d. Monitor vital signs; hematuria is expected. Report frank bleeding or clots.
   e. Use oral thermometer (no rectal treatments).
   f. Encourage patient to avoid straining. Encourage fluids and provide stool softeners.
   g. Observe for bladder spasms. Note if catheter is draining freely. Irrigate by syringe as ordered. Administer antispasmodics.
   h. Administer analgesic as needed for postoperative pain.
   i. Monitor intake and output; record all drainage tubes separately.
   j. Provide sitz bath for pain and inflammation if perineal prostatectomy was performed.
   k. Provide care instructions if patient is discharged with indwelling catheter.

Cancer of the Prostate

A. Definition: malignant tumor. No symptoms occur until it has become large or metastasized.
B. Cause: unknown; increased incidence with age (all men older than 40 years should have rectal examinations annually)
C. Signs and symptoms
   1. Early tumor has no symptoms.
   2. Subjective
      a. Back pain
      b. Frequency, nocturia, dysuria, urinary retention
   3. Objective: symptoms from metastasis
D. Diagnostic tests and methods
   1. Rectal examination
   2. Biopsy examination
   3. Acid phosphatase
   4. Transrectal ultrasonography
   5. Prostate-specific antigen (PSA) level
   6. Serum alkaline phosphatase level (elevated in bone metastasis)
   7. Bone scan to assess metastasis
   8. MRI, CT
E. Treatment
   1. Surgery: radical perineal prostatectomy (removal of prostate, capsule, and seminal vesicles)
   2. Bilateral orchiectomy (removal of both testes)
   3. TURP
   4. Estrogen therapy
   5. Agonists of luteinizing hormone (LH)–releasing hormone
   6. Radiation (external, interstitial, spot, brachytherapy [seed implant])
F. Nursing interventions
   1. See nursing interventions for a patient with benign prostatic hypertrophy.

2. Be supportive as concerns are expressed about a malignancy and feminization from estrogens. Answer questions; refer problems to physician.
3. Control pain for terminally ill patient. Hospice care may be considered.

Hydrocele

A. Definition: cystic mass filled with fluid that forms around the testis
B. Causes
   1. Infection
   2. Trauma
C. Signs and symptoms
   1. Swelling of testis
   2. Discomfort in sitting and walking
D. Diagnostic tests and methods: assessment by physical examination
E. Treatment
   1. Aspiration (usually only in children)
   2. Injection of a sclerosing solution
   3. Surgical removal of the sac (hydrocelectomy)
F. Nursing interventions
   1. Provide usual preoperative and postoperative care (see Chapter 2).
   2. Scrotal support (elevation) may be necessary during postoperative period.
   3. Be supportive regarding concerns expressed by patient.

Cancer of the Testes

A. Definition: uncommon malignancy; usually no systemic symptoms are present until metastasis occurs; can be diagnosed early only by examination and finding a hard, nontender mass (testicular self-examination should be done monthly); age of incidence is usually in early 30s.
B. Treatment
   1. Surgery: orchiectomy
   2. Radiotherapy
   3. Chemotherapy
   4. Possibly radical lymph node dissection
C. Nursing interventions related to treatment selected
D. Teach monthly preventive testicular self-examination.

FEMALE REPRODUCTIVE SYSTEM

ANATOMY AND PHYSIOLOGY

A. External genitalia
   1. Vulva
      a. Labia majora: two long folds of skin on each side of the vaginal orifice outside of the labia minora
      b. Labia minora: two flat, thin, delicate folds of skin that are highly sensitive to manipulation and trauma; enclose the region called the *vestibule,* which contains the clitoris, the urethral orifice (opening), and the vaginal orifice
      c. Clitoris: very sensitive erectile tissue; becomes swollen with blood during sexual excitement
      d. Vaginal orifice: opening into vagina. Hymen, fold of mucosa, partially closes orifice and commonly is ruptured during first sexual intercourse.
      e. Bartholin glands: located on posterior and lateral aspect of the vestibule of the vagina; secrete lubrication fluid
   2. Perineum: between vaginal orifice and anus; forms pelvic floor

B. Internal organs (Figure 5-17)
  1. Ovaries: main sex glands
     a. Located on either side in pelvic cavity
     b. Produce ova, which form in the graafian follicles
     c. Graafian follicle produces estrogen.
     d. Rupture of a follicle releases an ovum (ovulation).
     e. Ruptured follicles become glandular mass called *corpus luteum*.
     f. Corpus luteum secretes estrogen, but mainly progesterone.
  2. Fallopian tubes
     a. Extend from point near ovaries to uterus; no direct connection between ovaries and tubes
     b. Fimbriae: fingerlike extensions on tubes; pick up ova and transport into fallopian tubes
     c. Fertilization occurs in outer one third of the fallopian tubes.
  3. Uterus
     a. Upper portion rests on upper surface of bladder; lower portion is embedded in pelvic floor between the bladder and the rectum.
     b. Pear-shaped, hollow organ that expands tremendously to accommodate a fetus
     c. Divisions
        (1) Body: upper main part
        (2) Fundus: bulging upper surface of the body
        (3) Cervix: neck of the uterus
     d. Endometrium: uterine lining; sloughs off during menstruation
     e. Functions
        (1) Menstruation
        (2) Pregnancy
        (3) Labor
  4. Vagina
     a. Located between rectum and urethra
     b. Structure: wrinkled mucous membrane (rugae); capable of great distention
     c. Functions
        (1) Lower part of birth canal
        (2) Receives semen from male
        (3) Passageway for menstrual flow
C. Breasts (mammary glands)
  1. Located over pectoral muscles
  2. Size: depends on adipose tissue rather than glandular tissue
  3. Consist of lobes, lobules, and milk-secreting cells (acini)
  4. Ducts: lead to opening called the *nipple*
  5. Areola: pigmented area surrounding the nipple
D. Function
  1. Reproduction
  2. Production of estrogen and progesterone
E. Menstrual cycle (Figure 5-18)
  1. Phases: regulated primarily by hormonal control of pituitary gland, ovaries, and uterus
     a. One ovum discharged each month from an ovary, ripens in the graafian follicle. Follicle-stimulating hormone (FSH) from anterior lobe of pituitary stimulates the formation of the follicle.
     b. Estrogen produced by the follicle builds up the endometrium in expectation of a fertilized ovum.
     c. Ovum is discharged into the fallopian tube by LH from the anterior lobe pituitary. Follicle is converted into the corpus luteum.
     d. Postovulation: Corpus luteum secretes progesterone and estrogen for final preparation of the endometrium.
     e. Premenstrual: The gradual drop in progesterone and estrogen leads to menses.
  2. Length of cycle: usually 28 days; highly variable. Ovulation occurs midway.
  3. Menopause (climacteric): gradual cessation of menstrual cycle. Ability to bear children ends; occurs at approximately 45 years of age.
     a. Ovaries lose their ability to respond to hormones.
     b. Levels of estrogen and progesterone are decreased.
        (1) Failure to ovulate
        (2) Monthly flow is less, is irregular, and gradually ceases.
        (3) Reproductive organs atrophy.

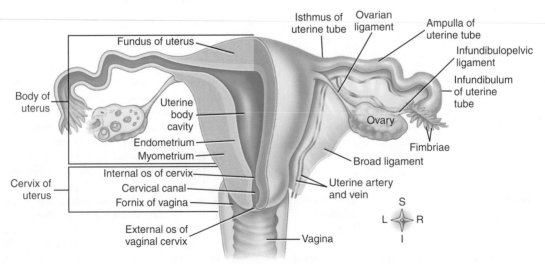

FIGURE 5-17 Female reproductive organs. (From Patton KT, Thibodeau GA: *Anatomy and physiology,* ed 8, St Louis, 2013, Mosby.)

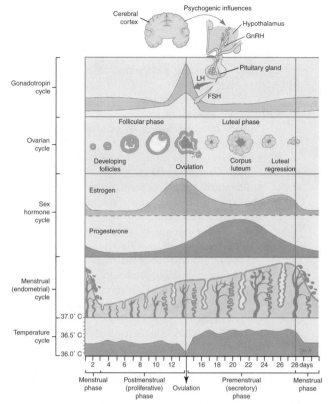

FIGURE 5-18 The human menstrual cycle. *FSH,* Follicle-stimulating hormone; *GnRH,* gonadotropin-releasing hormone; *LH,* luteinizing hormone. (From Thibodeau GA, Patton KT: *Anatomy and physiology,* ed 6, St Louis, 2007, Mosby.)

FEMALE REPRODUCTIVE SYSTEM CONDITIONS AND DISORDERS

Childbearing is the major physiological function of the female reproductive system. Disorders of this system are distressing to the patient because of interference with sexuality, conception, and self-image. The nurse plays an important role by clearly providing information to the concerned patient.

NURSING ASSESSMENT

A. Observations (objective data)
1. General appearance
2. Vital signs
3. Weight
4. Breasts
   a. Contour
   b. Skin dimpling
   c. Nodules
      (1) Size
      (2) Consistency
      (3) Mobile or fixed
   d. Nipples
      (1) Asymmetry
      (2) Retraction
      (3) Rash
      (4) Ulceration
      (5) Discharge

5. External genitalia
   a. Irritation
   b. Redness
   c. Excoriation
   d. Bulge
6. Introitus
   a. Irritation
   b. Redness
   c. Excoriation
   d. Nodules
7. Discharge
   a. Color
   b. Malodorous
   c. Consistency
B. Patient description (subjective data)
1. Lower abdominal pain and cramping
2. Backache
3. Stress incontinence
4. Urinary frequency and urgency
5. Urine or fecal material draining from vaginal tract
6. Breasts
   a. Tenderness
   b. Burning
   c. Swelling
   d. Pain
   e. Nipples: tenderness, burning
7. External genitalia
   a. Itching
   b. Burning
8. Introitus
   a. Burning
   b. Itching
   c. Tenderness
   d. Dyspareunia (painful intercourse)
9. Menstrual cycle
   a. Duration of cycles
   b. Number of days between cycles
   c. Associated symptoms
      (1) Pain
      (2) Headache
      (3) Irritability
      (4) Depression
      (5) Insomnia

DIAGNOSTIC TESTS AND METHODS

A. Serum laboratory studies
1. LH
   a. Stimulates progesterone secretion
   b. Diminished levels may relate to prolonged, heavy menses.
   c. Elevated levels may result in short, scanty menses.
2. FSH
   a. Stimulates estrogen secretion
   b. Diminished levels may relate to bleeding between cycles.
   c. Elevated levels may result in excessive uterine bleeding.
3. Thyroid function tests
   a. Used to rule out menstrual abnormality secondary to thyroid dysfunction
   b. Diminished thyroid hormone secretion may result in bleeding between cycles, irregular menses, or absence of menstrual flow.

4. Adrenal function tests
   a. Used to rule out menstrual abnormality secondary to adrenal dysfunction
   b. Elevated or decreased production of adrenal cortex hormone may result in amenorrhea.

B. Procedures
1. Pelvic examination: to inspect and assess the external genitalia, perineal and anal areas, introitus, vaginal tract, and cervix
   a. Have patient empty bladder.
   b. Place patient in the lithotomy position.
   c. Flex and abduct patient's thighs.
   d. Place patient's feet in stirrups.
   e. Extend patient's buttocks slightly beyond the edge of the examining table.
2. Laparoscopy: visualization of pelvic structures with a lighted laparoscope inserted through abdominal wall
3. Culdoscopy: visualization of ovaries, fallopian tubes, and uterus with a lighted instrument inserted through vaginal tract
   a. After procedure position patient on abdomen to expel air.
   b. Monitor for vaginal bleeding.
   c. Instruct patient to abstain from intercourse, douching, and using tampons until advised by physician.
4. Colposcopy: visualization of cervix with an instrument that magnifies tissue
5. Papanicolaou smear test (Pap smear): Sample of cervical scrapings is obtained for study under a microscope for evidence of malignant cell changes.
   a. Follow nursing actions as for a pelvic examination.
   b. Write patient's name on the frosted side of the slide, handling edges only.
   c. Smear the specimen on a glass slide.
   d. Place a drop of a fixative, dry, and send to laboratory.
   e. Reinforce importance of Pap smears as recommended by the American Cancer Society.
6. Cervical biopsy examination: removal of tissue to examine for presence of malignancy
   a. After procedure advise patient to rest and avoid strenuous activity for 24 hours.
   b. Leave packing in place until physician permits removal (usually 12 to 24 hours).
   c. Monitor for vaginal bleeding.
   d. Instruct patient to abstain from intercourse, douching, and use of tampons until advised by physician.
   e. Explain that a malodorous discharge that may last 3 weeks will occur; daily bath should help control this discharge.
7. Conization
   a. Removal of cone-shaped tissue of the cervix for analysis of cancerous cells
   b. Indicated for removal of diseased cervical tissue
   c. Nursing interventions
      (1) Maintain packing for 12 to 24 hours.
      (2) Monitor for bleeding.
      (3) Instruct patient to abstain from intercourse, douching, and using tampons until advised by physician.
8. Schiller test
   a. Application of a dye to the cervix to aid in detecting cancerous cells
   b. Normal vaginal cells stain a deep brown.

c. Abnormal cells do not absorb the dye.
d. Nursing intervention: Recommend to patient that a perineal pad be used to protect clothes from stain.
9. Ultrasonography
   a. Use of a sound frequency that reflects an image of the pelvic structures
   b. An aid in confirming ovarian and uterine tumors
10. Culture and sensitivity
    a. Culture of a specimen of exudate suspected of infection
    b. Sensitivity of an antibiotic to the microorganism
11. Dilation and curettage (D&C)
    a. A diagnostic and therapeutic procedure
    b. The cervix is dilated to scrape the lining of the uterine cavity with a curet.
    c. Nursing interventions
       (1) After procedure provide sterile perineal pads, and record amount of drainage.
       (2) Encourage voiding to prevent urinary retention.
       (3) Instruct patient to abstain from intercourse, douching, and using tampons until advised by physician.
12. Mammography: x-ray examination of the breasts to detect tumors. Screening test is done annually for women over age 40.
13. Thermography: infrared photography used to detect breast tumors
14. Xerography: x-ray examination of the breasts and skin that provides clear definition of the tissue
15. CT, MRI

FREQUENT PATIENT PROBLEMS AND NURSING CARE

A. Anxiety related to modesty
1. Keep patient's body covered at all times.
2. Provide privacy.
3. Speak with patient during the examination or procedure.
B. Deficient knowledge related to understanding of menstruation
1. Provide factual information related to the process of menstruation.
2. Describe abnormalities associated with menstruation.
3. Describe emotional changes associated with menstruation.
4. Teach menstrual hygiene.
   a. Change perineal pad or tampon every 3 to 4 hours.
   b. Remove napkin front to back.
   c. Alternate sanitary napkins and tampons daily to prevent toxic shock syndrome or backflow of menstruation.
C. Deficient knowledge related to menstrual abnormalities: Explain which menstrual symptoms are considered abnormal.
1. Flow occurring more frequently than every 21 days
2. Flow occurring less frequently than every 35 days
3. Duration of less than 3 days
4. Duration of more than 7 days
5. Use of 12 or more perineal pads per 24 hours
D. Acute pain related to menstruation
1. Assess location, duration, onset, and quality of pain.
2. Apply heating pad to the abdomen.

3. Provide warm liquids of patient's choice.
4. Provide massage to lumbar area.
5. Provide pain relief medication as ordered by physician.

E. Deficient knowledge related to breast self-examination (BSE)
1. Recommend that breasts be examined 7 days after onset of menstruation every month (Figure 5-19).
2. Instruct patient on technique of BSE.
   a. Inspect breasts in front of mirror with arms at sides.
   b. Observe breasts with arms raised above the head.
   c. With hands on hips, lean forward and contract chest muscles.
3. Lying supine, palpate each breast with flat part of fingers and continue in a circular movement to nipple.
4. Observations of the breasts
   a. Size
   b. Symmetry
   c. Skin texture
   d. Color
   e. Nipple position
   f. Nipple discharge

F. Deficient knowledge related to menopause
1. Describe accompanying symptoms associated with menopause.
   a. Irregular menses
   b. Hot flashes
   c. Night sweats
   d. Insomnia
   e. Depression
   f. Anxiety
2. Onset is usually after age 40 years.
3. Explain that menopause does not interfere with sexuality.
4. Recommend use of lubricant before intercourse.
5. Recommend use of contraception for 6 months after the last menstrual period.

Perform breast self-examination (BSE) monthly, approximately 1 week after the menstrual period, when breasts are not tender or swollen from hormonal changes. This is an ideal time to feel breasts for consistency in breast tissue. Perform BSE the same day each month so it becomes routine (you will be less likely to forget to do it).

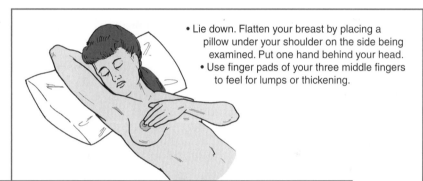

- Lie down. Flatten your breast by placing a pillow under your shoulder on the side being examined. Put one hand behind your head.
- Use finger pads of your three middle fingers to feel for lumps or thickening.

- Press firmly enough to distinguish different breast textures.
- Move around the breast in a set way. You can choose the circle movement, the up-and-down line, or the wedge movement.
- Use the same way each time to remember how the breast feels.
- Examine the other breast the same way. Compare what you feel in one breast with the other.

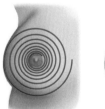
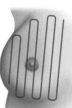

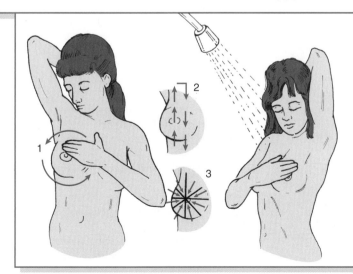
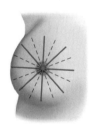

- Inspect your breasts while looking in the mirror with your hands at your sides. Look for noticeable dimpling of skin, swelling, reddening, asymmetry, or changes in the nipple.
- You may want to palpate your breasts while taking a shower, when the skin is wet and lumps may be easy to feel. Your soapy hands will glide over the wet skin, making it easy to check how your breast feels.
- Report any changes, such as lumps, dimpling, thickening of skin, or nipple discharge.

FIGURE 5-19 Breast self-examination. (From Leifer G: *Maternity nursing: an introductory text,* ed 11, St Louis, 2012, Mosby.)

MAJOR MEDICAL DIAGNOSES
Menstrual Abnormalities
Dysmenorrhea
A. Definition: intense pain at the time of menses
B. Cause: Uterine spasms cause cramping of the lower abdomen.
C. Signs and symptoms
   1. Subjective
      a. Headache, backache
      b. Abdominal pain
      c. Chills
      d. Nausea
   2. Objective
      a. Fever
      b. Vomiting
D. Diagnostic method: pelvic examination to rule out other physical disorders
E. Treatment
   1. Analgesics such as NSAIDs
   2. Local application of heat
   3. Pelvic exercises
   4. D&C
F. Nursing interventions
   1. Instruct patient on avoidance of fatigue and overexertion during menstrual period.
   2. Instruct patient on ingestion of warm beverages before onset of pain to prevent attack.

Premenstrual Syndrome (PMS)
A. Definition: large number of symptoms occurring a few days before menstruation
B. Cause: Cause is unclear; may be related to fluid retention combined with emotional tension; usually disappears with onset of menstruation.
C. Signs and symptoms
   1. Subjective
      a. Breast tenderness
      b. Headache
      c. Nausea
      d. Depression
      e. Insomnia
      f. Irritability
      g. Fatigue
   2. Objective: weight gain 2 to 10 days before onset of menstruation
D. Diagnostic method: assessment of specific symptoms and psychological health
E. Treatment
   1. Diuretics
   2. Mild sodium restriction
   3. Mild tranquilizers
   4. Well-balanced diet
   5. Exercise
F. Nursing interventions
   1. Help patient follow a diet with decreased sodium content.
   2. Instruct patient to decrease consumption of coffee, alcohol, and nicotine during latter half of menstrual cycle.

Amenorrhea
A. Definition: absence of menstrual periods
B. Causes
   1. Diabetes
   2. Debilitating illness
   3. Malnutrition; anorexia
   4. Obesity
   5. Extreme anxiety
   6. Anemia
   7. Oral contraceptives
   8. Chronic nephritis
   9. Tumors of the endocrine glands
C. Signs and symptoms
   1. Subjective: anxiety
   2. Objective
      a. Absence of menses by age 17 years (primary amenorrhea)
      b. Failure of a menstrual period (secondary amenorrhea)
D. Diagnostic tests and methods
   1. Pelvic examination
   2. LH level
   3. FSH level
   4. Thyroid function test
   5. Adrenal function test
E. Treatment: according to cause
F. Nursing interventions
   1. Encourage patient to follow prescribed orders to ensure success of therapeutic plan.
   2. Provide clear explanations related to cause of disorder to decrease anxiety.

Menorrhagia (Hypermenorrhea)
A. Definition: excessive menstrual flow (amount or duration)
B. Causes
   1. Uterine tumors
   2. Pelvic inflammatory disease (PID)
   3. Endocrine disturbances
C. Signs and symptoms
   1. Subjective
      a. Feeling of pelvic heaviness
      b. Fatigue
   2. Objective
      a. Profuse menstrual bleeding with clots
      b. Pale, tired appearance
D. Diagnostic tests and methods
   1. Pelvic examination
   2. LH level
   3. FSH level
   4. Thyroid function test
   5. Adrenal function test
   6. RBC count
E. Treatment
   1. According to cause
   2. D&C
F. Nursing interventions
   1. Encourage intake of foods high in iron content.
   2. Encourage planned rest periods.
   3. Instruct patient to count number of pads used during an abnormal period.
   4. Weigh each pad before and after use to estimate blood loss.

Metrorrhagia
A. Definition: bleeding between menstrual intervals
B. Pathology
   1. Causes are similar to those of menorrhagia.
   2. Breakthrough bleeding may occur with use of contraceptive pills.
   3. May be early symptom of cervical cancer.

C. Signs and symptoms
   1. Subjective
      a. Feeling of pelvic heaviness
      b. Fatigue
   2. Objective
      a. Spotting or bleeding between menstrual periods
      b. Tired appearance
D. Diagnostic tests and methods
   1. Pelvic examination
   2. LH level
   3. FSH level
   4. Thyroid function test
   5. Adrenal function test
   6. RBC count
   7. Pap smear
E. Treatment: according to cause
F. Nursing interventions
   1. Instruct patient about how to keep accurate records of bleeding episodes.
   2. Encourage continued medical follow-up because of possible cervical changes associated with cancer.

Vaginitis

A. Definition: inflammation of the vaginal mucosa
B. Pathology
   1. Invasion of virulent organisms permitted by changes in normal flora; pH becomes alkaline.
   2. Causes
      a. Trichomoniasis: parasitic organism
      b. *Candida albicans* (moniliasis): fungal organism
      c. Atrophic (senile): occurs in postmenopausal women because of atrophy of vaginal mucosa
      d. Bacterial: invasion by staphylococci, streptococci, *Escherichia coli, Chlamydia, or Gardnerella vaginalis*
      e. Foreign body
      f. Allergens or irritants
C. Signs and symptoms
   1. Trichomoniasis: thick, white or yellow, frothy, malodorous discharge causing itching, burning, and excoriation of vulva
   2. Monilial: thick or watery, white or yellow, curdlike discharge. Mucosa becomes reddened.
   3. Atrophic: blood-flecked discharge with burning and itching of vagina and dyspareunia
   4. Bacterial: profuse, yellow mucoid discharge with irritation to vulva and urethra; fishy or foul odor
   5. Foreign body: blood-tinged serosanguineous or purulent discharge; foul odor; may be thin or thick
   6. Allergens, irritants: increase in usual secretions, itching, burning, rash
D. Diagnostic tests and methods: culture and sensitivity, pelvic examination
E. Treatment
   1. Trichomoniasis: metronidazole (Flagyl), iodoquinol (Floraquin) tablets administered vaginally, and carbarsone suppositories administered rectally; sitz baths to relieve itching
   2. Candidiasis: nystatin (Mycostatin) or miconazole (Monistat) cream daily for 14 days; sitz baths to relieve itching
   3. Atrophic: antibiotics and estrogen therapy
   4. Bacterial: antibiotics and sulfonamide creams

5. Foreign body: removal of object; use of antibiotics
   6. Allergens or irritants: removal of cause; use of topical steroid ointment if necessary
F. Nursing interventions
   1. Reassure patient during vaginal examination to decrease anxiety.
   2. Instruct patient on perineal hygiene: cleansing front to back.
   3. In the event of trichomoniasis, instruct patient to abstain from intercourse or have partner wear a condom because this infection can be transmitted.
   4. Advise patient to use perineal pads because of increased discharge.
   5. Teach patient importance of compliance with treatment.

Uterine Cancer (Endometrium)

A. Definition: new growth of abnormal cells in uterine lining
B. Pathology
   1. Spreads to cervix, fallopian tubes, ovaries, bladder, and rectum
   2. Associated factors are age older than 50 years, obesity, diabetes, and hypertension.
   3. Prognosis is good if cancer is identified in early stages.
C. Signs and symptoms
   1. Subjective
      a. Postmenopausal bleeding
      b. Bleeding between cycles
      c. Bleeding after intercourse
      d. Watery vaginal discharge
   2. Objective
      a. Uterine enlargement
      b. Suspicious Pap test results
D. Diagnostic tests and methods
   1. D&C
   2. Tissue biopsy examination
E. Treatment
   1. Surgical intervention
      a. Panhysterectomy (removal of uterus and cervix)
      b. Oophorectomy (removal of ovaries)
      c. Salpingectomy (removal of fallopian tubes)
   2. Chemotherapy
   3. Radiation
F. Nursing interventions: See section on cancer of the cervix.

Uterine Fibroid Tumors

A. Definition: benign tumors located in the uterus
B. Pathology
   1. Develop slowly; symptoms occur only in relation to size, location, and number of tumors present.
   2. Occur in 25% of women older than 35 years
C. Signs and symptoms
   1. Subjective
      a. Menstrual disturbances
      b. Backache
      c. Frequent urination
      d. Constipation
   2. Objective: uterine enlargement
D. Diagnostic tests and methods
   1. Pelvic examination
   2. Laparoscopy

E. Treatment
1. Excision of the myoma is indicated for small tumors.
2. Hysterectomy (removal of uterus) with preservation of ovaries is indicated for large tumors.
F. Nursing interventions
1. Explain to patient that tumors may decrease in size after menopause.
2. Encourage patient to verbalize concerns.
3. If patient undergoes myomectomy, follow general postoperative nursing measures related to abdominal surgery for cancer of the cervix, p. 264.
4. If patient undergoes hysterectomy, follow nursing interventions for cancer of the cervix, p. 264.

Endometriosis

A. Definition: Tissue resembling the endometrial membrane grows in another location in the pelvic cavity
B. Pathology
1. During menstrual period, endometrial cells are stimulated by ovarian hormone.
2. Bleeding into surrounding tissue occurs, causing inflammation.
3. Condition may result in adhesions, fusion of pelvic organs, bladder dysfunction, stricture of bowel, or sterility.
C. Signs and symptoms: Symptoms usually appear in women older than 30 years.
1. Subjective
a. Discomfort of pelvic area before menses, becoming worse during menstrual flow and diminishing as flow ceases
b. Dyspareunia
c. Fatigue
2. Objective: infertility
D. Diagnostic tests and methods
1. Laparoscopy
2. Culdoscopy
E. Treatment
1. Hormonal therapy to suppress ovulation
2. Surgical intervention: hysterectomy, oophorectomy, or salpingectomy
F. Nursing interventions
1. Provide emotional support.
2. If patient is young, advise not to delay having a family because of risk of sterility.
3. Explain that hormonal drug may cause pseudopregnancy and irregular bleeding.
4. If patient is middle-aged, advise her that menopause may stop progression of condition.
5. Follow general postoperative nursing actions if patient undergoes surgical procedure.
a. Observe for vaginal hemorrhage, malodorous vaginal discharge, or vaginal discharge other than serosanguineous discharge.
b. Observe for urine retention, burning, frequency, or urgency to void.
c. Listen for renewed bowel sounds.
6. Provide patient teaching on discharge.
a. Heavy lifting, prolonged standing, walking, and sitting are contraindicated.
b. Sexual intercourse should be avoided until approved by physician.

Pelvic Inflammatory Disease

A. Definition: inflammation of the pelvic cavity
B. Pathology
1. Pathogenic organisms are introduced into the cervix.
2. PID may be confined to one or more structures: fallopian tubes, ovaries, pelvic peritoneum, pelvic veins, or pelvic tissue.
3. May result in adhesions, strictures, or sterility
4. Most common causative organism: gonococcus
5. Also caused by staphylococci or streptococci
C. Signs and symptoms
1. Subjective
a. Abdominal pain
b. Pelvic pain
c. Low-back pain
d. Nausea
2. Objective
a. Malodorous, purulent discharge
b. Fever
c. Vomiting
D. Diagnostic tests and method: culture and sensitivity test, CBC, pelvic examination, laparoscopy
E. Treatment
1. Antibiotic therapy
2. Analgesics
F. Nursing interventions
1. Provide nonjudgmental, accepting attitude.
2. Place patient in semi-Fowler position to provide dependent pelvic drainage.
3. Apply heat to abdominal area if ordered to improve circulation and provide comfort.
4. Patient teaching should include the following:
a. Take shower instead of tub bath.
b. Perform perineal hygiene; wipe from front to back.
c. Learn how to recognize if sexual partner is infected with gonococcus: discharge from penis of whitish fluid with painful urination (not all males are symptomatic).
d. Learn importance of routine physical examinations because gonococcal infection is asymptomatic in women.
e. Reinforce "safe sex" guidelines.

Vaginal Fistula

A. Definition: tubelike opening between two internal organs
B. Pathology
1. Causes include radiation therapy, gynecological surgery, or traumatic childbirth.
2. Impaired blood supply and sloughing of tissue result, leading to abnormal opening.
3. Four types affect female reproductive organs:
a. Ureterovaginal: between ureter and vagina. Urine leaks into vagina.
b. Vesicovaginal: between bladder and vagina. Urine leaks into vagina.
c. Urethrovaginal: between urethra and vagina. Urine leaks into vagina.
d. Rectovaginal: between rectum and vagina. Flatus and fecal matter leak into vagina.
C. Signs and symptoms
1. Subjective
a. Leakage of urine, flatus, and fecal matter
b. Pain in affected area

2. Objective
   a. Excoriation
   b. Malodor
D. Diagnostic methods
   1. Symptoms and physical examination
   2. Patient history of radiation therapy
   3. IVP
   4. Cystoscopy
E. Treatment
   1. Small fistula: may heal spontaneously
   2. Surgical excision
   3. Temporary colostomy for rectovaginal fistula
F. Nursing interventions
   1. Provide psychological support; offer reassurance and acceptance.
   2. Encourage patient to verbalize feelings; express empathy.
   3. Observe vaginal discharge, and record.
   4. Change perineal pad every 4 hours and p.r.n.
   5. Instruct on perineal hygiene.
   6. Provide sitz bath and irrigation solutions for hygiene if ordered.
   7. Follow general postoperative nursing actions if patient undergoes surgery.
      a. Monitor Foley catheter for drainage at all times.
      b. Caution patient not to strain when having a bowel movement.

Prolapsed Uterus

A. Definition: downward displacement of the uterus through the vaginal orifice
B. Pathology
   1. Result of weakened supporting muscles and ligaments of the pelvis
   2. Causes include childbirth injuries, repeated pregnancies with short intervals between, menopausal atrophy, and congenital weakness.
C. Signs and symptoms
   1. Subjective
      a. Pain in lower abdomen
      b. Feeling of pressure within pelvis
      c. Stress incontinence
      d. Dyspareunia
      e. Backache
   2. Objective
      a. Urinary stasis
      b. Elongated cervix
D. Diagnostic methods
   1. Signs and symptoms
   2. Pelvic examination
E. Treatment
   1. Placement of a pessary in the vagina to support uterus
   2. Surgical suspension of the uterus
   3. Hysterectomy if condition is postmenopausal
F. Nursing interventions
   1. Approach with a relaxed manner, demonstrate calmness, and encourage expression of feelings to decrease anxiety.
   2. Explain all procedures.
   3. Follow general postoperative nursing actions.
      a. Chart number of perineal pads used during 8-hour period.
      b. Observe for hemorrhage.

c. Observe for vaginal discharge other than serosanguineous fluid.
   d. Listen for renewed bowel sounds.
   e. Observe for urinary retention and pelvic congestion.

Cystocele and Rectocele

A. Definition
   1. Cystocele: abnormal protrusion of bladder against vaginal wall
   2. Rectocele: abnormal protrusion of part of rectum against vaginal wall
B. Pathology
   1. Result of weakened supporting muscles and ligaments of pelvis
   2. Causes include childbirth injuries, repeated pregnancies with short intervals between, menopausal atrophy, and congenital weakness.
C. Signs and symptoms
   1. Subjective
      a. Pelvic pressure, backache
      b. Stress incontinence, dysuria (cystocele)
      c. Constipation or incontinence of feces and flatus (rectocele)
   2. Objective
      a. Residual urine after voiding (cystocele)
      b. Hemorrhoids (rectocele)
D. Diagnostic methods
   1. Signs and symptoms
   2. Pelvic examination
E. Treatment
   1. Anterior colporrhaphy to adjust cystocele
   2. Posterior colporrhaphy to adjust rectocele
F. Nursing interventions
   1. Administer catheter care twice each day (bid) and p.r.n.
   2. Splint abdomen when coughing.
   3. Place in low-Fowler position or flat in bed to avoid pressure on suture line.
   4. Explain to patient that she should respond to bowel stimuli to avoid suture strain.
   5. After each bowel movement, clean perineum with warm water and soap; pat dry anterior to posterior.
   6. Apply heat lamp, anesthetic spray, or ice packs if ordered to relieve discomfort.
   7. Provide patient teaching.
      a. Heavy lifting and prolonged standing, walking, and sitting are contraindicated.
      b. Sexual intercourse should be avoided until approved by physician.
      c. Perform pelvic exercises.

Ovarian Tumors

A. Definition: mass of tissue growing on the ovary; usually asymptomatic until large enough to cause pressure
B. Pathology: two classifications
   1. Ovarian cyst: benign condition but may transform to a malignancy; may be small, containing clear fluid, or filled with a thick, yellow fluid; size varies.
   2. Malignant tumor: cancerous growth found on the ovary; can be primary site of the cancer or secondary site caused by metastasis from the GI tract, breast, pancreas, or kidneys

C. Signs and symptoms
  1. Subjective
    a. Pelvic pain
    b. Menstrual disturbances
    c. Abdominal distention
    d. Constipation
    e. Dyspareunia
  2. Objective: palpable mass
D. Diagnostic tests and methods
  1. Culdoscopy
  2. Ultrasonography
  3. Biopsy examination
E. Treatment
  1. Cyst may be observed for regression in size.
  2. Oophorectomy (removal of ovaries)
  3. Removal of all reproductive organs
  4. Estrogen replacement therapy
  5. X-ray therapy and chemotherapy
  6. Radiation therapy
F. Nursing interventions
  1. If patient undergoes oophorectomy, follow general post-operative nursing care related to abdominal surgery for cancer of the cervix (see the following section on cancer of the cervix).
  2. If patient undergoes surgery for removal of all abdominal reproductive organs, follow nursing interventions covered later for cancer of the cervix (see the following section on cancer of the cervix).
  3. Assist patient in dealing with changes in body image.

Cancer of the Cervix

A. Definition: new growth of abnormal cells in the neck of the uterus
B. Pathology
  1. Early stage confined to epithelial cervical layer
  2. Will continue to invade surrounding area such as bladder and rectum
  3. Metastasizes to lungs, bones, and liver
  4. Relationship exists between cervical cancer and smoking and infection with the human papillomavirus (HPV).
C. Signs and symptoms
  1. Subjective
    a. Asymptomatic in early stage
    b. Menstrual disturbances
    c. Postmenopausal bleeding
    d. Bleeding after intercourse
    e. Watery discharge
  2. Objective: suspicious Pap test result
D. Diagnostic tests and methods
  1. Pap smear
  2. Cervical biopsy examination
  3. Colposcopy
  4. Schiller test
  5. Conization
E. Treatment
  1. Panhysterectomy (excision of uterus and cervix)
  2. Radiation in advanced cases
  3. Chemotherapy
F. Nursing interventions
  1. Reassure patient and family that adjustment to illness can be slow.

  2. Acknowledge that patient must adapt to illness according to her age, developmental stage, and past life experiences.
  3. If patient is to receive internal radium implant:
    a. Provide isolation.
    b. Instruct her to maintain supine or side-lying position.
    c. Explain to patient and visitors that the amount of time spent with patient will be limited to avoid overexposure to radiation.
    d. Provide high-protein, low-residue diet to avoid straining of bowels, which may dislodge implant.
    e. Maintain high fluid intake: 2000 to 3000 mL daily.
    f. Insert Foley catheter to prevent bladder distention.
    g. Administer antiemetics as ordered.
  4. If patient undergoes surgery, follow general postoperative nursing actions.
    a. Observe for vaginal hemorrhage, malodorous vaginal discharge, or any vaginal discharge other than serosanguineous discharge.
    b. Observe for urinary retention.
    c. Change perineal pads every 3 to 4 hours and p.r.n.
    d. Listen for renewed bowel sounds.

Bartholin Cysts

A. Definition: tumorlike capsules formed from retained secretions
B. Pathology
  1. May develop as a consequence of an earlier bacterial infection of these glands
  2. Formation of these cysts results from obstruction in the outlet of these glands.
C. Signs and symptoms
  1. Subjective
    a. Pain on walking
    b. Dyspareunia
  2. Objective: mobile nodule
D. Diagnostic methods
  1. Pelvic examination
  2. Palpable nodule
E. Treatment
  1. Incision and drainage
  2. Antiseptic wound packing
F. Nursing interventions
  1. Reassure patient that normal function of the gland will be regained after the procedure.
  2. After surgery provide a sterile perineal pad every 4 hours and p.r.n.
  3. Provide sterile wound care as ordered.
  4. Instruct on perineal hygiene.
  5. Provide sitz baths for increased circulation and comfort.
  6. On patient's discharge from the hospital, explain that the surgical wound is susceptible to bacterial infection until healing has taken place.

Fibrocystic Breast Disease

A. Definition: fiberlike tumors of the breast tissue with cyst formation
B. Pathology
  1. Cause unknown; possible hormonal imbalance
  2. Occurs during reproductive years and disappears with menopause
  3. Benign condition affecting 25% of women older than 30 years of age

C. Signs and symptoms
  1. Subjective: breast tenderness and pain
  2. Objective: small, round, smooth nodules
D. Diagnostic tests and methods
  1. Mammography
  2. Thermomastography
  3. Xerography
E. Treatment: conservative
  1. Aspiration
  2. Biopsy examination to rule out malignancy
F. Nursing interventions
  1. Explain importance of monthly BSE.
  2. Encourage patient to seek medical evaluation if nodule forms because cystic disease may interfere with early diagnosis of breast malignancy.
  3. A dietary treatment limiting the amount of methylxanthines (coffee, tea, or cola) consumed may improve symptoms.

Cancer of the Breast
A. Definition: small, painless, fixed lump most frequently located in the upper, outer portion of the breast
B. Pathology
  1. Risk factors increase with age.
  2. Influenced by heredity
  3. Sites of metastasis: lymph nodes, lungs, liver, bone, brain
  4. Other risk factors
    a. Obesity
    b. Diet high in fat and protein
    c. Nulliparity
    d. Parity after 35 years of age
    e. Menarche before 11 years of age
    f. Menopause after 55 years of age
    g. History of cancer in one breast
C. Signs and symptoms
  1. Subjective: nontender nodule
  2. Objective
    a. Enlarged axillary nodes
    b. Nipple retraction or elevation
    c. Skin dimpling
    d. Nipple discharge
D. Diagnostic tests and methods
  1. Mammography
  2. Thermography
  3. Xerography
  4. Breast biopsy examination
E. Treatment
  1. Lumpectomy: removal of the lump and partial breast tissue; indicated for early detection
  2. Mastectomy
    a. Simple mastectomy: removal of breast
    b. Modified radical mastectomy: removal of breast, pectoralis minor, and some of adjacent lymph nodes (the pectoralis major is preserved)
    c. Radical mastectomy: removal of breast, pectoral muscles, pectoral fascia, and nodes
  3. Oophorectomy, adrenalectomy, or hypophysectomy to remove source of estrogen and hormones that stimulate breast tissue
  4. Radiation therapy to destroy malignant tissue
  5. Chemotherapeutic agents to shrink, retard, and destroy cancer growth
  6. Corticosteroids, androgens, and antiestrogens to alter cancer that depends on hormonal environment
F. Nursing interventions
  1. Provide atmosphere of acceptance, frequent patient contact, and encouragement in illness adjustment.
  2. Introduce a person who has successfully undergone the same experience: arrange contact from Reach to Recovery representative.
  3. Encourage grooming activities such as hair, nails, teeth, and skin.
  4. Arrange attractive environment.
  5. If patient is receiving radiation or chemotherapy, explain and assist her with potential side effects.
    a. Nausea and vomiting
    b. Anorexia
    c. Diarrhea
    d. Stomatitis
    e. Malaise
    f. Itching
    g. Hair loss (alopecia)
  6. If patient has undergone surgical intervention, the following postoperative nursing actions should be observed.
    a. Elevate affected arm above level of right atrium to prevent edema.
    b. Drawing blood or administering parenteral fluids or taking blood pressure on affected arm is contraindicated.
    c. Monitor dressing for hemorrhage; observe back for pooling of blood.
    d. Empty Hemovac and measure drainage every 8 hours.
    e. Assess circulatory status of affected limb.
    f. Measure upper arm and forearm twice daily to monitor edema.
    g. Encourage exercises of the affected arm when approved by physician; avoid abduction.
    h. Assist with brushing hair.
    i. Assist with squeezing ball.
    j. Assist with feeding self.
  7. Patient teaching on discharge
    a. Exercise to tolerance.
    b. Sleep with arm elevated.
    c. Elevate arm several times daily.
    d. Avoid injections, vaccinations, and taking blood pressure in affected arm.
    e. Never allow blood to be drawn from or an IV line started in affected arm.

Paget Disease of the Breast
A. Definition: cancer of the nipple
B. Pathology
  1. Rare occurrence affecting women older than 40 years of age
  2. Spreads from nipple to areola to part of the breasts; ulcerates
C. Signs and symptoms
  1. Subjective
    a. Itching
    b. Swelling
  2. Objective
    a. Blistering
    b. Discharge
    c. Nipple retraction

D. Diagnostic method: biopsy examination

E. Treatment: mastectomy

F. Nursing interventions: See nursing interventions for cancer of the breast.

SEXUALLY TRANSMITTED INFECTIOUS DISEASES

SYPHILIS

A. Description: caused by a spirochete, *Treponema pallidum;* appears in three stages; transmitted through sexual contact or warm blood

1. Primary stage: After an incubation period of 10 to 60 days (usually 3 weeks), during which no symptoms occur, an ulcer or chancre appears at the site of entry; it contains many organisms and is highly infectious. Minor local discomfort or mild generalized symptoms may occur (e.g., headache, lymph node enlargement). Without treatment the condition heals in 3 to 5 weeks.

2. Secondary stage: Three weeks later it appears as a mild rash on skin (usually palms of hands and soles of feet) and as papules on mucous membranes. All lesions contain organisms and are highly contagious. Symptoms may be mild or generalized (e.g., bone pain, sore throat, hair loss in patches, lymph node changes); lasts a few weeks and becomes dormant if not treated; patient is infectious for approximately 1 year.

3. Third or latent stage: Ten to 30 years later, the spirochetes, which have been deposited in tissues and organs, are in lesions (gummas); these destroy the tissue; common sites are the CNS, eyes, and aorta.

B. Signs and symptoms: relate to organ involved

C. Diagnostic tests and methods

1. Primary stage: microscopic examination of smear

2. Second and third stages: blood serum tests (e.g., Venereal Disease Research Laboratory [VDRL] and rapid plasma reagin [RPR])

D. Treatment: penicillin or tetracycline (patient and partner)

GONORRHEA

A. Definition: a highly communicable disease. Inflammation of the urethra occurs and spreads to other organs of the genital tract. Incubation period is 3 to 4 days.

B. Cause: *Neisseria gonorrhoeae;* transmitted by sexual contact

C. Signs and symptoms

1. Female patients may have no early symptoms or purulent vaginal discharge, dysuria, or urgency; untreated, it may spread to other organs in the pelvic cavity (see section on pelvic inflammatory disease).

2. Male patients have purulent urethral discharge and burning on urination; may develop urethral stricture, epididymitis, prostatitis.

D. Diagnostic tests and methods

1. Patient history and physical examination

2. Smear or culture

E. Treatment: penicillin or tetracycline; ceftriaxone (a cephalosporin) for penicillinase-resistant strains

HERPES GENITALIS

A. Description: Fluid-filled vesicles on genitalia form crusts, causing generalized symptoms such as elevated temperature and pain. Patient may have no symptoms. Recurrent episodes; causes problems in pregnancy; believed to predispose to cervical cancer

B. Cause: herpesvirus hominis type 2 (herpes simplex virus [HSV])

C. Treatment: symptomatic; topical or oral antiviral agents (acyclovir [Zovirax]); no cure

D. Recommend use of barrier forms of contraception

CHLAMYDIA TRACHOMATIS INFECTION

A. Definition: most common STD in the United States; causes symptoms similar to gonorrheal infections

B. Cause: *C. trachomatis*

C. Signs and symptoms

1. In men: urethritis, dysuria, frequency, watery mucoid discharge. Complications include epididymitis, prostatitis, and infertility.

2. In women: often asymptomatic; mucopurulent cervicitis, dysuria, frequency, local soreness. Complications include salpingitis, PID, ectopic pregnancy, and infertility.

D. Diagnostic tests and methods: urogenital smear analysis for enzyme or antibody

E. Treatment: antibiotic therapy (doxycycline, tetracycline, erythromycin)

CONDYLOMATA ACUMINATA

A. Definition: also referred to as *genital* or *venereal warts;* often seen with other STDs such as gonorrhea and trichomoniasis; highly contagious

B. Cause: HPV

C. Signs and symptoms: initially single, small papillary growths that grow into large cauliflower-like masses; profuse, foul-smelling vaginal discharge; bleeding; may progress to genital and cervical dysplasia, cancer

D. Diagnostic tests and methods: inspection of urinary meatus, vulva, labia, vagina, cervix, penis, scrotum, anus, perineum; culture and biopsy

E. Treatment

1. Cryotherapy with liquid nitrogen or cryoprobe

2. Laser therapy

3. Acid treatments

4. Surgery

5. Chemotherapy (5-FU)

TRICHOMONIASIS AND CANDIDIASIS

A. Definition: very common STDs; symptoms frequently seen only in women

B. Cause: *Trichomonas vaginalis* and *C. albicans,* respectively

C. Signs and symptoms: itching, discharge

D. Diagnostic tests and methods: culture and inspection of affected tissues

E. Treatment: antifungals, antiprotozoal drugs (metronidazole [Flagyl])

INTEGUMENTARY SYSTEM

ANATOMY AND PHYSIOLOGY

A. Structure of skin (Figure 5-20): includes epithelial, connective, and nerve tissue; consists of sweat and oil glands; is soft and has elasticity

1. Epidermis: outermost layer; cells flat and tough; no blood supply

a. Cells undergo constant cellular change by mitosis.

b. Contains pigment (melanin); amount of pigment varies among races and individuals.

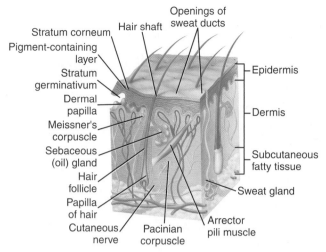

FIGURE 5-20 Structures of the skin. (From Herlihy B: *The human body in health and illness,* ed 3, St Louis, 2007, Saunders.)

2. Dermis: "true skin," the inner layer, composed of living cells
   a. Connective tissue framework
   b. Contains blood vessels, nerves, hair roots, and oil and sweat glands
   c. The ridges and grooves form the pattern for fingerprints, unique to each individual.
   d. Nerve endings provide sensation (touch).
      (1) Receptors: small, round bodies (tactile corpuscles)
      (2) Located in dermis; numerous in tips of fingers, toes, and tongue
      (3) Allow perception of heat, cold, and pain
3. Subcutaneous tissue: lies under dermis
   a. Contains fat cells, which give skin its smooth appearance
   b. Serves as shock absorber and insulates deeper tissues
4. Glands
   a. Sebaceous (oil glands)
      (1) Excrete oily substance (sebum)
      (2) Keep skin soft and moist
   b. Sudoriferous (sweat glands)
      (1) Secrete perspiration
      (2) Part of the heating and regulating equipment of the body
5. Appendages
   a. Hair: covers skin except on palms of hands and soles of feet; composed of dead keratinized cells
      (1) Shaft: hair above the skin
      (2) Follicle: a tiny sac from which hair root grows
   b. Nails: tightly packed cells of scaly epidermis
      (1) Roots are living cells; visible ends are dead cells.
      (2) They protect the tips of the fingers and toes.
      (3) The pink coloring comes from the blood supply in the nail bed.
B. Functions
   1. Protection: protects deeper tissues from pathogenic organisms and harmful chemicals
   2. Excretion: limited to water and urea; only a small amount of waste products eliminated
   3. Regulation: helps regulate body temperature and fluid content
   4. Sensory: contains millions of nerve endings that provide sensory reception to pressure, touch, pain, and temperature
   5. Vitamin D production—effect of sunlight
C. Effects of aging: skin, hair, nails (Table 5-7)

INTEGUMENTARY SYSTEM CONDITIONS AND DISORDERS

The skin is the barrier that protects the body from the environment. It prevents loss of body fluids and protects tissues and organs from external injury and organisms. Temperature regulation, sensation, and excretion of small amounts of water and sodium chloride are functions of the skin. Maximum health and healing of the skin are maintained by proper nutrition, hydration, electrolyte balance, exercise, and rest. Problems arise from systemic allergies (e.g., food and medication; exposure to external irritants such as chemicals, plants, and cosmetics) and exposure to sun, parasites, microorganisms, injury, and new growths.

The following terms are used to describe skin lesions:
- Atheroma: fatty patch or thickening on skin
- Bleb: blister filled with fluid
- Bulla: large blister filled with fluid such as occurs with burns
- Comedo: blackhead or acne
- Cyst: sac or capsule containing fluid or semisolid material (e.g., sebaceous cyst of scalp)
- Erythema: red area (e.g., sunburn)
- Excoriation: abrasion of outer layer of skin (e.g., friction, trauma)
- Exudate: fluid, usually containing pus, bacteria, and dead cells (e.g., fluid from infected wound)
- Fissure: groove, crack, or slit such as occurs with ulceration
- Furuncle: painful, erythematous raised lesion (e.g., boil)
- Hive: solid, raised, and itchy area (wheal), usually the result of allergy
- Macule: small, flat discolored area (e.g., freckle)
- Maculopapular: multiple lesions consisting of both macules and papules (e.g., early chickenpox)
- Mole: flat or raised pigmented growth (e.g., birthmark)
- Nevus: congenital, raised, pigmented growth (e.g., birthmark or mole)
- Nodule: small, solid mass (e.g., swollen lymph node)
- Papule: small, red, raised elevation (e.g., measles)
- Petechia: red pinpoint hemorrhage; seen in some blood diseases
- Pustule: small elevation on skin containing purulent fluid (e.g., acne)
- Ulcer: depression (e.g., open lesion on skin)
- Urticaria: hives (e.g., blood transfusion reaction)
- Vesicle: small sac containing serous or sanguineous fluid (e.g., pimple)
- Wheal: raised lesion, usually accompanied by itching (e.g., mosquito bite)

NURSING ASSESSMENT
A. Observations
   1. Skin
      a. Color: any deviation from normal (e.g., pallor, cyanosis, jaundice, blanching), general pigmentation, vascularity, bruising

Table 5-7	Changes from Aging in Skin, Hair, and Nails	
PARAMETERS	**OBSERVABLE CHANGES**	**CAUSE**
SKIN		
Color	Paleness in white skin	Decreased vascularity of dermis; loss of melanocytes
	Brown spots (senile lentigines)	Hyperpigmentation
	Purple patches (senile purpura)	Blood leaking from poorly supported, fragile capillaries
Moisture	Dry skin, decreased perspiration	Decreased sebaceous and sweat gland activity
Elasticity, turgor	Decreased elasticity	Loss of collagen and elastic fibers
	Loose folds and wrinkles	
	Decreased turgor	
Texture	Some rough areas	Environmental effects over time and decreased moisture
	Thinner, more transparent skin	Thinning of epidermis from decreased vascularity of dermis; loss of underlying tissue
HAIR		
Color	Grayness	Decreased number of melanocytes in hair
Consistency	Thinner on head and body	Decreased density and rate of hair growth
	Coarser in nose of men	Increased density of nasal hair
Distribution	Loss of hair on head and body	Decreased rate of hair growth; decreased hormones; decreased peripheral circulation
	Increased hair on face of women	Higher androgen/estrogen ratio
NAILS	More brittle	Slowing of nail growth; decreased peripheral circulation
	Longitudinal ridges	
	Thickening and yellowing of toenails	

Adapted from Monahan FD et al: *Phipps' medical-surgical nursing: health and illness perspectives,* ed 8, St Louis, 2007, Mosby.

b. Turgor: hydration, elasticity, and mobility
c. Lesions and rashes: size, location, color, drainage, crusts, pattern or shape, distribution
d. Skin temperature for inconsistency: areas cool or warm to the touch
e. Cleanliness and hygiene
f. Odor
g. Pressure areas for existing or potential decubitus ulcers
2. Hair and scalp
a. Unusual distribution or absence of scalp and body hair; lesions
b. Texture: smooth or coarse
c. Parasites: scalp and pubic
3. Nails
a. Cleanliness
b. Brittleness
c. Length
d. Pitting
e. Shape, contour, clubbing
f. Color, splinter hemorrhages
B. Patient description (subjective data)
1. History to include onset, changes, and presence of itching, pain, or burning
2. Factors that make condition worse or better
3. Allergies
4. Recent changes in environment and diet

5. Medications taken
6. Concerns about appearance, change in body image, and disfigurement
7. Changes in activities or lifestyle caused by disease
8. Environmental or occupational hazards (sun exposure, toxic chemicals, insect bites)
9. History of systemic disorders

FREQUENT PATIENT PROBLEMS AND NURSING CARE

A. Disturbed body image related to disfigurement
1. Show acceptance by being nonjudgmental.
2. Plan time to allow patient to express feelings.
B. Pain related to pruritus (itching)
1. Administer antipruritics and antihistamines (see Chapter 3).
2. Keep nails short.
3. Use cotton bedding and clothing; avoid rough fabrics.
4. Encourage use of cotton gloves when sleeping.
5. Bathe with tepid water; use minimal soap; pat dry using no friction.
6. Give oil, medicated, or starch baths.
C. Risk for infection or injury related to open lesions
1. Use aseptic technique in cleaning; teach handwashing.
2. Monitor for redness, swelling, elevated temperature.
3. Use dressings only when necessary, and apply loosely with gauze and nonallergenic tape.

D. Impaired skin integrity related to seborrhea: oily scalp with shedding of greasy scales
   1. Give frequent shampoos.
   2. Use medicated shampoos; rinse thoroughly.

MAJOR MEDICAL DIAGNOSES

Contact Dermatitis

A. Definition: inflammatory response of skin with redness, edema, thickening, and frequent scaling. Vesicles and papules may be present.
B. Cause: an allergic reaction or unusual sensitivity when a substance comes in direct contact with the skin (e.g., poison ivy, soaps, cleaning agents, fabrics)
C. Symptoms: pruritus, erythema
D. Diagnostic test and methods
   1. Allergy testing
   2. Patient history and assessment
E. Treatment
   1. Systemic medication: antihistamines, antipruritics, corticosteroids (see Chapter 3)
   2. Topical medication: corticosteroids (see Chapter 3)
   3. Removal of cause
F. Nursing interventions
   1. Prevent scratching.
   2. Give tepid baths.
   3. Cut nails.
   4. Administer p.r.n. medications as soon as possible.

Psoriasis

A. Definition: chronic condition in which patches of inflammation occur that are red and covered with silvery scales that are shed. These usually occur on elbows, knees, lower back, and scalp; they may cover the entire body.
B. Cause: unknown. There may be a family tendency. Symptoms increase during stress and high anxiety; other related factors are alcoholism, trauma, and infection.
C. Signs and symptoms
   1. Subjective
      a. Pruritus, mild to severe
      b. Depression related to appearance
   2. Objective
      a. Scratching
      b. Sharply demarcated scaling plaques
D. Diagnostic methods: patient history and physical appearance
E. Treatment (individual)
   1. Topical medication: coal tars, corticosteroids (see Chapter 3)
   2. Systemic medication: corticosteroids, methotrexate (in severe cases) (see Chapter 3)
   3. Exposure to ultraviolet light, photochemotherapy
   4. Anxiolytics
   5. Antimetabolites
F. Nursing interventions
   1. During bath gently remove scales with cloth or brush.
   2. Occlusive dressing may be wrapped in plastic.

Herpes Simplex (Cold Sore, Fever Blister) Type 1 (HSV-1)

A. Definition: group of blisters on a reddened base, usually on or near mouth or genitalia
B. Cause: viral infection precipitated by an upper respiratory tract infection or elevation of temperature from systemic infection; frequently related to emotional upset, menstrual cycle, or general immunosuppression
C. Signs and symptoms
   1. Pain and local discomfort
   2. Distress about appearance
D. Diagnostic methods: physical assessment, viral isolation by tissue culture
E. Treatment: lasts approximately 1 week; antiviral agents (acyclovir) administered topically or systemically
F. Nursing interventions: none indicated

Herpes Zoster (Shingles)

A. Definition: crops of vesicles and erythema following sensory nerves on the face and trunk; higher incidence in older adults
B. Cause: varicella zoster virus (chickenpox)
C. Signs and symptoms
   1. Subjective
      a. Severe pain
      b. Malaise
      c. Anorexia
      d. Pruritus
   2. Objective
      a. Elevation of temperature
      b. Results of diagnostic tests
D. Diagnostic methods: physical examination. Vesicles follow sensory nerve paths.
E. Treatment: no specific treatment (symptomatic only); analgesics may be used for pain; usually subsides in 3 weeks (pain may last for months); antivirals, corticosteroids, capsaicin (Zostrix) for temporary relief of pain
F. Nursing interventions
   1. Keep patient in isolation while vesicles are present.
   2. Apply topical lotions to lesions for itching.
   3. Give baths or compresses for cooling and soothing.
   4. Prevent scratching and secondary infection.
   5. Anticipate pain; medicate as needed.
   6. Provide small, frequent, well-balanced meals.
G. Varicella vaccine (Varivax)

Neoplasms

A. Definition: any new and abnormal growth; may be of varied size and location
B. Cause
   1. Benign: unknown
   2. Malignant: related to exposure to sun and chemical and physical irritants such as pipe smoking
C. Signs and symptoms: anxiety related to diagnosis and change in physical appearance; appearance of lesions
D. Diagnostic test: biopsy examination—high cure rate with early detection
E. Treatment: Table 5-8
F. Nursing interventions
   1. Assess all patients for skin lesions.
   2. Discuss with patient the importance of reporting any changes in moles.
   3. Give preoperative and postoperative instructions (see Chapter 2); surgery is usually on outpatient basis.
   4. Provide general care for patient receiving radiotherapy (see Chapter 2).
   5. Give general care for patient receiving chemotherapy (see Chapter 3).
G. Classification of common skin tumors (see Table 5-8)

| Table 5-8 | Classification of Common Tumors of the Skin |

CLASSIFICATION	DESCRIPTION	TREATMENT
Benign	Nevus, brown or black mole	Observe for changes: remove only if irritated or changes are observed
Premalignant or potentially malignant	Actinic keratosis: common, sun-induced, premalignant (precancerous) lesions; often on the face and backs of hands; irregular margins, increased vascularity, and rough-textured surface; becomes reddish and scaly	Cryosurgery; topical medication
	Senile keratosis; brownish scaly spots on face and hands of aging persons	Surgical removal or topical medication or cryosurgery
	Leukoplakia: shiny white patches on mucous membranes of mouth and female genitalia	Removal of irritating teeth; oral hygiene For genitalia: surgical excision; biopsy
	Moles (nevi) that bleed, grow, or are irritated or crusted Black, smooth moles	May become malignant and are surgically removed
Malignant	Squamous cell carcinoma: begins as a warty growth and grows and becomes ulcerated; found on exposed surfaces of the body (tongue, lip)	Early surgical removal
	Basal cell carcinoma: a slow-growing tumor; results from exposure to the sun	Chemosurgery, electrosurgery, or surgical removal
	Malignant melanoma: black tumor that has metastasized	Widespread excision

Burns

A. Definition: wound in which skin layers and underlying tissue are destroyed
B. Causes
   1. Heat: dry or moist (e.g., fire)
   2. Chemical (e.g., acids)
   3. Electrical (e.g., lighting fixtures, electrical wires)
   4. Radiation (e.g., sunlight)
   5. Mechanical (e.g., friction from rope)
C. Signs and symptoms: depend on depth (Table 5-9) and area involved
   1. Infection: destruction of body's first line of defense; time after burn (hypovolemic and diuretic stage)
   2. Loss of body tissue (protein)
   3. Loss of fluid and electrolytes (edema)
   4. Pain
   5. Respiratory distress
   6. Immobilization
   7. Disfigurement
   8. Impending shock resulting from circulatory collapse
D. Diagnostic methods: physical assessment
E. Treatment
   1. Respiratory evaluation, maintenance of airway, and possible tracheostomy. Edema of lung tissue from smoke inhalation may cause increased secretions.
   2. Replacement of fluids and electrolytes with large amounts of IV solutions: plasma, blood, dextran, and electrolytes
   3. Emergency wound care: removal of foreign material; avoidance of contamination
   4. Prevention of infection: tetanus immune globulin and antibiotics
   5. Analgesics for pain (see Chapter 3)

   6. Prevention of shock: using plasma expanders; keeping patient warm; monitoring vital signs, urine output
   7. Wound treatment method
      a. Open method exposure: Wound heals by epithelialization of eschar. This method requires reverse isolation; eschar must be removed by débridement (cutting away), whirlpool baths, and escharotomy (incision into eschar).
      b. Topical medications (see Chapter 3)
      c. Grafts: to minimize infection and fluid loss; may be temporary because they are frequently rejected. This method allows for growth of new tissue underneath the protection of the graft.
         (1) Autograft: transplantation of skin from patient's own body. Care must also be given to donor site. Skin can also be grown in test tube and then grafted.
         (2) Homograft (allograft): transplantation of tissue from living human
         (3) Heterograft: transplantation from animal (pig or cow xenograft)
         (4) Synthetic material used in grafting
      d. Cosmetic surgery may be performed during recovery phase.
F. Nursing interventions
   1. Anticipate and prevent respiratory distress. Maintain airway, monitor breathing hourly and then every 4 hours (see Chapter 2). Keep tracheostomy equipment available.
   2. Maintain fluid balance: Monitor IV fluids, monitor urine output hourly through indwelling catheter, monitor specific gravity hourly, weigh patient daily.

Table 5-9 Description of Burns

CLASSIFICATION	DEPTH	DESCRIPTION	POSSIBLE CAUSE
Superficial or shallow partial thickness	Epidermis	Red and dry; painful; may cause edema; no scarring	Sunburn
Deep partial thickness	Epidermis and some dermis	Mottled, pink-to-red blisters; painful; leaves scar	Hot oil
Partial full thickness	Epidermis, dermis, and subcutaneous tissue	Black or bright red eschar forms leathery covering; leaves scar; patient may have no pain	Fire
Deep full thickness	All of the above plus subcutaneous fat, fascia, muscle, and bone (nerve endings, hair follicles, and sweat glands destroyed)	Black; no pain	Fire

3. Anticipate infection: Maintain asepsis and reverse isolation, administer antibiotics, monitor temperature every 2 hours. Keep patient warm.
4. Anticipate pain: Give frequent sedation as ordered, especially before dressing change (administered intravenously during early phase of treatment).
5. Prevent dangers of immobilization (see Chapter 2): Provide proper alignment to prevent deformities (may be uncomfortable or painful), prevent skin surfaces from touching, use turning frames and cradles.
6. To enhance tissue repair, diet must be high in calories (6000 calories daily) and high in protein; tube feeding or TPN may be necessary.
7. Anticipate shock: Assess LOC and mental status; monitor pulse rate and blood pressure.
8. Anticipate Curling ulcer (stress ulcer): At end of first week assess for GI distress or bleeding.
9. Be aware of anxiety. Provide diversional activities. Allow time for patient to verbalize feelings; encourage contact with family. Involve patient as much as possible with planning and self-care; administer tranquilizers and sedation as necessary.

SENSORY SYSTEMS

VISUAL SYSTEM

Anatomy and Physiology (Figures 5-21 and 5-22**)**
A. Lies in a protective bony orbit in the skull
B. Eyebrows, eyelids, and lashes also protect the eye.
C. Sphere consists of three layers of tissue:
1. Sclera: thick, white fibrous tissue (white of eye). A transparent section over the front of the eyeball, the cornea, permits light rays to enter.
2. Choroid: middle vascular area; brings oxygen and nutrients to the eye. Choroid extends to ciliary body (two smooth muscle structures), which helps control shape of the lens. The front is a pigmented section (iris), which gives the eye color; in the center of the iris lies the pupil, the "window of the eye" (allows light to pass to lens and retina).
3. Retina: inner layer; physiology of vision takes place; contains receptors of optic nerve. Neurons are shaped as rods and cones; cones permit perception of color, rods permit perception of light and shade.
D. Chambers

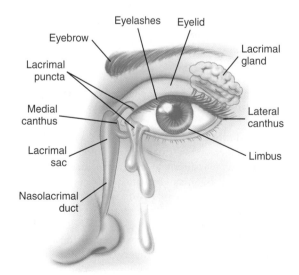

FIGURE 5-21 Horizontal section through the eyeball. (From Thibodeau GA, Patton KT: *Anatomy and physiology,* ed 6, St Louis, 2007, Mosby.)

FIGURE 5-22 Visual accessory organs. (From Herlihy B: *The human body in health and illness,* ed 4, St Louis, 2011, Saunders.)

1. Anterior: contains aqueous humor, maintains slight forward curve in cornea
2. Posterior: contains vitreous humor, maintains spherical shape of eyeball

E. Conjunctiva: mucous membrane that covers eyeball and eyelid; keeps eyeball moist
F. Lens: transparent structure behind iris; focuses light rays on retina
G. Lacrimal apparatus: gland located in upper, outer part of eye; produces tears to lubricate and cleanse; nasolacrimal duct located in nasal corner; tears drain into nose.
H. Normal intraocular pressure: 10 to 21 mm Hg

Conditions and Disorders of the Eye

Sight is the most important sense to most people. Visual acuity depends on general good health, CNS regulation of movement and conduction, and condition of the structures of the eye. Changes in vision frequently indicate systemic disease; routine examination of the eye can provide information about diseases in other systems. The nurse must assess the eyes of each patient under his or her care. Although the incidence of blindness and visual impairment increases with age, problems are seen in patients of all ages.

Nursing Assessment

A. Observations
   1. Glasses, contact lenses, or false eyes
   2. Tearing, discharge (clear or purulent), and color of sclera (white, yellow, or pink)
   3. Accuracy and range of vision
   4. Edema of eyelids; crusting; blinking, rubbing; redness
   5. Clouded appearance over pupil; protrusion or bulging of one or both eyes; pupil response to light; pupils equal, round, reactive to light, accommodation (PERRLA)
   6. Squinting or drooping (ptosis) of eyelid
   7. Symmetry
B. Patient description (subjective data)
   1. Double vision (diplopia), decreased or absent vision in one or both eyes, blurred or clouded vision
   2. Sensitivity to light (photophobia), spots, halos around lights, flashes of light, problems seeing in the dark
   3. Eye fatigue, itching, pain, tearing, burning, headache, dryness
C. Note patient history of:
   1. Stumbling.
   2. Trauma of face or eyes.
   3. Contact lenses or eye medication.
   4. Changes in vision and any related circumstances.
   5. Any systemic medications taken.

Diagnostic Tests and Methods

A. Ophthalmoscope: assessment of interior of eye
B. Tonometer: measurement of intraocular pressure; increased pressure may indicate early glaucoma; recommended every one to two years for individuals 40 years of age and over, especially if there is a family history of glaucoma.
C. Fields of vision: testing to measure sight on one or both sides (peripheral vision); perimetry
D. Refraction: measurement of light refraction and lenses required for visual acuity
E. Slit lamp: examination of intraocular structures with a high-intensity light beam (corneal abrasions, iritis)
F. Snellen chart: assessment of visual acuity (three times: left eye [OS], right eye [OD], both, or each eye [OU])
G. Retinal angiography: retinal vessels

Eye Care Professionals

A. Ophthalmologist (also called *oculist*): medical doctor who specializes in diagnosis, treatment, and surgery of the eyes, including prescribing glasses
B. Optometrist: educated and licensed to test for refractive problems; may prescribe and fit glasses; may, within limits, diagnose disease, prescribe medication, or treat eye diseases (laws vary among states)
C. Optician: fills prescription for corrective lenses as prescribed by physician; fits glasses properly

Frequent Patient Problems and Nursing Care

A. Anxiety and fear related to concerns about loss of vision, altered lifestyles, ability to function, employment, plans for future, and altered body image. Allow time for patient to express feelings.
B. Risk for infection related to drainage, use of eyedrops
   1. Clean as necessary with normal saline solution.
   2. Gently apply compresses to loosen if necessary.
   3. Use aseptic technique; wipe from inner canthus to outer canthus.
   4. If drainage is purulent, dispose of properly.
C. Risk for injury related to need for corrective lenses
   1. Glasses must be kept clean and in a protective case.
   2. Contact lenses are kept in a case marked with R and L to designate which eye the lens fits; obtain directions for soaking from patient.
   3. If patient depends on lenses, obtain permission for him or her to wear glasses or lenses when going for diagnostic tests.
D. Risk for injury related to photophobia
   1. Keep room dim and evenly lighted.
   2. Keep blinds adjusted to avoid glare.

Major Medical Diagnoses
Low Vision

A. Definition: defects that cannot be corrected with lenses
B. Cause: disease of the eye itself in the visual pathways to the brain or in receptors in the brain; macular degeneration
C. Signs and symptoms: Vision may be blurred and images distorted. Vision may be clear only at close range. Shades of color may not be distinguishable.

Total or Legal Blindness

A. Definition: Legal blindness is the ability to see at no more than 20 ft (6 m) what normally should be seen at a distance of 200 ft (60 m) (20/200). This may also refer to severe restrictions in peripheral fields of vision (when corrective lenses are used).
B. Pathology
   1. Macular degeneration, glaucoma, detached retina, diabetic retinopathy
   2. Trauma, laceration
   3. Inflammation, optic neuritis
   4. Vascular or hypertensive retinopathy
   5. Neoplasms of the brain or eye
   6. Cataract

C. Patient problems
   1. Inability to care for self (dependency)
   2. Frustration
   3. Occupational hazards
   4. Boredom
D. Nursing diagnoses
   1. Anxiety related to degree of visual impairment
   2. Risk for injury or trauma related to degree of visual impairment
   3. Disturbed body image
E. Nursing interventions
   1. Allow as much independence as possible. Help make use of existing vision. Encourage use of any visual aids recommended by physician (e.g., special lenses, large-type books, cane). Provide reading material in braille for the patient who has learned this method.
   2. Do not touch patient without talking. Always address patient by name, introduce yourself, and tell patient when you are leaving the room.
   3. Explain all care and treatments; encourage patient to participate in planning care.
   4. At mealtime indicate position of utensils and placement of food on dish by comparing it with numbers on a clock (e.g., "the potato is at 3 o'clock").
   5. Orient patient to room and entire unit. Point out hazards and obstacles (doors and windows); explain location of furniture, bathroom, call bell, telephone. Keep items in the same place.
   6. Leave bedside table, call bell, and personal items in close reach.
   7. Maintain safety. Keep unit uncluttered, floor clean and dry, bed in low position, and side rails up as necessary. Tell patient position of bed and side rails.
   8. Guide the ambulatory patient by placing his or her arm on your arm while walking slowly.
   9. Provide diversion: radio and audiobooks. Be aware of local agencies in the community; many libraries have braille books or audiobooks available.
   10. Be mindful of patient confidentiality and security.

Refractive Disorders

A. Definition: inability of the refractory media to make light rays converge and focus on retina
   1. Myopia (nearsightedness): Eyeball is too long; light rays focus at a point before reaching the retina.
   2. Hyperopia (farsightedness): Eyeball is shorter than normal; light rays focus beyond the retina.
   3. Presbyopia: Gradual loss of elasticity of the lens; ability to focus on near objects is decreased.
   4. Astigmatism: Unequal curve in shape of cornea or lens; vision is distorted.
B. Cause: unknown; may be inherited
C. Symptoms: diminished or blurred vision
D. Diagnostic tests and methods
   1. Patient history
   2. Refraction
E. Treatment: corrective lenses (glasses or contact lenses); keratorefractive surgery
F. Nursing interventions
   1. Encourage proper care of lenses.
   2. Encourage follow-up checkups as indicated.

Conjunctivitis

A. Definition: infection or inflammation of the conjunctiva
B. Causes: bacteria, usually staphylococci; allergens; chemical reactions; chlamydial or viral infections
C. Patient problems
   1. Very contagious (especially in young children); spread by direct contact with organisms
   2. Purulent drainage and itching
   3. Photophobia
   4. Tearing
D. Diagnostic method: physical assessment, culture and sensitivity of conjunctival scrapings
E. Treatment: ophthalmic antibiotics (see Chapter 3)
F. Nursing interventions
   1. Prevent transmission to others: encourage frequent handwashing.
   2. Provide warm compresses; cleanse eyelids; remove crusts before administering ophthalmic medications.
      a. Discourage rubbing of eyes.
      b. Isolate personal items (towels, washcloths, pillowcases).

Cataract

A. Definition: crystalline lens becomes clouded and opaque (not transparent).
B. Causes
   1. Trauma
   2. Congenital
   3. Related to diabetes
   4. High incidence in the elderly population (senile cataracts)
   5. Heredity
   6. Infections
   7. Excessive exposure to the sun or ultraviolet rays
C. Signs and symptoms
   1. Loss of vision
   2. Progressive blurring
   3. Haziness with eventual complete loss of sight
D. Diagnostic tests and methods
   1. Examination with ophthalmoscope
   2. Patient history
   3. Ultrasonography
E. Treatment: surgical removal of opaque lens, usually on an outpatient basis. After surgery, corrective lenses are necessary (glasses, contact lenses, or surgical implantation of an artificial [intraocular] lens [IOL])
F. Nursing interventions
   1. Give general preoperative care (see Chapter 2).
   2. Provide nursing care as for patient with low vision.
   3. Postoperative management depends on surgical procedure. Be careful to adhere to physician's order. General principles are to have patient avoid coughing, bending, or rapidly moving head; provide bed rest for a specified time (usually 2 hours); keep patient flat or in low-Fowler position; have patient deep breathe (avoid coughing); be sure that patient avoids straining (give stool softener); help patient avoid vomiting (an antiemetic will be ordered; administer as needed); observe dressing; report pain or bleeding; position patient with unoperated side down.

Glaucoma

A. Definition: Intraocular pressure increases because of a disturbance in the circulation of aqueous humor; there is an imbalance between production and drainage as the angle of drainage closes.

1. Acute (closed-angle) glaucoma: dramatic onset of symptoms. Immediate treatment, usually surgery, is required.
2. Chronic (open-angle) glaucoma: symptoms progress slowly and frequently are ignored. If disease is not detected early, it may lead to permanent loss of vision.

B. Pathology
1. Familial tendency
2. Related to age; incidence increases after 40 years of age
3. Secondary to injuries and infections

C. Signs and symptoms
1. Subjective
   a. Loss of peripheral vision (tunnel vision), halos around lights, permanent loss of vision (a leading cause of blindness)
   b. Pain, malaise, nausea
   c. Reduced visual acuity at night
2. Objective
   a. Pupils fixed and dilated
   b. Vomiting
   c. Results of diagnostic tests

D. Diagnostic tests and methods
1. History of symptoms
2. Measurement of visual fields
3. Measurement of intraocular pressure
4. Gonioscopy: measures angle of the anterior chamber
5. Tonometry

E. Treatment
1. Miotics to decrease intraocular pressure (see Chapter 3)
2. Surgery: iridectomy (an incision through the cornea to remove part of the iris to allow for drainage), laser trabeculoplasty (relieves excess intraocular pressure), trabeculectomy (new opening made to bypass obstruction and facilitate flow of aqueous humor), laser iridotomy
3. Continued medical supervision

F. Nursing interventions
1. Encourage patient to wear medical identification tag.
2. Administer eye medications on schedule.
3. Inform patient to avoid drugs with atropine; discourage straining and lifting.
4. Give preoperative and postoperative care according to that for a patient with a cataract; pay careful attention to specifics in physician's orders.

Detached Retina

A. Definition: Sensory layer of retina pulls away from pigmented layer; vitreous humor may leak into the space occupying the position the retina normally assumes.

B. Cause: usually unknown and spontaneous; may be related to sudden blow to the head or follow eye surgery (e.g., removal of cataract)

C. Signs and symptoms
1. Subjective
   a. Loss of vision in affected area (may be complete loss)
   b. Painless
   c. Visual disturbance (blurring)
   d. Spots and flashes of light
2. Objective: results of diagnostic tests

D. Diagnostic tests and methods
1. Patient history and physical assessment
2. Retinal examination with ophthalmoscope

3. Ultrasonography
4. Slit lamp

E. Treatment: depends on area of detachment
1. Bed rest
2. Prevention of extension of detachment by restriction of eye movements
3. Mydriatics
4. Surgical intervention: laser photocoagulation, cryopexy, diathermy, scleral buckling, pneumatic retinopexy, vitrectomy

F. Nursing interventions
1. Provide individual care according to location of detachment; physician's orders will be specific.
2. Maintain absolute rest; restrict activity. Patch eye to limit eye movement; may use eye shield. Patient position is based on location of retinal detachment.
3. Prepare patient for postoperative care. Inform patient that both eyes may be patched and that he or she may be unable to see.
4. Postoperative care: Position patient exactly as ordered. Maintain eye patch or patches. Have patient deep breathe and avoid coughing. Administer medication for pain. Provide care as needed for a person with limited sight.

G. Patient problems, nursing diagnoses
1. Anxiety related to possibility of permanent vision loss
2. Self-care deficit: bathing, dressing, feeding, toileting related to imposed activity restrictions
3. Acute pain related to surgical correction and unusual positioning

AUDITORY SYSTEM

Anatomy and Physiology (Figures 5-23 and 5-24)

A. External ear (pinna or auricle): outer, visible portion, shaped like a funnel; gathers sound and sends it into the auditory canal, which is lined with tiny hairs and secretes cerumen, a waxy substance. Canal extends to the eardrum, also called the *tympanic membrane.*

B. Middle ear: small, flattened space; contains three small bones called *ossicles:* malleus (hammer), incus (anvil), and stapes (stirrup). Bones are mobile and vibrate; conduct sound waves. Eustachian tube extends into nasopharynx and equalizes the pressure in middle ear to that of atmospheric pressure.

C. Internal ear (labyrinth): vestibule; cochlea, snail-shaped bony tube, contains organ of Corti (organ of hearing). Semicircular canals are the receptors for equilibrium and head movements.

D. Function
1. Transmission of sound waves; result is hearing.
2. Maintenance of equilibrium

CONDITIONS AND DISORDERS OF THE EAR

Hearing problems are not as obvious initially during assessment as are many other problems. Hearing loss may be misinterpreted. Many people associate hearing aids with dependency or disfigurement or signs of aging and refuse to wear them. However, the sense of hearing contributes to well-being and safety. This assessment (hearing) must be made for each patient.

Nursing Assessment

A. Observations
1. Difficulty hearing or understanding verbal communication
2. Not responding to loud or sudden noises
3. Use of hearing aid, lip reading, or sign language
4. Drainage, dried secretion, or deformities of the ear

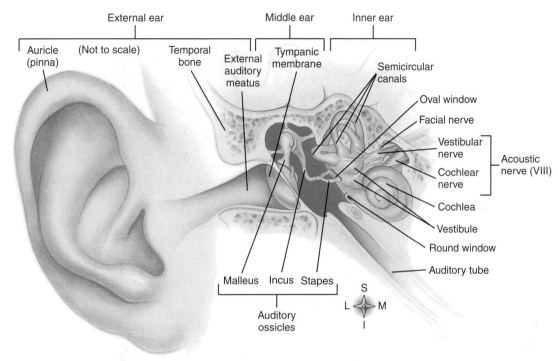

FIGURE 5-23 The ear. (From Patton KT, Thibodeau GA: *Anatomy and physiology,* ed 8, St Louis, 2013, Mosby.)

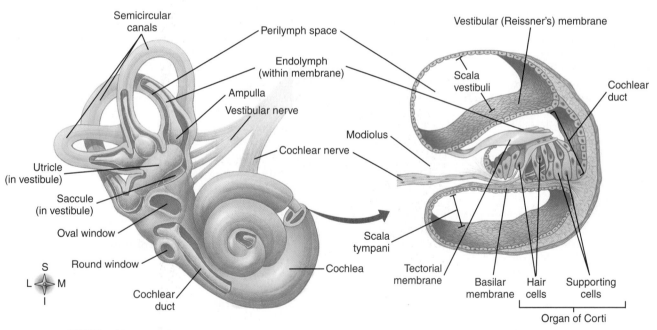

FIGURE 5-24 The inner ear. (From Thibodeau GA, Patton KT: *Anatomy and physiology,* ed 6, St Louis, 2007, Mosby.)

B. Patient description (subjective data)
   1. Earache or headache
   2. Difficulty hearing (or lack of hearing) in one or both ears
   3. Itching, drainage, pressure or full feeling
   4. Ringing, buzzing, popping, echoes
   5. Vertigo
   6. Medications taken
C. Note history of:
   1. Ear infections.
   2. Ear surgery.
   3. Head injury.
   4. Medications taken.

Diagnostic Tests and Methods

A. Audiometry: hearing test to determine ability to discriminate sounds, voices, degrees of loudness, and pitch
B. Otoscopy: visual examination of the ear canal and tympanic membrane
C. Weber test: A tuning fork is struck and placed midline on patient's forehead. Patient is asked where the sound is

heard; in this test of conduction, sounds should be heard equally well in each ear.

D. Rinne test: The tuning fork is struck and placed on the mastoid process of the skull behind the ear; the fork is removed, and patient indicates when the sound can no longer be heard. The still-vibrating fork is then placed near the external ear canal; normally the sound is heard longer through air conduction than through bone conduction.

E. Caloric stimulation test (CST): tests vestibular reflexes of inner ear that control balance

F. Electronystagmography: monitors eye movements; done with CST

Patient with Impaired Hearing

A. Definition
1. Conductive hearing loss occurs when injury or disease interferes with the conduction of sound waves to the inner ear (e.g., cerumen in canal).
2. Sensory hearing loss occurs when malfunction of the inner ear, auditory nerve, or auditory center in the brain (e.g., toxic effect to eighth cranial nerve from drugs [aspirin]) occurs.

B. Patient problems
1. Inability to communicate
2. Inability to hear hazards in the environment (e.g., automobiles)
3. Frustration, anxiety, anger, insecurity
4. Misinterpretation of communication

C. Treatment: according to cause (cochlear implants, stapedectomy); frequently none

D. Nursing interventions
1. Determine if a hearing aid can be fitted.
   a. Encourage patient to wear it.
   b. Test batteries for function.
   c. Make sure hearing aid is turned on.
   d. Protect hearing aid from breakage. Ask patient or family about usual care and storage.
2. Attract patient's attention before speaking.
3. Do not touch patient until he or she is aware that you are in the room.
4. Speak face to face; articulate clearly but not too slowly; move close to patient; avoid covering mouth with hand.
5. Provide alternate methods of communication.
   a. Find out if patient reads lips or uses sign language.
   b. Provide magic slate or pad and pencil.
6. Nursing interventions after surgery
   a. Give general preoperative and postoperative care (see Chapter 2).
   b. Report drainage immediately.
   c. Observe for facial nerve injury: inability to close eyes or pucker lips.
   d. Anticipate vertigo; provide safety.
   e. Be sure patient avoids blowing nose.
   f. Note specific instructions from physician for positioning, activity, and diet.

Major Medical Diagnoses
Ménière Syndrome

A. Definition: chronic disease with sudden attacks of vertigo and tinnitus (ringing in the ear) with progressive hearing loss; attacks last a few minutes to a few weeks; usually occurs in women older than 50 years

B. Cause: unknown; related to fluid in cochlea, either increased production or decreased absorption

C. Signs and symptoms
1. Vertigo
2. Nausea and vomiting
3. Ringing in the ears, hearing loss
4. Disequilibrium

D. Diagnostic tests and methods: patient history, physical examination, neurological assessment, CST, radiography, electronystagmography, audiogram

E. Treatment
1. Diuretics, low-sodium diet, vasodilators, antihistamines, antiemetics, vestibular depressants, adrenergic agents
2. Surgery: endolymphatic shunt (reduces pressure and controls vertigo), destruction of the labyrinth as a last resort

F. Nursing interventions
1. Provide bed rest; position of comfort.
2. Maintain quiet and safety.
3. Provide low-sodium diet.
4. Provide specific nursing care such as for patient with impaired hearing (this section).
5. Provide general preoperative and postoperative care (see Chapter 2).
6. Provide nursing care for patient after ear surgery (see this section on patient with impaired hearing).

Mastoiditis

A. Definition: infection of mastoid process; may be acute or chronic; not common because of antibiotics

B. Cause: extension of middle ear infection that was inadequately treated

C. Signs and symptoms
1. Subjective: headache, ear pain, tenderness over mastoid process
2. Objective
   a. Elevation of temperature
   b. Drainage from ear

D. Treatment
1. Antibiotics
2. Surgery
   a. Simple mastoidectomy: removal of infected cells
   b. Radical mastoidectomy: more extensive excision resulting in some degree of hearing loss

E. Nursing interventions
1. See discussion of patient with impaired hearing (this section).
2. Provide general preoperative and postoperative care (see Chapter 2).
3. Provide nursing care for patient after ear surgery (see this section on patient with impaired hearing).

Otosclerosis

A. Definition: progressive formation of new bone tissue around the stapes, preventing transmission of vibrations to the inner ear

B. Cause: unknown

C. Signs and symptoms
1. Loss of hearing
2. Ringing or buzzing (tinnitus)

D. Treatment
1. Hearing aid
2. Surgery; stapedectomy (removal of diseased bone and replacement with prosthetic implant)

E. Nursing interventions
1. Provide general care for patient who is hearing impaired.
2. Give general preoperative and postoperative care (see Chapter 2).
3. Follow specific orders from physician.
4. Provide general nursing care for patient after ear surgery (see patient with impaired hearing, p. 276).

Bibliography

Christensen BL, Kockrow EO: *Foundations of nursing*, ed 6, St Louis, 2010, Mosby.

deWit SC: *Fundamental concepts and skills for nursing*, ed 4, St Louis, 2014, Saunders.

deWit SC: *Medical-surgical nursing: concepts and practice*, ed 2, St Louis, 2013, Saunders.

Edmunds MW: *Introduction to clinical pharmacology*, ed 7, St Louis, 2013, Mosby.

Emergency Nurse's Association: *Sheehy's manual of emergency care*, ed 7, St Louis, 2013, Mosby.

Herlihy B, Maebius NK: *Human body in health and illness*, ed 4, Philadelphia, 2011, Saunders.

Hill SS, Howlett HS: *Success in practical/vocational nursing*, ed 7, St Louis, 2013, Saunders.

McKinney ES, et al: *Maternal-child nursing*, ed 4, St Louis, 2013, Saunders.

Monahan FD, et al: *Phipps' medical-surgical nursing: health and illness perspectives*, ed 8, St Louis, 2007, Mosby.

Morrison-Valfre M: *Foundations of mental health care*, ed 5, St Louis, 2013, Mosby.

Mosby's dictionary of medicine, nursing, and health professions, ed 9, St Louis, 2013, Mosby.

Nix S: *Williams' basic nutrition and diet therapy*, ed 14, St Louis, 2013, Mosby.

Patton KT, Thibodeau GA: *Anatomy and physiology*, ed 8, St Louis, 2013, Mosby.

Perry AG, Potter PA, Elkin MK: *Nursing interventions and clinical skills*, ed 5, St Louis, 2012, Mosby.

Potter PA, et al: *Basic nursing: a critical thinking approach*, ed 7, St Louis, 2011, Mosby.

Venes D: *Taber's cyclopedic medical dictionary*, ed 21, Philadelphia, 2010, FA Davis.

Wold GH: *Basic geriatric nursing*, ed 5, St Louis, 2012, Mosby.

REVIEW QUESTIONS

1. A patient who is to undergo a cardiac catheterization communicates to the nurse that he forgot to inform the physician that he is allergic to shrimp. What should the nurse do next?
1. Inform the physician of patient's allergy.
2. Prepare patient for the catheterization.
3. Ask patient what happens when he eats shrimp.
4. Place an allergy band around patient's wrist.

2. A nurse is observing a new graduate as she evaluates a patient with the Glasgow Coma Scale (GCS). What indicates that the new graduate understands the assessment criteria?
1. Posturing, reflexes, eye opening
2. Eye opening, verbal response, motor response
3. Voice commands, posturing, reflexes
4. Seizure activity, motor response, verbal response

3. A nursing assistant asks the nurse how a patient's wound has healed in such short a time. The nurse relates that through the process of _____ the wound has healed itself through primary intention.
1. Lysis
2. Mitosis
3. Osmosis
4. Crenation

4. The nurse administers an antitoxin to an individual who may have been exposed to tetanus. The patient asks the nurse what kind of immunity the shot provided. The nurse is correct in stating that the immunity is:
1. Active.
2. Passive.
3. Permanent.
4. Autoimmune.

5. A patient is admitted to the hospital with a possible diagnosis of otosclerosis. If the patient has the following presenting symptoms, which symptoms may indicate the diagnosis? Select all that apply.
_____ 1. Diplopia
_____ 2. Low-pitched tinnitus
_____ 3. Ear pain
_____ 4. Progressive hearing loss
_____ 5. Vertigo

6. A patient has fallen off a horse and is brought to the emergency department for evaluation for a closed head injury. Which assessment finding should the nurse report immediately to the physician?
1. Vomiting
2. Headache
3. Tremors
4. Pruritus

7. The nurse is teaching a fertility class to a group of individuals. The nurse correctly states that the ovaries produce which two hormones?
1. Estrogen and testosterone
2. Estrogen and progesterone
3. Progesterone and prolactin
4. Progesterone and testosterone

8. A patient is scheduled to have both of his testes removed because of testicular cancer. The nurse prepares the patient with the understanding that the patient may need to receive replacement:
1. Estrogen.
2. Progesterone.
3. Testosterone.
4. Aldosterone.

9. The nurse is caring for a patient with a new diagnosis of Parkinson disease. Which assessment data would best describe the symptoms of an individual with Parkinson disease? Select all that apply.
_____ 1. Diplopia
_____ 2. Headache
_____ 3. Shuffling gait
_____ 4. Tinnitus
_____ 5. Dysphagia

10. A patient with diverticulitis makes the following statements. Which statement would indicate to the nurse that further teaching is indicated?
1. "I can eat popcorn for a snack; the fiber is good for me."
2. "I should try to avoid constipation as much as possible."
3. "I should increase my fluids."
4. "I should take a stool softener every day."

11. A patient is scheduled to have a bowel resection. The patient inquires why he will need to be on total parenteral nutrition (TPN) after the surgery. What is the best response by the nurse?
    1. "The added nutrients are necessary because your small intestine may not be able to absorb as many nutrients."
    2. "The extra glucose in the TPN is necessary for proper body repair."
    3. "The TPN will help reestablish the normal flora of your small intestine."
    4. "Your liver will be incapable of processing nutrients because of the complexity of the surgery."

12. Which nursing measure would best alleviate the pruritus and burning that a patient has because of external hemorrhoids?
    1. Sitz bath
    2. Pillows
    3. Acetaminophen
    4. Tap-water enema

13. A patient who has had a cholecystectomy asks the nurse in what area his T tube has been "hooked." What is the correct response by the nurse?
    1. "It is inserted into the area where the gallbladder was to drain blood."
    2. "The T tube drains the juices from your liver."
    3. "It is inserted into the common bile duct to drain bile while your incision heals."
    4. "It drains stomach acid so it does not inflame your incisional area."

14. Which nursing diagnosis is of priority concern for a patient undergoing peritoneal dialysis?
    1. Risk for infection
    2. Deficient fluid volume
    3. Disturbed body image
    4. Feeding self-care deficit

15. A patient is scheduled to have his right labyrinth destroyed because of Ménière's disease. Which statement is true regarding this procedure?
    1. The patient may still have symptoms from the disease.
    2. The patient will be unable to hear on that side after the procedure.
    3. The symptoms will likely come back after the procedure.
    4. Symptoms will gradually decline after the procedure.

16. A patient in diabetic ketoacidosis has metabolic acidosis. Which pH level may indicate this condition?
    1. 7.41
    2. 7.40
    3. 7.36
    4. 7.30

17. A patient's abdominal incision is no longer approximated, and the nurse observes viscera protruding from the wound. Prioritize the order of the nurse's actions from first to last using the following interventions:
    1. Call the physician.
    2. Cover the viscera with sterile saline-soaked gauze.
    3. Assess vital signs.
    4. Notify the nursing supervisor.
    5. Remain calm.

18. A patient has been diagnosed with breast cancer in the early stage. Which surgical procedure would preserve the most breast tissue for this patient?
    1. Lumpectomy
    2. Mastectomy
    3. Needle biopsy
    4. Oophorectomy

19. A patient with hypertension lists the following foods in his food history. Which would be detrimental to his low-sodium diet?
    1. Bananas and apples each day
    2. Take-out Chinese food three times per week
    3. Fresh fish, including trout and bass, twice per week
    4. Garlic and rosemary herbs as seasonings for most foods

20. A patient returns from a tonsillectomy. Which task is the priority for the nurse at this time?
    1. Assessing pain status
    2. Assessing vital signs
    3. Assessing airway
    4. Assessing for hemorrhage

21. A patient is being prepared for a cholecystectomy. What would best prevent postoperative aspiration?
    1. Nothing by mouth status for 6 to 8 hours before surgery
    2. Reglan 10 mg IVPB over 1 hour before surgery
    3. Versed 5 mg 1 hour before surgery
    4. Nasogastric decompression during the surgery

22. A patient is diagnosed with a detached retina. Which symptom did the patient most likely report?
    1. Diplopia
    2. Painless loss of vision
    3. Tunnel vision
    4. Headache on affected side

23. Which assessment data would be included in an integumentary assessment? Select all that apply.
    _____ 1. Blood sugar levels
    _____ 2. Blood pressure
    _____ 3. Rashes
    _____ 4. Decubitus ulcer
    _____ 5. Bruises

24. Which symptom is associated with the diagnosis of glaucoma?
    1. Painless loss of vision
    2. Diplopia
    3. Tunnel vision
    4. Strabismus

25. A patient asks the nurse about the purpose of a miotic. What is the correct information to include in the answer?
    1. It makes pupils small and decreases intraocular pressure.
    2. It increases the diameter of your pupil to allow more free flow of fluid in the eye.
    3. It is used as a diuretic for the eye.
    4. It is used to treat detached retina.

26. A patient is being discharged after being treated for fractured ribs. Which discharge instructions are appropriate for this patient?
    1. Morphine p.r.n. for pain
    2. Oxygen 4 L per minute via nasal cannula
    3. Incentive spirometry 10 times per hour
    4. Cast care every 4 hours

27. A nurse is caring for a patient who has an injury to the left motor area of the cerebrum. Where would the nurse expect to see paralysis?
    1. Both arms and legs
    2. The left side of the body
    3. The right side of the body
    4. No paralysis should be observed.

28. A patient is receiving external radiation to treat bone cancer. What should be stressed during a patient teaching session?
    1. Use cocoa butter oil to lubricate the skin each day.
    2. Do not allow anyone to wash the markings off your skin.
    3. Try ice or heat packs if the area becomes sore.
    4. Go to the emergency department right away if the area becomes red.

29. A nurse assesses a patient with a positive purified protein derivative (PPD). What is true concerning this situation?
    1. The patient needs to be on contact isolation.
    2. The patient has antibodies to the tuberculosis (TB) bacillus.
    3. The patient has an active TB infection.
    4. This patient will need to be on antibiotics for 3 to 6 years.

30. A nurse on a skilled nursing unit needs to assess the following residents. Which resident should the nurse visit first?
    1. A resident who has just fallen from her wheelchair
    2. A resident who is requesting pain medication
    3. A resident with a glucometer reading of 302
    4. A resident who needs to go to the restroom

31. Which assessment data would indicate compromised neurovascular function? Select all that apply.
    _____ 1. Bounding pulse
    _____ 2. Capillary refill time of 6 seconds
    _____ 3. Cool extremity
    _____ 4. Complaints of pain
    _____ 5. Numbness and tingling
    _____ 6. Blue discoloration to the skin

32. A patient is diagnosed with a herniated nucleus pulposus. Which fact in the patient's history is significant with regard to the diagnosis?
    1. Has smoked one pack per day for 4 years
    2. Plants a garden each year
    3. Eats only two meals per day
    4. Works as a warehouse manager for a grocery store

33. The nurse is monitoring a patient immediately after a laminectomy. What suggests that the patient is experiencing a complication from the surgery?
    1. The patient complains of a headache when sitting upright.
    2. The patient complains of pain when sitting in a chair.
    3. The patient's incision line is wet.
    4. The patient complains of nausea.

34. A patient with diabetes is being managed on a split dose of 70/30 isophane insulin suspension (NPH insulin) at 7:30 AM and 4:30 PM. At 2:30 PM one afternoon the patient calls the nurses' station stating that she is not feeling well. On assessment the nurse notes that her skin is cool and clammy, her hands are shaking, and she appears very apprehensive. The glucometer blood sugar is 45 mg/dL. The most appropriate nursing intervention for the patient's current symptoms is to provide:

1. A cube of sugar.
2. A large candy bar.
3. 4 oz of fruit juice.
4. 12 oz of diet drink.

35. Which assessment data may indicate that a patient with an external fixation device has developed osteomyelitis?
    1. Chest pain, dyspnea
    2. Edema, pain, drainage
    3. Numbness, delayed capillary refill
    4. Paresthesia, bluish skin around the knee

36. A patient has undergone a craniotomy for removal of a meningioma. Which question would be the most appropriate in assessing a possible complication of this patient's surgery?
    1. "Have you noticed any salty or sweet-tasting drainage coming from your incision?"
    2. "Do you have any headache when you turn to your left side?"
    3. "Are you hungry or thirsty yet?"
    4. "Do you feel that you need to sleep more?"

37. When planning care for a patient with amyotrophic lateral sclerosis (ALS), a priority nursing intervention would include:
    1. Increased periods of exercise.
    2. Alternative means of communication.
    3. Clear airway maintenance.
    4. Means of adjusting to diagnosis.

38. The nurse observes that an older patient uses her diaphragm during inspiration and plans to teach her to do pursed-lip breathing, based on the understanding that older persons:
    1. Need to consciously think about taking deep breaths.
    2. Are more likely to develop chronic obstructive pulmonary disease.
    3. Experience a loss of elastic recoil of the lungs.
    4. Lose the use of their intercostal muscles.

39. A nurse is caring for a patient with a suspected diagnosis of osteoarthritis. What are common characteristics of osteoarthritis?
    1. Tenderness and crepitus
    2. Bilateral inflammation and immobility
    3. Pain resulting from destruction of supportive structures
    4. Fluid within the joint along with inflammatory tissue changes

40. A nurse is caring for a patient with insulin-dependent diabetes mellitus. The nurse finds the patient unconscious 2 hours after administration of 12 units of regular insulin. A blood glucose reading shows 30 mg/dL. What is the nurse's next course of action?
    1. Administer IV insulin.
    2. Sit the patient up and place a small amount of orange juice in her mouth.
    3. Place crushed crackers in the patient's mouth and help her swallow.
    4. Place concentrated glucose between the cheek and the gum and allow it to be absorbed.

41. A patient pulls out his chest tube. The nurse immediately places petroleum gauze over the puncture site. A dietary aide asks the nurse why she used that dressing. The nurse's most appropriate response is:
    1. "A dressing is used to prevent the patient from infecting the puncture site."

2. "The petroleum will allow the site to get air circulation."

3. "The occlusive dressing is used so air does not enter the lung."

4. "The dressing is used in case there is any leakage."

42. A patient underwent a right lower lobectomy at 10:00 AM. It is now 2:00 PM. The nurse knows that the best turning schedule for the patient is:
    1. Right side to back to left side to right side.
    2. Left side to back to left side to back.
    3. Back to left semiprone to back.
    4. Back to right semiprone to back.

43. The nurse is caring for a patient who has undergone a subtotal thyroidectomy. The nurse is aware that accidental removal of the parathyroid glands can occur and will closely monitor the patient for which of the following? Select all that apply.
    _____ 1. Low calcium levels
    _____ 2. Excess cortisol secretion
    _____ 3. High urine output
    _____ 4. Decreased gag reflex
    _____ 5. High thyroid-stimulating hormone (TSH) levels
    _____ 6. Tetany

44. A patient with a hiatal hernia and reflux syndrome reports having pain when he lies down to go to bed at night. An appropriate suggestion by the nurse would be:
    1. Remove high-acid food from the diet.
    2. Drink a hot cup of cocoa before retiring for the night.
    3. Abstain from food or drink before going to bed.
    4. Take a sleeping pill 1 hour before retiring for the night.

45. A patient has the following in his health history. Which would contribute most to the development of oral cancer?
    1. Alcohol abuse
    2. Poor dental hygiene
    3. Frequent bouts of tonsillitis
    4. Chewing smokeless tobacco

46. The nurse is teaching a patient newly diagnosed with diabetes mellitus about reducing the risk of hypoglycemia. What will be included in the health teaching? Select all that apply.
    _____ 1. "Exercise by walking on a regular basis."
    _____ 2. "Space your meals 5 to 6 hours apart."
    _____ 3. "Take your diabetes medicine in early afternoon."
    _____ 4. "Carry a form of rapid-acting sugar with you at all times."
    _____ 5. "Do not take any insulin on days that you feel nauseated or sick."
    _____ 6. "If your glucometer reading is low, make sure to double the next insulin dose."

47. A female patient receiving antibiotic therapy calls the clinic to speak with the nurse about new-onset symptoms. Which patient complaints would lead the nurse to suspect a secondary candidiasis infection?
    1. High fever and swollen lymph nodes
    2. Itching and white discharge from the vagina
    3. Chancres that develop on the outside of the vagina
    4. Excessive bleeding occurring in the absence of a period

48. In planning the nursing care of a patient with dysmenorrhea, the nurse suggests that the patient:
    1. Engage in strenuous exercise to relieve pain.

2. Eat protein-packed foods to delay painful cramps.
3. Drink warm beverages and use heat to relieve symptoms.
4. Apply ice packs to the abdomen twice per day.

49. A patient with Addison disease is being regulated with medication. The nurse knows that the primary goal of medication therapy is:
    1. Restoring electrolyte balance.
    2. Reducing the white blood cell (WBC) count.
    3. Increasing bone marrow functioning.
    4. Maintaining the red blood cell (RBC) count level.

50. A neighbor comes to your house after falling on an icy sidewalk. You note that the right forearm is angulated but the skin is intact. First-aid measures would include:
    1. Calling 911.
    2. Splinting the affected area.
    3. Wrapping the area in a warm compress.
    4. Keeping the affected area below the level of the heart.

51. A patient's sputum has suddenly become pink and frothy. The nurse has gathered the following data during her assessment. Which of the data are significant and need to be reported and documented? Select all that apply.
    _____ 1. Decreased appetite
    _____ 2. Complaints of dull headache
    _____ 3. Lung sounds with bibasilar crackles
    _____ 4. Blood pressure of 140/88 mm Hg
    _____ 5. Orthopnea
    _____ 6. Increased urination

52. A patient is scheduled for a pulmonary angiogram and wants to know what will happen. The nurse explains that:
    1. She will receive a local anesthetic, and a tube will be inserted through her nose.
    2. She will be placed in a big hollow tube and must remain completely still.
    3. She will wear a clip on her nose and breathe into a machine.
    4. A dye will be injected through an IV line, and an x-ray image will be taken.

53. Which subjective symptom from a patient would lead a nurse to suspect that he may have benign prostatic hyperplasia (BPH)?
    1. Inability to have intercourse
    2. Dizziness
    3. Decreased force of urine stream
    4. Testicular pain when voiding

54. What should be included in the plan of care for a patient undergoing a computed tomography scan with contrast? Select all that apply.
    _____ 1. Restricting fluids to 1000 mL 4 hours before the test
    _____ 2. Placing the patient on NPO status for at least 4 hours before the test
    _____ 3. Allowing the patient to have her usual meal
    _____ 4. Telling the patient that she will be on bed rest for 4 hours after the test
    _____ 5. Maintaining a prone position after the procedure
    _____ 6. Ascertaining allergies to seafood or iodine before the test

55. A patient experienced an acute episode of sharp chest pain, breathing difficulty, and change in breath sounds.

Which diagnostic procedure would the nurse expect the physician to order for the patient?
1. Ventilation-perfusion scan
2. Angiography
3. Pulmonary function tests
4. Arthroscopy

56. A patient is scheduled for a thoracentesis. The nurse's primary responsibility during this procedure is:
1. Handing the physician collection bottles.
2. Keeping the patient still and in proper position.
3. Arranging for follow-up x-ray studies.
4. Setting up the three-bottle drainage system.

57. The physician has ordered oxygen at 6 L per nasal cannula for his patient. The nurse prepares the humidifier bottle and tubing. The patient asks why the water bottle is necessary. The nurse's best response would be:
1. "The water helps you derive more benefit from the oxygen."
2. "The humidification keeps your nose from becoming dry."
3. "Most patients feel more comfortable when the oxygen is humidified."
4. "Humidity decreases the fire hazard of using oxygen."

58. A nurse is caring for a patient with cirrhosis. Which snack would help to prevent the development of hepatic coma?
1. Banana and mayonnaise sandwich
2. Cheese and crackers
3. Peanut butter and jelly sandwich
4. Milk and cookies

59. A patient has had a hydrocelectomy because of a severe bacterial infection. Which nursing measure may be necessary after surgery?
1. Scrotal elevation
2. Urinary retention catheter
3. Estrogen therapy
4. Wet-to-dry saline dressings

60. A nurse is cautioning a patient with diabetes mellitus about the dangers of developing diabetic ketoacidosis (DKA). Which situations should the nurse tell the patient can be a possible cause of DKA? Select all that apply.
_____ 1. Stress
_____ 2. Infection
_____ 3. Excess insulin
_____ 4. Insufficient calories in the diet
_____ 5. Too much exercise
_____ 6. Insufficient insulin

61. The nurse is teaching a patient about laryngitis. The patient asks if he will still be able to sing in the choir. The nurse's best response is:
1. "You should really rest your voice for a while."
2. "If you gargle with saltwater, you should be okay to sing."
3. "You should practice singing as much as possible before your performance."
4. "You should probably give up singing in the choir because of the laryngitis."

62. Which statement made by a patient with sinusitis would indicate to the nurse that further teaching is required?
1. "I use a warm mist humidifier at night."
2. "I take my decongestants when the doctor ordered."
3. "I will call the physician if my fever comes back."
4. "I will put ice packs on my nose three times each day."

63. Which statement made by a patient who has had a subtotal thyroidectomy may indicate that the patient is experiencing hypocalcemia? Select all that apply.
_____ 1. "I have a massive headache."
_____ 2. "My face feels numb."
_____ 3. "I feel nauseous."
_____ 4. "I got dizzy when I went to the bathroom."
_____ 5. "My hand shook when you took my blood pressure."
_____ 6. "I have to go to the bathroom all the time."

64. Which would be a priority nursing diagnosis for a patient who has AIDS?
1. Risk for infection
2. Risk for loneliness
3. Adult failure to thrive
4. Ineffective sexuality pattern

65. A patient with a head injury has been ordered mannitol intravenously. The patient is most likely receiving the mannitol because:
1. The chance for infection is increased.
2. He has increased intracranial pressure.
3. It will help him rest more comfortably.
4. He has a potential for seizures.

66. A patient diagnosed with chronic renal failure is becoming more confused. Because all previous laboratory test results were within normal range, what would be of concern to the nurse and should be reported at once? Select all that apply.
_____ 1. Potassium of 5.2 mEq/L
_____ 2. Glucose of 90 mg/100 mL
_____ 3. Platelet count of 100,000/mm³
_____ 4. Leukocyte count of 5500/mm³
_____ 5. Blood urea nitrogen (BUN) of 82 mg/dL

67. Which nursing intervention would discourage the development of edema in the arm of an individual who has had a mastectomy?
1. Administer diuretics as ordered
2. Elevate the arm above the level of the heart
3. Bind the affected arm to the patient's side
4. Assess circulatory status frequently

68. A patient is to have an autograft to a burn site on his left thigh. The nurse knows that the transplanted graft will contain tissue from:
1. A cadaver.
2. His own body.
3. A living relative.
4. An animal.

69. A nurse is caring for a patient who has undergone arthroplasty of the left knee. Which data, observed in the immediate postoperative period, must be reported immediately?
1. Nausea and vomiting
2. Slow capillary refill to left foot
3. Infiltration of IV fluids
4. Inability to cough productively

70. The nurse is preparing to receive a patient who has been diagnosed with blistered shingles. Which room would the nurse choose for the patient?
1. A room with a roommate who has had an arthroscopy
2. A room with a pediatric patient
3. An isolation room
4. It does not matter to what room the patient is assigned.

71. The nurse is caring for the stomal area of a patient who had a urinary diversion 2 weeks ago. Which action is most appropriate?
    1. Massaging the area two or three times per day
    2. Applying baby oil to the area and stoma
    3. Moistening the stoma and area with aloe lotion
    4. Cleansing the area with soap and water and patting dry

72. A patient has continuous bladder irrigation ordered on return from the operating room; 2500 mL of irrigation solution was used over an 8-hour period of time. The patient's total urinary output for that same period of time was 3650 mL. Calculate the amount of the patient's true urine output.
    Answer: _____ mL

73. The nurse assists an elderly patient who has had a hip replacement onto an elevated toilet seat. The patient asks the nurse why she must use this device. What is the nurse's best response?
    1. "The elevation will help the fracture heal properly."
    2. "The elevation will keep you from flexing your hip."
    3. "The other toilet causes too much pressure on your suture line."
    4. "We can keep your hip in better alignment using this seat."

74. A patient diagnosed with varicose veins is reluctant to have surgery to repair them. She asks the nurse what she can do to reduce the pain of the varicosities. The nurse suggests that the patient:
    1. Engage in 30 minutes of aerobic exercise every day.
    2. Wear knee-high trouser socks.
    3. Avoid sitting or standing for long periods.
    4. Ride a stationary bike each day.

75. In a patient with myasthenia gravis, which drug would the nurse question if it was ordered?
    1. Neostigmine (Prostigmin)
    2. Neomycin (Mycifradin)
    3. Prednisone (Deltasone)
    4. Pyridostigmine (Mestinon)

76. A nurse is preparing to administer an injection to a non-ambulatory patient. Which intramuscular (IM) injection site is appropriate for this patient, who has muscle atrophy of both upper and lower extremities?
    1. Deltoid
    2. Abdomen
    3. Ventrogluteal
    4. Gluteus maximus

77. A nurse is caring for a patient 2 days after an appendectomy. The patient experiences incisional pain on ambulation. The nurse suggests splinting the wound with a pillow based on the understanding that:
    1. Splinting allows for deeper respirations and coughing.
    2. Persons with abdominal incisions are hesitant to ambulate.
    3. An abdominal binder would restrict the patient's movements.
    4. Sustained stress disrupts wound layers and may impede tissue repair.

78. A patient with hypertension is upset that he has to undergo treatment and states, "I don't feel bad. Why is the doctor making such a fuss?" The best reply by the nurse is:
    1. "I will ask the doctor to see you in the morning."

2. "Why do you question our care? We are only trying to help you."
3. "What could I do to help you understand the seriousness of your disease?"
4. "What questions do you have regarding your care? Maybe I can answer them."

79. The nurse is assessing a patient for evidence of a hypoglycemic reaction. Which assessments indicate this reaction? Select all that apply.
    _____ 1. Polyuria
    _____ 2. Glycosuria
    _____ 3. Pale, clammy skin
    _____ 4. Ketonuria
    _____ 5. Irritability
    _____ 6. Hot flashes

80. Which device will assist the patient with a knee replacement to maintain the flexibility of the knee?
    1. A trochanter roll
    2. An abductor pillow
    3. A continuous passive range-of-motion (ROM) machine
    4. A Hemovac drainage device

81. A patient with arteriosclerosis obliterans asks the nurse how he can best control the pain in his extremity. Which suggestion should the nurse make?
    1. Wear support hose.
    2. Apply hot packs to the area.
    3. Wear warm clothing over the extremity.
    4. Apply ice to the area.

82. What is true when comparing Raynaud disease and Buerger disease?
    1. Raynaud disease affects primarily men.
    2. Buerger disease is not as serious as Raynaud disease.
    3. Raynaud disease is triggered by environmental cold.
    4. Buerger disease affects arteries only.

83. Nursing observations of a patient with severe liver dysfunction with accompanying jaundice would include:
    1. Dark stools, yellow sclera, dark urine
    2. Clay-colored stools, pruritus, dark urine
    3. Dark stools, pruritus, straw-colored urine
    4. Clay-colored stools, yellow sclera, blood-tinged urine

84. A patient has a thoracotomy tube in his left anterior upper thorax. The patient asks the nurse why no blood is draining from the tube. What is the nurse's best response?
    1. "You should probably ask your doctor."
    2. "The blood should begin draining any time now."
    3. "The tube was most likely placed to drain air, not blood."
    4. "Not all chest tubes drain blood."

85. A patient has had a coronary artery bypass graft (CABG). The patient's spouse wants to know why her husband has a tube coming from his chest. What is the nurse's best response to her question?
    1. "It drains blood from his lung."
    2. "It is a method for delivering oxygen."
    3. "It prevents a buildup of blood from around his heart."
    4. "It allows us to administer medications if needed."

86. During a care conference, the head nurse asks if the nursing diagnosis of ineffective airway clearance related to bronchial secretions is still appropriate for the patient. The nurse caring for this patient can best evaluate this by:
    1. Taking the patient's temperature.
    2. Checking the rate and strength of the patient's pulse.
    3. Counting the patient's respirations for 1 full minute.
    4. Ascertaining the effectiveness of the patient's cough.

87. The patient's left thoracotomy tube is connected to water-seal drainage and suction. The patient is to be transported to the x-ray department. How will the nurse transport the patient?
    1. Disconnect the suction; maintain the water-seal drainage
    2. Disconnect the chest tube from the water-seal drainage system
    3. Ask if the x-ray department can possibly do its procedure in the patient's room
    4. Obtain a portable suction machine from central supply to transport the patient

88. A patient has been diagnosed with carpal tunnel syndrome. What would help alleviate the pain the patient is experiencing?
    1. Type frequently to keep fingers mobile
    2. Perform range-of-motion exercises three times per day
    3. Wear a sling for 8 hours a day
    4. Wear hand splints during the day

89. A nurse is caring for a patient diagnosed with meningitis. The patient is extremely sensitive to light, and her mother sits at her bedside crying. What should the nurse include in this patient's plan of care?
    1. Maintaining a calm, relaxed environment
    2. Encouraging visitors to help stimulate patient interactions
    3. Providing for frequent interactions between the patient and her mother
    4. Placing her in a semiprivate room or ward to foster interaction and release tension

90. If 1000 mL of D5W is to infuse over 8 hours, and the drop factor for the tubing is 10 gtt/mL, how many gtt/min should the IV line infuse?
    Answer: _____ gtt/min

91. A patient with hypertension has complaints of headache and weakness. The nurse notes that the patient's face is flaccid on the left side. The nurse should continue to monitor the patient for:
    1. Angina.
    2. Hypertension.
    3. Myocardial infarction.
    4. Cerebrovascular accident.

92. The nurse is preparing to educate a group of students regarding measures in preventing the spread of hepatitis B. What does the nurse include in the lecture?
    1. Testing blood donors
    2. Avoiding blood donations
    3. Adding bleach to the water
    4. Avoiding consumption of all shellfish

93. A young patient with a diagnosis of Crohn disease has recently undergone an ileostomy. The patient asks the nurse what sports he should avoid when he returns to school. What would the nurse caution the patient to avoid?
    1. Track
    2. Football
    3. Shot put
    4. Swimming

94. A patient is suspected of having acute appendicitis. Which laboratory test would most support this diagnosis?
    1. High red blood cell count
    2. Low platelet count

    3. High serum albumin
    4. High white blood cell count

95. A nurse is preparing to educate a group of individuals concerning severe acute respiratory syndrome (SARS). What information should the nurse include in her education? Select all that apply.
    _____ 1. Illness is caused by a virus.
    _____ 2. Symptoms include fever, headache, and muscle aches.
    _____ 3. The syndrome resolves in 2 or 3 days with antibiotic therapy.
    _____ 4. Eighty percent of people can die from the disease.
    _____ 5. Frequent international travelers are at greater risk.
    _____ 6. SARS is a reportable condition to the Public Health Department.

96. A patient with leukemia tells the nurse that he is going to receive a stem cell transplant. The nurse understands that the stem cells may:
    1. Act as an antibiotic within the patient's bloodstream.
    2. Cause the cancer cells to destroy themselves.
    3. Grow new cells that are not cancerous.
    4. Take the place of the destroyed cancer cells.

97. The patient returning home after a right cataract extraction with an intraocular lens implant needs to be instructed to avoid:
    1. Excessive fluid intake.
    2. Straining at stool.
    3. Bathing.
    4. Standing near a microwave.

98. A patient who has had a tonsillectomy and adenoidectomy complains of having to swallow frequently and asks if she can have some more water to drink. The nurse is concerned because the patient:
    1. May be hemorrhaging.
    2. Should not be drinking that much water.
    3. Might damage her incision site by swallowing.
    4. Should not have discomfort after this surgery.

99. A patient is scheduled for an eye examination and receives mydriatic drops beforehand. After the examination the nurse advises the patient to:
    1. Wear a patch over her eye.
    2. Wear a pair of sunglasses for the next few hours.
    3. Avoid lifting anything heavier than 5 pounds.
    4. Avoid sleeping on that side of her head for 2 days.

100. A patient with the diagnosis of heart failure is being treated with furosemide (Lasix). The patient has complained to the nurse about frequent urination. Which nursing diagnosis is correct for this situation?
    1. Ineffective peripheral tissue perfusion
    2. Excess fluid volume
    3. Deficient knowledge
    4. Deficient fluid volume

101. A patient has had a hemorrhoidectomy. Which physician order would be appropriate for this individual?
    1. Encouraging warm showers
    2. Changing occlusive rectal dressings
    3. Using fecal tube to reduce gas pain
    4. Administering laxatives and stool softeners

102. Which assessment finding is an early sign of lymphoma?
    1. High fever
    2. Decreased urine output
    3. Dependent edema
    4. Painless swelling of lymph nodes

103. Which diet would be best for a patient with hyperthyroidism?
  1. Low-purine, high-fat, 1000-calorie diet
  2. Clear liquids in the form of six small feedings
  3. 2-g, low-sodium diet with an evening snack
  4. High-protein, high-calorie, high-carbohydrate diet with snacks

104. A patient with hypertension is being managed by medication, including a diuretic. Regarding the diet, the nurse would educate the patient to:
  1. Maintain a high-potassium diet.
  2. Drink at least 1 quart of liquids each day.
  3. Avoid spicy and high-fat, high-cholesterol foods.
  4. Refrain from caffeine and caffeine-containing products.

105. The nurse needs to obtain a sterile urine specimen for culture and sensitivity from a patient with an indwelling urinary catheter. Select all that apply.
  _____ 1. Disconnect the catheter from the drainage tubing and let the urine drip into the sterile bottle.
  _____ 2. Use a needle and syringe to withdraw urine from the tubing port.
  _____ 3. Inject the specimen from the syringe into the sterile bottle.
  _____ 4. Place a towel under the bag and open the drainage valve at the bottom of the drainage bag.
  _____ 5. Remove the old Foley catheter, using a straight catheter, and perform another catheterization.

106. The patient's wife is concerned because her husband, who had a cerebrovascular accident (CVA) 3 days ago, laughs and cries inappropriately. The nurse's best reply is:
  1. "This is a normal healing sign for someone who has had a CVA."
  2. "I ignore him when he starts acting like that."
  3. "He has what is called 'emotional lability.' This may occur after a stroke."
  4. "Men your husband's age like to tease us by acting this way."

107. A patient who had a cerebrovascular accident (CVA) 2 weeks ago has dysphagia. Based on these data, the nurse tells the aide to:
  1. Keep the patient in bed.
  2. Speak loudly when talking.
  3. Allow extra time for him to answer her.
  4. Make sure he swallows his food.

108. A nurse is discharging a patient who has hyperparathyroidism. The nurse advises the patient to contact the physician if she develops flank pain because:
  1. Flank pain can signal a worsening of her condition.
  2. Low calcium levels might be causing the pain.
  3. Kidney stones are a frequent complication of her disorder.
  4. Pain requires immediate surgical intervention.

109. The nurse observes that her patient, age 60, has stress incontinence each time she coughs or gets out of bed. The nurse understands that:
  1. Hormonal changes place older women at risk for stress incontinence.
  2. Her patient is not emptying her bladder completely.
  3. The nerves controlling the bladder are affected.
  4. Her patient's bladder is displaced in her pelvic cavity.

110. A patient sustained an injury to his spinal cord at the C2 level. Based on a spinal cord injury at this level, the nurse would most likely expect the patient to be treated with:
  1. Diuretics.
  2. Oxygen via ventilator.
  3. Oxygen via nasal cannula.
  4. Vasopressors.

111. Initial treatment for epistaxis includes:
  1. Applying pressure to the soft part of the nose with thumb and forefinger.
  2. Packing the anterior nares with sterile, saline-soaked gauze.
  3. Tilting the head back and closing the mouth while pinching the nose.
  4. Blowing nose until all blood is removed from both nares.

112. A patient complains of "skipping sensations" in her chest while she is working at home. The nurse would anticipate that the physician will order for the patient:
  1. A glucometer.
  2. Urine collection.
  3. A Holter monitor.
  4. A Doppler flow study.

113. Which is the priority nursing responsibility for a patient who has a tracheostomy?
  1. Suctioning as ordered
  2. Changing the dressing
  3. Maintaining a patent airway
  4. Allaying any anxiety

114. On the following illustration, indicate where the nurse would assess a pacemaker insertion site.

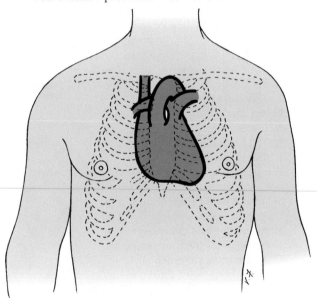

115. Which concern is a priority in a patient with an open head injury?
  1. Infection
  2. Hemorrhage
  3. Increased intracranial pressure
  4. Consciousness

116. A patient has been diagnosed with labyrinthitis. What was likely his primary complaint?
  1. Sinus pain
  2. Dizziness

3. Cephalgia
4. Diplopia

117. A patient with bilateral hearing aids complains of ear pressure and is subsequently diagnosed with impacted ear cerumen. Which physician orders will the nurse anticipate? Select all that apply.
    _____ 1. Remove hearing aids during the day.
    _____ 2. Provide hydrogen peroxide drops to ears twice each day for 7 days.
    _____ 3. Irrigate ears with normal saline once daily.
    _____ 4. Leave the right hearing aid out of the patient's ear.
    _____ 5. Do not put hearing aids in until further notice.

118. A patient is to receive 1000 mL of 5% dextrose in water plus 40 mEq potassium chloride in 8 hours. In checking the flow rate, how much should the patient receive per hour?
    Answer: _____ mL/hr

119. Diabetic ketoacidosis (DKA) is treated with:
    1. Oral antidiabetic agents.
    2. Glucose and water.
    3. Diuretics.
    4. Insulin.

120. Which intervention will the nurse anticipate implementing for a patient with a diagnosis of a myocardial infarction?
    1. Adjusting the bed to Trendelenburg position
    2. Maintaining prescription of complete bed rest for at least 5 days
    3. Providing clear, room-temperature liquids throughout hospitalization
    4. Administering a stool softener to prevent straining with bowel movements

121. A nurse is doing blood glucose screenings at a local mall. In addition to testing capillary blood, he or she inquires about possible symptoms of diabetes mellitus. What would the nurse include? Select all that apply.
    _____ 1. Polydipsia
    _____ 2. Cold extremities
    _____ 3. Polyphagia
    _____ 4. Excess urination
    _____ 5. Lack of appetite

122. A patient comes to the emergency department a few days after removing a tick from his skin. He complains of influenza-like symptoms and painful joints. The patient may have:
    1. Amyotrophic lateral sclerosis.
    2. Lyme disease.
    3. Encephalitis.
    4. Chronic fatigue syndrome.

123. A patient has Ménière's disease and is taking medication for the vertigo. The nurse is with the patient during a severe attack. What helps reduce the vertigo?
    1. Encouraging the patient to move slowly to a chair
    2. Taking an additional dose of meclizine (Antivert)
    3. Increasing fluid intake to 2000 mL/day
    4. Darkening the room

124. A patient has a seizure that is accompanied by incontinence. The patient sleeps for several hours afterward. What kind of seizure did the patient most likely have?
    1. Partial
    2. Focal
    3. Absence
    4. Tonic-clonic

125. A patient asks the nurse why she must lie flat after her lumbar puncture. The nurse correctly answers the patient by saying:

1. "You may get a bad headache if you sit up now."
2. "You may have leakage of spinal fluid if you sit up."
3. "Let me help you sit up; there's no reason why you can't."
4. "Your blood pressure will bottom out if you sit up now."

126. A nurse is presenting a class on hearing difficulties to a group of nursing assistants. Behavioral clues indicating difficulty in hearing and the need for evaluation by an otolaryngologist include:
    1. Complaining of ringing in the ears.
    2. Avoiding face-to-face contact.
    3. Changing body positions frequently.
    4. Speaking while others are talking.

127. In distinguishing between a sprain and a fracture, the nurse would be more suspicious of a fracture if which sign was present on assessment?
    1. Edema
    2. Deformity
    3. Limited movement
    4. Tenderness to palpation of the area

128. An adult patient is placed in Buck's extension traction to the left leg. The nurse is aware that this type of traction can be useful in which injury?
    1. Neck sprains
    2. Spinal fractures
    3. Shoulder dislocations
    4. Lower extremity and hip fractures

129. A patient has had a subtotal thyroidectomy. What should be available in the room of the patient at all times?
    1. Chest tube tray
    2. Spinal puncture tray
    3. Tracheostomy tray
    4. Transtracheal oxygen delivery

130. Using the illustration at right, trace the flow of urine in the proper order through the organs and body structures, beginning with the most superior organ.
    1. Ureter
    2. Kidney
    3. Meatus
    4. Bladder
    5. Urethra

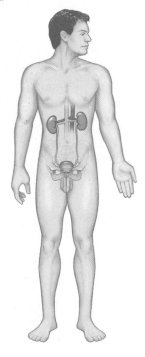

131. A patient is being treated for acute glomerulonephritis. Which fact in the patient's history may have precipitated the event?
    1. Antibiotic therapy
    2. Upper respiratory infection
    3. Frequent urinary tract infections
    4. Low fluid intake

132. A patient is being observed for increased intracranial pressure. Which classification of drugs, besides anticonvulsants and corticosteroids, would the nurse expect the physician to order?
    1. Narcotic analgesics
    2. Antiemetics
    3. Osmotic diuretics
    4. Antibiotics

133. The nurse is distributing health literature on prostate cancer. Which blood test is recommended by the American Cancer Society as a screening test for this type of cancer?
    1. Carcinogenic embryonic antigen
    2. Prostate-specific antigen
    3. Digital rectal examination
    4. Enzyme-linked immunosorbent assay

134. Which physician order would the nurse expect for a patient diagnosed with renal calculi?
    1. Whirlpool baths
    2. Limiting fluid intake
    3. Racking all urine
    4. Straining all urine

135. In teaching a patient who is experiencing migraine headaches, which of these behaviors indicates that patient teaching has been successful?
    1. The patient states that she needs to exercise daily.
    2. The patient states that she will wear sunglasses when outdoors.
    3. The patient states that she will take an aspirin daily to prevent the headache.
    4. The patient identifies the factors that trigger her headaches.

136. A nurse is caring for a patient with heart failure who has the symptoms of dyspnea, pedal edema, and increased abdominal girth. Indicate on the illustration which part of the heart is most likely failing.
    1. A
    2. B
    3. C
    4. D

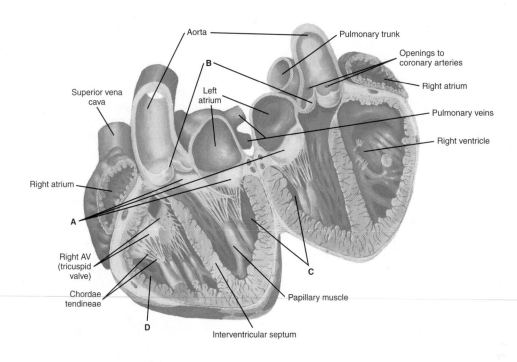

137. The nurse is assessing a patient who fell at home. If the patient has a hip fracture, which symptom(s) would you expect to find?
    1. Pain and numbness
    2. External rotation of the leg
    3. Large hematoma at the hip
    4. Lengthening of the extremity

138. A patient is admitted with transient ischemic attack (TIA). Which symptoms indicate this disorder? Select all that apply.
    _____ 1. Gradual loss of sensory function occurs.
    _____ 2. Temporary loss of motor or sensory function occurs.

    _____ 3. It results from a sudden lack of blood flow to the brain.
    _____ 4. Emergency treatment is required.
    _____ 5. The patient is at high risk for developing a cerebrovascular accident.

139. A patient has returned from having a myelogram in which metrizamide (water-based) dye was used. Which postprocedure action is most appropriate?
    1. Encourage fluids.
    2. Secure a bedside commode.
    3. Spray the room with a room deodorizer.
    4. Administer all drugs withheld before the procedure.

140. A patient is diagnosed with an abdominal aortic aneurysm. The nurse is planning the activity level for the patient. Which would be an appropriate activity for this patient?
    1. Bicycling
    2. Reading
    3. Jogging
    4. Tennis

141. A patient has been diagnosed with varicose veins. Which fact in the patient's history would predispose the patient to this disorder? Select all that apply.
    _____ 1. Pregnancy
    _____ 2. Obesity
    _____ 3. Many hours spent driving
    _____ 4. Mother who had varicose veins
    _____ 5. High blood pressure

142. A patient has had a cutaneous ureterostomy performed and has catheters (stents) inserted through the ureters to drain the renal pelvis. One of the nurse's main concerns is:
    1. Irrigating the stents.
    2. Maintaining patency of the stents.
    3. Testing urine for protein, blood, and glucose.
    4. Preventing contamination of the stents with stool.

143. The patient with type 2 diabetes mellitus may use which treatments to control his condition? Select all that apply.
    _____ 1. Insulin
    _____ 2. Oral antidiabetics
    _____ 3. Diet
    _____ 4. Exercise
    _____ 5. Glucometer monitoring

144. A patient has been newly diagnosed as having obstructive sleep apnea. The nurse is aware that the patient may be exhibiting which symptoms? Select all that apply.
    _____ 1. Daytime sleepiness
    _____ 2. Upper respiratory infections
    _____ 3. Personality changes
    _____ 4. Excessive snoring
    _____ 5. Hyperglycemia
    _____ 6. Tremors

145. Which is true concerning rheumatoid arthritis?
    1. Local joint disease
    2. Self-limited illness
    3. Disease of striated muscles
    4. Systemic disease

146. What is a first-line pharmacologic medication used in the treatment of rheumatoid arthritis?
    1. Muscle relaxants
    2. Narcotic analgesics
    3. Antiinflammatory agents
    4. Calcium channel blocking agents

147. A patient has had a bilateral oophorectomy. Which assessment finding would cause the nurse concern?
    1. Serosanguineous drainage from the vagina
    2. Changing the perineal pads every 3 to 4 hours
    3. Foley catheter draining clear yellow urine
    4. Malodorous vaginal discharge

148. A patient receives hemodialysis treatments through an arteriovenous (AVF) fistula in the left arm. What is included in the plan of care?
    1. Keeping the patient on bed rest
    2. Irrigating the fistula every 4 hours
    3. Taking the blood pressure on the right arm
    4. Monitoring input and output hourly

149. During the fifth day in coronary care, a patient with a diagnosis of myocardial infarction develops dyspnea; has blood-tinged, frothy sputum; and becomes very anxious. These symptoms may indicate:
    1. Emphysema.
    2. Pulmonary edema.
    3. Pulmonary embolism.
    4. Chronic obstructive pulmonary disease.

150. Which nursing care measures are appropriate for a patient diagnosed with gout? Select all that apply.
    _____ 1. Allopurinol twice daily
    _____ 2. Increased intake of organ foods
    _____ 3. Acid ash diet
    _____ 4. Blood glucose monitoring
    _____ 5. Alkaline ash diet

151. A nurse is assisting a physician in the application of a plaster cast to a foot and calf. What is the correct way for the nurse to handle the extremity?
    1. Instruct the patient to elevate the extremity
    2. Place a pillowcase under the cast to move the extremity
    3. Pick up the extremity in a cast, supporting it with the palms of the hands
    4. Instruct a nursing assistant to elevate the extremity by pulling up on the patient's toes

152. A patient with osteomyelitis of the right knee is admitted to an orthopedic unit. Which statement would indicate to the nurse that further teaching may be necessary?
    1. "I should only be in the hospital overnight."
    2. "I guess this infection could have come from the accident I had a few weeks ago with the staple gun."
    3. "I need to stay in bed for a while."
    4. "I guess I should expect my knee to hurt when I move it around."

153. A nurse is bathing a patient 1 day after total hip replacement. Which statement made by the patient would indicate understanding of the positioning required after this surgery?
    1. "I know I shouldn't point my toes."
    2. "I need to have lowered chairs."
    3. "It will be hard for me not to cross my legs."
    4. "I will have trouble not walking for a long time."

154. A nurse is caring for a patient with a diagnosis of possible rheumatoid arthritis. Which elevated laboratory values would support the patient's diagnosis?
    1. White blood cells (WBCs) and hematocrit (Hct)
    2. Uric acid and hemoglobin
    3. Erythrocyte sedimentation rate (ESR) and rheumatoid factor
    4. Lupus erythematosus (LE) and rheumatoid factor

155. A nurse is assisting a patient with an above-the-knee amputation (AKA) into a prone position. Which statement made by the patient would indicate that he or she understands the need for this positioning?
    1. "Lying prone will alleviate my phantom limb pain."
    2. "I have to lie this way to make sure that I have good circulation to my residual limb."
    3. "This position will allow me greater comfort than lying on my back."
    4. "I have to do this to make sure that my hip doesn't get a flexion contracture."

156. A patient who has undergone a hemigastrectomy has been diagnosed with pernicious anemia. The patient asks the nurse what might have caused her problem. What should be the nurse's best response?
    1. "You are no longer able to absorb vitamin B_{12} because of your surgery."
    2. "You are most likely not receiving enough folic acid in your low-fat diet."
    3. "Because you have less hydrochloric acid since your surgery, you will have difficulty absorbing vitamin B_{12}."
    4. "You can no longer use iron adequately in your body because of your surgery."

157. A patient asks the nurse about the purpose of a serum erythrocyte sedimentation rate (ESR). The nurse is correct in responding that:
    1. "This test will show if you have an infection in your body."
    2. "Elevation of the ESR signifies an inflammatory process."
    3. "This is a test to measure how well the kidneys are working."
    4. "Elevation of the ESR usually means that you have a blood dyscrasia."

158. A patient with chronic heart failure inquires why he does not become short of breath until he exercises or takes a shower. Which statement made by the nurse would best answer his question?
    1. "The shortness of breath is caused by your lung constricting."
    2. "You need to condition your heart to be able to tolerate exercise."
    3. "When you exercise your heart can no longer meet the oxygen needs of your body."
    4. "The blood vessels of your lungs constrict as you exercise, causing the shortness of breath."

159. An elderly patient has had a myocardial infarction of the right side of the heart. Which sign should the nurse anticipate when assessing for heart failure?
    1. Nausea
    2. Heart murmur
    3. Crackles in lungs
    4. Edema in feet and legs

160. A nurse is obtaining a history from a patient who has been admitted with a diagnosis of probable mitral insufficiency. Which fact in the patient's history would be most significant?
    1. Appendectomy 1 year ago
    2. One-pack-a-day smoker for 20 years
    3. History of rheumatic fever as a child
    4. History of a pacemaker insertion 5 years ago

161. The family of a patient who has just returned from an esophagogastroduodenoscopy attempts to feed the patient a milkshake. What should be the nurse's first course of action?
    1. Check the patient's diet order to see if a full liquid diet is ordered.
    2. Explain that the patient must wait at least 6 hours before eating.
    3. Monitor the procedure to ensure that the patient swallows the liquid.
    4. Ask the family to wait until you have checked the patient's gag reflex.

162. A patient is hospitalized with an acute exacerbation of systemic lupus erythematosus (SLE). Which part of the patient's recent history may have contributed to this hospitalization?
    1. Ate seafood the night before
    2. Went to the beach the day before
    3. Has been constipated for the last few days
    4. Began taking prednisone a few days ago

163. A patient recently diagnosed with cholecystitis arrives at an outpatient clinic complaining of severe right upper quadrant pain. Which data, obtained from the patient history, may have precipitated this problem?
    1. Spent 3 hours mowing the lawn
    2. Had a hamburger and French fries for lunch
    3. Took three acetaminophen tablets for a headache
    4. Had three beers and a bowl of pretzels after mowing the lawn

164. A nurse is teaching a patient the proper method for administering pancreatic enzymes. Which method would the nurse advise?
    1. "Take the enzymes between meals."
    2. "Take the enzymes only if eating a fatty meal."
    3. "Take the enzymes at the same time you eat the meal."
    4. "Take the enzymes before you retire to bed each night."

165. A nurse notes that a patient's nasogastric tube has not been draining as much as usual. The patient complains of nausea, and abdominal distention is noted. What is the nurse's next course of action?
    1. Remove the nasogastric tube
    2. Call the physician immediately
    3. Assess the patency of the tube
    4. Call for a portable abdominal x-ray unit

166. A physician tells a patient that he is going to correct a shoulder dislocation by closed reduction. The nurse is correct when she tells the patient that this procedure involves:
    1. Surgery.
    2. General anesthesia.
    3. Realigning the joint by manually pulling on bones.
    4. Realigning the bones by placement of an external fixation device.

167. Which assessment data may indicate that a patient has diabetes insipidus?
    1. Bounding pulse and low urine output
    2. Increased blood pressure and tachycardia
    3. Decreased fluid intake and high specific gravity of urine
    4. Increased fluid intake and low specific gravity of urine

168. Which measure would assist in ensuring that a patient with diabetes mellitus would receive proper care outside the hospital or clinic?
    1. Wearing a medical alert tag
    2. Carrying a rapid source of glucose
    3. Carrying a syringe full of insulin at all times
    4. Reporting condition to the local ambulance service

169. A nurse is caring for a patient with hyperpituitarism. Which nursing diagnosis may be appropriate for this patient?
    1. Impaired comfort
    2. Disturbed body image
    3. Deficient fluid volume
    4. Imbalanced nutrition: less than body requirements

170. A patient is admitted with a diagnosis of hyperglycemic hyperosmolar nonketotic coma (HHNC). The nurse is aware that HHNC differs from diabetic ketoacidosis (DKA) in that:
    1. HHNC is more difficult to treat.
    2. DKA includes the complication of metabolic acidosis.
    3. DKA is mostly found in patients who are not insulin dependent.
    4. HHNC includes elevated serum levels of glucose and ketones.

171. A frantic mother calls a health clinic and says that her son, who has diabetes, has a glucometer reading of 36. The child is conscious but nervous. What should the nurse suggest?
    1. Give the child a can of diet soda.
    2. Bring the child to the hospital immediately.
    3. Give the child some orange juice with sugar in it.
    4. Let the child eat some cheese and crackers.

172. A nurse is caring for a female patient who has had a conization. Which nursing intervention should the nurse expect to carry out for this patient?
    1. Instruct her to replace tampon every 3 hours
    2. Maintain vaginal packing for the first 12 to 24 hours
    3. Assist her in using a sitz bath twice per day
    4. Provide her with instructions on the use of a medicated, vaginal douche

173. A 47-year-old female patient who works as a nursing assistant comes to an outpatient clinic for a routine physical examination. The nurse collects the following group of data. Which of these findings needs to be addressed by the nurse?
    1. Gynecological examination 6 months ago
    2. Hepatitis B vaccine 4 months ago
    3. Last mammogram 8 years ago
    4. Last tuberculosis test 3 months ago after starting a new job

174. The nurse is educating a group of women on the correct technique for breast self-examination (BSE). Which method should the nurse recommend?
    1. "Examine your breasts when your period first starts."
    2. "Palpate your breasts for lumps while sitting at a table."
    3. "Use the palms of your hands to feel for lumps in your breasts."
    4. "Palpate the breasts while lying, sitting, and standing each month."

175. The nurse is caring for a patient who has developed a possible rectovaginal fistula after delivery of her fifth child. Which symptom would suggest that the patient has developed this fistula?
    1. Leakage of urine from the vagina
    2. Extreme pain after a bowel movement
    3. Passage of stool and flatus from the vagina
    4. White creamy discharge and extreme pruritus

176. A female patient visits an outpatient clinic because she is concerned that she may have gonorrhea. The patient states that her male partner was diagnosed but she has had no symptoms. What is the best response by the nurse?
    1. "I am sure there is no reason to worry if you have no symptoms."

2. "I think we should test you because gonorrhea can be asymptomatic in women."
    3. "You can return to the clinic whenever you have burning on urination or get a fever."
    4. "I think we can prescribe an antibiotic without even doing a culture because your partner is infected."

177. A nurse is preparing a patient for an upcoming panhysterectomy. What should the nurse caution the patient to expect after the surgery?
    1. The patient will have a catheter after surgery.
    2. The patient should expect to be on bed rest for at least 4 days.
    3. It is unlikely that the patient will resume a normal diet for a few days.
    4. Physical therapy will be an integral part of her rehabilitation process.

178. A nurse is educating a group of women on premenstrual tension. The nurse has the participants complete a survey of favorite foods. Which favorite food of the participants can aggravate premenstrual syndrome (PMS)?
    1. Pizza
    2. Mineral water
    3. Pasta and sauce
    4. Raw fruits and vegetables

179. A patient admitted with chronic obstructive pulmonary disease also has psoriasis. Which types of skin lesions does the patient have?
    1. Red patches with silver scales
    2. Large, pus-filled macules
    3. A bright red, blistered rash
    4. Large, ulcerated areas

180. A patient in the clinic has been diagnosed with asthma. Laboratory studies have been done and returned. The nurse knows that the primary antibody affected in asthmatic patients is:
    1. International normalized ratio (INR).
    2. Immunoglobulin E (IgE).
    3. Hepatitis C virus (HCV) antibody.
    4. Carcinoembryonic antigen (CEA).

181. A newly admitted patient has asthma and uses inhalers. He takes metaproterenol (Alupent), albuterol (Proventil), and beclomethasone (Vanceril). He complains that he does not like the side effects that these inhaled medications cause. The nurse instructs him that he:
    1. Must sit down when using inhalers.
    2. Is overdosing himself if he uses all three inhalers within 1 hour.
    3. Needs to use the metaproterenol and albuterol inhalers before the beclomethasone.
    4. Needs to stop using the inhalers until his next scheduled clinic appointment.

182. A patient is to begin medications for tuberculosis (TB). Which statement made by the patient would indicate that further teaching is required?
    1. "I should cover my mouth and nose when sneezing."
    2. "I won't ever be able to get a PPD again."
    3. "I am glad I will take these drugs for only a few months."
    4. "I can resume normal activity as long as I plan for rest periods."

183. The patient tells the nurse that the reason he came to the clinic is because he has been having difficulty breathing, especially at night. The nurse would be most correct in

documenting this information under which section of the admission sheet?
1. Chief complaint
2. Psychosocial history
3. Past medical history
4. Review of systems

184. A case of active tuberculosis (TB) has been confirmed in the nurse's neighborhood, and a neighbor asks how she might have been exposed. The nurse's reply states how TB is transmitted. This includes what?
1. By using the same door handle as the infected person
2. By an airborne route; the infected person coughing, sneezing, laughing
3. By touching a tissue that the person infected with TB used
4. By riding the bus after the person infected with TB rode it

185. A patient has a medical diagnosis of respiratory acidosis. His nursing diagnosis is ineffective airway clearance. Which activity is most directly aimed at his nursing diagnosis?
1. Encouraging fluid intake by offering fluids every 2 hours
2. Suctioning him every 2 hours and p.r.n.
3. Walking in the halls twice per day
4. Planning activities to provide rest periods between them

186. A patient has a possible diagnosis of mitral stenosis. Which symptoms correlate with this diagnosis? Select all that apply.
_____ 1. Heart murmur
_____ 2. Heart failure
_____ 3. Palpitations
_____ 4. Orthopnea
_____ 5. Pulmonary edema

187. Which patient history would relate to a diagnosis of bacterial endocarditis?
1. Previous heart catheterization
2. Strep throat 4 weeks earlier
3. Open reduction, internal fixation of the left hip last year
4. Smokes two packs per day

188. A patient is admitted to the clinic for a complete physical examination. To prevent injury during the otoscopic examination, which action should the nurse avoid?
1. Inserting the otoscope until it touches the eardrum
2. Tipping the patient's head away from the examiner
3. Bracing the examining hand against the patient's head
4. Pulling the ear being examined up and back

189. A patient has been diagnosed with pernicious anemia. What should be done for this patient on a monthly basis?
1. Administration of vitamin B_{12} PO
2. Vitamin K given intramuscularly
3. Therapeutic multivitamin given intravenously
4. Administration of injectable form of vitamin B_{12}

190. A male patient is being evaluated for chlamydia. Which symptom would cause the physician to suspect a *Chlamydia* infection?
1. Urethritis
2. A chancre
3. Anal itching
4. Papular warts

191. What is included in patient teaching before a barium enema? Select all that apply.
_____ 1. Nothing to eat for 2 hours before the test
_____ 2. Enemas before the examination
_____ 3. Laxatives after the examination
_____ 4. No meat for 4 days before the examination

192. A patient has stomatitis, and the nurse administers topical lidocaine to her mouth before her meal. The intent of the lidocaine is to:
1. Decrease the pain associated with chewing.
2. Keep the sores from becoming infected.
3. Avoid food becoming lodged in the sores.
4. Allow the patient to absorb the food more readily.

193. The nurse is monitoring a patient with recent bleeding esophageal varices. What is most likely in the patient's history?
1. Bronchitis
2. Esophageal cancer
3. Cirrhosis
4. Gastritis

194. A patient is unable to respond appropriately and clearly. He is also disoriented to time and is unable to follow commands. What best describes his level of consciousness (LOC)?
1. Oriented, arousable, difficult
2. Confused
3. Having periods of lethargy
4. In a stuporous state

195. What is the most common cause of autonomic dysreflexia?
1. Visitors
2. Full bladder
3. Taking tympanic temperatures
4. Taking an apical pulse

196. The nurse is assigned to a newly admitted patient who was burned in an apartment fire. The patient quickly develops edema. Which statement best addresses why the nurse is concerned about the edema?
1. Edema means that the patient's kidneys have shut down.
2. Edema means that frequent skin care is necessary.
3. Edema may lead to hypovolemic shock.
4. Edema indicates that the IV line is being infused too rapidly.

197. An aerobic instructor complains to the nurse that she often gets "heartburn" after her aerobic class. What would the nurse advise for the patient?
1. Drink a large amount of fluids before the class.
2. Limit the amount of bending over in the class.
3. Lie down for 30 minutes before the class.
4. Do not eat a large meal before the class begins.

198. New medications and combinations of medications are used to treat active tuberculosis disease. The most predominant side effect the nurse needs to look for with the use of tuberculosis drugs such as isoniazid (INH) is:
1. Changes in liver enzymes.
2. Sores in the mouth.
3. Increased urination.
4. Decreased saliva.

199. What is an appropriate short-term goal for a patient with the nursing diagnosis of acute pain related to humeral fracture?
1. Patient will be able to move arm freely without pain in 1 week.

2. Patient will report relief from pain before discharge.

3. Patient will state a reduction in pain during physical therapy sessions.

4. Patient will report reduction in painful stimuli 45 minutes after pain medication is given.

200. A patient returns to the unit after a suprapubic prostatic resection. He has an IV line and a three-way Foley catheter connected to continuous bladder irrigation. At the end of the shift, he had an intake of 725 mL fluids IV, 150 mL fluids PO, 3200 mL of irrigation fluid, and 4000 mL output. What is the patient's intake for the shift?

Answer: _____ mL

201. What patient teaching points should be included in the discharge teaching of a patient who is susceptible to urinary tract infections? Select all that apply.

_____ 1. Avoid sexual intercourse.

_____ 2. Avoid perfumed feminine hygiene products.

_____ 3. Take showers daily instead of tub baths.

_____ 4. Increase daily orange juice to eight 8-oz glasses.

_____ 5. Wipe perineum from front to back.

202. A patient with peptic ulcer disease says to the nurse, "I guess my stress has gotten the better of me." What is the nurse's most correct response?

1. "I know what you mean; we all need to decrease stress."

2. "Not all peptic ulcers are caused by stress; there are other factors."

3. "You probably have a streptococcal infection."

4. "Maybe I can get you into a stress-reduction workshop."

203. When providing care to a patient taking sulfa drugs for a urinary tract infection, the nurse should offer fluids frequently during the day to:

1. Prevent crystals from forming in the urine.

2. Provide comfort from the burning sensation.

3. Maintain constant blood levels of the medication.

4. Maintain sufficient urine output.

204. After an automobile accident, a 35-year-old patient is admitted with a Glasgow Coma Scale score that has ranged from 13 to 15 since the accident. The nurse knows that these scores indicate:

1. Coma.

2. Mild head injury.

3. Moderate head trauma.

4. Optimum cerebral functioning.

205. The nurse is planning her care for a patient who has edema of his legs after extensive burns to both lower extremities. The nurse knows that intracellular swelling after a severe burn is related to:

1. Decreased circulating immunoglobulin.

2. Increased cardiac output.

3. Increased metabolic demands.

4. Disruption in sodium and potassium at the cellular level.

206. A comatose patient has an intact airway and is being fed via a nasogastric tube. Which nursing diagnosis is a priority for this patient?

1. Ineffective airway clearance

2. Ineffective breathing pattern

3. Toileting self-care deficit

4. Risk for aspiration

207. A patient with asthma tells the nurse that he does not use his albuterol (Ventolin) inhaler because it is the same thing as his ipratropium (Atrovent). The nurse needs to teach him that both inhalers contain:

1. Medications that cause bronchodilation but in different ways; he should wait 5 minutes after using the one inhaler before using the next.

2. Medications that cause bronchoconstriction but in different ways; he should wait 15 minutes after using one inhaler before using the next.

3. Medications that are used for bronchospasm; he can use either one if he feels an attack coming on.

4. The same medication; the names are different because they are made by a different company. He is acting correctly.

208. Which situation best describes the potential of contracting a tuberculosis (TB) infection from a person who has active TB?

1. Lack of frequent handwashing practices in the work setting

2. Close, frequent, or extended contact

3. Sharing a computer at work

4. Sharing the same bathroom in a restaurant

209. A patient has had nasal surgery with the insertion of posterior nasal packing. Which nursing diagnosis is a priority for this patient?

1. Risk for injury

2. Risk for infection

3. Risk for aspiration

4. Ineffective breathing pattern

210. The laboratory results for a patient who is being treated for asthma have just arrived. Which results indicate the therapeutic blood level for theophylline?

1. 10 to 20 mcg/mL

2. 20 to 30 mcg/mL

3. 30 to 40 mcg/mL

4. 40 to 50 mcg/mL

211. A patient with respiratory failure has an ineffective breathing pattern as a nursing diagnosis. The patient is most likely experiencing:

1. Respiratory alkalosis.

2. Metabolic alkalosis.

3. Metabolic acidosis.

4. Respiratory acidosis.

212. The nurse is caring for a patient who has nosocomial pneumonia. According to the Centers for Disease Control and Prevention (CDC), the single most effective way to prevent the spread of disease is:

1. Using antibiotics.

2. Using Protective Isolation technique.

3. Washing hands frequently.

4. Using Standard Precautions.

213. Which symptoms indicate the diagnosis of pheochromocytoma? Select all that apply.

_____ 1. Blood pressure of 90/50 mm Hg

_____ 2. Diaphoresis

_____ 3. Heart rate of 50 beats/min

_____ 4. Blood pressure of 200/120 mm Hg

214. The nurse is instructing the patient with asthma about the importance of measuring peak flow rates. Which statement about the purpose of measuring peak flow rates is correct?

1. They help wean him off his bronchodilator.

2. They measure his response to bronchodilator therapy.
3. They eliminate the need for blood test monitoring of the drug level.
4. They determine when he may return to work.

215. With which data should the nurse be most concerned during assessment of a patient with pneumonia?
    1. Capillary refill of more than 3 seconds and buccal cyanosis
    2. An Hct of 47% and white blood cells of 5500/mL
    3. Nonproductive cough and clear lung sounds
    4. Potassium level of 3.7 mEq/L and clear, amber urine

216. Which is the most likely nursing diagnosis for a patient with an ileal conduit?
    1. Disturbed body image
    2. Ineffective sexual pattern
    3. Risk for impaired skin integrity
    4. Impaired physical mobility

217. A patient has a urinary tract infection, and the nurse encourages her to void every 2 to 3 hours to:
    1. Train the bladder.
    2. Reduce the possibility of reflex incontinence.
    3. Reduce urinary stasis and the risk of infection.
    4. Prevent fluid retention with overflow.

218. A patient is admitted for obstructive urinary retention. He is newly diagnosed with adult-onset diabetes mellitus. The nurse checked his blood glucose level before dinner; it was 45 mg/dL. The best action is to:
    1. Give 6 oz of orange juice to drink immediately.
    2. Administer regular insulin according to the sliding scale orders.
    3. Call the physician immediately.
    4. Call the dietary department to have them deliver his dinner as soon as possible.

219. A patient was admitted with second- and third-degree burns over 40% of her body after her house was destroyed by fire yesterday. The nurse is monitoring her condition. What would the nurse want to report immediately?
    1. Urine output of 200 mL in the last 6 hours
    2. Decrease of body temperature to 98.4° F in the last hour
    3. Edema formation in the upper airway
    4. Complaints of pain during dressing changes

220. A 42-year-old patient is recovering from cranial surgery. It is important to plan nursing interventions to prevent an increase in intracranial pressure (ICP). Which action best helps to decrease the possibility of increased intracranial pressure?
    1. Encouraging her to deep breath and cough
    2. Doing endotracheal suctioning every 4 hours or as needed
    3. Maintaining her bed in a high-Fowler (90-degree) position
    4. Spreading interventions evenly throughout the day

221. A patient is diagnosed with basal cell carcinoma of the scalp. He has the following histories listed. Which probably contributed to his condition?
    1. The patient uses Rogaine.
    2. The patient has a family history of colon cancer.
    3. The patient smokes cigarettes.
    4. The patient has a receding hairline.

222. A patient calls in to the clinic and states that he is having painless hematuria. What advice should the nurse give the patient?

1. Drink a large amount of fluids.
2. Try not to drink any reddish-colored fluids.
3. Make an appointment with your physician as soon as possible.
4. Go to the emergency department right away.

223. A nurse is attempting to gather information from a patient who has a sexually transmitted disease (STD). What is true regarding this situation?
    1. Most individuals speak freely about their sexual contacts.
    2. It is not necessary to know with whom the patient has had sex.
    3. Patients with asymptomatic STDs cannot transmit the disease.
    4. Individuals are often reluctant to discuss personal sexual information.

224. Thrombolytic agents are used to treat patients with myocardial infarction. What is the action of the thrombolytic?
    1. Dissolves fresh thrombi
    2. Prevents further thrombi from developing
    3. Thins the blood
    4. Keeps platelets from aggregating in the bloodstream

225. A patient has been placed on nitroglycerin. This medication treats angina by:
    1. Increasing blood flow to the myocardium.
    2. Lowering the patient's blood pressure.
    3. Dilating cerebral arteries.
    4. Decreasing the number of ectopic beats.

226. A patient calls a clinic and states that her stools have turned tarry black. She believes that she is bleeding internally. Which question should the nurse ask next?
    1. "Are you taking vitamin K?"
    2. "Do you have hemorrhoids?"
    3. "Do you take ferrous sulfate?"
    4. "Why don't you come to the clinic?"

227. Some anticancer medications depress the patient's bone marrow and require careful observation for:
    1. Increased platelet counts.
    2. Anemia.
    3. High levels of white blood cells (WBCs).
    4. Metastasis.

228. A patient is taking a vasodilator. He complains that he becomes dizzy when he stands. The patient is experiencing:
    1. Vertigo.
    2. Anemia.
    3. Bradycardia.
    4. Hypotension.

229. The physician orders butorphanol (Stadol), 2 mg IM stat. The pharmacy sends a vial that reads Stadol, 5 mg/mL. How much will the nurse give?
    Answer: _____ mL

230. A patient has had a myocardial infarction. He is most at risk for developing:
    1. Cardiogenic shock.
    2. Anaphylaxis.
    3. Hypertension.
    4. Vascular injury.

231. A patient asks why he cannot receive anything by mouth after his gastrointestinal (GI) surgery. The nurse is most correct in saying that this order has been given because:
    1. The patient is really not hungry after surgery.

2. He will become extremely nauseated afterward.

3. He might aspirate.

4. The GI tract is not working because of the anesthesia.

232. The nurse medicates a patient with a narcotic analgesic. Which nursing diagnosis is priority at this time?
1. Risk for falls
2. Ineffective breathing pattern
3. Acute pain
4. Risk for infection

233. A physician orders meperidine (Demerol), 50 mg IM, for a patient's postoperative pain. The nurse has meperidine, 100 mg/mL, on hand. How much will the nurse give?
Answer: _____ mL

234. A nurse is preparing to deliver nasogastric tube feedings. Which assessments should be carried out before delivery of the feedings? Select all that apply.
_____ 1. Assess bowel sounds
_____ 2. Assess lung sounds
_____ 3. Measure blood pressure
_____ 4. Measure heart rate
_____ 5. Ensure patency of tube

235. After a patient undergoes surgery to the upper respiratory tract, the priority assessment for which the nurse should monitor is:
1. Infection.
2. Patent airway.
3. Bleeding tendencies.
4. Septicemia.

236. The nurse is addressing a group of high school students regarding the use of tobacco. A student says, "I won't get lung cancer because I don't smoke; I chew snuff." What is the best response by the nurse?
1. "Well, you shouldn't do that either."
2. "You're right, you won't get lung cancer."
3. "You can get oral cancer from the smokeless tobacco."
4. "I don't think you understand the purpose of my speech!"

237. What structure or structures return oxygenated blood from the lungs?
1. Pulmonary artery
2. Pulmonary veins
3. Superior vena cava
4. Inferior vena cava

238. A nurse is teaching a patient about Buerger-Allen exercises. These exercises will help the patient who has a diagnosis of:
1. Pulmonary edema.
2. Thromboangiitis obliterans.
3. Thrombophlebitis.
4. Paget's disease.

239. Which patient teaching points should be included in the discharge planning of a patient who has heart failure? Select all that apply.
_____ 1. Weigh yourself every day.
_____ 2. Take your blood pressure before taking your digoxin.
_____ 3. Increase your carbohydrate intake.
_____ 4. Take your diuretic early in the morning.

240. A patient who is on a sodium-restricted diet is retaining fluid. She states that she has not been eating salt but has been eating at a lot of restaurants. Which type of restaurant would have food that is most likely to cause the fluid retention?
1. Vegetarian

2. Italian
3. Chinese
4. French

241. Which is true concerning ulcerative colitis?
1. Major symptoms are constipation and flatus.
2. It involves the stomach and duodenum.
3. It is caused by overuse of laxatives.
4. Symptoms are caused by inflammation of the colon.

242. Gigantism and acromegaly are caused by a disorder of the:
1. Thyroid gland.
2. Adrenal gland.
3. Pituitary gland.
4. Pancreas.

243. A physician orders midazolam (Versed), 3 mg IM before surgery, for a patient scheduled to have a bowel resection. The nurse has Versed, 10 mg/2 mL, on hand. How much will the nurse give?
Answer: _____ mL

244. A patient with insulin-dependent diabetes mellitus asks the nurse what the new "blood test" is that his physician wants him to have. If the patient is referring to the HgbA$_{1c}$, the nurse explains that this test:
1. Gauges how well the patient's blood sugar is controlled over a 3-month period.
2. Can show if the patient has been cheating on his diet.
3. Can measure the amount of insulin the patient uses over time.
4. Is routine before a pancreatic stem cell transplant.

245. The patient has a large accumulation of fluid in his abdominal cavity. The nurse surmises that this patient has a diagnosis of:
1. Peritonitis.
2. Cirrhosis.
3. Hepatitis.
4. Diverticulitis.

246. The physician's order reads to infuse 2000 mL of IV fluids over 10 hours. The drop factor of the administration set is 10 gtt/mL. How many drops per minute will the nurse infuse in the IV line?
Answer: _____ gtt/min

247. A patient has had a cholecystectomy. During discharge teaching, which foods would the nurse discourage her from consuming?
1. Raw vegetables
2. Fried foods
3. Tomatoes
4. Pasta

248. A patient is to receive three 8-oz cans of formula feeding via a tube-feeding pump. If the nurse infuses the feeding at 80 mL/hr, how long will it take to infuse the feeding?
Answer: _____ hours

249. A patient has a prolapsed uterus. What is the primary concern for this patient?
1. Hemorrhage
2. Dyspareunia
3. Urinary incontinence
4. Bowel incontinence

250. The primary problem in a patient with a vesicovaginal fistula is:
1. Elimination.
2. Infection.
3. Bleeding.
4. Respiratory difficulty.

ANSWERS AND RATIONALES

1. Analysis, planning, physiological integrity, (c).
   3. Many individuals react differently to foods. By finding out what his reaction entails, you can better inform the physician.
   1. Further action is indicated before the procedure.
   2. You should ascertain the nature of the allergy first.
   4. This will eventually be done but is not a priority.
2. Analysis, evaluation, health promotion and maintenance, (a).
   2. These are the identified components of the Glasgow Coma Scale (GCS).
   1. Posturing and reflexes are not components of the GCS.
   3. None of these are components of the GCS.
   4. Best motor response and best verbal response are parts of the GCS, but seizure activity is not.
3. Comprehension, assessment, physiological integrity, (a).
   2. The DNA molecules in the nucleus of a cell duplicate themselves, and the cell divides, forming two identical cells.
   1. Lysis is the swelling of red blood cells (RBCs) placed in a hypotonic salt solution.
   3. Osmosis is the movement of water through a permeable membrane.
   4. Crenation is the shrinking of RBCs placed in a hypertonic solution.
4. Application, implementation, health promotion and maintenance, (b).
   2. In acquiring passive immunity, the body of the recipient plays no active part in response to an antigen.
   1. In active immunity the resistance to a disease results from the development of antibodies within the body.
   3. Newborn babies receive short-term immunity as a result of the antibodies of their mother, but it is not considered permanent.
   4. Autoimmune immunity occurs when the body produces antibodies to its own tissues.
5. Analysis assessment, physiological integrity, (b).
   _____ 1. This is double vision and is not a symptom of this disorder.
   __X__ **2. Tinnitus may accompany the hearing loss.**
   _____ 3. Pain is not a common symptom of otosclerosis.
   __X__ **4. Loss of hearing of the affected ear is the most likely symptom.**
   __X__ **5. Vertigo may accompany the hearing loss.**
6. Analysis, assessment, physiological integrity, (b).
   1. Vomiting is a sign of increased intracranial pressure, which is a complication of head injury.
   2. A person with head trauma is likely to have a headache.
   3. Tremors are not directly related to closed head injury.
   4. Itching skin would not be a complication of closed head injury.
7. Application, implementation, health promotion and maintenance, (b).
   2. Estrogen and progesterone promote development of the female sex characteristics and sex organs; they also regulate menstruation for the purpose of reproduction.
   1. Testosterone is produced by male testes.
   3. Prolactin is produced by the pituitary gland.
   4. Progesterone is produced by the ovaries; testosterone is produced by the testes.
8. Application, implementation, physiological integrity, (a).
   3. The testes produce testosterone, which gives men their secondary sex characteristics.
   1. Estrogen is produced by the ovaries.
   2. Progesterone is produced by the ovaries.
   4. Aldosterone is produced by the adrenal cortex.
9. Analysis, assessment, health promotion and maintenance, (c).
   _____ 1. Individuals with Parkinson disease do not usually experience diplopia, although they do have tremors.
   _____ 2. Headache is not a common symptom, and ataxia (difficulty walking) may be found in the form of a shuffling walk.
   __X__ **3. A shuffling gait is a common symptom.**
   _____ 4. Tinnitus normally is not associated with Parkinson disease.
   __X__ **5. Difficulty swallowing or speaking is a common symptom.**
10. Analysis, evaluation, physiological integrity, (c).
    1. Popcorn has hulls and seeds, which precipitate a diverticular attack. More teaching about diet is needed.
    2, 3, 4. These are all correct teaching points for a patient diagnosed with diverticulitis.
11. Analysis, implementation, physiological integrity, (c).
    1. The small intestine contains villi that absorb most of the nutrients that are derived from the digestion of food. The surgery will disrupt the absorption.
    2. TPN does contain a lot of glucose, but protein is needed for body repair.
    3. TPN is a sterile IV fluid that does not assist in establishing normal flora.
    4. This may or may not be true. A bowel resection does not normally disrupt the action of the liver.
12. Application, planning, physiological integrity, (b).
    1. Sitz baths will soothe the patient's itching and burning skin.
    2. Pillows may provide comfort but do not soothe itching and burning.
    3. Acetaminophen (Tylenol) does not diminish itching and burning.
    4. A tap-water enema will further irritate the area.
13. Comprehension, implementation, physiological integrity, (c).
    3. T tubes are used to drain away bile from the incision site.
    1. Other types of devices are used to drain blood.
    2. The T tube is not inserted into the liver.
    4. The T tube is not positioned in such a way as to drain stomach acids.
14. Analysis, planning, physiological integrity, (c).
    1. Of the nursing diagnoses listed, infection is of paramount importance based on Maslow's hierarchy of needs because the catheter is inserted into the abdomen.
    2. Deficient fluid volume might be a nursing diagnosis; however, it is more likely that individuals undergoing peritoneal dialysis have excess fluid volume.

3. Many patients undergoing peritoneal dialysis have a disturbed body image, but this is not the priority nursing diagnosis.

4. Patients who undergo peritoneal dialysis do so at home and should not have a self-care deficit.

15. Comprehension, planning, physiological integrity, (c).

2. When a patient has his labyrinth destroyed, he will be unable to hear from that side.

1. The patient, although unable to hear, should be free from symptoms.

3. The symptoms should not come back after the procedure.

4. The symptoms should stop when the labyrinth is destroyed.

16. Analysis, assessment, physiological integrity, (b).

4. A pH level of 7.30 indicates metabolic acidosis.

1. This is a normal pH reading for the bloodstream.

2. 7.36 is a normal blood pH.

3. 7.40 is within the normal range for blood pH.

17. Analysis, implementation, physiological integrity, (c).

Correct order: 52314.

5. Remaining calm helps allay the patient's fears.

2. The organs then need to be covered by a sterile, saline-soaked gauze.

3. Vital signs need to be taken.

1. The physician needs to be notified (the physician will need to know the condition of the patient, including vital signs).

4. The nursing supervisor then needs to be made aware of the situation.

18. Application, implementation, physiological integrity, (c).

1. A lumpectomy is a surgical procedure designed to limit the size of breast tissue removed in patients with an early diagnosis.

2. A mastectomy, removal of the breast, would not preserve the most breast tissue.

3. A needle biopsy is a diagnostic examination and not a surgical procedure for removal of breast tissue.

4. An oophorectomy is removal of an ovary.

19. Application, implementation, physiological integrity, (b).

2. Soy sauce is high in sodium, which the patient should avoid.

1. Fresh fruits would be good for this patient and are relatively free from sodium.

3. Saltwater fish would be detrimental to the patient, but freshwater fish is a good food choice.

4. These herbs should have no adverse effects on the individual.

20. Analysis, assessment, physiological integrity, (c).

3. Airway is the priority concern after surgery for this patient.

1. Pain management is important but can impede the respiratory drive.

2. Vital signs are extremely important but come second to airway status.

4. Bleeding should be assessed for after the initial airway, and vital signs should be monitored.

21. Analysis, evaluation, physiological integrity, (c).

1. Having an empty stomach is the best way to prevent aspiration.

2. This does assist in preventing aspiration, but the best method is NPO status.

3. This does not assist in preventing aspiration.

4. Although this helps to decrease the risk for aspiration, it is not the most effective method.

22. Analysis, assessment, health promotion and maintenance, (c).

2. A painless loss of vision is one of the predominant symptoms in patients with a detached retina.

1. Double vision is not a common symptom.

3. Tunnel vision is common in patients with glaucoma.

4. Headaches are not a common symptom.

23. Application, assessment, health promotion and maintenance, (b).

_____ 1. Blood sugar levels would be part of an assessment of the endocrine system.

_____ 2. Blood pressure is considered part of assessment of the cardiovascular system.

__X__ 3, 4, 5. *Rashes, bruises, and decubitus ulcers are all data that are derived from assessing the skin and its appendages—the integumentary system.*

24. Application, assessment, health promotion and maintenance, (c).

3. Because individuals with glaucoma experience loss of peripheral vision, they have the symptom of tunnel vision.

1. Painless loss of vision is a common finding with detached retina.

2. Diplopia is not a common finding in patients with glaucoma.

4. Strabismus is more common in children and is not common in patients with glaucoma.

25. Comprehension, implementation, physiological integrity, (c).

1. Miotics are used to make the pupil smaller and increase the angle of Schlemm to allow fluid to flow from the eye, decreasing intraocular pressure.

2. Mydriatics increase the diameter of the pupil and are contraindicated in patients with glaucoma.

3. Although they reduce intraocular pressure, they are not a diuretic.

4. These medications are not used to treat detached retina.

26. Analysis, planning, physiological integrity, (c).

3. Breathing deeply several times per hour decreases the chances for the patient developing atelectasis, a frequent complication of fractured ribs.

1. Morphine inhibits breathing and is usually not prescribed for home use.

2. The patient should not need supplemental oxygen for this problem.

4. The patient will not have a cast.

27. Analysis, assessment, physiological integrity, (b).

3. The left motor control center in the brain controls the right side of the body because of the crossing of the nerve tracts within the brain.

1. Only one side of the body is affected if an injury is to only one side of the brain.

2. The left side of the body is controlled by the right side of the brain.

4. Normally some paralysis is observed when damage occurs to the motor control center of the brain.

28. Application, planning, physiological integrity, (c).
    2. The physician has placed the marks on the skin to guide the radiation beam to the tumor; removing the markings may cause inaccurate treatments.
    1. The patient should not apply any oils or lubricants over the skin.
    3. Ice and heat create further discomfort for the patient.
    4. The area that is irradiated will become red; it is an expected result.

29. Analysis, implementation, physiological integrity, (c).
    2. A positive test result indicates that the patient has TB antibodies.
    1. The patient would be placed in Droplet Isolation if the disease is active.
    3. The patient may or may not have an active infection.
    4. Drug therapy usually lasts 6 to 18 months.

30. Analysis, assessment, physiological integrity, (c).
    1. Any patient who falls must be immediately assessed.
    2. This patient does not take priority over the patient who fell; another nurse can administer the medication.
    3. Although this reading is high, it is not life-threatening, as the fall may be.
    4. The nurse should delegate this task to a nursing assistant and then assess the fallen patient.

31. Analysis, assessment, physiological integrity, (c).
    _____ 1. A bounding pulse indicates good arterial blood flow.
    __X__ **2. Capillary refill times (CRTs) longer than 3 seconds accompanied by cyanosis and numbness and tingling may signal neurovascular compromise.**
    _____ 3. A cool extremity may be a sign of decreased neurovascular status, but the patient may simply be cold.
    _____ 4. Complaints of pain are not usually associated with neurovascular impairment; numbness and tingling are more common.
    __X__ **5. CRTs longer than 3 seconds accompanied by cyanosis, numbness, and tingling may signal neurovascular compromise.**
    __X__ **6. CRTs longer than 3 seconds accompanied by cyanosis, numbness, and tingling may signal neurovascular compromise.**

32. Analysis, evaluation, physiological integrity, (c).
    4. Working in a warehouse, the patient would be required to bend and lift heavy objects, which is one of the predisposing factors for herniated disks.
    1. Although this is not a healthy lifestyle practice, it has little to do with a herniated nucleus pulposus.
    2. This practice should not contribute significantly to this disorder.
    3. This should have little bearing on this diagnosis.

33. Analysis, assessment, physiological integrity, (c).
    3. This observation may indicate the leakage of cerebrospinal fluid.
    1. This is a common complaint from a patient, and he or she should not be sitting upright at this time.
    2. Again, the patient will have difficulty sitting after the surgery.
    4. Nausea may accompany a headache in these individuals.

34. Analysis, implementation, physiological integrity, (c).
    3. This should raise the blood sugar to the desired level. The patient is alert and able to consume the juice.
    1. This is not a sufficient amount to raise the glucose level.
    2. This can cause the blood sugar to rise quickly and then fall quickly again.
    4. Diet drinks do not contain sugar and do not alter the blood sugar level.

35. Application, assessment, physiological integrity, (b).
    2. These are the classic symptoms of osteomyelitis.
    1. These symptoms can signal pulmonary emboli.
    3. These symptoms may indicate neurovascular impairment.
    4. These are symptoms of neurological impairment.

36. Application, assessment, physiological integrity, (c).
    1. Salty or sweet-tasting drainage from the operative area may indicate that cerebrospinal fluid is leaking.
    2. Headache is frequent after craniotomy, usually caused by stretching or irritation of scalp nerves during the operation. Position should not affect headache unless the left is the operative side.
    3. Neither hunger nor temporary anorexia would indicate a possible complication. The nurse would anticipate thirst after surgery.
    4. The patient has had general anesthesia so sleepiness is expected, but level of consciousness changes are critical.

37. Application, planning, physiological integrity, (c).
    3. A patient diagnosed with ALS needs to maintain a patent airway at all times, a priority for patients with ALS.
    1, 2. Periods of exercise are necessary, but they would not be increased. Adequate periods of rest are a necessity for this patient, as are alternative forms of communication. However, these are not a priority at this time.
    4. Providing counseling and other means to facilitate coping with the diagnosis also is important, although not as critical as No. 3.

38. Comprehension, planning, physiological integrity, (b).
    3. It is true that it takes longer to inspire or expire air because of age-related physiological changes.
    1. This is not a proven fact for older persons.
    2. This is not a proven correlation.
    4. Overall respiratory muscle structure and function decrease in older adults.

39. Analysis, assessment, physiological integrity, (b).
    1. Tenderness and crepitus are common characteristics of joints involved in osteoarthritis.
    2. Most joints involved in osteoarthritis are on one side of the body. These findings are consistent with rheumatoid arthritis.
    3. In osteoarthritis pain is caused by the loss of articular cartilage.
    4. Rheumatoid arthritis commonly causes these symptoms.

40. Application, implementation, physiological integrity, (c).
    4. Concentrated glucose can be absorbed between the buccal mucosa and gum; when patient fully awakens, give a fast-acting carbohydrate by mouth.

1. Insulin would further lower the blood glucose reading, and LPN/LVNs are not permitted to administer IV insulin.
2. This places the patient in danger for aspiration.
3. This action will most likely result in the patient choking and aspirating.

41. Analysis, implementation, physiological integrity, (c).
    3. ***This is standard practice. The petroleum gauze creates an occlusive dressing that does not allow air to flow into the lung.***
    1. Infection is not a priority at this time.
    2. The petroleum has the opposite effect.
    4. Although this is true, it is not the primary reason an occlusive gauze is used.

42. Application, implementation, physiological integrity, (b).
    1. ***A patient with a lobectomy may be turned to either side.***
    2. This does not allow for full expansion.
    3. This position does not facilitate drainage and expansion of the remaining lobes.
    4. These do not allow for full expansion and drainage of all remaining lobes.

43. Analysis, assessment, health promotion and maintenance, (c).
    __X__ 1. ***Accidental removal of the parathyroid glands can lead to hypocalcemia and result in tetany.***
    _____ 2. Cortisol is secreted by the adrenal gland and is not associated with a thyroidectomy.
    _____ 3. This is not associated with parathyroid removal.
    _____ 4. Although respiratory compromise is a potential problem with a thyroidectomy, loss of the gag reflex is not associated with parathyroid removal.
    _____ 5. TSH is secreted from the pituitary gland and should not be affected by parathyroid removal.
    __X__ 6. ***Accidental removal of the parathyroid glands can lead to hypocalcemia and result in tetany.***

44. Application, implementation, health promotion and maintenance, (b).
    3. ***Abstaining from food or drink decreases the chance of esophageal reflux when he lies down.***
    1. This suggestion does not reduce bedtime discomfort.
    2. This worsens the symptoms; chocolate is one of the aggravating factors for hiatal hernia.
    4. This causes a worsening of symptoms.

45. Analysis, assessment, health promotion and maintenance, (b).
    4. ***Smokeless tobacco or snuff is a precipitating factor for oral cancer.***
    1. Alcohol abuse is not a factor in oral cancer; however, it is for other conditions.
    2. Poor dental hygiene is not a predisposing cause for oral cancer.
    3. Frequent bouts of tonsillitis are not a precipitating cause for oral cancer.

46. Application, implementation, health promotion and maintenance, (b).
    __X__ 1. ***Walking is an acceptable activity for an individual with diabetes mellitus.***
    _____ 2. Meals should be spaced no further than 4 hours apart.
    _____ 3. Medication should be taken first thing in the morning.
    __X__ 4. ***Hypoglycemia can be countered with the ingestion of a rapid-acting sugar.***

_____ 5. The individual should contact his or her health care provider for instructions.
_____ 6. This would result in an even lower glucometer reading.

47. Analysis, assessment, health promotion and maintenance, (b).
    2. ***These are the common symptoms of candidiasis.***
    1. This is not common in candidiasis, but it is common in some systemic infections.
    3. This is common in genital warts.
    4. Although a cause for concern, these are not symptoms associated with candidiasis.

48. Application, implementation, physiological integrity, (b).
    3. ***The application of heat alleviates discomfort, and drinking warm beverages decreases the incidence of abdominal cramps.***
    1. This increases discomfort.
    2. This has no bearing on abdominal cramps.
    4. Applying ice does not alleviate discomfort.

49. Application, planning, physiological integrity, (c).
    1. ***Addison disease is a failure to produce the needed hormones by the adrenal cortex that help regulate electrolyte balance.***
    2. Addison disease does not affect the WBC count, and this goal would cause the patient to be unable to fight off infectious diseases.
    3. Because Addison disease does not affect the bone marrow, this would not be a goal of therapy.
    4. The RBC count is not affected in Addison disease, and this would not be a goal of therapy.

50. Application, implementation, physiological integrity, (b).
    2. ***Splinting protects the fracture, immobilizes the arm, and may prevent worsening of the situation.***
    1. Use 911 only in true emergencies.
    3. Warmth may actually cause an increase in edema and does not immobilize the fracture.
    4. The extremity should be elevated to prevent edema formation.

51. Application, implementation, health promotion and maintenance, (c).
    _____ 1. Decreased appetite is common in many disorders.
    _____ 2. Although the nurse will alert the physician about the headache, it is not of paramount importance.
    __X__ 3. ***Crackles with resulting orthopnea may be associated with left-sided heart failure.***
    _____ 4. This blood pressure is not at a dangerous level.
    __X__ 5. ***Crackles with resulting orthopnea may be associated with left-sided heart failure.***
    _____ 6. Usually pulmonary edema is not associated with increased urination.

52. Application, implementation, physiological integrity, (b).
    4. ***This is the correct definition.***
    1. This is the definition of a bronchoscopy.
    2. This is the definition of magnetic resonance imaging.
    3. This is the definition of spirometry.

53. Application, assessment, health promotion and maintenance, (c).
    3. ***Men with BPH complain of urgency, frequency, and diminished urine stream.***
    1. This is not a common problem with BPH.

2. Dizziness is a common symptom for many disorders but not BPH.

4. This is not a common finding.

54. Application, implementation, physiological integrity, (c).

_____ 1. Inappropriate. The patient should be on NPO status.

__X__ 2. *This is correct based on the use of the contrast medium (dye).*

_____ 3. Inappropriate. The patient should be on NPO status.

_____ 4. This is not necessary; the patient's activity has nothing to do with standard protocol for this test under normal circumstances.

_____ 5. This intervention is not indicated in this situation.

__X__ 6. *This is correct based on the use of the contrast medium (dye).*

55. Comprehension, assessment, physiological integrity, (c).

1. *This is used to determine areas of lung being ventilated because of an obstruction or clot in the pulmonary circulation. It is a common procedure for this diagnosis.*

2, 3. These are inappropriate tests for this medical diagnosis.

4. This is done for joint pain.

56. Application, implementation, physiological integrity, (c).

2. *The primary responsibility is for the nurse to reduce the risk of an accidental injury by keeping the patient still.*

1. This may be a secondary objective for the nurse; however, physicians usually handle this on their own.

3. This can be done before the procedure.

4. If this is indicated, the nurse will have completed the setup before the procedure begins.

57. Application, implementation, physiological integrity, (b).

2. *Oxygen is very drying when the flow rate is more than 4L/min; humidification is necessary.*

1. This is not really responsive to the patient's concern.

3. Although true, this response is incomplete in rationale.

4. Humidity does not increase safety factors when oxygen is in use; in addition, such a statement may be cause for patient concern.

58. Comprehension, planning, physiological integrity, (c).

1. *Protein is converted to ammonia, and a buildup of ammonia affects brain tissue. Protein should be restricted if ammonia levels rise. This snack is lowest in protein.*

2, 3, 4. These snacks are high in protein.

59. Application, planning, physiological integrity, (c).

1. *After a hydrocelectomy the scrotum is elevated to prevent edema.*

2. The patient may have a catheter, although this is not always true.

3. Estrogen therapy may be indicated for prostate cancer.

4. A wet-to-dry saline dressing normally is not indicated.

60. Application, evaluation, health promotion and maintenance, (c).

__X__ 1. *Stress can cause fluctuations to occur in blood sugar, usually in the form of elevations.*

__X__ 2. *Infection can cause fluctuations to occur in blood sugar, usually in the form of elevations.*

_____ 3. Excess insulin would cause hypoglycemia.

_____ 4. Insufficient calories in the diet would also cause hypoglycemia.

_____ 5. Too much exercise would cause hypoglycemia.

__X__ 6. *Insufficient insulin would contribute to hyperglycemia.*

61. Comprehension, planning, physiological integrity, (b).

1. *Patients with laryngitis should rest the voice.*

2. Resting the voice is a more effective treatment modality than is gargling with saltwater.

3. Treatment is aimed at resting the voice.

4. This would be very traumatic to tell a patient, and it may not be true.

62. Application, planning, physiological integrity, (c).

4. *Application of ice packs is not standard treatment for sinusitis, and this statement needs clarification for the patient.*

1. This is standard treatment for sinusitis.

2. Decongestants are a standard treatment.

3. These are standard discharge instructions for a patient with sinusitis.

63. Application, assessment, physiological integrity, (c).

_____ 1. A headache is not one of the warning signs of hypocalcemia.

__X__ 2. *Facial numbness is the first sign of hypocalcemia.*

_____ 3. Nausea is not a predominant symptom of hypocalcemia.

_____ 4. This can be caused by several factors and not merely hypocalcemia.

__X__ 5. *Carpopedal spasms also indicate hypocalcemia.*

_____ 6. Increased urination is not a factor in hypocalcemia.

64. Application, planning, physiological integrity, (c).

1. *Because of the destruction of T cells, opportunistic infections are the priority problem for these individuals.*

2. This is a concern for many patients; however, it is not the priority nursing concern based on Maslow's hierarchy of needs.

3. The wasting that takes place at the end of life for an AIDS patient is a problem, but it is not the priority problem at this time.

4. Although this may very well be a problem for patients with AIDS, it is not the priority based on Maslow's hierarchy of needs.

65. Comprehension, planning, physiological integrity, (c).

2. *Mannitol is an osmotic diuretic used to decrease intracranial pressure in patients with head injury.*

1. Mannitol is not an antibiotic.

3. Sedatives or pain medications would offer this action.

4. Although mannitol may indirectly reduce the chance of seizures by decreasing intracranial pressure, this is not the primary reason for giving this medication.

66. Analysis, implementation, physiological integrity, (b).

_____ 1. This laboratory value is within normal range.

_____ 2. This laboratory value is within normal range.

__X__ 3. *This is considered a low platelet count, which can predispose the patient for bleeding episodes.*

_____ 4. This laboratory value is within normal range.

__X__ 5. *An elevated BUN is associated with worsening renal failure.*

67. Application, implementation, health promotion and maintenance, (b).
   2. **This would promote venous return and decrease the swelling in the extremity.**
   1. A diuretic is not normally used for swelling caused by injury or surgery.
   3. This technique would not reduce swelling and would limit range of motion.
   4. Although this is done on a routine basis, it does not decrease edema formation.
68. Comprehension, implementation, physiological integrity, (b)
   2. **An autograft is tissue taken from the patient's own body.**
   1, 3, 4. These are all derived from substances other than the patient's own skin.
69. Application, assessment, physiological integrity, (b).
   2. **Changes in the circulatory status of the involved extremity indicate a complication.**
   1. This is not serious and may be a reaction to the anesthetic.
   3. This can be handled by the nurse in most cases and is not a serious complication of arthroplasty.
   4. This may not be of any concern; the patient may not have any sputum to produce; as long as he or she does incentive spirometry and deep-breathing exercises, pulmonary status should be maintained.
70. Analysis, planning, safe and effective care environment, (c).
   3. **This is the best choice, given that the patient's blisters are weeping and still infectious.**
   1. The chance of infection in the roommate makes this situation a bad choice.
   2. Pediatric patients are more susceptible to infection, and adults are not normally placed with a pediatric roommate.
   4. Choosing the room for the patient is important because of the chance of contamination.
71. Application, implementation, physiological integrity, (b).
   4. **This maintains cleanliness. Preventive skin care is important in maintaining the integrity of the skin and stoma.**
   1. Massaging may injure the delicate stoma and is unnecessary unless ordered by the physician.
   2. Oils may be irritating to the skin and stoma; they promote fungal infection.
   3. The lotion provides a medium for fungal growth and may irritate the stoma.
72. Application, implementation, physiological integrity, (b).
   Answer: 1150 mL
   Subtract the amount of irrigation solution (2500 mL) from the total amount of urine output (3650 mL); 1150 mL is the true urine output.
73. Comprehension, planning, physiological integrity, (b).
   2. **The elevated toilet seat does not allow the patient to flex her hip past 90 degrees, an activity that may dislocate the hip.**
   1. This does not cause the hip to heal properly, but it does prevent it from dislocating.
   3. Again, this may be true, but it is not the reason for use of the elevated seat.
   4. Once again, this may be true, but it is not the primary reason for using the seat.
74. Comprehension, implementation, physiological integrity, (b).
   3. **Standing and sitting for long periods cause varicose veins to develop and increase pain for the patient. In addition, blood stasis predisposes the patient to blood clots.**
   1. This activity would increase pain for the patient.
   2. These would not provide support for the patient, as would antiembolism or support stockings.
   4. This activity would not decrease the pain of varicose veins and may prompt further development.
75. Application, implementation, physiological integrity, (c).
   2. **This drug potentiates muscle weakness because of its effect on the myoneural junction.**
   1. This drug blocks the action of cholinesterase at the myoneural junction and allows acetylcholine to act. It is therapeutic.
   3. Corticosteroids are sometimes used as an adjunct therapy. They are therapeutic.
   4. This drug blocks the action of cholinesterase at the myoneural junction and allows acetylcholine to act. It is therapeutic.
76. Application, planning, physiological integrity, (c).
   3. **The ventrogluteal is a deep muscle located in the upper outer quadrant of the hip. It has few superficial blood vessels and makes a good injection site for someone who has muscle atrophy.**
   1. The deltoid is not a good choice because of the patient's muscle atrophy.
   2. IM injections are not given in the abdomen.
   4. The gluteus maximus is not a good choice because of the muscle atrophy.
77. Application, implementation, physiological integrity, (c).
   4. **Additional stress placed on the tissues by movement may disrupt the healing tissue. Splinting lessens the chance for this to occur.**
   1. This is true, but the question is specific to ambulation.
   2. This is too sweeping a statement. Although more pain is involved from movement with an abdominal incision, not all patients are hesitant to move.
   3. The binder would be a good choice for the patient if it were applied correctly.
78. Application, implementation, psychosocial integrity, (c).
   4. **This is an open-ended question that seeks to explore the patient's feelings. It is always best to allow the patient to express his or her views.**
   1. This does not address the patient's fears.
   2. This is defensive and will not help the patient cope.
   3. This statement appears to be patronizing. It is best to first ascertain what the patient's questions are.
79. Application, assessment, physiological integrity, (b).
   _____ 1. This is associated with hyperglycemia.
   _____ 2. This is associated with hyperglycemia.
   __X__ 3. **This is a low blood sugar (hypoglycemic) symptom.**
   _____ 4. This is a symptom of ketoacidosis.
   __X__ 5. **This is a low blood sugar (hypoglycemic) symptom.**
   _____ 6. Flushed, hot, dry skin is associated with hyperglycemia.
80. Application, implementation, health promotion and maintenance, (b).

     3. A continuous passive ROM machine allows the patient to regain flexibility of the knee very early after surgery.

     1. A trochanter roll would keep the patient's leg from rotating externally.

     2. An abductor pillow keeps the patient from adducting the legs after a hip replacement.

     4. A Hemovac drainage device does not promote flexibility of the knee.

81. Application, implementation, physiological integrity, (b).

     3. Treatment for this condition revolves around keeping the extremities warm with socks, mittens, and other warm layers.

     1. Support hose will not keep this patient from experiencing exacerbations.

     2, 4. Patients with this disorder worsen their condition by application of hot or cold to the areas affected.

82. Application, planning, health promotion and maintenance, (b).

     3. Raynaud phenomenon is triggered by contact with cold.

     1. This is not true; Raynaud disease affects primarily women.

     2. Both of these diseases cause considerable pain for patients.

     4. Buerger disease affects both types of blood vessels.

83. Application, assessment, physiological integrity, (c).

     2. Damaged parenchymal cells are unable to metabolize bilirubin, which gives the stool its normal color; bilirubin in the circulation causes jaundice, pruritus, and dark urine.

     1. Stools are clay-colored because of the inability of the liver to metabolize bilirubin.

     3. Clay-colored stools are common in advanced liver disease; urine is dark in color.

     4. Urine is not blood tinged but dark in color with liver dysfunction.

84. Analysis, implementation, physiological integrity, (c).

     3. Tubes that are placed high in the anterior part of the chest are placed primarily to reestablish normal pressure in the lung by creating an outlet for air.

     1. This is a trite response. The nurse should respond to the question with the correct answer.

     2. This statement is not true.

     4. Although this statement is true, it does not meet the learning needs of the patient.

85. Application, implementation, psychosocial integrity, (c).

     3. This is the correct response, presented in terms the wife can understand.

     1. This is not a correct response; thoracotomy tubes drain blood from the lung.

     2. A tracheotomy may be a means for delivery of oxygen.

     4. Medications are not normally administered through these tubes.

86. Application, evaluation, physiological integrity, (b).

     4. The nurse needs to establish whether the patient can clear his own airway.

     1. This would indicate an infection or dehydration or both.

     2. This is inappropriate for this nursing diagnosis.

     3. This would give the opportunity to assess the effort of breathing.

87. Application, planning, physiological integrity, (b).

     1. This is the only choice that maintains the water-seal drainage. The patient can be off suction for short periods.

     2. This would break the closed system and might create a pneumothorax.

     3. Although this is possible, and it would depend on the patient's condition, no harm exists in transporting the patient to the x-ray department.

     4. This would take much time, and no harm exists in transporting the patient.

88. Application, planning, physiological integrity, (b).

     4. Hand splints lessen wrist flexion, decreasing pain and numbness.

     1. This may assist somewhat, but typing aggravates the condition. Immobility is needed.

     2. Range of motion aggravates the problem.

     3. A sling does not provide immobility at the wrist.

89. Application, planning, psychosocial integrity, (c).

     1. A calm environment is important; these patients are usually in a hyperactive state.

     2. The number of visitors may need to be limited to avoid overtaxing the patient's energies.

     3. A supportive environment is necessary but does not overstimulate the patient.

     4. A private room ensures better control over the environment.

90. Application, implementation, physiological integrity, (c).

     Answer: 21 gtt/min

     $1000\,mL/8\,hr = 125\,mL/hr$

     $125\,mL/hr \times 10\,gtt \div 60\,min/hr = 20.83 = 21\,gtt/min$

91. Application, assessment, health promotion and maintenance, (b).

     4. Muscle weakness and personality changes herald the possibility of neurological problems.

     1. Chest pain on exertion is a symptom of angina; this patient does not exhibit this.

     2. The patient may have no symptoms at all or symptoms of fatigue and headache.

     3. The presenting symptoms indicate a potential neurological complication, not a cardiac one.

92. Application, planning, health promotion and maintenance, (b).

     1. Protecting the blood supply is a sound measure to prevent the transmission of hepatitis B and C and HIV.

     2. Blood donors cannot get a bloodborne disease by donating blood.

     3. This may reduce the risk of ingestion of some pathogens but not the hepatitis B virus.

     4. Shellfish are associated with contraction of hepatitis A.

93. Comprehension, planning, physiological integrity, (b).

     2. Contact sports that can result in blunt blows to the abdomen should be discouraged.

     1. This noncontact sport poses a reduced risk of injury.

     3. Although strenuous, this sport poses little risk of injury to the patient's stoma.

     4. If the patient feels comfortable swimming with an ileostomy, it should not be discouraged.

94. Application, assessment, health promotion and maintenance, (b).

     4. This is a common laboratory finding in appendicitis.

     1. This is found in polycythemia vera.

     2. A low platelet count is not consistent with appendicitis.

3. This is not common in appendicitis, but it is in chronic renal failure.

95. Application, implementation, health promotion and maintenance, (b).
   __X__ *1. SARS is caused by a coronavirus.*
   __X__ *2. SARS causes these symptoms.*
   _____ 3. Antibiotics may not be useful against the virus.
   _____ 4. Twenty percent of individuals will develop severe respiratory impairment.
   __X__ *5. Travelers are at increased risk for contact with those who are affected.*
   __X__ *6. Because of the highly infectious nature of this virus, it is a reportable condition.*

96. Application, planning, health promotion and maintenance, (b).
   3. Stem cells may begin to produce new cells that will be cancer free.
   1. Stem cells are given to stimulate growth of new cells.
   2. If the stem cells work, they will stimulate the growth of new bone marrow cells.
   4. Stem cells can stimulate new growth of noncancerous cells.

97. Analysis, planning, physiological integrity, (c).
   2. Straining at stool increases intraocular pressure and can damage the eye.
   1. Restricting fluids is unnecessary.
   3. Bathing is allowed, although showers may be prohibited.
   4. This has no bearing on the patient's surgery.

98. Analysis, assessment, physiological integrity, (c).
   1. Frequent swallowing is a sign that the patient may be swallowing blood from a hemorrhage.
   2. No restriction in water intake has been ordered.
   3. This normally is not a problem from swallowing, although swallowing after this surgery is difficult.
   4. This surgery is very uncomfortable for both children and adults.

99. Application, implementation, physiological integrity, (b).
   2. Mydriatics cause an enlarged pupil that would let too much light into the eye. The effects should last only a few hours, and sunglasses should help them.
   1. No need exists for a patch over her eye.
   3. This restriction is imposed on individuals who have had eye surgery.
   4. This is an unnecessary restriction.

100. Application, assessment, physiological integrity, (b).
   3. This patient has deficient knowledge about the desired action of diuretics.
   1. Altered tissue perfusion is not a concern for this patient.
   2. The patient may have excess fluid volume, but that information was not provided; the paramount concern in this situation is the deficient knowledge.
   4. The patient shows no indication of deficient fluid volume.

101. Application, planning, physiological integrity, (b).
   4. This will assist the patient with elimination and make the first bowel movement less painful.
   1. Sitz baths are more soothing to the rectum.
   2. Occlusive dressings are not normally used; rectal packing and loose dressings to collect drainage may be used.
   3. Gas formation is not a common problem with this procedure.

102. Comprehension, assessment, health promotion and maintenance, (b).
   4. The painless swelling of lymph nodes is one of the hallmarks of Hodgkin disease and non-Hodgkin lymphoma.
   1. This is not an early sign of the disorder.
   2. This is a common finding in renal disorders.
   3. This is frequently a problem in many disorders but not lymphoma.

103. Comprehension, planning, physiological integrity, (b).
   4. Diet should supply calories, protein, and carbohydrates to compensate for the increased metabolic demands imposed by the disease.
   1. Restriction of purine is not necessary, and calories in this diet are insufficient.
   2. This would provide insufficient calories; it will not meet the metabolic demands of the body.
   3. Restricting sodium is not necessary.

104. Application, planning, physiological integrity, (b).
   1. Many diuretics cause excretion of both sodium and potassium; maintaining adequate potassium levels is important for proper heart function.
   2. This may potentiate a fluid-retention problem.
   3. These foods would not be restricted because the patient is taking a diuretic.
   4. Caffeine is a natural diuretic and normally is not restricted in patients taking diuretics.

105. Application, implementation, safe and effective care environment, (c).
   _____ 1. This will not provide a sterile specimen.
   __X__ *2. This maintains an intact drainage system. It is less likely that the urine specimen will become contaminated.*
   __X__ *3. This maintains the sterility of the specimen.*
   _____ 4. This will not provide a sterile specimen.
   _____ 5. There is no need to have the patient endure a repeat and unnecessary catheterization.

106. Application, implementation, psychosocial integrity, (a).
   3. This is an emotional change that is common after a CVA. Emotional lability may or may not be appropriate to the situation.
   1. This is common but normal.
   2. This is inappropriate and encourages negative behavior modification technique. The patient has emotional lability.
   4. This is inappropriate. The patient is not acting this way on purpose.

107. Analysis, assessment, physiological integrity, (b).
   4. Dysphagia means difficulty swallowing. He may need to double swallow between bites.
   1. This is an inappropriate, unnecessary restriction.
   2. This is not necessary. No indication exists that the patient is hearing impaired.
   3. This is a good practice for any person who has had a CVA. However, it is not specific to this question.

108. Comprehension, implementation, health promotion and maintenance, (c).
   3. Flank pain would signal the presence of kidney stones.
   1. This is a trite reason to give; the patient needs more information.
   2. Usually high calcium levels are a problem in this disorder.
   4. Often kidney stones can be treated conservatively.

109. Comprehension, planning, physiological integrity, (a).
1. **This is true. Weakened pelvic muscles may also be a cause.**
2. This is an inappropriate assumption; this is called "residual" and is not usually a factor in stress inconvenience.
3. This is an inappropriate assumption; muscles and nerves are usually involved, not nerves alone.
4. This is an inappropriate assumption; this may be true, but other symptoms such as back pain would be evident.

110. Analysis, planning, physiological integrity, (c).
2. **Injuries above C3 cause respiratory paralysis and necessitate ventilatory support.**
1. Diuretics may be ordered, but a patent airway is a more pressing concern.
3. This would not maintain a patent airway for this patient.
4. These may also be indicated, but the patent airway is the immediate concern.

111. Application, implementation, physiological integrity, (b).
1. **This is the proper procedure for stopping the nosebleed.**
2. This does not stop the nosebleed and may increase the amount of blood.
3. This causes blood to run down the throat, possibly obstructing the airway.
4. Blowing the nose only increases the bleeding.

112. Analysis, evaluation, physiological integrity, (b).
3. **The Holter monitor records a tracing of the heart during various activities and is compared with activities that the patient is documenting.**
1. A glucometer evaluates capillary blood sugar levels.
2. Urine is used to evaluate various conditions but not heart activity during exertion.
4. This study evaluates blood flow through a carotid artery or extremity.

113. Comprehension, planning, physiological integrity, (c).
3. **Maintaining a patent airway is the primary concern based on the patient's medical diagnosis and Maslow's hierarchy of human needs.**
1. Suctioning clears the airway, maintaining patency; it is a means of maintaining a patent airway.
2. Changing the dressing around the tracheostomy would be a nursing skill to prevent infection. Airway is the primary concern.
4. Although this is important, airway is still the more immediate concern.

114. Application, assessment, physiological integrity, (a).

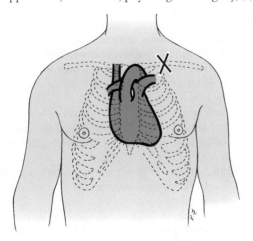

Pacemaker generator insertion sites are frequently found near the clavicle in the upper chest.

115. Analysis, assessment, safe and effective care environment, (c).
1. **Infection is the primary concern based on Maslow's hierarchy of needs. The patient's first line of defense is gone.**
2. Hemorrhage is a problem, but it is a lesser problem compared with the infection process.
3. Increased ICP is more of a problem with a closed head injury.
4. Consciousness would not be the primary concern, although it is a secondary concern.

116. Analysis, assessment, physiological integrity, (c).
2. **Because of pathological changes in the inner ear, patients with labyrinthitis frequently complain of dizziness.**
1. Sinus pain is not associated with labyrinthitis.
3. Cephalgia may be a complaint, but it is generally not the principal complaint.
4. Double vision is not a frequent complaint.

117. Application, planning, physiological integrity, (a).
_____ 1. No need exists to remove the hearing aids unless the patient is uncomfortable.
__X__ 2. **This is a standard treatment for patients with impacted cerumen.**
__X__ 3. **This is a standard treatment for patients with impacted cerumen.**
_____ 4. No need exists to remove the hearing aids unless the patient is uncomfortable.
_____ 5. No need exists to remove the hearing aids unless the patient is uncomfortable.

118. Application, planning, physiological integrity, (a).
Answer: 125 mL/hr
The patient should receive 1000 mL/8 hr, or 125 mL/hr.

119. Comprehension, implementation, physiological integrity, (b).
4. **Insulin must be given to patients with DKA to correct the hyperglycemia and ketosis.**
1. Oral antidiabetic agents do not correct DKA, although they are helpful in type 2 diabetes mellitus.
2. Glucose and water would create further problems for the patient with DKA.
3. Diuretics are used to treat hypertension or heart failure but not DKA.

120. Application, planning, physiological integrity, (b).
4. **This reduces the risk of constipation and straining, which may put a strain on damaged myocardium.**
1. This is not a standard of care for a patient having a myocardial infarction.
2. Prolonged bed rest is no longer advocated for patients with myocardial infarction.
3. This is no longer a standard of care.

121. Application, planning, health promotion and maintenance, (c).
__X__ 1. **This is a classic sign of diabetes mellitus.**
_____ 2. Cold extremities noted in individuals with impaired circulation could be seen in a patient with diabetes, but it is not considered a classic symptom.
__X__ 3. **This is a classic sign of diabetes mellitus.**
__X__ 4. **This is a classic sign of diabetes mellitus.**
_____ 5. This is not seen in patients with diabetes mellitus; anorexia can be the result of a variety of conditions, such as cancer.

122. Analysis, evaluation, physiological integrity, (a).
    2. These are the signs and symptoms of Lyme disease.
    1. The signs and symptoms and history do not point to a diagnosis of ALS.
    3. Patients with encephalitis experience photophobia and headache.
    4. Patients with chronic fatigue syndrome experience extreme fatigue.

123. Analysis, implementation, safe and effective care environment, (b).
    1. To prevent falling and to decrease vertigo sensation, the person has to be still and avoid all head movements that aggravate the spinning sensation.
    2. This would be appropriate only if p.r.n. medication had been ordered.
    3. Normal hydration is 2000 mL/day. At times, a diuretic may be prescribed to help decrease fluid volume of endolymph.
    4. This may increase the sensation of vertigo; however, bright, glaring lights should be avoided.

124. Application, evaluation, physiological integrity, (b).
    4. Tonic-clonic seizures are total body seizures that have the signs and symptoms exhibited by this patient.
    1. Partial seizures are not normally accompanied by incontinence.
    2. A focal seizure does not normally involve the entire body, resulting in incontinence or somnolence.
    3. An absence seizure is a trance or staring seizure that does not have these symptoms associated with it.

125. Application, implementation, physiological integrity, (b).
    1. Some patients experience a spinal headache after removal of cerebrospinal fluid.
    2. Leakage of spinal fluid can occur even if lying flat.
    3. This is an inappropriate response for the nurse to make; the nurse must know why the patient must lie flat.
    4. This is inappropriate. Blood pressure is affected by many factors and should not be affected directly by this procedure.

126. Application, assessment, health promotion and maintenance, (a).
    1. This may indicate a problem in the middle ear.
    2. It is important to frequently watch others' faces to read lips.
    3. This may be true if position changes were to lean forward to hear better.
    4. This behavior may result from a variety of factors that are not hearing related.

127. Application, assessment, physiological integrity, (b).
    2. Angulation, deformities, and shortening of a limb suggest a break in bone continuity.
    1. Edema is present with both sprains and fractures.
    3. Contused soft-tissue structures are tender, thus limiting mobility as well.
    4. Both types of injuries may evidence tenderness.

128. Application, planning, physiological integrity, (b).
    4. Traction is commonly used to reduce femoral fractures.
    1. Buck traction is not used to treat neck sprains.

2. Patients with spinal fractures normally are placed on Stryker frames.
3. Shoulder dislocations are treated with immobilization devices.

129. Application, planning, physiological integrity, (b).
    3. One of the complications of a thyroidectomy is swelling around the trachea, compromising the airway. A tracheostomy set must be in the room for quick intervention if this happens.
    1. A chest tube tray would not be necessary. No fear of fluid collection in the pleural space exists.
    2. A spinal tray should not be necessary.
    4. Transtracheal oxygen delivery would not be beneficial because the patient's upper trachea would be occluded.

130. Comprehension, assessment, physiological integrity, (a).
    Correct order: 21453.
    2. Kidney
    1. Ureter
    4. Bladder
    5. Urethra
    3. Meatus
    The urine passes from the kidney (2) to the ureters (1), urinary bladder (4), and urethra (5), and it exits through the meatus (3).

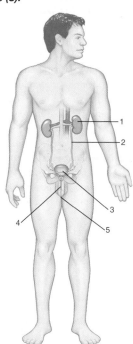

131. Application, evaluation, physiological integrity, (b).
    2. Many times glomerulonephritis is precipitated by an upper respiratory infection caused by Streptococcus bacteria. The antigen-antibody complex formed from the infection impairs kidney function.
    1. Antibiotic therapy is not a precipitating factor for this disorder.
    3. Upper respiratory infections are implicated in this disorder, not urinary tract infections.
    4. Although a low fluid intake is important to many other kidney disorders, it does not predispose a person to this disorder.

132. Comprehension, planning, physiological integrity, (c).
    3. These are also known as hyperosmolar drugs. Mannitol (Osmitrol) is an example. These agents draw water from the edematous brain.
    1. These should be used carefully; they may mask level of consciousness or cause respiratory depression.
    2. These may be ordered if nausea is present.
    4. These may be ordered if an open wound is caused by trauma.

133. Application, assessment, health promotion and maintenance, (a).
    2. This is recommended as an annual test for all men age 50 years and older.
    1. This is a blood test used as a monitoring tool to evaluate the response to treatment of a patient with cancer or for recurrence of the disease.
    3. This is a screening test for benign prostatic hyperplasia or prostate cancer; it is not a blood test. It is an examination recommended for all men older than the age of 40 years.
    4. This is one of the diagnostic tests for human immunodeficiency virus.

134. Analysis, planning, physiological integrity, (c).
    4. A common order for anyone admitted with nephrolithiasis would be straining urine to try to collect a stone specimen, which would then be sent to the laboratory for analysis.
    1. Whirlpool baths would not be beneficial to this patient and are not usually ordered. When patients have extracorporeal shock wave lithotripsy, they are immersed in a bath for this procedure.
    2. The opposite order would be given unless contraindicated. The patient needs to increase fluid intake.
    3. Racking urine is a physician order that was common for suspected hematuria. It entails placing urine in test tubes and allowing it to sit for hours until blood settles out.

135. Application, evaluation, psychosocial integrity, (a).

    4. Discovery of triggering factors demonstrates understanding of the disease process and preventive health habits.
    1. This is not directly related. However, it may relieve stress, which is frequently a trigger of headaches.
    2. No proof exists that sunlight triggers these types of headaches.
    3. Acetylsalicylic acid (aspirin) is seldom effective for classic migraine. Taking it as a preventive may not be a healthful habit.

136. Analysis, evaluation, physiological integrity, (c).
    Answer: D. Right ventricle problems cause a pooling and backup of blood entering the heart from the systemic circulation.

137. Application, assessment, physiological integrity, (b).
    2. Patients with a hip fracture generally have shortening and external rotation of the affected extremity.
    1. Pain and numbness may be present with sprains, contusions, and other problems.
    3. A large hematoma at the hip certainly may be present at the site of a hip fracture; however, the symptoms of No. 2 are more indicative of this event.
    4. Lengthening of the extremity is not seen in a hip fracture.

138. Application, evaluation, physiological integrity, (a).
    _____ 1. A TIA has a sudden onset.
    __X__ **2. This is consistent with a TIA.**
    __X__ **3. This statement is consistent with a TIA.**
    __X__ **4. This is consistent with a TIA.**
    __X__ **5. This statement is consistent with a TIA.**

139. Application, implementation, physiological integrity, (c).
    1. This aids in absorption of dye. Metrizamide dye is water soluble and does not need to be removed.
    2. This is not usually necessary.
    3. Common side effects of this dye include nausea, vomiting, and seizures, with the peak time of risk at 4 to 8 hours after the procedure.

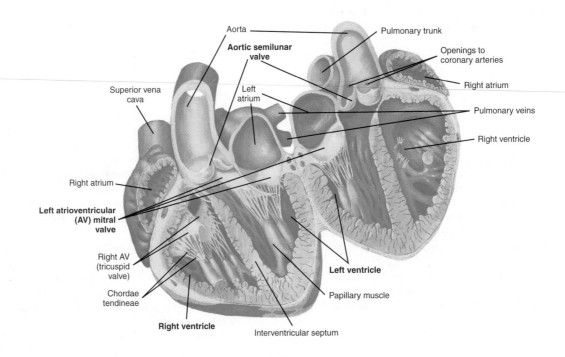

4. Phenothiazines, tricyclic antidepressants, central nervous system stimulants, and amphetamines should not be taken from 24 to 48 hours before or immediately after the procedure. These drugs lower seizure threshold.

140. Analysis, planning, health promotion and maintenance, (b).
2. Reading is a noncontact activity that would be the safest for the individual.
1. This activity can result in contact or would result in jarring of the abdomen, which may cause the aneurysm to rupture.
3. Jogging could jar the aneurysm, causing it to rupture.
4. Tennis is too physical an activity and could cause rupture in the patient.

141. Analysis, evaluation, health promotion and maintenance, (c).
__X__ **1. Pregnancy predisposes to the development of varicose veins because it causes pooling of blood in the extremities, which leads to incompetent valve development.**
__X__ **2. Obesity predisposes to the development of varicose veins because it causes pooling of blood in the extremities, which leads to incompetent valve development.**
_____ 3. This is a risk factor for deep-vein thromboses.
__X__ **4. This predisposes to the development of varicose veins.**
_____ 5. High blood pressure is not a causative factor of varicose veins; however, if uncontrolled, it can be a risk factor for several conditions such as stroke and kidney disease.

142. Application, planning, physiological integrity, (c).
2. Hydronephrosis can occur rapidly if obstruction occurs.
1. Stents are not irrigated.
3. This may be ordered but is not directly related to this situation.
4. The stents are not near the rectum.

143. Comprehension, planning, physiological integrity, (c).
__X__ **1. Oral antidiabetic medication may be used first, but insulin is used if oral medications cannot control the diabetes.**
__X__ **2. Oral antidiabetics may be part of the treatment plan for an individual with type 2 diabetes mellitus.**
__X__ **3. Diet is part of the treatment plan for an individual with type 2 diabetes mellitus.**
__X__ **4. Exercise is usually part of the treatment plan for an individual with type 2 diabetes mellitus.**
__X__ **5. Glucometer monitoring is part of the treatment plan for an individual with type 2 diabetes mellitus.**

144. Application, assessment, physiological integrity, (b).
__X__ **1. Daytime sleepiness is associated with obstructive sleep apnea.**
_____ 2. Sleep apnea does not normally cause upper respiratory infections.
__X__ **3. Personality changes are associated with obstructive sleep apnea.**
__X__ **4. Excessive snoring is associated with obstructive sleep apnea.**
_____ 5. Hyperglycemia is common in diabetes mellitus.
_____ 6. Tremors are not characteristic of sleep apnea.

145. Application, assessment, health promotion and maintenance, (b).
4. Disorder tends to progress, and involvement of other systems is common with advancement of the disorder.
1. This is characteristic of osteoarthritis.
2. The disease tends to be chronic in nature.
3. This does not describe rheumatoid arthritis.

146. Comprehension, planning, physiological integrity, (b).
3. These drugs reduce the inflammatory process.
1. These are not normally used as a first-line drug in treating rheumatoid arthritis.
2. These are not used as first-line drugs in treating rheumatoid arthritis.
4. These are not the drugs of choice for treating rheumatoid arthritis.

147. Analysis, assessment, physiological integrity, (a).
4. Malodorous discharge would signal a possible infectious process. It should be reported and investigated immediately.
1. This is a common occurrence after this surgery.
2. Again, it is to be expected that the patient will have some bleeding.
3. This is a normal, expected finding.

148. Application, implementation, physiological integrity, (a).
3. Taking the blood pressure in the left arm may cause compression or occlude the fistula or both. Any compression, tight clothing, or carrying of objects with arm bent should be avoided.
1. This is unnecessary; patients are discharged with this in place.
2. This is inappropriate and is not proper procedure.
4. Fluids may be restricted. Some patients may have fluid retention, although hourly monitoring usually is not appropriate.

149. Application, assessment, physiological integrity, (b).
2. These symptoms indicate pulmonary edema, a complication of myocardial infarction caused by heart failure.
1. These symptoms do not support a diagnosis of emphysema.
3. These symptoms do not support a diagnosis of pulmonary embolism.
4. COPD does not cause these symptoms.

150. Application, planning, physiological integrity, (c).
__X__ **1. This may be ordered and should be followed by the patient who has gout. Allopurinol is a medication used to control symptoms.**
_____ 2. Organ foods are high in purine, which contributes to uric acid formation.
_____ 3. An acid ash diet also contributes to uric acid formation.
__X__ **4. Patients who have gout may also be prone to diabetes.**
__X__ **5. An alkaline ash diet helps decrease uric acid tophi formation.**

151. Application, implementation, physiological integrity, (c).
3. By using the palms of the hands, the nurse is less likely to place indentations in the cast, which can compromise circulatory status when the plaster dries.
1. The patient will not be able to hold the extremity for a prolonged period.

2. The pillowcase will stick to the cast, causing excess pressure that will mold the cast.

4. Not only is this uncomfortable for the patient, but it also restricts adequate support of the extremity.

152. Analysis, evaluation, physiological integrity, (b).
     1. **Osteomyelitis most often requires extensive long-term antibiotic therapy.**
     2. This activity can have introduced pathogenic bacteria near the bone.
     3. In the acute phase mobility should be minimized to decrease the spread of the infection.
     4. Pain on movement is common in patients with osteomyelitis.

153. Analysis, evaluation, physiological integrity, (c).
     3. **Crossing the legs may result in displacement of the new femoral head.**
     1. No restriction on plantar flexion exists; this should be done to increase circulation to the legs.
     2. Low chairs would cause a greater than 90-degree hip flexion; elevated toilet seat and chairs are needed.
     4. Physical therapy, with limited weight bearing and ambulation, begins soon after surgery.

154. Analysis, assessment, physiological integrity, (b).
     3. **The presence of an elevated ESR and rheumatoid factor would indicate rheumatoid arthritis.**
     1. Although the WBCs are slightly elevated, the patient should not have an elevated Hct count.
     2. Uric acid is elevated in patients with gout.
     4. Although the rheumatoid factor is present, LE cells are present in patients with systemic LE.

155. Application, evaluation, physiological integrity, (b).
     4. **This is the correct rationale behind positioning.**
     1. The prone position does not alleviate phantom limb pain.
     2. Although important, this is not the primary reason for the positioning.
     3. Most patients do not feel that the prone position is the most comfortable. This is not the reason for the positioning.

156. Application, implementation, physiological integrity, (c).
     1. **Because of the patient's surgery, hydrochloric acid secretion and intrinsic factor are lacking; the patient is not able to absorb vitamin B_{12}, and this causes pernicious anemia.**
     2. A lack of folic acid does not cause pernicious anemia.
     3. Although technically correct, this question does not adequately explain the rationale to the patient.
     4. This is untrue; a lack of iron does not cause pernicious anemia.

157. Application, implementation, physiological integrity, (c).
     2. **This is the correct statement by the nurse.**
     1. This is incorrect information.
     3. The nurse is providing incorrect information to the patient.
     4. The patient is not likely to understand the term *dyscrasia,* and it is incorrect.

158. Analysis, implementation, physiological integrity, (c).
     3. **Exercise increases the oxygen demands of the body, which the failing heart is not able to accommodate.**
     1. Bronchi dilate with exercise.
     2. This may be true; exercise must be started gradually, but this statement does not answer the patient's questions.

4. The blood vessels of the heart and lungs dilate, increasing blood flow, which does not cause shortness of breath.

159. Application, assessment, physiological integrity, (c).
     4. **With right-sided heart failure, blood backs up in the systemic circulation, causing swelling of the lower extremities.**
     1. Nausea is not normally associated with heart failure.
     2. An extra heart sound may be heard (S3), but it is not the sound of a murmur.
     3. These are symptoms of left-sided heart failure.

160. Application, assessment, physiological integrity, (c).
     3. **Rheumatic fever and subsequent heart disease are the prominent causes of valvular insufficiency.**
     1. An appendectomy should not have any bearing on the patient's present diagnosis.
     2. Although significant for heart disease in general, the history of rheumatic fever is more significant.
     4. Although significant because of the possible introduction of bacteria into the heart, the history of rheumatic fever is more significant.

161. Application, implementation, physiological integrity, (c).
     4. **The nurse should first check to see that the patient's gag reflex has returned.**
     1. The patient will most likely return to his or her pre-test diet, but a gag reflex must be intact first.
     2. No time restrictions exist on this test; a gag reflex must be intact.
     3. This would be done after checking for an intact gag reflex.

162. Analysis, evaluation, health promotion and maintenance, (b).
     2. **Sunlight is one of the triggers for SLE. Going to the beach may have exposed the patient to too much sunlight.**
     1. Iodine in the seafood would not precipitate the attack.
     3. Constipation should not trigger an exacerbation.
     4. This should suppress an exacerbation, not cause one.

163. Application, assessment, physiological integrity, (b).
     2. **This high-fat meal may precipitate a gallbladder attack.**
     1. Physical activity does not normally cause or precipitate gallbladder pain.
     3. Taking acetaminophen does not normally precipitate pain in this area.
     4. Although alcohol may cause gastritis, it does not normally cause pain in the gallbladder region.

164. Application, planning, physiological integrity, (b).
     3. **Pancreatic enzymes are taken with meals.**
     1. The enzymes are not able to aid digestion if taken between meals.
     2. The enzymes need to be taken when any carbohydrates, proteins, or fats are eaten.
     4. This would not allow proper digestion to take place.

165. Analysis, evaluation, physiological integrity, (b).
     3. **Assess the patency of the tube by checking with an air bolus.**
     1. This may be contraindicated and is premature; assess patency first.
     2. Assess patency of tube before notifying the physician.
     4. This requires a physician's order; ascertain whether the tube is patent first.

166. Application, planning, physiological integrity, (b).
    3. The definition of a closed reduction is manually pulling on bones to realign the extremity. In some instances this is done in the emergency department, with pain medication given before the procedure.
    1. This would be an open reduction, internal fixation.
    2. This procedure does not involve general anesthesia.
    4. This would require a surgical procedure.

167. Analysis, assessment, physiological integrity, (b).
    4. Individuals with diabetes insipidus have an increased intake of fluids coupled with dilute urine.
    1. A bounding pulse and low urine output are signs of a hypervolemic state.
    2. Individuals who are hypovolemic have low blood pressure; tachycardia is a significant finding for dehydration.
    3. Individuals with diabetes insipidus have an increased urine output and a low urine specific gravity.

168. Analysis, planning, physiological integrity, (b).
    1. Wearing a medical alert tag ensures that others who are outside the hospital setting will respond appropriately.
    2. Although this is advisable, without the medical alert tag no one would know what to do with the glucose.
    3. This practice is not advisable and will not assist personnel unless a medical alert tag is present.
    4. Although this is a good idea, it does not ensure proper care in all locations.

169. Comprehension, planning, psychosocial integrity, (b).
    2. Patients with hyperpituitarism have structural alterations to their body, which can cause problems with self-esteem and body image.
    1. The problems that stem from excess pituitary hormone do not normally cause an alteration in comfort.
    3. Alteration in fluid and electrolytes is more common with Addison disease.
    4. This diagnosis is more common in hyperthyroidism.

170. Comprehension, assessment, physiological integrity, (b).
    2. Ketones cause metabolic acidosis in DKA.
    1. Both conditions are treated with insulin administration.
    3. HHNC is found primarily in patients who are non–insulin dependent.
    4. Serum ketones and glucose are elevated in DKA.

171. Analysis, implementation, physiological integrity, (b).
    3. The child should be given orange juice with sugar, which will increase his blood sugar level quickly.
    1. This will not increase the child's blood glucose because it contains no sugar.
    2. It will take too long for the child to go to the hospital, and this condition is treatable at home. Patient teaching in the prevention of hypoglycemic episodes should follow this occurrence.
    4. Cheese and crackers should be given after the orange juice; however, they will not elevate the glucose level quickly enough in this instance.

172. Comprehension, planning, physiological integrity, (b).
    2. Patients who have undergone conization normally have vaginal packing that needs to be maintained. The nurse should also anticipate monitoring for bleeding.

    1. The patient should not use tampons until instructed to do so by her physician.
    3. This may disrupt the site and can encourage bleeding.
    4. Patients should not douche until instructed to do so by their physician.

173. Analysis, assessment, health promotion and maintenance, (b).
    3. Mammograms are recommended annually for individuals older than 40 years of age.
    1. Gynecological examinations should be done on an annual basis.
    2. Hepatitis B vaccine is indicated for this individual because she works in a high-risk occupation.
    4. Tuberculosis tests should be done on an annual basis.

174. Analysis, implementation, health promotion and maintenance, (b).
    4. Breasts should be palpated in a variety of positions to ensure that all areas are assessed.
    1. BSEs should be conducted 7 days after onset of menstruation.
    2. This can be done, but breasts also need to be palpated while lying and standing.
    3. The pads of the fingers should be used to feel for lumps.

175. Comprehension, assessment, physiological integrity, (b).
    3. Patients with rectovaginal fistulas have leakage of fecal matter and flatus from the vagina. This condition causes extreme anxiety in the patient.
    1. This occurs in a ureterovaginal, vesicovaginal, or urethrovaginal fistula.
    2. This is common with hemorrhoids.
    4. These are common findings in a patient who has *Candida albicans* infection.

176. Application, implementation, health promotion and maintenance, (b).
    2. Women rarely have any early symptoms of gonorrhea. The patient should be tested because her partner is infected.
    1. This is not true; gonorrhea does not always cause symptoms in women.
    3. The patient should be tested immediately.
    4. The patient should be tested before being given antibiotics; she may not be infected.

177. Application, implementation, physiological integrity, (c).
    1. Because of the nature of the surgery and the proximity to the urethra, an indwelling catheter is placed during the surgery and will remain for a few days.
    2. Because of the complications of immobility, patients are ambulated early after surgery, even surgeries involving internal organs.
    3. The patient will most likely resume a normal diet after the bowel sounds have returned.
    4. Unless the patient has a preexisting condition, physical therapy would not necessarily be a part of her postsurgical care.

178. Analysis, implementation, physiological integrity, (b).
    1. Pizza is high in sodium and would aggravate PMS symptoms.
    2. Mineral water should not aggravate the condition. Beverages with caffeine would worsen the symptoms.
    3. Pasta and sauce should not aggravate the condition unless the sauce contains excessive amounts of salt.

4. Raw fruits and vegetables are a healthy snack and should not aggravate PMS.

179. Comprehension, assessment, physiological integrity, (b).
    1. *Patients with psoriasis experience reddened patches with silvery scales that sometimes slough off; they are very self-conscious about this problem.*
    2. Large pus-filled macules normally are not found in patients with psoriasis.
    3. This may be a sign of impetigo or another infectious disease.
    4. These normally are not present in psoriasis.

180. Comprehension, assessment, physiological integrity, (c).
    2. *IgE is the antibody most often associated. Many persons with asthma have an allergic component to their disease.*
    1. INR is a calculated measure as part of a coagulation profile (blood clotting).
    3. The HCV test is performed to detect the hepatitis C virus and to determine the antibody level.
    4. CEA is a measure that may be increased with various cancers such as cancer of the colon, liver, and pancreas. CEA levels may also be increased in persons who are long-term cigarette smokers and those who have inflammatory bowel disorders.

181. Application, planning, physiological integrity, (c).
    3. *This is proper technique. Corticosteroid inhalers should be used last because they require gargling after use to prevent oral candidiasis.*
    1. This may help; it depends on the side effects he is experiencing. Sitting may calm the patient, reduce a sense of panic, and maximize chest expansion.
    2. He should be using as prescribed. A few to 5 minutes are generally recommended between medications.
    4. If he is concerned, he needs to call the clinic and make an appointment. He should not stop taking these medications on his own.

182. Application, implementation, physiological integrity, (b).
    3. *Usually the patient with tuberculosis takes medications for as long as needed, generally 6 to 18 months or longer.*
    1. The patient understands infection control.
    2. This statement conveys understanding that once a PPD is positive it will always test positive.
    4. The patient understands the importance of rest in recovery from TB.

183. Application, implementation, safe and effective care environment, (c).
    1. *The reason for coming as perceived by the patient is defined as the chief complaint. The physician first looks to this part of the admission sheet as a basis for setting priorities of treatment and care.*
    2. This section refers to environmental, spiritual, and cultural aspects and family dynamics.
    3. The past medical history may be important. The reason for seeking treatment today warrants attention. Frequently the information in this section is not always accurate, depending on the reliability of the memory of the person supplying the information.
    4. The review of systems is a thorough body-system approach of assessment and data gathering. The physician or nurse practitioner fills out this section.

184. Analysis, implementation, physiological integrity, (b).
    2. *This bacillus is transmitted in the droplet nuclei formed when the person with active TB coughs, sings, talks, laughs, or sneezes.*
    1. This would indicate contact exposure; TB is transmitted by droplet.
    3. Once again, this signifies contact exposure.
    4. Inspiring the droplet in these situations is highly unlikely. Prolonged contact is necessary.

185. Application, implementation, physiological integrity, (b).
    2. *These actions ensure that the patient has a patent airway.*
    1. Fluids would thin secretions, enhancing airway clearance, but this is not the best choice.
    3. This does not directly relate to his nursing diagnosis.
    4. Although this is important, it does not directly relate to the nursing diagnosis.

186. Application, assessment, physiological integrity, (b).
    __X__ 1. *This symptom is caused by the stricture of the mitral valve.*
    _____ 2. Heart failure may be a complication of this malady; however, it is not a symptom of it.
    __X__ 3. *This symptom is caused by the stricture of the mitral valve.*
    __X__ 4. *This symptom is caused by the stricture of the mitral valve.*
    __X__ 5. *This symptom is caused by the stricture of the mitral valve.*

187. Application, evaluation, physiological integrity, (b).
    2. *Bacterial endocarditis is generally associated with an upper respiratory infection caused by Streptococcus bacteria.*
    1, 3, 4. These are not generally associated with bacterial endocarditis, although a heart catheterization may predispose the patient to other infections.

188. Application, implementation, physiological integrity, (a).
    1. *This is unsafe and can cause damage to the eardrum. This would also cause discomfort. It is best if the otoscope is held in a superior position.*
    2. This helps to visualize the eardrum.
    3. This steadies the examiner as he or she views the eardrum.
    4. This is correct technique for this type of examination.

189. Application, planning, physiological integrity, (b).
    4. *Because the patient cannot absorb vitamin B_{12}, he or she must be injected with it.*
    1. Vitamin B_{12} usually cannot be given by mouth because it is broken down by gastric juice.
    2. This is not associated with pernicious anemia.
    3. This is not associated with pernicious anemia.

190. Application, assessment, health promotion and maintenance, (b).
    1. *In men with chlamydia, urethritis, conjunctivitis, arthritis, and mucocutaneous lesions (Reiter syndrome) are the common symptoms.*
    2. This is present in syphilis.
    3. This is usually not present in sexually transmitted diseases.
    4. This is a manifestation of genital warts.

191. Application, assessment, physiological integrity, (b).
    __X__ 1. *The patient should be on NPO status before the examination.*

__X__ **2. The patient is given enemas and may also be given laxatives to cleanse the bowel before the examination.**

__X__ **3. After the examination, laxatives are given to remove any residual barium that would be left behind.**

_____ 4. Eating or not eating meat does not affect examination results. Preparation begins, at most, the day or evening before the examination, not 4 days in advance.

192. Application, planning, physiological integrity, (b).
 1. The lidocaine numbs the mouth, making it easier for the patient to chew and swallow.
 2, 3, 4. Topical lidocaine does not act as an antibiotic or a barrier, nor does it aid in absorption of the food because that takes place in the small intestine.

193. Comprehension, assessment, health promotion and maintenance, (b).
 3. Patients with cirrhosis generally have portal hypertension, which predisposes the patient to esophageal varices.
 1. Bronchitis is not a predisposing factor to bleeding esophageal varices.
 2. Esophageal cancer may cause irritation and some bleeding, but not of this type.
 4. Gastritis may cause peptic ulcer disease, which could result in bleeding, but not esophageal bleeding.

194. Application, implementation, physiological integrity, (a).
 2. LOC is defined by both the character of consciousness and the arousal level. Confusion is defined by having the described behaviors in addition to agitation and irritability. Disorientation to time occurs first, followed by place and person.
 1. "Difficult" is a value judgment.
 3. Lethargy is reflective of a patient who is unable to be aroused spontaneously but requires some external stimuli such as touch or voice. Confusion may also be present.
 4. Stupor indicates a patient who is in a deep sleep or unresponsive. Arousal occurs only with vigorous and continuous stimulation.

195. Analysis, assessment, physiological integrity, (b).
 2. Although any stimulation can cause this phenomenon to occur, the most common are stimulations such as a full bladder, full bowel, or wrinkled sheets.
 1. Visitors may accidentally cause a reaction, but their presence does not normally do this.
 3. This should not stimulate autonomic dysreflexia.
 4. Any skin stimulation could cause this reaction, but assessing an apical pulse does not normally cause it.

196. Comprehension, planning, physiological integrity, (b).
 3. Hypovolemic shock may occur as a result of intravascular volume depletion as fluid moves into the intracellular spaces. Observing and planning for shock are critical. This is a priority. The greatest initial threat to a patient with a major burn is hypovolemic shock.
 1. Monitoring urine output would better indicate kidney status.
 2. Skin care and comfort are important.
 4. A too-rapid IV line would increase intravascular volume.

197. Application, planning, physiological integrity, (b).
 4. If the patient eats a large meal before the class, she is more likely to have symptoms because of the increased abdominal pressure she experiences while exercising.
 1. This will increase the problem for the patient.
 2. This would be rather difficult to do in an aerobics class! It is unrealistic.
 3. This is likely to contribute to increased heartburn symptoms.

198. Application, assessment, physiological integrity, (b).
 1. The nurse needs to assess for hepatitis, because risk increases with the age of the patient. Hepatic enzymes are measured before and during therapy.
 2. This is common when taking antineoplastic medications.
 3. This is common when taking diuretics.
 4. This is common when taking diuretics.

199. Application, planning, physiological integrity, (b).
 4. A short-term goal for pain should have a very short time frame, given the severity of the pain. The only one of these distracters that is associated with pain and is of short duration is No. 4.
 1. This is a more a long-term pain goal associated with impaired mobility.
 2. This is a long-term pain goal.
 3. This is not a realistic goal for any nursing diagnosis because most patients have increased pain during and after physical therapy.

200. Application, implementation, physiological integrity, (b)
 Answer: 875 mL
 The IV and PO intake equals 875 mL.

201. Application, planning, physiological integrity, (c).
 _____ 1. Avoiding sex is unnecessary. Voiding before and after sex is recommended.
 __X__ **2. Using scented feminine hygiene products may contribute to urinary tract infections.**
 __X__ **3. Showers do not usually contribute to urinary tract infections; tub baths do contribute to urinary tract infections.**
 _____ 4. Orange juice has too much sugar to recommend this amount per day, and it does not decrease the incidence of urinary tract infections.
 __X__ **5. The perineum should be wiped from front to back.**

202. Comprehension, evaluation, psychosocial integrity, (c).
 2. This statement is both knowledgeable and truthful.
 1. This statement signifies that no further teaching is needed.
 3. _Streptococcus_ has not been implicated in peptic ulcer disease; _Helicobacter pylori_ has been.
 4. This may be very helpful to the individual, but further teaching is required.

203. Application, implementation, physiological integrity, (a).
 1. Fluid intake is especially important, at least eight 8-oz glasses per day. Encouraging fluid decreases the potential of the adverse effect of crystal formation.
 2. This decreases pain but is not the main reason.
 3. This is important and best achieved by giving the drug as scheduled.
 4. Although important, decreasing the formation of crystals is the most important reason.

204. Analysis, assessment, physiological integrity, (b).

    4. The higher the number rating on this scale, which ranges from 0 to 15, the better will be the prognosis and the likelihood of optimal cerebral functioning.

    1. A score of 1 to 3 may indicate coma.
    2. This score would be lower than 13.
    3. Moderate head trauma would result in a score somewhere below 13.

205. Comprehension, planning, physiological integrity, (b).

    4. A disruption of the transmembrane potential at the cellular level causes sodium-potassium pump impairment, resulting in intracellular swelling.

    1. Decreased immunoglobulins would affect the immune status and not third-tissue spacing.
    2. The cardiac output would be decreased.
    3. The hypermetabolic state increases the oxygen consumption.

206. Analysis, assessment, physiological integrity, (c).

    4. Risk for aspiration is the most pressing concern for this patient, given the nasogastric tube feedings.

    1, 2. These could be of concern if the patient had a problem with a patent airway or if pneumonia or congestive heart failure were present.
    3. The tube feedings may cause diarrhea, but it is not the most pressing concern at this time.

207. Application, implementation, physiological integrity, (b).

    1. The reason stated is correct. In addition, remind him to shake the inhalers before using and to hold his breath for 10 seconds after inhaling the medications.

    2, 3, 4. These statements give incorrect rationales and information. Albuterol is a beta-adrenergic agonist that stimulates beta-adrenergic receptors, producing bronchodilation. Ipratropium is an anticholinergic that acts by blocking acetylcholine, resulting in bronchodilation.

208. Comprehension, implementation, physiological integrity, (a).

    2. This describes the person who is at greatest risk.

    1. TB is spread by droplet.
    3. It is highly unlikely that the bacillus lives long enough on a computer at work for it to be inhaled.
    4. The spread is by the airborne route. It is highly unlikely that the bacillus lives long outside the host or that a casual contact is a high-risk situation.

209. Application, implementation, physiological integrity, (b).

    4. Packing in the posterior pharynx may obstruct the patient's airway. Use a flashlight when assessing the back of the throat.

    1. Injury may occur if the packing dislodges.
    2. It is more likely that the patient will have an ineffective breathing pattern than a risk for infection.
    3. The patient is more likely to obstruct his airway than to aspirate.

210. Comprehension, implementation, physiological integrity, (b).

    1. Individuals metabolize xanthines at different rates. Dosage is determined by monitoring response, tolerance, pulmonary function, and serum theophylline levels. Serum theophylline concentrations should range from 10 to 20 mcg/mL; toxicity has been reported with levels above 20 mcg/mL.

    2, 3, 4. These levels may be considered toxic. The patient needs to be assessed for theophylline toxicity.

211. Analysis, assessment, physiological integrity, (c).

    4. Carbon dioxide (CO_2) is trapped in the alveoli; the basic problem in emphysema. Respiratory acidosis occurs when the lungs cannot exhale CO_2 adequately. As a result, the partial pressure of carbon dioxide in the arterial blood and carbonic acid increase, and pH decreases.

    1, 3. These are potential effects of emphysema, not the basic cause of acidosis.
    2. This is an abnormal condition characterized by a significant loss of acid in the body (as a result of excessive vomiting or insufficient replacement of electrolytes) or by increased levels of base bicarbonate (as a result of ingestion of excessive amounts of antacids or excessive volumes of IV fluids containing high concentrations of bicarbonate).

212. Comprehension, implementation, safe and effective care environment, (b).

    3. Handwashing for at least 15 to 20 seconds is still considered the best means of preventing disease transmission.

    1, 2. These should be used only when medically indicated.
    4. Handwashing is part of Standard Precautions. Potential for exposure to blood and body fluids determines the need for protective equipment.

213. Application, assessment, physiological integrity, (b).

    _____ 1. This is a symptom of hemorrhage.

    __X__ *2. Excessive sweating along with headache, flushing, palpitation, nervousness, nausea or vomiting, and syncope are also present.*

    _____ 3. Bradycardia is not common in this tumor formation.

    __X__ *4. High blood pressure caused by excessive catecholamine secretion results from this disorder.*

214. Comprehension, planning, physiological integrity, (b).

    2. Serial measurements of peak flow rate provide objective data regarding the therapeutics of drug response.

    1. The results of the peak flow rate may indicate appropriate response.
    3. Blood test monitoring should be done while the person is on bronchodilator therapy.
    4. This may be an indirect result of the peak flow rate level.

215. Application, assessment, physiological integrity, (b).

    1. These indicate decreased tissue oxygenation.

    2. These are normal laboratory findings.
    3. These are normal assessment findings.
    4. A normal potassium level and clear amber urine would not cause concern in the patient with pneumonia.

216. Application, planning, physiological integrity, (b).

    3. Ileal conduits may allow leakage of urine onto the skin, altering skin integrity.

    1, 2. These may be a result of the ileal conduit; however, alteration in skin integrity is the primary concern.
    4. No alteration in mobility should occur from the conduit.

217. Application, planning, physiological integrity, (b).

    3. Voiding this often, in addition to having adequate fluid intake, has been shown to reduce the possibility of urinary stasis and reinfection.

1. This is true for patients who need bladder training such as those with incontinence.
2. Reflex incontinence is seen in neurogenic disorders; it is the loss of urine caused by detrusor hyperreflexia or involuntary urethral relaxation or both in the absence of the desire to void.
4. This is dribbling of urine by reason of the inability of the bladder to empty itself. The cause of this problem should be determined. This problem may lead to urinary tract infections.

218. Application, implementation, physiological integrity, (c).
    1. Orange juice is a simple source of carbohydrate, which would increase his glucose level quickly. Remember that the normal glucose level needs to be 60 to 99 mg/dL.
    2. This is unsafe. This action would increase his potential for insulin shock.
    3. The immediate notification of the physician is unnecessary; however, the physician should be made aware of action taken and the patient's response.
    4. This action may be appropriate, but it is not the first action.

219. Application, implementation, physiological integrity, (b).
    3. This is the most life-threatening.
    1. This is a normal urine output.
    2. Hypothermia may result because of fluid evaporation from open wounds.
    4. Patient comfort is important. Pain medication may be necessary before dressing changes.

220. Application, implementation, physiological integrity, (b).
    4. ICP is the pressure produced by the brain tissue, cerebrospinal fluid, and blood volume within the skull. Allowing the patient to rest between nursing activities helps to keep the ICP between 5 and 15 mm Hg. Too many activities may increase metabolic demands that would alter the balance of the three components that determine ICP and the inherent compensatory capability of the brain.
    1, 2. Coughing, suctioning, lying flat, bearing down, or the Valsalva maneuver may cause ICP to rise.
    3. Neck and hip flexion should be avoided. Maintaining the patient's neck, hips, and knees in alignment promotes venous flow. A high-Fowler position causes flexion. A semi-Fowler position improves cerebral perfusion and allows for gravity to drain fluid from the brain.

221. Analysis, evaluation, physiological integrity, (c).
    4. This is the only answer that includes a possible link to skin cancer. The patient with thinning hair and a receding hairline has more potential for a sunburned scalp, which increases the risk for this cancer.
    1, 2, 3. None of these distracters has been shown to increase the risk of skin cancer.

222. Analysis, planning, physiological integrity, (b).
    3. Because the hematuria may be a sign of bladder cancer, the patient should be directed to visit his physician as soon as possible.
    1. This is good advice if the patient is having symptoms of a urinary tract infection.
    2. This would not affect the color of the patient's urine.

4. This would be good advice if it is not given in an urgent manner. This matter is urgent, but the patient might be frightened with this advice.

223. Comprehension, assessment, psychosocial integrity, (b).
    4. Sexual contact information is extremely personal, and many patients are not willing to disclose this information.
    1. This is generally not the case.
    2. Knowing who the contacts are is required so that proper screening and treatment can begin.
    3. This is not true; patients who do not have symptoms can still transmit the disease.

224. Comprehension, evaluation, physiological integrity, (a).
    1. The action of a thrombolytic agent is to dissolve fresh thrombi that have formed.
    2. This is an action of heparin or warfarin (Coumadin).
    3. This drug does not thin the blood; platelet inhibitors keep platelets from adhering to the walls of the blood vessels.
    4. The action of a thrombolytic is to dissolve fresh thrombi. Clopidogrel (Plavix) inhibits platelets.

225. Comprehension, planning, physiological integrity, (c).
    1. This is the correct action of this medication.
    2. Although this drug does lower the blood pressure, this does not alleviate angina.
    3. Although this medication may dilate cerebral arteries, this is only a side effect.
    4. This is the action of antiarrhythmics.

226. Application, implementation, physiological integrity, (c).
    3. This medication would contribute to tarry stool color.
    1. Vitamin K does not contribute to the formation of tarry stools.
    2. Bleeding from hemorrhoids is generally bright red in color, not tarry.
    4. This may be the nurse's next advice; however, the nurse wants to determine if a reason exists for the stool color before making an appointment.

227. Analysis, evaluation, physiological integrity, (c).
    2. Anemia is a common problem in patients who take antineoplastic agents. Suppression of red blood cell formation of bone marrow is the primary reason.
    1. Antineoplastics can cause decreased platelet counts.
    3. Leukemia causes an increase in immature WBCs.
    4. Metastasis is always a concern in a patient with cancer but is not normally caused by antineoplastics.

228. Analysis, evaluation, physiological integrity, (b).
    4. Patients taking vasodilators often experience a drop in blood pressure when quickly rising from a seated position.
    1. The dizziness experienced by the patient is secondary to the decrease in blood pressure.
    2, 3. There is no indication that the patient is anemic or has a slow pulse rate.

229. Application, implementation, physiological integrity, (c).
    Answer: 0.4 mL
    Dosage/On hand=Quantity
    2 mg/5 mg × 1=0.4 mL

230. Analysis, assessment, physiological integrity, (b).
    1. Cardiogenic shock may develop in patients who have had a myocardial infarction in which a large

portion of the left ventricle has been affected by the infarction.

2. Anaphylaxis stems from an antibody-antigen reaction.

3. Hypertension may contribute to having a myocardial infarction but is not usually caused by one.

4. Vascular injury is not associated with having had a myocardial infarction.

231. Comprehension, implementation, physiological integrity, (c).

4. This is the only correct information of which the nurse can be aware. Anesthesia slows peristalsis, and eating after surgery would likely result in emesis.

1. This may be true; however, it is not the correct response for everyone. Although a patient may be hungry after surgery, food is prohibited until return of peristalsis.

2. This is very true, but the most valid response for not giving food is response No. 4.

3. The risk of aspiration is high when a person has emesis but is not the primary reason why food is prohibited after surgery.

232. Application, assessment, health promotion and maintenance, (c).

2. Narcotics such as meperidine hydrochloride and morphine sulfate, in general, suppress the central nervous system, slowing respirations, which predisposes the patient to ineffective breathing patterns.

1. Although this is a valid response, based on Maslow's hierarchy of needs it is less important than respiration.

3. Acute pain is the diagnosis for which the narcotic is given. If the analgesic is effective, the pain diagnosis should cease to be a problem for the time being.

4. No data in the situation support this diagnosis.

233. Application, implementation, physiological integrity, (b).
Answer: 0.5 mL
Dose/On hand=Quantity
50 mg/100 mg/mL × 1=0.5 mL

234. Analysis, implementation, safe and effective care environment, (c).

__X__ *1. Assessments made on the bowel sounds would confirm peristalsis. This ensures the safety of the procedure.*

__X__ *2. Lung sounds would alert the nurse to any adventitious sounds (possible aspiration). This ensures the safety of the procedure.*

_____ 3. Measuring blood pressure is not a necessary assessment before a nasogastric tube feeding.

_____ 4. Measuring heart rate is not a necessary assessment before a nasogastric tube feeding.

__X__ *5. Ensuring the patency of the tube is imperative before each feeding because it confirms proper placement of the tube.*

235. Analysis, assessment, physiological integrity, (b).

2. Airway is always the primary assessment to be made after surgery.

1, 3, 4. These assessments should be made; however, airway remains the most important.

236. Application, implementation, health promotion and maintenance, (b).

3. This is the only true teaching response that is nonjudgmental and meets the needs of the adolescent.

1. This is demeaning and not helpful to the teen.

2. This is true but needs to be expanded with further information.

4. This is argumentative and is not helpful to the learning needs of the adolescent.

237. Knowledge, assessment, physiological integrity, (b).

2. The four pulmonary veins return blood from the lungs to the left atrium of the heart.

1. The pulmonary artery carries deoxygenated blood to the lung.

3. The superior vena cava transports deoxygenated blood from above the diaphragm into the right atrium of the heart.

4. The inferior vena cava transports deoxygenated blood from below the diaphragm into the right atrium of the heart.

238. Comprehension, planning, physiological integrity, (b).

2. Thromboangiitis obliterans is Buerger disease. These exercises are designed to assist the individual in promoting arterial circulation to his extremities.

1. The exercises are designed to increase circulation to the extremities.

3. These exercises would be contraindicated in someone with thrombophlebitis.

4. Paget disease is a condition of the bone, and these exercises would not help this disorder.

239. Application, planning, physiological integrity, (c).

__X__ *1. The patient can assess any fluid retention by weighing himself daily.*

_____ 2. The patient should be instructed to take his pulse before taking his digoxin.

_____ 3. Increasing carbohydrates does not affect the patient's heart failure and may contribute to weight gain.

__X__ *4. The patient should also take his diuretic in the morning to decrease the chance that he will have nocturia.*

240. Analysis, planning, health promotion and maintenance, (c).

3. Chinese food usually contain monosodium glutamate (MSG), which should be avoided on a salt-restricted diet.

1. Vegetarian diets contain little meat and few dairy products, which are high in sodium.

2. Italian foods are not especially high in salt or MSG.

4. French cooking is not especially high in salt or MSG.

241. Comprehension, assessment, physiological integrity, (c).

4. This is the only true statement concerning ulcerative colitis.

1. The patient's major symptoms are likely to be cramps and diarrhea.

2. The colitis involves the large intestine.

3. This syndrome is not caused by an overuse of laxatives; it may be an autoimmune disorder.

242. Comprehension, assessment, physiological integrity, (b).

3. The pituitary gland secretes growth hormone, which is the hormone malfunction in these two disorders.

1. The thyroid gland secretes thyroxine and calcitonin.

2. The adrenal gland secretes catecholamines.

4. The pancreas secretes the hormones insulin and glucagon.

243. Application, implementation, physiological integrity, (b).
Answer: 0.6 mL
Dosage/On hand=Quantity
3 mg/10 mg × 2 mL=0.6 mL

244. Comprehension, implementation, physiological integrity, (c).
    1. *HgbA$_{1c}$ is a marker that measures how well individuals have controlled their blood sugar over a 3-month period. It is much more accurate than fasting blood glucose level.*
    2. Although this may be true, it is not an adequate explanation.
    3. This test cannot measure the amount of insulin a patient has been using.
    4. This really has nothing to do with the question; it is not necessarily indicated before this treatment, and whether the patient is being prepared for one is unknown.

245. Analysis, assessment, physiological integrity, (c).
    2. *Cirrhosis creates changes in oncotic pressure within the portal system; this creates ascites, an accumulation of fluid within the abdomen.*
    1. Peritonitis is an infection of the peritoneum and results in abdominal distention and slowed peristalsis.
    3. Hepatitis may cause this problem, but it is much more likely that it will occur with cirrhosis.
    4. Diverticulitis contributes to cramping, constipation, and pain but does not result in ascites.

246. Application, implementation, physiological integrity, (c).
    Answer: 33 gtt/min
    Calculation: Amount of infusion/Time to deliver = Milliliters per hour
    Milliliters per hour × gtt factor/60 min
    2000 mL/10 hr = 200 mL/hr
    200 mL/hr × 10 gtt/min/60 min = 33 gtt/min

247. Application, planning, physiological integrity, (b).
    2. *Fried foods would stimulate the gallbladder to contract to release its bile. Eating a large, fatty meal after a cholecystectomy may cause the patient to have painful diarrhea.*
    1. Raw vegetables should not create a problem for the patient.
    3. Vegetables are acidic; they do not cause excess bile to be released.
    4. Pasta is a carbohydrate but has little fat; therefore it should not create a problem.

248. Application, implementation, physiological integrity, (c).
    Answer: 9 hours
    8 oz = 240 mL
    240 mL × 3 cans = 720 mL
    720 mL/80 mL/hr = 9 hr to infuse

249. Analysis, planning, physiological integrity, (c).
    1. *Hemorrhage is the primary risk in the patient who has a prolapsed uterus.*
    2. Although this may be a concern, it is not the primary problem.
    3. Although this may be a problem, it is not the primary problem.
    4. This should not be a problem for this patient.

250. Analysis, planning, physiological integrity, (c).
    2. *The patient has the potential for multiple urinary tract infections because of the fistula.*
    1, 3, 4. These problems should not develop in this patient.

Objectives

After studying this chapter, the student should be able to:

1. Define ego defense mechanisms; name five examples.
2. Compare and contrast therapeutic communication techniques and ineffective responses, citing five examples of each.
3. Describe three types of anxiety disorders, including their characteristics.
4. Explain mood disorders and the role of the interventions appropriate to the specific form.
5. Describe thought disorders, citing three examples and their symptoms.

The licensed practical nurse/licensed vocational nurse (LPN/LVN) must understand basic mental health nursing principles to practice nursing safely. Basic mental health concepts are useful in understanding responses to disease and dysfunction, both physically and socially. Each person responds to disease and disorder according to his or her own basic personality, past experiences, intelligence, and coping skills. These concepts are explored and studied in mental health nursing.

HOLISM

A. Definition: This concept of health holds that illness results from a complex interaction among the mind, body, spirit, and the environment, a concept that views an individual as more than the sum of his or her parts.
B. Approaches to treatment: Multifaceted approaches are used to treat disturbances rather than simply relying on treatment aimed at specific symptoms. We are no longer content to treat the illness; we are learning to treat the whole person. Approaches include the following dimensions:
   1. Physical
   2. Emotional
   3. Intellectual
   4. Sociocultural
   5. Spiritual

MENTAL HEALTH CONTINUUM

A. Mental health and mental illness are seen as opposite poles on a continuum.
B. The precise point at which an individual is deemed mentally ill is determined by the specific behavior exhibited and the context in which the behavior is seen.
C. Some behaviors that are considered inappropriate in one setting may be considered normal in another setting.
D. Variations are based on culture, the time or era, personality, and other variables.
E. Behaviors of mentally ill people are often exaggerations of normal human behaviors.

MENTAL HEALTH

A. Definition: an individual's ability to cope with problems in life and draw satisfaction from living throughout various life stages
B. Individuals may experience times of greater or lesser satisfaction with life; during times of lesser satisfaction they may seek the assistance of a therapist or counselor.
C. No clear set of characteristics specific to mental health can be identified.
   1. All behavior is considered meaningful and may be interpreted as the individual's effort to adapt to or cope with the environment.
   2. At times some adaptations fail; others are continued long after the need for them has passed; still others may be directed to an undesired end.

MENTAL ILLNESS

A. Definition: a pattern of behavior that is disturbing to the individual or the community in which the individual resides; behaviors may interfere with daily activities, impair judgment, or alter reality. A mental illness is a disturbance of a person's ability to cope effectively, which results in maladaptive behaviors and impaired functioning.
   1. The person who is mentally ill may act in ways that seem unrelated to current reality. (Depressed individuals may not exhibit this type of behavior.)
   2. Relationships with family and friends are frequently disturbed.
   3. The person's ability to function effectively and contribute to his or her own welfare may be impaired.
   4. The person often experiences subjective discomfort.
   5. The person may exhibit symptoms such as delusions, hallucinations, paranoia, hopelessness, passive-aggressive behavior, or compulsions.
B. Historical perspective of mental illness
   1. Early history
      a. Mentally ill people were thought to be possessed by supernatural forces, evil spirits, or demons.
      b. Mentally ill people were removed from society, frequently mistreated in other ways, and often jailed.

c. These beliefs and practices have lasted many years; some are still practiced today.

2. Classical era (Greco-Roman)
   a. Early Greek physicians began to see nature as a healing force.
   b. This early scientific interest led to various classification systems.
   c. The idea of divine possession was rejected in favor of the humoral theory of disease.
   d. Humors were thought to be basic internal fluids capable of controlling behavior.
   e. The terms *melancholia* and *hysteria* are derived from these ancient beliefs.

3. The Middle Ages, Renaissance, and Protestant Reformation eras saw some reform; however, in general:
   a. Society returned to the idea of divine possession or spiritual explanations for mental illness.
   b. The mentally ill person was often mistreated by incarceration.

4. Individuals responsible for instituting reforms in the modern era
   a. Eighteenth century
      (1) Phillipe Pinel freed the mentally ill from chains.
      (2) Benjamin Rush, known as the Father of American Psychiatry
   b. Nineteenth century
      (1) Florence Nightingale, known as the founder of modern nursing
      (2) Dorothea Dix promoted legislation to establish mental hospitals.
      (3) Linda Richards was the first psychiatric nurse.
   c. Twentieth century
      (1) Clifford Beers wrote the book *The Mind That Found Itself,* which generated public concern for the mentally ill.
      (2) Adolf Meyer founded the mental hygiene movement.
      (3) Emil Kraepelin classified mental disorders.
      (4) Eugene Bleuler coined the term *schizophrenia* and classified it into types.
      (5) Sigmund Freud developed psychoanalytical theory.
      (6) Carl Jung developed the personality theory that included introversion and extroversion.
      (7) Karen Horney theorized that culture influences mental illness.

5. Modern developments
   a. Discovery of phenothiazines (the major tranquilizers such as chlorpromazine [Thorazine]) in the 1950s
   b. Community mental health: 1960s; still in use today. The aim is to provide care of mentally ill people in their own communities rather than in large institutions. Primary goals of the community mental health concept are to return patients to their home as quickly as possible and foster the development of culturally appropriate support systems in the community.
   c. Deinstitutionalization: In the late 1970s a large number of mentally ill people were released from long-term hospitals into communities where they often did not receive treatment either because they did not seek it or because adequate types of services were not available. Some people believe that this process led to an increase of street people and homelessness.
   d. Community mental health centers were established to provide comprehensive treatment within the community.
   e. Development of more effective psychotropic medications has helped to decrease treatment costs.

C. Common mental health terms: The following terms are not defined in other sections of this chapter
   1. Egocentric—self-centered
   2. Hysteria—the unconscious conversion of anxiety into physical symptoms; somatization
   3. Kinesics—body communication via movements, posture, expression, gesture
   4. Narcissistic—self-absorption to an extreme degree
   5. Paralinguistics—the voice quality; volume, tone, speed, flow, inflection, and other audible sounds other than words, for example, laugh, cry, moan
   6. Proxemics—manner in which individuals relate to space and distance with others; influenced by culture
   7. Self-esteem—an individual's assessment of self-worth and value

NURSING ROLE

A. The nursing process
   1. Assessment: The LPN/LVN gathers subjective and objective data through observation, interview, and examination. Data are obtained through:
      a. Health history.
      b. Mental status examination.
         (1) General description—appearance, speech, motor activity
         (2) Affect and mood
         (3) Intellect and sensorium—consciousness, memory
         (4) Thought content and processes—what is thought (e.g., delusions, phobias) and how one thinks (e.g., blocking, flight of ideas)
         (5) Insight—patient's understanding of the condition
      c. Psychological testing.
         (1) Intelligence testing—standardized tests administered by psychologists, designed to assess intellectual capacity
         (2) Personality testing—standardized tests administered by psychologists, designed to assess specific personality traits
      d. Self-assessment (e.g., stress scale, decision-making trees).
      e. Physical examination.
   2. Diagnosis: Nurses diagnose and treat human responses to illness. The nursing diagnosis is formulated by the registered professional nurse; the LPN/LVN contributes to this phase of the nursing process by collecting objective and subjective data. Potential nursing diagnoses identify the problem and etiological factors of the problem; actual nursing diagnoses identify the problem, origin, and signs and symptoms. The North American Nursing Diagnosis Association International (NANDA-I) listing is used. Examples of actual and potential nursing diagnoses used in mental health nursing include the following (these are examples, not a complete listing):

a. Anxiety (panic) related to family rejection; exhibited by chest discomfort, palpitations, dizziness, diaphoresis, and trembling

b. Impaired social interaction related to negative role modeling; exhibited by verbalized and observed discomfort in social situations

c. Risk for self-directed violence related to history of suicide attempts

d. Risk for trauma related to muscular incoordination.

It is critical for nurses to consider many areas when formulating nursing diagnoses for patients experiencing mental health issues and to identify the ones that will best meet all the needs of a particular patient. These areas include:

a. Promotion of both mental and physical health and well-being

b. Overall functional ability of the individual

c. Differences in the individual's thinking, understanding, and communication skills

d. Behaviors of the individual that, combined with mental health issues, increase the risk of danger to self or others

e. Effects of emotional stress on the individual in light of current circumstances

f. Management of unwarranted symptoms (side effects) from medications and ordered treatments

g. Barriers that could interfere with treatment and overall recovery of the individual

h. Changes in the individual's concept of self, including that of body image

i. Physical symptoms that could result from the individual's mental status

j. Psychological symptoms that may be due to changes in physical needs

k. Factors that influence the individual, the family, or the community (social, religious, cultural, environmental)

l. Factors that could affect the individual's recovery (financial security/job, family/community support, housing)

Consideration of these areas will be advantageous when moving into the planning phase of the nursing process.

3. Planning: Plan of care is based on the nursing diagnosis. Specific nursing interventions are devised to attain specifically stated goals. When possible, goals should be developed jointly with the cooperation of patient or family or both. They may be short-term or long-term goals; all goals should be prioritized, emphasizing reduction or elimination of the identified problem. They usually include the anticipated length of time for accomplishment and the standard for judging whether the goal has been met.

4. Implementation: Planned nursing actions that assist patient in achieving the identified goal (e.g., health teaching, assist with activities of daily living [ADLs], other prescribed treatments, medications). This phase is ongoing, and reactions to treatment are observed and documented so the care plan may be modified periodically as goals are met.

5. Evaluation: Outcome achievement and the factors that affected the goal being met, partially met, or not met are identified. This process is followed by the decision to continue, modify, or terminate the plan. After evaluation of goal achievement, the entire nursing process and care plan are reviewed, modified, or updated to reflect new nursing diagnoses.

B. Critical thinking: The application of critical thinking in the delivery of nursing care is essential. The concept incorporates the sum total of the nurse's knowledge, experience, assessments, and clinical judgment. The nurse questions assumptions and continuously seeks the highest level of nursing practice. It is probing and creative in assessment. Thoughtful, outcome-oriented, and prudent, critical thinking contributes greatly to optimum outcomes for the patient. Critical thinking has been defined by Wilkenson (2001) as "careful, goal-oriented, purposeful thinking that involves many mental skills, such as determining which data are relevant, evaluating the credibility of sources and making inferences."

C. Principles of mental health nursing: The nurse must:

1. Provide for and maintain a therapeutic environment, called *milieu therapy.*

2. Understand own inner needs, thoughts, and feelings and be aware of how these affect patients.

3. Be aware of own resources and limitations so as to function effectively in mental health nursing.

4. Respect patient as a person; take time to listen to what is said.

5. Be considerate of patient's dignity; show patience and understanding.

6. Establish a trusting relationship, which requires an accepting, nonjudgmental, and nonthreatening approach.

7. Be honest.

8. Reassure patients by being available, allaying fears, and being consistent.

9. Explain routines, rules, and regulations when appropriate.

10. Maintain a calm, hopeful attitude.

11. Encourage reality orientation, and avoid entering into patient's unrealistic thinking.

12. Emphasize strengths that patient displays by acknowledging healthy behavior and offering warm understanding. Do not encourage overdependency or intimacy.

13. Remember that all staff members are role models and are often viewed as authority figures by patients.

14. Help reduce anxiety by making as few demands as possible on patients.

15. Explain to patient what is happening in simple, understandable language.

16. Remain objective but do not display aloofness or distance; maintain awareness of patient's humanity and dignity.

17. Maintain a nurse-patient relationship that is always realistic and professional.

18. Remember that a reason exists for all behavior.

19. Note that behavior is changed through emotional experience rather than through rational means.

20. Patients must be allowed to exercise all of their basic human rights.

21. Use the least-restrictive method or methods of controlling behavior such as effective communication.

22. Respect the confidentiality of the patient.

D. Communications in mental health nursing
1. Communication: complex activity consisting of a series of events, each interdependent on the others, which results in a negotiated understanding between two or more people in a given situation
   a. Communication is not merely the exchange of information.
   b. Each message (input) generates an extremely complex reaction that eventually leads to a selective response (output), which in turn becomes a new input for the communicators.
2. Modes of communication
   a. The most apparent form is verbal (written or spoken language) communication; spoken communication is the tool frequently used in mental health nursing.
   b. Spoken communication is always accompanied by at least one of the following additional communication forms:
      (1) Paralanguage: voice quality, tones, grunts, and other nonword vocalizations
      (2) Kinesis: facial expression, gestures, and eye and body movements
      (3) Proxemics: the spatial relationship between people
      (4) Touch and messages to other sensory organs: aromas and cultural artifacts (jewelry, clothing, hairstyle)

c. Effective communication includes:
   (1) Efficiency: messages are simple, clear, and timed correctly.
   (2) Appropriateness: messages are relevant to the situation.
   (3) Flexibility: communication is open to alteration based on perceived response.
   (4) Receptivity: feedback is allowed (checking and correcting by either or both parties).
3. Therapeutic communication (Box 6-1)
4. Blocks to communication (Table 6-1)
E. Nurse-patient relationship
1. One-on-one relationship between a nurse and a patient
2. Patient centered
3. Goal directed
4. Not for nurse's satisfaction
5. Focus on modification of patient behavior, increasing patient's self-worth, and improving patient's coping strategies
6. Therapeutic, not social, relationship
7. Phases
   a. Preorientation (preparation): about patient; self-analysis of attitudes, biases, and perceptions by the nurse
   b. Orientation: two to ten sessions. Nurse and patient become acquainted; trust and rapport are established;

Box **6-1**   Therapeutic Communication Techniques

LISTENING
Definition: an active process of receiving information and examining reactions to the messages received
Example: maintaining eye contact and receptive nonverbal communication
Therapeutic value: nonverbally communicates to the patient the nurse's interest and acceptance

BROAD OPENINGS
Definition: encouraging the patient to select topics for discussion
Example: "What are you thinking about?"
Therapeutic value: indicates acceptance by the nurse and the value of the patient's initiative

RESTATING
Definition: repeating the main thought the patient expressed
Example: "You say that your mother left you when you were 5 years old."
Therapeutic value: indicates that the nurse is listening and validates, reinforces, or calls attention to something important that has been said

CLARIFICATION
Definition: attempting to put into words vague ideas or unclear thoughts of the patient to enhance the nurse's understanding, or asking the patient to explain what he or she means
Example: "I'm not sure what you mean. Could you tell me about that again?"
Therapeutic value: helps clarify feelings, ideas, and perceptions of the patient and provides an explicit correlation between them and the patient's actions

REFLECTION
Definition: directing back the patient's ideas, feelings, questions, and content
Example: "You're feeling tense and anxious, and it's related to a conversation you had with your husband last night?"
Therapeutic value: validates the nurse's understanding of what the patient is saying and signifies empathy, interest, and respect for the patient

HUMOR
Definition: the discharge of energy through the comic enjoyment of the imperfect
Example: "That gives a whole new meaning to the word *nervous*"; said with shared kidding between the nurse and patient
Therapeutic value: can promote insight by making conscious repressed material, resolving paradoxes, tempering aggression, and revealing new options and is a socially acceptable form of sublimation

INFORMING
Definition: the skill of information giving
Example: "I think you need to know more about how your medication works."
Therapeutic value: helpful in health teaching or patient education about relevant aspects of patient's well-being and self-care

FOCUSING
Definition: questions or statements that help the patient expand on a topic of importance
Example: "I think that we should talk more about your relationship with your father."
Therapeutic value: allows the patient to discuss central issues and keeps the communication process goal directed

---

Box 6-1 Therapeutic Communication Techniques—cont'd

SHARING PERCEPTIONS

Definition: asking the patient to verify the nurse's understanding of what the patient is thinking or feeling

Example: "You're smiling, but I sense that you are really very angry with me."

Therapeutic value: conveys the nurse's understanding to the patient and has the potential for clearing up confusing communication

THEME IDENTIFICATION

Definition: underlying issues or problems experienced by the patient that emerge repeatedly during the course of the nurse-patient relationship

Example: "I've noticed that in all of the relationships that you have described, you've been hurt or rejected by the man. Do you think this is an underlying issue?"

Therapeutic value: allows the nurse to best promote the patient's exploration and understanding of important problems

SILENCE

Definition: lack of verbal communication for a therapeutic reason

Example: sitting with a patient and nonverbally communicating interest and involvement

Therapeutic value: allows the patient time to think and gain insights; slows the pace of the interaction and encourages the patient to initiate conversation while conveying the nurse's support, understanding, and acceptance

SUGGESTING

Definition: presentation of alternative ideas for the patient's consideration relative to problem solving

Example: "Have you thought about responding to your boss in a different way when he raises that issue with you? For example, you could ask him if a specific problem has occurred."

Therapeutic value: increases the patient's perceived options or choices

Modified from Stuart GW, Laraia MT: *Principles and practice of psychiatric nursing,* ed 9, St Louis, 2009, Mosby.

Table 6-1 Ineffective Responses That Hinder Therapeutic Communication

RESPONSE	DISCUSSION	NONTHERAPEUTIC RESPONSE	THERAPEUTIC RESPONSE
Offering false reassurance	In an effort to be supportive and make the patient's pain disappear, the nurse offers reassuring clichés. This response is not based on fact. It brushes aside the patient's feelings and closes communication. It is often the result of the nurse's inability to listen to the patient's negative emotions. No one can predict the outcome of a situation.	"Don't worry; everything will be okay." "Things will be better soon; you'll see."	"I know you have a lot going on right now. Let's make a list and begin to discuss the concerns one at a time. Working toward solutions will help you get through this."
Not listening	The nurse is preoccupied with other work that needs to be done, is distracted by noise in the area, or is thinking about personal problems.	"I'm sorry, what did you say?" "Could you start again? I was listening to the other nurse."	"That's interesting. Please elaborate." "I really hear what you're saying; it must be difficult."
Offering approval	How a patient feels about what he or she said or did is most important. The patient must approve of his or her own actions.	"That's good." "I agree; I think you should have told him."	"What do you think about what you said to him?" "How do you feel about it?"
Minimizing problem	The nurse may use this when facing the enormity of a particular problem. It is an effort to make the patient feel better. It cuts off communication.	"That's nothing compared to that other patient's problem." "Everyone feels that way at times; it's not a big deal."	"That is a very difficult problem for you." "That sounds pretty important for you to handle."
Offering advice	This response undermines patients' ability to solve their own problems. It renders them dependent and helpless. If the solution provided by the nurse doesn't work, the patient may blame the nurse for the outcome. Patients do not take responsibility for developing outcomes. The nurse maintains control and at the same time devalues the patient.	"I think you should…" "In my opinion, it would be wise to…" "Why don't you do…" "The best solution is…"	"What do you think you should do?" "There can be several alternatives; let's talk about some. However, the final decision must be yours." "I'll listen to your problem and help you see it clearly." "We can develop a pros and cons list, which may assist you in solving the problem."

Continued

Table 6-1   Ineffective Responses That Hinder Therapeutic Communication—cont'd

RESPONSE	DISCUSSION	NONTHERAPEUTIC RESPONSE	THERAPEUTIC RESPONSE
Giving literal responses	The nurse feeds into a patient's delusions of hallucinations and denies the patient the opportunity to see reality. This doesn't provide a healthy response toward growth.	Patient: "That TV is talking to me." Nurse: "What is it saying to you?" Patient: "There is nuclear power coming through the air ducts." Nurse: "I'll turn off the A/C for a while."	"The TV is on for everyone." "Cool air is blowing from the vents. It's the A/C system."
Changing the subject	The nurse changes the topic at a crucial time because the discussion is too uncomfortable. It negates what the patient seems interested in discussing. Communication will remain superficial.	Patient: "My mother always puts me down." Nurse: "That's interesting, but let's talk about…"	"Tell me about that."
Belittling	The nurse puts down patient's expressed feelings to avoid having to deal with painful feelings.	Patient: "I don't want to live anymore now that my child is gone." Nurse: "Anyone would be sad; but that's no reason to want to die."	"The death must be very difficult for you. Tell me a little more about how you're feeling."
Disagreeing	The nurse criticizes the patient who is seeking support.	"I definitely do not agree with your view." "I really don't believe that."	"Let's talk about the way you see that." "It seems hard to believe. Please explain further."
Judging	The nurse's responses are filled with his or her own values and judgments. This demonstrates a lack of acceptance of the patient's differences. It provides a barrier to further disclosures.	"You are not married. Do you think having this baby will solve your problems?" "This is certainly not the Christian thing to do." "You are thinking about divorce when you have three children?"	"What will having this baby provide for you?" "What do you think about what you're attempting to do?" "Let's discuss this option," or "Let's discuss other options."
Excessive probing	This controls the nature of the patient's responses. The nurse asks many questions of patients before they are ready to provide the information. This is self-protective to the nurse because it allows him or her to avoid the anxiety of uncomfortable silences. The patient feels overwhelmed and may withdraw.	"Why do you do this?" "What do you think was the real cause?" "Do you always feel this way?" "Why do you think that way?"	"Tell me how this is upsetting you." "Tell me what you believe to be the cause." "Tell me how you feel when that happens." "Explain your thinking on this if you can."
Challenging	This stems from the nurse's belief that if patients are challenged regarding their unrealistic beliefs, they will be coerced into seeing reality. The patient may feel threatened when challenged, holding onto the beliefs more strongly	"you're not the Queen of England." "If your leg is missing, how can you walk this hall?"	"You sound like you want to be important." "It seems to you like you are missing a leg. Tell me more about that."
Superficial comments	The nurse gives simple or meaningless responses to patients. It suggests a lack of understanding regarding the patient as an individual. The interactions remain superficial, maintaining distance between nurse and patient. Nothing of significance is communicated.	"Great day, huh!" "You should be feeling good; you're being discharged today." "Keep the faith; your doctor should be coming anytime now."	"What kind of day are you having?" "How are you feeling about leaving the hospital today?" "You look worried. Your doctor called and said he would be here within the hour."

Table 6-1	Ineffective Responses That Hinder Therapeutic Communication—cont'd			
RESPONSE	**DISCUSSION**	**NONTHERAPEUTIC RESPONSE**	**THERAPEUTIC RESPONSE**
Defending	The nurse may believe that he or she must defend himself or herself, the staff, or the hospital. He or she may not take the time to listen to the patient's concerns. Efforts need to be made to explore the patient's thoughts and feelings.	"You have a good doctor. He would never say that." "We have a very experienced staff. They would not ever do that."	"What has you so upset about your doctor?" "Tell me what happened on the evening shift."
Self-focusing	The nurse focuses attention away from the patient by thinking about and sharing his or her own thoughts, feelings, problems. The focus is taken away from the patient who is seeking help. The nurse is more interested in what to say next instead of actively listening to the patient.	"That may have happened to you last year, but it happened to me twice this month, which hurt me a great deal and…" "Excuse me, but could you say that again? I want to answer, but I want to be sure of what you said."	"Tell me about your incident and how it might relate to your sadness now." "If I heard you accurately, you said…"
Criticism of others	The nurse puts down others.	Patient: "The staff members on the day shift let me smoke two cigarettes." Nurse: "The day shift is always breaking the rules. On this shift we follow the one-cigarette policy." Patient: "My daughter is hateful to me. "Nurse: "She must be just awful to live with."	"The policy is one cigarette, which we must follow." "It sounds like you're having a rough time now with your daughter."
Premature inter-pretation	The nurse doesn't wait until the patient fully expresses thoughts and feelings related to a particular problem, which rushes the patient and disregards his or her input. The nurse may miss what the patient wants to explain.	"I think this is what you really mean." "You may think that way consciously, but your unconscious believes…"	"What do you think this means?" "So you think…"

Modified from Fortinash KM, Holoday Worret PA: *Psychiatric–mental health nursing*, ed 4, St Louis, 2008, Mosby.

parameters of the relationship are also established; discussions are contracted; patient problems are identified. The plan is built on patient's strengths.

c. Working begins when patient demonstrates responsibility to uphold terms of the contract. Establish priorities and goals with patient. Help patient achieve behavior change (e.g., discussion, role playing). Focus on the present. Reinforce the contract terms as necessary.

d. Termination begins during orientation phase; purpose is to conclude the relationship. Focus on patient growth, and help patient with expression of feelings about relationship closure.

Note: Some authors and models list three phases: orientation, maintenance, and termination.

F. Settings of mental health nursing
   1. Community mental health center
   2. Partial hospitalization setting: day or night hospitals
   3. Mental health clinic
   4. Liaison: use of mental health workers in the general hospital setting
   5. Alcohol and drug abuse facilities and clinics
   6. Inpatient units
   7. Crisis intervention centers
   8. Health maintenance organizations
   9. Group homes
   10. Specialty hospitals

PERSONALITY DEVELOPMENT

A. Definition: the sum total of unique components (i.e., thoughts, feelings, physical composition, behavioral traits, and attitudes) that distinguish one individual from another

B. Heredity
   1. Personality is influenced by inherited characteristics, both physical and psychological.
   2. Controversy exists regarding the extent of genetic influence on specific human behaviors.

C. Environment
   1. The environment is a strong determining factor in the individual's development.
   2. Environment includes the intrauterine environment and all of the external factors that influence the individual after birth.

D. Physical basis: Personality can develop normally if the necessary physical basis is present.

1. The brain is the major organ of thought and is vital to the development of personality.
2. The endocrine system strongly influences behavior as well.

E. Major theorists: comparison of Freud, Sullivan, Erikson, and Piaget (Table 6-2)
F. Elements of personality (Freud)
   1. Levels of consciousness
      a. The unconscious: always outside the awareness of the individual; influences actions in ways the individual may not understand; thought to include dreams
      b. The preconscious: usually outside awareness; available to the conscious mind in special circumstances such as under hypnosis or during therapy
      c. The conscious: ordinary awareness
   2. Structures: Some theorists refer to *personality structures.*
      a. Freud: ego, id, and superego
      b. Berne: child, adult, and parent
         (1) Eric Berne was the psychiatrist best known as the founder of Transactional Analysis; he labeled the three ego states as *child, parent,* and *adult* as opposed to *id, ego,* and *superego.*
            (a) The child interactions reflect feelings and desires—for example, "I'm afraid."
            (b) The parent interactions focus on aspects such as values, moral concepts, and rules—for example, "Please shut the door," "Be quiet in church."
            (c) In adult interactions the individual uses learned concepts and prior knowledge—for example, "The stove is hot," "A broken clock is right twice a day."
         (2) Berne also established the concept of *strokes,* which can be either positive or negative.
         (3) He believed that individuals receiving positive strokes will thrive and be encouraged to have positive interactions. (Morrison-Valfre)
   3. Functions: Each structure is thought to perform specific functions (Freud).
      a. Id (child): basic, innate psychic energy; emotional
      b. Ego (adult): mediates between person's perception and objective reality; always rational
      c. Superego (parent): incorporates societal values; judgmental and critical
G. Development levels: Various theorists describe levels of development.
   1. Freud (infant, child): oral, anal, phallic, latency, genital
   2. Erikson (incorporates levels across the life span): basic trust versus mistrust; autonomy versus shame and doubt; initiative versus guilt; industry versus inferiority; identity versus role diffusion; intimacy versus isolation; generativity versus stagnation; ego integrity versus despair
H. Development of the self-concept
   1. Development through experience with other people (e.g., parents, siblings, relatives, peers, teachers, other adults)
      a. Feelings of adequacy or inadequacy
      b. Feelings of acceptance or rejection
      c. Opportunities for identification
      d. Expectations of values, goals, and behaviors
   2. Self-concept consists of:
      a. Body image: one's perception of one's body.
      b. Self-ideal: one's idea of what is good behavior.
      c. Self-esteem: personal judgment of one's own worth.
      d. Role: one's perception of how one fits into the society.
      e. Identity: the combination of all of these factors into a unified whole.

STRESS

In 1956 Hans Selye defined *stress* as wear and tear on the body. All people are continuously exposed to varieties of stress: physical, chemical, psychological, and emotional. Almost any situation, pleasant or unpleasant, that requires change leads to some level of stress. Stress produces a clearly identifiable response called the *general adaptation syndrome;* it is associated with concomitant physical and chemical changes that commonly occur in the body. How individuals adapt to stressors can affect both their psychological and their physical health.

EGO DEFENSE MECHANISMS

Ego defense mechanisms are basic psychological tools that individuals use at various times to manage life's crises. These mechanisms may also be referred to as *ego defenses, defense mechanisms,* or *protective mechanisms.* As such they defend the ego or self from untoward anxiety, help resolve conflicts, and return the individual to a point of psychological homeostasis or comfort. These mechanisms are usually outside conscious awareness and are not considered pathological in and of themselves; they should not be removed or challenged until the individual is ready and has adequate strength to tolerate the stressful situation. Common defense mechanisms are listed in Table 6-3.

DIAGNOSTIC AND STATISTICAL MANUAL OF MENTAL DISORDERS (DSM-5)

The DSM-5 (approved May 2013) is the 5th edition and is widely used by physicians to establish the diagnosis of patients in mental health. The document DSM-IV was revised and further developed by the American Psychiatric Association to become the accepted standard within the profession.

Although several changes have been made in DSM-5, the most notable of these changes include the elimination of Asperger syndrome as a separate classification and the elimination of subtype classifications for variant forms of schizophrenia. Additional notable changes include eliminating the "bereavement exclusion" for depressive disorders, a revision in the treatment of gender identity issues, and the addition of a new gambling disorder.

ANXIETY DISTURBANCES AND RESOURCES

ANXIETY

A. Definition: a state of alertness or apprehension, tension or uneasiness; a major component of many mental disturbances. Anxiety is an internal state that the individual experiences when a perceived threat to the physical body or the psychological integrity of the person exists. It interferes with concentration, focusing attention on the perceived threat. In its mild form anxiety serves to alert the person to danger and prepare the body to react to danger; in its severe form it is debilitating and may immobilize the person and interfere with activities. Anxiety is usually described in degrees or levels.
B. Process: coping behaviors
   1. Adaptive coping: The problem creating the anxiety is resolved.

Table 6-2   Comparison of the Development Stages Postulated by Freud, Sullivan, Erikson, and Piaget

FREUD	SULLIVAN	ERIKSON	PIAGET

I. Oral stage (0-18 mo)
  A. The mouth is a source of satisfaction
  B. Two phases
    1. Passive
      • Only interests are satisfying hunger and sucking
      • Completely helpless, security the greater need
      • Narcissistic and egocentric, operates on pleasure principle
      • Omnipotent feelings are prevalent
    2. Active
      • Biting is a mode of pleasure
      • Continuous experimentation and associations
      • Sensory discrimination
      • Differentiation between mental images and reality
      • Differentiation of others and discovery of self
 	
II. Anal stage (1½-3yr)
  A. Primary activity is on learning muscular control association with urination and defecation (toilet-training period)
  B. Exhibits more self-control; walks, talks, dresses, and undresses
  C. Negativism—assertion of independence
  D. Introduction of reality principle, ego development
  E. Superego begins to develop
  F. Engages in parallel play
	I. Infancy (0-18 mo)
	  A. The mouth is a source of satisfaction
	  B. Mouth—takes in (sucking), cuts off (biting), and pushes out (spitting) objects introduced by others
	  C. Crying, babbling, and cooing are modes of communication used by the infant to call attention of adults to self
	  D. Satisfaction response (pleasure principle); infant's biological needs are met, and a mutual feeling of comfort and fulfillment is experienced by mother and infant (mother gives and infant takes)
	  E. Empathic observation—capacity to perceive feelings of others as his or her own immediate feelings in the situation
	  F. Autistic invention—state of symbolic activity in which the infant believes that he or she is master of all he or she surveys
	  G. Experimentation, exploration, and manipulation are methods used to acquaint self with environment
	
	II. Childhood (1½-6yr)
	  A. Begins with the capacity for communicating through speech and ends with a beginning need for association with peers
	  B. Uses language as a tool to communicate wishes and needs
	  C. Anus is power tool used to give or withhold a part of self to control significant people in his environment
	  D. Emergence and integration of self-concept and reflected appraisal of significant persons
	  E. Awareness that postponing or delaying gratification of one's wishes may bring satisfaction
	  F. Begins to find limits in experimentation, exploration, and manipulation
	  G. More aggressive
	  H. Uses parallel play and curiosity to explore environment
	  I. Uses exhibitionism and masturbatory activity to become acquainted with self and others
	  J. Demonstrates a beginning ability to think abstractly
		I. Oral-sensory stage (0-12 mo)
		  A. The mouth is a source of satisfaction and a means of dealing with anxiety-producing situations
		  B. Focus is on the development of the basic attitudes of trust versus mistrust
		  C. Attitudes are formed through mother's reaction to infant needs
		
		II. Anal-muscular stage (1-3yr)
		  A. Learns the extent to which the environment can be influenced by direct manipulation
		  B. Focuses on the development of the basic attitudes of autonomy versus shame and doubt
		  C. Exerts self-control and willpower
			I. Sensorimotor stage (0-12 mo)
			  A. Emphasis is on preverbal intellectual development
			  B. Learns relationships with external objects
			  C. Focus is on physical development with gradual increase in ability to think and use language
			
			II. Preoperational stage (2-7yr)
			  A. Learns to use symbols and language
			  B. Learns to imitate and play
			  C. Displays egocentricity
			  D. Engages in animistic thinking—endowment of objects with power and ability

III. Phallic stage (3-6yr)
A. Libidinal energy focus on the genitals
B. Learns sexual identity
C. Superego becomes internalized
D. Sibling rivalry and manipulation of parents occurs
E. Intellectual and motor facilities are refined
F. Increased socialization and associative play

IV. Latency (6-12yr)
A. Quiet stage in which sexual development lies dormant, emotional tension eases
B. Normal homosexual phase
 • For boys, gangs
 • For girls, cliques
C. Increased intellectual capacity
D. Starts school
E. Identifies with teachers and peers
F. Weakening of home ties
G. Recognizes authority figures outside home, age of hero worship

III. Genital-locomotor stage (3-6yr)
A. Learns the extent to which being assertive will influence the environment
B. Focus is on the development of the basic attitudes of initiative versus guilt
C. Explores the world with senses, thoughts, and imagination
D. Activities demonstrate direction and purpose
E. Engages in first real social contracts through cooperative play
F. Develops conscience

IV. Latency (6-12yr)
A. Learns to use energy to create, develop, and manipulate
B. Focus is on the development of basic attitudes of industry versus inferiority
C. Able to initiate and complete tasks
D. Understands rules and regulations
E. Displays competence and productivity

III. Juvenile stage (6-9yr)
A. Learns to form satisfactory relationship with peers
B. Peer norms prevail over family norms
C. Engages in competition, experimentation, exploration, and manipulation
D. Able to cooperate and compromise
E. Demonstrates capacity to love
F. Distinguishes fantasy from reality
G. Exerts internal control over behavior

IV. Preadolescence (9-12yr)
A. Learns to relate to a friend of the same sex—chum relationship
B. Concerned with group success and derives satisfaction from group accomplishment
C. Shows signs of rebellion— restlessness, hostility, irritability
D. Assumes less responsibility for own actions
E. Moves from egocentricity to a more full social state
F. Uses experimentation, exploration, manipulation
G. Seeks consensual validation

III. Concrete operations stage (7-11yr)
A. Deals with visible concrete objects and relationships
B. Increased intellectual and conceptual development—uses logic and reasoning
C. More socialized and rule conscious

Continued

Table 6-2 Comparison of the Development Stages Postulated by Freud, Sullivan, Erikson, and Piaget—cont'd

FREUD	SULLIVAN	ERIKSON	PIAGET
V. Genital stage (12 yr–early adulthood) A. Appearance of secondary sex characteristics, reawakening of sex drives B. Increased concern over physical appearance C. Striving toward independence D. Development of sexual maturity E. Identity crisis F. Identification of love object of opposite gender G. Intellectual maturity H. Plans future	V. Early adolescence (12-14 yr) A. Experiences physiological changes B. Uses rebellion to gain independence C. Fantasizes, overidentifies with heroes D. Discovers and begins relationships with opposite gender E. Demonstrates heightened levels of anxiety in most interpersonal relationships VI. Late adolescence (14-21 yr) A. Establishes an enduring intimate relationship with one member of the opposite sex B. Self-concept becomes stabilized C. Attains physical maturity D. Develops ability to use logic and abstract concepts VII. Adulthood (21 yr and older) A. Assumes responsibility relevant to station in life B. Maintains balance and involvement among self, family, and community C. Further develops creativity D. Reaffirms values in life	V. Puberty and adolescence (12-18 yr) A. Demonstrates an ability to integrate life experiences B. Focuses on the development of the basic attitudes of identity versus role diffusion C. Seeks partner of the opposite gender D. Begins to establish identity and place in society VI. Young adulthood (18-35 yr) A. Primarily concerned with developing an intimate relationship with another adult B. Focus is on the development of the basic attitudes of intimacy and solidarity versus isolation	IV. Formal operations stage (11-15 yr) A. Develops true abstract thought B. Formulates hypotheses and applies logical tests C. Experiences conceptual independence V. Adulthood (35-65 yr) A. Primarily concerned with establishing and maintaining a family B. Focus is on the development of the basic attitudes of generativity versus stagnation C. Displays a marked degree of creativity D. Adjusts to circumstances of middle age E. Reevaluates life accomplishments and goals VI. Maturity (older than 65 yr) A. Accepts lifestyle as meaningful and fulfilling B. Focuses on the development of basic attitudes of ego integrity versus despair C. Remains optimistic and continues to grow D. Adjusts to limitations E. Adjusts to retirement F. Adjusts to reorganized family patterns G. Adjusts to losses H. Accepts death with serenity

Table 6-3   Ego Defense Mechanisms

DEFENSE MECHANISM	EXAMPLE
Compensation: process by which a person makes up for a perceived deficiency by strongly emphasizing a feature that he or she regards as an asset	A businessman perceives his small physical stature negatively. He tries to overcome this by being aggressive, forceful, and controlling in business dealings.
Denial: avoidance of disagreeable realties by ignoring or refusing to recognize them; probably the simplest and most primitive of all defense mechanisms	Mrs. P has just been told that her breast biopsy indicates a malignancy. When her husband visits her that evening, she tells him that no one has discussed the laboratory results with her.
Displacement: shift of emotion from a person or object to another, usually neutral or less dangerous, person or object	A 4-year-old boy is angry because his mother just punished him for drawing on his bedroom walls. He begins to play war with his soldier toys and has them battle and fight with each other.
Dissociation: the separation of any group of mental or behavioral processes from the rest of the person's consciousness or identity	A man is brought to the emergency department by the police and is unable to explain who he is and where he lives or works.
Identification: process by which a person tries to become like someone he or she admires by taking on thoughts, mannerisms, or tastes of that individual	Sally, 15 years old, has her hair styled similarly to that of her young English teacher whom she admires.
Intellectualization: excessive reasoning or logic used to avoid experiencing disturbing feelings	A woman avoids dealing with her anxiety in shopping malls by explaining that she is not engaging in the frivolous waste of time and money by not going into them.
Introjection: intense type of identification in which a person incorporates qualities or values of another person or group into his or her own ego structure; one of the earliest mechanisms of the child and is important in formation of conscience	Eight-year-old Jimmy tells his 3-year-old sister, "don't scribble in your book of nursery rhymes. Just look at the pretty pictures," thus expressing his parents' values to his little sister.
Isolation: splitting off of emotional components of a thought, which may be temporary or long term	A second-year medical student dissects a cadaver for her anatomy course without being disturbed by thoughts of death.
Projection: attributing one's thoughts or impulses to another person; through this process one can attribute intolerable wishes, emotional feelings, or motivations to another person	A young woman who denies that she has sexual feelings about a co-worker accuses him without basis of being a "flirt" and says he is trying to seduce her.
Rationalization: offering a socially acceptable or apparently logical explanation to justify or make acceptable otherwise unacceptable impulse, feelings, behaviors, and motives	John fails an examination and complains that the lectures were not well organized or clearly presented.
Reaction formation: development of conscious attitudes and behavior patterns that are opposite to what one really feels or would like to do	A married woman who feels attracted to one of her husband's friends treats him rudely.
Regression: retreat in face of stress to behavior characteristic of any earlier level of development	Four-year-old Nicole, who has been toilet trained for more than a year, begins to wet her pants again when her new baby brother is brought home from the hospital.
Repression: involuntary exclusion of a painful or conflictual thought, impulse, or memory from awareness; the primary ego defense, and other mechanisms tend to reinforce it	Mr. R does not recall hitting his wife when she was pregnant.
Splitting: viewing people and situations as either all good or all bad; failure to integrate the positive and negative qualities of oneself	A friend tells you that you are the most wonderful person in the world one day and how much she hates you the next day.
Sublimation: acceptance of a socially approved substitute goal for a drive whose normal channel of expression is blocked	Ed has an impulsive and physically aggressive nature. He tries out for the football team and becomes a star tackle.
Suppression: a process often listed as a defense mechanism but really a conscious counterpart of repression; intentional exclusion of material from consciousness	A young man at work finds that he is thinking so much about his date that evening that it is interfering with his work. He decides to put it out of his mind until he leaves the office for the day.
Undoing: act or communication that partially negates a previous one; primitive defense mechanism	Larry makes a passionate declaration of love to Sue on a date. On their next meeting, he treats her formally and distantly.

Modified from Stuart GW, Laraia MT: *Principles and practice of psychiatric nursing,* ed 9, St Louis, 2009, Mosby.

2. Palliative coping: The problem creating the anxiety is not resolved but rather temporarily reduced; the problem can return at a later date.
3. Maladaptive coping: Energy is channeled toward reducing the anxiety, and no effort is made to solve the problem.
4. Dysfunctional coping: The problem is not solved, and the anxiety not reduced.

C. Levels of anxiety (Table 6-4)
   1. Minimal (0)
   2. Mild (1)
   3. Moderate (2)
   4. Severe (3)
   5. Panic (4)

D. Assessment (Table 6-4)

E. Interventions
   1. Remain with the highly anxious patient; leaving him or her alone increases anxiety.
   2. Maintain a calm milieu, which reduces stimuli.
   3. Remain in control and calm; patient fears losing control and needs to feel secure.

Table 6-4   **Levels of Anxiety**

SEVERITY OF ANXIETY	PHYSICAL	INTELLECTUAL	SOCIAL AND EMOTIONAL
Minimal (near 0)	Basal levels of: Pulse Respiration rate Oxygen consumption Pupillary constriction Muscles relaxed	Cognitive activity minimal Disregard for external environmental stimuli; no attempt to actively process information Focus typically on single, nonthreatening mental image States of altered consciousness	No social interaction No attempt to deal with environmental stimuli Minimal emotional activity Feelings of indifference, invulnerability, and contentment prevail
Mild (+1)	Low-level sympathetic arousal Moderate-to-low skeletal muscle tension Body relaxed Voice calm, well modulated	Perceptual field open; able to shift focus of attention readily Passively aware of external environment Self-referent thoughts positive; low concern for unexpected or negative outcomes	Behavior primarily automatic; habitual patterns and well-learned skills Positive feeling of security, confidence, and satisfaction dominate Solitary activities
Moderate (+2)	Sympathetic nervous system activation Increased blood pressure Increased pulse rate Increased respiratory rate Pupillary dilation Sweat glands stimulated Peripheral vascular constriction Increased muscular tension Heightened performance of well-learned skills Rate of speech increased, pitch heightened Increased alertness	Narrowing of perception; attentional focus on specific internal or external stimuli Conscious effort in processing of information; optimal level for learning Self-referent thoughts—mixed; some concern about personal ability or available resources necessary to solve problems; probability of positive outcomes increasingly uncertain	Increased skill in learning and refining of skills, analyzing problematic situations, integrating cognitive and motor domains Feelings of challenge; drive to resolve problems or dilemmas Mixed sense of confidence or optimism with fear, lowered self-esteem, and potential inadequacy
Severe (+3)	Fight-or-flight response Stimulation of adrenal medulla Increased catecholamines, accelerated heart rate, palpitations Increased blood glucose Increased blood flow to digestive system Increased blood flow to skeletal muscles Muscles extremely tense Hyperventilation Physical actions increasingly agitated; pacing, wringing of hands, fidgeting, trembling May experience loss of appetite, nausea, "cold sweats" Rapid, high-pitched speech Facial expression: poor eye contact, fleeting eye movements	Perceptual capacity restricted; exclusive attention to singular stimuli (internal or external) or multifocal, fragmented processing of stimuli Problem solving inefficient, difficult Some threatening stimuli disregarded, minimized, denied Disorientation in terms of time and place Expected likelihood of negative consequences or outcomes high; estimates of personal self-efficacy low	Flight behavior may manifest as withdrawal, denial, depression, somatization Feelings of increasing threat; need to respond to situation is heightened Dissociating tendency; feelings are denied

Continued

Table 6-4	Levels of Anxiety—cont'd		
SEVERITY OF ANXIETY	**PHYSICAL**	**INTELLECTUAL**	**SOCIAL AND EMOTIONAL**
Panic (+4)	Continued physiological arousal Actions disorganized, directionless; unable to execute simple motor tasks; fumbling, gross motor agitation, flailing May strike out verbally or physically; may attempt to withdraw from situation Eventual depletion of sympathetic neurotransmitters Blood redistributed throughout body Hypotension May feel dizzy, faint, or exhausted Appears pale, drawn, weary Facial expression: aghast, grimacing, eyes fixed Voice louder, higher pitched	Perception severely restricted, may be impervious to external stimuli Thoughts are random, distorted, disconnected, logical processing impaired Unable to solve problems; limited tolerance for processing novel stimuli (verbal, auditory, or visual) Preoccupied with thoughts of highly probable negative outcomes; conclusions may be drawn, negative consequences seen as inevitable	Emotionally drained, overwhelmed Reliance on earlier, more primitive coping behaviors: crying, shouting, curling up, rocking, freezing Feelings of impotence, helplessness, agony and desperation dominate; may be experienced as horror, dread, defenselessness; may be converted to anger, rage

4. Communicate with clear, simple, short sentences because patient's ability to deal with complex, abstract statements is compromised. Similarly, ask questions requiring brief, concise responses.

5. Use of as-necessary (*pro re nata* [p.r.n.]) medications may be needed to decrease patient anxiety to a manageable level (e.g., benzodiazepines, such as lorazepam [Ativan] or alprazolam [Xanax]).

6. Encourage use of relaxation and other stress-reduction techniques, such as guided imagery or deep-breathing exercises.

7. When appropriate, assist patient with recognizing early signs of anxiety and developing effective ways to prevent its escalation.

8. Provide opportunities for discussing the relationship of thoughts and emotions to anxiety.

9. More restrictive interventions such as seclusion, restraints, or both may be necessary if patient is a danger to self or others.

PHOBIAS

A. Definition: irrational, continual fears of an activity, situation, object, or event that are obsessive

B. Types (examples, not inclusive)
   1. Agoraphobia (literal meaning: fear of the marketplace) without panic attacks: fear of being away from a safe environment or person from which escape may not be readily available
   2. Social phobia: irrational fear of exposure to the scrutiny of others
   3. Simple or specific phobia: disabling fear of some specific object or situation such as the fear of animals (zoophobia) or of being in a high place (acrophobia)

C. Assessment data
   1. History and physical examination, including family history
   2. Panic or anticipatory anxiety or both
   3. Recognition of phobia as irrational
   4. Defense mechanisms of displacement and repression

   5. Avoidance behaviors
   6. Interference with demands of daily activities
   7. Social history such as alcohol, caffeine use or intake

D. Interventions
   1. Accept patient and his or her fears.
   2. Encourage involvement in activities that do not increase anxiety.
   3. Help patient recognize that his or her behavior is an attempt to cope with anxiety.
   4. Use a calm, nonauthoritative approach.
   5. Reassure patient that he or she will not be made to confront the phobia in treatment until ready to do so.
   6. Use systematic desensitization.

OBSESSIVE-COMPULSIVE DISORDER (OCD)

A. Definition: obsessive thoughts (troublesome, persistent thoughts) usually triggered by anxiety and compulsions (ritualistic behaviors) that are repetitive and represent an attempt to reduce anxiety

B. Assessment data
   1. Compulsive, ritualistic behavior
   2. Obsessive thoughts
   3. Alterations in normal functioning
   4. Fear of loss of control
   5. Feelings of guilt
   6. Suicidal thoughts or feelings
   7. Rumination (preoccupation with specific thoughts)
   8. Insight impairment
   9. Feelings of worthlessness
   10. Decreased self-esteem

C. Interventions
   1. Always follow patient's behavioral support and modification plan regarding the behavioral rituals exhibited.
   2. If permitted by the plan, allow patient time to perform rituals. Limit but do not interrupt the compulsive act because it may increase anxiety.
   3. Ensure that basic daily needs are met.
   4. Redirect rumination positively.

5. Do not initially call attention to or interfere with the compulsive act.
6. Demonstrate concern for and interest in the patient.
7. Encourage verbalization of concerns and feelings.
8. As anxiety decreases and patient feels comfortable talking with the staff, encourage him or her to talk about his or her behavior and thoughts.
9. Encourage patient to try to reduce the frequency of compulsive behavior.
10. Observe patient response to ordered medications such as antianxiety or antidepressant agents.

POSTTRAUMATIC STRESS DISORDER

Posttraumatic stress disorder (PTSD) is the development of certain characteristic symptoms after a psychologically traumatic event; these symptoms can include numbness of responses, frequent reliving of the event, dreams, depression, and anxiety.

PERCEPTION

A. Definition: awareness acquired through the five senses
B. Alterations: thought to be pathological conditions resulting from anxiety
  1. Illusion: an actual stimulus in the environment that is misinterpreted or misperceived
  2. Hallucination: a sensation without an external stimulus; it may be:
     a. Auditory: hearing nonexistent voices or sounds.
     b. Olfactory: smelling nonexistent odors or aromas.
     c. Visual: seeing nonexistent things, people, or animals.
     d. Tactile: feeling somatic sensations.
     e. Gustatory: experiencing flavors or tastes.
  3. Delusion: false belief, not based in fact, that cannot be changed by reasoning
     a. Delusions of grandeur: feelings of greatness
     b. Delusions of persecution: feelings of being mistreated
     c. Delusions of sin or guilt: feelings of deserving punishment; may have religious basis
     d. Somatic delusions: feelings about the body or part of the body
C. Ideas of reference: feeling that certain events or words have special meaning for self

THOUGHT DISORDERS

Schizophrenia is considered to be the psychiatric manifestation of a thought disorder. This group of illnesses represents the largest number of severely mentally ill people (some authors list depression and generalized anxiety disorder as more prevalent). Schizophrenia affects approximately 1% of the population. The diagnosis requires continuation of symptoms for 6 months or more, generally occurring before 45 years of age.
A. Types of schizophrenia
  1. Disorganized: includes frequent incoherence, nonsystematic delusions, and inappropriate affect
  2. Catatonic: includes stupor, negativity, rigidity, excitement, and posturing
  3. Paranoid: includes persecutory delusions, grandiosity, delusional jealousy, and hallucinations; may include aggressive, argumentative, or hostile behaviors
  4. Undifferentiated: does not fit criteria of other categories or combines them; delusions, hallucinations, or both are prominent

5. Residual: presence of residual symptoms (e.g., marked social isolation, inappropriate affect, odd beliefs) without delusions, hallucinations, or gross disorganization of thought
B. Assessment data
  1. History and physical, including family history
  2. Delusions of being controlled
  3. Somatic delusions (grandiosity, religious, or nihilistic)
  4. Persecutory delusions accompanied by hallucinations
  5. Auditory hallucinations of a running commentary on behavior or thought
  6. Auditory hallucination on several occasions with content of more than one word
  7. Incoherence, looseness of association, illogical thinking with a deterioration in function
C. Interventions
  1. Milieu therapy
  2. Establish trust.
  3. Do not enter into patient's delusions; maintain own view of reality without demeaning patient's view of reality. This is done by letting patient know that what he or she is experiencing is real to him or her but that you are not experiencing it.
  4. Do not argue about hallucinations; the patient views them as real.
  5. Offer reassurance: most patients are experiencing pain and fear from their symptoms.
  6. Touch only with permission; the thought-disordered patient may have a distorted sense of his or her own person and may easily misinterpret the actions of others.
  7. If you are afraid, be aware that the patient senses this; be sure that you have sufficient backup for your own safety and comfort.
  8. Maintain patient safety; reassess frequently for potential for harm to self or others.
  9. Medicate as ordered. Observe patient for therapeutic effect and side effects (e.g., extrapyramidal symptoms [EPSs], or neuroleptic malignant syndrome); see Chapter 3.

AFFECTIVE DISORDERS

Disturbances in feeling or affective disorders are classified as either depressive disorders or bipolar disorders.

DEPRESSIVE DISORDERS

A. Major depression is the predominant mental illness in the United States and Canada, with ranges from 7% to 12% in the male population and 26% to 30% in the female population.
B. Assessment data
  1. History and physical examination, including family history, to rule out medical causes contributing to patient's condition
  2. Persistent sadness, hopelessness, or tearfulness
  3. Loss of interest in some or all usual activities (anhedonia), fatigue, inability to concentrate
  4. Change in appetite: usually decreased
  5. Changes in weight: usually a loss in weight
  6. Sleep disturbances: usually insomnia but may be sleeping more during the day

7. Withdrawal from family and friends; feeling guilty and unworthy

8. Hopelessness and helplessness that may become profound and lead to delusions or fantasies of ending it all

9. If left in this pattern, patient eventually might justify how nonexistence may solve the problems.

10. Patient may start to dwell on death and devise a plan of self-destruction.

11. Self-destruction becomes the goal; this is suicidal ideation.

C. See discussion of suicide prevention and suicide intervention.

BIPOLAR DISORDERS

A. Category used when one or more manic episodes are noted, whether or not a depressive episode is or has been experienced

B. Mania characterized by unstable, elevated, or irritable mood; pressured speech; irritability; and increased motor activity. Patient often displays racing thoughts, impulsivity, attention-seeking or agitated behavior, psychosis, and alterations in sleep.

C. Interventions
   1. Demonstrate sincere interest.
   2. Accept patient's feelings. Anger may be directed at the nearest safe object, often the nurse, and should not be taken personally.
   3. Allow patient to express feelings (e.g., crying) in a dignified environment.
   4. Be aware of patient's limited ability to control his or her behavior, and encourage expression of feelings (e.g., crying) only within a safe context.
   5. If patient is overactive, limit-setting or reduction of stimuli may be necessary to allow him or her to regain self-control and increase focus.
   6. Avoid power struggles: use force only if necessary to protect patient or others in the environment.

EATING DISORDERS

A. Obesity and compulsive overeating: consuming more than the required number of calories, which results in weight gain; not burning as many calories as consumed. The person is usually considered obese when weight is 20% more than is recommended for his or her height.

B. Anorexia nervosa: an eating disorder characterized by refusal to maintain a minimally normal body weight. It is most often seen in adolescent women (may occur with bulimia or separately).

C. Bulimia: an eating disorder characterized by episodes of binging and then purging. Person may not appear overweight or underweight. With nonpurging bulimia the person uses laxatives, diuretics, fasting, or exercise to control his or her weight. Bulimia often leads to other symptoms such as menstrual irregularities, gastric dilation, aspiration pneumonia, dental caries (caused by frequent vomiting), and esophagitis.

D. Interventions: Treatment of these disorders will vary; however, it is centered around the following goals:
   1. Stabilizing existing medical conditions
   2. Establishing appropriate nutrition
   3. Resolving existing emotional and psychological problems

PERSONALITY DISORDERS

Personality disorders are long-standing, maladaptive patterns of behaving and relating that result in continual difficulties with interpersonal relationships.

A. The American Psychiatric Association in its DSM-5 classifies personality disorders as follows:
   1. Eccentric Personality Disorders
      a. Paranoid Personality Disorder: characterized by suspicion, rigidity, secretiveness, oversensitivity and alertness, distortions of reality, and the use of projection as a major defense mechanism
      b. Schizoid: limited emotional expression, distant, seemingly detached in social situation and interactions
      c. Schizotypal: often considered strange because of behaviors, appearance, excessive anxiety, illogical or confused speech, odd beliefs and ideas of reference; prefer to be alone and avoid social interactions
   2. Erratic Personality Disorders
      a. Antisocial Personality Disorder: characterized by lack of remorse and willingness to exploit others for personal gains; use dishonest methods and tactics to achieve desired outcomes; disregard rights of others, laws, and social norms but expect others to conform to the same; persist in dishonest and unlawful behaviors without regret, remorse, or concern for their victims; can be charming, clever, and entertaining in their efforts to deceive
      b. Borderline Personality Disorder: at times moderately neurotic; at other times overtly psychotic; extremely difficult to treat and often unstable after numerous treatment attempts; lack emotional control and the ability to form and maintain relationships with others; can engage in self-injurious behaviors (SIBs) and suicidal gestures when fearful of separation or rejection; social relationships characterized by highs and lows (love and hate), which drives away those with whom they desire relationships; split staff by allegations and manipulation
      c. Histrionic Personality Disorder: have highly emotional responses, short attention spans; are superficial, lack depth; seek attention, affection, and approval of others.
      d. Narcissistic Personality Disorder: seek approval and admiration of others and use attention-seeking behaviors; demonstrate little empathy and can be grandiose; see themselves as special, deserving of special consideration; demonstrate a sense of entitlement and seem arrogant
   3. Fearful/Anxious Personality Disorders
      a. Avoidant Personality Disorder: fear rejection; avoid social relationships, yet desire the closeness they avoid out of fear; see themselves as social misfits, uninteresting, and less acceptable than others; can also be depressed and anxious and dwell on health concerns
      b. Dependent Personality Disorder: fear separation and being left alone because they believe that they cannot survive alone; have a clinging manner, seek others to care for day-to-day matters, avoid personal responsibility and submit to others in most matters; tolerate unhappy and even abusive relationships in an effort to prevent separation; disorder often found in individuals who are disabled or have ongoing medical conditions

c. Obsessive-Compulsive Personality Disorder: fear uncertainty, lack of total control, disorder, unpredictability and delegation; are focused on rules, regulations, procedures, lists, and organization; are devoted to tasks, work, and process, but drive for perfection prevents accomplishment; personal relationships can be superficial and controlled in spite of real affection for others

B. Interventions
1. Be honest with patient.
2. Help patient increase coping skills.
3. These patients are often manipulative and attention seeking, requiring a firm, consistent response by staff. Limit-setting is very important here.
4. They tend to view people or situations in extremes such as all good or all bad.
5. Patients need to begin developing meaningful relationships in which they can begin to trust.
6. Consistency is important; patients may split the staff to play one staff member against another.
7. Patients need to take responsibility for their behaviors and the consequences of these behaviors.

C. Codependency: meeting goals successfully by relying on another person for the answers. Characteristics of the codependent person include the following:
1. Partners are dependent on each other to make a whole relationship.
2. One of the partners in this relationship assumes a passive role.
3. One or both may have low self-esteem.
4. One or both may have poor self-image.
5. One or both may have an addictive disorder (e.g., alcohol, drugs).
6. They tend to be manipulative—a constant conflict exists, either between them or within the family.
7. They tend to operate in a series of delusions.
8. Because of delusions, they tend to promote their version of any story as the absolute truth.
9. They exhibit poor boundaries (limits) in relationships.
10. They are somewhat to totally insensitive to others' emotions and feelings.
11. If the codependency exists within a family, it is highly likely that a dysfunctional family unit will emerge and the children will become part of the codependency.
12. Codependency may be generational and therefore cyclical.
13. In helping the dependent individual, the codependent can become an enabler—especially by helping a chemically dependent person escape the consequences of his or her addiction.
14. The treatment of codependent people is designed to identify the underlying emotions that are fostering the codependency.

D. Substance abuse disorders: pattern of pathological use of substances that entails factors such as the need for daily use, loss of control, efforts to control use, overdoses, impairment of social functioning, family disruptions, and legal problems. Abuse is distinguished from dependency by tolerance of the substance (increasing use requires increasing doses to achieve the same effect) and the presence or absence of a withdrawal syndrome.
1. Alcoholism
a. Abuse is distinguished from recreational use by features such as daily drinking; frequent need for the chemical; blackouts; social impairment; and evidence of decreased ability to function, such as job loss, driving while intoxicated, and arrests.
b. A pattern of acute alcohol ingestion may result in a condition formerly known as *delirium tremens* (DTs), now known as *acute alcohol withdrawal syndrome;* key features are hallucinations, extreme agitation, and disorientation; treatment includes anxiolytics (benzodiazepines), anticonvulsants, and hydration.
c. Long-term use may lead to peripheral neuropathy; Wernicke syndrome (confusion, ataxia, abnormal eye movements); or Korsakoff syndrome (alcoholic amnesia syndrome), which manifests with memory loss and confabulation. Confabulation can be the primary component. These effects are largely caused by deficiency of thiamine and may be partially reversed by provision of thiamine. Korsakoff syndrome is usually irreversible but may be arrested by thiamine replacement therapy and cessation of alcohol abuse.
2. Barbiturate and sedative abuse (barbiturates or minor tranquilizers—e.g., diazepam, benzodiazepines)
a. Cross-tolerant with alcohol
b. May be used by street addicts when they are unable to obtain opiates
c. Second most abused substance after alcohol in the United States
d. Intoxication is similar to that from alcohol.
e. A withdrawal syndrome occurs that is similar to, and as serious as, that from alcohol withdrawal.
3. Opiates (heroin, morphine)
a. Used by street addicts who inject intravenous (IV) heroin and medical addicts who use various prescribed substances such as codeine and other pain medications
b. IV drug users are at a high risk for acquired immunodeficiency syndrome (AIDS).
c. Intoxication includes pupil constriction, poor attention span, apathy, slurred speech, euphoria, and psychomotor retardation.
d. A physical withdrawal syndrome occurs.
4. Cocaine
a. Stimulant
b. Increasing use among the middle class
c. Considered a social drug; many people believe that it is not addictive.
d. May be snorted or smoked as freebase or as crack
e. Intoxication includes poor judgment; poor impulse control; feeling of confidence; euphoria; talkative, rapid speech; pacing; elevated heart rate and blood pressure; dilated pupils; nausea; and sweating.
f. May lead to hallucinations with prolonged use; severe depression occurs after substance use is stopped, leading to strong psychological craving.
g. A true withdrawal syndrome may not occur.
5. Amphetamines, including methamphetamine, with a very high abuse potential, are becoming a major problem as their use increases.
a. Abuse may begin in an effort to control weight or stay awake for long periods.
b. They may be combined with other drugs such as heroin or barbiturates or used intravenously by addicts for a rush.

c. Intoxication includes elevated heart rate and blood pressure, dilated pupils, chills, perspiration, nausea, and vomiting.

d. Truck drivers often abuse amphetamines to facilitate driving coast to coast without sleep.

e. Bath salts

(1) An amphetamine-like chemical

(2) A dangerous synthetic stimulant

(3) Several names such as "Ivory Snow," "Pure Ivory," "White Lightening," "Bliss."

(4) Hallucinations, delusions, extreme agitation, and hyperactivity are known to occur from their use.

(5) Causes life-threatening conditions such as chest pain, tachycardia, hypertension, cerebrovascular accident (CVA), and death.

(6) Long-term effects are being assessed in this new designer drug.

(7) A white powder; can be inhaled, injected, or ingested

(8) Illegal in many states but sold, mainly in convenience stores, in other states.

6. Hallucinogens (e.g., lysergic acid diethylamide [LSD], mescaline)

a. Used much less than in the early 1970s

b. Use leads to altered perceptions and hallucinations; distorted perception of colors; illusions and delusions; unpredictable effects.

c. Intoxication includes perceptual changes; dilated pupils; increased pulse, sweating, anxiety, tremors; feelings of paranoia; and poor judgment.

7. Cannabis (marijuana, hashish)

a. Widely used by various groups, usually smoked or eaten

b. Intoxication includes increased pulse rate, bloodshot eyes, increased appetite, dry mouth, distorted perception of time, euphoria, and apathy.

c. May precipitate panic attacks

d. Used with medical approval in some places—counteracts side effects of some chemotherapy

8. Inhalants

a. Primary users are teens

b. Can be obtained legally as solvents, spray or aerosol cans, glue, and anesthetic agents

c. Rapid acting and short-lived, producing lightheadedness, euphoria, diminished judgment, and delusions and hallucinations

d. Respiratory, liver, cardiac, brain and renal damage can result from their use, which can be irreversible and lethal.

9. Caffeine

a. Widely consumed as the active ingredient in soft drinks, coffee, and tea

b. A central nervous stimulant

c. Can cause gastrointestinal distress, tachycardia, and insomnia

10. Nicotine

a. Active ingredient in products containing tobacco such as cigarettes, cigars, nicotine gum and patches

b. Addictive

c. Multiple health problems associated with its use and for those exposed to its "secondhand" effects

11. Substance abuse interventions

a. Severe denial is a common defense mechanism.

b. Keep patient focused on the purpose of treatment.

c. Manipulation may be used in an attempt to obtain a substance for abuse.

d. The nurse must remain nonjudgmental; intervention focuses on acting as a therapeutic agent.

e. These patients may require repeated attempts at treatment before they can conquer their addiction.

f. Adequate diet, rest, and vitamin supplements are helpful in restoring physiological health.

g. Long-term success is often achieved through a lifelong affiliation with abstinence programs such as Alcoholics Anonymous (AA) and Narcotics Anonymous (NA).

h. Alcoholism is usually treated in several steps, the first being detoxification; in detoxification the person with alcoholism is withdrawn from the chemical through the use of a cross-tolerant substance, usually a benzodiazepine, which is administered for 3 to 5 days in decreasing doses.

(1) Detoxification should occur in a controlled (monitored) setting because it may become-life threatening.

(2) After the acute detoxification period of 3 to 5 days, intense counseling occurs.

(3) Patient may find that continuing in a peer group setting on a regular, full- or part-time schedule is beneficial. Referral to AA or other support groups is often helpful, especially for long-term recovery.

(4) Halfway houses may be suggested to extend treatment an additional 6 to 12 months.

i. Other forms of substance abuse are treated similarly, with combinations of detoxification, if needed, and supportive long-term treatment settings. Opiate abusers may also be treated with methadone maintenance in attempts to prevent heroin use and allow the addict to return to more socially acceptable behavior patterns (see Critical Thinking Challenge box).

? Critical Thinking Challenge

Drug Abuse

A nurse working in a drug rehabilitation clinic is beginning the admission process by interviewing the patient, Jenny, an 18-year-old being admitted for her repeated use of cocaine over the past 10 months. Her mother is present during the process but does not seem interested in what is going on. However, she also exhibits extreme anxiety because she feels this reflects negatively on her as a mother. Jenny is being uncooperative and completely ignores both her mother and the nurse. How can the nurse best handle this situation and still meet the needs of both Jenny and her mother?

Because Jenny is 18 years old and legally considered an adult, arrange for the mother to talk with a colleague who can help identify the cause of the mother's extreme anxiety. By doing so, the nurse interviewing Jenny will be able to give Jenny her full attention and begin to develop an accepting relationship that will create an environment in which Jenny will feel safe and hopefully more cooperative. This is important because the end goal is for Jenny to be successful in the program. Overall assessment includes obtaining a history of the patient's substance abuse, learning of any relevant medical and psychiatric history, and determining whether or not there are any existing psychosocial issues to be considered. This all takes time and may not be gathered in one or two sessions. Knowing what must be done helps the nurse, in conjunction with the health care team and Jenny, develop an ongoing plan of care.

PHYSICALLY BASED MENTAL DISORDERS

A. Organic brain syndrome (dementia) may result from vascular disorders of the brain, brain infections, trauma, altered metabolism, poisoning, endocrine disorders, and deficiencies.
1. Global involvement: Confusion is often seen in delirium and dementia.
2. Selective involvement: may be limited to portions of the personality (e.g., amnesia, hallucinations, psychosomatic disorders)
3. Functional impairment: has the features of psychosis (e.g., paranoia, depression, mania). Patients with dementia have progressive problems with memory, judgment, and abstract thinking, with abilities eventually declining to difficulty with ADLs.
4. Special needs of the older adult (elderly people): special consideration is given to the role of declining physical attributes.
   a. Prejudices regarding older adults may be present.
   b. Most older adults are not senile.
   c. Apparent senile-type behavior may be the result of depression, delirium, other forms of illness (e.g., alcoholism).
   d. The reaction to drugs of all types may be idiosyncratic (unusual response) among older adults.
   e. Special techniques
      (1) Life review
      (2) Group work aimed at socialization such as remotivation
      (3) Touch: Many older adults are deprived of touch in the usual manner because of relationship losses.
      (4) Medication history review
      (5) See Chapter 9 for special needs of the aging adult.
B. Mental retardation: subaverage intelligence. Numerous causes have been discovered, including inherited defects in metabolism, genetic defects, birth injuries, and developmental anomalies.
1. Classified as follows, with interventions geared accordingly:
   a. Profoundly retarded: needs total nursing care in early stages; may later develop rudimentary ability to care for self; always requires some care
   b. Severely retarded: may be able to care for self in protected environment; requires monitoring
   c. Moderately retarded: usually capable of self-care but requires supervision when under stress
   d. Mildly retarded: usually self-supporting; may require support of family or others when under stress
2. Special needs of children and adolescents: Many similarities and some differences exist in the therapeutics for children and adolescents.
   a. Services in hospitals are usually short and aimed at assessment and evaluation.
   b. Most ongoing treatment is on an outpatient basis.
   c. Treatment is action oriented, with use of such modalities as play therapy, art therapy, and behavioral therapy.
   d. Many issues of trust versus mistrust are present.
   e. Issues of self-image, limit testing, and developmentally specific concerns exist.
   f. Treatment is selected based on the child's mental age, not his or her physical age.

Note: See Chapter 8 regarding autism and related developmental disabilities, which are diagnosed in childhood.

C. Other somatic manifestations of mental disturbance: Several conditions, some of which are listed here, have defined or suggested psychological bases.
1. Ulcers
2. Bowel disorders
3. Cardiovascular disorders
4. Asthma
5. Allergies
6. Eating disorders: anorexia, bulimia
7. Headaches
8. Certain endocrine disorders (e.g., hyperthyroidism, hypothyroidism)

DEATH AND DYING

Nursing intervention is aimed at ensuring the transition of the patient through each of the stages listed in this section. Nurses must be aware of their own attitudes about death and ensure that they are meeting the patient's needs and not their own. Being nonjudgmental and allowing the expression of emotions by the patient are also essential. The patient's defenses are necessary in accepting his or her own death and should not be challenged. Elisabeth Kübler-Ross describes dying as a process that proceeds through the following stages:

A. Shock and denial: Patient cannot actually accept or believe that he or she is going to die. He or she may repress information, seek to escape the truth by seeking other opinions, and be unable to hear the real message.
B. Anger and rage: Patient becomes angry with the terrible truth of impending death; he or she may be hypercritical of others, demanding, and resentful. Health care workers often bear the brunt of a patient's rage because they represent cure for others but not for him or her.
C. Bargaining: Acceptance has begun, and the patient begins to bargain for more time or for some specific request. During this stage wills may be finalized and legacies of various kinds bestowed. If possible, requests should be granted because they bring comfort to the dying person.
D. Depression: After acceptance of the inevitable has begun, the person feels sad and alone. He or she may speak little and cry often. Quiet acceptance is often the most helpful kind of intervention in this stage.
E. Acceptance: Once this occurs, the person is often seen as tranquil and at peace with himself or herself. Again, he or she may speak little because most of what he or she has to say to others has been said. Although still sad, the patient has made his or her peace with death and has accepted the inevitable. This phase may last for months or longer.

GRIEVING

In 1964 George Engel defined grieving as a process of sequential steps similar to those in the dying process.

A. Shock and disbelief: The person refuses to accept the loss and may feel stunned or numbed; it is similar to the first stage of dying.
B. Developing awareness: The person may experience varying degrees of physical symptoms such as nausea, vomiting, and loss of appetite. Crying is common, and anger may be felt and expressed toward the lost person for the act of desertion. Anger may be self-directed, and recriminations may be made.

C. Restitution (resolution): Acceptance occurs and is aided by the culturally approved modes of grieving such as funerals and wearing black.

D. The process of grieving may take more than 1 year. All stages must be experienced for grief to be completed successfully. If grieving is not successful, it may lead to one of the following:
   1. Delayed reaction: a later reaction to the loss. Delay is caused by repressing reality; it may result in more painful experiences than the normal immediate reaction.
   2. Distorted reactions: Symptoms similar to those of the lost person (e.g., medical illnesses, social isolation, agitated depression, and increased use of alcohol or other drug) may develop.

CRISIS INTERVENTION

In general, all crisis situations have common components. Based on this, strategies are developed to assist people through a crisis and minimize its detrimental effects.

A. A crisis is an event that disturbs the equilibrium of the individual or family.

B. A major aspect of crisis is the concept of a loss. This can be an actual loss such as health, life, property, or job or a perceived loss. This can be an individualistic response. A crisis for one person may not be for another.

C. The disturbance leads to development of certain symptoms, most notably anxiety and depression.

D. These feelings continue until a need is felt to reduce or alleviate them.

E. If the person or family has adequate coping mechanisms, the problem is resolved, and balance is restored.

F. Without coping mechanisms, anxiety and depression increase to intolerable levels.

G. Interventions are aimed at providing short-term therapy to increase coping behaviors.

H. Most crises are resolved within 6 to 8 weeks.

I. Intervention entails:
   1. A thorough assessment of the situation.
   2. Planned strategies that do not attempt to rearrange a person's life.
   3. Strategies that increase intellectual understanding, explore current feelings, offer coping mechanisms, and support existing ties and helpful relationships.

CRISIS OF RAPE OR INCEST

Assisting survivors of rape or incest requires substantial time. Intervention begins when the victim calls for help in any form or seeks treatment. This type of violence has two possible phases. One is the acute or immediate phase, during which the victim exhibits fear, confusion, disorganization, and restlessness. The second phase is a long-term process of reorganization and usually begins weeks after the attack.

A. Early relevant feelings include:
   1. Physical pain.
   2. Anger.
   3. Fear of another attack.
   4. Outrage at the perpetrator.
   5. Total violation of (emotional) space.
   6. Fear of involvement with anyone of the same gender as the perpetrator.
   7. Emotional drain.
   8. Helplessness.
   9. Fear of pregnancy.
   10. PTSD—related to certain sights, smells, places.

B. If these immediate feelings are not externalized and dealt with, the result may be serious psychological damage, including but not limited to the following psychosexual dysfunctions:
   1. Sexual arousal disorders
   2. Sexual deviations (several varieties)
   3. Sexual aversions
   4. Delusions of violent sexual behavior, which can then be incorporated in patient's lifestyle

C. Interventions include the following:
   1. Assess victim's safety: "Are you in a safe place?" "Is there help for you?" to address a primary goal of preventing further violence.
   2. Listen and accept what is said.
   3. Respond as appropriate. Strong support, gentle understanding, and nonjudgmental acceptance all aid in the victim's recovery.
   4. Refer patient to appropriate agency.

SUICIDE PREVENTION

Suicide ranks as a leading cause of death in the United States. Specific indicators assist in assessing suicidal risk.

A. Risk factors include:
   1. Age and gender: more women attempt suicide; more men are successful.
   2. Rising adolescent suicide rates.
   3. Higher risk for men older than 35 years of age. Most suicides occur in men aged 35 to 50 years; another 20% occur in Caucasian men older than 65 years.
   4. Anxiety and depression. Many potential suicide victims report increasing anxiety and depression; most significant is a recent change in these feelings.
   5. Past coping pattern does not work in the current situation.
   6. A past suicide attempt, which is always considered a high-risk factor.
   7. Alcohol or drug abuse.
   8. Concrete plan. If a plan is in place, considerations include the following:
      a. Is it set in a current time frame?
      b. Is it lethal?
      c. Does the potential victim have the necessary resources to carry out the plan?
   9. Significant others. A suicide is often committed to communicate with others.

B. Interventions include the following:
   1. Focus on clear and present danger.
   2. Reduce present hazards.
   3. Give clear directions for patient to follow.
   4. Assign constant monitoring in a hospital.
   5. Mobilize significant others when possible.
   6. Mobilize past coping mechanisms.
   7. Assign concrete specific tasks.
   8. Explore positive alternatives to suicide.
   9. Teach problem-solving techniques.
   10. Contract with patient for safety.

SUICIDE INTERVENTION

Intervention becomes critical at the point of suicidal ideation. If intervention does not occur, suicide is highly likely. The patient may be having underlying feelings of hopelessness, helplessness, and impending doom. Frequently the patient verbalizes the need to end it all.

A. Always ask:
  1. "Do I understand that you want to hurt yourself?" (This confirms suicide ideation.)
  2. "Do you have a plan of how you will hurt yourself? Will you share your plan with me?" (Suicidal gesturing may be evident.)
  3. If the specific plan calls for using an enabling device or instrument: "May I have the _____ that is included in the plan?" (Specify item [e.g., knife, razor, or rope].)
B. Ordinarily a loud cry for help can be heard before the suicide occurs if others are perceptive enough to hear it.

Note: Severely depressed patients are often so physically impaired that they rarely have the energy to commit suicide. As the depression begins to lift, the potential to commit suicide increases as the energy level increases; this is especially problematical if the patient has communicated the need to end it all.

TREATMENT MODALITIES

PSYCHOTHERAPY

A. Individual psychotherapy: one-on-one relationship between a therapist (physician, psychologist, social worker, nurse clinician) and a patient. Sessions of 45 to 50 minutes are usually held weekly or more often; the aim is to improve the person's functioning. It is most effective with the neuroses and in patients who have good verbal skills and high intelligence.
B. Family group therapy: A family is seen as a group by a therapist, based on the premise that disturbance arises as a function of family interactions and that treatment must be aimed at the family as a whole.
C. Group therapy: Treatment is provided to a group of people related by age, symptom, or other commonality; it occurs on a weekly or biweekly basis and may include more than one therapist.
D. Behavior modification: Techniques are based on conditioning; undesired behaviors are ignored, and desired behaviors are rewarded.

MILIEU THERAPY

Milieu therapy is the use of a controlled environment to influence the treatment of a patient.

A. Interactions between patient and staff and interpatient relationships are used as a basis for treatment.
B. Therapeutic communications: Behavior modeling and some behavior-modification techniques are often used.

THERAPEUTIC COMMUNITY

Therapeutic community is a method of establishing a milieu for treatment in which all members (staff and patients) have assigned responsibilities and defined roles in the community. The reasoning is that this type of democratic environment prepares the patient for release into the larger community.

ELECTROCONVULSIVE THERAPY

Use of electroconvulsive therapy (ECT, shock therapy) has recently increased for patients with severe depression who have not responded to other therapies. ECT is the application of an electrical current through the brain, resulting in a grand mal seizure. Some patients experience a short-term memory loss as a result of the treatment. A physician, using general anesthesia, gives the treatments; the treatment can be given on an outpatient or inpatient basis. Some patients with severe depression can control further episodes with regular periodic treatments.

PSYCHOPHARMACOLOGICAL THERAPY

Psychopharmacological agents are used in treating mental health disorders. *Note:* When administering medication to the mental health patient, remember to use a tongue blade to examine the interior of the mouth if there is a suspicion that the patient is "cheeking," or hiding the medication in his or her mouth.

A. EPSs: EPSs are unusual muscle movements that involve the fine muscles of the body. These symptoms (dystonia, akinesia, akathisia, tardive dyskinesia) are acute and tonic or dystonic reactions to the antipsychotic medication.
  1. Frequently EPSs appear in the tongue or in the muscles of the upper chest, jaw, neck, and shoulders.
  2. Medications used to reverse the muscular side effects of the antipsychotics are diphenhydramine hydrochloride (Benadryl) and benztropine mesylate (Cogentin).
B. See Chapter 3 for greater detail regarding drugs that are commonly used to treat mental illness. Drugs used to treat psychiatric disorders:
  Antianxiety drugs
  Antidepressants:
  Tricyclic agents
  Monoamine oxidase inhibitors (MAOIs)
  Selective serotonin reuptake inhibitors (SSRIs)
  Antipsychotics and second-generation antipsychotics
  Antimanic agents
  Antiepileptic drugs

ADJUNCTIVE THERAPIES

A. Occupational therapy: use of vocational tasks to encourage patients' expressions of various underlying feelings
B. Recreational therapy: use of recreational activities to allow patients to express feelings
C. Art therapy: use of the various artistic media to express feelings
D. Other therapies: may include vocational counseling, bibliotherapy (writing or reading), and dance therapy

LEGAL AND ETHICAL CONSIDERATIONS IN PATIENT CARE

A. In most places patients may sue institutions under habeas corpus proceedings for their release from treatment.
B. Laws guarantee rights to patients.
C. Nurses and other staff members may be sued for assault and battery for forcing treatments on patients. Close attention must be paid to legal guidelines.
D. Wrongful death suits have followed certain circumstances in which a patient has died.

E. A narrow line exists between therapeutic treatment and abuse; nurses may restrict privileges based on noncompliance with plan of care, but they must be careful that these restrictions are not viewed or used as threats and that required approvals are in place.

F. Local laws vary in different parts of the United States, and nurses should be aware of local statutes.

G. Confidentiality, now stressed in all of health care by way of Health Insurance Portability and Accountability Act (HIPAA) laws, is essential in mental health nursing.

H. Communications between a patient and a nurse may be considered privileged, whereas most medical records are open to subpoena.

I. Documents should contain only factual material, not conjecture (opinion).

J. If a patient threatens bodily harm to others, such information is no longer considered privileged and is required to be reported to the authorities.

K. Aversive treatment may infringe on a patient's rights, and nurses should be aware of their responsibilities in such situations.

L. If the patient has information and chooses not to comply, he or she is noncompliant; the nurse has allowed the patient his or her rights if the information was provided and questions answered. The nurse cannot force a patient to accept treatment.

PATIENTS' RIGHTS

A. Although patients in psychiatric settings are ill, they retain their civil rights and are often specifically protected under special sections of the law.

B. In most jurisdictions, commitment removes only the patient's right to leave the hospital or terminate treatment.

C. Legal decisions indicate that patients may expect treatment and may not simply be detained where no active treatment is available.

D. In recent years patient and former-patient groups have formed and demanded access to records of treatment rationales.

CARE AND TREATMENT OF PATIENTS

The basic needs of patients in psychiatric settings are similar to those of other patients; usually psychiatric patients do not have the accompanying impairments of the physically ill patient.

A. Most patients are ambulatory.

B. The nurse's role is to guide, encourage, and teach by example.

C. Patients may be socially and functionally impaired, requiring assistance in tasks such as ADLs and time management.

D. Interventions such as encouragement and praise are helpful in guiding patients in these activities.

Bibliography

Alfaro-LeFevre R: *Critical thinking, clinical reasoning, and clinical judgment: a practical approach*, ed 5, St Louis, 2013, Mosby.

American Psychiatric Association (APA): *Diagnostic and statistical manual of mental disorders*, ed 5, text revision (DSM-V-TR), Washington, DC, 2013, APA.

Asperheim Favaro MK, Favaro J: *Introduction to pharmacology*, ed 12, St. Louis, 2012, Saunders.

Christensen BL, Kockrow EO: *Foundations of nursing*, ed 6, St Louis, 2010, Mosby.

Edmunds MW: *Introduction to clinical pharmacology*, ed 7, St Louis, 2013, Mosby.

Fortinash KM, Holoday Worret PA: *Psychiatric-mental health nursing*, ed 5, St Louis, 2012, Mosby.

Goodenough A, Zezima K: An alarming new stimulant, legal in many states, *New York Times* , July 16, 2011.

Keltner NL, Bostrom CE, McGuinness T: *Psychiatric nursing*, ed 6, St Louis, 2011, Mosby.

Morrison-Valfre M: *Foundations of mental health care*, ed 5, St Louis, 2013, Mosby.

Stuart GW, Laraia MT: *Principles and practice of psychiatric nursing*, ed 10, St Louis, 2013, Mosby.

Varcarolis EM, Halter MJ: *Essentials of psychiatric mental health nursing*, ed 2, St Louis, 2013, Saunders.

Varcarolis EM, Halter MJ: *Foundations of psychiatric mental health nursing*, ed 6, St Louis, 2010, Saunders.

Volkow ND: *Bath salts: emerging and dangerous products*, February, 2011, National Institute on Drug Abuse Website. Available at http://www.drugabuse.gov/about-nida/directors-page/messages-director/2011/02/bath-salts-emerging-dangerous-products.

REVIEW QUESTIONS

1. The nurse is assigned to work with a depressed patient and wants to make sure that her initial contact does what?
   1. Addresses the root of depression
   2. Keeps communication open
   3. Establishes trust
   4. Raises the patient's spirits

2. Which reasons would cause a psychiatric patient to be hospitalized involuntarily? Select all that apply.
   _____ 1. Homelessness
   _____ 2. Threat to self
   _____ 3. Threat to others
   _____ 4. Low income

3. A patient was given both verbal and written instructions before his discharge. He verbalized an understanding of his instructions but has made no attempt to take his medication as ordered or to return for a follow-up visit. He may be labeled as:
   1. Delusional.
   2. Stuporous.
   3. Noncompliant.
   4. Confabulating.

4. In caring for the suicidal patient, the nurse is aware that all are true *except*:
   1. It is harmful to discuss the subject of suicide because you might give the patient the idea.
   2. Depressed people often show improved mood and attitude once the decision to commit suicide has been made.
   3. Every threat of suicide is serious.
   4. Suicidal behavior is the leading cause of psychiatric hospitalization for young children.

5. The nurse is admitting a schizophrenic patient who has not eaten in 3 days. The nurse arranges for food to be brought to the patient before she begins the admission paperwork. This action best meets which level of Maslow's hierarchy of needs?
   _____ 1. First
   _____ 2. Second

_____ 3. Third

_____ 4. Fourth

6. In what step of the nursing process do the patient and nurse develop the goals?
   1. Data gathering
   2. Planning
   3. Implementation
   4. Evaluation

7. A patient approaches the nurse and says, "I am omnipotent. Someday soon I'm going to take over this unit, you'll see." The appropriate nursing intervention should be to:
   1. Call a code.
   2. Tell the patient that no one is omnipotent and to calm down.
   3. Help the patient find a distraction.
   4. Ask the patient why he thinks he is omnipotent.

8. In what phase of the nurse-patient relationship does termination begin?
   1. Presentation
   2. Orientation
   3. Working
   4. Termination

9. Suicide is most likely to occur:
   1. On admission.
   2. On discharge.
   3. As the depression deepens.
   4. As the depression lifts.

10. Select all the following interventions that may positively affect a patient with obsessive-compulsive disorder (OCD).
    _____ 1. The nurse shows concern for the patient.
    _____ 2. The nurse assists with activities of daily living.
    _____ 3. The nurse hurries the patient through the ritual.
    _____ 4. The nurse makes a point of calling attention to the repetitive act.
    _____ 5. The nurse encourages the patient to reduce the frequency of the behavior.

11. A patient who hallucinates indicates that he smells "something funny." The nurse knows this type of hallucination as:
    1. Tactile.
    2. Auditory.
    3. Gustatory.
    4. Olfactory.

12. To help a patient cope with death, the nurse must first know:
    1. How she feels about death.
    2. How the patient feels about dying.
    3. How the family feels about the patient's illness.
    4. The meaning of death.

13. The patient is being admitted to the psychiatric unit and is extremely agitated and pacing the floor. Which nursing intervention would have priority at this time?
    1. Placing the patient in a quiet area away from other patients
    2. Encouraging the patient to participate in a group activity
    3. Setting firm limits on the patient's behavior
    4. Orienting the patient to his room and the nursing unit

14. The nurse was told in report that she is to observe a particular patient for extrapyramidal side effects, which include:
    1. Dry mouth.
    2. Gastrointestinal upset, constipation.
    3. Heart palpitations.
    4. Muscle rigidity, tremors.

15. A nurse working in a hospice overhears one of the patients talking with the physician, begging to be kept alive just 1 more year. The nurse recognizes this as what stage of the grief process?
    1. Denial
    2. Bargaining
    3. Depression
    4. Acceptance

16. The patient yells at the nurse after talking on the phone with his spouse. The nurse recognizes this as what type of defense mechanism?
    1. Identification
    2. Displacement
    3. Sublimation
    4. Conversion

17. Which sign or symptom would the nurse *not expect* to see in a patient experiencing alcohol withdrawal syndrome?
    1. Restlessness
    2. Tachycardia
    3. Febrile state
    4. Diaphoresis

18. Which statement by the nurse would gain the most information from a patient who is going through a family crisis?
    1. "Do you hate your spouse?"
    2. "Do you and your family get along?"
    3. "Do you see your family often?"
    4. "What is it like with you and your family?"

19. What symptom/s may be seen in a patient diagnosed with anxiety? Select all that apply.
    _____ 1. Pacing
    _____ 2. Hyperventilation
    _____ 3. Muscle tension
    _____ 4. Loss of appetite
    _____ 5. Hypotension
    _____ 6. Calmness

20. What patient complaints and observations may a nurse note in a patient experiencing a panic attack? Select all that apply.
    _____ 1. Feels faint
    _____ 2. Complains of being "dizzy"
    _____ 3. Is able to problem solve
    _____ 4. Has increased attention span
    _____ 5. Is agitated

21. The nurse is caring for a patient returning to his room following electroconvulsive therapy (ECT). What behavior should the nurse expect the patient to exhibit?
    1. The patient complains to the nurse that someone is poisoning his food.
    2. The patient goes to the game room to play pool.
    3. The patient is unable to recall the date.
    4. The patient prepares to go on a field trip.

22. The nurse caring for a depressed patient would expect to see all *except*:
    1. Elevated mood.
    2. Isolation.
    3. Ambivalence.
    4. Overdependence.

23. Patients who abuse alcohol may become tremulous and have hallucinations when they stop drinking. This is known as:
    1. Tolerance.
    2. Abstinence.
    3. Withdrawal.
    4. Dementia.
24. The nurse would suspect that the patient is becoming toxic from his lithium therapy if he begins complaining of: Select all that apply.
    _____ 1. Ringing in ears
    _____ 2. Constipation
    _____ 3. Euphoria
    _____ 4. Nausea
    _____ 5. Tremors
25. Which priority nursing interventions should the nurse use during the manic phase of bipolar disorder? Select all that apply.
    _____ 1. Decrease environmental stimuli
    _____ 2. Ensure a safe environment
    _____ 3. Pace activities to keep patient busy
    _____ 4. Monitor drug levels daily
26. Which items indicate major depression? Select all that apply.
    _____ 1. Hopelessness
    _____ 2. Sadness
    _____ 3. Motivation
    _____ 4. Increased self-esteem
    _____ 5. Weight loss
27. When the nurse gathered admission data on a patient, it was determined that the patient is on the health end of the mental health–mental illness continuum. Which statement best supports these findings?
    1. The patient is in an abusive marriage.
    2. The patient describes her life as boring.
    3. The patient is satisfied with her life.
    4. The patient is being checked for terminal disease.
28. The nurse has noted substantial changes in the behavior of a suicidal patient. Which intervention by the nurse would be most therapeutic?
    1. Document the observations
    2. Ask co-workers if they have also noticed the changes
    3. Ask the patient, "Are you thinking of suicide?"
    4. Restrict the patient's privileges
29. For the patient diagnosed with obsessive-compulsive disorder (OCD), criteria for obsessions include which of the following? Select all that apply.
    _____ 1. The person attempts to suppress or ignore the problematical thoughts.
    _____ 2. Repetitive behaviors are used to reduce anxiety.
    _____ 3. The person denies that such thoughts exist.
    _____ 4. Flashbacks are a frequent occurrence.
    _____ 5. The person recognizes that the thoughts are a product of his own mind.
30. A nurse is caring for a mentally ill patient who is convinced that his wife is trying to kill him. No evidence exists to support this belief. The nurse recognizes that the patient is suffering from:
    1. Delusions.
    2. Hallucinations.
    3. Illusions.
    4. Compensation.

31. A nurse is caring for a patient with bulimia. The patient tells the nurse that she has been bulimic for the last 5 years. When assessing the patient, the nurse hears about the following complaints:
    1. Gastrointestinal upset
    2. Toothache
    3. Diarrhea
    4. Sore throat
32. Paranoid thinking is characterized by feelings of:
    1. Anger and aggression.
    2. Suspicion and jealousy.
    3. Self-pity and self-centeredness.
    4. Simultaneous hero worship and hero hating.
33. The nurse is caring for a patient who is undergoing electroconvulsive therapy (ECT). When planning care for this patient, what should the nurse expect?
    1. The patient will be incontinent.
    2. The patient will be at risk for suicide.
    3. The patient will cry and be depressed.
    4. The patient will be confused and experience a temporary loss of recent memories.
34. An irrational fear is known as a(n):
    1. Flashback.
    2. Hallucination.
    3. Compulsion.
    4. Phobia.
35. A patient admitted with chronic depression has not responded to antidepressant medications. The physician has ordered electroconvulsive therapy (ECT) treatments. The patient has signed the permission slip and is asking the nurse what to expect after the treatment. Which response is most appropriate for the nurse to give the patient?
    1. "ECT changes your chemical messengers."
    2. "ECT changes your subconscious thoughts."
    3. "ECT causes you to have seizure activity."
    4. "ECT helps to alleviate your depression."
36. Which findings would contribute to a diagnosis of anxiety? Select all that apply.
    _____ 1. Follows directions easily
    _____ 2. Apprehension
    _____ 3. Uneasiness
    _____ 4. Decreased concentration
    _____ 5. Pays attention to details
    _____ 6. Waits patiently for a turn
37. A patient approaches the nurse and says, "With all my troubles, I feel worthless. I would like to end this misery. Everyone would be better off if I were gone." The nurse's most appropriate response to this statement would be:
    1. "Tell me more."
    2. "Are you thinking of killing yourself?"
    3. "I can see that you're very upset."
    4. "I have to take blood pressures right now, and then we can talk."
38. A patient exhibiting which signs and symptoms would be diagnosed with a paranoid personality disorder? Select all that apply.
    _____ 1. Is suspicious of others
    _____ 2. Is jealous of his or her spouse
    _____ 3. Has strong social support
    _____ 4. Is able to control his or her temper

39. A 42-year-old patient was admitted to the unit for alcohol rehabilitation. The patient tells the nurse that he often cannot remember what he does while he is drinking. The nurse asks him additional questions and determines that he is experiencing:
    1. Psychosis.
    2. Blackouts.
    3. Denial.
    4. Alcoholism.
40. A patient tells the nurse that the television is cursing her. The idea of the television cursing at the patient is an example of:
    1. Persecutory delusion.
    2. Visual hallucination.
    3. Incoherence.
    4. Flight of ideas.
41. Nurses working on the admissions unit of a psychiatric facility frequently care for aggressive patients. The best nursing intervention in most cases when caring for an aggressive patient is to:
    1. Apply restraints until the patient calms down.
    2. Take away privileges if behavior is inappropriate.
    3. Schedule activities with limited stimuli.
    4. Plan a variety of activities to keep the patient occupied.
42. The nurse assessing the patient with anorexia nervosa would expect to see which of the following? Select all that apply.
    _____ 1. Excessive use of diuretics and laxatives
    _____ 2. Disinterested in body shape and size
    _____ 3. Amenorrhea
    _____ 4. Eating behaviors perceived as a source of self-esteem
43. If codependency exists within a family unit, how may the family be labeled?
    1. Abusive
    2. Neurotic
    3. Dysfunctional
    4. Psychotic
44. Poor impulse control, confidence, rapid speech, and hypertension are all signs and symptoms of which type of intoxication?
    1. Cocaine
    2. Alcohol
    3. Opiate
    4. Hallucinogenic
45. A patient rushes up to the nurse and says, "They're after me. They want to torture and kill me." What is the most appropriate response?
    1. "Tell me who they are."
    2. "There's no one here except you and me."
    3. "I need to go look for myself."
    4. "you'resafe here. Can you tell me more?"
46. The nurse is caring for a patient experiencing extrapyramidal side effects from antipsychotic medications. All of the following medications are ordered. Which one should the nurse administer for the side effects?
    1. Furosemide (Lasix)
    2. Benztropine mesylate (Cogentin)
    3. Prochlorperazine (Compazine)
    4. Acetaminophen (Tylenol)

47. Why is it important that detoxification for substance abuse occur in a hospital setting?
    1. Adequate rest and nutrition are needed.
    2. Panic attacks may occur.
    3. It may become life-threatening.
    4. Other substances can be substituted for the substance of abuse.
48. Select the nursing intervention that should take priority in a crisis.
    1. Allow friends to visit.
    2. Provide a safe environment.
    3. Rearrange the patient's schedule.
    4. Make decisions for the patient.
49. A patient complains of trouble with control of his tongue. The neck muscles are also beginning to tighten, and the patient is having difficulty keeping his head in an upright position. The nurse's first response should be to:
    1. Check the medication administration record.
    2. Call the physician.
    3. Draw blood per standing order.
    4. Fill out an incident report.
50. A 46-year-old patient is admitted to the psychiatric unit of the hospital because of an increasingly depressed mood. After a few weeks of treatment the nurse observes that the patient has started putting on large amounts of makeup, has become seductive with male patients, and stays up very late pacing the floor. The nurse might conclude that the patient:
    1. Was initially diagnosed incorrectly.
    2. May be having a manic episode as part of her illness.
    3. Is showing signs of recovery.
    4. May be having side effects of the medication.
51. Characteristics often associated with dementia include which of the following? Select all that apply.
    _____ 1. Difficulty concentrating
    _____ 2. Insomnia
    _____ 3. Symptoms that are permanent and progressive
    _____ 4. Lethargy
    _____ 5. Sudden onset
52. Extreme mood swings ranging from deep depression to high activity levels are most often seen in:
    1. Paranoid disorders.
    2. Bipolar disorders.
    3. Schizophrenia.
    4. Eating disorders
53. The nurse is completing discharge instructions for a patient being discharged on disulfiram (Antabuse) to help avoid using alcohol. Which statement should the nurse include in the teaching?
    1. "You will need biweekly blood work to determine blood levels of the medication."
    2. "The disulfiram can cause you to be sensitive to sunlight."
    3. "This drug causes sedation; do not operate heavy equipment."
    4. "The disulfiram can stay in your system as long as 14 days after you stop taking the medication."
54. If a nurse were to select a single identifying characteristic of the patient with obsessive-compulsive disorder (OCD), it would be:
    1. Desire for seclusion.
    2. Aggression.
    3. Orderliness.
    4. Instant gratification.

55. A nurse is caring for a patient experiencing manic behavior who is too distracted to eat. The most appropriate nursing intervention should be to:
    1. Plan mealtime as a social event.
    2. Plan for meals that include the patient's favorite foods.
    3. Offer finger foods that the patient can eat on the go.
    4. Provide a calm mealtime.
56. Which group of people listed here should the nurse expect to be most likely to abuse inhalants?
    1. Adolescents, particularly in groups
    2. Middle-aged men
    3. Older men
    4. Pregnant females
57. A patient tells the nurse that he is depressed over the recent death of a parent. Which response is the best communication intervention for this patient?
    1. Say nothing.
    2. "Wouldn't you rather talk about something else?"
    3. "I have some time. Tell me more about your feelings."
    4. "I don't have time for sad people."
58. What illegal drug is often snorted to obtain confidence and euphoria?
    1. Heroin
    2. Cocaine
    3. Marijuana
    4. LSD
59. The nurse is preparing a patient for discharge. Which statement by the patient diagnosed with anxiety would indicate that he understands his diagnosis?
    1. "Wine with my meals may help me cope better with my anxiety."
    2. "I understand that anxiety sometimes will help me perform better."
    3. "As long as I take my antianxiety medication, I can continue to work 16 to 18 hours per day."
    4. "I understand that my life will be great from now on."
60. A nurse working on an inpatient psychiatric unit is also responsible for operating a 24-hour emergency telephone line. During a short time four potential suicide calls have come in. Which caller should the nurse rank at greatest risk for carrying out his or her suicide threat?
    1. An adolescent who is thinking of cutting his wrist
    2. A young adult who has agreed to go to the emergency department
    3. A young man who plans to use a gun
    4. A young woman who is talking of overdosing on pills
61. What defense mechanism do nurses commonly see used by patients admitted for drug abuse?
    1. Substitution
    2. Rationalization
    3. Identification
    4. Denial
62. A patient on a psychiatric unit makes all of the following comments. Which comment suggests that the patient may be suffering from mania?
    1. "I get messages from my dead mother."
    2. "Leave me alone while I'm playing solitaire."
    3. "I don't need to sleep."
    4. "My health is very important to me."
63. In assessing suicidal risk, what is a high-risk factor?
    1. Long psychotherapeutic treatment
    2. A concrete plan that is relatively lethal
    3. Past attempts, because these usually mean that the person is now able to cope better with stresses
    4. Deviance in the person's background
64. If a nurse forces treatment on a patient against his or her will, the nurse may be sued for:
    1. False imprisonment.
    2. Assault and battery.
    3. Wrongful death.
    4. Habeas corpus.
65. The nurse understands that the patient who has been committed to the hospital may:
    1. Have length of hospitalization determined by the court.
    2. Lose all of his or her civil rights.
    3. Not have access to his or her records.
    4. Not make any decisions regarding his or her care.
66. The physician slams the chart down and leaves in a huff shortly after meeting with a young patient to discuss her terminal diagnosis. This is an example of which defense mechanism?
    1. Rationalization
    2. Undoing
    3. Displacement
    4. Compensation
67. The nurse recognizes the communication technique of receiving information and examining responses to the message as:
    1. Restating.
    2. Listening.
    3. Reflection.
    4. Clarification.
68. The nurse encourages the patient to expand on a given topic, using:
    1. Restating.
    2. Broad openings.
    3. Reflection.
    4. Silence.
69. Which statement is most true about the difference between a delusion and a hallucination?
    1. Delusions are false beliefs; hallucinations are false sensory perceptions.
    2. Delusions are systems; hallucinations are beliefs.
    3. Delusions are always true; hallucinations are always false.
    4. Delusions are based on fact; hallucinations are based on belief.
70. The nurse states, "don't worry, everything will be all right." This is an example of what type of communication?
    1. Offering false reassurance
    2. Offering approval
    3. Minimizing the problem
    4. Offering advice
71. When a patient makes a statement that negates what he said to the nurse earlier in the day, the nurse recognizes that the patient is using the defense mechanism of:
    1. Rationalization.
    2. Projection.
    3. Regression.
    4. Undoing.

72. The chief defense mechanism used by the alcoholic (addict) is:
    1. Denial.
    2. Compensation.
    3. Reaction formation.
    4. Sublimation.
73. In a crisis the aim of intervention is to:
    1. Rearrange life elements of the people involved.
    2. Provide treatment for as long as possible.
    3. Offer support and explore alternatives.
    4. Avoid old ties because these led up to the crisis.
74. The nurse is explaining a diagnostic test to the patient. The patient is very anxious about the test. What should the nurse do to reduce the patient's anxiety?
    1. Explain the details of the procedure to the patient
    2. Explain the treatment the test provides
    3. Explain the patient's nothing by mouth (NPO) status
    4. Assure the patient that the test is very accurate in identifying health problems
75. Which question by the nurse would best determine if her patient is a victim of abuse?
    1. Are you being abused?
    2. Are the children being abused?
    3. Have neighbors or relatives witnessed any abuse?
    4. Can he or she make a home visit to determine if any abuse is occurring?
76. In a psychiatric setting a nurse would understand that patients diagnosed with posttraumatic stress disorder (PTSD) commonly report:
    1. Auditory hallucinations.
    2. Recurring nightmares.
    3. Displaced anger.
    4. Depression.
77. A patient on suicide precautions reports a recent positive change in mood. The nurse knows that:
    1. This is a high-risk factor.
    2. The crisis has probably passed.
    3. The patient may be manic-depressive.
    4. The patient is responding to the added attention of the precautions.
78. Posttraumatic stress disorder (PTSD) is seen not only in the military, but also in people:
    1. Raised in foster care.
    2. With a genetic weakness.
    3. With work-related failures.
    4. Who have survived a catastrophe.
79. What complication might the nurse expect in a patient withdrawing from alcohol?
    1. Bleeding
    2. Jaundice
    3. Polyphagia
    4. Seizures
80. A severely depressed patient tells the nurse, "There is no reason for me to continue living." Which response by the nurse would be the most appropriate?
    1. "Are you thinking about suicide?"
    2. "There are a lot of people worse off than you."
    3. "What would your family do?"
    4. "You have a lot to live for."
81. For the nurse to accept the alcoholic patient's behavior, he or she must first:
    1. Look at the patient's motives.
    2. Look at his or her own feelings about alcoholism.

3. Compare normal and abnormal behavior.
4. Take a course in crisis management.
82. Which nursing action takes priority when administering medications to a depressed patient?
    1. Make sure that the patient drinks plenty of water.
    2. Make sure that the patient swallows the medication.
    3. Give the medication on an empty stomach.
    4. Give the medication exactly on time.
83. The nurse is caring for a patient with dementia and memory loss. Which communication technique would be most effective?
    1. Talk loudly
    2. Repeat everything three times
    3. Use short sentences
    4. Use written communications
84. A middle-aged male patient is in the waiting room of the physician's office. He has come to get the results of his prostate biopsy. He is overheard laughing loudly and telling inappropriate jokes. The nurse should:
    1. Ask the patient to be quiet.
    2. Ignore the patient's behavior.
    3. Move the patient to an examination room as soon as possible.
    4. Recognize that the patient is expressing his anxiety.
85. Patients diagnosed with major depression commonly display signs of:
    1. Anxiety.
    2. Agitation.
    3. Energy.
    4. Hopelessness.
86. The nurse collects objective and subjective data from a newly diagnosed mental health patient. What is a good example of subjective data?
    1. Stares into space blankly
    2. Looks sad
    3. Appears in no acute distress
    4. States, "I have no energy and have to drag myself out of bed."
87. What type of coping mechanism is used when anxiety is resolved?
    1. Adaptive
    2. Palliative
    3. Maladaptive
    4. Dysfunctional
88. What is likely to happen when the nurse leaves a highly anxious patient to go and check on another patient?
    1. The patient understands that the nurse has other patients to check.
    2. The patient becomes depressed.
    3. The patient becomes more anxious.
    4. The patient seeks someone else with whom to talk.
89. A schizophrenic patient who appears to be in a stupor may be:
    1. Paranoid.
    2. Catatonic.
    3. Incoherent.
    4. Suspicious.
90. Characteristics of delirium usually include all except:
    1. Slow, insidious onset.
    2. Affects consciousness.
    3. Frequently reversible.
    4. Delusions and hallucinations.

91. A mentally retarded child who demonstrates academic skills at the second-grade level, can attend to personal care with supervision, and adapts well to community life in a supervised environment would likely be classified as having:
    1. Profound mental retardation.
    2. Severe mental retardation.
    3. Moderate mental retardation.
    4. Mild mental retardation.

92. The nurse is caring for a patient recently diagnosed with a severe, rare form of bone cancer. At what stage of the grief process would the nurse expect the patient to be more demanding and resentful?
    1. Bargaining
    2. Anger
    3. Denial
    4. Acceptance

93. The nurse doing medication discharge teaching for a patient receiving monoamine oxidase inhibitor (MAOI) antidepressants would be sure to include which guidelines? Select all that apply.
    _____ 1. Advise to have medication blood levels checked regularly.
    _____ 2. Advise regarding dietary restrictions, especially with foods high in tyramine.
    _____ 3. Advise to watch for temperature elevation as an indication of neuroleptic malignant syndrome (NMS).
    _____ 4. Advise that even over-the-counter medications require physician approval because of possible drug interactions.

94. The nurse is preparing to do the discharge teaching for a patient recently started on antianxiety medication. The physician has left a prescription for the patient. What is the first step in the teaching process?
    1. Give the patient the prescription.
    2. Provide the patient with written drug information.
    3. Assess the patient's knowledge about the new medication.
    4. Explain common side effects of the medication.

95. Prioritize the four phases of the nurse-patient relationship.
    1. Working phase
    2. Orientation phase
    3. Termination phase
    4. Preorientation phase

96. The nurse recognizes that a patient who was raised by an abusive mother and then describes that relationship as "ideal, warm, and nurturing" is demonstrating which defense mechanism?
    1. Projection
    2. Regression
    3. Reaction formation
    4. Displacement

97. The patient has benztropine mesylate (Cogentin) ordered for extrapyramidal side effects (EPSs). Which of the medications that the patient is receiving is most likely causing these reactions?
    1. Valproic acid (Depakene)
    2. Fluoxetine (Prozac)
    3. Lithium
    4. Haloperidol (Haldol)

98. After a co-worker is overlooked for a promotion he thought he deserved, he begins coming in late; leaving tasks undone; and turning in sloppy, incomplete work. This response could be labeled as:
    1. Passive-aggressive behavior.
    2. Battery.
    3. Substitution.
    4. Undoing.

99. The preparation phase of the therapeutic relationship includes which tasks? Select all that apply.
    _____ 1. Building trust
    _____ 2. Collecting data from chart and significant others
    _____ 3. Having the patient try out new behaviors
    _____ 4. Examination by the nurse of her own feelings and reactions to this patient and his problems

100. A mental status examination would include assessing which of the following? Select all that apply.
    _____ 1. Health history data from the chart
    _____ 2. Thought processes and content
    _____ 3. Level of consciousness
    _____ 4. Mood
    _____ 5. Identification of patient's strengths
    _____ 6. Motor activity

ANSWERS AND RATIONALES

1. Application, planning, psychosocial integrity, (b).
   3. Trust is essential when working with a depressed patient.
   1, 4. These are ongoing processes.
   2. This is not the first priority.

2. Comprehension, implementation, psychosocial integrity, (a).
   _____ 1. Although this is not grounds for hospitalization, homelessness may be an end product of chronic mental illness.
   __X__ 2. **This is a reason to hospitalize a person for further evaluation and treatment to decrease the threat.**
   __X__ 3. **This is a reason to hospitalize a person for further evaluation and treatment to decrease the threat.**
   _____ 4. Low income may contribute to noncompliance with treatment but is not a reason to institutionalize someone.

3. Knowledge, assessment, psychosocial integrity, (a).
   3. This patient is noncompliant: the situation presented clearly demonstrates an informed decision by the patient not to adhere to treatment.
   1. This represents a false belief unchanged by reasoning or explanation.
   2. This is a level of consciousness that requires stimulation to stay awake.
   4. This is filling in memory losses with untrue statements.

4. Application, implementation, psychosocial integrity, (b).
   1. The interest and concern expressed offer acceptance and emotional support.
   2, 3, 4. These are all often true for suicidal patients.

5. Application, implementation, psychosocial integrity, (b).
   __X__ 1. **First level applies to physiological needs (air, water, food, shelter, rest and sleep, activity, and temperature maintenance)**
   _____ 2. Second level applies to safety and security.
   _____ 3. Third level applies to love and belonging.
   _____ 4. Fourth level applies to esteem needs.

6. Comprehension, planning, psychosocial integrity, (b).
   2. *Patient and nurse work together to set goals in this phase.*
   1. Much of this phase may occur before the nurse sees the patient.
   3. In this phase the interventions are carried out.
   4. In this phase they are evaluating whether the goals worked.
7. Analysis, implementation, psychosocial integrity, (c).
   3. *This is the most appropriate option; briefly acknowledge the patient's feelings and then distract him by offering a less-threatening topic or activity.*
   1. Measures to reduce anxiety should be started at the first sign of anxiety or discomfort.
   2. Never challenge the patient's delusion system; he will have to defend it.
   4. This reinforces the delusion, and the patient is further from reality.
8. Application, assessment, psychosocial integrity, (b).
   2. *In this phase the nurse meets the patient and discusses the nurse's involvement.*
   1. This occurs before the nurse meets the patient.
   3. The patient upholds the terms of the contract, which establishes goals and priorities of treatment.
   4. The patient may be angry if the nurse does not let him know in advance when the relationship will end.
9. Comprehension, assessment, psychosocial integrity, (b).
   4. *Most authorities agree that as depression lifts, the patient is at greatest risk for committing suicide.*
   1. He will not likely attempt suicide during the admission process.
   2. A patient who is suicidal will not be discharged.
   3. As depression deepens, he will not have energy to commit suicide.
10. Application, implementation, psychosocial integrity, (b).
    __X__ 1. *This is therapeutic.*
    _____ 2. This has no effect on the ritual.
    _____ 3. The nurse should allow time for the ritual.
    _____ 4. The nurse should not call attention to the act.
    __X__ 5. *This is therapeutic.*
11. Comprehension, assessment, psychosocial integrity, (a).
    4. *This involves a smell, odor, or aroma.*
    1. This involves touch sensation.
    2. This involves hearing.
    3. This involves flavor or taste.
12. Analysis, assessment, psychosocial integrity, (b).
    1. *Nurses must first be in touch with their feelings.*
    2. This is nursing's second priority.
    3. Nurses should also consider this, but knowing their own feelings about death is a priority.
    4. This is not a priority.
13. Application, implementation, psychosocial integrity, (b).
    1. *Remove the patient from added stimuli so he can better cope.*
    2. The patient does not need added stimuli at this time.
    3. The patient cannot control his anxiety.
    4. Added stimuli are contraindicated.
14. Analysis, evaluation, physiological integrity, (b).
    4. *These are common extrapyramidal side effects.*
    1. This is considered an anticholinergic side effect.
    2, 3. These are not considered abnormal involuntary movement disorders.

15. Comprehension, assessment, psychosocial integrity, (a).
    2. *This is common in the bargaining phase.*
    1. In this phase the patient says, "No, not me."
    3. In depression he quietly sits in the dark.
    4. He is calm and peaceful.
16. Comprehension, assessment, psychosocial integrity, (b).
    2. *Displacement means that feelings for an object or person are transferred to a less threatening object or person.*
    1. Identification refers to taking on the characteristics of another.
    3. Sublimation refers to channeling unacceptable behaviors into socially acceptable ones.
    4. Conversion refers to channeling anxieties into physical symptoms.
17. Comprehension, assessment, physiological integrity, (b).
    3. *Typically, a febrile state is not identified with alcohol withdrawal.*
    1, 2, 4. Restlessness, tachycardia, and diaphoresis are classic symptoms of a person withdrawing from alcohol.
18. Application, implementation, safe and effective care environment, (b).
    4. *The nurse should encourage the patient to express his feelings.*
    1, 2, 3. These are not appropriate because they are closed questions that will elicit only a yes-or-no response.
19. Application, assessment, psychosocial integrity, (b).
    __X__ 1. *This symptom is usually seen in varying degrees.*
    __X__ 2. *This symptom is usually seen in varying degrees.*
    __X__ 3. *This symptom is usually seen in varying degrees.*
    __X__ 4. *This symptom is usually seen in varying degrees.*
    _____ 5. Hypertension may be seen but not hypotension.
    _____ 6. The patient is more likely to be aggressive.
20. Comprehension, assessment, psychosocial integrity, (a).
    __X__ 1. *This is expected in panic-attack victims.*
    __X__ 2. *This is expected in panic-attack victims.*
    _____ 3. This is incorrect; the patient is unable to solve problems.
    _____ 4. Decreased attention span is seen.
    __X__ 5. *This is expected in panic-attack victims.*
21. Application, evaluation, physiological integrity, (b).
    3. *Amnesia is common after ECT.*
    1. Paranoid behavior is not seen with ECT.
    2. The patient is probably sedated.
    4. The patient is more likely to be sedated.
22. Knowledge, assessment, psychosocial integrity, (a).
    1. *Elevated and expansive mood is usually seen in a patient experiencing the manic phase of a bipolar illness.*
    2, 3, 4. These are classic symptoms often seen with the depressed patient.
23. Knowledge, assessment, physiological integrity, (a).
    3. *Symptoms occur after stopping the drug.*
    1. Tolerance means increasing doses are required to achieve effects.
    2. To abstain is to avoid drinking.
    4. Dementia is unrelated.

24. Application, assessment, psychosocial integrity, (b).
    _X_ 1. Ringing in ears is a typical symptom of lithium toxicity.
    _____ 2. Diarrhea, sometimes severe, frequently accompanies lithium toxicity.
    _____ 3. This is a symptom of an acute manic episode but is not seen with lithium toxicity.
    _X_ 4. Nausea is a typical symptom of lithium toxicity.
    _X_ 5. Tremors are a typical symptom of lithium toxicity.
25. Application, implementation, psychosocial integrity, (b).
    _X_ 1. This is therapeutic.
    _X_ 2. This is therapeutic.
    _____ 3. Patients in the manic phase are already extremely active.
    _____ 4. They are not monitored daily but usually biweekly initially and then every 2 to 3 months after becoming stable.
26. Application, assessment, psychosocial integrity, (b).
    _X_ 1. This is a classic symptom.
    _X_ 2. This is a classic symptom.
    _____ 3. Decreased motivation is noted.
    _____ 4. Decreased self-esteem is noted.
    _X_ 5. This is a classic symptom.
27. Comprehension, assessment, psychosocial integrity, (a).
    3. This is a healthy response.
    1. This is unhealthy.
    2, 4. These move toward the illness end of the continuum.
28. Application, implementation, psychosocial integrity, (b).
    3. Be direct; ask the patient what the nurse needs to know.
    1. This takes no action related to the nurse's suspicions.
    2. This does nothing to allay the nurse's concerns.
    4. This may make the patient feel worse or unworthy.
29. Comprehension, assessment, psychosocial integrity, (a).
    _X_ 1. The person recognizes that the obsessive thoughts are of his own creation but cannot avoid acknowledging them.
    _____ 2. These define compulsions, the behaviors in which the patient engages when trying to lessen the produced anxieties from the obsessive thoughts.
    _____ 3. Far from denying, the patient readily acknowledges the problematical thoughts but has difficulty not acting on them.
    _____ 4. Flashbacks are common with posttraumatic stress disorder, not with OCD.
    _X_ 5. The person recognizes that the obsessive thoughts are of his own creation but cannot avoid acknowledging them.
30. Application, assessment, psychosocial integrity, (b).
    1. A delusion is a false fixed idea.
    2. A hallucination is a sensory experience.
    3. An illusion is a misrepresentation.
    4. Compensation is a defense mechanism.
31. Application, assessment, psychosocial integrity, (b).
    2. Erosion of tooth enamel is common.
    1, 3, 4. These complaints are not as common as toothache.
32. Comprehension, assessment, psychosocial integrity, (b).
    2. Suspicion and jealousy are the predominant thoughts of the paranoid patient.
    1. Paranoid patients are so preoccupied with suspicion and jealousy that these are not substantial possibilities.

3. Self-pity and self-centeredness are more closely associated with the depressed patient who is trying to blame himself or herself or relieve feelings of guilt.
    4. This is the definition of ambivalence.
33. Application, planning, psychosocial integrity, (b).
    4. Temporary amnesia is expected after ECT.
    1. This is not an expected outcome after ECT.
    2. ECT patients are not usually suicidal.
    3. ECT treats depression.
34. Knowledge, assessment, psychosocial integrity, (a).
    4. Phobia is the correct response.
    1. *Flashback* refers to reliving a traumatic event, often seen in posttraumatic stress disorder.
    2. The term *hallucination* refers to an alteration in perception, involving any of the five senses.
    3. *Compulsion* refers to behaviors designed to decrease anxiety resulting from obsessive thoughts.
35. Application, implementation, psychosocial integrity, (b).
    4. This is the desired effect of the treatment and can be more effective than medications; for this patient, this is the most appropriate response.
    1. This is the primary effect of antidepressant medications, although some people believe that ECT causes changes in monoamine neurotransmitter systems.
    2. Although ECT may cause a brief period of amnesia, it does not last. This affects conscious thinking.
    3. This occurs during the treatment.
36. Comprehension, assessment, psychosocial integrity, (b).
    _____ 1. This is incorrect; anxious people have difficulty with details.
    _X_ 2. This is a symptom of anxiety.
    _X_ 3. This is a symptom of anxiety.
    _X_ 4. This is a symptom of anxiety.
    _____ 5. This is incorrect; the person finds details difficult.
    _____ 6. This is incorrect; anxious people are usually impatient.
37. Application, implementation, safe and effective care environment, (b).
    2. Identify the plan and then intervene; be direct.
    1. "Tell me more" may not identify the plan.
    3. Although this is true, it does not address the plan.
    4. This response is incorrect; if anyone approaches the nurse with statements such as the ones in this question, he or she should find out if the person has a plan.
38. Application, assessment, psychosocial integrity, (b).
    _X_ 1. Suspicion is seen in paranoia.
    _X_ 2. Jealousy is seen in paranoia.
    _____ 3. This is incorrect; the person may lack social support.
    _____ 4. This is incorrect; the person has trouble controlling temper.
39. Comprehension, evaluation, psychosocial integrity, (b).
    2. A blackout is the inability to remember what was done while under the influence of alcohol.
    1. Psychosis would include short-term and long-term memory loss.
    3. Denial is a part of the grieving process.
    4. He may be alcoholic, but this does not explain the memory loss.
40. Analysis, assessment, psychosocial integrity, (c).
    1. In a persecutory delusion the television actually does not curse the patient; she feels persecuted by it.
    2. This is not a visual hallucination.

3. This is not incoherent but structured thought.

4. This is not flight of ideas.

41. Application, implementation, psychosocial integrity, (b).

    3. Excessive stimuli can agitate the patient.

    1. Restraints would be a last resort.

    2. Behavior modification may not be appropriate on an admissions unit.

    4. This would provide too many stimuli.

42. Application, assessment, psychosocial integrity, (b).

    _____ 1. Bulimic patients typically abuse these, not anorexic ones.

    _____ 2. Anorexic patients are fixated, or unduly focused, on body size and shape, often misperceiving themselves as fat even when emaciated.

    __X__ 3. **This is a classic symptom of anorexia. The amenorrhea occurs over several months.**

    __X__ 4. **This is a classic symptom of anorexia. Control over eating is desirable in the anorexic patient.**

43. Comprehension, assessment, psychosocial integrity, (a).

    3. The family may be labeled as dysfunctional.

    1. This refers to intentional misuse of another.

    2, 4. These refer to an individual's maladaptive coping.

44. Knowledge, assessment, psychosocial integrity, (a).

    1. These are seen with cocaine use.

    2. These do not indicate alcohol abuse.

    3. These are not common with opiates.

    4. These are not seen with hallucinogenic drug use.

45. Application, assessment, psychosocial integrity, (b).

    4. Assurance and willingness to listen are key to therapeutic relations.

    1. The nurse's knowledge may intimidate the patient; do not buy into their false beliefs.

    2. Be nonjudgmental and nonthreatening.

    3. Avoid buying into a false belief.

46. Application, planning, physiological integrity, (b).

    2. This is the drug of choice.

    1. This is a diuretic.

    3. This is used as a sedative for nausea.

    4. Acetaminophen is an analgesic.

47. Comprehension, planning, psychosocial integrity, (b).

    3. Life-threatening events may occur.

    1. A person does not have to be hospitalized to get adequate rest and food.

    2. This is not usually seen with withdrawal and detoxification.

    4. This is not necessary.

48. Application, implementation, psychosocial integrity, (b).

    2. Safety is always a priority.

    1. This may not be appropriate during the crisis.

    3. This is not a good time to attempt to make a change.

    4. This is not a priority at this time.

49. Analysis, evaluation, physiological integrity, (c).

    1. This is the correct answer; the patient may be experiencing the beginning effects called extrapyramidal side effects or symptoms (EPSs). These symptoms are associated with the administration of antipsychotic medications. An anti-EPS medication will probably be ordered to reverse the EPSs.

    2, 3. These are not appropriate as a first response.

    4. This should not be a first response but may be required at some point in the event.

50. Analysis, assessment, psychosocial integrity, (b).

    2. The behavioral changes indicate mania.

    1. This may not be true; diagnosis was accurate for the presenting symptoms.

    3. This is not true; the change is too rapid and extreme.

    4. This is unrelated.

51. Application, implementation, psychosocial integrity, (b).

    __X__ 1. **This is typically apparent with dementia, notably Alzheimer type.**

    _____ 2. Sleep patterns are often unchanged.

    __X__ 3. **This is typically apparent with dementia, notably Alzheimer type.**

    _____ 4. Activity levels are often normal.

    _____ 5. Symptoms are usually slow in onset, especially Alzheimer type.

52. Comprehension, assessment, psychosocial integrity, (a).

    2. Mood swings are the characteristics of bipolar disorder; manic (elation) and depression are two phases.

    1. Paranoid disorders generally do not involve mood swings.

    3. Schizophrenia is characterized by disorganized thinking.

    4. People with eating disorders do not experience mood swings.

53. Application, evaluation, physiological integrity, (b).

    4. This is a true statement.

    1. Toxic blood levels are not a concern.

    2. Photosensitivity is not a problem.

    3. Sedation is not a side effect.

54. Comprehension, assessment, psychosocial integrity, (a).

    3. Orderliness is the single feature of the patient with OCD; activities are usually performed as rituals.

    1. The patient with OCD is so busy thinking and doing that a time for seclusion would not exist.

    2. Aggression is not an obsessive-compulsive characteristic.

    4. Instant gratification is related to poor impulse control; the patient with OCD has an overwhelming need to perform activities that release the underlying feelings.

55. Application, planning, physiological integrity, (b).

    3. During the manic phase, patients have trouble being still but may eat on the go.

    1. This will not make the patient comply.

    2. This will not make the patient able to comply.

    4. The patient will still be experiencing difficulty in focusing.

56. Comprehension, assessment, psychosocial integrity, (a).

    1. Inhalants are most commonly abused by individuals of this age, particularly in group settings.

    2, 3. These groups are not commonly seen abusing inhalants.

    4. This group most commonly abuses nicotine, alcohol, and marijuana, although opiate usage is increasing.

57. Application, implementation, psychosocial integrity, (b).

    3. An open-ended question, with ample time to listen, is the best therapeutic technique in this situation.

    1. The nurse should indicate an interest in what the patient has said; saying nothing is the wrong intervention.

    2. The pressing issue is death of parents; diversion of discussion is not appropriate.

    4. This is inappropriate, and it is insulting.

58. Comprehension, evaluation, psychosocial integrity, (a).
    2. Cocaine increases confidence and decreases judgment; it causes euphoria.
    1. Heroin causes euphoria and slurred speech.
    3. Marijuana causes euphoria and increased appetite.
    4. LSD (lysergic acid diethylamide) alters perception and causes paranoia.
59. Analysis, evaluation, psychosocial integrity, (c).
    2. Anxiety is sometimes a healthy response to problems.
    1. Alcohol is not effective in managing anxiety.
    3. Leisure time is necessary for a healthy lifestyle.
    4. The patient will still have good and bad days.
60. Analysis, assessment, psychosocial integrity, (b)
    3. A gun would be a very serious weapon.
    1. The patient is thinking of it but has no exact plan or weapon.
    2. This individual is seeking help.
    4. The patient does not necessarily have pills.
61. Comprehension, assessment, psychosocial integrity, (a).
    4. Drug users frequently deny they have a problem.
    1. This is not commonly used by drug abusers.
    2. This is not seen as often as denial.
    3. This is not frequently seen.
62. Comprehension, assessment, psychosocial integrity, (a).
    3. This is common among patients with mania.
    1. This behavior is not seen in manic patients.
    2. The patient probably would not be focused enough to remain still to play cards.
    4. This attitude is not associated with mania.
63. Application, assessment, psychosocial integrity, (b).
    2. A concrete, lethal plan is a very high–risk factor.
    1. Treatment duration is usually unrelated.
    3. The presence of past attempts is high risk but not for the reason stated.
    4. This is unrelated.
64. Application, implementation, psychosocial integrity, (b).
    2. Forcing treatment on a patient may result in assault and battery charges.
    1. This refers to the patient being held against his or her will.
    3. This applies if the patient dies because of a treatment error.
    4. Patients use this to petition the court for their release.
65. Comprehension, evaluation, psychosocial integrity, (b).
    1. If the patient were committed by the court, length of stay and treatment regimens require court approval.
    2. The patient does not lose his or her civil rights.
    3. Many people request access to records.
    4. The patient can make some decisions.
66. Comprehension, evaluation, psychosocial integrity, (a).
    3. The physician is frustrated over the diagnosis and was not able to express this with the patient.
    1. No explanation was given.
    2. Nothing was undone.
    4. He did not try to make up for a deficiency.
67. Application, assessment, psychosocial integrity, (b).
    2. Active listening is being defined.
    1. This is repeating what was said.
    3. This is giving back what was said.
    4. This means to explain using other words.
68. Application, implementation, psychosocial integrity, (b).
    2. This helps the patient expand on what he or she is saying.
    1. This is repeating what the patient has said.
    3. This is directing what the patient said back to him or her.
    4. This is a lack of communication.
69. Comprehension, assessment, psychosocial integrity, (a).
    1. These are definitions of the respective terms.
    2. Although both are beliefs, hallucinations are based on misconceptions, and delusions are not based on anything real.
    3. Delusions are always false, as are hallucinations.
    4. Both are real to the patient; hallucinations have triggers.
70. Comprehension, implementation, psychosocial integrity, (b).
    1. This is an example of offering false hope, which is never therapeutic.
    2. Offering approval does nothing to make the patient feel better about what was said. An example of this would be, "That's good."
    3. Minimizing a problem cuts off communication and does not help build nurse-patient relationships. An example of this would be, "That's okay. It's not a big deal."
    4. Offering advice is not allowing patients to make their own decisions. An example of this would be, "I think you should…"
71. Application, assessment, psychosocial integrity, (b).
    4. Undoing is undoing (negating) previous declarations.
    1. Rationalization is offering a socially acceptable explanation.
    2. Projection puts thoughts and actions on others.
    3. Regression is retreating to an earlier level of development.
72. Comprehension, assessment, psychosocial integrity, (a).
    1. Denial is the chief defense mechanism used by an addict; an addict can always find a reason to drink.
    2. The addiction is the weakness and has an underlying cause that is uncompensated.
    3. Although underlying feelings of guilt and sadness are relieved by the addiction, these feelings return once the drug wears off. The addiction is not the expression of an opposite attitude; it is relief from the underlying feelings.
    4. Sublimation does not fit in the discussion of addiction.
73. Application, implementation, psychosocial integrity, (b).
    3. A new observer is often helpful in sorting out complexities and offering useful solutions.
    1. This is not a goal.
    2. Treatment is always time limited.
    4. Old ties are often strengthened.
74. Application, implementation, physiological integrity, (b).
    1. The more the patient knows, the less anxious he should be.
    2. The treatment may vary, depending on test results.
    3. This may not be all the patient needs to know before the test.
    4. Do not offer false assurance.
75. Comprehension, assessment, psychosocial integrity, (b).
    1. Asking directly is the best approach.
    2. Asking about the children does not answer the question about the patient.
    3. This would be secondhand information, not proof.
    4. The nurse would not want to leave the patient in a potentially dangerous situation until he or she were able to visit.

76. Comprehension, assessment, psychosocial integrity, (b).
    2. Recurring nightmares about the traumatic event are common.
    1. Hallucinations are not common, especially auditory ones.
    3. Displaced anger is not common in PTSD.
    4. Depression is not a common concern in PTSD.
77. Analysis, assessment, psychosocial integrity, (c).
    1. This is high risk: mood change may signal behavior change.
    2. The nurse should not assume that the crisis has passed.
    3. This is a medical diagnosis, and nurses do not make medical diagnoses.
    4. This is not necessarily true.
78. Comprehension, assessment, psychosocial integrity, (b).
    4. Any major trauma can lead to PTSD.
    1. This is not a reason for trauma.
    2. Genetics is not related to PTSD.
    3. Work-related failures are not necessarily traumatic.
79. Comprehension, assessment, psychosocial integrity, (b).
    4. Seizures are common during alcohol withdrawal.
    1. Bleeding is not commonly seen in alcohol withdrawal.
    2. Jaundice is usually seen in liver failure.
    3. Excessive hunger is not seen; the person usually drinks and does not eat.
80. Application, evaluation, psychosocial integrity, (b).
    1. This obtains the necessary information.
    2, 3. These are examples of a nontherapeutic technique using a stereotyped response.
    4. This is a nontherapeutic technique of giving reassurance.
81. Comprehension, assessment, psychosocial integrity, (b).
    2. The nurse should first understand her own feelings.
    1, 3, 4. These do not help the nurse accept the patient's behavior.
82. Application, implementation, physiological integrity, (b).
    2. The patient may hoard the medication, which is undesirable.
    1. This is not a priority related to administration of medication.
    3. Some medications are to be taken with food.
    4. A window of time is allowed; the nurse cannot give each patient's medication exactly on time.
83. Application, implementation, psychosocial integrity, (b).
    3. Using short sentences may help the patient comprehend.
    1. The patient does not have a hearing problem.
    2. Hearing the words three times will not help the patient comprehend.
    4. He will not comprehend written instructions any better than he would verbal ones.
84. Analysis, assessment, psychosocial integrity, (b).
    4. His loud behavior is a common sign of anxiety.
    1. He is probably not aware that he is so loud and inappropriate; it is the anxiety.
    2. He needs attention; he may upset or offend other patients.
    3. This gets him away from other patients but is not the best way to address the problem.
85. Application, assessment, psychosocial integrity, (b).
    4. Hopelessness is a classic symptom of depression.
    1. This is another medical diagnosis and may accompany depression.
    2. Agitation is more frequently seen with anxiety.
    3. Depressed people are more likely to be fatigued.
86. Comprehension, assessment, psychosocial integrity, (b).
    4. Subjective remarks come from the patient.
    1, 2, 3. These are the nurse's observations and can be considered objective data.
87. Comprehension, assessment, psychosocial integrity, (a).
    1. If the patient adapts, he deals with the problem and resolves the anxiety.
    2. Palliative coping may decrease the anxiety.
    3. Maladaptive behavior may make the patient more anxious.
    4. The problem will not be solved, and the anxiety will not be reduced.
88. Comprehension, assessment, psychosocial integrity, (b).
    3. Leaving the patient alone will make him more anxious.
    1. An anxious patient cannot understand that the nurse must care for others.
    2. Nothing in the question supports depression.
    4. No data exist to support another person being sought out.
89. Comprehension, assessment, psychosocial integrity, (a).
    2. In a catatonic state the patient appears in a stupor and is rigid.
    1. Paranoid patients are jealous and suspicious.
    3. *Incoherent* means not making sense.
    4. Suspicion accompanies paranoia.
90. Comprehension, assessment, psychosocial integrity, (b).
    1. Rapid or sudden onset is typically seen with delirium.
    2, 3, 4. These are generally true of delirium and often improve as the underlying condition is addressed.
91. Comprehension, assessment, psychosocial integrity, (a).
    3. These behaviors are associated with moderate mental retardation.
    1. People with profound mental retardation are unable to care for themselves without much assistance.
    2. People who are severely mentally retarded can learn only select "survival" words.
    4. People who are mildly mentally retarded can attain skills of sixth-grade level and live in the community successfully.
92. Analysis, assessment, psychosocial integrity, (b).
    2. In the anger phase the patient is most likely to be demanding.
    1. In this phase he is requesting more time.
    3. In denial he does not think he has the illness.
    4. When the patient reaches acceptance, he is at peace.
93. Application, implementation, psychosocial integrity, (b).
    _____ 1. Blood levels are done with lithium therapy, not with MAOIs.
    _X_ 2. This is essential with patient education because the hypertensive crisis that can occur can be life-threatening.
    _____ 3. NMS can occur with use of antipsychotics, not MAOIs.
    _X_ 4. This is essential patient education because the hypertensive crisis that can occur can be life-threatening.
94. Application, assessment, physiological integrity, (b).
    3. Assessment is always first.
    1. This does not teach.
    2. This alone does not teach.
    4. Other information is required first.

95. Comprehension, assessment, psychosocial integrity, (a).
    Correct order: 4213.
    4. Preorientation phase
    2. Orientation phase
    1. Working phase
    3. Termination phase
96. Application, assessment, psychosocial integrity, (b).
    3. Reaction formation by definition is expressing the opposite of what occurred.
    1. Projection is putting one's thoughts or feelings on another.
    2. Regression is returning to a more secure stage.
    4. Displacement is redirecting energies to another.
97. Analysis, evaluation, physiological integrity, (b).
    4. Antipsychotic medications, such as haloperidol, have a high incidence of causing EPSs.
    1. Valproic acid is an antimanic with side effects of drowsiness and dizziness.
    2. Fluoxetine is a selective serotonin reuptake inhibitor with numerous side effects; however, the EPSs are generally associated with antipsychotics.
    3. Lithium side effects are frequently associated with symptoms of toxicity.
98. Analysis, assessment, psychosocial integrity, (c).
    1. This is behavior that involves indirect expressions of anger as shown by the individual in this situation.
    2. Battery refers to use of force on another.
    3. Substitution is a defense mechanism involving replacing unacceptable with acceptable behavior.
    4. Undoing is a defense mechanism in which unacceptable behavior is followed by an attempt to rectify.

99. Application, planning, safe and effective care environment, (b).
    _____ 1. Building trust occurs in the orientation phase.
    __X__ **2. The preparation phase is one of data gathering from a variety of sources that allows the caregiver to prepare for the relationship.**
    _____ 3. Having the patient try out new behaviors occurs during the working phase.
    __X__ **4. Examining and understanding his or her own feelings are also critical for the nurse to establish a relationship with the patient.**
100. Application, implementation, psychosocial integrity (b).
    _____ 1. Reviewing health history data is an early stage of therapeutic relationship development but not part of mental status assessment.
    __X__ **2. Thought processes (i.e., delusions) are part of the assessment protocol for a mental status examination.**
    __X__ **3. Consciousness (alert, oriented) is part of the assessment protocol for a mental status examination.**
    __X__ **4. Mood, expressed both verbally and via behaviors, is part of the assessment protocol for a mental status examination.**
    _____ 5. Assessing patient strengths is a goal for the orientation stage.
    __X__ **6. Motor activity (lethargy or hyperactivity) is part of the assessment protocol for a mental status examination.**

Objectives

After studying this chapter, the student should be able to:

1. Correctly use terminology appropriate in maternal child nursing.
2. Identify the signs and symptoms of labor in all three stages.
3. Using the nursing process, describe the care required for a "pregnant family" in all four trimesters of pregnancy.
4. Develop a nursing care plan for both the normal postpartum family and families experiencing complications of pregnancy.
5. Describe causes of high-risk pregnancy and the nursing interventions involved.
6. Explain the nursing care involved in the entire process of labor.

The aim of obstetrics is to offer health services to the childbearing mother, her baby, and her family that will ensure a normal pregnancy and a safe prenatal labor and delivery and postnatal experience. This chapter reviews components of the nursing process. Each topic presents pertinent information helpful in planning the nursing assessment and determining the nursing needs of the family. Nursing management is outlined, giving options for selecting appropriate plans for action. The evaluation of whether outcomes and goals of maternity nursing have been met completes the nursing process.

EVOLUTION OF MODERN OBSTETRICS

Modern obstetrics has seen influences as far back as the Middle Ages, early Christianity, Judaism, and the Renaissance. Western European influences include the use of forceps, texts on obstetrical practices, the importance of asepsis (handwashing), and the discovery by Pasteur of *Streptococcus* as a causative organism in puerperal fever.

A. Contributors in the United States:
1. Anne Hutchinson (1634): midwife who delivered many babies of early settlers
2. William Shippen: established first lying-in hospital and midwifery school in the United States in 1762
3. Oliver Wendell Holmes (1809-1894): stressed cleanliness and handwashing before caring for new mothers
4. Margaret Sanger Research Bureau (1923): first organization to address question of contraception and planned parenthood
B. U.S. legislation affecting mothers and children
1. 1921: Sheppard Towner Act: promoted health and welfare for mothers and children
2. 1936: First Social Security benefits; later to include entitlement benefits for mothers and their dependent children
3. 1943: Emergency Maternal and Infant Care Act to assist families of soldiers during World War II
4. 1973: Supreme Court legalized abortion.

5. 1974: Women, Infants, and Children (WIC) Program: federally funded nutritional program providing supplementary food to eligible pregnant, lactating, or postpartum women; their infants; and children under 5 years of age
6. 1995-1996: Several states enacted legislation to lengthen a postpartum stay to 48 hours for a vaginal delivery and 96 hours for a caesarean birth; early discharge would be voluntary.

DEFINITIONS COMMONLY USED IN OBSTETRICS

STATISTICS

Birth rates: number of live births per 1000 population
Fetal death (stillborn): fetus of 20 weeks or more gestational age who dies in utero before birth
Infant mortality rate: number of deaths before the first birthday per 1000 live births
Maternal mortality rate: number of mothers dying in or because of childbirth per 100,000 live births
Neonatal death: death within first 4 weeks of life
Neonatal death rate: number of deaths within the first 4 weeks of life per 1000 live births
Note: Statistics are important to identify problem areas and trends in the health care setting.

ABBREVIATIONS (LIMITED LISTING)

ABC: alternative birthing center
AIDS: acquired immunodeficiency syndrome
ARM, AROM: artificial rupture of membranes
CPD: cephalopelvic disproportion
CS: caesarean section
DIC: disseminated intravascular coagulation
EDC: estimated date of confinement; due date for birth
EDD: estimated date of delivery
FHR: fetal heart rate
FHT: fetal heart tone
G: gravida; number of pregnancies

GH: gestational hypertension (formerly known as *pregnancy-induced hypertension* [PIH])

GTPAL: gravida, term, premature, abortions, living children; identification of pregnancy status

hCG: human chorionic gonadotropin

HELLP: hemolysis, elevated liver enzymes, low platelet count; extension of pathological factors related to severe preeclampsia

HIV: human immunodeficiency virus

LDRP: labor, delivery, recovery, postpartum: All phases of maternal and child care occur in the same room with the same staff member.

LGA: large for gestational age

LMP: last menstrual period

P: para; number of viable births

PROM: premature rupture of membranes

Q: quadrant; one of four equal parts into which abdomen is divided to designate position of fetus in uterus

RhoGAM: antibody against Rh factor given early prenatally or within 72 hours postpartum to mother

SGA: small for gestational age

TORCHES: a group of intrauterine infections, including toxoplasmosis, rubella, cytomegalovirus, herpes, and syphilis; commonly associated with high infant mortality

COMMON OBSTETRICAL TERMINOLOGY

Advanced maternal age: age older than 35 years of age for a woman giving birth to her first child

Ante: prefix meaning *before*, e.g., antepartum: time before delivery

Apgar score: method of evaluating infant immediately after delivery; usually determined at 1 minute and 5 minutes

Braxton-Hicks contractions: painless uterine contractions felt throughout pregnancy, becoming stronger and more noticeable during second and third trimesters

Caput: head; cephalic portion of infant

Cyesis: pregnancy

Dystocia: long, painful labor and delivery

Gestation: developmental time of embryo, fetus in utero

Grand multipara: having had more than five children

Gravida: any pregnancy, regardless of duration, including the present one

High risk: describes a pregnant woman with preexisting problems that can jeopardize the pregnancy, the fetus, or herself; younger than 18 years of age or older than 35 years of age with no prenatal care (any one or more of these conditions)

Lightening: moving of the fetus and uterus downward into the pelvic cavity during the last 2 weeks before EDC (usually just before labor in multiparas)

Low birth weight: weight less than 5½ pounds (2500 g) because the baby is preterm (premature) or because of intrauterine growth retardation

Low risk: describes a pregnant woman with normal history between ages 18 and 34 years with no medical, psychological, or other preexisting problems and under good prenatal care

Meconium: first bowel movement of the newborn—thick, tarlike, greenish-black substance

Multigravida: a woman who has been pregnant more than one time

Multipara: a woman who has given birth to more than one child

Para: number of births after 20 weeks' gestation, whether infants were born alive or dead

Postmature infant: an infant born after 42 weeks' gestation

Premature infant: an infant born any time before 37 weeks' gestation

Primigravida: a woman who is pregnant for the first time

Primipara: a woman who is giving birth to her first child

Pseudocyesis: false pregnancy

Quickening: first movements of the fetus felt by the mother (16 to 18 weeks' gestation)

Secundines: afterbirth of placenta and membranes

Term infant: an infant born between 38 and 42 weeks' gestation

Vernix caseosa: cheesy material covering the fetus and newborn that acts as a protection to the skin

Viable: capable of developing, growing, and sustaining life, such as a normal human fetus at 24 weeks' gestation. The current legal age of viability is 24 weeks.

Vis a tergo: external pressure on the fundus to assist in the delivery of the infant

TRENDS

A. Cost containment: Rising health care costs are a national concern. Increased home care, shortened stays, and increased emphasis on prenatal care are interventions to help control cost and maintain quality. Regionalization of services for high-risk childbearing families and managed care are newer methods to attempt to control costs.

B. Prenatal care: Emphasis must be placed on improving access to prenatal care, particularly for low-income women. Prenatal care can avoid many conditions (complications) that can be prevented with adequate monitoring during pregnancy.

C. Legislation has been passed at a federal level that guarantees women who give birth vaginally a minimum stay of 48 hours. Women who have a caesarean birth are guaranteed 72 hours.

D. High-technology care: Technological developments, including fetal surgery, ultrasonography, and genetic testing, have often outpaced society's ability to determine ethical implications of their use. Advancements in technology have enabled many infants to survive today who would not have done so in the past.

E. Changing demographics: Women are waiting longer in life to have their first babies; nurses need to be familiar with effects of pregnancy on older women.

F. Teen pregnancy: Nurses need to identify and implement strategies to decrease incidence of adolescent pregnancy.

G. Changing cultures: Nurses need to be sensitive to ideas and health practices of different cultures. Examples in which culture plays an important part include pain expression, choice of support person, and preference for a female health care provider. Many cultures view childbirth as a natural experience; therefore it does not require any special care. Specific cultural and genetic groups are associated with different genetic conditions. An example of this would be sickle cell anemia, which is common in African Americans.

H. Prepared childbirth experience: Mother and father (or alternate) jointly attend childbirth education classes to prepare for the child and for the childbearing and childbirth experience.

I. Alternative birth centers (ABCs)
Birthing centers outside of hospital:
Individual's home: The number of home births has remained small in the United States.

Use of the birthing chair instead of traditional table

Birthing room: Labor, delivery, and postpartum hospital stay are incorporated into one cheerful, homelike room set up with necessary labor and delivery equipment.

J. Variety of positions used to assist labor and delivery (e.g., squat, side position)

K. Showering during first or second stage of labor; some hospitals have whirlpool for early labor.

L. Inclusion of father or alternate: Support person stays in labor and delivery area for both vaginal and caesarean deliveries.

M. Rooming-in: allows newborn in room with mother for the day; fathers allowed unlimited visiting time

N. Sibling visits: designated hours that children may visit and see baby

O. Use of midwives: Many hospitals and birthing centers throughout the United States now have nurse-midwives as the primary care person conducting prenatal, labor, delivery, and follow-up care.

P. Caesarean deliveries: more frequent now because of sophisticated fetal monitoring. The practice is controversial because the number has been increasing in recent years.

Q. Breast-feeding: accepted and encouraged. Societies such as La Leche League and the popularity of natural foods encourage breast-feeding. Lactation practitioners are available in many facilities to assist women with nursing.

R. Genetic counseling: Increasingly accurate, safe amniocentesis and advances in genetics encourage counselors to advise couples with genetic concerns. The human genome project is an effort to identify the genes that can cause genetic disorders. Identification and replacement of genes are still not routine.

S. In vitro method of fertilization to assist pregnancy and fetal development: usually chosen by couples with fertility problems after exploring various methods, including fertility drugs and other insemination practices. Newborn screening is standard in many countries.

T. Sex selection: available before conception by separating sperm. Many ethical concerns surround this practice.

U. Students are advised to review U.S. Department of Health and Human Services: *Healthy People 2020: National Health Promotion and Disease Prevention Objectives,* http://www.healthypeople.gov/2020/default.aspx.

PROCEDURES TO DIAGNOSE MATERNAL AND FETAL PROBLEMS

A. Alpha-fetoprotein (AFP) test
1. Screening procedure, not diagnostic
2. Serum from maternal blood sample tested; best results if sample is taken at 16 to 18 weeks' gestation; identifies unrecognized high-risk pregnancies
3. Elevated levels in maternal serum: indicate 5% to 10% of open neural tube defects (spina bifida) in developing fetus
4. Recommend two samples be tested, followed by ultrasound and amniocentesis to confirm findings; genetic counseling availability if confirmed
5. Other causes of elevated AFP levels: multiple gestation, missed abortions, other abnormalities (elevated levels may indicate Down syndrome)

B. Hemoglobin electrophoresis identifies presence of sickle cell trait in women of African or Mediterranean descent.

C. Ultrasound: can be performed endovaginally or abdominally
1. Performed when high risk of fetal loss is suspected
2. Used to evaluate pregnancy and determine the age of the fetus

D. Amniocentesis: invasive procedure during which a needle is inserted through abdomen and uterus to withdraw amniotic fluid; usually done after fourteenth week
1. Used for determining gender, defects in fetus (e.g., Down syndrome, Tay-Sachs disease), and fetal status (Rh isoimmune problem, fetal maturity, other tests as listed in this section)
2. Lecithin/sphingomyelin ratio (L/S ratio): used to determine fetal lung maturity by testing surfactant by thirty-fifth week of pregnancy; lecithin level two times greater than sphingomyelin level indicates that lungs are mature.
3. Creatinine level: used to test fetal muscle mass and renal function; 0.2 mg/100 mL amniotic fluid at 36 weeks is normal level; large amount may also indicate a large fetus such as the fetus of the mother with diabetes.
4. Bilirubin level: used for determination of fetal liver maturity; should decrease as term progresses.
5. Cytological testing: determines percentage of lipid globules present in amniotic fluid; indicates fetal age

E. Chorionic villi test
1. Permits first-trimester testing for biochemical and chromosomal defects; invasive and high-risk procedure during which a plastic catheter is inserted vaginally into the uterus; ultrasound guides catheter to chorionic frondosum.
2. Can be done 9 to 11 weeks after LMP
3. Done earlier than amniocentesis. Recent evidence shows that test may increase risk of babies born with missing toes and fingers or shortened digits.

F. Fetoscopy: invasive procedure involving transabdominal insertion of metal cannula into abdomen; visualization of fetus and placenta for developing abnormalities and to obtain fetal skin or blood samples
1. High-risk procedure; complications include spontaneous abortion and premature labor.
2. Limited usage, only if defect cannot be detected otherwise

G. Umbilical cord technique: evaluates condition of fetus
1. Superior technique because fetal blood can be analyzed as early as eighteenth week of gestation
2. Can evaluate blood count, liver function, blood gases, acid-base status
3. Invasive procedure; limited use because of risk of injury to fetus

H. Estriol level study: 24-hour urinalysis of urine from mother; determines estriol level to ascertain fetal well-being and placental functioning
1. Performed at third trimester (32 weeks)
2. Level of 12 mg of estriol in 24 hours is good; below 12 mg indicates that infant is in jeopardy (related to decreased placental functioning).
3. Decreasing estriol levels can be used in combination with other diagnostic tests to indicate a compromised placenta or fetus.

I. Heterozygote testing (mother's blood): done to detect clinically normal carriers of mutant genes
1. Tay-Sachs disease: common fatal genetic disease affecting children of Ashkenazi Jews (Eastern Europe)
2. Sickle cell anemia: common disorder among black Americans of African descent; 1 in 10 African Americans is a carrier.

3. Cooley anemia (β-thalassemia): genetic disorder frequent among Mediterranean ethnic groups: Italians, Sicilians, Greeks, Turks, Middle Eastern Arabs, Asian Indians, Pakistanis

J. Contraction stress test (CST): late-trimester test to measure placental insufficiency and fetal reaction to uterine contractions (potential fetal compromise)
1. Usually done after EDC has passed
2. Invasive procedure during which intravenous (IV) oxytocin is administered; baseline recorded on monitor; takes 20 to 60 minutes
3. Breast stimulation techniques done in some health care settings in place of oxytocin infusion during a CST
4. Results: Late decelerations during contraction for at least three contractions indicate a positive test result. No decelerations during three successive contractions within 10 minutes indicate a negative test result. Occasionally inconsistent decelerations indicate suspicious conditions.

K. Nonstress test (NST): assesses and evaluates FHT response to uterine movement or increased fetal activity

L. Ultrasound procedure: use of high-frequency sound waves to determine fetal size, estimate amniotic fluid volume, detect neural tube defects, assess for limb abnormalities, evaluate fetal presentation, and diagnose breech presentation
1. Usually a second-trimester procedure
2. Procedure is noninvasive and relatively comfortable.
3. Acoustic sound waves can be used to help stimulate an inactive fetus during an NST.

M. Biophysical profile: Using ultrasound and an NST, this profile evaluates five fetal variables—breathing movements, body movements, muscular tone, qualitative amniotic fluid volume, FHR.

N. Doppler flow studies: use of ultrasound techniques to evaluate blood flow studies in deep-lying vessels. These are particularly useful in managing high-risk pregnancies.

O. Fetal movement: noninvasive method of determining fetal well-being. Patterns that deviate from normal pattern may be an indication for further studies.

ANATOMY AND PHYSIOLOGY OF REPRODUCTION

OBSTETRICAL PELVIS

A. Types (Figure 7-1)
1. Gynecoid: "true" female pelvis—considered the ideal pelvis for a vaginal birth
2. Anthropoid: narrow from side to side
3. Android: male pelvis (not adequate for vaginal delivery)
4. Platypelloid: flat pelvis that is narrow from front to back (not adequate for vaginal delivery)

B. Components
1. Ilium: flat or lateral, flaring part of pelvis or hip. Iliac crest is top part of ileum.
2. Ischium: inferior dorsal or lower part of hip bone. The ischial spines, sharp projections of the ischium, are important in obstetrics because they are landmarks to measure progress of presenting part of fetus.
3. Sacrum: triangular bone between the two hip bones; flat part of the lower back (spine)
4. Coccyx: two to five rudimentary vertebrae that are fused and attached to lower part of sacrum (tailbone)

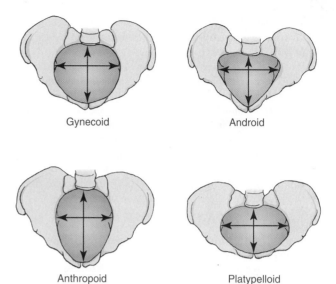

Gynecoid Android

Anthropoid Platypelloid

FIGURE 7-1 Female pelvis: pure types. (From Leifer G: *Maternity nursing: an introductory text,* ed 11, St Louis, 2012, Mosby.)

The physician will measure the pelvis to determine the adequacy of the birth canal. Sonograms can be used as well for more accuracy.

FERTILIZATION AND IMPLANTATION

A. Definitions
1. Fertilization: occurs when the sperm and ovum join, usually at the distal third of the fallopian tube within 12 to 48 hours after intercourse
2. Zygote: product of the union of a sperm and ovum
3. Implantation: occurs when zygote burrows into the endometrium of the uterus, approximately 7 days after fertilization
4. Nidation: completion of implantation

B. Processes
1. Mitosis: rapid cell division
2. Blastoderm: first division of the zygote
3. Morula: ball-like structure of the blastoderm; sometimes referred to as mulberry-like
4. Blastocyst: The ball-like structure (morula) becomes the blastocyst as it enters the uterus.
5. Trophoblast: As blastocyst implants in the uterus, the wall becomes the trophoblast.
6. Chorionic villi: Trophoblasts develop villi that become fetal portion of the placenta.
7. Decidua: Endometrium undergoes a change when pregnancy occurs.
8. Decidua vera: portion of the decidua that becomes the lining of the uterus, except for around implantation site
9. Decidua basalis: where implantation occurs and chorionic villi become frondosum, or the beginning of the placental formation
10. Decidua capsularis: covers blastocyst and fuses to form fetal membranes
11. Amnion: inner membrane, which comes from the zygote and blends with the cord
12. Chorion: outer membrane, which comes from the zygote and blends with the fetal portion of the placenta

DEVELOPMENT OF HUMAN ORGANISM

A. Ovum stage: preembryonic stage from conception until the primary villi appear (first 14 days)

B. Embryo: end of ovum stage to 8 weeks from LMP; period of rapid cellular development. Disruption causes developmental abnormality.

C. Fetus: from end of embryonic stage (8 weeks) to term

D. Placenta: membrane weighing approximately 1 pound (450 g); develops cotyledons that act as areas for nourishing fetus; maternal surface beefy and red; fetal surface shiny and gray

E. Amnionic cavity: fills with fluid (1000 mL) that is replaced every 3 hours; shelters and protects fetus

GENDER DETERMINATION

A. Normal sperm; carries 22 autosomes and 1 sex chromosome (either an X or a Y chromosome)

B. Normal ovum: carries 22 autosomes and 1 sex chromosome (always an X chromosome)

C. Combined number of chromosomes: 44 autosomes and 2 sex chromosomes (at conception)

D. Genetic component of sperm determines gender of child (Box 7-1).

E. Chromosome carries genes plus deoxyribonucleic acid (DNA) and proteins

F. Genes: factors in chromosomes carrying hereditary characteristics

PHYSIOLOGY OF THE FETUS

A. Membranes and amniotic fluid
   1. Protect from blows and bumps mother may experience
   2. Maintain even heat to fetus
   3. Act as an excretory system
   4. Supply oral fluid for fetus
   5. Allow free movement of fetus

B. Placenta
   1. Transport organ: passes nutrients from mother to fetus and relays excretory material from fetus to mother
   2. Formation completed by 3 months.
   3. Functions: acts as kidneys, lungs, stomach, and intestines during fetal life
   4. Requirement: adequate oxygen from mother to function well

C. Weekly development
   1. Embryonic stage (first to eighth weeks)
      a. Beginning: pulsating heart, spinal canal formation: no eyes or ears; buds for arms and legs
      b. By end: just more than 1 inch (2.5 cm) long; eyelids fused; distinct divisions of arms, legs; cord formed; tail disappears

---

Box 7-1 | Gender Determination

Sperm supplies 22 autosomes and an X sex chromosome.
Ovum supplies 22 autosomes and an X sex chromosome.
Result: 44 autosomes and an XX = female

Sperm supplies 22 autosomes and a Y sex chromosome
Ovum supplies 22 autosomes and an X sex chromosome
Result: 44 autosomes and an XY = male

---

c. The yolk sac begins feeding stem cells to the liver in the fifth week. The actual formation of blood begins in the fetal liver during the sixth week.

d. The liver and biliary tract develop during the fourth week of gestation.

e. The respiratory system begins development during the embryonic stage and continues through childhood.

f. The kidneys form during the fifth week and begin to function approximately 4 weeks later.

g. The nervous system originates from the ectoderm during the third week after fertilization. The open neural tube forms during the fourth week. It usually closes at what will be the junction of the brain and the spinal cord. The neural tube further delineates during the fifth week. The structures that will become the brain and the spine are formed.

h. The thyroid gland develops along with structures in the head and neck during the third and fourth weeks.

2. Fetal stage (ninth week to term)
   a. Between 20 and 24 weeks is considered the legal threshold for viability, the age at which the fetus is capable of surviving outside of the uterus. Infants with 22 to 23 weeks of gestation have a better chance of surviving owing to advances in medical care.

   b. The embryo or fetus is most vulnerable to damaging effects of teratogenic agents during the first trimester (12 weeks); tetracycline, caffeine, and many over-the-counter drugs are examples of drugs that are teratogenic. The fetus is vulnerable to central nervous system (CNS) depressants during the entire pregnancy.

   c. At 3 months: 3 inches (7.5 cm) long; weighs 1 oz (28 g); fully formed arms, legs, fingers; distinguishable sex organs.

   d. At 4 months: development of muscles, movement; mother feels quickening; 6 to 7 inches (15 to 17.5 cm) long; weighs 4 oz (112 g); lanugo over body; head large. Until 17 weeks the skin is thin and wrinkled with blood vessels visible. The skin begins to thicken and all layers are present at term. At 32 weeks, subcutaneous fat begins to be deposited.

   e. At 5 months: 10 to 12 inches (25 to 30 cm) long; weighs ½ to 1 pound (225 to 450 g); internal organs maturing; lungs immature; FHT heard on examination; eyes fused; rarely survives more than several hours The fetus is able to distinguish taste by the fifth month.

   f. At 6 months: 11 to 14 inches (27.5 to 35 cm) long; weighs 1 to 1½ pounds (450 to 675 g); wrinkled "old man" appearance; vernix caseosa covers body; eyelids separated; eyelashes and fingernails formed.

   g. At 7 months: begins to store fat and minerals; 16 inches (40 cm) long; may survive with excellent care The fetus can see. Eyes with both rods and cones are formed in the seventh month.

   h. At 8 months: beginning of month weighs 2 to 3 pounds (900 to 1350 g); by end of month, 4 to 5 pounds (1800 to 2250 g); continues to develop; loses wrinkled appearance

   i. At 9 months: 19 inches (47.5 cm) long; weighs 7 pounds (3200 g) (girl) or 7½ pounds (3400 g) (boy); more fat under skin; vernix caseosa; has stored vitamins, minerals, and antibodies; fully developed

D. Fetal circulation
  1. Special structures
     a. Ductus venosus: passes through liver; connects umbilical vein to inferior vena cava (IVC); closes at birth
     b. Ductus arteriosus: shunts blood from pulmonary artery to descending aorta; closes almost immediately after birth
     c. Foramen ovale: valve opening that allows blood to flow from right to left atrium; functionally closes at birth. All three fetal structures previously listed allow blood to bypass the fetal lungs and liver.
     d. Umbilical arteries (two): transport blood from the hypogastric artery to the placenta; functionally close at birth
     e. Umbilical vein (one): transports oxygenated blood from the placenta to the ductus venosus and liver, and then to the IVC; closes at birth
  2. Fetal circulation (Figure 7-2)
     a. Oxygenated blood from the placenta goes through the umbilical vein, bypassing the portal system of the liver by way of the ductus venosus.
     b. From the ductus venosus it goes to the ascending vena cava (inferior) to the heart, right auricle.

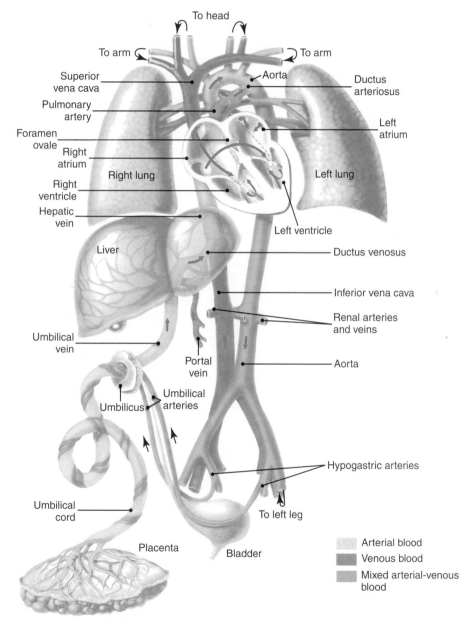

FIGURE 7-2 Fetal circulation. Before birth: Arterialized blood from the placenta flows into the fetus through the umbilical vein and passes rapidly through the liver into the inferior vena cava; it flows through the foramen ovale into the left atrium, soon to appear in the aorta and arteries of the head. A portion bypasses the liver through the ductus venosus. Venous blood from the lower extremities and head passes predominantly into the right atrium, the right ventricle, and then into the descending pulmonary artery and ductus arteriosus. Thus the foramen ovale and the ductus arteriosus act as bypass channels, allowing a large part of the combined cardiac output to return to the placenta without flowing through the lungs. Approximately 55% of the combined ventricular output flows to the placenta; 35% perfuses body tissues; and the remaining 10% flows through the lungs. After birth: The foramen ovale closes, the ductus arteriosus closes and becomes a ligament, the ductus venosus closes and becomes a ligament, and the umbilical vein and arteries close and become ligaments. (Used with permission of Ross Products Division, Abbott Laboratories, Columbus, Ohio.)

c. It goes from the right auricle through the foramen ovale.

d. It goes to the left auricle and then to the left ventricle.

e. Blood leaves the heart through the aorta to the arms and head.

f. It then returns to the heart, passing through the descending vena cava (superior).

g. It goes to the right auricle and then to the right ventricle.

h. It leaves the heart through the pulmonary arteries, bypassing the lungs.

i. It goes through the ductus arteriosus to the aorta and down to the trunk and lower extremities.

j. It then goes through the hypogastric arteries to the umbilical arteries on to the placenta, carrying carbon dioxide and waste materials.

Note: The fetus is able to feel and requires anesthesia for invasive procedures that may be necessary during this time.

NORMAL ANTEPARTUM (PRENATAL)

PHYSIOLOGICAL CHANGES DURING PREGNANCY

A. Reproductive system
1. External changes
   a. Perineum: increased vasculature; enlarges
   b. Labia majora: change especially in parous woman; separate and stretch
   c. Anal and vulvar varices: caused by increased pelvic congestion
2. Internal changes
   a. Uterus: enlarges to accommodate growing fetus; walls thicken first trimester; Hegar sign (soft lower lip of uterus)
   b. Cervix: Goodéll sign (thickens, softens) 6 weeks from LMP because of vascular changes
   c. Vagina: Chadwick sign (bluish-violet color); mucosal changes approximately 8 weeks from LMP. Estrogen activity may cause thick vaginal discharge.
B. Other body system changes
1. Breasts
   a. Increased size, tingling sensations, heavy
   b. Increased pigmentation, darkened areolae
   c. Montgomery tubercles on areolae
2. Cardiovascular changes
   a. Slight enlargement of heart resulting from increased blood volume
   b. Increased circulation (47%)
   c. Cardiac output increases 30% first and second trimesters, then levels off until term; increases during labor and delivery; approximately 13% above normal during postpartum period.
3. Hematological changes
   a. Increased red blood cell (RBC) count; decreased hemoglobin level
   b. Increased tendency for blood to coagulate during pregnancy
   c. Coagulation factors return to normal during postpartum period, increasing likelihood of thromboembolism.
4. Respiratory and pulmonary changes: enlarging uterus presses on diaphragm, causing difficulty breathing

5. Skin: increased pigmentation
   a. Linea nigra: darkening line from below breast bone (sternum) down midline of abdomen to symphysis pubis
   b. Chloasma gravidarum (mask of pregnancy): dark, frecklelike pigmentation over nose and cheeks; disappears after delivery
   c. Striae gravidarum: stretching of skin with silvery to reddish, bluish stretch marks on breasts, abdomen, thighs; never disappears completely. Lotion, cocoa butter lubricants may help.
6. Urinary system changes
   a. Traces of sugar in urine resulting from activity of lactiferous ducts
   b. Even though glucosuria is common in pregnancy, all women should be screened for diabetes.
   c. Transitory albumin: may be indication of pending GH
   d. Cystitis: frequent because ureters lose some compliance or elasticity
7. Endocrine system
   a. Variable production of insulin during pregnancy
   b. Mother's cells become more insulin resistant.
   c. Thyroid gland increases in size, resulting in increased basal metabolic rate (BMR).
8. Digestive system
   a. Morning sickness: nausea and vomiting common during first trimester
   b. Increased appetite after first trimester
   c. Indigestion (heartburn): caused by increasing upward pressure of enlarging uterus or by relaxin hormone, which slows metabolism and keeps food in stomach longer in pregnant women
   d. Constipation: caused by changes in organ positions; pressure of growing uterus on sigmoid colon
9. Musculoskeletal system
   a. Normal lumbar curve becomes more pronounced as weight of pelvic contents tilts the pelvis forward.
   b. Extra weight may lead to backache experienced in late pregnancy.
10. Weight gain: total weight gain varies from 25 to 30 pounds (12 to 13.5 kg) (Table 7-1).

DURATION OF PREGNANCY

A. Length in terms of time
1. 9 calendar months
2. 10 lunar months
3. 280 days (266 days from time of ovulation)
4. 40 weeks
B. Nägele rule: to calculate EDC, count back 3 months from the month of the LMP and add 7 days to the first day of LMP.

Example

First day of LMP was July 17
Seventh month (July) 17, minus 3 months, plus 7 days
Fourth month (April) 24=EDC (April 24)

SIGNS AND SYMPTOMS OF PREGNANCY

A. Presumptive signs (subjective: mother usually notices)
1. Missed menstrual period
2. Breast changes: nipples tingle; fuller, darker areola in approximately 6 weeks

Table 7-1 Distribution of Weight Gain during Pregnancy

DISTRIBUTION	POUNDS	GRAMS
Fetus	7½	3400
Placenta	1	450
Amniotic fluid	2	900
Uterus	2½	1125
Increased blood volume	3-4	1350-1800
Breasts	2-3	900-1350
Mother's gain (e.g., fat, tissue)	4-8	1800-3600
Total weight gain	21-28 pounds	9.5-12.7 kg

3. Frequency of urination increases in approximately 6 weeks
4. Morning sickness: nausea and vomiting in 4 to 6 weeks
5. Skin changes: chloasma, linea nigra, striae (some authors call this a "probable" sign)

B. Probable signs (objective examiner usually notices)
1. Uterus: enlarges; shape changes at 12 to 16 weeks; Hegar sign: 8 weeks
2. Cervix: Goodell sign
3. Vagina: Chadwick sign
4. Implantation site: softens, enlarges (von Fernwald sign) at 6 to 7 weeks
5. Laboratory tests
    a. Immunological: widely used today; faster, 90% accurate. Beta subunit of hCG can be used even before missed period.
    b. Commercially sold pregnancy test: Home pregnancy tests are uncomplicated and convenient, producing results in as little as 4 minutes; should be confirmed by a physician.
6. Braxton-Hicks contractions
7. Ballottement

C. Positive signs (by examiner)
1. Palpate: can feel fetal parts
2. Hearing: FHT
    a. Electronic Doptone scope (audible at 8 to 11 weeks)
    b. Sonogram (can ascertain at 12 weeks)
    c. Auscultation (17 to 24 weeks) with fetoscope (head scope) or Leff stethoscope
3. Ultrasonographic (echographic) evidence of pregnancy visualized on screen
4. Fetal movement palpable after 20 weeks

PRENATAL CARE

A. Importance
1. Regular assessments and monitoring detect early signs and symptoms disrupting normal, healthy pregnancy.
2. Early evaluation of problem permits development of an appropriate plan of action based on findings.

B. Visits and examinations
1. Initial visits: establish diagnosis of pregnancy
2. Laboratory work drawn during prenatal visits
    a. AFP measurements in maternal serum are used for early diagnosis of fetal neural tube defects such as spina bifida and anencephaly.
    b. Estriol levels are assessed as part of a triple marker test; in the presence of a fetus with Down syndrome, the AFP levels, estriol levels, and hCG levels are low. These tests in combination with maternal age are used to calculate the risk.
    c. Human placental lactogen (HPL): a placental hormone that may be deficient in certain abnormalities of pregnancy

3. Complete medical history
    a. General personal health, habits, diseases, and medical or surgical problems
    b. History of communicable diseases, especially scarlet fever, measles, rubella, streptococcal infections; kidney conditions that might adversely affect pregnancy; sexually transmitted diseases; HIV status; tuberculosis
    c. Psychosocial history: assessment of substance use or abuse (including alcohol, tobacco, illegal prescription drugs, or over-the-counter drugs), social support, physical abuse, stress, employment, physical activity, cultural influences, and sibling adjustment. Siblings of the baby should be provided with explanations of pregnancy appropriate for the child's age.
    d. Previous pregnancies, miscarriages, abortions, blood transfusions, gynecological problems
    e. Family health status: diabetes, tuberculosis, heart disease, cancer, epilepsy, allergies, mental problems

4. Complete examination to include:
    a. Routine laboratory tests.
        (1) Matching blood type and Rh factor
        (2) Antibody screen (rubella, sickle cell) if appropriate
        (3) Complete blood count, including hemoglobin and hematocrit
        (4) Venereal Disease Research Laboratory (VDRL) test (for syphilis)
        (5) Herpes simplex virus 1 and 2 tests
        (6) HIV testing for the AIDS virus
        (7) Hepatitis A and B tests
        (8) Papanicolaou (Pap) smear
        (9) Purified protein derivative test used for tuberculosis
        (10) Cervical culture to check for group B streptococci
    b. Physical examination, including:
        (1) Pelvic examination and measurements
        (2) Abdominal palpation
        (3) Examination of breasts, nipples
        (4) Vital signs: blood pressure (BP), weight, temperature, respirations
        (5) Urinalysis for sugar and albumin
        (6) Smears (Papanicolaou [Pap] test) for cytology, gonorrhea, *Chlamydia*

5. Usual schedule for prenatal visits
    a. Every month for 28 weeks
    b. Every 2 weeks thereafter to thirty-sixth week
    c. Every week from thirty-seventh week to term
    d. Adjusted to individual needs

6. Usual routine for prenatal visits
    a. Perform urinalysis each visit for sugar, acetone, albumin.
    b. Perform capillary blood testing on a glucose oxidase strip for gestational diabetes mellitus (GDM), followed by plasma glucose testing at 12 weeks' gestation for all high-risk pregnancies.
    c. Check vital signs (especially BP).
    d. Check weight gain every visit.

(1) First trimester: 3 to 4 pounds (1.5 to 2 kg) total
(2) Second trimester: 1 pound (0.5 kg) per week; 12 to 14 pounds (6 to 7 kg) total
(3) Third trimester: 1 pound (0.5 kg) per week; 8 to 10 pounds (4 to 5 kg) total

e. Measure height of fundus to evaluate growth of fetus (Figure 7-3).
f. Listen to FHT and FHR by Doptone or auscultation.
g. Ask about fetal activity, attitude of family; answer parents' questions, fears.
h. Recommend childbirth education classes.

C. Promotion of positive health
1. Nutritional counseling
a. Fetus receives all nourishment from mother.
b. Teenage pregnant mother requires extensive counseling (nutritional pattern poor); focus is on positive effect of good nutrition on adolescent and fetus.
c. In the past, sodium restriction was advised to help prevent edema, retention of fluids, and GH; research has shown that sodium intake during pregnancy helps maintain normal and expanded fluid levels during the pregnancy. Women may be told to limit foods high in sodium.
d. Direct relationship exists between maternal nutrition and mental development of the child.
e. Megavitamins should be avoided during pregnancy; they can be dangerous for the developing fetus.
f. Long-term users of oral contraceptives may have depleted bodily reserves of vitamin B_6 and folate.
g. High folic acid intake may disguise vitamin B_{12} deficiency (pernicious anemia), which can lead to neurological damage; folic acid intake should not exceed 400 mcg/day.

h. Energy needs during pregnancy increase little (300 kilocalories/day {kcal/day}) compared with the increased need for nutrients.
i. A fluid intake of six to eight glasses of water per day is recommended to maintain body temperature and to prevent constipation.
j. Calcium and iron supplements may be ordered to prevent complications.
k. Proper (20 mg for a term infant) intake of docosahexaenoic acid (DHP, an omega fatty acid) is recommended for proper brain development.
l. Women who are pregnant should avoid swordfish, shark, and king mackerel because of toxic levels of mercury.
m. A dietician's orders should be sought for women on special diets (e.g., vegetarian) to ensure adequate intake of nutrients.
2. Nutritional needs during pregnancy
a. See Table 7-2.
b. See Chapter 4.
3. General health teaching
a. Daily baths for cleanliness; showers during last 6 weeks for safety's sake
b. Moderate exercise, especially walking
c. Douching only on advice of physician
d. Sexual intercourse is permissible as long as it is not uncomfortable, cervix is closed, and membranes are intact.
e. Good support bra
f. Unrestrictive comfortable clothing, hose
g. Good mental attitude; discuss ambivalent feelings.
h. Smoking: Nicotine retards growth of fetus, constricts blood vessels in mother, decreases placental function, and may cause premature labor. Growing evidence shows that secondary smoke has damaging effects on the mother, fetus, children, and spouses. Research has shown a relationship between mothers who smoke excessively and the incidence of pneumonia and bronchitis in babies at 6 to 9 months of age.
i. Alcohol: Research has yet to determine minimum safe amounts of alcohol (if any) that can be consumed in pregnancy.
j. Caffeine: Caffeine has been shown to cause teratogenic effects in animals. Pregnant women should be counseled to avoid foods containing caffeine (found in coffee, tea, chocolate, colas, and some analgesics). Newer evidence indicates a higher incidence of sudden infant death syndrome (SIDS) in infants of mothers who consumed significant amounts of caffeine during pregnancy.
k. Drugs: may pass placental barrier and affect fetus. Greatest danger is during first trimester, but effects may not be evident until years after birth. New evidence shows that crack or cocaine may cause significant complications for mother and newborn. Pregnant women should be counseled to avoid over-the-counter or prescription medications without the advice of a physician. Pregnant women should be counseled about their regular use of vitamins and warned against taking megadoses.
4. Childbirth and parent education classes
a. Various methods are available, including Bradley and Lamaze. These methods are specifically designed to educate and prepare expectant parents for all phases

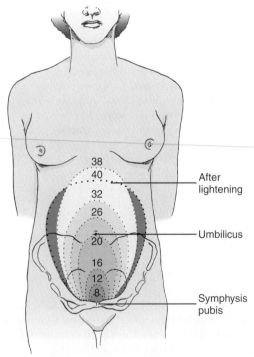

FIGURE 7-3 Height of fundus by weeks of normal gestation with a single fetus. (Modified from Leifer G: *Maternity nursing: an introductory text,* ed 9, St Louis, 2005, Saunders.)

Table 7-2	Nutritional Needs during Pregnancy			
NUTRIENT	**NONPREGNANT WOMAN**	**PREGNANT WOMAN**	**USAGE**	**FOOD SOURCE**
Protein	44 g	74-100 g; needs twice as much	Growth of fetus Placental growth During labor and delivery During lactation	Milk, cheese, eggs, meat, grains, legumes, nuts
Calcium	800 mg	1200 mg; needs 1½ times as much	Fetal skeleton Fetal tooth buds Calcium metabolism in mother	Milk, cheese, whole grains, leafy vegetables, egg yolk
Phosphorus	800 mg	1200 mg; needs 1½ times as much		Milk, cheese, lean meats
Iron	18 mg	30- to 60-mg supplement; needs almost two to three times as much	Increased maternal blood volume Fetus stores iron in third trimester	Liver, meats, eggs, leafy vegetables, nuts, legumes, whole wheat
Vitamin C (not stored in body so pregnant mother should have at least one serving per day)	60 mg	80 mg	Tissue formation Increased iron absorption	Citrus fruits, berries, melon, tomatoes, green peppers, green leafy vegetables, broccoli
Vitamin D	5-10 mcg; 200-400 international units	10-15 mcg; 400-600 international units; needs almost twice as much	Tooth buds Mineralizes bone tissue Aids absorption of calcium and phosphorus	Fortified milk Fortified margarine
Folic acid	180 mcg	400 mcg	Increases red blood cell formation Prevention of macrocytic and megaloblastic anemia and neural tube defects	Green leafy vegetables, oranges, broccoli, asparagus, liver

of childbirth and through the postpartum period. Parents are encouraged to use any combination of exercise that works for them.

b. Lamaze method (American Society for Prophylaxis in Obstetrics [ASPO]; psycho-prophylactic method [PPM], 1960): combines breathing techniques with preparation for childbirth by training mother to anticipate various stages of labor and meet each stage with practiced relaxation and breathing methods. Coach supports mother and directs her if necessary.

c. Breathing techniques are more effective if learned before labor. If a woman and her partner are using a technique effectively, do not interfere.

5. Nonpharmacological techniques can be used to augment pain relief; these include breathing, distraction, skin stimulation. Practitioners must be trained in these techniques before implementing them with patients.

6. Teaching of danger signs (those that must be reported to physician immediately)
   a. Persistent, severe vomiting beyond first trimester
   b. Epigastric or abdominal pain
   c. Edema: face, fingers; especially in the morning
   d. Visual disturbances: blurring, double vision, spots
   e. Frequent or continuous headaches
   f. Bleeding or leakage of fluid from vagina
   g. Absence of fetal movements (after quickening)
   h. Chills and fever (signs of infection)
   i. Rapid weight gain (signs of possible preeclampsia)

NORMAL DISCOMFORTS OF PREGNANCY
See Table 7-3.

ABNORMAL ANTEPARTUM

HYPERTENSIVE STATES
A. Definition: group of conditions that occur during pregnancy, usually after 20 weeks' gestation. Symptoms range from high BP to headaches, blurred vision, and convulsions with ensuing coma.
   1. Frequent in high-risk mothers
   2. Greater likelihood during first pregnancies
   3. Incidence: 5% to 7% of all pregnancies
B. Types
   1. GH: increase of BP to or above 140/90 mm Hg
      a. Increased BP only symptom
      b. Disappears within 10 days after delivery

Table 7-3 Normal Discomforts of Pregnancy

DISCOMFORT	PROBABLE CAUSE	RELIEF MEASURES
FIRST TRIMESTER		
Breasts: painful	Hypertrophy of glandular tissue Increased blood flow to area Hormonal effects	Firm, supportive bra, even a nursing bra
Urinary frequency	Pressure on bladder from expanding uterus reduces bladder capacity; increased vascular content	Pads if necessary
Yawning (tired, sleepy)	Whether result of relaxin hormone is questionable; possibly caused by sudden chemical changes in body	Frequent rest periods Balanced diet to prevent anemia
Nausea and vomiting	Hormonal changes Ambivalent feelings regarding pregnancy	Small, frequent meals Limited fluids Dry crackers with tea Avoidance of greasy, fried foods
SECOND TRIMESTER		
Heartburn (acid taste in mouth)	Relaxin hormone effect Enlarging uterus displaces stomach upward	Avoidance of fatty foods Antacids: milk of magnesia, Gelusil, Maalox, Amphojel
Pigmentation	Hormonal	Reassuring the mother that it is temporary and will disappear after delivery
Leg cramps	Calcium-phosphorus imbalance	Position relief Calf stretching Calcium supplements, milk
Constipation	Hormonal: slowing down of peristaltic movements Compression of colon by uterus and baby	Adequate fluids, fruits, foods with roughage Exercises Stool softener but no mineral oil
THIRD TRIMESTER		
Urinary incontinence	Lightening or dropping of fetus into pelvic cavity pushes presenting part on bladder	Pelvic floor exercises (Kegel): tighten perineal muscles, relax, then repeat
Hemorrhoids	Pressure from fetal presenting part	Increased vascular activity Knee-chest (elevate hips): Kegel exercises Comfort measures: frequent rest periods; sitting in warm tub; supporting legs with pillows
Low back pain	Increased pressure Fatigue Poor weight distribution	Pelvic exercises Pushing, stretching Comfort massaging Good posture
Insomnia	Increased fetal movements Muscular cramping Urinary frequency Dyspnea	Adequate rest periods Warm milk at bedtime Relaxing shower Support with pillows Deep breathing
Varicosities (leg, vulva)	Hereditary disposition Pelvic vasocongestion Pull of gravity Pressure of uterus Forcing stool (constipation)	Support stockings Changing position frequently Abdominal support Keeping legs uncrossed
Edema (legs, feet)	Immobility (staying in one position for a prolonged time)	Periodic resting Moving around Support stockings Elevating legs Plenty of fluids (to serve as a diuretic)

Table 7-3	Normal Discomforts of Pregnancy—cont'd	
DISCOMFORT	**PROBABLE CAUSE**	**RELIEF MEASURES**
Dyspnea (shortness of breath)	Pressure on diaphragm from expanding uterus	Sitting erect Deep breathing Putting arms above head Keeping weight down
Leaking of colostrum	Increased blood supply Prominent nipples	Support bra Pads if necessary (keep clean and dry)
Supine hypotension syndrome (feeling faint)	Pressure on ascending vena cava by uterus	Lying on left side with legs flexed or semisitting position
Vaginal discharge	Hormonal	No douching Keeping area clean, dry (perineal care)

2. Preeclampsia: an acute hypertensive condition resulting in elevated BP (increased systolic BP [30 mm Hg] or increased BP [15 mm Hg] over baseline) and proteinuria; edema may also be present.
   a. Mild preeclampsia
      (1) BP 140/90 mm Hg
      (2) Proteinuria 1+
      (3) Rapid weight gain
   b. Moderate-to-severe preeclampsia
      (1) Hospitalize immediately.
      (2) BP 160/110 mm Hg
      (3) Proteinuria 2 to 4
      (4) Persistent, severe headaches with visual disturbances
      (5) Epigastric pain (late sign)
      (6) Hyperactive deep-tendon reflexes (DTRs), clonus: an abnormal pattern of neuromuscular activity, characterized by rapidly alternating involuntary contraction and relaxation of skeletal muscle
3. Eclampsia
   a. Definition: most severe form of the hypertensive state, characterized by hypertensive crisis, shock, then grand mal seizure and possibly coma
   b. Signs and symptoms
      (1) Alarming weight gain
      (2) Scanty urine (less than 30 mL/hr)
      (3) Proteinuria 4+, RBCs in urine
      (4) BP 200/100 mm Hg or higher
      (5) Edema of retina; can cause blindness
      (6) Severe epigastric pain
      (7) Hyperactive DTRs
      (8) Convulsions: tonic and clonic

Note: May start labor prematurely; infant may be severely compromised and die.

4. HELLP (hemolysis, elevated liver function, and low platelet level) syndrome: a severe form of GH that involves multiple organ damage. The exact cause is unknown; HELLP syndrome is thought to arise as a result of changes occurring with preeclampsia. Arteriolar vasospasm, endothelial damage, and platelet aggregation lead to decreased tissue perfusion and organ damage.
C. Treatment and nursing management
   1. According to classification and severity of symptoms; varies from home care precautions to absolute bed rest in a hospital with patient lying on left side

2. Reduce stimuli.
3. Take seizure precautions.
4. Selective antihypertensive and diuretic therapy may be ordered (e.g., hydralazine hydrochloride [Apresoline], furosemide [Lasix], magnesium sulfate, mannitol, labetalol); nurse should know effects and untoward symptoms.
5. Monitor edema, BP, FHT, levels of consciousness, DTRs, impending labor signs.

HYPEREMESIS GRAVIDARUM

A. Definition: pernicious vomiting of pregnancy lasting into second trimester. It is a rare complication of pregnancy.
B. The cause is unknown. Theories include an adverse reaction to the elevated levels of the hormone hCG during pregnancy. Recent research shows that there may be a genetic component.
C. Signs and symptoms
   1. Excessive nausea, vomiting
   2. Considerable weight loss
   3. Severe dehydration
   4. Depletion of essential electrolytes (sodium and potassium)
   5. Vitamin, glucose, protein deficiencies
   6. Ketone bodies in urine: proteinuria 1+
   7. Elevated hemoglobin level, RBC count, hematocrit
D. Treatment and nursing management: if untreated, leads to death of mother or fetus or both
   1. Hospitalize in well-ventilated, private, pleasant environment.
   2. Restrict visitors.
   3. Allow nothing by mouth (NPO) first 48 hours.
   4. Record intake and output (I&O).
   5. If vomiting occurs, antiemetic medications may be administered.
   6. Provide IV fluids to replace losses in nutrition.
   7. Provide gradual servings of attractive, small portions of food on china dishes, starting with dry toast and tea.
   8. Present nonjudgmental nursing attitudes.
   9. Refer for psychotherapy when appropriate.

HEMORRHAGIC CONDITIONS

A. Abortion (early-pregnancy bleeding)
   1. Definition: the expulsion of uterine contents before viability of the fetus for medical reasons or spontaneously

2. Types
   a. Induced abortion
      (1) Termination of pregnancy (therapeutic): legal aborting of the fetus for medical or psychological reasons by a licensed physician under controlled, aseptic conditions
      (2) Criminal: an abortion performed under illegal, unsafe conditions
   b. Spontaneous abortion
      (1) Definition: an abortion that occurs naturally (usually in the first trimester)
      (2) Possible causes: hormonal deficiencies, abnormalities of the fetus, incompetent cervix, abnormalities of the reproductive organs, emotional shock, physical injury, acute infections, growths

3. Terminology of abortions
   a. Habitual abortion: three or more consecutive spontaneous abortions for unknown reasons
   b. Threatened abortion: minimal signs and symptoms of abortion such as bleeding and cramping but with no loss of uterine contents
   c. Imminent abortion: considerable blood loss, severe contractions; urge to push that, without treatment, results in loss of uterine contents
   d. Inevitable abortion: bleeding, contractions, rupture of membranes, and cervical dilation in which the uterine contents are lost. Treatment concentrates on the mother.
   e. Incomplete abortion: Part or parts of uterine contents are retained, necessitating administration of oxytocin to accelerate expulsion of remaining contents or dilation and curettage (D&C; a minor surgical intervention) to prevent prolonged bleeding.
   f. Complete abortion: Entire uterine contents are expelled.

4. Signs and symptoms of abortion
   a. Vaginal bleeding: scant to profuse
   b. Abdominal cramping: slight to severe
   c. Contractions: intermittent, steady, mild, or severe

5. Treatment and nursing management
   a. Prompt and immediate bed rest
   b. Hospitalization when appropriate
   c. Prevention of blood loss and shock
   d. Replacement blood treatment if necessary
   e. Checking of vital signs and temperature for 24 hours
   f. After an abortion, an Rh-negative woman should receive RhoGAM.
   g. Surgical intervention when appropriate: Shirodkar operation (purse-string suturing) for known incompetent cervix
   h. Psychotherapy when appropriate
      (1) Prepare for grieving process.
      (2) Provide assistance for burial regulations.
      (3) Let mother vent feelings of love, loss, guilt.
      (4) Provide quiet, supportive, compassionate nursing care.

B. Ectopic pregnancy (early pregnancy bleeding)
   1. Definition: extrauterine pregnancy in which the products of conception are implanted outside the uterine cavity; 90% occur in the fallopian tube (right tube more frequent). Other sites include the abdomen or the ovary.

2. Signs and symptoms
   a. Abnormal or missed menstrual period
   b. Slight uterine bleeding or spotting
   c. Possible mass on affected side; pain, tenderness, rigid abdomen
   d. If tube ruptures, may be little bleeding externally but massive internal hemorrhaging, with accompanying severe shock
   e. A diagnosis via transvaginal ultrasound is possible before tube ruptures. If diagnosis is made before rupture, laparoscopy is done to remove portion of the tube; goal is to remove ectopic pregnancy and preserve reproductive function; may also treat with methotrexate.

3. Treatment and nursing management
   a. Hospitalize immediately.
   b. Treat shock (warm, quiet; replacement therapy—IV fluids, oxygen).
   c. Cross-match and do other blood work: prepare for transfusion.
   d. Support mother, who will be extremely frightened.
   e. If tube is not ruptured, an effort is made to save the fallopian tube.
   f. Arrange for baptism of fetus when appropriate.
   g. Provide postsurgical care with IV fluids, medications, other appropriate treatments (RhoGAM if necessary).
   h. Provide emotional support to mother and family; get assistance of clergy when requested.

C. Gestational trophoblastic neoplasm (formerly known as *hydatidiform mole*)
   1. Definition: rare degeneration of chorionic villi into a benign neoplasm in which the villi fill with clear viscous fluid and form grapelike clusters; the neoplasm fills the decidua and expands the uterus to larger than normal for gestational age.

2. Signs and symptoms
   a. Enlarging uterus, greater than for normal gestation
   b. Missed period; spotting to profuse bleeding
   c. Several shiny, tapioca-like "grape clusters" escaping through vaginal tract
   d. Nausea and vomiting
   e. Signs of GH; usually before 20 weeks' gestation
   f. No FHT
   g. No fetal structures on ultrasound examination
   h. Laboratory findings: hCG titers up to 1 to 2 million (normally 350,000 to 400,000 at 8 weeks)

3. Treatment and nursing management
   a. Termination as soon as diagnosis confirmed
   b. Blood transfusion if indicated
   c. Assistance in grieving process of mother and family
   d. Follow-up very important
      (1) Contraceptive advice (nothing oral because hCG titers are distorted)
      (2) hCG titers for at least 6 months

D. Placenta previa (third-trimester bleeding)
   1. Definition: abnormal implantation of a normal placenta for unknown reasons, usually in the lower segment of the uterus. Condition usually occurs in multiparas, and incidence appears to increase with age; may also be caused by fibroids.
   2. Types (Figure 7-4)

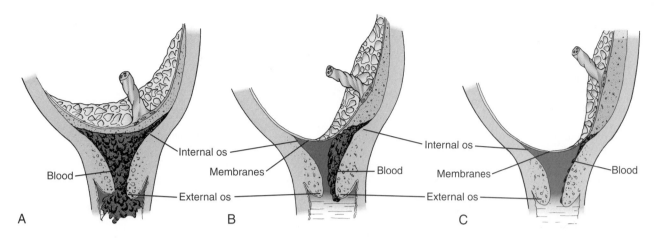

FIGURE 7-4 Types of placenta previa after onset of labor. **A,** Complete, or total. **B,** Incomplete, or partial. **C,** Marginal or low lying. (From Lowdermilk DL, et al: *Maternity and women's health care,* ed 10, St Louis, 2012, Mosby.)

a. Partial (incomplete): incomplete coverage of the uterine os
b. Complete (total): entire uterine os completely covered
c. Marginal (low lying): located in lower uterine segment but away from the os

3. Signs and symptoms
   a. Painless uterine bleeding: may be intermittent or occur in gushes; scanty to severe; bright red
   b. Third-trimester occurrence

4. Treatment and nursing management
   a. Diagnosis confirmed by ultrasound or x-ray examination
   b. Avoidance of vaginal examinations
   c. Immediate hospitalization
   d. Quiet environment; fetus uncompromised; station high
   e. Fowler position (head at 30-degree angle)
   f. Tocolytic therapy with use of magnesium sulfates to manage uterine irritability under certain circumstances
   g. Have double setup ready so that if vaginal examination is imperative, emergency caesarean equipment is available and blood is ready for transfusion.
   h. Foley catheter if condition is severe. Provide shock care.
   i. Count pads to determine amount, color, duration of bleeding.
   j. Monitor vital signs, especially BP.
   k. Monitor FHT and FHR.
   l. IV fluids; monitor
   m. Support patient and family; keep them informed.

E. Abruptio placentae (third-trimester bleeding)
   1. Definition: premature separation of a normally implanted placenta before the birth of the fetus
   2. Causes
      a. Trauma
      b. Chronic maternal disease
      c. Grand multipara
      d. Unknown
   3. Types (Figure 7-5)
      a. Complete: separation of the placenta from the uterine wall before birth of the fetus
      b. Partial: separation of a portion of the placenta from the wall of the uterus before the birth of the fetus
   4. Signs and symptoms
      a. Severe abdominal pain; sometimes called *exquisite* or *unrelenting*
      b. Patient is distressed and depressed, and she exhibits signs of shock.
      c. Painful bleeding: moderate to severe; internal or external; dark red, not clotted; varying amount
      d. Abdomen tense, boardlike; nurse unable to feel contractions; uterus irritable
      e. Hypovolemic shock possibly resulting in renal failure

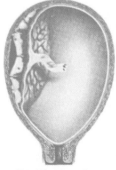
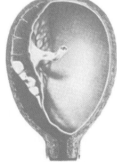
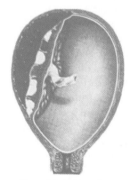

Partial separation (concealed hemorrhage)   Partial separation (apparent hemorrhage)   Complete separation (concealed hemorrhage)

FIGURE 7-5 Abruptio placentae. Premature separation of normally implanted placenta. (From Lowdermilk DL, et al: *Maternity and women's health care,* ed 10, St Louis, 2012, Mosby.)

f. Sudden change in heartbeat or bradycardia, or absence of FHT

5. Treatment and nursing management
   a. Depends on stage and intensity of condition; for reasons not clearly understood, partial abruptio placentae may seal off bleeding spontaneously, and labor proceeds normally.
   b. Check coagulation profile: fibrinogen and fibrin, platelets
   c. Prevent hypovolemic shock and fetal hypoxia.
   d. Cross-match, type, readiness for transfusions
   e. Monitor contractions, FHT, and vital signs.
   f. Slight or moderate bleeding may indicate ARM (or AROM) and thus a need to hasten delivery or seal off bleeding.
   g. Severe bleeding (dark red) may indicate immediate caesarean section.
   h. Support mother and family.
   i. Continued bleeding after delivery may necessitate hysterectomy.

F. DIC
   1. Cause
      a. Unknown
      b. Coincidental with abruptio placentae, postabortal infection, amniotic fluid emboli, placenta previa, and uterine atony
   2. Pathology: not clearly understood; massive clotting and depletion of coagulant factors. Factors that stimulate clotting and factors that prevent clotting are both activated at the same time.
   3. Signs and symptoms: excessive bleeding at placental site, incisional site, nose, mouth, gums
   4. Treatment and nursing management
      a. Halting or reversal of DIC by early detection of excessive bleeding (e.g., injection sites, gums)
      b. Elimination of cause
      c. Immediate delivery
      d. Blood replacement
      e. IV fibrinogen, heparin

MEDICAL AND INFECTIOUS CONDITIONS

A. Chickenpox (varicella)
   1. Causative agent: herpesvirus; varicella zoster virus (VZV)
   2. Effect on mother
      a. May manifest as herpes zoster (shingles)
      b. May be fatal if severe
      c. May cause abortion
   3. Effect on fetus
      a. May cause defects of skin, bones, hydrocephalus if contracted during first trimester
      b. Fetal death

B. German measles (rubella or 3-day measles)
   1. Causative agent: virus
   2. Effect on mother
      a. Rash, fever, photophobia
      b. Possible abortion
   3. Effect on fetus if infected during first trimester
      a. Rubella syndrome: heart defects, blindness, deafness, mental retardation
      b. Delayed effect on brain (15 to 20 years of age)

C. Genital herpes
   1. Causative agent: herpes simplex virus 2
   2. Effect on mother
      a. Vaginal discharge
      b. Genital blisters, ulcers
      c. Fever
      d. Painful inguinal lymph nodes
   3. Effect on fetus
      a. Abortion or premature birth
      b. Neonatal infections
      c. Survivors may have CNS symptoms.

D. Group B streptococcal infection
   1. Causative agent: *Streptococcus* bacterium found in the lower genital tract or rectum of 10% to 30% of all healthy pregnant women.
   2. Effect on mother
      a. Asymptomatic carriers
      b. Increased risk of abnormal vaginal discharge, urinary tract infection (UTI), endocarditis
   3. Effect on fetus
      a. Pneumonia and sepsis, which can result in death in 12 to 24 hours
      b. Blindness, deafness, mental retardation
   4. Treatment
      a. Prenatal screening: If cultures are positive, the drug of choice is penicillin G.
      b. High-risk women should be offered prophylactic antibiotics in labor.

E. Hepatitis A
   1. Causative agent: virus
   2. Effect on mother
      a. Abortion
      b. Liver failure
   3. Effect on fetus
      a. First-trimester infection: fetal anomalies
      b. Premature birth
      c. Neonatal hepatitis

F. Hepatitis B (serum hepatitis)
   1. Causative agent: hepatitis B virus (HBV); contact with blood and through sexual intercourse
   2. Effects on mother
      a. May be asymptomatic
      b. Low-grade fever, fatigue, joint pain, nausea, vomiting
      c. Liver and spleen enlargement, cirrhosis
      d. Vaccine available for high-risk women and health care workers
   3. Effect on fetus
      a. Avoid exposure of newborn to blood of mother.
      b. Preterm at birth
      c. May be asymptomatic at birth
      d. May exhibit signs of acute hepatitis
      e. Possible carrier
      f. Infants born to women who have hepatitis B should receive appropriate vaccinations.

G. Influenza
   1. Causative agent: virus
   2. Effect on mother
      a. Pneumonia
      b. Abortion
      c. Premature labor
   3. Effect on fetus

a. Abortion or premature birth

b. Fetal death

4. Vaccine for pregnant women available; live viral vaccine can infect fetus.

H. Gonorrhea ("clap")

1. Causative agent: *Neisseria gonorrhoeae* bacterium

2. Effect on mother

a. Vaginal discharge

b. Cervical tenderness

c. Dysuria

d. Affects ovaries, tubes, causing sterility

3. Effect on fetus

a. Ophthalmia neonatorum

b. Conjunctivitis

c. Mild-to-severe infections

I. Syphilis (lues)

1. Causative agent: *Treponema pallidum* bacterium

2. Effect on mother (if untreated)

a. Primary chancre

b. Secondary skin rash

c. Latent or tertiary CNS problems

3. Effect on fetus

a. Rhagades of the corners of mouth and anus

b. Snuffles

c. Maceration of palms of hands and soles of feet

d. Congenital syphilis (symptoms appearing later in life)

e. Death (stillborn)

J. Cytomegalovirus infection (CMV)

1. Causative agent: CMV of the herpes group, transmitted by close body and sexual contact

2. May be transmitted by asymptomatic woman to fetus, causing fetal damage, retardation, or fetal death

3. The infant may acquire the virus by exposure to cervical mucus during vaginal birth.

4. No satisfactory treatment is available for maternal or neonatal CMV.

K. Chlamydia

1. Causative agent: bacterial microorganism *Chlamydia trachomatis* (CT); transmitted by close body and sexual contact

2. May initiate pelvic inflammatory disease (PID), leading to ectopic pregnancy and infertility

3. Some evidence suggests relationship between CT and PROM, preterm labor and delivery, low birth weight, increased perinatal mortality, and late-onset endometritis.

4. Treatment is extended erythromycin.

5. Transmission from infected birth canal may result in conjunctivitis or pneumonia or both.

L. Cardiac disease

1. Classification

a. Class I: no limitation of activity

b. Class II: slight limitation of activity

c. Class III: considerable limitation of even ordinary activity

d. Class IV: symptoms of cardiac insufficiency even at rest

2. Treatment and nursing management

a. Close medical and nursing supervision

b. Watch for signs and symptoms of fatigue, dyspnea, coughing, palpitations, tachycardia.

c. Promote rest.

d. Hospitalize at end of second trimester.

e. Breast-feeding is contraindicated.

f. Provide contraceptive education.

g. Nutrition: Offer foods high in iron and protein. Avoid raw deep-green vegetables because these foods may interfere with clotting.

h. Prevent infections: Report first signs of exposure.

i. Teach comfortable positions: Use pillows, support left side.

j. During labor and delivery: Use epidural or caudal anesthesia block to minimize discomfort on bearing down.

k. Watch for cardiac decompensation (pulse rate more than 100 beats/min; respirations more than 25/min).

l. Vaginal delivery preferred.

(1) Episiotomy, low forceps

(2) Oxygen to decrease pulmonary edema

(3) Medication to regulate heart rate

(4) Diuretic to reduce fluid retention

m. Postpartum care

(1) Hospitalization longer than normal to stabilize cardiac output

(2) Application of abdominal binder (because of rapid change in intraabdominal pressure)

(3) Bed rest with progressive bathroom privileges dependent on progress

(4) Prevention of overdistention of bladder

(5) Encourage bonding. Nurse should hold baby at eye level to allow mother to touch and talk to baby.

(6) Inform mother and family of progress.

M. Diabetes mellitus

1. Definition: inborn error in the transportation and metabolism of carbohydrates

2. Classification: See Table 7-4.

3. Effects of diabetes on pregnancy

a. Difficult to control because of changing patterns of fetal growth and development and maternal demands

b. Fluctuating insulin requirements

c. Tendency to develop acidosis (diabetic coma) from lack of insulin

Table 7-4 Classifications of Diabetes

CLASSIFICATION	CHARACTERISTICS	TREATMENT DURING PREGNANCY
Type 1: insulin-dependent diabetes mellitus (IDDM)	Usually juvenile onset; prone to ketosis	Diet control and insulin
Type 2: non–insulin-dependent diabetes mellitus (NIDDM)	Usually adult onset; ketosis resistant; insulin may be required for hyperglycemia during stress; insulin required during pregnancy	Diet control and insulin
Other: gestational diabetes mellitus (GDM)	Develops during pregnancy	Diet control alone or insulin

    d. Increased tendency to infection (urinary tract, vaginal tract), preeclampsia, and polyhydramnios

    e. Increased incidence of premature labor

    f. Macrosomia (oversized baby)

    g. Possibility of dystocia

    h. Increased danger of placental deterioration causing hypoxia in fetus

    i. Tendency toward abruptio placentae

4. Changing insulin requirements during pregnancy

    a. First trimester: insulin requirement decreased

    b. Second trimester: insulin requirement increased

    c. Third trimester: careful regulation (blood sugar); evaluation of placenta, oxytocin challenge test (CST)

    d. Intranatal: Labor depletes glycogen.

    e. Postpartum: Insulin reaction results from sudden drop in need.

    f. Watch for hypoglycemia, shock, infection, bleeding.

    g. Insulin is not needed 24 to 48 hours after delivery.

    h. Hospitalize until insulin balance is restored.

5. Early recognition of insulin reaction and diabetic coma

6. Treatment and nursing management

    a. Weekly prenatal visits

    b. Regulation of insulin dosage and dietary management

    c. Mother taught to test blood three or four times per day

    d. Testing for placental adequacy: CST (stress test) measures fetal response to uterine contractions; late deceleration indicates problem.

    e. Teach good nutrition.

    f. Help allay fears and anxieties.

N. Addiction and pregnancy

1. Drug addiction

    a. Effect on mother

      (1) Abortion

      (2) Premature birth

      (3) Stillbirth

    b. Effect on neonate: see section on drug addiction in newborns, p. 382.

2. Alcohol and pregnancy

    a. Effect on mother

      (1) Poor nutritional habits

      (2) Poor hygiene

      (3) Physical, psychosocial deterioration

    b. Effect on neonate: see section on abnormal newborn, p. 377.

3. Treatment and nursing management

    a. Supervised withdrawal

    b. Substitute therapy

ACQUIRED IMMUNODEFICIENCY SYNDROME

A. Transmission of HIV to the unborn fetus has been confirmed via anal or vaginal intercourse, sharing of needles among drug addicts, and contaminated blood transfusions. Transmission to the fetus or neonate can occur transplacentally and via breast milk. Caesarean delivery does not appear to totally prevent the transmission of the virus.

B. Treatment and nursing management

1. If an HIV-positive pregnant woman is not already on a combination of antiretroviral medications, she should be started on them immediately. During labor the physician may elect to administer IV zidovudine (INN) or azidothymidine (Retrovir) or (AZT). Babies may receive antiviral medications as well.

2. Pregnant HIV-infected women should receive Pneumovax and influenza and hepatitis vaccines and be screened for sexually transmitted diseases; results are confidential.

3. HIV-positive women need counseling to practice safe sex to decrease risk of repeatedly exposing fetus.

4. Infants need to be observed and tested for a minimum of 2 years to determine if they have the disease.

5. Strict adherence to Standard Precautions is required.

TUBERCULOSIS

A. Tuberculosis is an increasingly prevalent health problem throughout the world. This can be attributed to homelessness, drug abuse, poverty, and HIV.

B. The major avenue of transmission is via the airborne route.

C. Treatment can be preventative or immediate.

1. Preventive therapy; postponed until after delivery

2. A pregnant woman with active disease needs immediate treatment with two or three antituberculosis drugs.

3. Breast-feeding is permitted; however, infant needs to undergo prophylactic treatment.

ASTHMA

A. Definition: chronic lung disease in which airways are overly responsive to stimuli such as allergens, pollutants, exercise, and cold air

1. Asthma occurs in approximately 1% of all pregnant women.

2. The incidence of preeclampsia is higher in patients with asthma.

B. Signs and symptoms: cough, wheezing, dyspnea, chest tightness

C. Treatment and nursing management

1. Pulmonary function tests to monitor lung function

2. NSTs to monitor fetal well-being

3. Avoidance of allergens

4. Pharmacological therapies

5. Breast-feeding to provide some neonatal protection against respiratory allergens

PREMATURE LABOR

A. Definition: labor occurring before 37 to 38 weeks' gestation

B. Effect on family (focus on psychosocial problems)

1. Mother not ready for delivery: apprehensive and frightened; feelings of guilt

2. Family plus professional staff: restrained, quiet, anticipating complications

C. Effect on fetus: see section on preterm (premature) infant in discussion of abnormal newborn, p. 377.

D. Treatment and nursing management

1. PROM usually precedes premature labor; test fluid with Nitrazine paper: if alkaline, positive for amniotic fluid.

2. If membranes are intact and cervix is undilated, halt labor if possible; magnesium sulfate and terbutaline are frequently used to halt premature labor.

3. Immediate bed rest is required.

4. Monitor maternal pulse and BP.

5. Know untoward effects of medications.

6. Prevent infection.

7. Offer constant emotional support to mother and family: inform, reassure, encourage mother and family.

NORMAL INTRAPARTUM (LABOR AND DELIVERY)

A. Fetal head (passenger)
　1. Two parietal bones: one on each side of head
　2. Two temporal bones: one on each side of head near temple
　3. Two frontal bones: one on each side of forehead
　4. One occipital bone: lower back of head
　5. Sutures: membranous spaces between bones
　　a. Sagittal suture: separates parietal bones and extends longitudinally back to front
　　b. Frontal suture: between two frontal bones, continuation of the sagittal suture
　　c. Coronal suture: as a crown; separates frontal and parietal bones
　　d. Lambdoid suture: separates occipital bone from two parietal bones
　6. Fontanels: formed by intersection of sutures; allow head bones to override and accommodate to birth passage
　　a. Anterior fontanel: membranous, diamond-shaped space (bregma) formed by intersection of sagittal, frontal, and coronal sutures; called *soft spot;* closes within 12 to 18 months
　　b. Posterior fontanel: small, membranous, triangular space between occipital bone and two parietal bones; closes within 6 to 8 weeks
　7. Principal measurements of the fetal head
B. Presentations, positions, station
　1. Presentation
　　a. Definition: refers to that part of the passenger (fetus) that enters the passage (true pelvis, uterine os, vaginal canal) first
　　b. Types of presentations
　　　(1) Cephalic: head, vertex, occiput (93%)
　　　(2) Breech: buttocks, sacrum, one or both legs, one or both feet (3%)
　　　(3) Shoulder: scapula (3%)
　2. Lie (Figure 7-6)
　　a. Definition: refers to the relationship between the long axis of the passenger and the long axis of the mother
　　b. Types
　　　(1) Longitudinal (99%)
　　　(2) Transverse (sideways)
　3. Position (Figure 7-7)
　　a. Definition: way in which the presenting part of the fetus lies in relation to the four quadrants of the mother's pelvis and to her back (posterior) and front (anterior)
　　b. To determine position, fetal reference points are used; these are:
　　　(1) Occiput (back of fetal head): O.
　　　(2) Chin (mentum): M.
　　　(3) Brow (bregma): B.
　　　(4) Buttocks (sacrum): S.
　　　(5) Shoulder (scapula): Sc.
　　c. Types of positions with occiput presentations: left occiput anterior (LOA); left occiput transverse (LOT); left occiput posterior (LOP); right occiput anterior (ROA); right occiput transverse (ROT); right occiput posterior (ROP) (Figure 7-7)

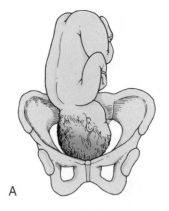

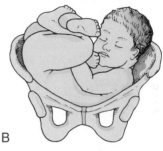

A

B

FIGURE 7-6 **A,** Longitudinal lie. **B,** Transverse lie. (From Phillips CR: *Family-centered maternity and newborn care: a basic text,* ed 4, St Louis, 1996, Mosby.)

　4. Attitude
　　a. Definition: relationship of the various fetal parts to one another or of the fetal extremities to the fetal body (trunk)
　　b. Normal attitude: flexed; fetal head on sternum, arms folded against chest; knees bent, pressing abdomen; legs flexed so toes touch arm
　5. Station
　　a. Definition: degree to which presenting part is located in the true pelvis. Points of reference are the ischial spines, which are designated as 0 (zero).
　　b. Levels
　　　(1) Minus: as in −1, −2, −3 station, means that presenting part is above the ischial spines
　　　(2) Plus: as in +1, +2, +3 station, means that the presenting part is below the ischial spines
　　　(3) −5=floating; +5=presenting part on perineum; or −3 to −5=floating; +3 to +5=presenting part on perineum. Check with agency for the numbers used.
C. Mechanisms and stages of labor: Labor cannot progress without power.
　1. Definition: the steps or maneuvers the fetus must undertake to accommodate to the passage and be delivered
　2. Process (mechanisms) (Figure 7-8)
　　a. Engagement: passage of the passenger into the pelvic inlet
　　b. Descent: continuous slow progress of the fetus through the pelvis and birth canal
　　c. Flexion: Head slowly adapts to birth canal by flexing chin.
　　d. Internal rotation: Fetal head turns in corkscrew maneuver so the long diameter of the head is parallel to the longest diameter of the pelvic outlet.

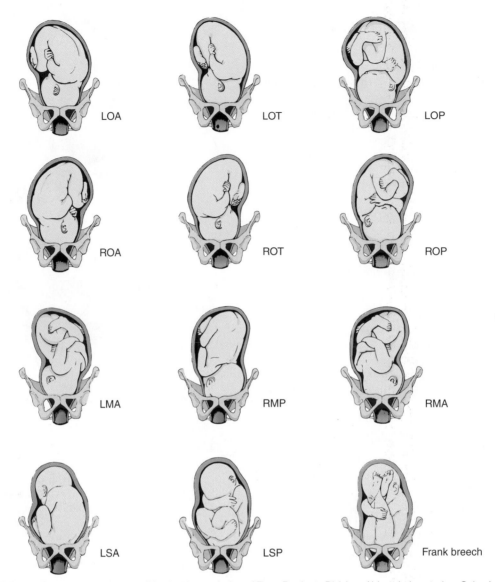

FIGURE 7-7 Categories of presentations. (Used with permission of Ross Products Division, Abbott Laboratories, Columbus, Ohio.)

e. Extension: The back of the fetal head goes under the pubic arch; the spine of the fetus extends to adapt itself to the curvature of the birth canal, and the head is delivered.

f. Restitution: As the head emerges, it rotates back 45 degrees to its position before internal rotation, which helps the shoulders accommodate to the outlet.

g. External rotation: The shoulders drop down and turn to the anteroposterior position, and the head slowly turns so both head and shoulders are aligned.

h. Expulsion: The posterior (underneath) shoulder is delivered by lateral flexion (upward motion); then the anterior upper shoulder slides out (downward motion) from under the pubic arch, and the body is easily expelled.

3. Stages of labor

a. First stage: begins with the first true labor contraction; ends with complete dilation and effacement of the cervix; consists of three phases (latent, active, and transition)

b. Second stage (expulsion): from complete effacement and dilation to expulsion of the infant

c. Third stage (placental): from delivery of the infant to delivery of the placenta and membranes (5 to 20 minutes)

d. Fourth stage: from delivery of the secundines and repair of the perineum to 1 hour thereafter

D. Fetal evaluation during labor and delivery and immediately after

1. During labor

a. Fetal monitoring devices

(1) Phonotransducer: amplifies fetal heart activity

(2) Doppler transducer: ultrasonic device

b. Special stethoscopes for monitoring FHT

(1) Head scope (fetoscope): stethoscope on a head device; FHT conducted through monitor's frontal bone

(2) Leff stethoscope: stethoscope with large, heavy conductor

(3) External fetal monitor (EFM): applied to abdomen; FHT monitored electronically

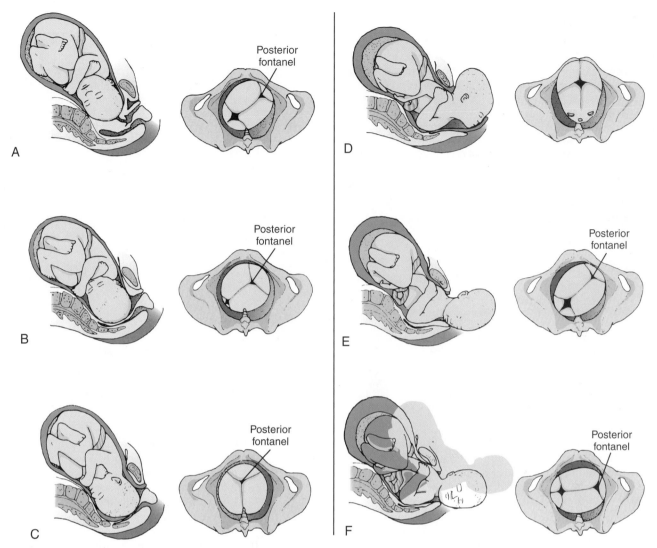

FIGURE 7-8 Mechanism of labor in left occipitoanterior (LOA) presentation. **A,** Engagement and descent. **B,** Flexion. **C,** Internal rotation to occipitoanterior (OA). **D,** Extension. **E,** Restitution. **F,** External rotation.

c. Direct fetal monitoring: an electrocardiogram (ECG). A fetal scalp electrode (FSE) is placed directly on the fetal head.
2. Evaluation immediately after delivery
   a. Establishment of patent airway
   b. Apgar scoring (Table 7-5): system of evaluating newborn response 1 and 5 minutes after birth
   c. Observation for any visible anomalies
E. Nursing assessment
   1. Premonitory (impending) signs and symptoms of labor
      a. Lightening: descent of fetus down pelvic cavity
      b. Braxton-Hicks contractions: painless contractions more frequent, irregular
      c. Breathing easier; heartburn disappears; hungry
      d. Weight loss (decrease in water retention)
      e. Frequency (pressure on bladder by presenting part)
      f. Bloody show (slight pinkish discharge with or without discharge of mucus plug)
      g. Bag of waters (BOW) ruptures spontaneously without prior contractions.
   2. Differences between true and false labor

   a. False labor
      (1) Contractions irregular
      (2) No progress in interval or duration of contractions
      (3) Some abdominal discomfort
      (4) No bloody show
      (5) Relief with walking
      (6) No cervical change
      (7) Discomfort mostly in front (lower abdomen)
   b. True labor
      (1) Contractions regular and progressive
      (2) Not relieved by walking
      (3) Cervical changes
      (4) Progressive discomfort starting in back, going around lower abdomen, indentable fundus
   3. Spontaneous rupture of membranes
      a. Note time, amount, and color of fluid; note FHTs.
      b. Prevent infection (handwashing, good hygienic practice).
      c. Observe for prolapsed cord (notify physician immediately).
      d. If leakage minimal, spontaneous resealing may occur.
      e. If close to EDC, contractions may begin, usually within 4 to 16 hours.

Table 7-5	**Apgar Scoring System**

The Apgar scoring system provides a quick and accurate way of evaluating a baby's physical status right at birth, regardless of any combination of weaknesses or debilities. The physician or nurse observes the five signs and records the score for each. Each sign is evaluated according to the degree to which it is present: 0 (poor), 1 (fair), or 2 (good). The five scores are then added together. Apgar scores ranges from 0 to 10. A score of 10 means the baby is in the best possible condition. A score of 9 or 8 indicates good condition; 7, 6, 5, or 4 indicates fair condition. A score of 3, 2, 1, or 0 indicates poor condition and the need for prompt diagnosis and treatment of specific disorders.

SIGN	0	1	2	SCORE
Heart rate: strong and steady?	Not detectable	Slow (less than 100)	Above 100	
Respiratory effort: breathing frequently and regularly?	Absent	Slow, irregular	Good; crying	
Muscle tone: kicking feet and making fists?	Flaccid	Some flexion of extremities	Active motion	
Reflex irritability: lusty cry elicited if catheter is pushed up one nostril or soles of feet are prodded?	No response	Grimace	Cry; cough or sneeze	
Color: pink all over, or hands and feet bluish?	Blue, pale	Body pink, extremities bluish	Completely pink or absence of cyanosis	
			TOTAL	

From Price DL, Gwin JF: *Pediatric nursing,* ed 10, St Louis, 2008, Saunders.

F. Nursing interventions
  1. Nursing management during first stage of labor
    a. Admit patient to labor room.
    b. Establish rapport. Ask pertinent questions regarding labor. Observe reaction to labor process.
    c. Offer bedpan frequently (keep bladder empty).
    d. Usually an IV line is started to keep a vein open. (Prepare equipment, solutions.)
    e. Monitor contractions, FHR.
      (1) Hook up to fetal monitoring device.
      (2) Check every 30 to 60 minutes (depending on progress).
      (3) Frequency, duration, and intensity of uterine contractions are assessed to help determine the progress of labor.
      (4) When ominous FHR patterns occur (e.g., late decelerations, lack of variability), the nurse must document interventions and subsequent fetal response.
    f. Keep mother, father informed about status and progress.
      (1) Monitor effacement, dilation, station.
      (2) Encourage father to follow monitor readout.
      (3) Encourage father to use comfort measures for mother.
  2. Nursing management during second stage of labor
    a. Uterine muscles bring about effacement and dilation. Abdominal muscles bring fetus down after dilation and effacement are complete. Levator muscles assist in pushing and expelling fetus.
    b. All monitoring equipment is removed from mother.
      (1) Explain procedures.

      (2) Clean perineal area according to hospital policy.
      (3) Computers are frequently used to monitor FHR. EFM, fetoscope, or both are also used. Inform physician of rate, strength, position.
      (4) Check BP every 15 minutes as necessary.
      (5) Prepare necessary equipment for delivery readiness and reception of baby.
      (6) Instruct mother to push with contractions when indicated.
      (7) When infant is delivered completely, note time.
      (8) Establish patent airway.
      (9) Encourage mother and father to see, touch, and speak to infant.
      (10) Carefully place prophylactic drops in each eye.
      (11) Follow proper identification routine.
      (12) Transfer infant into warm crib for further evaluation and care.
  3. Nursing management during third stage (placental)
    a. Be sure that cord blood specimen is taken.
    b. Placenta is delivered within 5 to 20 minutes from expulsion of infant.
    c. Note time and which side of placenta is delivered.
      (1) Maternal side, raw and meaty: Duncan delivery
      (2) Fetal side, shiny and neat: Schultze delivery
    d. Administer oxytocin immediately after delivery of placenta to contract uterus and prevent hemorrhage.
    e. Check BP every 15 minutes.
    f. Check fundus for firmness; soft, boggy indicates possible hemorrhaging.
    g. Check and clean perineal area; apply sanitary napkin.
    h. Mother may experience knees shaking, teeth chattering.

(1) Sudden changes in abdominal pressure plus hormonal changes trigger these symptoms.

(2) Place several warm blankets over mother.

(3) Reassure mother and family that it is a normal physiological phenomenon.

   i. Transfer mother to recovery area (if not in birthing room).

4. Nursing management during fourth stage of delivery
   a. Critical hour after delivery; watch for complications, especially hemorrhaging.
   b. Perform fundal check every 5 minutes; massage gently if necessary.
   c. Check BP and vital signs every 10 to 15 minutes until stable.
   d. After approximately 1 hour, when vital signs are stable:
      (1) Offer warm drink, toast, or even meal tray if mother wishes and physician approves.
      (2) Offer bedpan frequently to prevent bladder distention, which impedes involution. If mother is unable to void, catheterization is usually a standing order.
      (3) Give sponge bath to refresh and clean body.
      (4) Teach perineal care with Peri-Bottle.
      (5) Transfer to postpartum room.
      (6) Advise mother to request help the first time she wishes to use the bathroom.

5. Commonly used medications during labor and delivery: Prepared childbirth has greatly diminished use of analgesics and anesthetics during labor and delivery. Patients who experience dystocia may need some medication for relief from exhaustion, fright, or prolonged pain.
   a. Amnesic
   b. Tranquilizer
   c. Analgesic
   d. Regional anesthesia
      (1) Paracervical block: anesthetizes cervical area
      (2) Pudendal block: peripheral nerve block; may also block urge to push for 30 minutes
      (3) Caudal block (spinal): used during first and second stages; continuous or one dose
      (4) Saddle block: third, fourth, or fifth lumbar interspace; anesthetizes saddle area (inner groin, perineal area)
      (5) Epidural: also administered into lumbar interspace; uses less anesthetic than caudal; blocks urge to push
      (6) Spinal block: most commonly used for caesarean birth
   e. Nursing management
      (1) Encourage urination; encourage fluids.
      (2) Observe for postspinal headache. Treatment includes bed rest, ibuprofen, IV caffeine. The definitive treatment is a blood patch.
   f. General anesthesia: rare

ABNORMAL INTRAPARTUM

DYSTOCIA

A. Definition: prolonged, difficult, painful labor or delivery involving one or more problems with any of the three *P*s: passage, power, and passenger

B. Problems with passage
   1. Inadequate pelvis
   2. Soft-tissue deviation: A full bladder is the most common cause.

C. Problems with the power (uterine contractions)
   1. Primary uterine inertia: inefficient contractions from the beginning
   2. Secondary uterine inertia: well-established labor with good contractions at first; then progress of labor suddenly or gradually slows and stops altogether
   3. Hypotonic contractions (atonic uterus): most common; no progress in effacement or dilation
   4. Hypertonic uterine contractions
      a. Intense, titanic
      b. No interval between contractions
   5. Dystonic contractions
      a. Painful
      b. Ineffective
      c. Asymmetrical (contractions in different segments of the uterus)

D. Problems with passenger (fetus)
   1. Excessive size
   2. Fetal anomaly
   3. Fetal malposition or malpresentation
      a. Occiput posterior (most common)
      b. Breech presentation
      c. Transverse lie
      d. Face presentation
      e. Soldier (military) presentation
   4. CPD
      a. Accommodation impossible
      b. May note unusual contour of uterus or abdomen

E. Complications
   1. PROM
   2. Predisposition to infection
   3. Trauma
   4. Hemorrhage
   5. Prolapse of cord
   6. Hypoxia of fetus
   7. Severe molding of fetal head: danger of intracranial hemorrhage
   8. Extreme backache (posterior positions)
   9. Flowering of anus early because of pressure of occiput on lower sacral region, with consequence of hemorrhoids
   10. Extreme fatigue

F. Treatment and nursing management
   1. Electronic monitoring of fetus and mother
   2. Frequent confirmation of cervical progress
   3. Sterile techniques during vaginal examination
   4. Check status of BOW.
   5. Check vital signs.
   6. Observe condition of mother.
      a. Need for pain relief
      b. Sometimes after a medicated sleep or rest, dystocia disappears.
   7. Support physical and psychological needs.
   8. Watch for dehydration.
   9. Spontaneous rotation toward end of transition may occur in occiput posterior presentations.

SUPINE HYPOTENSIVE SYNDROME

A. Definition: condition caused by compression of vena cava by heavy uterus for a prolonged period; caused by mother's staying in one position for a long time
B. Signs and symptoms
  1. Pallor
  2. Light-headedness
  3. Dizziness
  4. Slight nausea
C. Treatment and nursing management: Turn patient on left side to relieve pressure. Advise frequent turning and changing of position.

RUPTURED UTERUS

A. Causes
  1. Tetanic, pauseless, or continuous contractions
    a. Possible cause: unmonitored oxytocin (Pitocin) infusion
    b. Unknown
  2. Stretching of uterine walls by extensive, rapid growth of hydatidiform mole
  3. Attempted vaginal birth after caesarean (VBAC) and uterine scar ruptures during labor
  4. CPD
  5. Forceps delivery
B. Treatment and nursing management
  1. Prepare for emergency caesarean delivery.
  2. Monitor for signs of hypovolemic shock and fetal distress.
  3. Prepare for all anticipatory nursing responsibilities, surgical and medical.

PROLAPSED CORD

A. Definition: displacement of the cord below the presenting part and into the vaginal passage before delivery of fetus
B. Causes
  1. Spontaneous rupture of the membranes before engagement
  2. Breech presentations
  3. Prematurity
  4. Polyhydramnios
  5. Abnormal presentations
C. Signs and symptoms
  1. Cord may be seen, felt, or palpated.
  2. Fetal heart pattern is abnormal (baseline bradycardia with decelerations).
D. Treatment and nursing management
  1. Call for immediate help.
  2. Do not compress cord; do not try to reposition it.
  3. Use sterile saline compress to keep cord moist and protected from infection.
  4. Place mother in knee-chest or Trendelenburg position so the presenting part is pushed away from cord by gravity.
  5. Prepare for caesarean delivery, blood cross-match, IV fluids, and so on.
  6. Check FHR or use continuous external fetal monitoring.
  7. Support frightened mother and family.
  8. If not a standing order, obtain an order for the mother to receive oxygen by mask.

MULTIPLE PREGNANCIES

A. Definition: simultaneous gestation; twins, triplets, quadruplets, quintuplets, sextuplets, septuplets
B. Signs and symptoms
  1. History of multiple gestation (female lineage)
  2. Hearing two FHTs, each with own rate
  3. Disclosure of multiple limbs, heads, by palpation
  4. Larger than normal uterus for time of gestation
  5. Weight gain increased more than in normal gestation
  6. Striae gravidarum more noticeable early in the pregnancy
  7. Confirmation by sonogram
  8. X-ray examination may be done but only in the third trimester.
C. Types (Figure 7-9)

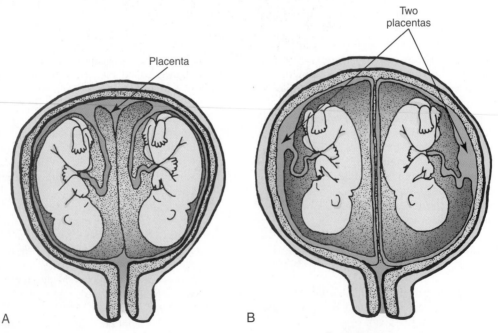

FIGURE 7-9 Multiple pregnancies. **A,** Identical (monozygotic) twins: two sacs, one placenta. **B,** Fraternal (dizygotic) twins: two sacs, two placentas. (From Phillips CR: Family-centered maternity and newborn care: a basic text, ed 4, St Louis, 1996, Mosby.)

1. Single-ovum twins (monozygotic, identical)
   a. Union of one sperm with one ovum
   b. During mitosis divides into two embryos
   c. One placenta, two amniotic sacs
   d. Same gender
   e. Heredity a factor
2. Fraternal twins (dizygotic, nonidentical)
   a. Union of two sperm with two separate ova
   b. Two amniotic sacs
   c. Separate or fused placenta
   d. Same or different gender
   e. Do not look identical
   f. Age of mother a factor. Older women tend to release more than one ovum.
3. Formation of triplets and so on varies.
D. Treatment and nursing management
   1. Prenatal care
      a. Visits are increased.
      b. Observe for signs and symptoms of preeclampsia.
      c. Premature labor is common.
      d. Backaches are common: support girdle, longer rest periods.
      e. Varicosities are common.
      f. Watch for complications resulting from position, presentation, lie of fetuses.
      g. Size of fetuses may cause problems.
      h. Be alert for possible caesarean delivery.
   2. Intrapartal care
      a. Be prepared for premature labor and premature babies.
      b. High-risk second stage
   3. Third and fourth stages
      a. There is a possibility of hemorrhage because of oversize uterus.
      b. Blood loss is greater than that for single births.
      c. Oxytocin is not administered to mother until all babies delivered.
      d. Risk of infection is greater than that in normal single births.
      e. Perinatal mortality is greater than that in single deliveries.

INDUCTION OF LABOR

A. Definition: use of medication (oxytocin) to stimulate contractions before spontaneous onset
B. Indications
   1. Overdue fetus (over 42 weeks' gestation)
   2. Fetal death
   3. Prolonged rupture of membranes (over 24 hours) if uterine contractions have not begun
   4. PROM
   5. Mother with diabetes
   6. Severe preeclampsia (exercise extreme caution)
   7. Steeply rising Rh titer
C. Contraindications
   1. CPD
   2. Fetal distress
   3. Previous caesarean delivery
   4. Multiple births
   5. Heart conditions
   6. Prematurity
   7. Unengaged presenting part
   8. Placenta previa

9. Abnormal fetal position (breech or transverse lie)
10. Active genital herpes
D. Treatment and nursing management
   1. Monitor contractions carefully with EFM.
   2. If there are no intervals between contractions, stop medication drip and call physician immediately.
   3. Monitor FHR and report any changes immediately.
   4. Check BP: Gradual elevation warrants immediate discontinuation of medication and prompt notification of physician.
   5. Keep family and mother informed of progress and procedure.
   6. Monitor vital signs, I&O.
   7. The physician or nurse-midwife assesses for cervical dilation as needed and observes for the resting tone of the uterus before increasing the oxytocin (Pitocin) dose.

AUGMENTATION OF LABOR

A. Definition: use of medication to enhance existing contractions
B. Uses
   1. Uterine inertia: primary or secondary
   2. Atonic or hypotonic uterine contractions (may be enhanced by a boost of oxytocin)

OPERATIVE OBSTETRICS

A. Episiotomy
   1. Definition: surgical incision of the perineum during delivery to enlarge the vaginal outlet
   2. Types (Figure 7-10)
   3. Indications
      a. To prevent tearing
      b. To shorten second stage of labor
      c. Fetus or mother in jeopardy
   4. Treatment and nursing management
      a. Provide comfort measures (to promote healing); sitz bath and ice pack first 12 hours.
      b. Encourage Kegel exercises (to lessen pain, promote healing).
      c. Apply witch hazel pads to perineal area (to decrease swelling, promote healing).
B. Forceps deliveries
   1. Definition: operative procedure using various instruments to deliver the presenting part

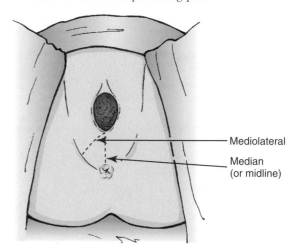

FIGURE 7-10 Types of episiotomies. (From Lowdermilk DL, et al: *Maternity and women's health care,* ed 10, St Louis, 2012, Mosby.)

2. Indications for use
   a. To shorten second stage
   b. To assist in descent of presenting part when poor progress or fetal distress occurs
   c. Maternal exhaustion
   d. When rotation (of head) is necessary (e.g., left occiput posterior [LOP] to occiput anterior [OA])
   e. To save fetus in jeopardy
3. Requirements for application
   a. No CPD
   b. Presenting part engaged and below ischial spines
   c. Full dilation and effacement
   d. Ruptured membranes
   e. Emptied bladder
   f. FHR checked before and after application
4. Complications
   a. Lacerations and tears
   b. Hemorrhage
   c. Rupture of uterus
   d. Facial marks or facial paralysis of fetus
   e. Intracranial hemorrhage or brain damage to fetus
C. Vacuum extraction
   1. Definition: Soft, flexible cup is placed over the fetal head as a machine exerts suction; allows practitioner to turn or pull the fetal head to assist delivery; an alternative to the use of forceps.
   2. Problems for the fetus can be observed at the attachment site, including caput succedaneum or cephalhematoma.
D. Caesarean section; also called *caesarean birth* or *caesarean delivery*
   1. Definition: operative procedure to deliver the fetus through a surgical incision made through the abdominal and uterine walls
   2. Indications
      a. CPD
      b. Fetal distress
      c. Prematurity
      d. Dystocia
      e. Prolapsed cord
      f. Oversize infant (macrosomia)
      g. Positions and presentations undeliverable through the vagina
      h. Some hypertensive states, placenta previa, abruptio placentae, prolapsed cord abnormalities
      i. Maternal exhaustion
   3. Types
      a. Elective
         (1) Anticipated difficulties: for example, inadequate pelvis or vaginal deliveries inadvisable because mother has AIDS or herpes
         (2) Previous caesarean deliveries (selective)
      b. Emergency
         (1) Sudden fetal distress (e.g., rupture of the uterus)
         (2) Accident
         (3) Breech presentation, shoulder presentation (transverse lie)
   4. Treatment and nursing management
      a. Perform routine surgical preoperative and postoperative care plus normal postpartum care.
      b. Promote involution.
      c. Provide perineal care.
      d. Monitor lochia (color, amount) same as for vaginal delivery.
      e. Support mother and family; allay fears.
      f. Watch for signs and symptoms of infection (chills, fever).
   5. VBAC: Vaginal delivery after a caesarean may be encouraged; depends on reason for caesarean.

NORMAL POSTPARTUM

A. Definition: period from end of fourth stage of labor to 6 weeks after day of delivery
B. Immediate care after delivery
   1. Continue checking vital signs.
   2. Encourage urination.
      a. Full bladder impedes involution.
      b. Full bladder may cause excessive bleeding.
   3. Offer food: If policy permits, offer food and drink to mother after vital signs are stable.
   4. Care of fundus
      a. Check for firmness. Place cupped hand under the umbilicus and press on abdomen firmly. Fundus feels like a grapefruit in the beginning. Measure number of fingerbreadths below the umbilicus.
      b. Check lochia for color, amount, and presence of clots.
   5. Provide perineal care and care of breasts.
   6. Check incision (episiotomy or abdominal).
   7. General hygiene: Shower may be permissible to clean, refresh mother after vital signs are stable (policies vary).
   8. Encourage putting infant to breast for feeding and bonding.
C. Physiological changes during puerperium
   1. Reproductive organs
      a. Uterus: involution (return of uterus to normal size and function)
         (1) Walls of uterus return to normal in 3 to 4 weeks.
         (2) Menstruation may return in 3 to 4 weeks.
         (3) Nursing mothers: Menstruation may be delayed several months.
         (4) Fundus involution is one finger width every day if umbilicus is used as point of reference (Figure 7-11).

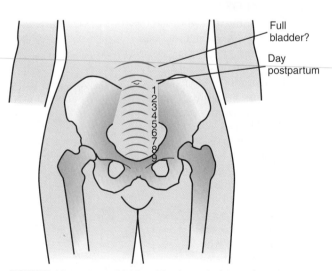

FIGURE 7-11 Involution. Height of fundus as it descends to prepregnant levels postpartum. (From Lowdermilk DL, et al: *Maternity and women's health care,* ed 10, St Louis, 2012, Mosby.)

b. Vagina
   (1) Returns to normal within 3 to 6 weeks after delivery, depending on factors such as type of delivery, length of labor, lacerations, and healing process
   (2) Caesarean deliveries: vaginal recovery rapid
c. Perineal area
   (1) Should be intact and clean
   (2) Requires 5 to 7 days for complete healing

2. Return to normal of body system and functions
   a. Hormonal recovery begins immediately.
   b. Lochia: vaginal discharge coming from decidual lining of uterus after delivery
      (1) Lochia rubra: dark red to bright red; occasional clots. Flow lasts 2 to 3 days.
      (2) Lochia serosa: pale pink to brownish lochia; lighter flow, dependent on ambulation; lasts 2 to 5 days
      (3) Lochia alba: yellowish, creamy discharge consisting of leukocytes and dead cells; lasts 5 to 10 days
      (4) Prolonged or recurring bleeding may indicate a medical problem.
   c. Vascular system
      (1) Average loss of blood at delivery: 250 to 400 mL
      (2) Hemorrhage: blood loss of 500 mL or more
   d. Urinary tract
      (1) Perineal soreness may temporarily reduce voiding reflexes.
      (2) Marked diuresis occurs 8 to 12 hours postpartum.

D. Treatment and nursing management for postpartum care
   1. Objectives for daily care
      a. Assist in normal process of involution; examples include assessing the fundus and promoting urination.
      b. Assist in preventing infection; examples include proper handwashing and promoting proper breastfeeding technique.
      c. Promote infant bonding with mother and family; examples include sibling visits when appropriate and encouraging partner to participate in care.
   2. Nursing techniques for postpartum care
      a. Vital signs: Watch for symptoms of hypovolemic shock and hemorrhage (fainting). Stay with mother who is out of bed for the first time since delivery.
      b. Check breasts.
         (1) Breasts should be soft until milk comes in.
         (2) Encourage daily cleansing in shower.
         (3) Perform daily breast examination to note any complications. Nodules may be felt second or third day as milk production begins. Teach breast self-examination; report any abnormalities.
      c. Engorgement
         (1) Nursing usually prevents this; breast pump; nipple shield.
         (2) Nonnursing mother
            (a) Cold compresses or ice bag on breasts
            (b) Supportive bra
            (c) Follow steps (a) and (b) only if requested.
      d. Infections
         (1) Redness, warmth, pain, elevated temperature 100.4° F (38° C) or more after 24 hours

(2) Minor surgical intervention may be required to release drainage
   e. Check fundus.
      (1) Height and firmness for proper involution
      (2) Relaxed fundus may indicate problem (hemorrhage or infection).
   f. Check lochia: color, amount, odor.
   g. Check perineal area: healing and cleanliness.
   h. Check legs: pain, tenderness, swelling (thrombi); Homans sign.
   i. Check urination: overdistention (subinvolution).
   j. Bowels: Keep open (encourage fluids with balanced diet). Administer stool softener (e.g., dioctyl sodium sulfosuccinate [Colace]).
   k. Afterpains: involution
   l. Postpartum blues ("baby blues"): possible hormonal transitory depression; usually noted after discharge

3. Teaching: important component of postpartum nursing management
   a. Personal hygiene
   b. Weight loss
      (1) Immediately after delivery, 7- to 10-pound weight loss
      (2) Total loss of pregnancy weight may take 6 weeks to 6 months or more to achieve.
   c. Phenylketonuria (PKU) tests: requirement by law to test for inborn error of metabolism involving the absence of phenylalanine hydroxylase, which converts the amino acid phenylalanine to tyrosine. Mental retardation would result if left untreated. The test is most accurate when performed 24 hours after birth. This allows time for phenylalanine to build in the bloodstream.
   d. Discuss with mother and father:
      (1) Importance of bonding.
      (2) Readiness for parenthood.
   e. Postpartum exercises
   f. Review methods of holding, bubbling, or burping baby.

See Critical Thinking Challenge box.

? Critical Thinking Challenge

A patient has delivered a healthy 8-pound baby boy. The nurse is responsible for admitting her to the postpartum unit. She is 1 hour postdelivery. Identify the goals and interventions required immediately and on an ongoing basis to provide safe, high-quality care for her and her family.

As a patient advocate it is essential the nurse identify goals and interventions for the well-being of her patient and her family. The goals include the prevention of infection and excessive bleeding throughout the postpartum period and beyond if necessary. Interventions (nursing actions) include monitoring the patient's vital signs, assessing the perineum for possible complications, monitoring uterine tone and position, monitoring for possible Homans sign, monitoring patient voiding to prevent bladder distention, and monitoring for normal bowel habits. Additional interventions include encouraging adequate rest, comfort, good nutrition, and fluid intake; promoting and encouraging breast feeding; and monitoring the parents' interaction with their newborn.

ABNORMAL POSTPARTUM

POSTPARTUM INFECTION

A. Definition: any infection in the reproductive organs during labor, delivery, or up to 1 month postpartum
B. Signs and symptoms
1. Chills, fever, localized back pain (kidney involvement)
2. Malaise
3. Lower abdominal tenderness, lower back pains
4. Foul-smelling lochia (retained placental infection)
5. Abnormal fundal height changes
C. Treatment and nursing management in general
1. Administration of appropriate antibiotics on time and as directed
2. Comfort measures appropriate to discomfort
3. Check of vital signs every 4 hours
D. Specific infections
1. UTI (cystitis, pyelitis)
   a. Cause: trauma (stretching or tearing) or by an organism
   b. Signs and symptoms
      (1) Three days postpartum
      (2) Low back pain
      (3) Localized pain (pyelitis)
      (4) Chills, high fever, apprehension
      (5) Frequency and burning urination (cystitis)
      (6) Discomfort
   c. Treatment and nursing management
      (1) Bed rest until symptoms subside (1 day)
      (2) Drugs (antibiotics)
      (3) Forced fluids
      (4) Careful handwashing by mother and nursing staff
2. Mastitis
   a. Definition: inflammation of the glands in one or both breasts; can lead to abscess complications if untreated
   b. Cause
      (1) *Staphylococcus* infection
      (2) Stasis of milk (usually occurs 2 to 4 weeks postpartum)
      (3) Bruising of breast tissue
      (4) Open cuts in nipple or areola
   c. Signs and symptoms
      (1) High fever (103° F [39.5° C])
      (2) Chills
      (3) Red, tender, painful, hard
   d. Treatment and nursing management
      (1) Support bra
      (2) Antibiotic therapy
      (3) Checking of incision for drainage
      (4) Heat to area
      (5) Increased fluid intake
      (6) Reassurance of mother
      (7) Continuation of breast-feeding if permitted by health care provider
3. Thrombophlebitis
   a. Definition: clot (thrombus) formed in response to an inflammation of the vessel wall
   b. Signs and symptoms
      (1) Local tenderness: femoral vein
      (2) 1 to 2 weeks postpartum
      (3) Swelling, chills, fever
   c. Treatment and nursing management

(1) Administration of anticoagulant
(2) Bed rest
(3) Antibiotic therapy
(4) Elevation of legs
(5) Warm, wet compresses every 15 to 30 minutes
(6) Massage contraindicated

POSTPARTUM HEMORRHAGE

A. Definition: any loss of 500 mL or more of blood during first 24 hours after delivery
B. Types
1. Early: resulting from uterine atony (1 to 3 days)
2. Late: resulting from subinvolution (inability of the uterus to involute or return to its prepregnant state) or placental infection
C. Causes
1. Uterine atony
2. Retained placental fragments
3. Overdistention of the uterus
4. Grand multiparity
5. Lacerations
6. Trauma of the uterus caused by forceps delivery
7. Inversion of the uterus (an abnormal condition in which the uterus is turned inside out)
D. Signs and symptoms
1. Visible blood loss
2. Shocklike symptoms: pale, clammy, hypotensive, apprehensive
E. Treatment and nursing management
1. NPO status, warm covers, oxygen as ordered
2. IV fluids (ordered medications; examples include oxytocin [Pitocin] and methylergonovine maleate [Methergine])
3. Replacement transfusion if ordered
4. Massage boggy uterus until firm.
5. Offer assurance and support to family and mother.
6. Medical management of cause (repair of laceration, possible D&C)

HEMATOMAS

A. Definition: local accumulation of blood caused by injury to a blood vessel from the following:
1. Undue pressure of heavy gravid uterus
2. Bearing down inappropriately
3. Long second stage
4. Primigravida's prolonged pushing
B. Signs and symptoms
1. Severe pain in perineal area
2. Visible vaginal hematoma
3. Vulvar hematoma
4. Large blood-filled sac visible
C. Treatment and nursing management
1. Ice to area for 24 hours (for a small hematoma)
2. Antibiotics if ordered; analgesics if ordered
3. Incision or ligation if necessary; vaginal packing and retention catheter
4. Comfort measures similar to episiotomy care (i.e., sitz bath)

SUBINVOLUTION

A. Definition: inability of the uterus to return to its normal size after delivery; failure to involute; diagnosed 4 to 6 weeks postpartum

B. Causes
1. Retention of placental pieces
2. Infection (endometrium)
C. Signs and symptoms
1. Involution process abnormal
2. Boggy uterus (not firm); foul odor
3. Lochia rubra continues for 2 weeks or longer.
D. Treatment and nursing management
1. Surgical intervention (D&C) (for retained placenta)
2. Support and reassurance to mother and family
3. Administration of medications to facilitate involution and cure infection

POSTPARTUM DEPRESSION

A. Postpartum depression is a form of clinical depression that can affect women typically after childbirth. There is no known cause.
B. Risk factors include a history of depression, smoking, low self-esteem.
C. Symptoms
1. Sadness
2. Fatigue
3. Changes in sleeping or eating habits
4. Decreased libido
5. Irritability
D. Nurses need to be aware of these symptoms. There is a matter of degree between "baby blues" and clinical depression. Any concerns should be reported to the charge nurse or supervisor for follow-up.

NORMAL NEWBORN

A. Immediate care after delivery
1. Maintain patent airway.
2. Apply cord clamp, check for bleeding, follow procedure for daily cord care.
3. Maintain warmth.
   a. Wrap in prewarmed receiving blankets, or
   b. Place in preheated crib.
4. Preventive care
   a. Instill prophylactic eyedrops in each eye as required by law to treat CT infection and prevent ophthalmia neonatorum.
   b. Commonly used prophylactic drugs: erythromycin, penicillin ointments or drops. Silver nitrate (frequently used in the past) is no longer as common.
   c. Administer intramuscular injection of vitamin K to reduce likelihood of hemorrhagic disease of the newborn.
   d. Hepatitis B vaccination is recommended for all neonates, regardless of hepatitis B surface antigen (HBsAg) status (first dose within 12 hours of birth, second dose at 1 month of age, third dose at 6 months of age).
5. Identification procedures
   a. Complete identification bands as required.
   b. Record footprints of baby and pointer fingerprint of mother.
6. Apgar scoring
7. Initial observation of newborn
   a. Initial observation is the primary responsibility of physician, pediatrician.
   b. Nurse should wear gloves when handling newborn during immediate care and until initial bath; regulations differ for daily routines.
   c. Nurse also makes quick observation, checking for visible anomalies such as cleft lip, cleft palate, extra digits, and anomalies of spinal column, limbs, skin, head.
   d. Reflexes that nurse may check include Moro, sucking, rooting, blinking, grasping.
8. Encourage bonding.
   a. After initial delivery room care, wipe off excess blood and debris from baby; wrap securely in clean, warm receiving blanket and let parents hold baby.
   b. Allow time for mother and father to look at, touch, and hold infant. Allow time to initiate breast-feeding if mother desires.
B. Normal physiology of newborn
1. Vital signs
   a. Temperature
      (1) Axillary: 97.7° to 98.6° F (36.5° to 37° C)
      (2) Rectal: 97.7° to 99° F (36.5° to 37.3° C)
      (3) Rectal temperatures taken only on initial reading or if temperature elevated to avoid damage to the large intestine
      (4) Tympanic temperatures not accurate on the newborn
   b. Pulse rate: 120 to 160 beats/min
      (1) Apical pulse rate
      (2) Irregular in rate and cadence (normal)
   c. Respirations: abdominal and irregular, 30 to 60/min
2. Measurements
   a. Weight
      (1) Girls: 7 pounds (3100 g)
      (2) Boys: 7½ pounds (3300 g)
      (3) 5½ to 9 pounds (3000 to 4500 g) considered normal
      (4) 5% to 10% weight loss in first 2 to 3 days
      (5) Regain of birth weight in 5 to 7 days
   b. Length: 18 to 22 inches (45 to 55 cm)
   c. Head circumference: 13 to 14 inches (33 to 35 cm)
   d. Chest circumference: 12 to 13 inches (30 to 33 cm)
3. Skin
   a. Milia: small, white sebaceous glands visible about nose, forehead, chin
   b. "Stork bites": telangiectasis or capillary hemangiomas
   c. Red nevi: discoloration, circumscribed, blanch on touch, prominent during crying, disappear in 6 to 12 months
   d. Mongolian spots: bluish, bruiselike spots on buttocks, back, shoulders; disappear by toddler or preschool age; found in babies of Hispanic, African-American, Slavic, or Asian background
   e. Erythema toxicum neonatorum (newborn rash): appears as scratches and pimples; may be nosocomial (hospital-based) infection
   f. Nevus vasculosus (strawberry mark): bright red or dark capillary hemangiomas with raised, rough surfaces; usually disappear by school age
   g. Nevus flammeus (port-wine stain): reddish-purple, raised capillary hemangiomas; do not blanch on pressure and may not disappear
   h. Lanugo: soft, downy hair on top of skin on ears, forehead, neck, shoulders; disappears in weeks

i. Vernix caseosa: cheeselike protective material coating fetus, especially under arms, beneath knees, and in folds of thighs and groin

j. Acrocyanosis: bluish color present for several hours after delivery (hands and feet)

k. Physiological jaundice: jaundice caused when excessive amounts of hemoglobin needed for intrauterine life decrease to extrauterine levels. The immature liver cannot process the bilirubin fast enough, and jaundice results.

(1) Fifty percent of normal newborns and 80% of premature newborns have some level of jaundice.

(2) Treatment includes bilirubin test, increased formula, possible phototherapy.

4. Elimination

a. Urine: three or four times per day for first few days; usually urinates after every feeding

b. Bowel movement: five or six times per day for first week

(1) Meconium: expelled within 2 to 12 hours; black, tarry, thick, unformed stool

(2) Transient stool: blackish or greenish stool expelled after first few feedings

c. Breast-fed infant's stool: yellow, odorless, slightly runny

d. Bottle-fed infant's stool: formed, brownish-yellow, distinct odor

e. Each infant establishes own pattern of stool movement.

5. Hyperestrogenism and its effect on the newborn

a. Swelling of the breasts in male or female infant because of hormones from mother. The ensuing discharge is called *witch's milk*.

b. Swelling of the male scrotum: large, with rugae; disappears within days

c. Pseudomenses with female infant

6. Reproductive organs of the male newborn

a. Cryptorchidism: Testes have not descended into scrotum; often present in premature infants.

b. Occasionally testes are in inguinal sac at birth but descend within hours or more; if undescended after 1 month, pediatrician should evaluate.

c. The foreskin should not be retracted until at least 3 years of age if newborn is uncircumcised.

7. Circulatory system: pulmonary circulation established within minutes of birth

8. Digestive system: immature at birth but can metabolize nutrients except fats

9. Visual capabilities: immature coordination and muscle control

10. Hearing capabilities: acute hearing within 2 minutes of birth

11. Taste perception: can distinguish sweet and sour in 1 to 3 days

12. Smelling perception: can distinguish smell of mother at 5 days

13. Sleep patterns

a. Unstable for 6 to 8 hours after birth

b. Has regular and irregular sleep cycles

14. Newborn reflexes

a. Sucking, rooting, swallowing, extrusion reflexes

b. Tonic neck (fencing) should disappear in 3 to 4 months.

c. Grasping (palmar) and plantar lessen in 3 to 4 months.

d. Moro (startle) disappears in 2 months.

e. Stepping disappears in 3 to 4 weeks.

f. Babinski (plantar): Absence indicates CNS damage.

g. Blinking, sneezing

15. Immunity in the newborn

a. Has 3-month supply (passive immunity) from mother if baby is term

b. Begins own synthesis (active immunity) by 3 months of age

C. Daily observation and nursing care

1. Newborn nursery care and observation

a. Constant, careful observation

b. Place infant in warmer until vital signs are stable.

c. Check temperature; follow agency policy (e.g., rectal, axilla).

(1) Infant is placed under warmer to prevent cold stress.

(2) Heat production becomes normal in 2 to 3 days.

(3) Newborn loses heat through convection, conduction, radiation, and evaporation.

d. Check respirations.

e. Place infant on right side to promote expansion of lungs and drain excess mucus.

f. Observe for signs and symptoms of respiratory distress syndrome (RDS).

g. Cord

(1) Cord clamp is removed within 8 to 24 hours.

(2) Observe carefully for signs of infection.

h. Check eyes and ears for abnormal drainage.

2. Daily nursery routine

a. Monitoring of daily weight and vital signs, especially temperature

b. Observation and recording of condition of skin, cord, eyes, elimination

c. Daily care and changing of crib linen

d. Daily cord care

e. General observations of cry and behavior

f. Observation of infant-mother bonding during feeding routine

3. Teaching mothers care of newborn: Mothers' classes should incorporate the care, handling, and dressing of the newborn in addition to procedures for and demonstrations of sponge baths, tub baths, and cord care.

4. Daily bath routine

a. Purpose

(1) Cleansing

(2) Exercise time

(3) Play, social time with parents (bonding time)

b. Prepare environment: select safe, convenient, warm area.

c. Select and prepare equipment.

(1) Utensils for sponge bath

(2) Necessary articles for procedure

(3) Clean clothing

d. Sponge baths: recommended for babies with cord intact

e. Tub baths: recommended for babies whose cord has fallen off—10 to 14 days after birth

5. Cord care: If drainage persists, cleanse with alcohol and notify pediatrician.
6. Diaper rash
   a. Change diapers frequently.
   b. Wash area with warm tap water.
   c. May apply A&D Ointment as a preventive and protective measure.
   d. Lay infant on abdomen and expose buttocks to air
   e. Apply Desitin or Balmex if A&D Ointment does not help.
7. Circumcision
   a. Definition: surgical cutting and removal of foreskin; usually done 1 to 3 days after birth
   b. Treatment and nursing management: The nurse should:
      (1) Observe for bleeding, edema.
      (2) Treatment may include petroleum jelly (Vaseline) for 3 days, depending on the type of instrument used for circumcision.
      (3) Check and record first voiding after procedure.
   c. Complications: rare
8. Facts about feeding the newborn
   a. Newborn metabolic rate twice that of adult
   b. Carbohydrates: needed for brain growth and as source of energy
   c. Protein: needed for building tissue. Inadequacy results in infection, slow growth, flabby muscles.
   d. Fat: difficult to digest and metabolize but needed to maintain integrity of skin
   e. Iron: Continuous supply needed for growth and development; storage from mother depleted in 4 to 6 months
   f. At birth can take 1 to 2 oz (30 to 60 mL) per feeding
   g. By 1 to 2 weeks can nurse 4 oz (120 mL) per feeding
   h. Gradual increase to 6 to 8 oz (180 to 240 mL) per feeding in 1 month
9. Facts about breast milk
   a. Less protein than cow's milk; easier to digest
   b. More lactose than cow's milk, which facilitates metabolism and is good for bones
   c. Lactoferrin decreases dangers of infection.
   d. Sucking stimulates posterior pituitary of mother to trigger letdown reflex, which allows milk to flow.
10. Guidelines for breast-feeding
    a. A general rule of thumb is to nurse until breasts are soft once milk is established.
    b. To ensure a good supply of breast milk, the mother should:
       (1) Obtain adequate rest.
       (2) Drink sufficient fluids.
       (3) Eat a balanced, nutritious diet.
       (4) Maintain psychological equilibrium (maternal-infant bonding).
11. The length of time for breast-feeding varies considerably from infant to infant and is normally 10 to 30 minutes. Limiting the time of nursing on each breast is no longer considered effective in preventing sore nipples; it is more important to use correct technique and empty the breasts completely.
12. Contraindications to breast-feeding
    a. Mother with AIDS
    b. Baby with galactosemia, PKU

ABNORMAL NEWBORN

PRETERM (PREMATURE) INFANT

A. Definition: a baby born before 37 weeks' gestation and weighing less than 5½ pounds (2500 g)
B. Infants may be SGA because they are preterm or from genetic or intrauterine causes.
C. Statistics
   1. Of all live births, 7% are premature.
   2. Incidence of prematurity increases to 10% in some minority populations.
   3. Prematurity is leading cause of death in infants in the United States.
D. Cause
   1. Young, adolescent mothers
   2. Elderly primigravidas
   3. Multiple births
   4. Poor prenatal care
   5. Congenital anomalies
   6. Diseases or conditions that compromise fetus
      a. GH
      b. Diabetes
      c. Heart disease
      d. Nutritional deficits
      e. Preterm labor
      f. Drug or alcohol addictions
      g. Smoking
      h. Placental insufficiency
E. Characteristics of a premature infant
   1. CNS
      a. Poor muscle tone
      b. Poor reflexes
      c. Limp
      d. Assumption of froglike position
      e. Weak, feeble cry
      f. Unstable heating mechanism: temperature fluctuates from 94° to 96° F (34° to 36° C)
      g. Poor sucking reflexes
      h. Weak gagging and sucking reflexes
   2. Respiratory system
      a. Insufficient surfactant
      b. Immature lungs, rib cage, muscles
      c. Prone to respiratory distress system (RDS)
      d. Poor oxygenation
   3. Digestive system: immature gastric system; decreased ability to convert protein and fat to energy; able to digest simple sugars
   4. Integumentary system
      a. Harlequin pattern observed (temporary flushing of the skin on the lower side of the body with pallor on the upward side); commonly seen in normal infants and disappears as the child matures
      b. Veins and capillaries visible
      c. Lanugo prominent
      d. Vernix prominent
      e. Decreased subcutaneous fat, thinner skin
      f. Skin tight, shiny, taut
   5. Circulatory system
      a. Fragile capillaries
      b. Susceptible to hemorrhages (intracranial)
   6. Renal system
      a. Inability to urinate properly

b. Easily dehydrated (decreased concentrated urine leading to fluid retention)

c. Fragile electrolyte balance (metabolic acidosis, sodium bicarbonate decreased, and excretion of drugs decreased)

7. Immune system

a. Too young to have obtained any immunity from mother

b. Vulnerable to infection

8. Endocrine system: A common complication is hypoglycemia.

9. Head

a. Fontanels large

b. Suture lines prominent

c. Old looking

F. Treatment and nursing management

1. Maintain patent airway.

2. Frequently monitor blood gases to determine oxygen need.

3. Maintain body temperature by placing infant in heater.

4. Conserve energy: basic care only.

5. Provide adequate nutrition.

a. Nasogastric feedings

b. Special soft nipples

c. Parenteral fluids

6. Prevent infection.

a. Prevent skin breakdown: change positions.

b. Keep dry and clean.

7. Length of hospitalization: usually until a weight of 5 ½ pounds (2500 g) is reached

8. Mothering stimulation taught and practiced

a. Encourage parents to stroke, cuddle, talk.

b. Feed, diaper infants.

c. Play soft music.

d. Encourage tapping on Isolette and talking.

9. Listen to concerns of mothers and fathers.

POSTTERM INFANT

A. Definition: infant born after more than 42 weeks' gestation

B. Cause: unknown

C. Characteristics of postmature infant

1. Old looking

2. No vernix; no lanugo

3. Color: yellow-green or meconium stained

4. Desquamation of hands (palms) and feet (soles)

5. May have respiratory problems

D. Nursing management

1. Observe for hypoglycemia.

2. Observe for RDS.

3. Look for birth injuries.

4. Provide symptomatic nursing care.

NEONATAL RESPIRATORY DISTRESS SYNDROME

A. Definition

1. A series of symptoms signifying respiratory distress

2. Synonyms: RDS, hyaline membrane disease (HMD)

B. Statistics

1. Common in premature babies

2. Leading cause of death in infants in the United States

C. Causes

1. Lack or loss of surfactant in lungs

2. Immaturity

3. Hypoxia

4. Hypothermia

D. Signs and symptoms

1. Appears within minutes to hours after birth

2. Grunting, rib retraction, nasal flaring (RDS symptoms)

3. Inadequate oxygen: 60 or more respirations per minute

E. Diagnosis: X-ray examination shows collapsed portions of lungs; arterial blood gases reveal hypoxia.

F. Treatment and nursing management

1. Transfer to intensive care unit and Isolette care.

2. Initiate oxygen therapy: 60%; hood is best.

a. Intermittent positive-pressure breathing (IPPB)

b. Continuous positive airway pressure (CPAP)

c. Positive end-expiratory pressure (PEEP)

d. Surfactant replacement

e. Monitor blood gases

3. Endotracheal tube if necessary

4. IV hydration and nutrition and antibiotic therapy

5. Elevate head of bed slightly.

G. Complication

1. Retinopathy of prematurity

2. Causes

a. High arterial oxygen levels

b. Retinal vascular immaturity

BIRTH INJURIES

A. Normal deviations of the head

1. Caput succedaneum (Figure 7-12)

a. Definition: edema (swelling) of soft tissues of scalp

b. Cause: continuous pressure of the fetal head on cervix

c. Signs and symptoms

(1) Crosses suture lines

(2) Appears at birth

(3) Disappears in 3 or 4 days

d. Treatment: none

2. Cephalhematoma (Figure 7-12)

a. Definition: blood between the periosteum and bone

b. Cause: pressure during delivery (forceps; prolonged labor)

c. Signs and symptoms

(1) Never crosses suture lines

(2) Appears several hours to several days after birth

(3) Disappears within 3 to 6 weeks

d. Treatment: none

3. Molding (Figure 7-13)

a. Definition: changes in the shape of the head

b. Cause: accommodation of fetal bones to birth canal during labor and delivery

c. Signs and symptoms: visual

d. Treatment: disappears without treatment in 3 days

4. Soft-tissue injuries (subcutaneous fat necrosis)

a. Definition: pressure necrosis

b. Signs and symptoms: purplish, movable mass

c. Treatment: resolves spontaneously

B. Subconjunctival hemorrhage (scleral or retinal)

1. Definition: rupture of small capillaries in eye

2. Cause: increased intracranial pressure of birth

3. Signs and symptoms: small, red pin dots in white of sclera or hemorrhaging in retina

4. Resolves without treatment in 5 days

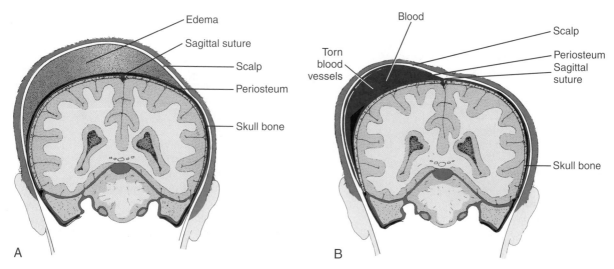

FIGURE 7-12 Differences between caput succedaneum and cephalhematoma. **A,** Caput succedaneum: Edema of scalp noted at birth; crosses suture line. **B,** Cephalhematoma: Bleeding between periosteum and skull bone appears within first 2 days; does not cross suture lines.

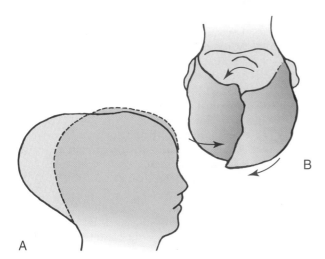

FIGURE 7-13 **A,** Various types of molding. **B,** Bones overlapping during molding. (From Hamilton PM: *Basic maternity nursing,* ed 6, St Louis, 1988, Mosby.)

C. Ecchymosis, petechiae, edema
　1. Definition: blood within tissues; does not blanch with pressure
　2. Cause: forceps, manipulation, pressure
　3. Signs and symptoms: visual in affected areas
　4. Resolves without treatment in 2 days
D. Skeletal injuries
　1. Skull fracture: rare, and unless blood vessels are involved, heals without treatment
　2. Fracture of the clavicle: most common fracture; usually caused by shoulder impaction; dystocia
　　a. Treatment: Handle infant with care.
　　b. Prognosis: good
　3. Fracture of the humerus or femur: rare
　　a. Cause: dystocia and difficult delivery
　　b. Treatment
　　　(1) Immobilize
　　　(2) Heals rapidly
　　c. Complications: rare

E. Neurological injuries
　1. Brachial paralysis of upper arm: Erb-Duchenne paralysis (Erb palsy)
　　a. Definition: traumatic injury to the upper brachial plexus with damage to one or more cervical nerve roots
　　b. Causes
　　　(1) Difficult labor
　　　(2) Shoulder impaction; dystocia
　　　(3) Malposition of forceps
　　c. Treatment: Immobilize with brace or splint.
　　d. Nursing management
　　　(1) Skin care as necessary
　　　(2) Gentle range-of-motion exercises after healing
　2. Brachial paralysis of lower arm: Klumpke paralysis (palsy)
　　a. Definition: nerves of hand and wrist crushed or severed
　　b. Treatment
　　　(1) Padding of wrist and fingers
　　　(2) Corrective surgery
　　　(3) Gentle massage after surgery
　　　(4) Range-of-motion exercises when appropriate
　　c. Prognosis: good
　3. Facial paralysis
　　a. Definition: crushed or severed nerves of face that cause grimacing and distortion, especially when crying; asymmetrical paralysis
　　b. Cause: misapplication of forceps
　　c. Treatment: condition transitory. Reassure parents.
F. CNS injuries
　1. Definition: injuries causing intracranial hemorrhaging
　2. Causes
　　a. Prematurity
　　b. Large full-term babies
　　c. Dystocia
　　d. Hypoxia
　　e. Hypovolemia
　3. Types
　　a. Within the brain itself
　　b. Subdural hematoma

4. Signs and symptoms
   a. Suture line separation
   b. Bulging anterior fontanel
   c. High-pitched cry
   d. Abnormal respirations
   e. Cyanosis
   f. Irritability or lethargy
   g. Twitching, convulsions
5. Treatment and nursing management
   a. Head higher than hips
   b. Warmth
   c. Oxygen
   d. IV therapy
   e. Minimal handling
   f. Surgical aspiration (if appropriate)
   g. Measurement of head size weekly
   h. Convulsion precautions

INFECTIONS OF THE NEWBORN

A. Causes
   1. Dystocia
   2. PROM of 24 hours or more (sepsis neonatorum)
   3. Clinical amnionitis
   4. Maternal infection (toxoplasmosis, syphilis, rubella)
   5. Nosocomial infection (usually *Staphylococcus*)
   6. *Monilia* or yeast infection in mother's vagina
B. Signs and symptoms
   1. Appears within first 48 hours
   2. Vague symptoms
   3. Lethargy, irritability, lack of appetite
   4. Low-grade temperature
   5. Diarrhea
   6. Jaundice
C. Treatment and nursing management
   1. Take cultures of blood, urine, throat.
   2. Administer antibiotic therapy.
   3. Keep warm.
   4. Administer oxygen therapy if necessary.
   5. Isolate if appropriate.
   6. Weigh daily.
   7. Watch for signs of jaundice.
   8. Keep parents informed of progress.

CONGENITAL MALFORMATIONS

A. Perinatal signs
   1. Polyhydramnios: excessive amniotic fluid; may occur with other congenital anomalies
   2. Oligohydramnios: scant amniotic fluid; indicates urinary tract anomalies and renal disturbances
B. Postnatal congenital malformations
   1. Choanal atresia (gastrointestinal anomaly)
      a. Definition: blockage between the nose and throat; can be unilateral or bilateral
      b. Signs and symptoms
         (1) Cyanotic at rest
         (2) Color improves when crying
         (3) Snorts when feeding
      c. Treatment and nursing management
         (1) Physician may pierce obstruction with a probe if it is only a membrane.
         (2) Minor surgical repair if bone involved; prognosis is excellent.

   (3) Feeding problems; positioning is important.
   (4) Gavage feeding may be necessary.
   (5) Watch closely for aspiration.
2. Esophageal atresia: Refer to Chapter 8.
3. Congenital laryngeal stridor (laryngomalacia)
   a. Definition: abnormal condition around larynx that causes noisy respiration, especially a crowing sound on inspiration
   b. Causes
      (1) Flabby epiglottis
      (2) Supraglottic aperture
      (3) Relaxation of laryngeal wall
      (4) Absence of tracheal rings
      (5) Deformity of vocal cords
   c. Signs and symptoms
      (1) Noisy respirations on inspiration
      (2) Most noticeable when crying
      (3) Mild-to-severe intercostal or supraclavicular retractions
      (4) Cyanosis
      (5) Dyspnea
   d. Treatment and nursing management
      (1) Depends on cause
      (2) Mild stridor may subside in 6 to 18 months.
      (3) Position baby upright for feeding.
      (4) Feed slowly, pausing to let infant catch his or her breath.
      (5) Use small nipple.
      (6) Watch for aspiration of feedings.
      (7) Prevent respiratory complications.
      (8) Keep infant warm, dry, away from drafts.
      (9) Have oxygen in readiness.
      (10) Prepare for tracheotomy.
   e. Prognosis: good
4. Cleft lip and cleft palate
   a. Definition: bilateral or unilateral fissure or opening on the palate or the upper lips resulting from failure of the bony and soft-tissue structures to unite
   b. Cause: developmental failure during the embryonic stage because of heredity, age, or a variety of other factors such as radiation or viral infections
   c. Signs and symptoms
      (1) Visual on lips
      (2) Palate more difficult to notice sometimes
      (3) Occurs more frequently in male infants
      (4) Difficulty feeding
      (5) Choking
      (6) Drooling
      (7) Milk may drain through nostrils.
   d. Treatment
      (1) Cleft lips may have butterfly adhesive taping as initial treatment; may be helpful in feeding so milk does not continually drain through fissure.
      (2) Cleft lip may be surgically repaired at 1 to 2 weeks of age or 12 pounds (5.5 kg).
      (3) Cleft palate: first repair usually by 18 months
   e. Nursing management
      (1) Feeding precautions
         (a) Use soft duck nipple, medicine dropper with rubber tip.
         (b) Place nipple away from cleft side.
         (c) Feed slowly.

(d) Bubble frequently.

(e) Rinse mouth after feedings.

(f) Watch for aspiration, respiratory distress, gastrointestinal disturbances.

(2) Mouth care: Prevent cracks, fissures on lips.

(3) Provide postoperative care for cleft lip.

    (a) Place infant on side.

    (b) Mouth care is important because of Logan bar applied to prevent stretching of sutures.

    (c) Prevent crying.

    (d) Check swelling (tongue, nose, mouth).

    (e) Watch for hemorrhage.

    (f) Apply elbow restraints.

    (g) Prevent crust formation.

    (h) Feed on opposite side of surgery.

    (i) Use rubber-tipped dropper (3 weeks).

5. Diaphragmatic hernia

  a. Definition: herniation of abdominal viscera into the thoracic cavity as a result of incomplete development during embryonic stage, ranging from minimal to complete herniation

  b. Signs and symptoms

    (1) Constant respiratory distress

    (2) Bowels distended

    (3) Bowel sounds heard in chest

    (4) Asymmetrical chest contour

  c. Treatment and nursing management

    (1) Early recognition and prompt surgery

    (2) Usual preoperative and postoperative management

  d. Prognosis guarded, depending on severity

6. Omphalocele: See Chapter 8.

7. Imperforate anus: See Chapter 8.

C. Congenital anomalies of the CNS

1. Spina bifida occulta

  a. Definition: defect in vertebral column without protrusion of spinal cord and meninges. This is one of three types of spina bifida, which is a malformation of the spine, most common in the lumbosacral region, in which the posterior portion of the vertebrae fails to close.

  b. Signs and symptoms

    (1) Dimple in lower lumbosacral skin

    (2) Hair over area (occasionally)

    (3) X-ray film confirmation

  c. Treatment and nursing management: No treatment is necessary unless neurological symptoms occur.

2. Meningocele

  a. Definition: defect in spinal cord with protrusion of meninges through an opening in spinal canal; no paralysis present; cosmetic problem

  b. Surgical correction

3. Myelomeningocele

  a. Definition: Both spinal cord and meninges protrude through defective bony rings in spinal cord; possible paralysis below sac more serious, paralysis is mild to severe; depends on level of sac that is protruding.

  b. Signs and symptoms

    (1) Look for visual signs.

    (2) Observe for change in intracranial pressure.

    (3) Check head measurements for hydrocephalus.

    (4) Report signs and symptoms of CNS involvement.

  c. Preoperative management

    (1) Flat on abdomen with sterile gauze, petroleum jelly (Vaseline), Telfa pad, normal saline

    (2) No diapers

    (3) Keep clean.

    (4) Use care to prevent sac from breaking.

    (5) Prevent infection; use sterile technique.

    (6) Prevent deformity.

    (7) Prevent injury.

  d. Postoperative management

    (1) Vital signs

    (2) Symptoms of shock

    (3) Oxygen readiness

    (4) Head measurements

    (5) Cast care if necessary; sometimes casts applied to legs

    (6) Importance of good nutrition

    (7) Orthopedic and urological habilitation

    (8) Encourage normal use of functions.

    (9) Minimize disabilities.

    (10) Paralysis (if present) may not be alleviated, but further damage can be prevented. Aim of surgery is to give infant opportunity for optimal growth and development.

    (11) Use Credé maneuver to keep bladder empty and free from infection.

4. Hydrocephalus: Refer to Chapter 8.

D. Congenital anomalies of the musculoskeletal system (limited)

1. Congenital dislocation of the hip: Refer to Chapter 8.

2. Talipes equinovarus (clubfoot): Refer to Chapter 8.

3. Phocomelia

  a. Definition: developmental congenital anomaly in which only stubs or parts of arms and legs are present. Degree of severity varies.

  b. Cause: interference with embryonic development of long bones; rare and seen as a result of the drug thalidomide taken during early pregnancy to relieve nausea

  c. Treatment and nursing management

    (1) Psychosocial problems for family and infant

    (2) Body surface limited, so heating mechanism overheats rest of body, causing diaphoresis

    (3) Personal hygiene; frequent baths

    (4) Special education imperative

4. Polydactyly

  a. Definition: supernumerary fingers or toes

  b. Cause: possibly hereditary

  c. Treatment and nursing management

    (1) Usually no bone or nerve involvement

    (2) Tie digit with silk suture in newborn nursery; it falls off.

    (3) Surgical intervention is necessary with bone involvement; x-ray examination is done first to ensure that no bone or ligaments are present.

E. Congenital anomalies of the male genitourinary system

1. Hypospadias: Refer to Chapter 8.

2. Epispadias: Refer to Chapter 8.

HEMOLYTIC DISEASE OF NEWBORN

A. Pathological jaundice

1. Cause: Rh factor incompatibility; occurs only when mother is Rh negative and fetus is Rh positive

2. Pathophysiology: The Rh-negative mother is exposed to and develops antibodies against the Rh antigen (sensitization). Sensitization to Rh-positive blood can be caused by exposure to the antigen during amniocentesis or when a transplacental bleed occurs during a miscarriage or abortion. The most common time for sensitization to occur is birth.

3. Signs and symptoms
   a. Jaundice
   b. Anemia
   c. Enlarged liver and spleen
   d. Generalized edema
   e. If untreated, "yellow bodies" travel to brain, causing brain damage, heart failure, kernicterus, and death.

4. Treatment and nursing management
   a. Blood types of mother and father are important for anticipatory guidance.
   b. First babies usually do not present a problem.
   c. If baby's bilirubin is above 10 or 12 mg/dL, phototherapy may be applied to reduce jaundice; exchange transfusions may be necessary.
   d. After birth of Rh-positive baby, an unsensitized Rh-negative mother is given RhoGAM, a specific gamma globulin that prevents the production of Rh antibodies; this must be given within 72 hours after delivery. The effect is the assurance that subsequent pregnancies will not be harmful to the baby.
   e. Rh-antibody titers can be monitored throughout pregnancy (prenatal).
   f. Amniocentesis reveals by indirect Coombs test if mother has antibodies circulating in the maternal plasma or serum.

B. Erythroblastosis fetalis (hydrops)
   1. Definition: most severe form of fetal hemolysis
   2. Rarely seen since the development of RhoGAM
   3. Signs and symptoms include anemia, congestive heart failure, and ascites.

C. ABO incompatibility
   1. Definition: incompatibility of blood groups A and B because of the presence of antigens developed and passed on to the fetus by a type O mother
   2. Signs and symptoms
      a. Jaundice: mild, occurring during first day or two
      b. Slight enlargement of liver and spleen
   3. Treatment and nursing management
      a. Phototherapy
      b. If bilirubin is above 20 mg/dL, an exchange transfusion with group O and appropriate Rh type
      c. Observe for progressive lethargy.
      d. Monitor level of jaundice (visual and laboratory).
      e. Observe color of urine.
      f. Observe for edema.
      g. Observe for convulsions.
      h. Provide symptomatic nursing care.

DOWN SYNDROME (TRISOMY 21)

Refer to Chapter 8.

DRUG ADDICTION IN NEWBORNS

A. Definition: secondary addiction caused by drugs being ingested or injected by addicted mother. Drugs cross the placental barrier and create a drug-dependent newborn (immature liver unable to excrete drug rapidly during fetal life).

B. Signs and symptoms
   1. Low birth weight
   2. Premature
   3. Immature
   4. Withdrawal symptoms within 48 to 72 hours. Watch for:
      a. Sneezing.
      b. Respiratory distress.
      c. Excessive sweating.
      d. Feeding problems.
      e. Frantic sucking of fists.
      f. High-pitched cry.
      g. Irritable, hyperactive, tremors.
      h. Fever.
      i. Diarrhea.

C. Treatment and nursing management
   1. Prevent infection.
   2. Promote good nutrition.
   3. Keep quiet (quiet, darkened environment).
   4. Offer loving, soothing, cuddling care.
   5. Give medications on time.
   6. Monitor vital signs.
   7. Keep warm.
   8. Protect from injury because child is hyperactive.
   9. Provide good skin care because of excessive sweating and diarrhea.
   10. Provide adequate fluids (prevent dehydration).
   11. Encourage mother to assist in care.
       a. Teach holding, diapering, talking, bathing.
       b. Encourage visits.

INFANTS OF MOTHERS WITH DIABETES

A. Complications
   1. Delivery date may be recommended before EDC or at approximately 36 to 37 weeks' gestation to prevent the following:
      a. Oversize baby (macrosomia)
      b. High-risk infant (babies with diabetes have high rate of infant mortality).
   2. Neonatal hypoglycemia, which is common
   3. RDS complications
   4. Hyperbilirubinemia (severe jaundice)
   5. Intracranial hemorrhage (birth trauma, LGA)
   6. Congestive heart failure
   7. Congenital anomalies in 5% of infants
   8. Hypocalcemia

B. Signs and symptoms
   1. Lethargic
   2. Plump, puffy face
   3. Long and heavy
   4. Respiratory problems
   5. Enlarged heart, liver, and spleen
   6. Symptoms of hypoglycemia
   7. Symptoms of hypocalcemia (tremors)

C. Treatment and nursing management
   1. Medical management is difficult because of rapid, changing growth patterns; nutritional demands; illness.
   2. Parents must be taught techniques for blood glucose monitoring.
   3. Short-acting insulin is best (easier to control).
   4. Treat hypoglycemia and hypocalcemia.
   5. Provide oral feedings when tolerated and when blood sugar levels are stable.

CRETINISM (CONGENITAL HYPOTHYROIDISM)

Refer to Chapter 8.

FAMILY PLANNING

A. Trends
1. Smaller families (except for the poor and disadvantaged)
2. Delayed parenthood by choice
   a. Career women
   b. Desire for higher education
   c. Alternate living arrangements
3. Single parents
   a. High divorce rate
   b. Expanding role of father as single parent because custody of children, traditionally awarded to mother, is now sometimes being awarded to fathers
   c. Lessening barriers for adoption by single men and women
   d. Cultural and ethnic acceptance of unmarried mothers
   e. Opportunities to continue education for pregnant adolescent without pressure of forced marriage
B. Communes: labor and delivery in communal community homes
C. Early sexual encounters (teenage pregnancies)
1. Need for referrals to family planning centers for guidance and counseling
   a. Teach use of condoms (controversial).
   b. Practice of abstinence
2. Problems originating from early sexual encounters
D. Surrogate mothers
1. In vitro transplantation of embryo in the uterus of a woman who agrees to carry a full-term pregnancy for another woman
2. Has moral and legal implications

POSSIBLE INFLUENTIAL FACTORS

A. Sex education: incorporation of sex education in public and parochial schools at an early age
B. Freedom of choice
1. Availability of over-the-counter pregnancy tests
2. Availability of over-the-counter contraceptives
3. Abortions mandated as legal by the U.S. Supreme Court in 1977
C. Postponement of family: use of available contraceptive devices
D. Economic factor: High cost of medical care forces young people to consider waiting until affluent enough to afford a family.

COMMON METHODS OF BIRTH CONTROL (CONTRACEPTION)

A. Natural
1. Rhythm (calendar) method
   a. Based on the principle that ovulation occurs during midcycle of a menstrual period (i.e., in a 28-day cycle, ovulation would occur on the fourteenth day)
   b. Accordingly the most fertile days are considered to be 3 to 4 days before and 3 to 4 days after ovulation.
2. Basal metabolism method: Daily monitoring of early morning temperature for a period of several months and entering it on a graph (Figure 7-14) establish an

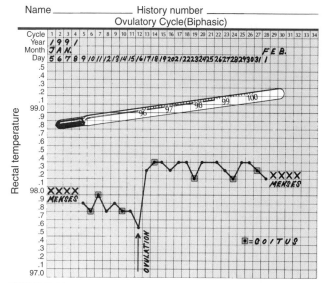

FIGURE 7-14 Basal temperature record shows drop and sharp rise at time of ovulation. (From Lowdermilk DL, et al: *Maternity and women's health care,* ed 10, St Louis, 2012, Mosby.)

ovulation time. Safe and fertile times can be determined, and mother can be advised on use of this method.

B. Coitus interruptus
1. Penis withdrawn from vagina just before ejaculation
2. Least effective of all methods
C. Condom (sheath, snakeskin, rubbers): thin rubber or plastic sheath that fits over penis and acts as barrier, preventing sperm from entering the vagina
D. Diaphragm: mechanical barrier placed at mouth of cervix; used with contraceptive cream or jelly to be effective; may engage in intercourse immediately after placement; should be left in place for 6 hours after intercourse. Spermicide must be added each time intercourse occurs.
E. Chemical agents: Foam, creams, jelly, vaginal suppositories, and sponges form a chemical barrier in the vagina and render the area unsafe for sperm.
F. Intrauterine devices (IUDs)
1. Devices come in various shapes made of memory plastic inserted in the uterine cavity immediately after the woman's menstrual cycle.
2. Mode of action unclear; thought to interfere with implantation by creating peristaltic waves
3. Disadvantages
   a. Excessive bleeding during menstrual cycle
   b. Extremely controversial. Dalkon Shield was taken off the market because of permanent sterility and multiple gynecological problems.
   c. Possible contamination from IUD string hanging in vaginal orifice
4. Advantage: once IUD has been inserted, only periodic checking (usually monthly) to confirm it is still intact
G. Oral contraceptive (birth control pill)
1. Most widely used
2. Considered 90% or more effective
3. Prevents anterior pituitary from releasing follicle-stimulating hormone (FSH); artificially raises estrogen and progesterone levels and prevents ovulation

4. Stimulates endometrium, creating hostile environment for sperm
5. Minor side effects, lasting a few weeks to months: nausea, weight gain, full breasts
6. Major side effects: thrombophlebitis, hypertension, embolism, cardiovascular disturbances

H. Cervical cap
1. Small rubber cap fitted over the cervix to prevent sperm from entering the cervical canal
2. More comfortable than the diaphragm
3. May be left safely on the cervix for longer periods and remain effective

I. Female condom
1. A sheath secured by two rings that cover the cervix and vulva; coated with a spermicide preparation
2. Protects against both pregnancy and disease
3. May cause a decrease in sensation during intercourse

J. Hormonal injection
1. Injectable form of progestin
2. Provides protection for 3 months

K. Hormone implants
1. Small capsules placed in upper arm release progestin.
2. Provide protection for up to 5 years

L. Transdermal patch—provides effective contraception similar to that of oral contraceptives

M. Operative sterilization
1. Vasectomy
   a. Removal of a portion of both vasa deferentia; prevents the transport of sperm into the seminal fluid
   b. Temporary birth control should be used for 2 to 3 months until a semen analysis determines that no viable sperm are present.
   c. Reversal may be possible using microsurgery.
2. Tubal ligation (bilateral partial salpingectomy)
   a. Fallopian tubes are clipped, cut, or cauterized.
   b. Sexual activity can resume whenever woman is comfortable enough.
   c. Reversal is possible; however, the probability of regaining fertility is seriously decreased.

Bibliography

Edmunds MW: *Introduction to clinical pharmacology*, ed 7, St Louis, 2013, Mosby.

Leifer G: *Introduction to maternity and pediatric nursing*, ed 6, St Louis, 2011, Mosby.

Leifer G: *Maternity nursing: an introductory text*, ed 11, St Louis, 2012, Mosby.

Lowdermilk DL, et al: *Maternity and women's health care*, ed 10, St Louis, 2012, Mosby.

McKinney ES, et al: *Maternal-child nursing*, ed 4, St Louis, 2013, Saunders.

Nix S: *Williams' basic nutrition and diet therapy*, ed 14, St Louis, 2013, Mosby.

Online References

American Academy of Pediatrics: www.aap.org.

American College (Congress) of Obstetricians and Gynecologists: www.acog.org.

Health Resources and Services Administration: Maternal and Child Health: http://mchb.hrsa.gov.

Healthy People 2020: www.healthypeople.gov.

March of Dimes Foundation: www.modimes.org.

National Center for Education in Maternal and Child Health: www.ncemch.org.

National Perinatal Information Center: www.npic.org.

REVIEW QUESTIONS

1. Identify the urinary bladder in the following diagram:

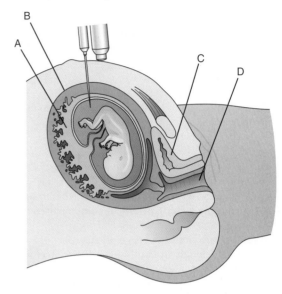

1. A
2. B
3. C
4. D

2. To confirm a patient's pregnancy, the nurse should give which instructions regarding the required urine specimen?
1. Give a voided specimen during her first visit.
2. Instruct her on how to give a sterile specimen in the office.
3. Tell her to withhold fluid intake during the night and bring in the first voided specimen in the morning.
4. Tell her a catheterized specimen will be required.

3. The communicable (childhood) disease most likely to affect pregnancy, with harmful effects to the fetus, is:
1. Chickenpox.
2. Rubella.
3. Varicella.
4. Rubeola.

4. In the following diagram, indicate at what station the baby's presenting part is.

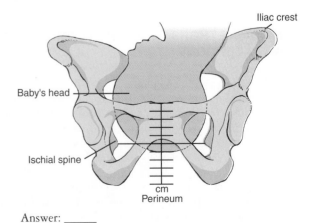

Answer: _____

5. The basal metabolic rate (BMR) of a prenatal patient generally increases. An explanation of this would be that:
   1. Hormone production is increased.
   2. The thyroid gland increases in size.
   3. Cardiac output and rate increase.
   4. The baby causes a need for excess energy.

6. A couple asks why it is so important to the fetus for both of them to stop smoking. The nurse responds:
   1. "Smoking and secondhand smoke cause decreased oxygenation to the fetus."
   2. "Pregnant women who smoke or who are around smoke tend to have larger babies."
   3. "Pregnant women who smoke tend to have babies who have diabetes."
   4. "Pregnant women who smoke tend to have babies with cardiac anomalies."

7. A couple of Eastern European–Jewish heritage is referred for genetic counseling. Which condition would be of most concern to this couple?
   1. Sickle cell anemia
   2. Tay-Sachs disease
   3. Thalassemia
   4. Cystic fibrosis

8. Which fetal position indicates a right occipital anterior (ROA) position?

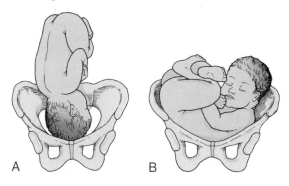

A   B

   1. A
   2. B

9. A baby is born with the following characteristics: a heart rate of 110; a loud, strong cry; well-flexed extremities; coughing when stimulated; and slightly cyanotic extremities. Using the following chart, determine his Apgar score.

SIGN	0	1	2	SCORE
Heart rate: strong and steady?	Not detectable	Slow (less than 100)	Above 100	
Respiratory effort: breathing frequently and regularly?	Absent	Slow, irregular	Good; crying	
Muscle tone: kicking feet and making fists?	Flaccid	Some flexion of extremities	Active motion	
Reflex irritability: lusty cry elicited if catheter is pushed up one nostril or soles of feet are prodded?	No response	Grimace	Cry; cough or sneeze	
Color: pink all over, or hands and feet bluish?	Blue, pale	Body pink, extremities bluish	Completely pink or absence of cyanosis	
			TOTAL	

Answer: _____

10. A woman in her first trimester tells the nurse that she is disappointed that she will not be able to go back to school as planned. The nurse should:
    1. Reassure the mother that feelings of ambivalence are not unusual in the first trimester.
    2. Tell her that she has everyone in the family to help her.
    3. Instruct her that she made the baby and she has to take full responsibility for it.
    4. Reassure her that as her pregnancy progresses her feelings will become more positive.

11. A patient in a prenatal class asks about whether Kegel exercises are beneficial in pregnancy. The most appropriate response by the nurse would be:
    1. "Absolutely not! They are dangerous to your heart."
    2. "They help some people, but the benefit is minimal."
    3. "Yes, they can help tighten the pelvic floor muscles."
    4. "Yes, these exercises help with leg cramps."

12. A primigravida in the sixth month of pregnancy is complaining of indigestion. The nurse explains that this is caused by:
    1. A growing uterus pushing on the diaphragm.
    2. Eating small, frequent meals that increase gastric acid secretion.
    3. An increasing basal metabolic rate, leading to increased appetite.
    4. Increased nausea and vomiting, common in this trimester.

13. A patient is a chain smoker. The prenatal nurse has taught her the effect of nicotine and hazards of passive smoke. In addressing the abuse of tobacco, the nurse would stress that:
    1. "It is a dirty, nasty habit that yellows your teeth, can cause lung cancer, and can offend nonsmokers."
    2. "It is becoming socially unacceptable and has widespread negative effects on both children and adults."

3. "It may cause adverse physiological effects on the fetus."

4. "It retards fetal growth, constricts blood vessels in the mother, decreases placental function, and may cause premature labor."

14. A nurse is advising a couple who is trying very hard to have a baby. Using the following graph, identify which day provides the best opportunity for conception to take place.

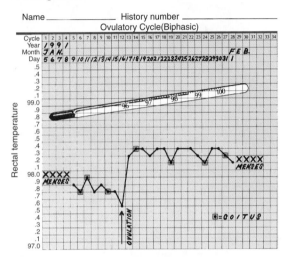

Answer: Day _____

15. Identify traits of the transition phase of labor. Select all that apply.
   _____ 1. Contractions occurring every 5 to 19 minutes
   _____ 2. Feeling like she has to have a bowel movement
   _____ 3. Doubting her ability to cope
   _____ 4. Irritability
   _____ 5. A feeling of warmth
   _____ 6. Nausea and vomiting

16. Prenatal care is considered the primary means of circumventing complications during pregnancy. Which complication would the nurse consider to be most affected by good prenatal care?
   1. Placenta previa
   2. Hyperemesis gravidarum
   3. Gestational hypertension
   4. Abortion

17. The symptom that is often considered a warning sign of an impending convulsion in the mother with eclampsia is:
   1. Headache.
   2. Severe epigastric pain.
   3. Scotoma.
   4. Puffy face.

18. A patient is diagnosed with abruptio placentae. The physician orders fibrinogen levels every 15 minutes. The patient's husband is frightened and asks the nurse why the physician has to withdraw so much blood. The nurse's best response should be:
   1. "You may ask the physician yourself."
   2. "Would you like me to inquire for you?"
   3. "This test determines the status of the clotting factor."
   4. "The physician is determining whether to give her a transfusion or operate."

19. During a nutritional assessment a nurse is concerned when the patient makes which statement?

1. "I love vegetables, especially broccoli."
2. "Some days I'm so busy that I eat fast food."
3. "I take a lot of different vitamins."
4. "I hate milk, but I guess I need it for the baby."

20. What would not be a routine assessment at 10 weeks' gestation?
   1. Goodell sign felt by the examiner
   2. Complaints of nausea and vomiting
   3. Feelings of quickening by the mother
   4. Increased feelings of tingling in the breast

21. A nurse is teaching a parenting class. She is asked, "When is it appropriate to give my baby a tub bath?" Which statement by the nurse is the most appropriate response?
   1. "A sponge bath or a tub bath is fine at any time, as long as you hold him carefully and support his head."
   2. "A tub bath is fine at any time after the cord falls off, usually in 3 to 5 days."
   3. "A tub bath is fine any time after the cord falls off in 10 to 14 days."
   4. "A tub bath is fine as soon as he can maintain a sitting position."

22. A primigravida who is at 30 weeks' gestation is admitted to the maternity unit after having been involved in an automobile accident. She is complaining of dull pain in her lower abdomen. Which assessment would be of the most concern to the nurse?
   1. A fetal heart rate (FHR) of 140 to 160 beats/min
   2. Complaints of irregular contractions relieved by walking
   3. Regular contractions occurring at intervals and unrelieved by walking
   4. Complaints of shortness of breath

23. A prenatal patient who has had diabetes for 2 years is admitted to a maternity unit because of hyperglycemia. She is 9 weeks pregnant and admits to the nurse that she does not always take her diabetes medications. What would most likely be ordered for this patient?
   1. Oral hypoglycemics
   2. Regular insulin to cover elevated blood sugar
   3. Oral antibiotics to protect against infection
   4. NPH and regular insulin

24. A newly arrived immigrant woman pregnant with her first child is being seen by the health care provider for the first time. The health care provider is concerned because she is complaining of fever, weight loss, night sweats, and a persistent cough. A diagnosis of active tuberculosis is made. The most appropriate course of action for this patient at this time should be to:
   1. Begin a drug treatment regimen according to drug susceptibility and patient's response to treatment.
   2. Do nothing until the pregnancy is over because of the risk of injury to the fetus.
   3. Start with a mild drug and monitor the pregnancy carefully for any signs of complications.
   4. Monitor the pregnancy carefully and begin treatment in the third trimester after the major fetal structures are complete.

25. A prenatal patient is diagnosed with group B *Streptococcus* infection. The treatment should be to:
   1. Obtain cultures to identify the organism responsible.
   2. Treat with a course of penicillin.
   3. Wait until labor and then treat with antibiotic.

4. Educate the patient on how to prevent future infection.

26. A patient in her twentieth week is admitted with hyperemesis gravidarum. The priority nursing intervention should be:
    1. Providing diversion to decrease pain.
    2. Monitoring accurate intake and output.
    3. Weighing the patient daily.
    4. Providing attractive, nourishing meals.

27. What should be of most concern to the nurse caring for a newborn?
    1. A newborn who has not voided in 24 hours
    2. A newborn whose hands and feet are slightly cyanotic
    3. A newborn who passes greenish, tarry stool
    4. A newborn who seems to sleep all the time

28. A staff nurse is concerned that the father of the baby is very quiet and does not seem to want to participate in the baby's care. The first priority in this case should be to:
    1. Make a special effort to cuddle and care for the baby to set an example for the parents.
    2. Insist that the father sit and hold the baby.
    3. Identify the cultural norms of the couple.
    4. Refer the couple to social services for counseling sessions.

29. New parents ask why antibiotic ointment is placed in the baby's eyes. The most appropriate response by the nurse is:
    1. "It is administered to prevent gonorrhea from being transmitted."
    2. "It is state law."
    3. "It is administered to prevent infection."
    4. "It prevents blindness caused by infection."

30. The nurse takes an axillary temperature of a 6-hour-old newborn. The most appropriate action for a reading of 96° F (35.6° C) is to:
    1. Place the newborn under the warmer until the temperature stabilizes at 97.6° to 99° F (36.4° to 37.2° C).
    2. Double wrap the infant and place a hat on his head.
    3. Recheck the temperature in 1 hour.
    4. Do nothing; this is a normal reading.

31. Newborn parents are concerned because their baby's eyes seem to be crossed at times. The most appropriate response for the nurse at this time should be:
    1. "This is normal. Newborns' eyes often seem uncoordinated for the first few days."
    2. "We have called the eye doctor in for a consultation."
    3. "This is often caused by the ointment that we put in their eyes at birth."
    4. "New parents worry about everything."

32. Cocaine is addictive to newborns because of:
    1. The inability of the newborn's immature liver to excrete the drug rapidly.
    2. The mother's long-term use of drugs before conception.
    3. The mother's ingestion of several different drugs, making it doubly addictive to the newborn.
    4. The mother's impaired uterine growth, resulting in the newborn having respiratory distress syndrome (RDS) after birth

33. What Apgar score would be given to a newborn who exhibited the following?
    Heart rate: below 100 beats/min
    Respiratory effort: weak cry
    Muscle tone: some flexion
    Reflex response: cough or sneeze
    Color: body pink; extremities blue
    Answer: _____

34. A newborn is exhibiting the following signs: His sclera is yellow, his bilirubin index is 17, and he is not nursing well. If the newborn's index continues to rise, the nurse should:
    1. Tell the mother that the baby will probably need an exchange transfusion and plan a teaching module of pros and cons.
    2. Prepare unit for possible exchange transfusion procedure; obtain supplies, review procedure, wait for physician's orders.
    3. Place the baby under phototherapy light for longer periods; offer water every 2 hours until jaundice begins to fade.
    4. Suggest that the entire family be tested for proper blood type.

35. During a vaginal examination the health care provider states that the fetus is engaged. The nurse explains to the patient that this means that the:
    1. Fetus is at the ischial spines.
    2. Fetus is floating high in the perineum.
    3. Presenting part is crowning.
    4. Infant has passed into the pelvic inlet.

36. The health care provider is evaluating whether the second stage of labor has begun. The nurse knows that this would be when the:
    1. Woman feels the urge to push.
    2. Fetus is at station 1.
    3. Cervix is fully dilated at 10 cm.
    4. Placenta is delivered.

37. After the birth of an infant the physician examines the umbilical cord carefully. The nurse understands that the physician is checking for the normal pattern, which is:
    1. Two arteries and one vein.
    2. Two veins and one artery.
    3. One vein and one artery.
    4. Two veins and two arteries.

38. The nurse is evaluating a woman during the fourth stage of labor. For a normal spontaneous vaginal delivery, which interventions are required? Select all that apply.
    _____ 1. Vital signs × 1
    _____ 2. Monitoring the fundus q15min × 4
    _____ 3. Monitoring bowel sounds
    _____ 4. Monitoring urinary output
    _____ 5. Checking lochia every 15 minutes
    _____ 6. Checking episiotomy every 15 minutes

39. To relieve supine hypotensive syndrome in a patient, the nurse should:
    1. Massage her leg.
    2. Instruct her to breathe deeply.
    3. Turn her on her left side.
    4. Advise her to walk slowly and carefully.

40. Which interventions would be appropriate for the first stage of labor? Select all that apply.
    _____ 1. Giving instructions for pushing
    _____ 2. Monitoring heart tone
    _____ 3. Orienting patient and significant others to environment
    _____ 4. Offering warm blankets for comfort

_____ 5. Checking fundus every 15 minutes
_____ 6. Noting time and delivery of placenta

41. After the placenta has been delivered and episiotomy suturing is completed, the nurse notes that the patient has begun to shiver. What should the nurse suspect as the probable cause of the shivering?
    1. The sudden emptying of the uterine contents plus the return of the body chemistry and hormones to the prepregnant state cause a certain shock to the system.
    2. Loss of blood, length of labor, and a certain fatigue cause lowering of the body temperature; the warm blankets will help.
    3. Oxytocin (Pitocin) is given after the delivery of the placenta and may cause the body to respond by shivering.
    4. The shiver is a normal reaction because she has been swallowing ice chips and is covered only with a thin sheet.

42. Using the following diagram, indicate by which method the baby is losing heat.

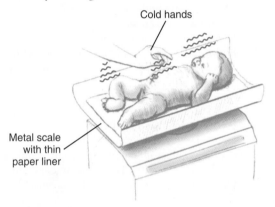

Cold hands

Metal scale with thin paper liner

    1. Evaporation
    2. Conduction
    3. Convection
    4. Radiation

43. A patient is admitted to the maternity care department. The mother-to-be has been having contractions intermittently at 10- to 20-minute intervals for the last 12 hours. The contractions are relieved by ambulation. Her estimated date of confinement (EDC) is 2 weeks away. The physician examines her and finds her to be 0 cm dilated and just slightly effaced. The nurse should determine that these contractions are most likely:
    1. True labor and will progress rapidly.
    2. True labor and will progress differently for every woman.
    3. False labor because they are relieved by activity.
    4. False labor that most likely will change to true labor in 24 hours.

44. A patient is admitted to the emergency department in active labor. She delivers a baby girl spontaneously after one contraction. The nurse is still alone with the patient. The first responsibility is to:
    1. Ascertain whether the fundus is likely to hemorrhage.
    2. Establish an airway for the baby by milking the trachea and maintaining the head lower than the body.
    3. Quickly tie and cut the umbilical cord.

    4. Look for the uterus to rise, watch the perineum for a trickle of blood, and deliver the placenta.

45. After reviewing prenatal care with a patient, the nurse should instruct the patient to notify the physician immediately if she experiences:
    1. Abdominal pain, bright red bleeding, chills, fever.
    2. Blood-streaked mucus, Braxton-Hicks contractions.
    3. Constipation, urgency, hemorrhoids.
    4. Quickening, varicosities, discomfort.

46. A patient who is in her third trimester of pregnancy suddenly notices that she is bleeding. At first the bleeding was scanty, but it has become heavier. She reports that she has no pain. A nurse should suspect:
    1. Abruptio placentae.
    2. Placenta previa.
    3. Ruptured uterus.
    4. Vasa previa.

47. In looking over a patient's chart a nurse sees that the patient's hemoglobin is 9.5 g/dL. The patient is at 32 weeks' gestation. What does this mean to the nurse?
    1. The patient is anemic and needs immediate treatment.
    2. This is probably resulting from increased blood volume of pregnancy.
    3. This must be her baseline.
    4. Z-track iron should be administered to this patient.

48. A patient who is 38 weeks pregnant is admitted to the maternity ward complaining of headaches and "blind spots" for approximately 1 week. She complained of upper abdominal pain in the morning. Emergency services brought her to the hospital immediately. After viewing the admitting record (see following illustration), the admitting nurse, knowing the situation, would place her in:

Patient Record

Admitting Record

BP: 140/112 mm Hg

Albumin: 4

FHT: 140 strong

Cervix: effaced, dilated 3 cm

Presenting part: station 0

Membranes: intact

    1. A semiprivate room with plenty of sunlight and air.
    2. A semiprivate room, darkened and quiet; restricted visitors.
    3. A single, darkened room; no visitors; close to nurses' station.
    4. A single room, plenty of sunlight; no visitors; away from the nurses' station.

49. A patient who is 2 months pregnant asks the nurse if it is all right to exercise during pregnancy. The nurse's most appropriate answer is:
    1. "It depends on your previous exercise patterns."
    2. "Absolutely. It will help you and your baby feel better."
    3. "Do not do any exercise that will jar the baby such as horseback riding or skydiving."

4. "Make certain that you let your physician know if you experience any pain or discomfort."

50. A patient delivered her first baby, a boy, several hours ago. She has been admitted to her postpartum room in stable condition and is euphoric over her successful implementation of the Lamaze techniques. The nurse finds her uterus firm, slightly above the umbilicus. She has saturated one pad with lochia rubra. Her episiotomy appears clean, but her labia and perineal area are swollen and slightly ecchymotic. The nurse's first priority in nursing care should be to:
    1. Apply an ice glove to the perineal area.
    2. Massage her uterus so it will go down below the umbilicus.
    3. Administer a tranquilizer because she is so euphoric.
    4. Watch for hemorrhage because her lochia is so red.

51. A home care nurse is interviewing and assessing a mother who gave birth 10 days ago. What should be reported to the physician?
    1. A fundus that is not palpable
    2. Reports by the mother of problems with constipation
    3. Reports by the mother of periods when she just cannot stop crying
    4. Reports by the mother of dark red lochia with small clots

52. A patient had a cesarean birth 2 days ago. She is of Asian heritage. Because her bowel sounds are positive, she is advanced to a clear liquid diet. She is refusing to drink any clear liquids except for hot water, hot tea, and a special broth that her mother brings her from home. Which intervention is appropriate for the nurse at this time?
    1. Insist that the patient consult a dietitian for additional clear liquids
    2. Sit the patient up and assist as needed with the clear liquids she will drink
    3. Speak with the family about encouraging the patient to drink more of a variety of clear liquids
    4. Explain to the patient that hospital clear liquids are healthier

53. For the last 3 days a patient who gave birth by cesarean 5 days ago has been experiencing frequent episodes of diarrhea. She is extremely weak and diaphoretic. She is breast-feeding and bonding well with the baby. For infection-control purposes, which intervention would be most appropriate?
    1. Have the patient placed on strict respiratory isolation
    2. Discontinue breast-feeding and have the baby remain in the nursery
    3. Have the baby remain in the room with the mother and have one nurse care for both
    4. Contact the physician for blood, sputum, and stool cultures

54. The nurse evaluates when it is appropriate to let a patient out of bed after epidural anesthesia. The most appropriate time is:
    1. As soon as the catheter has been removed from the epidural space.
    2. When full sensation has returned to the patient's legs.
    3. When the baby is born and she feels up to it.
    4. After her first meal.

55. Identify features that would distinguish a premature infant from an infant born full term. Select all that apply.
    _____ 1. Wrinkled skin
    _____ 2. Thin skin
    _____ 3. Excessive subcutaneous fat
    _____ 4. A lack of lanugo
    _____ 5. Prominent fontanels
    _____ 6. Poor muscle tone

56. A nurse is caring for a woman in active labor. Indicate signs that would be a cause for concern. Select all that apply.
    _____ 1. Contractions less than 2 minutes apart
    _____ 2. Contractions lasting longer than 45 seconds
    _____ 3. Excessive bleeding and hypotension
    _____ 4. Intermittent back pain
    _____ 5. Contractions that come at more frequent intervals
    _____ 6. Late decelerations of fetal heart rate

57. A couple is admitted to the family birthing center. They are from a culture with which the nurse is not familiar. Identify questions that would be both appropriate and effective in helping the nurse plan appropriate care. Select all that apply.
    _____ 1. "Have you attended childbirth classes?"
    _____ 2. "Is your husband going to participate in the birthing process?"
    _____ 3. "What religion are you?"
    _____ 4. "If the child is a male, are you going to have him circumcised?"
    _____ 5. "What type of infant feeding are you planning?"
    _____ 6. "Who should be present during your physical examinations?"

58. Although rare, a spinal headache is often treated conservatively. If conservative treatment is not adequate, which intervention may be attempted?
    1. Epidural anesthesia
    2. Transcutaneous electrical nerve stimulation
    3. A blood patch
    4. Antibiotics

59. Which finding in a 10-day postpartum patient would indicate that involution is proceeding at a normal rate?
    1. The uterus is firm, midline, and three fingers below the umbilicus.
    2. The uterus is firm, deviated to the right, and three fingers below the umbilicus.
    3. The uterus is no longer palpable in the abdominal cavity.
    4. The uterus is firm and at the umbilicus.

60. A nurse is teaching a new mother how to breast-feed. The nurse is concerned because the woman is very quiet and appears discouraged. The nurse asks the patient if something is troubling her. The patient replies, "I'm worried that my baby isn't getting enough to eat." The most appropriate response by the nurse is:
    1. "When he falls asleep after nursing, he is satisfied."
    2. "If he nurses at least 10 minutes on each side, he is satisfied."
    3. "If he urinates six to eight times per day, he is adequately nourished."
    4. "If he gains weight on a regular basis, he is fine."

61. Which assessment would be of most concern to the nurse in a patient 2 days after giving birth?
    1. A firm fundus two fingers below the umbilicus
    2. Frequency and burning on urination

3. Breasts that are firm and engorged
4. Lochia rubra with small clots

62. A patient is admitted to the nurse's medical-surgical unit after having delivered a full-term infant who was stillborn. The husband says to the nurse, "I will see my baby and take care of the arrangements. I don't want anyone to say anything to my wife about what happened." The most appropriate action of the nurse should be to:
    1. Reassure the husband that his wishes will be respected.
    2. Explain to the husband that no one will initiate the specific topic with his wife but they will not stop her from talking about it.
    3. Encourage the husband to talk with his wife so that they can support each other through the grieving process.
    4. Explain politely to the husband that his wife is the patient and it is the nurse's responsibility to encourage communication in every way possible.

63. An adolescent who is 1 day postpartum is discussing future birth-control methods with the nurse. She states that she is busy and forgetful and doesn't want to think about it every day. The most appropriate method for the nurse to recommend would be:
    1. Abstinence.
    2. Estrogen patch.
    3. Condoms.
    4. Depo-Provera injection.

64. A nurse is completing her assessments on a postpartum patient. The patient asks the nurse why she had to dorsiflex her foot. Which statement is the most appropriate response for the nurse?
    1. "It is a precautionary assessment to be certain that your circulation is healthy."
    2. "Pain in your inner calf may be an indication of a blood clot."
    3. "Women have extra clotting factors to minimize blood loss during pregnancy."
    4. "Exercise is good for the extremities to help prevent blood clots."

65. A patient in her third trimester is complaining of shortness of breath when she is trying to rest. The most appropriate intervention for the nurse to suggest is to:
    1. "Rest during the day whenever you have a chance."
    2. "Elevate your legs above the level of your heart."
    3. "Use two pillows when you are trying to sleep."
    4. "Avoid eating too close to your bedtime."

66. A woman is diagnosed with an ectopic pregnancy. Identify all possible causes. Select all that apply.
    _____ 1. Chronic vaginal infections
    _____ 2. Placenta previa
    _____ 3. A history of drug abuse
    _____ 4. Inflammation of fallopian tubes
    _____ 5. Congenital inflammation of the fallopian tube
    _____ 6. A history of infection in the fallopian tube

67. The initial assessment of a primigravida documents the following information: The patient is alert and talkative and is 2 cm dilated with mild contractions every 15 minutes lasting 20 to 30 seconds. The nurse knows from these data that the patient is in the:
    1. First stage of labor (latent phase).
    2. First stage of labor (active phase).

3. First stage of labor (transition phase).
4. Stage of dilatation and effacement.

68. Newborns must be protected against infection because:
    1. The immune system of the infant is not fully developed and takes time to do so.
    2. The portals of entry of infection are much more vulnerable than those of an adult.
    3. An infection that is minor in an adult might kill a child.
    4. Babies who are not breast-feeding do not receive protective antibodies from the mother.

69. A pregnant woman is lying on her back during an examination. She begins to complain of light-headedness and dizziness. The most appropriate nursing intervention at this point would be:
    1. Have the patient change to a sitting position.
    2. Turn patient on her left side.
    3. Elevate the patient's legs.
    4. Elevate her to semi-Fowler position.

70. A nurse is caring for a high-risk mother who is 8 months pregnant who states that her membranes ruptured and she is having contractions. The nurse suspects that a prolapsed cord may have occurred. After calling for emergency help, the priority action for the nurse is to:
    1. Place the woman in high-Fowler position to decrease pressure.
    2. Support the cord to prevent repositioning.
    3. Place the mother in knee-chest position.
    4. Monitor the fetal heart rate.

71. A woman is admitted to the maternity unit with a diagnosis of severe gestational hypertension (GH). Which medication would the nurse expect to be ordered?
    1. Furosemide (Lasix)
    2. Acetylsalicylic acid (ASA)
    3. Magnesium sulfate
    4. Calcium gluconate

72. The nurse is concerned because a 12-hour-old infant has a bilirubin level of 14 mg/dL. On assessment the infant would show:
    1. Signs of jaundice.
    2. Irritability.
    3. Signs of infection.
    4. A weak cry.

73. A woman who gave birth 1 hour ago is getting out of bed for the first time. Prioritize the items below for teaching purposes during the next 48 hours from highest priority to lowest.
    1. Breast-feeding techniques
    2. Proper perineal care
    3. The importance of good nutrition
    4. Prevention of infection for herself and her baby
    5. Infant care techniques
    6. Methods to cope with sibling rivalry

74. Identify signs of distress in a neonate. Select all that apply.
    _____ 1. Slight cyanosis in the extremities
    _____ 2. Positive Babinski reflex
    _____ 3. Nostrils flaring on inspiration
    _____ 4. Irritability
    _____ 5. Poor feeding
    _____ 6. Urinating six to eight times per day

75. Identify items that are characteristic of abruptio placentae. Select all that apply.

_____ 1. An abnormally placed placenta
_____ 2. Cramplike to severe pain
_____ 3. Soft, nondistended abdomen
_____ 4. Risk of maternal mortality
_____ 5. Tender-to-rigid abdomen and uterus

76. Identify contributing factors that would be warning signs for possible postpartum depression. Select all that apply.
_____ 1. Too many family members discussing the baby's future
_____ 2. A history of depression
_____ 3. Anger exhibited toward partner
_____ 4. Difficulty with breast-feeding
_____ 5. Taking a great deal of time over her own appearance

77. A nurse is teaching a newborn care class. Indicate items that would need to be taught. Select all that apply.
_____ 1. Safety needs of the newborn
_____ 2. The importance of giving a tub bath every day
_____ 3. Maintaining a specific schedule for bathing the newborn
_____ 4. Recommended lotions and powders to be used on the baby
_____ 5. The age appropriateness of having siblings help in the newborn care
_____ 6. The importance of maintaining the warmth of the baby

78. Indicate the order of priority for the nursing interventions in the following situation. A woman is admitted to the birthing center in active labor. She is feeling the urge to push. There is no history of prenatal care. Place the interventions in order from highest priority to lowest priority.
   1. Ascertain her knowledge of the childbirth process.
   2. Assess the viability of the fetus by placing a monitor on the mother.
   3. Place ordered oxygen on the mother.
   4. Do a vaginal examination to determine effacement and dilation.
   5. Quickly teach the mother appropriate breathing techniques.
   6. Determine if there are any preexisting medical problems.

79. A new mother asks the nurse about the bruises on her baby's back. The nurse replies:
   1. "These are not bruises; they are called mongolian spots."
   2. "These are bruises from the birth process, and they will fade."
   3. "These are mongolian spots and are caused by pigment-producing cells."
   4. "I will make certain the pediatrician is informed of these areas."

80. A woman is gravida 3, para 0. The nurse knows that this patient will require:
   1. No special support because she has been pregnant before.
   2. A careful assessment to find out the mother's feelings about the pregnancy.
   3. Immediate intervention to help her deal with her anxiety.

   4. A careful history to determine the outcomes of the previous pregnancies.

81. A mother asks the nurse about the "little white pimples" on her baby's cheeks. Which response is the most appropriate reply by the nurse?
   1. "The doctor will order a mild antibiotic cream."
   2. "Wash it very well with soap and water; this will clear up the rash."
   3. "We will keep an eye on the rash to make sure that it does not spread."
   4. "They are normal on a newborn and do not require any special intervention."

82. A woman at her second prenatal visit is 8 weeks pregnant. She confides to the nurse that she is worried about her ability to be a mother. The nurse replies:
   1. "Many pregnancies are unplanned."
   2. "It is normal to have concerns about the pregnancy at this point."
   3. "Don't worry; these feelings will pass."
   4. "Your partner will help you work through these anxieties."

83. A patient in the physician's office complains of increased vaginal discharge. The most appropriate nursing intervention would be to:
   1. Advise her to decrease sexual intercourse.
   2. Encourage her to wear only cotton underwear.
   3. Ask her if the discharge burns or itches.
   4. Ask her physician to prescribe a douche.

84. A newborn receives an Apgar score of 9 at 1 minute after birth. The reason for this would be:
   1. A heart rate of 110 beats/min.
   2. Active spontaneous motion.
   3. A strong, lusty cry.
   4. Slight cyanosis of the extremities.

85. Decreases in fetal heart rate during labor are called:
   1. Accelerations.
   2. Decelerations.
   3. Baseline rate.
   4. Variability.

86. Which is an incorrect statement comparing the differences between true and false labor?
   1. True labor discomfort is usually felt in the lower back and lower abdomen.
   2. In false labor walking tends to relieve or decrease contractions.
   3. In false labor bloody show is often present.
   4. In true labor contractions gradually develop a regular pattern.

87. Early decelerations are noted on the external fetal monitoring strip of a patient in active labor. The first nursing action is:
   1. No intervention is required; this is a reassuring pattern.
   2. Reposition the patient on her left side.
   3. Give the patient 2 L of oxygen.
   4. Notify the physician to obtain an order for an IV line.

88. A woman in labor asks the nurse why she and her partner have to keep walking around the hall. All reasons are appropriate, except:
   1. Walking helps to use gravity in the baby's descent.
   2. Walking decreases back pain.

3. Walking helps the membranes rupture.

4. Walking stimulates contractions.

89. A nurse is teaching a student how to palpate contractions. The correct position of the examiner's hand is:
    1. On the symphysis pubis.
    2. In the vagina.
    3. On the fundus of the uterus.
    4. On the woman's umbilicus.

90. A primigravida calls the physician's office and gives the nurse the following information. She is having regular contractions every 8 minutes, and her membranes have not ruptured. The most appropriate intervention for the nurse would be to advise her to:
    1. Walk around in her house and come to the hospital when her contractions are 5 minutes apart.
    2. Call an ambulance, and come to the hospital immediately.
    3. Have someone drive her to the hospital quickly and safely.
    4. Come to the physician's office for further assessment.

91. Which assessment would be of most concern 24 hours after birth?
    1. A moderate amount of lochia with a dime-sized clot
    2. A firm fundus deviated to the right
    3. A severely bruised perineum
    4. An intact, slightly reddened perineum

92. A woman in labor states that she feels like she has to push. The initial intervention by the nurse would be to:
    1. Reassure the woman that this is a normal sensation in labor.
    2. Monitor the contractions to assess the duration.
    3. Assess the perineum for signs of bulging.
    4. Call the physician in preparation for delivery.

93. A newborn is diagnosed with caput succedaneum. During an assessment, the nurse would expect to see:
    1. Depressed fontanels.
    2. Swelling of the scalp.
    3. A swelling on one side of the scalp.
    4. Bulging fontanels.

94. Identify risk factors for preterm labor. Select all that apply.
    _____ 1. History of preterm labor
    _____ 2. Primigravida
    _____ 3. Short cervix
    _____ 4. Vaginal infections between weeks 22 and 37
    _____ 5. Hypotensive episodes
    _____ 6. Cigarette smoking

95. What treatment is required for a cephalhematoma?
    1. No treatment is required; it disappears in 3 to 4 days.
    2. Gently massage twice per day.
    3. No treatment is required, and it will disappear in 3 to 6 weeks.
    4. Monitor carefully to be certain that it does not get larger.

96. A major concern for women with premature rupture of membranes (PROM) is:
    1. Dystocia.
    2. Hemorrhage.
    3. Infection.
    4. Hypertension.

97. Indicate the appropriate position for the fundus of a woman who is postpartum day 1.

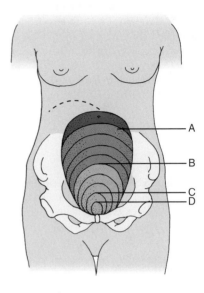

1. A
2. B
3. C
4. D

98. Oligohydramnios may indicate which anomaly in the newborn?
    1. Abnormalities of the gastrointestinal tract
    2. Cardiac abnormalities
    3. Neurological abnormalities
    4. Urinary tract abnormalities

99. HELLP (hemolysis, elevated liver enzymes, low platelets) is defined as:
    1. A severe form of anemia that needs to be treated in pregnancy.
    2. A mild form of gestational hypertension (GH) that needs close monitoring.
    3. A severe syndrome that occurs with GH.
    4. This is not specifically associated with hyperemesis gravidarum.

100. Which mother is at the highest risk for postpartum infection?
    1. A woman who delivered a baby precipitously
    2. A woman who delivered via cesarean section
    3. A woman with premature rupture of membranes (PROM)
    4. A woman with a prolonged labor

101. An infant is in the ninetieth percentile for weight. This would classify the baby as:
    1. Appropriate for gestational age.
    2. Overweight.
    3. Small for gestational age.
    4. Large for gestational age.

102. Women with diabetes are more prone to urinary tract infections because:
    1. They have to limit their fluid intake.
    2. Increased amounts of glucose are in their urine.
    3. Their babies tend to be larger and put more pressure on the bladder.
    4. Their insulin requirements fluctuate in pregnancy.

103. A woman and her partner are embarrassed about being sent home because of false labor. The best response of the nurse would be:
    1. "Don't be upset; it happens all the time."
    2. "Next time wait until your contractions are 5 minutes apart."
    3. "Do not hesitate to come to the hospital with any concern."
    4. "Wait until your membranes rupture."

104. A woman is admitted in labor. Her mother and her husband are with her. The woman wants her mother to be with her, and the husband states that he will wait in the waiting room. The most appropriate intervention for the nurse is:
    1. Tell the husband that he will regret not being present at his baby's birth.
    2. Explore the reasons behind the couple's request.
    3. Explain to the husband that he will be at the mother's head and will not have to see any blood.
    4. Respect the woman's wishes.

105. The primary reason for having a Foley catheter inserted before a cesarean birth is to:
    1. Make certain that the urinary output is adequate during surgery.
    2. Prevent infection.
    3. Keep the bladder empty so it does not interfere with surgery.
    4. Eliminate the need for early ambulation after surgery.

106. A primigravida in her second trimester is planning a long driving vacation with her spouse. The most pertinent advice for the nurse to give is:
    1. "Bring plenty of nutritious snacks so you won't get hungry."
    2. "Elevate your legs at night to decrease edema."
    3. "Let your husband do most of the driving to avoid leg cramps."
    4. "Stop at least every 3 hours and elevate your legs."

107. A woman gave birth 3 hours ago. The nurse observes the patient trying to care for the baby. The woman states, "I'm just too tired." She returns to bed. The best action for the nurse at this point is:
    1. Complete the newborn's care quietly and allow the mother to rest.
    2. Encourage the mother to complete the care.
    3. Complete the care but put in a consultation request to social services.
    4. Instruct the mother on completing the care while she is resting.

108. During a postpartum examination the nurse assesses a small hematoma on the vulva. The most appropriate intervention (with a standing order) would be:
    1. Ice pack.
    2. Bath.
    3. Spray.
    4. Lamp.

109. A young couple wants to know when the gender of the fetus is determined. The correct answer is:
    1. At birth.
    2. At conception.
    3. During amniocentesis.
    4. From results of blood work after first prenatal visit.

110. The physician is concerned because the baby has a nuchal cord. The nurse knows this means that the cord is:
    1. Coming out before the head.
    2. Too long.
    3. Around the baby's neck.
    4. Too high.

111. The hormone that stimulates uterine contractions and helps keep the uterus contracted after birth is:
    1. Prolactin.
    2. Oxytocin.
    3. Estrogen.
    4. Progesterone.

112. A patient tells the nurse that she is interested in using herbal medicines to ease some of the common discomforts of pregnancy. The best response by the nurse would be:
    1. "Most herbal medicines are natural and safe."
    2. "Check with the physician before taking any medicine."
    3. "Just be certain to watch your dose."
    4. "The safety of most of these medicines has not been determined for pregnancy."

113. After examination, a woman is 5 cm dilated and 50% effaced. The nurse knows that she is in the:
    1. Second stage.
    2. First stage—latent phase.
    3. First stage—transition phase.
    4. First stage—active phase.

114. Which contraction pattern would be characteristic of the transition phase of labor?
    1. 8:00 AM, end 8:00 AM and 30 seconds; 8:05 AM, end 8:05 AM and 30 seconds
    2. 8:00 AM, end 8:01 AM; 8:03 AM, end 8:04 AM
    3. 8:00 AM, end 8:00 AM and 20 seconds; 8:15 AM, end 8:15 AM and 20 seconds
    4. Irregular contractions lasting 45 to 60 seconds with no spaced pattern

115. Which pregnant woman might find working until full term the most difficult?
    1. A self-employed accountant
    2. A hair stylist
    3. A book editor
    4. A real estate agent

116. Indicate possible reasons for a cesarean section. Select all that apply.
    _____ 1. Precipitous delivery
    _____ 2. Breech
    _____ 3. Cephalopelvic disproportion
    _____ 4. Diabetes in the mother

117. What initial advice should be given to the pregnant woman to relieve constipation?
    1. Increase fluid intake to eight glasses of water per day
    2. Obtain a prescription for a stool softener
    3. Increased exercise increases peristalsis
    4. Use a natural laxative

118. Which snack for a pregnant patient would be of most concern to the nurse?
    1. Cafe latte at 3:00 PM
    2. Ice cream at 9:00 PM
    3. Low-fat yogurt at 11:00 AM
    4. Gelatin for dessert

119. A Native-American family asks permission to perform a ceremony blessing their newborn. What further information is needed before an answer can be given?
    1. Is the woman in a private room?
    2. What exactly is involved in the ceremony?
    3. What supplies need to be provided by the hospital?
    4. Will hospital staff be permitted to attend the ceremony?

120. A patient is in the transitional phase of labor. Which best describes her behavioral pattern?
    1. Happy and talkative
    2. Anxious and uncomfortable
    3. Irritable and introverted
    4. Relaxed and receptive

121. Using the accompanying diagram, determine what the fetal heart rate is.

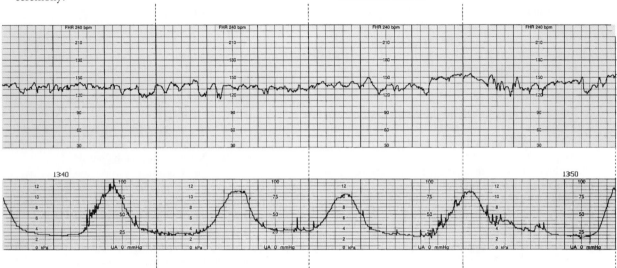

Answer: Approximately _____ beats/min

122. Identify which fetal heart rate deceleration is indicated in the accompanying tracing.

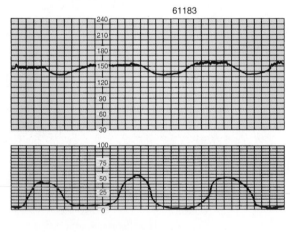

    1. Late deceleration
    2. Early deceleration
    3. Variable deceleration
    4. Intermittent deceleration

123. The nurse evaluates her patient teaching concerning sibling rivalry as successful when her patient states the following:
    1. "I need to make sure that I spend special time with each of my children."
    2. "My oldest can help with babysitting chores."
    3. "They need to understand that the baby will occupy a great deal of my time."
    4. "Thank goodness that my 5-year-old is starting kindergarten in the fall."

124. The second trimester is most commonly noted for which behavior in the woman?
    1. Introversion—questioning her role as a mother
    2. Separating the fetus from herself and making concrete plans
    3. Acceptance of the fetus as part of her body image
    4. Ambivalent feelings concerning being a mother

125. Late decelerations during labor:
    1. Are of concern because they may indicate the fetus is not getting enough oxygen.
    2. Are expected and not of any concern.
    3. Indicate that the fetus is tolerating the stress of labor.
    4. Are of concern because they indicate that the labor is progressing faster than expected.

126. Which statement by a primigravida indicates the need for further teaching?
    1. "Fast food is okay as long as I make healthy choices."
    2. "I am really nervous about the pain of childbirth."
    3. "I know the signs of impending labor and when to call the doctor."
    4. "I had a miscarriage 2 years ago."

127. A nurse is teaching a 14-year-old primigravida how to bathe her baby. Which statement would be of most concern?
    1. "I will make sure that I bathe the baby after I feed her."
    2. "The baby does not have to be on any special schedule."
    3. "Sometimes I get so frustrated when she cries and cries and cries."
    4. "My boyfriend said he will help me sometimes."

128. Which statement by a new mother best indicates that she understands the needs of a newborn during bath time?
    1. "Sometimes my partner can help me with the bath."
    2. "I don't have to be on a rigid schedule."

3. "I must never take my hands off the baby during bath time."

4. "I will feed my baby after I bathe him."

129. Which is the best suggestion to give new parents to prevent postpartum baby blues?
1. "You have to be strong and take responsibility for your baby."
2. "Keep your strength up with plenty of nutritious snacks."
3. "Be certain to spend time with each other and communicate your feelings."
4. "Call your physician if you are feeling sad and depressed."

130. The first nursing intervention immediately after the membranes rupture is:
1. Assessing the maternal blood pressure.
2. Assessing the maternal pulse.
3. Assessing the fetal heart rate.
4. Assessing the interval between contractions.

131. The most appropriate instruction that should be given to help prevent a urinary tract infection is:
1. Limit fluid intake to between meals.
2. Drink at least eight glasses of water per day.
3. Try to avoid emptying your bladder until it's really necessary.
4. Drink cranberry juice at least once each day.

132. If the nurse is uncertain whether the fluid is amniotic fluid, the proper intervention is to:
1. Send a sample to the laboratory.
2. Consult with the physician.
3. Arrange for a stress test.
4. Test the fluid with Nitrazine paper.

133. Identify signs of illness in a newborn. Select all that apply.
_____ 1. Refusal of a feeding
_____ 2. A pulse rate of 180 beats/min
_____ 3. A temperature of less than 97° F (36.1° C)
_____ 4. A positive Babinski reflex
_____ 5. Fewer than four voidings per day

134. A postpartum patient calls the maternity unit with a question about feeding. Her bottle-fed infant has only had two stools in the last 24 hours. The nurse advises her to call the physician and also gives her the following suggestion:
1. Try switching to a formula with increased iron.
2. Feed the infant on a strict schedule.
3. Increase the amount of fluid in the infant's diet.
4. Two stools per day are not unusual for a newborn.

135. One of the dangers of cold stress in a newborn is that the newborn is:
1. Prone to reverse peristalsis.
2. Prone to swallowing air and crying during feeding.
3. At risk for hypoglycemia.
4. At risk for infection.

136. Which are examples of heat loss by evaporation? Select all that apply.
_____ 1. The moisture present on the baby immediately after birth
_____ 2. Cold hands
_____ 3. Wet diapers
_____ 4. A draft from an open door
_____ 5. The bassinet against a cold radiator
_____ 6. Blanket loose or off

137. One benefit of breast-feeding over bottle-feeding is that the infant:
1. Receives passive immunity for some viral and bacterial infections.
2. Receives a supply of vitamin K.
3. Receives a supply of iron.
4. Is less likely to have problems with constipation.

138. Which reflex is most important in encouraging the newborn to eat?
1. Gag
2. Moro
3. Pupillary
4. Rooting

139. A positive Babinski response in a full-term infant:
1. Is abnormal and may indicate a spinal cord abnormality.
2. Is normal and indicates an intact central nervous system.
3. Is unusual but occurs as a genetic trait in some nationalities.
4. Occurs when an object is placed in the infant's hand.

140. A key difference that distinguishes baby blues from postpartum depression is:
1. The woman cannot distinguish reality from fantasy.
2. The woman is unable to care for her baby or the rest of her family.
3. The woman has crying spells for no apparent reason.
4. Feelings of sadness are more transient.

141. One reason adolescents have a special need for nutritional counseling is that:
1. They are influenced by their peers to eat the wrong food.
2. They like to eat a lot of fast food because of their busy lifestyle.
3. Their food may not include enough choices of healthy nutrients.
4. They tend to eat too few calories to avoid gaining a lot of weight.

142. Postpartum hemorrhage can cause which type of shock?
1. Hypovolemic shock
2. Anaphylactic shock
3. Septic shock
4. Physiological shock

143. A pregnant woman is classified as nonimmune to rubella. The appropriate action at this point is:
1. Counsel the patient that an abortion may need to be considered.
2. Advise the patient to avoid situations in which she may be exposed.
3. Arrange for appropriate diagnostic tests to detect possible fetal abnormalities.
4. Arrange for the vaccine to be administered immediately.

144. A patient is being cared for in a prenatal clinic. She tells the nurse that she is a vegetarian. What follow-up information is required at this point?
1. To what degree is the woman a vegetarian?
2. How long has she been a vegetarian?
3. Is the baby going to be a vegetarian?
4. Is she going to eat meat during the pregnancy?

145. A gravida 2, para 1 patient asks her physician about the possibility of a vaginal birth after cesarean (VBAC) for her second child. Which reason would rule out this possibility?
1. Her first baby was a breech.

2. A transverse lower-abdominal incision
3. A current diagnosis of placenta previa
4. A history of maternal heart disease

146. Which interventions are required for a cesarean birth mother and not for a mother who had a vaginal delivery? Select all that apply.
_____ 1. Checking for vaginal bleeding
_____ 2. Checking for urinary drainage in catheter
_____ 3. Encouraging deep breathing
_____ 4. Checking the dressing for drainage
_____ 5. Checking the episiotomy
_____ 6. Checking for hematomas

147. Which of these conditions would be a contraindication for discontinuing an IV line in a cesarean patient?
1. The patient is afebrile.
2. The patient has faint bowel sounds.
3. The patient is complaining of nausea.
4. The patient is tolerating clear liquids.

148. A nurse is counseling a woman and her partner. They are considering having a baby in the near future. The woman is 23 years old. She states that she eats "pretty healthy," although she does like to eat junk food once in awhile. She is approximately 5 pounds overweight for her height. Which suggestions would be appropriate for the nurse to make to this couple? Select all that apply.
_____ 1. Lose 10 pounds before you think about getting pregnant.
_____ 2. Make sure that you have your blood pressure checked frequently before getting pregnant.
_____ 3. Take folic acid supplements before and during pregnancy.
_____ 4. Select an obstetrician carefully and form a relationship with him or her.
_____ 5. Make healthy food choices before and after pregnancy. Obtain education from professionals to assist you with this.
_____ 6. Avoid consuming junk food before and during pregnancy.

149. A student nurse is observing in the nursery. She asks why the PKU test is not done immediately after birth. The nurse responds:
1. It is more adequate 24 hours after birth.
2. Severe effects are rare because of early screening.
3. Time must be allowed to ensure that the newborn has ingested sufficient levels of phenylalanine.
4. Important enzymes need time to develop.

150. A nurse is counseling a mother of Hispanic origins on different techniques of breast-feeding. The mother has a beginning knowledge of English. Her partner is assisting in the translation. The mother successfully demonstrates attachment techniques and burping positions. She seems increasingly confused and a little frustrated when the nurse mentions the "football" hold. A possible explanation for this might be:
1. She is uncomfortable holding the baby at her side.
2. She is worried about the possibility of injuries associated with football
3. Her mother told her that there is only one safe position for breast-feeding
4. Cultural influences may give another meaning to the word.

ANSWERS AND RATIONALES

1. Knowledge, assessment, physiological integrity, (a).
   3. The urinary bladder is label C.
   1. The placenta is label A.
   2. The uterus is label B.
   4. The vagina is label D.

2. Application, implementation, health promotion and maintenance, (b).
   3. These are the correct instructions.
   1. This is acceptable for a routine urinalysis.
   2. Pregnancy tests do not require a sterile specimen.
   4. This is untrue.

3. Comprehension, assessment, health promotion and maintenance, (a).
   2. German measles have a devastating effect on fetal growth: physical abnormalities, mental retardation, hearing impairment or deafness, blindness.
   1. Chickenpox may have a more severe action on the mother but does not cause fetal physiological defects or problems.
   3. This is a synonym for chickenpox.
   4. This is regular measles; it does not affect the unborn.

4. Application, implementation, physiological integrity, (b).
   Answer: +1. The baby's head or presenting part is at +1 station. Station is defined as the relationship of the presenting parts of the fetus to the pelvic ischial spine.

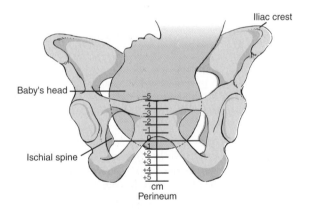

5. Comprehension, planning, health promotion and maintenance, (b).
   2. Increased thyroid hormones cause an increase in basal metabolic rate (BMR).
   1. This is true but is not specific enough.
   3. This is true; however, it does not answer the question.
   4. Increased caloric energy is needed, but this is not the cause of the increased BMR.

6. Application, planning, health promotion and maintenance, (a).
   1. Smoking causes vasoconstriction and decreased oxygenation.
   2. Women who smoke actually tend to have smaller babies.
   3, 4. No documented connection exists.

7. Comprehension, planning, health promotion and maintenance, (b).
   2. This is an inherited neurodegenerative disease of lipid metabolism.
   1. This is an anemia that is more common in African Americans.

3. This is an anemia common in people from the Mediterranean area.

4. This is more common in Caucasians and is a disorder of fat metabolism.

8. Comprehension, assessment, physiological integrity, (c).

   1. The correct answer is A, right occipital anterior (ROA). Position *is defined as relationship of fetal presenting part to the mother's pelvis.*

   2. Position B is a transverse lie.

9. Analysis, evaluation, physiological integrity, (c).

   Answer: 9. Slight cyanosis of the extremities is normal when an infant is first born. The Apgar score is an assessment of the newborn's respiratory and circulatory system at 1 and 5 minutes after birth.

10. Analysis, planning, psychosocial integrity, (b).

    1. In the first trimester the mother generally thinks more about herself and how the pregnancy will affect her life.

    2. This is fine, but it does not answer her concerns.

    3. This is judgmental and does not offer therapeutic communication.

    4. This is what is hoped for; however, it is not guaranteed.

11. Application, implementation, physiological integrity, (b).

    3. This is the correct use of Kegel exercises.

    1. They are not dangerous to the heart.

    2. This is not a correct statement.

    4. Range-of-motion exercises help with leg cramps.

12 Application, planning, physiological integrity, (b).

   1. The growing uterus leaves less space for the stomach; therefore food sometimes remains there longer.

   2. This does not cause heartburn; it is sometimes recommended to decrease symptoms.

   3. This does not cause heartburn.

   4. These symptoms are not common in this trimester and if present may indicate hyperemesis gravidarum.

13. Application, planning, psychosocial integrity, (b).

    4. This is the correct answer. It gives the mother specific information that directly addresses the harmful effects of nicotine on her unborn child. Pregnancy can be a very motivating factor to stop smoking.

    1. These are all true. However, they are all reasons that the mother knew before pregnancy, and there is no reason to believe that they would motivate her now any more than they did before she was pregnant.

    2. This is also true but is not the best answer to motivate a pregnant woman.

    3. This is too vague; it is not the best answer to provide motivation.

14. Analysis, evaluation, health promotion and maintenance, (b).

    Answer: Day 12. If the mother takes her temperature every day, she will note a slight drop when ovulation occurs. This is the most likely window for conception to happen.

15. Analysis, assessment, physiological integrity, (b).

    _____ 1. This is more characteristic of the active phase of the first stage.

    __X__ **2. The woman feels as if she has to have a bowel movement because of the pressure of the presenting part on the floor of the perineum.**

    _____ 3. This is more characteristic of the active phase of the first stage.

    __X__ **4. The transition phase of labor is from 7 to 10 cm. The woman is using her energy for**

the laboring process and has little patience with distraction.

   __X__ **5. The woman is perspiring heavily because of increased expenditure of energy. This leads to a feeling of warmth.**

   __X__ **6. Nausea and vomiting are a result of pressure on the intestines.**

16. Comprehension, assessment, health promotion and maintenance, (b).

    3. This is the correct answer; early, frequent, and continual testing of urine and blood pressure would signal early signs that can be addressed rapidly and appropriately.

    1. This is usually a third-trimester complication and would not be considered a preventable condition.

    2. This is not exactly preventable but can be helped by easing discomfort, teaching, and advising on care.

    4. Spontaneous abortions might have some early signs and symptoms that alert the physician to pending conditions, but this is not the best answer.

17. Comprehension, assessment, physiological integrity, (b).

    2. This is the significant symptom of an impending convulsion and is caused by hepatic alterations, which include enlargement of the liver and tension on the liver capsule.

    1. This is a sign of change in blood pressure, preeclampsia.

    3. Eye changes would not be noted by the mother.

    4. This is not necessarily a sign of impending convulsions, but rather of fluid retention.

18. Application, planning, psychosocial integrity, (c).

    3. The nurse is explaining procedure and giving reassurance.

    1. This response is rude and curt and did not answer the question.

    2. The physician was in the room, but he asked the nurse.

    4. This answer creates unnecessary anxiety with no explanation.

19. Application, assessment, physiological integrity, (b).

    3. Megadoses of vitamins can be teratogenic.

    1. This is okay as long as the diet is balanced.

    2. This is okay as long as healthy choices can be made.

    4. Alternatives can be offered for milk.

20. Comprehension, assessment, health promotion and maintenance, (a).

    3. Fetal movement is normally felt at approximately 16 weeks.

    1. The cervix thickens and softens; this is normally felt by 6 weeks.

    2. This is normal during the first trimester.

    4. This is normal.

21. Application, planning, health promotion and maintenance, (a).

    3. This is correct, and the cord generally does fall off in 10 to 14 days.

    1. Babies should always be held carefully with the head supported.

    2. This is partially correct, but the cord does not fall off in 3 to 5 days.

    4. This is not a requirement for a tub bath.

22. Application, assessment, health promotion and maintenance, (b).

    3. This is one sign of true labor.

    1. This is a normal range for FHR.

2. Contractions relieved by walking are Braxton-Hicks contractions.

4. This is normal in the beginning of the third trimester, caused by a growing baby putting pressure on the diaphragm.

23. Comprehension, planning, health promotion and maintenance, (c).

   4. A combination of types of insulin with different durations allows for a steadier therapeutic level of insulin in the body.

   1. Oral hypoglycemics are contraindicated during pregnancy because their effect on the fetus is uncertain.

   2. Regular insulin is short acting and therefore would not act on a long-term basis.

   3. The question has no mention of infection.

24. Application, implementation, physiological integrity, (b).

   1. A pregnant woman with active disease needs effective treatment to protect her and her fetus.

   2. Preventive therapy can be postponed until after pregnancy; the risk of doing nothing in active disease is too great.

   3. Treatment for active disease includes a minimum of two or three drugs.

   4. Risk to the mother and fetus is too great to wait until the third trimester.

25. Comprehension, implementation, physiological integrity, (b).

   2. Treatment before birth of the infant is preferred; it decreases the chance of the infant's exposure to the organism.

   1. This has already been done.

   3. This is an option for high-risk women; however, treatment should not wait if a diagnosis has been made.

   4. This is also important; treatment takes priority.

26. Application, implementation, physiological integrity, (b).

   2. Monitoring the IV line and urinary output is the priority.

   1. Patients need quiet; pain is not usually present.

   3. A baseline is important, but this is not a priority.

   4. Small meals may be provided after the intestinal tract has had the opportunity to rest.

27. Analysis, assessment, health promotion and maintenance, (b).

   1. This is a priority and should be reported to the physician.

   2. This is normal.

   3. This is normal and called *meconium*.

   4. For newborns to sleep many hours is not unusual.

28. Application, assessment, safe and effective care environment, (b).

   3. This may be the way that they were brought up in their culture. The father may be very proud of the infant and show it privately.

   1. This is fine, but further information is needed first.

   2. This is not appropriate.

   4. This is very premature until a great deal of additional information is gathered.

29. Application, evaluation, health promotion and maintenance, (b).

   3. This is factual without causing undue alarm.

   1. This is true, but it may be insulting.

   2. This is true; however, it does not answer the question.

   4. This causes undue alarm.

30. Application, implementation, physiological integrity, (b).

   1. Cold stress is dangerous for infants; this is the appropriate action.

   2. This can be done after the infant has spent time in the warmer.

   3. This should also be done after the first two interventions are completed.

   4. This is incorrect.

31. Application, evaluation, health promotion and maintenance, (b).

   1. This is correct, reassuring information.

   2. This is not necessary and alarming.

   3. This is incorrect information.

   4. This is a demeaning statement.

32. Comprehension, evaluation, psychosocial integrity, (c).

   1. This is the correct answer. Because all newborns have an immature liver, putting a drug into the system jeopardizes the infant.

   2. Prolonged use of a drug by the mother just before conception does not necessarily cause newborn addiction unless the mother continues the habit from conception throughout pregnancy to term.

   3. This answer in itself is not correct; usage must be continued during pregnancy.

   4. Drugs may affect uterine growth because the addictive mother seldom has good nutritional habits; however, if carried through term, the infant does not necessarily have RDS.

33. Analysis, evaluation, health promotion and maintenance, (b).

   Answer: 6. The Apgar score is 6 as shown below:
   Heart rate: 1
   Respiratory effort: 1
   Muscle tone: 1
   Reflex response: 2
   Color: 1

34. Analysis, planning, physiological integrity, (c).

   2. This is the best response. Preparation is started; thus if the procedure is ordered, time is not lost. These are signs of pathological jaundice.

   1. Responsibility is not assumed until order is given by physician.

   3. Unless a standing order is in place, this would not be appropriate.

   4. Alarming the family without proper teaching or preparation is inadvisable.

35. Application, implementation, health promotion and maintenance, (b).

   4. This is the definition of engagement.

   1. This is station 0.

   2. This means that the baby is high in the pelvis.

   3. This means that the presenting part is visible to the health care provider.

36. Comprehension, evaluation, health promotion and maintenance, (a).

   3. Stage 2 is from full dilation of the cervix until birth of the fetus.

   1. Pushing before full dilation can be dangerous to the fetus and exhausting to the mother.

   2. This is still too high.

   4. This is stage 3.

37. Comprehension, evaluation, health promotion and maintenance, (b).

   1. This is the normal pattern.

2, 3, 4. Any deviations may indicate fetal anomalies.

38. Analysis, evaluation, physiological integrity, (b).

_____ 1. Checking vital signs×1 is not sufficient. Every 15 minutes is indicated to detect potential complications.

__X__ 2. **The fundus should be firm and at or just below the umbilicus immediately after delivery.**

_____ 3. Monitoring bowel sounds is not indicated in a vaginal delivery.

_____ 4. Mothers are not necessarily expected to void within 1 hour after birth.

__X__ 5. **Lochia needs to be monitored for potential hemorrhage. It should be moderate and rubra.**

__X__ 6. **The episiotomy should be checked for potential dehiscence.**

39. Application, implementation, physiological integrity, (b).

3. Simply relieving pressure by changing positions will correct the situation.

1. The symptoms are pallor, light-headedness, dizziness, and slight nausea; rubbing the legs does not correct the syndrome.

2. This is incorrect; it is caused by the heavy uterus exerting pressure on the inferior vena cava and hampering good circulation; determine the cause and effect first, and then plan the intervention.

4. Know the cause and effect; because the patient is dizzy, the nurse would not recommend walking.

40. Analysis, implementation, health promotion and maintenance, (b).

_____ 1. Instructions for pushing are given during the second stage of labor.

__X__ 2. **Baseline fetal heart tones are essential to detect any complications.**

__X__ 3. **Knowledge and reassurance decrease anxiety.**

_____ 4. Women often experience chills during the fourth stage of labor related to fluid loss and excitement.

_____ 5. This is important to prevent hemorrhage after birth.

_____ 6. This is an appropriate intervention in the fourth stage of labor.

41. Comprehension, planning, physiological integrity, (b).

1. This is the correct answer.

2. This does not explain the physiological dynamics.

3. Oxytocin (Pitocin) is an oxytocic that acts on the uterus.

4. This does not explain the physiological dynamics of immediate postpartum phenomenon.

42. Comprehension, implementation, physiological integrity, (a).

2. Conduction occurs when the infant comes into contact with cold objects.

1. Evaporation of heat can occur during birth or bathing from moisture on the skin.

3. Convection occurs from drafts in the room.

4. Radiation cooling occurs when the infant is placed near a cold surface.

43. Comprehension, assessment, health promotion and maintenance, (a).

3. False labor is generally relieved by activity.

1. True labor will have a regular interval between contractions, and progress is shown in effacement and dilation of cervix.

2. True labor does progress differently; however, this is not true labor.

4. No way is known to determine when true labor will occur after an episode of false labor.

44. Application, implementation, health promotion and maintenance, (b).

2. First priority is to establish a patent airway so the baby can breathe, cry, and fill her lungs with oxygen.

1. This is not first priority.

3. Umbilical cord can be left attached; no danger exists in delaying the cutting of the cord while tasks with a higher priority are performed.

4. The delivery of the placenta may take from 5 to 20 minutes because it must separate from the walls of the uterus; therefore this is not the top priority.

45. Comprehension, planning, health promotion and maintenance, (a).

1. These are reportable signs and symptoms that should be taught to the patient.

2. These are usual signs and symptoms and are normal.

3. These are nonemergency signs and symptoms, which can be addressed during regular visits.

4. These are later signs and symptoms and are not emergencies.

46. Analysis, assessment, physiological integrity, (c).

2. This is the correct answer; signs and symptoms are bright red clots first and then light, painless bleeding.

1. In abruptio placentae pain is present, and bleeding may or may not occur; if bleeding is present, it is dark red and usually not clotted.

3. Bleeding would be bright red in variable amounts with pain.

4. The patient would experience painless vaginal bleeding with bloody amniotic fluid.

47. Analysis, assessment, physiological integrity, (b).

2. This is the correct statement and correct answer.

1. The nurse would consider doing follow-up tests to determine precise findings, and the physician would consider what medical treatment is needed.

3. This is a false assumption.

4. Making this kind of determination is not a part of the nursing process.

48. Analysis, evaluation, physiological integrity, (c).

3. Intent is to prevent convulsions and be able to respond immediately.

1. A mother who is severely eclamptic should not be in a semiprivate room and certainly not in a sunny room with visitors.

2. The room must be quiet, with absolutely no visitors.

4. Bright sunshine aggravates the central nervous system, and being far from the nurses' station hampers emergency nursing care.

49. Application, implementation, physiological integrity, (b).

1. Exercise is generally safe during pregnancy if the woman has exercised previously; otherwise it may be necessary to begin slowly.

2, 3. These are true; however, they do not completely answer the question.

4. A physician should be consulted before starting exercise. A patient should not wait until pain is experienced.

50. Application, implementation, physiological integrity, (a).
    1. **This reduces perineal swelling and ecchymosis.**
    2. This is the normal location of the fundus a few hours after delivery.
    3. A natural reaction is to be happy over an apparently successful birthing experience.
    4. One pad saturated with red lochia several hours after delivery is normal and not a sign of hemorrhage.

51. Application, implementation, physiological integrity, (b).
    4. **Return of lochia rubra after its initial cessation may indicate uterine subinvolution or hemorrhage.**
    1. At 10 days postpartum the fundus has returned to its position as a pelvic organ and is no longer palpable.
    2. Mothers commonly experience constipation; simple interventions can be suggested.
    3. Postpartum blues occur most commonly during the third to tenth day postpartum.

52. Comprehension, planning, physiological integrity, (b).
    2. **In many cultures drinking hot liquids after childbirth is important to restore the balance of nature.**
    1. A clear liquid diet is fairly self-explanatory; a dietitian can basically offer the same items as the nurse can.
    3. The patient is able to decide what she will drink or not drink according to her likes and desires.
    4. This is not true and is judgmental.

53. Comprehension, implementation, safe and effective care environment, (b).
    3. **Bonding and breast-feeding can continue with minimal exposure to other patients and staff.**
    1. Standard Precautions and gown and gloves for direct care are appropriate.
    2. If the baby is breast-feeding well, there is no reason to discontinue; there is also no reason to expose other babies in the nursery to potential infection.
    4. Diagnosis is important, but precautions can start before that.

54. Application, evaluation, physiological integrity, (b).
    2. **In addition, she has to be able to support herself.**
    1. It takes time for sensation to return after the catheter has been removed.
    3. Further assessments need to be made other than these.
    4. It is helpful for the patient to eat something, but it is not the only criterion.

55. Comprehension, assessment, physiological integrity, (b).
    X 1. **The preterm infant's skin is wrinkled and delicate because the skin has not had time to develop.**
    X 2. **The preterm infant's skin is wrinkled and delicate because the skin has not had time to develop.**
    X 3. Premature newborns have little subcutaneous fat and are very susceptible to cold stress.
    ___ 4. They usually have a tremendous amount of lanugo, which is used for protection in the womb.
    X 5. **Prominent fontanels indicate a musculoskeletal system that is not fully developed.**
    X 6. **Poor muscle tone also indicates a musculoskeletal system that is not fully developed.**

56. Application, implementation, physiological integrity, (b).
    X 1. **Conractions less than 2 minutes apart and lasting 45 to 90 seconds would compromise both fetal and maternal integrity.**
    ___ 2. This is a normal assessment finding in labor.
    X 3. **Excessive bleeding would result in decreased BP and again put fetus and mother at risk.**
    ___ 4. This is a normal assessment finding in labor.
    ___ 5. This is a normal assessment finding in labor.
    X 6. **Late decelerations that do not respond to positional change could indicate fetal compromise.**

57. Analysis, planning, health promotion and maintenance, (c).
    X 1. **It is always important to know a person's baseline level of knowledge concerning his or her health care situation.**
    ___ 2. This makes a value judgment. A better way to word the question would be, "Who is going to be your support person in labor?"
    ___ 3. A person's religion may or may not be an indication of birth practices.
    X 4. **Many different factors are considered when deciding whether to circumcise a child, and culture is definitely one of them.**
    X 5. **Infant feeding practices are influenced by a person's culture.**
    X 6. **Who should be present during physical examinations and at the birth is influenced by a person's culture.**

58. Comprehension, planning, physiological integrity, (b).
    3. **This procedure attempts to form a small clot to stop the leaking fluid.**
    1. This is done before childbirth and involves invading the epidural space.
    2. This is done for chronic pain.
    4. Infection is not a cause.

59. Application, evaluation, health promotion and maintenance, (a).
    3. **This would indicate a healthy involution.**
    1. This would be normal for 2 to 3 days after birth.
    2. If the uterus is deviated to the right, the bladder needs to be emptied.
    4. This is healthy immediately after birth.

60. Analysis, evaluation, physiological integrity, (b).
    3. **This evaluation is the most accurate way of ensuring that the baby is receiving adequate nourishment and is not becoming dehydrated.**
    1. Many babies fall asleep partway through a feeding and need to be stimulated to feed a little longer.
    2. Time is no longer considered relevant for nourishment or to prevent complications.
    4. This is a measurement but not on a short-term basis.

61. Comprehension, assessment, health promotion and maintenance, (a).
    2. **This may indicate a urinary infection.**
    1, 3, 4. These are normal at this time.

62. Application, implementation, psychosocial integrity, (c).
    3. **This answer allows for communication that encourages the couple to deal with their pain as a family unit and allows for more effective coping with grief.**

1. The patient is an adult who cannot have her rights for appropriate standards of care taken away from her.
2. Nurses should implement therapeutic methods of communication as an appropriate standard of care.
4. Patients exist as part of a family unit; family member's needs should be considered.

63. Application, implementation, health promotion and maintenance, (b).
   4. This provides 3 months of protection without daily attention.
   1. This would be ideal, but it is not realistic.
   2. This requires at least weekly attention.
   3. Condoms rely on the partner's attention.

64. Application, implementation, health promotion and maintenance, (b).
   1. This is accurate information that does not produce undue anxiety.
   2. This is true; however, it produces anxiety in the patient.
   3. This is also true but does not answer the question.
   4. This is also true, but this intervention was for assessment purposes.

65. Comprehension, implementation, physiological integrity, (a).
   3. This allows for greater expansion of the diaphragm and easier breathing.
   1. This is important but does not ease the shortness of breath.
   2. This improves circulation but does not decrease shortness of breath.
   4. Unless the meals are unusually large, this does not affect shortness of breath.

66. Comprehension, assessment, physiological integrity, (b).
   _____ 1. Vaginal infections do not cause ectopic pregnancies.
   _____ 2. Placenta previa is an abnormally implanted placenta.
   _____ 3. Substance abuse during pregnancy may cause fetal anomalies, but they do not cause ectopic pregnancies.
   __X__ 4, 5, 6. Ectopic pregnancies are caused by abnormalities in the fallopian tubes.

67. Analysis, assessment, physiological integrity, (b).
   1. These are the appropriate characteristics of the latent phase of the first stage of labor.
   2. In the active phase of the first stage of labor, contractions occur approximately every 5 minutes and last 30 to 45 seconds; dilatation of the cervix progresses from 4 to 7 cm during this phase.
   3. In the transition phase of the first stage of labor, contractions are more frequent (approximately every 2 to 3 minutes) and last 60 seconds; dilatation of the cervix progresses from 7 to 10 cm (full dilatation).
   4. In general the first stage of labor is referred to as the _stage of dilatation and effacement_ and encompasses all three phases as described above.

68. Application, implementation, health promotion and maintenance, (b).
   1. The infant's immune system does take time to produce antibodies fully.
   2. The portals of infection are the same for an infant as they are for an adult.

3. This is true; however, it does not answer the question.
4. This is also true; however, these antibodies do not fully protect breast-fed infants from infection.

69. Application, implementation, health promotion and maintenance, (c).
   2. This relieves pressure on the vena cava by the uterus.
   1. Having the patient sit does not relieve uterine pressure on the vena cava.
   3. This improves circulation.
   4. Having the patient sit up does not relieve pressure on the vena cava. This would be appropriate if the woman were feeling short of breath because it would allow for greater expansion of the diaphragm.

70. Application, implementation, health promotion and maintenance, (c).
   3. This position or the Trendelenburg position would push the presenting part away from the cord by gravity.
   1. This does not use gravity to help the presenting part.
   2. Compressing or manipulating the cord can cause further distress to the fetus.
   4. This should be done on a continual basis.

71. Comprehension, planning, physiological integrity, (b).
   3. Magnesium sulfate is given to lower blood pressure and as an anticonvulsant.
   1, 2. These have not been shown to be effective in GH.
   4. Calcium gluconate is the antidote for magnesium therapy and should be available if magnesium levels become toxic.

72. Analysis, assessment, health promotion and maintenance, (b).
   1. A high bilirubin within the first 24 hours of life indicates pathological jaundice, which is not normal and needs to be reported.
   2. This may be a sign of drug withdrawal.
   3. Elevated bilirubin is not an indication of infection in an infant.
   4. A weak cry may be an indication of respiratory distress.

73. Application, planning, health promotion and maintenance, (b).
   Correct order: 241536.
   2. Proper perineal care
   4. Prevention of infection for herself and her baby
   1. Breast-feeding techniques
   5. Infant care techniques
   3. The importance of good nutrition
   6. Methods to cope with sibling rivalry.
   Although all of these items are important and need to be discussed immediately after birth, the mother needs to rest and meet her own basic needs. Proper perineal care is really the only item that needs to be discussed at this time.

74. Knowledge, assessment, physiological integrity, (a).
   _____ 1. This is a normal finding on assessment of the newborn.
   _____ 2. This is a normal finding on assessment of the newborn.
   __X__ 3. Flaring nostrils indicate that the infant is having trouble obtaining adequate amounts of oxygen.
   __X__ 4. Irritability may indicate an infection.

X 5. Poor feeding may mean that the infant has a gastrointestinal virus. Neonates become dehydrated very quickly.

_____ 6. This is a normal finding on assessment of the newborn.

75. Comprehension, assessment, physiological integrity, (b).
_____ 1. This is a characteristic of placenta previa.
X 2. *This is a characteristic of abruptio placentae.*
_____ 3. This is a characteristic of placenta previa.
_____ 4. Fetal distress or fetal death may occur.
X 5. *This is a characteristic of abruptio placentae.*

76. Comprehension, planning, psychosocial integrity, (b).
_____ 1. Having too many family members concerned with the baby is not usually a concern unless the mother is unable to control the situation or feels left out.
X 2. *It is impossible to predict this condition all of the time. Individuals with a history of psychiatric conditions are at higher risk for depression.*
X 3. *Anger may be an indication of feelings of lack of support from her partner and therefore directed toward the baby.*
X 4. *Difficulty breast-feeding may lead to feelings of low self-esteem.*
_____ 5. Taking extra care with her appearance is normal after giving birth.

77. Comprehension, implementation, safe and effective care environment, (b).
X 1. *Safety and warmth are priorities in infant care.*
_____ 2. Babies do not necessarily need a bath every day.
_____ 3. There is no need to have a specific schedule for the baby's bath. The nurse should actually teach the opposite to the parents. The parents do not need to add stress to their lives by trying to keep to a specific schedule or give their baby a complete bath every day.
_____ 4. Babies also do not need a tremendous amount of lotions or powders.
X 5. *Sibling rivalry is a safety issue, and having siblings help in caring for the infant assists in having a happy family.*
X 6. *Cold stress is a danger for infants.*

78. Analysis, implementation, safe and effective care environment, (c).
Correct order: 324561.
3. *Oxygen is needed for the fetus immediately and helps improve the viability.*
2. *Determining the status of the fetus is vital to determine exactly how quickly this delivery has to be done. There may be a need for a cesarean if the fetus is in acute distress.*
4. *A vaginal examination is required to determine exactly how far the labor has progressed. However, the condition of the fetus has to come first.*
5. *This is an intervention that will promote comfort and decrease stress. It is not a lifesaving intervention.*
6. *Ascertaining any preexisting medical complications will help predict possible complications.*

1. *Finding out her knowledge of the childbirth process is also beneficial, but lifesaving interventions have to come first.*

79. Comprehension, assessment, physiological integrity, (b).
3. *This answers concerns and gives information.*
1. This does not answer the question.
2. This is inaccurate information.
4. The pediatrician will assess and note on the record.

80. Application, planning, physiological integrity, (b).
4. *Knowing what happened is important because feelings might differ if the pregnancies were voluntarily or spontaneously terminated.*
1. The para of this patient indicates that additional support may be required.
2. All women require careful assessments to determine their feelings about the pregnancy.
3. An assessment of anxiety must be made before an intervention can be effective.

81. Comprehension, implementation, physiological integrity, (a).
4. *These are called* milia *and disappear spontaneously.*
1. No antibiotic cream is needed.
2. Extra washing is not needed.
3. This is anxiety producing and does not answer the question.

82. Application, implementation, health promotion and maintenance, (b).
2. *This gives reassurance without dismissing anxieties.*
1. This is true, but it does not address concerns.
3. This also may be true—feelings normally improve in the second trimester—but it does not address concerns.
4. This also may be true, but the partner has concerns of his own. Hopefully they will work out their feelings together.

83. Application, implementation, health promotion and maintenance, (a).
3. *This can be an indication of infection.*
1. This is not necessary unless advised by the physician.
2. This is helpful and would promote comfort. It would not cure any infection.
4. Douching is not usually recommended in pregnancy.

84. Comprehension, assessment, health promotion and maintenance, (a).
4. *For extremities to be slightly cyanotic at birth is not unusual.*
1, 2, 3. These are acceptable findings and would receive scores of 2.

85. Knowledge, assessment, physiological integrity, (a).
2. *Decelerations are rate decreases during contractions.*
1. Accelerations are rate increases during contractions.
3. This is the rate between contractions.
4. This describes fluctuations in the heart rate from baseline.

86. Comprehension, assessment, physiological integrity, (b).
3. *In true labor bloody show is often present.*
1. In false labor discomfort is often felt in the abdomen and groin.
2. In true labor walking increases contractions.
4. In false labor contractions are irregular.

87. Application, implementation, health promotion and maintenance, (c).
    1. *This pattern indicates that the fetus is receiving adequate oxygenation.*
    2. This would be appropriate for late decelerations caused by supine hypotension.
    3. This would be appropriate for late decelerations and supine hypotension.
    4. This may be needed for late decelerations.
88. Comprehension, application, physiological integrity, (b).
    3. *No evidence exists that this helps the membranes rupture.*
    1, 2, 4. These are benefits of walking.
89. Application, implementation, physiological integrity, (b).
    3. *This is the proper position. The fundus is the uppermost portion of the uterus. It is where the contractions are most accurately felt by the examiner.*
    1. The symphysis pubis is part of the pelvis. The contractions would not be felt here. Above the symphysis pubis would be appropriate to determine bladder distention.
    2. Vaginal examination is appropriate for advanced practitioners to determine the extent of dilation and effacement.
    4. The umbilicus would not allow for accurate determination of the contractions of the uterus.
90. Analysis, implementation, health promotion and maintenance, (b).
    3. *Regular contractions 8 minutes apart indicate the end of the latent phase of labor; she needs to be assessed.*
    1. Five minutes apart is the beginning of the active phase of labor. She can walk in the hospital.
    2. An ambulance is not required at this point.
    4. The hospital is appropriate at this point.
91. Application, assessment, physiological integrity, (b).
    3. *Slight bruising is normal. Ice is used for 12 to 24 hours; after that, heat may be comforting.*
    1. This is normal.
    2. This is a concern. However, have the mother void and reassess.
    4. The episiotomy should be intact. A slight redness related to the inflammatory process is normal.
92. Application, assessment, physiological integrity, (b).
    3. *Bulging indicates that the woman may be fully dilated and ready to push.*
    1. The urge to bear down usually indicates that the first stage is ending and the birth of the baby is imminent.
    2. These should be done throughout the labor process.
    4. This should be done, but the assessment in No. 3 is required first.
93. Comprehension, assessment, physiological integrity, (b).
    2. *Caput succedaneum is a swelling of the soft tissues of the head.*
    1. This indicates dehydration.
    3. This indicates cephalhematoma.
    4. Bulging fontanels indicate increased intracranial pressure, which can be caused by a variety of conditions.
94. Analysis, planning, health promotion and maintenance, (c).
    __X__ 1. *The exact cause of preterm labor is not known, but a previous history of preterm labor is a risk factor for a current pregnancy. Preterm labor has been associated statis-*

tically with lack of prenatal care and substance abuse. It is also seen in hypertensive states because of the damage caused to the mother's circulatory system.
    _____ 2. There is no documented relationship between a woman having her first baby and premature labor.
    __X__ 3. *A short cervix may not allow the woman to carry the baby to term.*
    __X__ 4. *The presence of fibronectin in vaginal secretions between 22 and 37 week's gestation and the presence of bacterial vaginosis are also considered to be risk factors for preterm labor.*
    _____ 5. Hypotension does not lead to premature labor.
    __X__ 6. *Cigarette smoking and substance abuse have long been considered high risk factors for preterm labor and growth restriction of the fetus.*
95. Comprehension, assessment, health promotion and maintenance, (b).
    3. *This will disappear spontaneously in this time frame.*
    1. This is the time frame for caput succedaneum.
    2. This is not required.
    4. It should be monitored, but this does not answer the question.
96. Comprehension, assessment, health promotion and maintenance, (a).
    3. *Infection is a possibility once the membranes have ruptured.*
    1. Dystocia can increase the chances of infection.
    2. The possibility of hemorrhage does not increase with PROM.
    4. The possibility of hypertension does not increase with PROM.
97. Comprehension, assessment, physiological integrity, (b).
    1. *The fundus descends approximately 1 fingerbreadth per day (see the following figure).*
    2. This would be the height on day 5 postpartum.
    3. This would be the height on day 8 postpartum.
    4. This would be the height on day 9 postpartum. By the tenth to twelfth day it has resumed its position as a pelvic organ and can no longer be palpated.

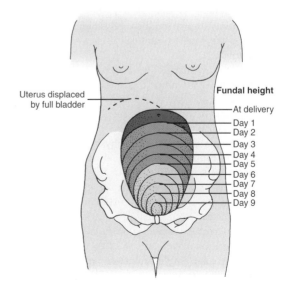

Uterus displaced by full bladder

Fundal height

At delivery
Day 1
Day 2
Day 3
Day 4
Day 5
Day 6
Day 7
Day 8
Day 9

98. Knowledge, assessment, physiological integrity, (b).
    4. This is an indication of urinary or renal anomalies, which can be determined by ultrasound before birth.
    1, 2, 3. These assessments would be made postnatally.
99. Knowledge, assessment, health promotion and maintenance, (b).
    3. HELLP is a severe form of gestational hypertension (GH).
    1. This is not an anemic condition.
    2. This is not a mild form of GH.
    4. This is not specifically associated with hyperemesis gravidarum.
100. Comprehension, planning, health promotion and maintenance, (a).
    3. PROM leaves the birth canal and the newborn more vulnerable to infection.
    1. A quick delivery does not predispose to infection.
    2. This does not increase the chances of infection.
    4. Exhaustion is common but does not increase risk of infection.
101. Comprehension, assessment, health promotion and maintenance, (a).
    4. This is the correct classification.
    1. In newborns a certain weight range is appropriate for gestational age. This is incorrect.
    2. No such classification exists.
    3. Newborns under 2500 g are termed SGA.
102. Comprehension, assessment, health promotion and maintenance, (b).
    2. Glucose provides an environment conducive to infection.
    1. This is not true.
    3. Their babies do tend to be larger, but this is not the primary reason for infection.
    4. This is true, but it does not answer the question.
103. Application, implementation, physiological integrity, (b).
    3. This is the safest comment and is reassuring to the couple.
    1. This does not answer their concern.
    2. This occurs very late in labor.
    4. This occurs late in labor and may predispose her to infection.
104. Application, implementation, physiological integrity, (b).
    4. This may be a cultural belief and should be respected.
    1. This may or may not be true, but it is judgmental.
    2. This may be appropriate, but their rights need to be respected.
    3. This may or may not be true, but the nurse does not know that this is the reason.
105. Application, implementation, physiological integrity, (b).
    3. This is the correct reason. A full bladder may impede the surgery.
    1. No need exists to monitor the output of a healthy patient. In an emergency situation a catheter would be inserted.
    2. Catheterizations are a major source of infection.
    4. Ambulation is vital after surgery.
106. Comprehension, implementation, health promotion and maintenance, (b).
    4. This is important in the prevention of thrombophlebitis.

1. This is valuable advice anytime, not just when driving.
2. This is true; however, it does not help during driving.
3. Stretching legs helps with cramps anytime.
107. Analysis, implementation, health promotion and maintenance, (a).
    1. The mother needs time to rest after birth.
    2. This is anxiety producing and not appropriate at this time.
    3. This is premature at this point.
    4. This is generally not effective at this time. The mother needs time to rest.
108. Application, implementation, physiological integrity, (a).
    1. This is usually the treatment of choice for small hematomas. Surgical excision may be needed for larger hematomas.
    2. Baths help with episiotomy discomfort and hemorrhoids.
    3. Sprays assist with episiotomy discomforts.
    4. Lamps may be used for generalized perineal discomfort.
109. Knowledge, application, physiological integrity, (a).
    2. The gender of the child depends on whether the X chromosome from the woman joins with an X or a Y chromosome from the man.
    1. This may be first known at birth, but it is determined at conception.
    3. This is or can be learned during an amniocentesis.
    4. Blood work does not determine gender.
110. Knowledge, assessment, health promotion and maintenance, (b).
    3. This is the correct definition of nuchal cord. A nuchal cord means that the cord is around the baby's neck. This can lead to lack of oxygen for the fetus.
    1. This is the correct definition for *prolapsed cord*.
    2. If the cord is too long it may be an indication of a possible genetic condition, but it is not the correct definition of a *nuchal cord*.
    4. The cord is supposed to follow the baby after birth. It cannot be defined as coming out too high.
111. Knowledge, planning, physiological integrity, (a).
    2. This is produced by the posterior pituitary gland and also stimulates milk ejection during breast-feeding.
    1. This prepares the breasts for lactation.
    3. This is responsible for enlargement of the uterus, breasts, and genitalia, among many other functions.
    4. This promotes development of the breasts for lactation, among other functions.
112. Application, implementation, health promotion and maintenance, (b).
    4. This is true, and many commonly used herbs have been shown to be harmful in pregnancy.
    1. This is not true, particularly in pregnancy.
    2. This is always a wise precaution, but further information is needed in this case.
    3. Herbs do not have doses and can be toxic with minimal or normal amounts.
113. Comprehension, assessment, physiological integrity, (a).
    4. First stage, active phase—4 to 7 cm
    1. Second stage—10 cm to birth of the baby
    2. First stage, latent phase—0 to 4 cm
    3. First stage, transition phase—7 to 10 cm

114. Comprehension, assessment, physiological integrity, (b).
   2. In transition, contractions last 60 to 90 seconds and come every 2 to 3 minutes.
   1. In the active phase, contractions occur every 5 minutes, lasting 30 to 45 seconds.
   3. In the latent phase, contractions occur every 10 to 15 minutes, lasting 15 to 20 seconds.
   4. These are Braxton-Hicks contractions.

115. Application, planning, health promotion and maintenance, (b).
   2 This requires a great deal of time standing.
   1, 3, 4. These allow for more rest periods and flexibility of hours.

116. Comprehension, planning, safe and effective care environment, (a).
   _____ 1. A *precipitous delivery* means the baby is delivered very rapidly. Often this may occur outside the hospital setting. These mothers are at risk for infection.
   __**X**__ **2. Breech babies are usually delivered by cesarean to decrease the stress on the baby. If a part other than the head is delivered first, it is possible that the baby may undergo severe respiratory distress if there is difficulty delivering the head.**
   __**X**__ **3. If the head is too big for the pelvis, the baby is delivered by cesarean to prevent fetal distress.**
   _____ 4. Although women with diabetes may have big babies, it is not always an indication for cesarean delivery.

117. Comprehension, implementation, physiological integrity, (a).
   1. Fluids (with the exception of caffeine and carbonated beverages) increase the amount of fluids in stools, leading to easier passage.
   2. This may be needed, but dietary changes should be made first.
   3. Assessment of exercise pattern is needed first.
   4. No laxative should be given without a physician's permission.

118. Application, implementation, health promotion and maintenance, (b).
   1. Cafe latte contains caffeine.
   2. Unless weight control is a concern, this snack would be appropriate.
   3. This is an appropriate snack.
   4. This does not give any nutrients; however, it is not a danger. Fruit may be a better choice.

119. Comprehension, planning, physiological integrity, (b).
   2. As long as no potential for danger exists, cultural ceremonies should be allowed.
   1. A private room might be preferable, but this is not the primary information.
   3. This is not a primary concern.
   4. This might be educational, but it is not a primary concern.

120. Application, assessment, physiological integrity, (b).
   3. This transitional phase is the last phase of the first stage of labor. The woman needs to use all of her energy to cope with labor.
   1. This is characteristic of the latent phase of labor (0 to 4 cm).
   2. This is from 4 to 7 cm and comes in part from ill-defined doubts and fears as well as anxious feelings due to increasing strength of contractions.
   4. In the third stage after the birth of the baby, the woman is usually relaxed and receptive to care.

121. Application, assessment, physiological integrity, (b).
   Answer: 120. The baby's heart rate is approximately 120 beats/min. This is within the normal range for a fetus and a newborn.

122. Analysis, assessment, physiological integrity, (c).
   1. Late deceleration occurs when the fetal heart rate declines at the end of the mother's contraction. It commonly indicates placental insufficiency and is an ominous sign.
   2. Early decelerations are also a concern and commonly indicate head cord compression.
   3. Variable decelerations indicate umbilical cord compression.
   4. Intermittent or occasional decelerations can occur with any pattern.

123. Analysis, evaluation, psychological integrity, (b).
   1. Each child needs to know that he or she is special and equally loved.
   2. This may or may not be true, depending on the child's age, but being taken for granted may cause problems.
   3. Depending on developmental level, this may or may not be possible.
   4. A 5-year-old still needs special attention.

124. Comprehension, assessment, psychological integrity, (b).
   3. This is the developmental task in the second trimester.
   1. This is most common in the first trimester.
   2. This is characteristic of the third trimester.
   4. This is most common in the first trimester.

125. Comprehension, assessment, health promotion and maintenance, (b).
   1. Decreased oxygen from the placenta is the most common cause of late decelerations.
   2. Late decelerations are always of concern.
   3. Early decelerations, which return to baseline, would indicate this.
   4. No relationship exists between length of labor and decelerations.

126. Analysis, evaluation, psychological integrity, (b).
   2. The person may benefit from learning breathing techniques and nonpharmacological methods of pain relief to increase her feelings of control.
   1. This is true.
   3. This is important for her to know. The nurse should review these with her.
   4. This would require further assessment, not necessarily teaching.

127. Analysis, evaluation, psychological integrity, (b).
   3. This may indicate ineffective coping.
   1. Feeding is preferable after bathing, but this is easily corrected with teaching.
   2. This is a true statement.
   4. This is fine; a father should be involved with his baby's care.

128. Analysis, evaluation, physiological integrity, (b).
   3. Safety comes first. Even young babies can roll off a platform.

1. This is a good way for a partner to help.
2. This is also true; babies do not tell time.
4. This is the preferred method because the bath provides stimulation and exercise and the feeding promotes sleep.

129. Application, implementation, psychosocial integrity, (b).
    3. Communication and spending time with your partner allow for emotional support and reassurance.
    1. This is true, but the parents' feelings need to be recognized as well.
    2. Nutritious food is always important as a part of overall good health.
    4. Depression is a serious medical condition that needs physician intervention. Depression lasts much longer than baby blues, which tend to have more of a transient nature.

130. Application, implementation, health promotion and maintenance, (b).
    3. This is the priority action because the danger of a prolapsed cord is greatest at this point. Pressure of the presenting part causes decreased oxygen flow to the fetus. Assessing the fetal heart rate is essential to detect any compromise in fetal circulation. A prolapsed cord is often an indication for an emergency delivery.
    1, 2. These can be done at the regular intervals required by hospital protocol. Assessing the maternal vital signs should be done, but at the moment the fetus is the priority.
    4. This is also done on an ongoing basis. This is called assessing the frequency of contractions and is done for all mothers in labor.

131. Application, implementation, health promotion and maintenance, (a).
    2. Adequate fluids are important to prevent urinary stasis.
    1. This is unnecessary.
    3. Keeping the bladder as empty as possible prevents urinary stasis and allows the bladder to rest.
    4. Cranberry juice is healthy, but water is the most vital.

132. Application, assessment, physiological integrity, (a).
    4. Nitrazine paper is used to assess the fluid for a pattern called ferning, which is a positive indication for amniotic fluid.
    1. This is not required.
    2. The physician should be notified when membranes have ruptured.
    3. Stress tests are done before labor to assess the status of the fetus

133. Comprehension, assessment, physiological integrity, (b).
    _____ 1. Refusal of two or more feedings may be an indication of illness.
    _____ 2. 180 beats/min may occur when the infant is excited.
    _X_ 3. A temperature below 97° F (36.1° C) is reason for concern, and a physician should be notified.
    _____ 4. A positive Babinski reflex is normal in an infant up to 1 year of age.
    _X_ 5. Fewer than six voidings in a 24-hour period is reason for concern, and a physician should be notified.

134. Comprehension, implementation, health promotion and maintenance, (b).
    3. Fewer than two stools per day indicates possible constipation, and fluid intake needs to be increased.
    1. Iron can cause constipation.
    2. Infants do not need a strict schedule, and this has nothing to do with constipation.
    4. A bottle-fed infant should produce three or four stools each day.

135. Comprehension, planning, health promotion and maintenance, (c).
    3. Cold stress can decrease stores of glycogen in the liver.
    1. Weak abdominal muscles make newborns prone to reverse peristalsis.
    2. Babies need to be burped frequently to eliminate swallowed air.
    4. Newborns are susceptible to infection for a variety of reasons.

136. Analysis, planning, physiological integrity, (b).
    _X_ 1. A loss of heat occurs as the water is converted to a vapor.
    _____ 2. Cold hands are an example of heat loss through conduction.
    _X_ 3. A loss of heat occurs as the water is converted to a vapor.
    _____ 4. A draft from an open door is an example of heat loss through convection.
    _____ 5. Placing the infant on a cold surface is another example of heat loss through conduction.
    _____ 6. A loose blanket or no blanket at all is another example of heat loss through convection.

137. Comprehension, planning, health promotion and maintenance, (a).
    1. The infant receives passive (3 to 5 months) immunity for any condition for which the mother has developed antibodies.
    2. The infant receives a vitamin K injection until bacterial synthesis begins.
    3. Some iron may be stored in the baby's liver, but this is present at birth.
    4. No relationship exists between breast-feeding or bottle-feeding and constipation.

138. Knowledge, implementation, physiological integrity, (a).
    4. Rooting is a normal response of the newborn to touch along the side of the mouth, resulting in turning of the head toward the stimulus.
    1. The gag reflex is caused by stimulation of the uvula, causing reverse peristalsis.
    2. The Moro reflex is caused by sudden jarring or movement; also called the *startle reflex*.
    3. The pupillary response is constriction of the pupil when stimulated by bright light.

139. Knowledge, assessment, health promotion and maintenance, (b).
    2. The Babinski reflex is elicited when the sole of the foot is stroked and the toes are hyperextended and fanned out. It disappears at approximately 1 year.
    1. Absence is abnormal in a newborn.
    3. This is not true.
    4. This is characteristic of the palmar reflex.

140. Comprehension, assessment, psychosocial integrity, (b).
    2. If the feelings are interfering with her life, medical intervention is needed to help relieve the depression.
    1. This is characteristic of postpartum psychosis.
    3. This is characteristic of baby blues.
    4. This is also characteristic of baby blues.

141. Comprehension, implementation, health promotion and maintenance, (b).
    1. Adolescents are highly influenced by their peers.
    2. Women of all ages have busy lifestyles. Correct choices can be made in fast-food restaurants.
    3, 4. These can be true of women at any age.

142. Knowledge, assessment, health promotion and maintenance, (a).
    1. This is the type of shock caused by a tremendous loss of blood.
    2. This shock is a severe allergic reaction.
    3. This shock is related to infection.
    4. This is a term not specifically related to shock.

143. Comprehension, implementation, health promotion and maintenance, (b).
    2. This is appropriate at this time. A history of possible exposure may be needed.
    1. No evidence of exposure exists; this choice is very premature.
    3. This may be needed at a later time if evidence of exposure exists.
    4. The vaccine is contraindicated during pregnancy.

144. Analysis, planning, health promotion and maintenance, (b).
    1. Some vegetarians eat eggs, cheese, fish, or any combination. These are adequate sources of complete protein.
    2. This is not relevant.
    3. Babies need complete sources of protein. Education may be needed at a later point to ensure that the baby has adequate nutrition.
    4. If she is a strict vegan, alternative sources of complete protein are available.

145. Comprehension, planning, physiological integrity, (b).
    3. Placenta previa is a placenta implanted in the lower third of the uterus, and a vaginal birth is contraindicated.
    1. The position of the second child needs to be determined.
    2. A transverse incision poses a decreased risk for uterine rupture.
    4. This could be an indication for a cesarean section because of the potential stress of labor on the heart.

146. Analysis, implementation, physiological integrity, (c).
    _____ 1. Although there may be less lochia for a cesarean mother, it is still a necessary assessment.
    X   2. Vaginal delivery mothers do not routinely have urinary catheters.

X   3. Deep breathing is important for any surgical patient.
X   4. Vaginal delivery mothers do not have dressings.
_____ 5. There is no episiotomy.
_____ 6. Hematomas are a complication of vaginal birth.

147. Application, assessment, health promotion and maintenance, (a).
    3. IV lines should be maintained until the patient is tolerating fluids well.
    1. Being without a fever is a positive sign.
    2. Bowel sounds mean peristalsis is returning.
    4. Tolerating clear fluid is a positive sign.

148. Analysis, implementation, health promotion and maintenance, (b).
    _____ 1. Being slightly overweight is not a serious concern. Being underweight can be dangerous as the patient may not be receiving the necessary nutrients.
    _____ 2. Her blood pressure will require the same monitoring as for any other patient unless a concern is indicated.
    X   3. Folic acid supplements are especially important for pregnant women and women of childbearing years. They have been shown to help prevent neural tube defects.
    X   4. An effective relationship with an obstetrician or nurse practitioner will facilitate the education, counseling, and support this couple will require for a positive outcome.
    X   5. It is always important to make the most effective use of calories.
    _____ 6. This may be ideal, but it is completely unrealistic. It is extremely difficult to completely change established food habits.

149. Comprehension, implementation, health promotion and maintenance, (c).
    3. This is correct. The test is most accurate if there is phenylalanine built up from formula or breast milk.
    1, 2. These are true. However, they do not answer the question.
    4. This test measures the lack of an enzyme. The enzyme will not develop over time.

150. Analysis, implementation, health promotion and maintenance, (a).
    4. Using terms with which the patient is familiar is important for effective learning. Everywhere in the world except for the United States, "football" means soccer.
    1, 2, 3. All of these may be true and require further clarification and education.

Objectives

After studying this chapter, the student should be able to:

1. Explain the developmental changes that occur in each age group from birth through adolescence.
2. Describe two congenital defects or hereditary disorders for each major body system.
3. List three major infections (fungal or bacterial) commonly seen in children.
4. Explain three disorders specific to each age group (e.g., infancy, toddler) as presented under each major body system.
5. List three common poisonous substances accounting for deaths in young children (ages 1 to 4).
6. Identify recommended immunizations given during the first 2 years of life.
7. Differentiate between the types of traction and their uses.
8. Discuss factors that affect nursing care of the hospitalized child.

Pediatric nursing includes the care of both well and sick children and covers both preventive health care and restorative nursing care. This chapter is divided into the following age groups: infancy, toddlerhood, preschool age, school age, and adolescence. The areas covered include normal growth and development, psychosocial development, health promotion, and health problems specific to each age group. Other topics discussed include battered child syndrome, hospitalization and the child, and nursing care of the hospitalized child. The information provided in this chapter presents both the physical and psychosocial aspects of care necessary in providing pediatric nursing care.

ASSESSMENT OF CHILD AND FAMILY

A. Functions and structure of family
   1. The functions and structure of the family are vital to the normal growth and development of the child.
   2. Three primary functions of the family
      a. Providing physical care such as food, clothing, shelter, safety; illness prevention; and care during illness
      b. Educating and training: language, values, morals, and formal education
      c. Protecting psychological and emotional health
B. Physical assessment of child
   1. Obtaining family health history, including the child's history and current complaints or problems, is done by the nurse, physician, or nurse practitioner.
   2. Assessing of child's physical growth and developmental level is done by the physician or nurse practitioner.
C. Concepts of child development (Table 8-1)
   1. Freud's theory of development is based on the child's psychosexual development.
   2. Erikson's theory of development is based on psychosocial development as a series of developmental tasks.

3. Piaget's theory of development is based on intellectual (cognitive) development: how the child learns and develops his or her intelligence.
4. Kohlberg's theory of moral development is based on the concept that the acceptance of values and rules of society shapes a child's behavior.

CONGENITAL DEFECTS AND HEREDITARY DISORDERS

Most congenital defects and hereditary disorders are identified during the initial assessment of the newborn.

Gastrointestinal System
Cleft Lip and Palate

A. Definition: abnormal openings in the lip or palate. The defects may occur unilaterally or bilaterally.
B. Symptoms: A cleft lip has a notched vermilion border, which may involve the alveolar ridge and dental abnormalities. A cleft palate includes a midline or bilateral cleft with variable extension from the uvula, soft and hard palates, exposed nasal cavities, and nasal distortion.
C. Diagnosis: based on observation and examination at birth; may also be diagnosed by in utero ultrasound
D. Treatment and nursing interventions: based on the severity of the defect
   1. Modified techniques for feeding are used to promote adequate nutrition and growth.
   2. Surgery to repair the cleft lip is done as early as possible, usually at age 3 to 6 months.
   3. Surgery to repair the cleft palate depends on the deformity and size of the child and is usually done by 1 year of age.
   4. Recurrent otitis media is treated as needed.
   5. Parent-child bonding is promoted, and emotional support is provided for parents throughout the process.

Table 8-1   Concepts of Child Development

AGE	DEVELOPMENTAL STAGE	FREUD'S THEORY	ERIKSON'S THEORY	PIAGET'S THEORY	KOHLBERG'S THEORY (MORALITY)
4 wk-1 yr	Infancy	Oral stage	Trust versus mistrust	Sensorimotor phase	Preconventional morality (stage 0)
1-3 yr	Toddlerhood	Anal stage	Autonomy versus shame and doubt	Preoperational phase	Preconventional morality (stage 1)
3-5 yr	Preschool age	Oedipal stage Latency stage	Initiative versus guilt	Preoperational phase continued	Preconventional morality (stages 1-2)
6-12 yr	School age	Latency stage continued Genital stage	Industry versus inferiority	Concrete operational phase Formal operational phase	Conventional morality (stages 3-4)
13-18 yr	Adolescence	Genital stage continued	Identity versus identity confusion	Formal operational phase continued	Morality of self-accepted moral principles

6. Other practitioners involved in the care of these children may include ear, nose, and throat specialist; speech and occupational therapists; psychologist; audiologist; orthodontic surgeon and dentist.

Gastroesophageal Reflux

A. Definition: regurgitation of gastric contents into the esophagus. It can be physiological (infrequent emesis), functional (frequent emesis after meals), or pathological (failure to thrive [FTT], aspiration pneumonia, coughing, choking, dyspnea, frequent emesis).

B. Symptoms: Emesis after meals, hiccups, and recurrent otitis media from secretions pooled in the nasopharynx are common to all types of gastroesophageal reflux (GER). Other manifestations include FTT, respiratory infections, weight loss, and irritability.

C. Diagnosis: After other illnesses have been ruled out, GER may be confirmed by barium swallow, upper gastrointestinal (GI) study, ultrasound, or endoscopy.

D. Treatment and nursing interventions: based on symptoms
   1. Provide small frequent feedings of predigested infant formula (Nutramigen, Pregestimil) or hydrolyzed formula in which protein content has been broken down.
   2. Position infant in prone position with head slightly elevated or in right side-lying position (these positions are considered appropriate for infants with GER).
   3. For infants with pathological reflux, antacids, H₂-receptor antagonists, mucosal protectants, and other medications may be used (see Chapter 3).
   4. Surgery (fundoplication) to prevent future reflux may be done in up to 15% of infants with GER.

Hirschsprung Disease

A. Definition: distention of a portion of the lower colon caused by a congenital lack of nerve cells in the wall of the colon just below the distended section (Figure 8-1)

B. Symptoms: constipation (including a lack of meconium stool in the newborn in the first 24 hours), abdominal distention, bile-stained mucus and emesis, inadequate weight gain

C. Diagnosis: based on the symptoms, results of barium enema, rectal biopsy, anorectal manometry, or any combination

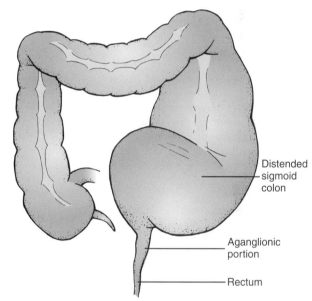

Distended sigmoid colon

Aganglionic portion

Rectum

FIGURE 8-1 Hirschsprung disease. (From Hockenberry MJ, Wilson D: *Wong's nursing care of infants and children*, ed 9, St Louis, 2011, Mosby.)

D. Treatment and nursing interventions: based on the type of surgery (bowel resection, sometimes with temporary colostomy); surgery performed in two or three stages
   1. Preoperative
      a. Observation of stools: color, amount, and consistency
      b. Intravenous (IV) fluids and electrolytes as ordered; if infant is malnourished, total parenteral nutrition (TPN) may be given before surgery.
   2. Postoperative.
      a. Nasogastric (NG) tube to low-suction or gravity drainage
      b. General postoperative care
      c. Routine colostomy care as necessary (*pro re nata* [p.r.n.])
      d. Monitor vital signs as ordered. Axillary temperatures should be taken; avoid taking rectal temperatures.
      e. IV fluids as ordered
      f. Maintain nothing by mouth (NPO) status. Resume diet as ordered.

g. Record intake and output (I&O) every shift (Foley catheter may be necessary).

h. Observe stools and record amount and characteristics.

i. Observe for rectal bleeding and abdominal distention.

j. Teach parents to provide care at home (colostomy care, dressing changes, skin care).

Omphalocele

A. Definition: Abdominal organs protrude through an abnormal opening in the abdominal wall and form a sac lying on the abdomen.

B. Diagnosis: based on symptoms and physical examination findings

C. Treatment and nursing interventions
   1. Preoperative
      a. Keep the omphalocele covered with sterile gauze moistened with normal saline and a plastic drape until surgery can be performed; minimize movement of the infant and the intestines.
      b. Maintain sterile technique as much as possible in caring for the omphalocele.
      c. Maintain proper body temperature; a warmer or an Isolette may be used.
   2. Postoperative
      a. Surgery: The organs are returned to the abdominal cavity, and the abdominal wall is closed.
      b. General postoperative care, including mechanical ventilation for several days; care of NG tube; pain management
      c. Parenteral nutrition for several days
      d. Observe stools and record amount and characteristics.

Imperforate Anus

A. Definition: Rectal pouch ends blindly at a distance above the anus. In some cases no anal opening is present. Various forms of this defect have been found.

B. Symptoms: no stools in the first 24 hours after birth. Rectal thermometer cannot be inserted properly.

C. Diagnosis: made by digital rectal examination, intestinal x-ray examination, and endoscopy, or antegrade endoscopic transillumination

D. Treatment and nursing interventions
   1. Surgical procedure to reconnect the ends of the rectum and form an anal opening
   2. General postoperative nursing care

Esophageal Atresia, Tracheoesophageal Fistula

A. Definition: Upper end of the esophagus ends in a blind pouch; lower end may also end in a blind pouch or may be connected to the trachea by fistula defect (tracheoesophageal fistula) (Figure 8-2).

B. Symptoms: excessive salivation and drooling, coughing and choking during feedings, regurgitation of all feedings

C. Diagnosis: based on symptoms and passage of an NG tube or catheter down the esophagus to test for patency. Exact anomaly is determined by x-ray film studies.

D. Treatment and nursing interventions
   1. Maintenance of NPO status with administration of IV fluids as ordered
   2. Suctioning of nose and mouth as needed
   3. Insertion of an NG tube to drain mucus and fluid from the blind pouch
   4. Antibiotic therapy as ordered (for probable aspiration pneumonia)
   5. Surgical repair to correct the defects and reconnect the ends of the esophagus
   6. Emotional support for the family; parent or caregiver teaching for home care

Intussusception

A. Definition: telescoping of one portion of the bowel into a distal portion; ileocecal valve most common site; usually occurs between 3 and 12 months of age

B. Symptoms: appear suddenly; pallor, sharp colicky pain that causes infant to draw up legs and cry out (this occurs every 5 to 10 minutes), vomiting, stools with blood and mucus ("red currant jelly" stools), signs of shock

C. Diagnosis: based on symptoms; definitive diagnosis made radiographically with barium enema

D. Treatment and nursing interventions: This is an emergency that requires immediate treatment. The initial treatment of choice is hydrostatic reduction by enema with water-soluble contrast or barium and air pressure; if this is not effective, surgery is necessary.
   1. Preoperative
      a. Careful observation and frequent recording of vital signs
      b. IV fluids with electrolytes as ordered
      c. Maintenance of NPO status
      d. NG tube to remove gastric contents

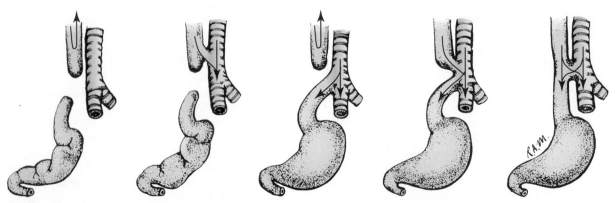

FIGURE 8-2 The five most common types of esophageal atresia and tracheoesophageal fistula. (From Hockenberry MJ, Wilson D: *Wong's nursing care of infants and children,* ed 9, St Louis, 2011, Mosby.)

e. Emotional support for parents; explanation of all procedures; answering questions

f. Observation for passage of normal brown stool (indicates the intussusception has reduced itself); report to physician immediately.

2. Postoperative
   a. Provide general postoperative care.
   b. IV fluids as ordered. Maintain NPO status.
   c. Record I&O.
   d. Auscultate for return of bowel sounds.
   e. Observe all stools and record.
   f. Resume feedings slowly as ordered.

Nervous System
Hydrocephalus

A. Definition: disorder caused by an obstruction of cerebrospinal fluid (CSF) drainage or impaired absorption of CSF in the subarachnoid space; characterized by an excess of CSF within the cranial cavity, which causes an enlarged head and potential brain damage or retardation. It occurs in association with several other anomalies (developmental defects; complication of meningitis, tumor, or hemorrhage) (Figure 8-3).

B. Symptoms: bulging of the anterior fontanel, enlargement of the head, irritability, lethargy, setting-sun sign (sclera can be seen above the iris because of increased intracranial pressure), lower extremity spasticity, opisthotonus

C. Diagnosis: based on the symptoms, frequent measurements of head circumference, computed tomography (CT), and magnetic resonance imaging (MRI)

D. Treatment and nursing interventions
   1. Surgical repair is necessary to relieve the obstruction or to shunt the CSF from the ventricles of the brain into the abdomen (ventriculoperitoneal shunt).
   2. Postoperative care includes frequent position changes to prevent pressure on the head, care of the shunt, general postoperative care, and observation for complications (infection, shunt malfunction, return of increased intracranial pressure).
   3. Measure head circumference daily.

Down Syndrome

A. Definition: an abnormality caused by extra chromosome 21 (trisomy 21). Children with Down syndrome (DS) are born to women of all ages. The risk is usually higher in women age 35 years and over, but some statistics indicate that more infants with DS are born to women age 35 years and under simply because that age group has more pregnancies. The incidence of DS in women age 40 years and older is approximately 1 in 100, however, one source indicated that women age 45 years have a 1 in 35 chance of having an infant with DS.

B. Symptoms: hypotonia; small, low-set ears; slanted eyes; protruding tongue; small, flattened nose; short, broad neck; single transverse palmar (simian) crease; dry, cracked skin; congenital heart defects; and mental retardation

C. Diagnosis: based on the physical defects. Chromosome studies are done to determine specific defects.

D. Treatment and nursing interventions
   1. Provide emotional support for parents; they expected a "normal" infant.
   2. Assist family in preventing physical problems (respiratory, integumentary, nutrition).
   3. Promote the child's developmental progress, and help parents set realistic goals for the child.
   4. Encourage activity and intellectual stimulation for the child through early intervention programs and school.
   5. Provide genetic counseling for the parents.

Genitourinary System
Epispadias and Hypospadias

A. Definition: congenital conditions in male infants in which the urethra ends on the underside (hypospadias) or the top side (epispadias) of the penis rather than at the end

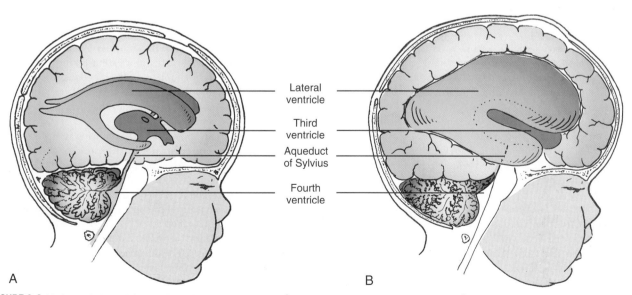

Lateral ventricle
Third ventricle
Aqueduct of Sylvius
Fourth ventricle

A   B

FIGURE 8-3 Hydrocephalus: a block in flow of cerebrospinal fluid. **A,** Patent cerebrospinal fluid circulation. **B,** Enlarged lateral and third ventricles caused by obstruction of circulation and stenosis of aqueduct of Sylvius. (From Hockenberry MJ, Wilson D: *Wong's nursing care of infants and children,* ed 9, St Louis, 2011, Mosby.)

B. Symptoms: obvious physical defects evident on physical examination; abnormal stream of urine

C. Diagnosis: based on physical examination findings

D. Treatment and nursing interventions
1. The surgery to extend the urethra to the end of the penis is usually done in several stages when the child is 6 to 18 months of age; the infant should not be circumcised because foreskin may be needed for later surgery.
2. Postoperative care includes inspection of the operative site for bleeding, catheter care, emotional support for the child and parents, and general postoperative care.

Cryptorchidism

A. Definition: failure of one or both testes to descend into the scrotal sac. Sterility may result if not treated.

B. Symptoms: Testes not palpable in the scrotal sac on physical examination.

C. Diagnosis: based on symptoms

D. Treatment and nursing interventions
1. The testes usually descend by 1 year of age (in 75% of affected infants).
2. Hormonal therapy (human chorionic gonadotropin [hCG]) may be used at an early age to promote descent of the testes into the scrotum.
3. Surgical intervention (orchiopexy), usually done at 6 to 24 months of age, is often necessary to bring the testes down the inguinal canal and into the scrotum. Postoperative care is routine.

Wilms Tumor (Nephroblastoma)

A. Definition: tumor in the kidney region

B. Symptoms: sometimes asymptomatic, discovered on routine examination; occasional occurrence of hematuria and elevated blood pressure; swelling or mass in the abdomen

C. Diagnosis: often palpable through the abdominal wall; occurs most often in children younger than 2 years and is usually found by the caregiver before the child reaches the age of 3 years

D. Treatment and nursing interventions
1. Surgery to remove the tumor is performed within 48 hours of diagnosis. Routine postoperative care is given.
2. Radiation therapy is given after surgery as ordered (for children with large tumors, metastasis, or recurrence).
3. Chemotherapy is given as ordered. The most effective agents are actinomycin D and vincristine.
4. Emotional support and education for parents are provided.

E. Prognosis is good with early diagnosis and treatment for children under 2 years of age.

F. *Alert:* Do not palpate abdomen preoperatively as this may cause trauma to the mass and release cancer cells into the patient's system.

Musculoskeletal System
Congenital Clubfoot (Talipes Equinovarus)

A. Definition: defect in which the entire foot is inverted, heel is drawn up, and front of foot is adducted; can affect one or both feet (Figure 8-4)

B. Symptoms: obvious physical defect evident on physical examination

C. Diagnosis: based on the presence of the physical defect on examination

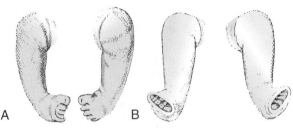

FIGURE 8-4 Feet in casts for correction of bilateral congenital talipes equinovarus. **A,** Before correction. **B,** Undergoing correction in plaster casts. (From Brashear HR, Raney RB: *Handbook of orthopaedic surgery,* ed 10, St Louis, 1986, Mosby.)

D. Treatment and nursing interventions
1. The deformity is usually repaired in stages. The type of treatment depends on the severity of the defect.
2. Various methods of treatment include manipulation and serial casting, splints, and surgery when necessary to repair the deformities. Nursing care depends on the method chosen.

Developmental Dysplasia of the Hip

A. Definition: group of disorders related to abnormal development of the hip in which a shallow acetabulum, subluxation, or dislocation is present; may result from laxity of the supporting capsule or an abnormality of the acetabulum

B. Symptoms: limited hip abduction, apparent shortening of femur, asymmetry of gluteal and thigh folds (Figure 8-5)

C. Diagnosis: symptoms found on physical examination by the physician or nurse practitioner

D. Treatment and nursing interventions
1. Treatment is started as soon as the defect is diagnosed. The hip is manipulated into proper position, and an abduction device (Pavlik harness, Figure 8-6) or hip spica cast is applied. Modified Bryant traction or modified Buck extension may also be used.
2. Nursing care includes parent teaching regarding application of the harness and cast care.

Cardiovascular System
Congenital Heart Defects (Cyanotic and Acyanotic)

A. Atrial septal defect (ASD): abnormal opening in the septum between the two atria, or a patent foramen ovale, that causes left-to-right shunting of the blood (acyanotic)

B. Ventricular septal defect (VSD): abnormal opening in the septum between the two ventricles that causes left-to-right shunting of the blood (acyanotic)

C. Patent ductus arteriosus (PDA): condition in which ductus arteriosus remains open after birth instead of closing off as normal, causing an overload of the left heart and a slight murmur (acyanotic)

D. Coarctation of the aorta: constriction of the aortic arch, causing hypertension in the upper body and hypotension in the lower body (acyanotic)

E. Tetralogy of Fallot: consists of four congenital defects—pulmonary stenosis, VSD, overriding of the aorta, and right ventricular hypertrophy (cyanotic)

F. Classic symptoms of congenital heart defects: dyspnea, difficulty with feeding, clubbing of fingers, cyanosis (in certain defects), heart murmurs, rapid pulse, recurrent respiratory infections, edema

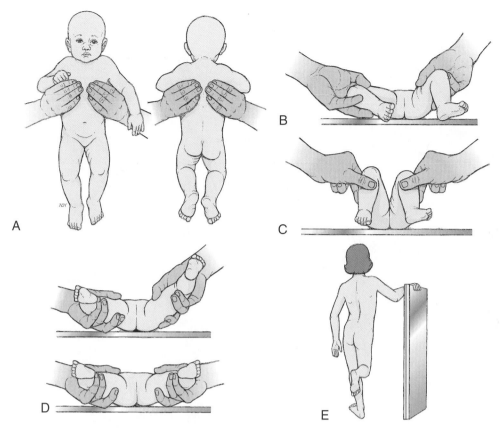

FIGURE 8-5 Signs of developmental dysplasia of the hip. **A,** Asymmetry of gluteal and thigh folds. **B,** Limited hip abduction, as seen in flexion. **C,** Apparent shortening of the femur, as indicated by the level of the knees in flexion. **D,** Ortolani click (if infant is younger than 4 weeks). **E,** Positive Trendelenburg sign or gait (if child is weight bearing). (From Hockenberry MJ, Wilson D: *Wong's nursing care of infants and children,* ed 9, St Louis, 2011, Mosby.)

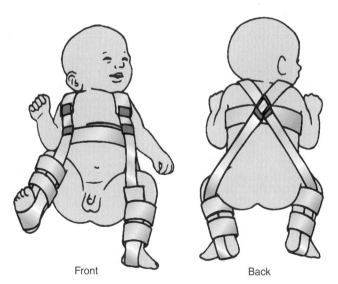

Front   Back

FIGURE 8-6 Child in Pavlik harness. (From Ball JW: *Mosby's pediatric patient teaching guides,* St Louis, 1998, Mosby.)

G. Diagnosis: based on symptoms, electrocardiograms, echocardiograms, cardiac catheterizations, and chest x-ray examinations

H. Treatment and nursing interventions
1. Most defects must be corrected by surgical intervention, often in stages. Some symptoms can be treated with medications as ordered.

2. Nursing care measures depend on the type of treatment or surgery. Most often, immediate postoperative care is given in intensive care units.
3. Patient and parent teaching should include instructing parents to help the child conserve energy without being overprotective.

Sickle Cell Anemia

A. Definition: autosomal disease occurring mainly in African Americans and occasionally in Caucasians of Mediterranean descent; causes breakdown of red blood cells (RBCs) carrying an abnormal hemoglobin S, which leads to a severe hemolytic anemia. The disease may not be recognized until the toddler or preschool period.

B. Symptoms: appear only in children who inherit the trait from both parents; fatigue, anorexia, decreased hemoglobin. Sickle cell crisis may occur, causing severe joint pain, abdominal pain, fever, and firm, distended abdomen (Figure 8-7). Because children with sickle cell disease do not have a properly functioning spleen, they are more susceptible to infection and sepsis.

C. Diagnosis: based on the symptoms; family history of the disease; and results of specific blood tests, including the sickle cell slide preparation, sickle turbidity test (Sickledex), and hemoglobin electrophoresis (fingerprinting)

D. Treatment and nursing interventions
1. IV fluids and fluids by mouth (PO) as ordered
2. Oxygen therapy, especially during sickle cell crisis

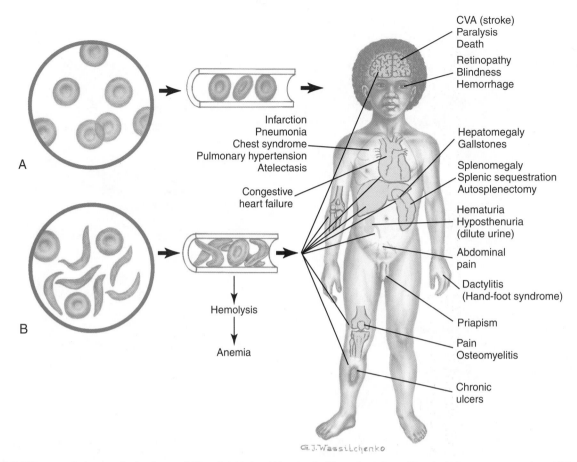

FIGURE 8-7 Differences between effects of normal (**A**) and sickled red blood cells (**B**) on circulation with selected consequences in a child. *CVA,* Cerebrovascular accident. (Modified from Hockenberry MJ, Wilson D: *Wong's nursing care of infants and children,* ed 9, St Louis, 2011, Mosby.)

3. Bed rest
4. Electrolyte replacement
5. Analgesics for pain as ordered
6. Blood transfusions as ordered (packed RBCs)
7. Prophylactic antibiotic therapy as needed
8. Education and genetic counseling for parents
9. Proper nutrition as tolerated, including folic acid
10. Avoidance of exposure to people with colds and infections
11. Avoidance of exercise at high altitudes because oxygen concentration in the blood is already severely reduced

Endocrine System
Hypopituitarism (Dwarfism)
A. Definition; growth retardation resulting from deficiency of the growth hormone (GH)
B. Symptoms: short stature, well-nourished appearance, delayed physical development
C. Diagnosis: based on family history, child's growth patterns, physical examination findings, x-ray film studies, and endocrine studies
D. Treatment and nursing interventions
   1. Replacement of the GH by subcutaneous injections
   2. Early diagnosis and treatment to help prevent many physical and emotional problems that occur later in childhood
   3. Provision of emotional support for the child and parents during diagnostic procedures and early stages of treatment (even after GH therapy is started, growth will be slower than normal)

Congenital Hypothyroidism (Cretinism)
A. Definition: lack of thyroid function resulting from failure of the embryonic development of the thyroid gland
B. Symptoms: usually do not appear until 6 to 12 weeks of age in bottle-fed infants and after weaning in breast-fed infants and include feeding problems; inactivity; anemia; thick, dry, mottled skin; bradycardia; relaxation of the abdominal muscles; and delayed development of the nervous system, which leads to mental retardation
C. Diagnosis: based on the symptoms and results of tests of thyroid function, such as initial measurement of the newborn's thyroxine (T_4) and thyroid-stimulating hormone (TSH) levels
D. Treatment and nursing interventions
   1. Early diagnosis and treatment are essential in preventing retardation and other severe physiological symptoms.
   2. Treatment is lifelong replacement therapy of the thyroid hormone.
   3. Teach parents concerning administration of the thyroid hormone, including signs and symptoms of thyroid overdose.

Respiratory System
Cystic Fibrosis
A. Definition: an autosomal-recessive hereditary disease of the exocrine glands causing those glands to produce abnormally thick secretions of mucus, increased sweat electrolytes, and increased activity of the autonomic nervous system causing

obstruction. The glands most often involved are those in the lungs and pancreas and the sweat glands. The disorder is diagnosed in infancy or early childhood.

B. Symptoms
   1. In newborns: meconium ileus, bile-stained emesis, distended abdomen, no stools, salty "taste" to the skin resulting from increased sodium in the perspiration
   2. In infants and children: harsh, dry cough; frequent bronchial infections; malnutrition; distended abdomen; barrel chest; clubbed fingers; bulky, greasy, foul-smelling stools (steatorrhea)

C. Diagnosis: based on family history, a history of FTT, the symptoms, lung changes revealed on chest x-ray films, an elevated sweat chloride level (increased sodium in the perspiration), and stool analysis for fat and enzymes

D. Treatment and nursing interventions
   1. Pancreatic enzymes given as ordered with food to improve digestion of fats and proteins
   2. High-carbohydrate, high-protein, low-fat diet
   3. Increased amounts of salt and water-soluble vitamins
   4. Inhalation therapy: nebulizer treatments of bronchodilators (see Chapter 3) and recombinant human deoxyribonuclease (DNase) to decrease the viscosity of the mucus
   5. Daily routine of chest physiotherapy and postural drainage to help in expectoration of mucus
   6. Physical exercise to stimulate mucus secretion; avoid use of cough suppressants
   7. Antibiotics for all pulmonary infections
   8. Parent teaching regarding diet, medications, and inhalation therapy for proper home care after discharge
   9. Referral to the Cystic Fibrosis Foundation for education and financial or emotional support
   10. Genetic counseling for parents

INFANCY (AGES 4 WEEKS TO 1 YEAR)

NORMAL GROWTH AND DEVELOPMENT
Physical Development
A. 1 month
   1. Physical
      a. Weight: gains approximately 5 to 7 ounces (150 to 210 g) weekly during first 6 months of life
      b. Height: gains approximately 1 inch (2.5 cm) per month for first 6 months of life
   2. Motor
      a. May lift head temporarily but generally needs support
      b. Holds head parallel with body when placed prone
      c. Can turn head from side to side when prone or supine
      d. Domination of asymmetrical posture such as tonic neck reflex
      e. Primitive reflexes still present and strong (grasp, Moro, tonic neck).
   3. Sensory
      a. Follows a light to midline
      b. Eye movements coordinated most of the time
      c. Visual acuity: 20/100 to 20/50
      d. Quiet when hears a voice
   4. Socialization and vocalization
      a. Smiles indiscriminately
      b. Makes small throaty sounds
      c. Watches parent's face when he or she talks to infant

B. 2 to 3 months
   1. Physical: posterior fontanel closed
   2. Motor
      a. Holds head erect for a short time and can raise chest supported on forearms
      b. Can carry hand or an object to the mouth at will
      c. Reaches for attractive objects but misjudges distances
      d. Grasp, tonic neck, and Moro reflexes fading
      e. Can sit when the back is supported; knees flexed and back rounded
      f. Disappearance of step or dance reflex
      g. Plays with fingers and hands
   3. Sensory
      a. Follows a light to the periphery
      b. Has binocular coordination (vertical and horizontal vision)
      c. Locates sounds by turning head in direction of the sound
   4. Socialization and vocalization
      a. Smiles in response to a person or object
      b. Coos and gurgles; shows pleasure in making sounds
      c. Stops crying when parent enters the room

C. 4 to 5 months
   1. Physical: Drooling begins because salivary glands are functioning, but the child does not have sufficient coordination to swallow saliva.
   2. Motor
      a. Balances head well in a sitting position
      b. Sits with little support; holds back straight when pulled to a sitting position
      c. Predomination of symmetrical body position
      d. Can sustain a portion of own weight when held in a standing position
      e. Reaches for and grasps an object with the whole hand
      f. Can roll over from back to side
      g. Lifts head and shoulders at 90-degree angle when prone
      h. Disappearance of primitive reflexes (e.g., grasp, tonic neck, Moro)
   3. Sensory
      a. Recognizes familiar objects and people
      b. Beginning eye-hand coordination
   4. Socialization and vocalization
      a. Laughs aloud
      b. Definitely enjoys social interaction with people
      c. Vocalizes displeasure when an object is taken away

D. 6 to 7 months
   1. Physical
      a. Weight: gains approximately 3 to 5 ounces (90 to 150 g) weekly during second 6 months of life; weight doubles by 6 months
      b. Height: gains approximately ½ inch (1.25 cm) per month
      c. Teething may begin with eruption of two lower central incisors, followed by upper incisors (Figure 8-8).
   2. Motor
      a. Can turn over equally well from stomach or back
      b. Sits fairly well unsupported, especially if placed in a forward-leaning position
      c. Hitches or moves backward when in a sitting position
      d. Can transfer a toy from one hand to the other
      e. Can approach toy and grasp it with one hand
      f. Plays with feet and puts them in mouth

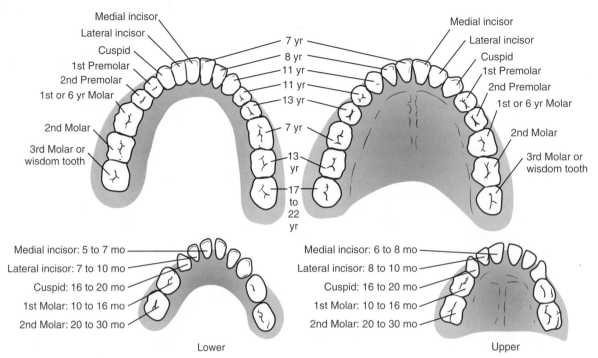

FIGURE 8-8 Eruption of permanent and deciduous teeth. (From Price DL, Gwin JF: *Pediatric nursing: an introductory text,* ed 11, St Louis, 2012, Saunders.)

g. When lying down, lifts head as if trying to sit up

h. Transfers everything from hand to mouth

3. Sensory
   a. Has taste preferences; will spit out disliked foods
   b. Responds to own name

4. Socialization and vocalization
   a. Begins to differentiate between strange and familiar faces and shows "stranger anxiety"
   b. Makes polysyllabic vowel sounds (baba, dada)
   c. Plays peek-a-boo
   d. Responds to word "no"

E. 8 to 9 months

1. Motor
   a. Sits steadily alone
   b. Has good hand-to-mouth coordination
   c. Develops pincer grasp, with preference for use of one hand over the other
   d. Crawls and then creeps (creeping is more advanced because the abdomen is supported off the floor)
   e. Can raise self to a sitting position but may require help to pull self to feet

2. Sensory
   a. Depth perception beginning to develop
   b. Displays interest in small objects

3. Socialization and vocalization
   a. Shows anxiety with strangers by turning or pushing away and crying
   b. Definite social attachment is evident: stretches out arms to loved ones
   c. Is voluntarily separating self from mother by desire to act on own
   d. Reacts to adult anger: cries when scolded
   e. Dislikes dressing, diaper change
   f. No true words as yet but comprehends words such as "bye-bye, no-no"

F. 10 to 12 months

1. Physical
   a. Has tripled birth weight by 1 year
   b. Eruption of upper and lower lateral incisors for total of six to eight teeth
   c. Head and chest circumferences equal
   d. Development of lumbar curve; lordosis evident when walking

2. Motor
   a. Stands alone for short times
   b. Walks with help; moves around by holding onto furniture
   c. Can sit down from a standing position without help
   d. Can eat from a spoon and drink from a cup but needs help; prefers using fingers
   e. Can play pat-a-cake
   f. Can hold a crayon to make a mark on paper
   g. Helps in dressing such as putting arm through sleeve

3. Sensory
   a. Visual acuity: 20/50
   b. Possible amblyopia with lack of binocularity
   c. Discriminates simple geometrical forms

4. Socialization and vocalization
   a. Shows emotions such as jealousy, affection, anger
   b. Enjoys familiar surroundings and will explore away from mother
   c. Fearful in strange situation or with strangers; clings to mother
   d. May develop habit of "security" blanket
   e. Can say three to five words besides "dada" or "mama"
   f. Understands simple verbal requests such as "Give it to me"
   g. Knows own name

Psychosocial Development

A. Infants are in Erikson's stage of "trust versus mistrust"; infants develop a sense of trust or mistrust, depending on how their needs are met by their parents (or other caregivers).

B. As infants grow, they slowly realize that they are separate from their environment and that they influence their environment with their actions.

C. Infants' early activities are mostly reflexes (e.g., crying, sucking, kicking). As the months progress, they learn to move in certain ways, follow with their eyes, and smile in response to a smile and soft words.

HEALTH PROMOTION

A. Immunizations should be given on schedule (Figure 8-9).

B. Nutrition appropriate to the age and needs of the infant should be provided.
1. Human milk is the most desirable complete diet for the first 6 months of life.
2. Introduction of strained foods may begin at 6 months of age, starting with strained fruits.
3. Solid foods should be introduced slowly, in small amounts and one at a time, to determine the infant's likes and dislikes. This also helps detect possible allergies to certain foods. Allow 4 to 7 days between the introduction of each new food. Honey should be avoided during the first 12 months because of the risk of botulism.
4. Weaning from breast or bottle to a cup can begin at 5 to 6 months of age, although the infant cannot be weaned completely until 12 to 24 months of age.

C. Safety and accident prevention includes a safe home environment, safe toys, use of car seats, and close attention to the infant who is crawling or walking.

HEALTH PROBLEMS
Nutritional Disorders
Failure to Thrive

A. Definition: state of inadequate growth resulting from inability to obtain or use calories; leads to malnutrition

B. Symptoms: below normal weight and height (below fifth percentile for age), listlessness, poor feeding habits, unresponsive to holding and attention, voluntary regurgitation, prolonged periods of sleep

C. Diagnosis
1. Based on symptoms and a continued deviation from an established growth curve
2. Three general categories of FTT
   a. Organic: result of a physical cause such as congenital defects of GI system or heart
   b. Nonorganic: unrelated to a disease; usually caused by psychosocial factors
   c. Idiopathic: unexplained cause; may be grouped with nonorganic FTT

D. Treatment and nursing interventions (directed at correcting the malnutrition)
1. Correction of organic causes if possible
2. Development of a structured routine
3. Sensory stimulation
4. Adequate food for weight gain; may include NG feedings and bottle feedings during early treatment
5. "Tender loving care" (TLC): holding and cuddling, talking to the infant

6. Teaching and encouraging the mother and father regarding feeding, infant care, and parenting skills
7. Family counseling when needed

Colic

A. Definition: paroxysmal abdominal pain or cramping that is exhibited by crying and drawing the legs up to the abdomen. Colic is most commonly seen in infants under the age of 3 months.

B. Symptoms: episodes of loud crying accompanied by abdominal cramping. Despite obvious indications of pain, the infant usually tolerates feedings well and gains weight.

C. Diagnosis: based on symptoms reported by parents or caregivers

D. Treatment and nursing interventions
1. Take a thorough history of the infant's daily activities, including the infant's and breast-feeding mother's diets; time of day when colic occurs; characteristics of crying; and activity before, during, and after crying.
2. If child is bottle-fed, investigate possibility of cow's milk allergy; substitution of another formula (e.g., casein hydrolysate [Nutramigen]) may be tried.
3. Comfort measures that can be used by the parents and caregivers
   a. Place infant prone over a covered hot-water bottle or covered heating pad (ensure that hot water bottle is warm, not hot).
   b. Massage infant's abdomen.
   c. Change infant's position frequently.
   d. Provide smaller, frequent feedings; burp infant during and after feedings, and place infant in an upright seat after feeding.
   e. Introduce pacifier for added sucking.
4. Pharmacological agents such as sedatives, antispasmodics, antihistamines, and antiflatulents are sometimes recommended.

Respiratory Disorders
Upper Respiratory Infection

A. Definition: viral or bacterial infection affecting the upper respiratory tract. Nasopharyngitis or the "common cold" is particularly common in children of all ages.

B. Symptoms: fever, sore throat, sneezing, nasal congestion, occasional cough, irritability, anorexia

C. Diagnosis: based on symptoms

D. Treatment and nursing interventions
1. Bed rest until free of fever
2. Encourage oral fluids
3. Antipyretics for fever (acetaminophen, ibuprofen; not aspirin)
4. Nose drops to relieve nasal congestion
5. Oral decongestants as ordered
6. Adequate nutrition for age. Infants and young children can better tolerate high-calorie fluids and soft foods.
7. Cool-air humidifier for moistened air (to assist in decreasing congestion)

Acute Otitis Media

A. Definition: infection and effusion in the middle ear; frequently caused by nasopharyngeal infections that travel through the infant's shortened, widened eustachian tubes. Causative organisms include *Streptococcus pneumoniae* and *Haemophilus influenzae*.

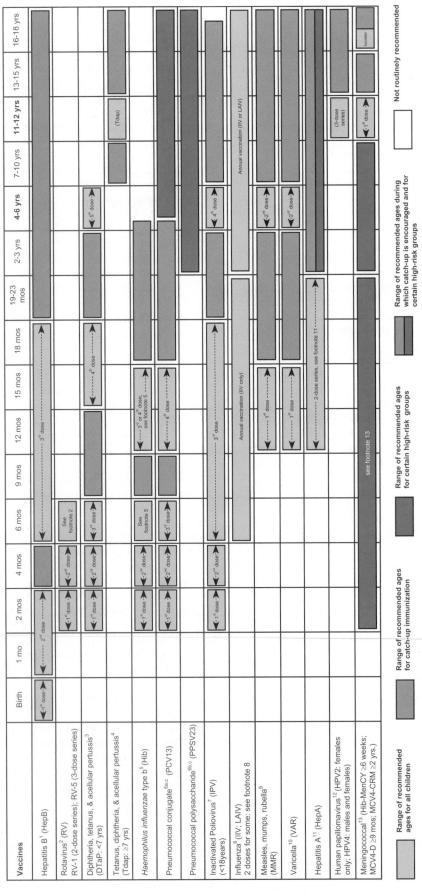

FIGURE 8-9 Recommended immunization schedule for persons aged 0 through 18 years—2013. See http://www.cdc.gov/vaccines/schedules/ for footnotes that accompany this schedule and for any updates to the schedule. (From Centers for Disease Control and Prevention: Recommended immunization schedules for persons aged 0 through 18 years, United States, 2013.)

B. Symptoms: fever, irritability, restlessness, pulling or rubbing of the ears, loss of appetite, and purulent drainage if the tympanic membrane is perforated. Otoscopic examination reveals a bright red, bulging tympanic membrane.

C. Diagnosis: based on the symptoms and history of recent upper respiratory infections (URIs)

D. Treatment and nursing interventions
1. Provide antipyretics for fever.
2. Provide analgesics or antipyretics for discomfort (acetaminophen, ibuprofen).
3. Encourage oral fluids.
4. Promote rest and quiet environment.
5. Antibiotics may be ordered if symptoms do not subside or if infant is at high risk for infection because of immunosuppression; amoxicillin is usually the antibiotic of choice.
6. Myringotomy and insertion of polyethylene tubes are performed by the physician to allow for drainage of fluid.
7. Observe for drainage. Keep ears clean.

Lower Respiratory Infections
Respiratory Syncytial Virus, Bronchiolitis

A. Definition
1. Bronchiolitis: acute viral infection that occurs primarily in winter and spring and is most common in infants and children up to 2 years of age. It causes the bronchioles to become plugged with mucus and the bronchiole mucosa to swell. The mucus traps the air in the lungs, making it difficult for the infant to expel it.
2. Respiratory syncytial virus (RSV): related to the parainfluenza virus. It is responsible for at least 50% of the diagnosed cases of bronchiolitis. The peak incidence for RSV infection is 2 to 5 months of age. It is transmitted predominantly through direct contact with respiratory secretions. RSV has been known to survive for hours on countertops, gloves, and cloth and for 30 minutes on skin.

B. Symptoms
1. Usually begins with a URI. Symptoms include rhinorrhea, coughing, sneezing, pharyngitis, wheezing, and intermittent fever.
2. With progression of the disease, increases in coughing and wheezing, air hunger, tachypnea, retractions, and cyanosis occur.
3. Symptoms of severe illness include tachypnea of more than 70 breaths/min, listlessness, poor air exchange, apneic spells, and oxygen saturation less than 95%.

C. Diagnosis
1. Based on clinical symptoms
2. Can be identified by various tests done on nasal or nasopharyngeal secretions to detect RSV antigen

D. Treatment and nursing interventions
1. Provide humidified oxygen inhalation (to relieve dyspnea and hypoxia).
2. Elevate head of crib.
3. Monitor vital signs and oxygen saturation (via pulse oximeter).
4. Provide adequate fluid intake, including IV fluids as needed for hydration.
5. Allow infant to rest as much as possible.

6. Medical therapy for bronchiolitis has not proved to be effective; however, ribavirin (Virazole), an antiviral agent, may be used specifically for RSV infection.
   a. Ribavirin is administered by nebulization via an oxygen hood, tent, or mask for 12 to 20 hours per day, for 1 to 7 days.
   b. Ribavirin is most commonly used in children with RSV infection who are at high risk for complications caused by other conditions, including chronic lung conditions, immunodeficiency, and certain neurological diseases (e.g., severe cerebral palsy).

E. Prophylactic treatment
1. Palivizumab (Synagis), a monoclonal antibody, has been used successfully in reducing hospitalizations caused by RSV.
2. Monthly injections of palivizumab are recommended for infants and children under 2 years of age with chronic lung disease; these injections are given throughout the RSV season (October through April).

Viral Pneumonia

A. Definition: inflammation of the lung characterized by interstitial pneumonitis with inflammation of the mucosa and walls of bronchi and bronchioles

B. Symptoms: fever, cough, rapid respiratory rate, listlessness

C. Diagnosis: based on the symptoms and results of chest x-ray examination

D. Treatment and nursing interventions
1. Elevate the head of the crib.
2. Provide croup tent for humidified oxygen inhalation.
3. Perform chest physiotherapy and postural drainage.
4. Administer antibiotics as ordered (for bacterial pneumonia).
5. Administer antipyretics for fever.
6. Monitor vital signs frequently.
7. Encourage clear fluids PO.
8. Allow infant to rest to prevent dyspnea.

Gastrointestinal Disorders
Infectious Gastroenteritis

A. Definition: diarrhea and vomiting that may be caused by viral or bacterial infections

B. Symptoms: frequent, loose stools, irritability, vomiting, abdominal distention. Serious symptoms include dehydration, sunken fontanel, poor skin turgor, weak rapid pulse.

C. Diagnosis: based on symptoms. Specific bacterial cause can be isolated via a stool culture (most commonly *Escherichia coli* or rotavirus in the infant). An evaluation of stool for ova and parasites may also be done.

D. Treatment and nursing interventions
1. Oral rehydration therapy (with commercially prepared solutions such as Pedialyte); amount is based on infant's weight and percentage of dehydration.
2. IV fluids with electrolytes as ordered, if oral rehydration therapy is not effective (or if dehydration is severe); take special care to maintain the infant's IV line.
3. Return to normal diet (including formula, cow's milk, and age-appropriate solids) should be started as soon as it is tolerated; the "BRAT" diet (bananas, rice cereal, applesauce, tea and toast) is contraindicated for the infant with acute diarrhea because it has little nutritional value.
4. Note amount, color, and consistency of stools and emesis.

5. Keep accurate I&O record (if necessary, weigh diapers to measure urine output).
6. Maintain proper isolation technique (Enteric Precautions).
7. Provide good skin care to buttocks and perineum after each diaper change. Cleanse well. Leave area open to air when possible. Apply ointments as ordered.
8. Provide time for stimulation, holding, and cuddling.
9. Antidiarrheal drug therapy is contraindicated in infants and young children because of possible adverse side effects and toxicity.

Hypertrophic Pyloric Stenosis

A. Definition: hypertrophy of the pyloric muscle fibers and narrowing of the pylorus, which is at the distal end of the stomach (Figure 8-10)
B. Symptoms: usually appear between 3 and 8 weeks of age; projectile vomiting of formula and mucus, irritability, weight loss, and dehydration. The physician can often palpate the olive-size pyloric mass in the abdomen.
C. Diagnosis: based on the symptoms, physical examination, and, if necessary, upper GI radiographic or ultrasound studies
D. Treatment and nursing interventions
   1. Preoperative
      a. IV fluids with electrolytes as ordered
      b. NPO status unless ordered to feed
      c. NG tube is often inserted to remove excess stomach contents immediately before surgery (pyloromyotomy).
   2. Postoperative
      a. Position the infant on right side or abdomen or in infant seat to prevent aspiration.
      b. Maintain NPO status. First feeding begins within the first 24 hours after surgery (clear liquids with glucose and electrolytes); amounts are increased slowly. Administer small frequent feedings as ordered. Formula is started 24 hours after surgery if clear fluids are retained.
      c. NG tube may remain in place for several hours.
      d. Provide general postoperative nursing care.

Nervous System Disorders
Febrile Seizures

A. Definition: seizures caused by high fever (102° to 105° F [38.8° to 40.5° C]); most often seen between 6 months and 3 years of age
B. Symptoms: seizures characterized by stiffening of the body with jerking movements of the extremities and face, ending with a lapse of consciousness
C. Diagnosis: based on evidence of seizure activity preceded by high fever
   1. Simple febrile seizures are brief and generalized.
   2. Complex febrile seizures are prolonged and may have focal features.
D. Treatment and nursing interventions
   1. Anticonvulsant (phenobarbital [Luminal]) and antianxiety (diazepam [Valium]) medications to control the seizures; antipyretics (ibuprofen or acetaminophen) to control fever (see Chapter 3)
   2. Padded side rails
   3. Airway and suction equipment at bedside
   4. During seizure do not restrain the infant; turn his or her head to the side to allow saliva to drain out of the mouth. Do not try to insert a seizure stick or airway in the infant's mouth during a seizure. Observe the seizure and protect the infant from harm.
   5. Documentation: Note the kinds of movements; behavior before the seizure (if known); duration of the seizure; skin color and vital signs during and after the seizure; and medications given during the seizure, including the infant or toddler's reaction to the medications.
   6. Parent teaching should include care of the infant during a seizure.

Meningitis

A. Definition: infection of the meninges and fluid; caused by several viruses and bacteria, including *H. influenzae* type B, *Neisseria meningitidis,* and *S. pneumoniae;* may also occur secondary to other infections or as a complication of trauma and neurosurgery

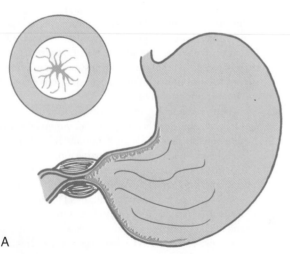
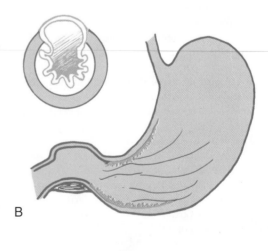

A

B

FIGURE 8-10 Hypertrophic pyloric stenosis. **A,** Enlarged muscular tumor nearly obliterates pyloric channel. **B,** Longitudinal surgical division of muscle down to submucosa establishes adequate passageway. (From Hockenberry MJ, Wilson D: *Wong's nursing care of infants and children,* ed 9, St Louis, 2011, Mosby.)

B. Symptoms: elevated temperature, irritability, poor feeding, high-pitched cry, nuchal rigidity, seizures, bulging fontanel

C. Diagnosis: based on the symptoms and the presence of cloudy spinal fluid when lumbar puncture is performed (increased white blood cell [WBC] count; decreased glucose level and increased protein level in the spinal fluid; increased CSF pressure) (Figure 8-11)

D. Treatment and nursing interventions
   1. Acute bacterial meningitis is a medical emergency. Early recognition and immediate treatment are required to avoid residual complications and prevent death; therefore treatment is started before the causative agent is identified.
   2. Isolation from other children (for bacterial meningitis) for at least 24 hours after antibiotics started
   3. IV antibiotics as ordered for bacterial meningitis
   4. Monitor vital signs, neurological status, and level of consciousness frequently.
   5. IV fluids as ordered
   6. Diet: infant possibly NPO at first until liquids can be tolerated
   7. Antipyretics to reduce elevated temperature
   8. Infant handled as little as possible when irritable and uncomfortable; quiet room necessary
   9. Seizure precautions (padded side rails)
   10. IV dexamethasone for management of increased intracranial pressure (recommended for treatment of *H. influenzae* type B meningitis)
   11. Treatment for viral meningitis is symptomatic and supportive.

Integumentary Disorders

Infantile Eczema

A. Definition: atopic dermatitis caused by an allergic reaction to some irritant; usually begins between 2 and 6 months of age and undergoes spontaneous remission around age 3 years

B. Symptoms: reddened, raised rash starting on cheeks and spreading to arms and legs; itching, oozing of vesicles

C. Diagnosis: based on the history and symptoms. The cause of the eczema (the allergen) must also be determined so further episodes can be controlled.

D. Treatment and nursing interventions
   1. Provide good skin care; keep affected areas clean.
   2. Provide tub baths with tepid water, baking soda, and cornstarch to relieve the itching.
   3. Keep skin well hydrated. Various lubricants or moisturizing lotions may be ordered.
   4. Encourage antihistamines and topical steroids as ordered to control itching.
   5. Use mittens to prevent scratching.
   6. Use elbow restraints to prevent scratching (only if necessary).
   7. Provide for sensory stimulation, holding, and cuddling at frequent intervals.

Impetigo

A. Definition: infection of the skin caused by *Streptococcus* or *Staphylococcus* bacteria; occurs in nurseries when strict handwashing technique is not followed (impetigo neonatorum); also occurs in preschool- and school-aged children, often during recovery from a URI

B. Symptoms: reddened, vesicular lesions (pustules) with honey-colored crusts

C. Diagnosis: based on the symptoms. Specific bacterial cause can be determined by culture of the draining lesions.

D. Treatment and nursing interventions
   1. Isolation of infant (child) for 24 to 48 hours after treatment started
   2. Strict handwashing technique by all persons coming in contact with the infant
   3. Warm saline compresses to lesions, followed by a gentle cleansing and topical antibiotic ointment
   4. Systemic antibiotics may be necessary for infants or children with widespread lesions.

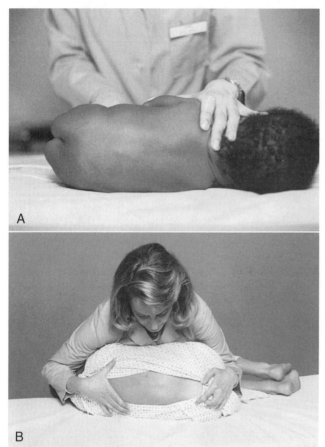

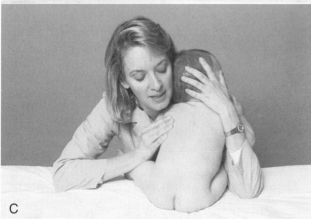

FIGURE 8-11 A, Modified side-lying position for lumbar puncture. **B,** Older child in side-lying position. **C,** Infant in sitting position allows for flexion of lumbar spine. (From Hockenberry MJ, Wilson D: *Wong's nursing care of infants and children,* ed 9, St Louis, 2013, Mosby.)

Burns.

Burns are covered in detail in Chapter 5 of this text. The "rule of nines" that is used to determine percentage of body affected by the burn in older children and adults is not applicable in smaller children and infants because of their smaller body proportions. See Figure 8-12 for estimated distribution of burns in children. See Critical Thinking Challenge box.

❓ Critical Thinking Challenge

A 6-year-old is admitted with deep partial thickness burns over approximately 25 to 30% of his body from hot oil after he accidently knocked over a skillet from the stove. The affected areas include primarily his chest, his abdomen, and the anterior surface of both thighs. The mother had just turned away from the stove for a second when the child reached for the skillet. Explain the initial and long-term nursing interventions and goals appropriate to the care of this child. Discuss ways that will help relieve the anxiety and guilt of the mother.

RECOMMENDATION

Initial nursing interventions include maintaining an open airway, monitoring respiratory efforts, and preventing shock. Oxygen will be administered and closely monitored. Shock results from capillary leakage of circulating fluid into surrounding tissues, therefore IV infusion with Ringers Lactate is started and will also be closely monitored. A Foley catheter is inserted to monitor success of fluid volume restoration. Once the child is stabilized, transfer to the burn unit will be necessary. Major goals and appropriate nursing interventions will include prevention of infection, pain management, management of adequate nutrition to enhance the healing process, and means by which the psychological needs of both the parent and child are met. Involving the child and the parent(s) in these goals and interventions is absolutely critical to the overall recovery process and will help to relieve the anxiety and guilt of the mother.

Sudden Infant Death Syndrome

A. Definition: sudden death of an infant under 1 year of age that remains unexplained after a complete postmortem examination, including an investigation of the death scene and a review of the infant's clinical history; the third leading cause of death in children 1 to 12 months of age. The peak age for sudden infant death syndrome (SIDS) is 2 to 4 months; 95% of cases occur by the age of 6 months.

B. Research: Numerous theories have been proposed regarding the cause of SIDS, but the exact cause is unknown. Many researchers believe that it may be related to a brainstem abnormality in the regulation of cardiorespiratory control. Other studies have demonstrated that infants sleeping in the prone position are at an increased risk for SIDS; because of these findings, the American Academy of Pediatrics recommends that healthy infants up to 6 months of age sleep on their backs.

C. Infants at risk for SIDS include those with a history of apnea requiring vigorous stimulation or cardiopulmonary resuscitation (CPR), preterm infants who continue to have apnea after hospital discharge, and siblings of two or more SIDS victims.

D. Emotional support for the parents
1. Parents always feel guilty and must be reassured that SIDS is not their fault.
2. Encourage them to allow an autopsy to try to determine a specific cause of death, which helps allay their guilt and feelings that they might have prevented it.

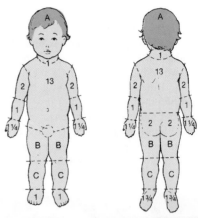

RELATIVE PERCENTAGES OF AREAS AFFECTED BY GROWTH

AREA	BIRTH	AGE 1 YR	AGE 5 YR
A = ½ of head	9½	8½	6½
B = ½ of one thigh	2¾	3¼	4
C = ½ of one leg	2½	2½	2¾

A

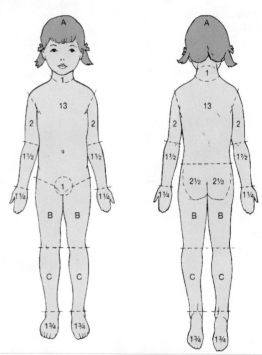

RELATIVE PERCENTAGES OF AREAS AFFECTED BY GROWTH

AREA	AGE 10 YR	AGE 15 YR	ADULT
A = ½ of head	5½	4½	3½
B = ½ of one thigh	4½	4½	4¾
C = ½ of one leg	3	3¼	3½

B

FIGURE 8-12 Estimation of distribution of burns in children. **A,** Children from birth to age 5 years. **B,** Older children. (From Hockenberry MJ, Wilson D: *Wong's nursing care of infants and children,* ed 9, St Louis, 2011, Mosby.)

3. Allow parents to spend some time with the child to say good-bye.
4. Refer the parents to the SIDS Foundation for counseling and support.
5. After the parents return home from the hospital, emotional support should continue to be provided for them by qualified health care professionals.

TODDLERHOOD (AGES 1 TO 3 YEARS)

NORMAL GROWTH AND DEVELOPMENT
Physical Development
A. Toddlerhood includes a decrease in the rate of growth but an increase in the rate of development.
B. Toddlers gain approximately 4 to 6 pounds (1.8 to 2.7 kg) and add 3 inches (7.5 cm) in height per year.
C. They have learned, and continue to learn, to walk between 1 and 2 years of age.
D. Visual acuity of 20/20 is achieved during the toddler years.
E. Anterior fontanel closes between 18 and 24 months of age.
F. Toddlers continue to learn to talk, learning new words and phrases; their favorite word is "no!"

Psychosocial Development
A. Behavior in the toddler is characterized by several aspects.
   1. Negativism: Toddlers say "no!" to almost everything; this is part of the child's becoming an individual person who is separate from parents.
   2. Ritualism: Toddlers develop and follow certain patterns of behavior to create their own security.
   3. Temper tantrums: Toddlers like to do everything for themselves; when they cannot do certain things, they're frustrated, and this frustration leads to temper tantrums. Tantrums should be ignored as much as possible, and the child should be dealt with after the "storm" is over.
B. Toddlers are in Erikson's stage of "autonomy versus shame and doubt"; they need to develop a sense of autonomy and self-control. To do so, they must be able to make some choices and learn to function within the limits set for them. They are in Kohlberg's stage 1 of preconventional morality; they obey rules to avoid punishment.
C. Discipline and limit-setting must be consistent to be effective; it is important to remember to criticize the behavior, not the child.
D. Toilet training is an important part of the socialization process in toddlers. They should be praised when they use the potty chair or toilet properly rather than being punished for not using it. Toilet training should begin only when the toddler is physically capable of controlling bowel and bladder (18 to 24 months).

HEALTH PROMOTION
A. Nutrition needs change because of change in growth rate. Toddlers need less food, and their appetites decrease (18 months of age).
   1. Teach parents that the decrease in food intake is normal.
   2. The child is more autonomous now and should be allowed to feed himself or herself as much as possible; "finger foods" are ideal.
   3. Snacks should be nutritious; cheese, fruit, and crackers are good choices.
   4. Desserts should not be used as rewards; this practice gets the toddler into a habit of expecting something sweet whenever he or she does something good.
B. Prevention of accidents is a major responsibility with toddlers. Keep dangerous items (sharp objects, medications, cleaning supplies) out of their reach; they should not be left unattended near a bathtub, swimming pool, whirlpool bath, or hot objects such as pans on the stove or open flames.
C. Teaching the toddler good oral hygiene habits is necessary to prevent early tooth decay and problems with gums.
   1. Brushing the teeth should begin at 12 to 18 months of age.
   2. Dental checkups with the dental hygienist or dentist should begin at approximately 1 year of age.
   3. Proper nutrition helps prevent a large amount of early dental caries.

HEALTH PROBLEMS
Respiratory Disorders
Epiglottitis
A. Definition: severely inflamed epiglottis, which begins abruptly and progresses rapidly into severe respiratory distress; usually caused by *H. influenzae* bacteria (unlike croup, which is viral and progresses more slowly than epiglottitis)
B. Symptoms: fever, sore throat, difficulty swallowing. Child insists on sitting up, leaning forward with chin thrust out, mouth open, and tongue protruding. Drooling is common.
C. Diagnosis: based on the symptoms and visualization of enlarged reddened epiglottis on careful throat examination and enlarged epiglottis on lateral neck x-ray examination
D. Treatment and nursing interventions
   1. Do not examine throat unless immediate intubation can be performed if necessary.
   2. Keep child as quiet as possible; allow child to sit up in bed or on lap of parent.
   3. Keep emergency tracheostomy tray (and intubation tray) with patient at all times.
   4. Administer IV fluids and antibiotics as ordered.
   5. Monitor child closely.

Cardiovascular Disorder
Kawasaki Disease (Mucocutaneous Lymph Node Syndrome)
A. Definition: acute inflammation of the vascular system; cause unknown; most common in children under 5 years of age, with peak incidence seen in the toddler age group; diagnosed in every racial group but most common in Japanese children; most cases diagnosed in late winter and early spring. Without proper treatment 20% of children develop cardiac complications, including damage to the cardiac blood vessels and the heart muscle itself. Kawasaki disease (KD) is the major cause of acquired heart disease in children in the United States.
B. Symptoms and diagnosis: child must exhibit five of the following six criteria, including fever:
   1. Fever for 5 or more days
   2. Bilateral conjunctival inflammation
   3. Changes in the oral mucous membranes, including dryness and erythema
   4. Changes in the extremities such as erythema and peeling of the palms and soles and peripheral edema
   5. Cervical lymphadenopathy
   6. Polymorphous rash
C. Treatment and nursing interventions
   1. High-dose IV immune globulin (IVIG) to decrease the fever and incidence of coronary artery damage
   2. Salicylate therapy to control fever and symptoms of inflammation
   3. I&O, daily weight (to assess for signs of congestive heart failure)
   4. Mouth care

5. Careful observation of the IV site
6. Quiet environment and proper rest
7. Emotional support for the child and family
8. Long-term follow-up should include monitoring of heart disease risk factors (abnormal blood pressure and cholesterol levels) and promotion of a heart-healthy lifestyle (proper nutrition, exercise, avoidance of smoking).

Gastrointestinal Disorder

Celiac Disease (Gluten Enteropathy)

A. Definition: defect of metabolism precipitated by the ingestion of wheat or rye gluten, leading to impaired fat absorption; exact cause unknown
B. Symptoms: usually appear between 1 and 5 years of age; chronic diarrhea with bulky, greasy, foul-smelling stools; malnutrition; anorexia; unhappy disposition; retardation of growth; distended abdomen; muscle wasting, especially of extremities and buttocks
C. Diagnosis: laboratory tests, including stool analysis for fecal fat; blood studies for anemia, hypoproteinemia, and serum iron; definitive diagnosis based on these tests, the symptoms, and a jejunal biopsy to demonstrate changes in the jejunal mucosa
D. Treatment and nursing interventions
  1. Provide gluten-free, low-fat diet; rice cereal for infants. Children with celiac disease may also be lactose intolerant.
  2. Provide parent teaching regarding diet and specific foods to avoid.
  3. The child should be protected from respiratory infections, which may lead to exacerbations of the disease known as *celiac crisis* (characterized by severe vomiting and diarrhea, dehydration, and acidosis).

Neurosensory Disorders

Eye Disorders

Strabismus

A. Definition: failure of the eyes to direct and focus on the same object at the same time
B. Symptoms: deviation of one eye to the center (esotropia) or to the other corner (exotropia)
C. Diagnosis: based on the symptoms
D. Treatment and nursing interventions
  1. Patching of unaffected eye to increase visual stimulation of weaker eye
  2. Eyeglasses and exercise to help improve vision
  3. Surgery to correct the muscle defects; often necessary when conservative treatment is ineffective
  4. Preoperative and postoperative nursing care as indicated

Amblyopia ("Lazy Eye")

A. Definition: reduced visual acuity in one eye, usually caused by strabismus. The eyes are unable to focus and work together, and blindness may occur in the weaker eye if left untreated.
B. Symptoms: blurred vision, double vision, development of a "blind spot"
C. Diagnosis: based on results of Snellen eye test and the symptoms
D. Treatment and nursing interventions: patching of the unaffected eye so the child is forced to use and focus the weaker eye. Early childhood the best time for treatment

Cerebral Palsy

A. Definition: group of nonprogressive disorders caused by a malfunction of the motor centers of the brain. Oxygen deprivation (anoxia) damages the motor centers of the brain prenatally, during or immediately after delivery, or during childhood after an accident or disease.
B. Symptoms: abnormal muscle tone and coordination, delays in development, hearing and vision impairment, seizures, mental retardation (in some cases)
C. Diagnosis: based on the mother's prenatal history, birth history, history of an accident or disease, presence of delays in growth and development, abnormal neurological examination findings (Table 8-2)
D. Types of cerebral palsy
  1. Spastic: hypertonicity with poor control of posture, balance, and coordination; impaired motor skills; hypertonicity of muscles and tendon reflexes, which leads to development of contractures
  2. Dyskinetic (athetoid): abnormal involuntary movement; athetosis, characterized by slow, writhing movements that involve extremities, trunk, neck, facial muscles, and tongue
  3. Ataxic: wide-based gait; disintegration of movements of the upper extremities when the child reaches for objects
  4. Mixed type: combination of spasticity and athetosis
E. Treatment and nursing interventions
  1. Treatment and care are supportive to ensure optimal level of development for the child.
  2. Physical and occupational therapy help the child learn some control over muscle movements.
  3. Braces or splints are used as needed to hold extremities in correct positions of function.
  4. Wheelchairs, walkers, and crutches are used as needed for ambulation and locomotion.
  5. Speech therapy or assistance with feeding is provided as needed.
  6. Treatment for respiratory problems, seizures, or contractures is provided as needed.
  7. Emotional support is provided for the family and child. Approximately 50% of children with cerebral palsy are of normal intelligence and have only physical disabilities; the remaining 50% have some degree of mental retardation.
  8. The child is encouraged to live as normal a life as possible. The family is referred to supportive groups such as Easter Seals.

Autism

A. Definition: a complex developmental disorder of the brain; three types—autistic disorder (classic autism), Asperger syndrome, and pervasive developmental disorder (atypical autism); cause unknown, although genetics, environmental factors, vaccines, and complications of pregnancy are thought to increase risk.
B. Symptoms: Child exhibits bizarre behavior; temper tantrums; does not maintain eye contact; delayed language development; often uses repetitive language; repetitive motor movements (rocking); lives in his or her own world; may have some degree of mental retardation. Some children may show exceptional talent in certain areas (music, memory, mathematics).

Table 8-2	Cerebral Palsy: Predisposing Factors and Known Causes

RISK FACTORS	ASSOCIATED CAUSES
PRENATAL	
Maternal	Metabolic diseases Nutritional deficiencies (e.g., anemia) Twin or multiple births Bleeding Toxemia Blood incompatibilities Exposure to radiation Infection (e.g., rubella, toxoplasmosis, cytomegalic inclusion disease) Premature labor
Prematurity	Asphyxia leading to cerebral hemorrhage
Genetic factors	Absence of corpus callosum, aqueductal stenosis, cerebellar hypoplasia
Congenital anomalies of the brain	Unknown causes not evident on clinical examination
PERINATAL	Anesthesia or analgesia during labor and delivery Mechanical trauma during delivery Immaturity at birth Metabolic disorders (e.g., hyperbilirubinemia, hypoglycemia, amino acid disorders, hyperosmolality) Electrolyte disturbances (e.g., hypernatremia, hypoglycemia)
POSTNATAL	Head trauma Infections (e.g., meningitis, encephalitis) Cerebrovascular accidents Toxicosis Environmental toxins (e.g., lead ingestion, methyl mercury ingestion from contaminated fish)

From McCance KL, Huether SE: *Pathophysiology: the biologic basis for disease in adults and children,* ed 6, St Louis, 2010, Mosby.

C. Diagnosis: developmental screening at 9, 18, 24 or 30 months to evaluate basic learning skills and identify any delays. If delays are noted, a comprehensive diagnostic evaluation should be done, including a review of the child's behavior, an interview of the parents, vision and hearing screenings, genetic testing, and additional medical testing as deemed appropriate.

D. Treatment: prognosis not promising, with many autistic children needing lifelong care. Medications used will not cure autism but will help manage high energy levels, depression, the inability to focus, or seizures. The U.S. Food and Drug Administration (FDA) has approved risperidone and aripiprazole (antipsychotics) for children who experience severe tantrums, aggression, and self-injurious behavior. In addition, treatment can include special behavioral and communication approaches, dietary approaches, and complementary and alternative therapies.

E. Nursing interventions
1. Support families and caregivers to conform with developmental and/or medical needs of the child.
2. Provide information on various means of diagnosis and appropriate referral sources.
3. Promote high-quality care for patients with autism by being an advocate in acute care and other medical settings.
4. Implement basic nursing interventions to decrease anxiety and pain for all involved.

Accidents

A. Accidents are the major cause of death in children aged 1 to 14 years, chiefly because of their ability to walk and move more freely than during infancy, along with their unawareness of danger within the environment.

B. Accident prevention during toddlerhood is a major task that requires the involvement of both parents and other family members. Following are several basic suggestions for accident prevention:
1. Supervise play, especially around dangerous areas such as cars, swimming pools, and open flames or hot appliances.
2. Use well-designed, safe car seats or restraints (use rear-facing car seat in the middle of the back seat for infants).
3. Turn all handles of pots and pans in toward the stove, away from the child's reach.
4. Cover electrical outlets with protective plastic caps.
5. Do not allow the child to play with the bathtub faucets; do not leave the child unattended in the bathroom.
6. Keep all medications and poisonous substances out of the child's reach (preferably in a locked cabinet).
7. Know the number and location of the nearest poison control center and hospital.
8. Put up gates at the top and bottom of stairwells.
9. Choose well-made toys appropriate for the child's age, without sharp edges or small removable pieces.
10. Store all guns and dangerous tools and equipment in a locked cabinet.

11. Teach the toddler about common dangers such as "hot" items, looking "both ways" before crossing the street, and water safety.
12. Provide bicycle helmets for toddlers to wear every time they ride a bike.

PRESCHOOL AGE (AGES 3 TO 5 YEARS)

NORMAL GROWTH AND DEVELOPMENT

Physical Development

A. Growth is slow during the preschool years; children gain approximately 5 pounds (2.3 kg) and 2 to 3 inches (5 to 7.5 cm) in height each year.
B. Deciduous teeth are being replaced by permanent teeth. Proper dental hygiene and regular dental checkups are definitely needed at this age level and throughout childhood.
C. Language development of preschoolers is rapid; 3-year-olds talk to themselves and their toys; 4-year-olds begin to talk and communicate more with other people.

Psychosocial Development

A. Preschoolers are in Erikson's stage of "initiative versus guilt"; at this age level they learn how to interact with other children and adults. They also learn the difference between proper and improper behavior and the rewards and disciplines associated with each. Without proper adult guidance, preschoolers can learn improper behavior and develop a sense of guilt and inferiority rather than a sense of initiative and accomplishment.
B. Preschoolers begin to develop their imaginations. They use "magical thinking" and have difficulty distinguishing fantasy from reality.
C. Preschoolers become acutely aware of their sexuality, including their roles as boys or girls and their sex organs. Parents must work with their children in a positive way to help them develop healthy attitudes toward themselves and their bodies.
D. Preschoolers continue to learn through play. They still use parallel play but also begin to use associative play (play with other children) and imitative play (play by imitating the actions of adults or other children).
E. Preschoolers are in stage 2 (preconventional morality) of Kohlberg's "theory of moral development"; they conform to rules to obtain rewards.

HEALTH PROMOTION

A. Immunizations started in infancy and toddlerhood should continue according to schedule (Figure 8-9).
B. Nutrition should be appropriate to age, keeping in mind that growth is slow during this period. Preschoolers should be eating foods from all four basic food groups.

HEALTH PROBLEMS

Communicable Diseases

See Appendix B.

Respiratory Disorders

Tonsillitis and Adenoiditis

A. Definition: inflammation of the tonsils and adenoids caused by chronic URIs
B. Symptoms: sore throat, difficulty in swallowing and breathing ("mouth breathers"), hoarseness, harsh cough
C. Diagnosis: based on symptoms and presence of swelling and redness of tonsils and adenoids on examination
D. Treatment and nursing interventions
1. Acute infections are treated with antibiotics as ordered, increased oral fluids, and warm saltwater gargles.
2. If chronic infections continue after antibiotic treatment, surgery is often indicated (tonsillectomy and adenoidectomy); however, surgery is less common today than it was in the past.
3. Postoperative nursing care measures include keeping the child in a prone position with head to the side until fully awake; monitoring vital signs frequently; checking the throat and nares for active bleeding; keeping the suction equipment at the bedside for emergency use; observing the child for frequent swallowing (this may indicate oozing of blood in the nasopharynx or pharynx); providing analgesic and antipyretic drugs for discomfort; and encouraging cool, clear oral fluids after the nausea has subsided (synthetic juices are less irritating than natural juices). Warm saltwater gargles may be used beginning 1 week after the surgery.
4. Teach the child not to cough, clear the throat, or blow the nose to help decrease risk of bleeding. Provide written instructions to parents regarding postoperative care and possible complications.

Genitourinary Disorders

Nephrotic Syndrome

A. Definition: several different types of kidney conditions resulting in massive proteinuria, hypoalbuminemia, hyperlipemia, and edema; the most common glomerular injury in children. It can be classified as primary (restricted to glomerular injury) or secondary (when it develops as part of a systemic illness).
B. Symptoms: edema of the face, extremities, and abdomen; proteinuria; hypoalbuminemia; respiratory distress; malnutrition; irritability; increased susceptibility to infection
C. Diagnosis: based on decreased serum protein levels; increased proteinuria, edema, and hypocholesterolemia; and results of a renal biopsy
D. Treatment and nursing interventions
1. Nephrotic syndrome is a chronic disorder with remissions and exacerbations, usually lasting 12 to 18 months. Treatment measures continue for an extended period.
2. Corticosteroids are ordered to reduce the edema.
3. An oral alkylating agent, usually cyclophosphamide (Cytoxan), alternating with prednisone (Deltasone), is ordered to reduce the relapse rate and induce long-term remission.
4. Frequent urine testing for protein and albumin
5. Recording of I&O
6. Daily weights
7. Diuretics as ordered (not always effective)
8. Low-salt diet during exacerbations
9. Antibiotics as ordered during exacerbations
10. Proper care of the skin to avoid breakdown caused by the edema
11. Parent teaching for home care regarding medications, diet, and follow-up

Acute Glomerulonephritis

A. Definition: inflammation of the glomeruli and nephrons of the kidney. It may occur as a primary event or as a reaction to an infection (most often streptococcal, pneumococcal, or viral).

B. Symptoms: edema of the face and eyes, anorexia, dark-colored ("tea") urine, oliguria, listlessness, irritability, headache, abdominal discomfort, vomiting, slightly elevated blood pressure, proteinuria. If the disease occurs as a result of a systemic infection, the symptoms occur approximately 10 days after the infection.

C. Diagnosis: based on the symptoms and a positive recent history of streptococcal or other infection

D. Treatment and nursing interventions
   1. Regular activity with rest periods as needed
   2. Antibiotics as ordered (see Chapter 3)
   3. Regular, low-salt diet
   4. Measurement of I&O, observation of color of urine
   5. Frequent checking and recording of blood pressure
   6. Urine testing for protein and specific gravity
   7. Daily weights
   8. Antihypertensives and diuretics for elevated blood pressure as ordered

Circulatory Disorders

Hemophilia

A. Definition: group of bleeding disorders resulting from a congenital deficiency of certain coagulation proteins; X-linked recessive in nature; typed according to which clotting factor is affected

B. Symptoms: prolonged bleeding and clotting times; easy bruising and bleeding into tissues and joints; joint pain

C. Diagnosis: based on symptoms, family health history, and prolonged clotting time

D. Treatment and nursing interventions
   1. Observations for any signs of internal bleeding and shock
   2. Transfusions as ordered with the missing clotting factor
   3. Frequent laboratory tests such as partial thromboplastin time (PTT), clotting time, complete blood count (CBC); screening for human immunodeficiency virus (HIV) and hepatitis (from receiving contaminated transfusions or clotting factors)
   4. Corticosteroids and nonsteroidal antiinflammatory drugs as ordered
   5. Exercise and physical therapy to strengthen muscles around joints
   6. Protection of the child from injuries as much as possible
   7. Emotional support and counseling for the child and parents
   8. Parent teaching regarding follow-up physical examinations, protecting the child from physical harm, the need for immediate care if any injury occurs, and administering the clotting factor to the child
   9. Referrals to community resources such as the National Hemophilia Foundation
   10. Genetic counseling for parents

Leukemia

A. Definition: broad term given to a group of malignant diseases of the bone marrow and lymphatic system; an unrestricted proliferation of immature WBCs in the blood-forming tissues of the body; classified according to its predominant cell type and level of maturity. Acute lymphocytic leukemia (ALL) is the most common (80%) childhood leukemia.

B. Symptoms: The three main consequences of bone marrow dysfunction are anemia, infection, and bleeding. Other symptoms include lethargy, pallor, anorexia, fever, and pain in the bones and joints; petechiae, easy bruising, and sores in the mouth; and decreased RBCs and WBCs.

C. Diagnosis: made on the basis of history, the symptoms, an elevated WBC count, and presence of immature leukocytes and blast cells in a bone marrow biopsy or aspiration specimen

D. Treatment and nursing interventions
   1. Leukemia is a chronic, sometimes fatal, disease with remissions and exacerbations. The child and family need a great deal of emotional support from the physician and nursing staff.
   2. Chemotherapy drugs and corticosteroids as ordered (see Chapter 3)
   3. IV fluids and blood transfusions as ordered
   4. Administration of pain medications as ordered. Joint pain during exacerbations may be severe, especially in the more advanced stages; higher than normal doses are often required.
   5. Proper skin and mouth care
   6. Provision of proper nutrition as the child's condition allows
   7. Prevention of infections whenever possible. Chemotherapy drugs lower the WBC count, which in turn decreases the child's resistance to infection.
   8. Observation for possible side effects of chemotherapy drugs
   9. Bone marrow transplants may be ordered for patients with certain types of leukemia to replace unhealthy bone marrow; an exact match is often difficult to find.
   10. Immunotherapy, passive or active, is a new treatment with the goal of increasing immune response to cancer cells.

Musculoskeletal Disorder

Muscular Dystrophy

A. Definition: group of hereditary muscle diseases (recessive trait) characterized by gradual degeneration of muscle fibers, which is evidenced by muscle wasting and weakness and increasing disability and deformity

B. Symptoms: gradual muscle weakness, including difficulty walking and standing up, a "waddle" gait, and mild mental retardation. Most symptoms appear in children aged 3 to 5 years.

C. Diagnosis: based on the history of the symptoms, family history, muscle biopsy (to determine muscle degeneration), electromyography (EMG), and serum enzyme (creatine phosphokinase [CPK]) measurement

D. Treatment and nursing interventions
   1. No cure has been discovered for muscular dystrophy (MD); thus treatment is supportive. The primary goal is to maintain function in the unaffected muscles for as long as possible.

2. Encourage the child to be as active and lead as normal a life as possible.
3. Provide range-of-motion exercises and physical therapy as ordered to prevent contractures.
4. Use walkers, crutches, braces, and wheelchairs as needed.
5. Provide emotional support for the parents and child; this is a progressive disease, and the family requires ongoing support by the health care team.
6. Frequent medical checkups are necessary to observe for progressive symptoms such as respiratory distress.
7. Genetic counseling for the parents and referral to the Muscular Dystrophy Association for education and community services are advised.

Psychosocial Disorder
Attention-Deficit/Hyperactivity Disorder
A. Definition: Attention-deficit/hyperactivity disorder (ADHD) is the most common chronic behavioral disorder of children; it is associated with problems in attention and concentration, impulse control, and overactivity.
B. Symptoms: behaviors in the categories of inattention (e.g., carelessness, difficulty attending to work and play, easily distracted, does not listen) and impulsivity and hyperactivity (e.g., fidgeting with hands, feet, or hair; difficulty concentrating on quiet activities; excessive talking; unable to remain seated for long periods)
C. Diagnosis: based on the reports of the child, parent, and teacher or teachers. The behavior or symptoms must be present in two out of three areas (home, school, social situations) to support the diagnosis. The American Psychiatric Association requires that a child must exhibit six or more of the common behaviors to be diagnosed with ADHD.
D. Treatment and nursing interventions: The goal of treatment of ADHD is to decrease the frequency and intensity of negative behaviors.
1. Setting realistic expectations for the child when attempting to change behaviors
2. Working with the parents to adapt the environment and develop strategies that support positive behaviors
3. Behavioral therapy and psychotherapy for the child and family
4. Psychostimulant medications (e.g., methylphenidate [Ritalin], dextroamphetamine [Dexedrine], dextroamphetamine and amphetamine [Adderall]) as a possible part of the treatment plan
5. Parent or caregiver education about the disorder and treatment methods

SCHOOL AGE (AGES 6 TO 12 YEARS)

NORMAL GROWTH AND DEVELOPMENT
Physical Development
A. Growth is slow in children between the ages of 6 and 10 years; the child gains 42 to 62 pounds (2 to 3 kg) and 2 inches (5 cm) per year.
B. Bone growth is slow; the cartilage is replaced by bone at the bone epiphyses.

C. Middle childhood (ages 6 to 12 years) is the stage of development when deciduous teeth are shed.

Psychosocial Development
A. School-aged children are in Erikson's stage of "industry versus inferiority"; an eagerness to develop new skills and interests and the processes of cooperating and competing with other children are characteristics of this age that engender a sense of accomplishment rather than a sense of inferiority and poor self-worth.
B. School-aged children are in Kohlberg's stage of conventional morality (level 2); the child conforms to rules to please others.
C. Children ages 7 to 10 years start to become more influenced by their peer group than by their parents; they develop "best friends" and start to separate into boy and girl groups.
D. The most significant skill acquired during the school-age period is the ability to read.

HEALTH PROMOTION
A. Communicable disease prevention is accomplished by timely immunizations, proper rest and diet, and frequent medical and dental checkups.
B. Accident prevention remains a major factor at this age level. Safety measures should include rules for bicycle and skateboard safety (helmets and pads for safety in competitive sports such as baseball, football, and soccer).
C. Sex education should begin at this age level and should be presented by the parents in simple, honest terms. Audiovisual aids such as books and pictures are available to assist parents in presenting the information on the child's level.
D. Education about the dangers of drug and alcohol abuse should begin at this age level.
E. Promotion of a balanced diet continues to be important at this age level; high-calorie, low-nutrition snacks are popular with school-aged children but often lead to excess weight gain.

HEALTH PROBLEMS
Respiratory Disorders: Allergic Conditions
Asthma
A. Definition: chronic inflammatory disorder of the airways, associated with airflow limitation or obstruction caused by edema of the bronchial mucosa, increased mucus production, and bronchial muscle contraction. It is often caused by an allergic response to allergens ("triggers") such as pollen; animal fur; food; or irritants such as tobacco smoke, exercise, cold air, respiratory infections, and changes in the weather. It is the most common chronic disease of childhood.
B. Symptoms: irritability; restlessness; tightness in the chest; hacking, nonproductive cough; dyspnea; and wheezing. Asthma is classified into four categories—mild intermittent, mild persistent, moderate persistent, and severe persistent.
C. Diagnosis: based on the symptoms, physical examination findings, the child's history, family history, and chest x-ray examination that rule out other respiratory diseases and pulmonary function studies (including peak expiratory flow rate)

D. Treatment and nursing interventions
1. Pharmacological therapy used in a stepwise approach based on the child's asthma severity classification; medications categorized as long-term control (preventive) and quick relief
2. Bronchodilator medications as ordered (administered by inhalation, mouth, or injection) (see Chapter 3)
3. Antiinflammatory medications, either corticosteroids (prednisone) or nonsteroidal agents (cromolyn sodium), administered by inhalation, mouth, or injection
4. Chest physiotherapy
5. IV fluids as ordered
6. Liquid diet progressing to a regular diet
7. Identification and removal of the allergens if possible
8. Parent and child teaching regarding home care, including medications, use of nebulizer or metered-dose inhaler (MDI), removal of any potential triggers, use of peak flow meter to measure peak expiratory flow rate, and follow-up examinations

Allergic Rhinitis (Hay Fever)
A. Definition: inflammation of nasal passages caused by sensitivity to some pollen, dust, or animal fur
B. Symptoms: sneezing; runny nose; postnasal drip; and watery, itchy eyes
C. Diagnosis: based on symptoms and results of allergy testing done to discover specific allergen
D. Treatment and nursing interventions
1. Find and remove the allergen if possible.
2. Provide antihistamines or decongestants as ordered.
3. Immunotherapy may be necessary if symptoms cannot be controlled.

Gastrointestinal Disorders
Appendicitis
A. Definition: inflammation of the appendix, often after an infection elsewhere in the body
B. Symptoms: localized abdominal tenderness in the right lower quadrant (increased on rebound during palpation), abdominal rigidity, decreased bowel sounds, fever, nausea and vomiting, constipation
C. Diagnosis: based on the symptoms, physical examination findings, and WBC count (usually elevated); abdominal ultrasound and CT scan may also be used.
D. Treatment and nursing interventions
1. Removal of the inflamed appendix (appendectomy), preferably before it ruptures and spreads the infection throughout the abdomen, causing peritonitis
2. Routine postoperative care, including monitoring vital signs, frequently observing the incision or dressing for bleeding, careful recording I&O, and administering IV fluids as ordered
3. Administration of antibiotics as ordered because of possible infection or a ruptured appendix
4. Administration of pain medication as ordered

Pinworms
A. Definition: worms that affect the intestine. The worms or eggs are swallowed and spread easily from person to person by the hands, linen, or food.
B. Symptoms; itching around the anus (especially at night), sleeplessness, anorexia, and diarrhea

C. Diagnosis: made by the cellophane tape test. The eggs are captured from the anal area during the night or early morning hours by placing a tongue blade covered with cellophane tape at the anal opening; the worms come out of the intestine at night to lay their eggs, and the eggs are picked up on the tape.
D. Treatment and nursing interventions
1. Use good handwashing technique to prevent spread of the worms and reinfection; keep fingernails short.
2. Frequently change underwear and linen.
3. Medication of choice is mebendazole (Vermox) for children over 2 years of age.
4. Examine and treat all family members because pinworms are easily transmitted.

Nervous System Disorder
Epilepsy
A. Definition: chronic seizure disorder with recurrent and unprovoked seizures. Although many causes can be found for seizures, most are idiopathic.
B. Symptoms: classification of seizures (Box 8-1)
C. Diagnosis: based on the evidence of seizures; differentiation of the type of seizure by physical examination, neurological assessment, patient history, and changes in the electroencephalogram (EEG) (changes in the brain wave patterns)
D. Treatment and nursing interventions
1. Anticonvulsant medications as ordered (see Chapter 3)
2. Parent and child education regarding medications and the necessity of taking them as prescribed, safety factors, actions to take if the child has a seizure at home, and the importance of follow-up physical examinations and laboratory work (to measure blood levels of anticonvulsants)
3. In some children with poorly controlled seizures, a ketogenic diet (either with or without the use of anticonvulsants) has been tried with moderate success. Children on this strict diet must be observed closely by a dietitian, neurologist, and pediatrician. The diet is adhered to for 1 to 3 years.
4. Community referrals to support groups such as the Epilepsy Foundation of America

Musculoskeletal Disorder
Scoliosis
A. Definition: lateral S-shaped curvature of the spine; can be congenital or caused by a variety of conditions but most often has no known cause (idiopathic); most often seen in young girls and most noticeable at the time of the preadolescent growth spurt
B. Symptoms: poor posture, uneven length of legs, asymmetry of shoulder and hip height, pelvic obliquity
C. Diagnosis: based on symptoms, x-ray examination, and physical examination
D. Treatment and nursing interventions
1. A brace (Milwaukee brace or Boston brace) or splint is often used along with exercises to prevent an increase in the degree of curvature; this may be the only treatment, or it may be used before surgery.
2. Spinal fusion may be necessary to correct severe scoliosis. Provide postoperative care as indicated.

| Box **8-1** | Classification of Seizures and Epilepsy Syndromes |

PARTIAL SEIZURES

Simple Partial Seizures with Motor Signs

Characterized by:

- Localized motor symptoms
- Somatosensory, psychic, autonomic symptoms
- Combination of these
- Abnormal discharges remain unilateral.

Manifestations:

- Aversive seizure (most common motor seizure in children)—Eye or eyes and head turn away from the side of the focus; awareness of movement or loss of consciousness
- Rolandic (Sylvan) seizure—Tonic-clonic movements involving the face, salivation, arrested speech; most common during sleep
- Jacksonian march (rare in children)—Orderly, sequential progression of clonic movements beginning in a foot, hand, or face and moving, or "marching," to adjacent body parts

Simple Partial Seizures with Sensory Signs

Uncommon in children under 8 years of age
Characterized by various sensations, including:

- Numbness, tingling, prickling, paresthesias, or pain originating in one area (e.g., face, extremities) and spreading to other parts of the body
- Visual sensations or formed images
- Motor phenomena such as posturing or hypertonia

Complex Partial Seizures (Psychomotor Seizures)

Observed more often in children from 3 years through adolescence
Characterized by:

- Period of altered behavior
- Amnesia for event (no recollection of behavior)
- Inability to respond to environment
- Impaired consciousness during event
- Drowsiness or sleep usually after seizure
- Possible prolonged confusion and amnesia
- Complex sensory phenomena (aura)—Most frequent sensation is strange feeling in the pit of the stomach that rises toward the throat and is often accompanied by odd or unpleasant odors or tastes; complex auditory or visual hallucinations; ill-defined feelings of elation or strangeness (e.g., déjà vu, a feeling of familiarity in a strange environment); strong feelings of fear and anxiety; a distorted sense of time and self; and in small children, emission of a cry or attempt to run for help

Patterns of motor behavior:

- Stereotypic
- Similar with each subsequent seizure
- May suddenly cease activity, appear dazed, stare into space, become confused and apathetic, and become limp or stiff or display some form of posturing
- May be confused
- May perform purposeless, complicated activities in a repetitive manner (automatisms) such as walking, running, kicking, laughing, or speaking incoherently; most often followed by postictal confusion or sleep; may exhibit

oropharyngeal activities such as smacking, chewing, drooling, swallowing, and nausea or abdominal pain followed by stiffness, a fall, and postictal sleep; rage or temper tantrums rare; aggressive acts uncommon during seizure

GENERALIZED SEIZURES

Tonic-Clonic Seizures

Formerly known as *grand mal seizures*
Most common and most dramatic of all seizure manifestations
Occur without warning
Tonic phase: lasts approximately 10 to 20 seconds
Manifestations:

- Eyes roll upward
- Immediate loss of consciousness
- If standing, falls to floor or ground
- Stiffens in generalized, symmetrical tonic contraction of entire body musculature
- Arms usually flexed
- Legs, head, and neck extended
- May utter a peculiar piercing cry
- Apneic; may become cyanotic
- Increased salivation and loss of swallowing reflex
- Violent jerking movements as the trunk and extremities undergo rhythmical contraction and relaxation
- May foam at the mouth
- May be incontinent of urine and feces

As event ends, movements less intense, occurring at longer intervals and then ceasing entirely
Status epilepticus: series of seizures at intervals too brief to allow the child to regain consciousness between the time one event ends and the next begins

- Requires emergency intervention
- Can lead to exhaustion, respiratory failure, and death

Postictal state:

- Appears to relax
- May remain semiconscious and difficult to arouse
- May awaken in a few minutes
- Remains confused for several hours
- Poor coordination
- Mild impairment of fine motor movements
- May have visual and speech difficulties
- May vomit or complain of severe headache
- When left alone, usually sleeps for several hours
- On awakening is fully conscious
- Usually feels tired and complains of sore muscles and headache
- No recollection of entire event

Absence Seizures

Formerly called *petit mal seizures* or lapses
Characterized by:

- Onset usually between 4 and 12 years of age
- More common in girls than boys
- Usually cease at puberty
- Brief loss of consciousness
- Minimal or no alteration in muscle tone

Box 8-1   Classification of Seizures and Epilepsy Syndromes—cont'd

- May go unrecognized because of little change in child's behavior
- Abrupt onset; suddenly develops 20 or more attacks daily
- Event often mistaken for inattentiveness or daydreaming
- Events possibly precipitated by hyperventilation, hypoglycemia, stresses (emotional and physiologic), fatigue, or sleeplessness

Manifestations:
- Brief loss of consciousness
- Appear without warning or aura
- Usually last about 5 to 10 seconds
- Slight loss of muscle tone that may cause child to drop objects
- Ability to maintain postural control; seldom falls
- Minor movements such as lip smacking, twitching of eyelids or face, or slight hand movements
- Not accompanied by incontinence
- Amnesia for episode
- May need to reorient self to previous activity

Atonic and Akinetic Seizures

Also known as *drop attacks*

Characterized by:
- Onset usually between 2 and 5 years of age
- Sudden, momentary loss of muscle tone and postural control
- Events recurring frequently during the day, particularly in the morning hours and shortly after awakening

Manifestations:
- Loss of tone causing child to fall to the floor violently
- Unable to break fall by putting out hand
- May incur a serious injury to the face, head, or shoulder
- Loss of consciousness only momentary

Myoclonic Seizures

A variety of seizure episodes

May be isolated as benign essential myoclonus
May occur in association with other seizure forms

Characterized by:
- Sudden, brief contractures of a muscle or group of muscles
- Occur singly or repetitively
- No postictal state
- May or may not be symmetrical
- May or may not include loss of consciousness

Infantile Spasms

Also called *infantile myoclonus, massive spasms, hypsarrhythmia, salaam episodes,* and *infantile myoclonic spasms*

Most commonly occur during the first 6 to 8 months of life

Twice as common in boys as girls

Numerous seizures during the day without postictal drowsiness or sleep

Poor outlook for normal intelligence

Manifestations:
- Possible series of sudden, brief, symmetrical muscular contractions
- Head flexed, arms extended, and legs drawn up
- Eyes sometimes rolling upward or inward
- May be preceded or followed by a cry or giggling
- May or may not include loss of consciousness
- Sometimes flushing, pallor, or cyanosis

Infants who are able to sit but not stand:
- Sudden dropping forward of the head and neck with trunk flexed forward and knees drawn up—the "salaam" or "jack-knife" seizure
- Less often: alternate clinical forms observed
- Extensor spasms rather than flexion of arms, legs, and trunk and head nodding
- Lightning events involving a single, momentary, shocklike contraction of the entire body

From Hockenberry MJ, Wilson D: *Wong's essentials of pediatric nursing,* ed 9, St Louis, 2013, Mosby.

Integumentary Disorders

Ringworm

A. Definition: fungal infection transferred from person to person or from animal to person. It can occur on the scalp (tinea capitis), the body (tinea corporis), or the feet (tinea pedis) (Figure 8-13).

B. Symptoms: small papules that have a distinct red ring with a clear center; dry, scaly skin; and itching on the affected part

C. Diagnosis: based on the symptoms

D. Treatment and nursing interventions
  1. Washing the affected areas with soap and water and removal of crusts
  2. Applying antifungal ointment to affected areas as ordered
  3. Antifungal oral medication as ordered (see Chapter 3); tinea capitis treated orally for 1 month

Pediculosis

A. Definition: infestation by lice of the scalp and hairy areas of the body

B. Symptoms: severe itching in the affected area, appearance of lice on the hair or clothing

C. Diagnosis: based on the symptoms

D. Treatment and nursing interventions

  1. Pediculicide shampoo to hair or scalp as ordered; remaining nits are removed with an extra-fine-toothed comb.
  2. Systemic trimethoprim-sulfamethoxazole (Bactrim) used to treat resistant head lice
  3. Washing of all linens and clothing in hot water to destroy the nits (small lice) and eggs of the lice
  4. Emphasis on importance of follow-up treatment to prevent reinfestation
  5. Examination and treatment of other family members (if affected)
  6. Reporting to school or day-care facility

Hives (Urticaria)

A. Definition: allergic reaction on the skin, usually caused by an allergy to food or drugs

B. Symptoms: bright red, raised wheals on the skin and itching of the affected areas

C. Diagnosis: based on the symptoms; allergy testing to determine the specific allergen

D. Treatment and nursing interventions
  1. Determination and removal of the allergen
  2. Antihistamines as ordered to decrease the swelling and inflammation

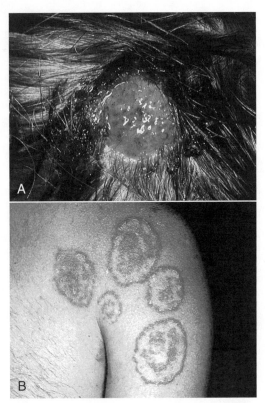

FIGURE 8-13 **A,** Tinea capitis. **B,** Tinea corporis. Both infections are caused by *Microsporum canis,* the "kitten" or "puppy" fungus. (From Habif TP: *Clinical dermatology: a color guide to diagnosis and therapy,* ed 4, St Louis, 2004, Mosby.)

3. Cool-water soaks to the affected areas to decrease the itching
4. Local soothing antipruritic lotions to affected areas as ordered
5. Keeping the child's nails short to avoid scratching and possible infection

Rheumatic Fever

A. Definition: autoimmune reaction to a group A beta-hemolytic streptococcal pharyngitis (strep throat); involves the joints, skin, brain, and heart
B. Symptoms: begin 2 to 6 weeks after the initial streptococcal infection; lethargy, anorexia, muscle and joint pain, fever, polyarthritis, chorea (muscle tremors and emotional upset), and carditis (Figure 8-14)
C. Diagnosis is based on symptoms utilizing the Jones Criteria which requires that two major or one major and one minor criteria are present in addition to definite evidence of a previous streptococcal infection, such as a positive throat culture for Group A beta-hemolytic streptococci or recent scarlet fever.

Major criteria include the following:
1. Carditis that involves all layers of cardiac tissue.
2. Polyarthritis of knees, ankles, elbows, and wrists.
3. Chorea which are abrupt purposeless movements (Sydenham chorea).
4. Non-pruritic rash (erythema marginatum) affecting the trunk and proximal extremities.
5. Subcutaneous nodules which are firm and painless occurring over bones or tendons.

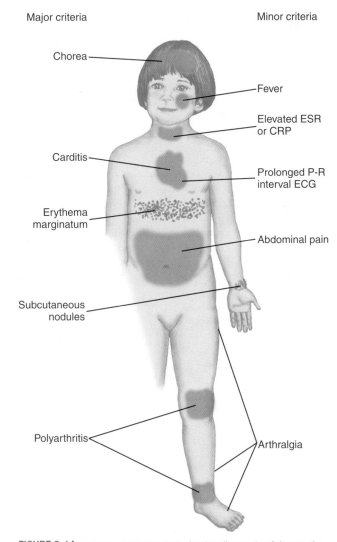

FIGURE 8-14 Major and minor criteria for the diagnosis of rheumatic fever. (From Price DL, Gwin JF: *Pediatric nursing: an introductory text,* ed 11, St Louis, 2012, Saunders.)

Minor criteria include fever, arthralgia, history of rheumatic fever or rheumatic heart disease, prolonged P-R interval on ECG, and acute phase reactants (leukocytosis and elevated ESR and C-reactive protein).
D. Treatment and nursing interventions
1. Bed rest to decrease the workload on the heart and help prevent or ease the carditis
2. Feeding meals to the child during strict bed rest
3. Medications as ordered, including salicylates for pain, steroids to decrease inflammation of the muscle and connective tissue, and antibiotics to fight infection (penicillin is the drug of choice) (see Chapter 3)
4. Emotional support and nonstressful diversion for the child during bed rest
5. Monitoring frequent laboratory tests, including the WBC count and the erythrocyte sedimentation rate (ESR) (elevated in inflammatory diseases)
6. Parent and child teaching for home care, including the need for rest, proper nutrition, proper administration of medications, and prophylactic antibiotic therapy before dental work and invasive procedures

Diabetes Mellitus

A. Definition: In type 1 diabetes the beta cells of the pancreas stop producing insulin, which is necessary for the metabolism of fats, carbohydrates, and proteins. Peak incidence is 10 to 15 years of age

B. Symptoms: rapid onset of symptoms, including easy fatigability, polydipsia (excessive thirst), polyphagia (increased appetite), polyuria (increased urine output), glycosuria (glucose in the urine), and weight loss

C. Diagnosis: based on symptoms, blood glucose levels, and presence of glucose and ketones in the urine

D. Treatment and nursing interventions

   1. Daily insulin administration by subcutaneous injections (usually twice per day) or by means of a portable insulin pump (see Chapter 3)

   2. Meal plan that includes three meals and between-meal snacks as planned by a dietitian, based on the child's age, weight, blood sugar levels, and normal eating pattern

   3. Routine blood sugar monitoring: Chemstrips, Accu-Chek, or one-touch glucometers commonly used for this purpose

   4. Routine urine testing for glucose and ketones

   5. Child and parent teaching regarding insulin injection technique, diet, exercise, urine testing, blood glucose monitoring, signs of hypoglycemia and hyperglycemia, sick day rules, long-term complications, and need for regular follow-up visits to the pediatrician

   6. Support group for parents and child

ADOLESCENCE (AGES 13 TO 19 YEARS)

NORMAL GROWTH AND DEVELOPMENT

Physical Development

A. During the adolescent period a growth spurt takes place; this accelerated growth includes an increase in both height and weight. In girls this occurs at 10 to 12 years of age; in boys it occurs at 12 to 14 years of age.

B. Secondary sex characteristics also develop during early adolescence.

   1. In girls the pelvis widens, the breasts develop and enlarge, and body hair starts to appear.

   2. In boys the penis and scrotum enlarge, and pubic and facial hair start to appear. Puberty in boys officially begins with the first nocturnal emission.

Psychological and Emotional Development

A. Adolescence is the time of transition from childhood to adulthood. Adolescents are in Erikson's stage of "identity versus role confusion"; they are in the process of developing a self-image or a sense of identity about who they are and what they want in life. If they do not develop a positive self-image and identity, they may develop a sense of inferiority, or a negative self-image.

B. Adolescents are in Kohlberg's stage of morality known as self-accepted moral principles (level 3); the focus is on individual rights and principles of conscience, with a concern for what is best for all.

C. Development of a positive self-image and healthy personality depends a great deal on the adolescents' relationships with their peer group and family.

D. Body image is a major part of adolescents' self-concept; sexuality and sexual feelings are a new part of their body image. Physical appearance is important to how they perceive themselves as being accepted by their peer group.

   1. Boys' responses to puberty include pleasure at becoming a "man" as evidenced by enlargement of the sex organs, being able to shave, and the sexual feelings they begin to have during this stage. Because of their strong sex drive, they often masturbate to relieve themselves of strong sexual tension.

   2. Girls' responses to puberty include a developing awareness of their body changes, both internal and external (e.g., hormonal changes, menstruation). The sex drive in girls is usually not as strong as it is in boys.

HEALTH PROMOTION

A. Immunizations and physical examinations should continue according to schedule (Figure 8-9, *B*).

B. Counseling and sex education, especially concerning acquired immunodeficiency syndrome (AIDS), venereal disease, and birth control, should continue to be made available to all adolescents.

C. Counseling regarding drug and alcohol abuse should continue to be presented and readily available to all adolescents who are in need of it.

D. Emotional stress is high during adolescence; psychiatric counseling is necessary for some adolescents to work through their stresses and fears.

E. Proper nutrition needs may not be met because of increased snacking, especially on high-calorie, high-fat foods; nutritional counseling may be helpful.

HEALTH PROBLEMS

Substance Abuse (Drugs, Alcohol)

A. Definition: abuse of alcohol or mood-altering drugs, usually because of peer pressure or increased tension and stress

B. Signs of abuse: increased school absences, poor academic performance, changes in behavior patterns, wearing dark glasses inside, wearing long-sleeved shirts or blouses every day, and having a sloppy, unclean appearance; signs often dependent on the drug being used

C. Diagnosis: based on the symptoms (signs of abuse)

D. Substances abused

   1. Alcohol

   2. Narcotics

   3. Psychedelic drugs (lysergic acid diethylamide [LSD], marijuana, phencyclidine [PCP])

   4. Depressants (barbiturates, methaqualone [Quaalude])

   5. Minor tranquilizers (diazepam [Valium])

   6. Hallucinogens (marijuana, LSD, PCP)

   7. Analgesics (codeine)

   8. Opiates (heroin, morphine, methadone)

   9. Organic solvents (e.g., glue, cleaning fluids)

   10. Stimulants (amphetamines ["speed"]; cocaine; 3,4-methylenedioxy-*N*-methylamphetamine [MDMA] ecstasy; rohypnol—"date rape" drug)

   11. Inhalants

   12. Tobacco

E. Treatment and nursing interventions

   1. Prevention of the problem is the best treatment.

   2. Perform emergency measures when necessary (e.g., CPR, gastric lavage)

3. Provide psychiatric counseling as needed for the adolescent and family. Identify reason or reasons for drug abuse.
4. Provide follow-up health care, group support, and counseling as needed for adolescent and family.

Suicide

A. Definition: act of taking one's own life voluntarily
B. Etiology: Suicide usually does not occur without warning. The adolescent usually has a history of emotional problems; difficult relationships; and emotional upsets, including factors such as divorce in the family, death of a family member or friend, or a self-identity crisis.
C. Treatment and nursing interventions
   1. Prevention is the best treatment. Listen for verbal clues such as, "After tomorrow, it won't matter anymore." Watch for warning signs such as giving away favorite possessions.
   2. Provide psychiatric counseling to determine the reasons for the adolescent's actions; this should also include the family members.
   3. Provide follow-up medical care as needed.
   4. Provide emotional support and counseling for the family members, especially during the crisis stages.

Anorexia Nervosa and Bulimia

A. Definition (eating disorders can occur together or separately)
   1. Anorexia nervosa: eating disorder characterized by a refusal to maintain a minimally normal body weight; most often seen in female adolescents
   2. Bulimia: eating disorder characterized by repeated episodes of "binge eating," followed by inappropriate compensatory measures such as self-induced vomiting; misuse of laxatives, diuretics, or other medications; fasting; or excessive exercise
B. Symptoms
   1. With anorexia nervosa, three basic psychological disturbances occur: the inability to correctly perceive body size, the absence of hunger or inability to perceive hunger, and feelings of inadequacy or lack of self-esteem. Other symptoms include amenorrhea, constipation, dry skin, low blood pressure, anemia, and lanugo (fine, soft hair) on the back and arms.
   2. With bulimia, as the disease progresses, the frequency of binges increases; the adolescent loses control over the binge-purge cycle. Other symptoms include loss of tooth enamel, dental caries, esophageal varices.
C. Diagnosis: based on symptoms, family history, and psychological evaluation
D. Treatment and nursing interventions
   1. The adolescent is usually hospitalized to correct the malnutrition and identify and treat the psychological cause.
   2. Behavior-modification techniques are often used to assist in changing the adolescent's behavior (e.g., privileges or visitors are withdrawn until the adolescent begins to gain weight).
   3. Psychological counseling is provided for the adolescent and family members to determine the cause.

Crohn Disease

A. Definition: chronic, recurrent inflammatory disorder of the intestines; occurs most often in upper-middle-class men and women aged 15 to 35 years
B. Symptoms: regional ileitis causing acute low abdominal pain, fever, chronic diarrhea, weight loss, abdominal tenderness and distention, anemia, and failure to grow
C. Diagnosis based on the symptoms, x-ray films of the intestine (barium enema), endoscopy, and mucosal biopsy of the intestines
D. Treatment and nursing interventions
   1. Goal of treatment: relieve symptoms and discomfort
   2. Adequate rest and relaxation to alleviate stress
   3. High-protein, high-calorie, low-fiber diet
   4. Corticosteroids as ordered to decrease inflammation of the intestines
   5. Sulfasalazine as ordered (because this interferes with the absorption of folic acid, folic acid may be ordered)
   6. Antidiarrheal drugs as ordered
   7. Antispasmodic drugs as ordered to relieve intestinal spasms
   8. Emotional support and psychological counseling as needed to decrease the stress level

Mononucleosis

A. Definition: acute infectious viral disease, causing an increase in mononuclear WBCs and signs of general infection; usually thought to be only mildly contagious and is spread by oral contact; Epstein-Barr virus principal cause
B. Symptoms: general malaise; sore throat; fever; enlarged lymph glands; lack of energy; headache; red, flat rash on the body; tonsillitis
C. Diagnosis: based on the symptoms, an elevated WBC count, and a positive Monospot blood test result, which indicates increased agglutinins in the blood count
D. Treatment and nursing interventions
   1. Antibiotics as ordered
   2. Antipyretics to relieve fever and discomfort
   3. Increased oral fluids; possible IV fluids for severe dehydration
   4. Gargles or lozenges as ordered for sore throat
   5. Adequate rest and sleep
   6. Diet as tolerated. If the patient can tolerate only fluids, high-calorie fluids are provided.
   7. Patient teaching regarding follow-up care, including the need for adequate rest and sleep

Acne Vulgaris

A. Definition: disorder of the sebaceous glands. The glands become irritated with the secretion of sebum and the interaction of the sebum with the hormones; the glands become impacted with sebum and form comedones (noninflamed) and papules and pustules (inflamed).
B. Symptoms: the appearance of the comedones, papules, and pustules on the face; they can also appear on other places on the body such as the chest and back.
C. Diagnosis: based on the symptoms
D. Treatment and nursing interventions
   1. Clean the affected areas with soap or soap substitute and water daily.
   2. Diet should be low in greasy foods, chocolate, and nuts to help decrease the amount of oil in the skin while avoiding other foods that tend to exacerbate the condition.
   3. Nonprescription topical creams and lotions (e.g., benzoyl peroxide, tretinoin [Retin-A]) have limited

effectiveness; retinoic acid (Accutane) is reserved for severe acne that has not responded to other treatments. A pregnancy test should be done before a patient begins taking Accutane.

4. Encouraging the adolescent to keep stress levels to a minimum when possible may help in keeping acne to a minimum.

5. Provide patient teaching: Papules and pustules should not be squeezed; they can become infected and spread.

6. Provide counseling for the adolescent to maintain a positive body image.

Acquired Immunodeficiency Syndrome

A. Definition: an immune disorder caused by the retrovirus HIV

1. The AIDS virus is known to be transmitted by blood and other body fluids containing blood (semen; saliva) (see Chapters 5 and 7).

2. Three primary modes of transmission of the AIDS virus in children are prenatal exposure to infected mothers, blood transfusion, and engaging in high-risk activities (sexual or IV drug use, specifically with adolescents).

3. As of June 2000 more than 8800 children younger than 13 years with AIDS had been reported to the Centers for Disease Control and Prevention (CDC); however, estimates suggest that 1.4 million children younger than 15 years are living with HIV/AIDS. The majority of children with HIV are younger than 7 years. The number of adolescents with HIV continues to increase. AIDS is the ninth leading cause of death in the United States for people aged 15 to 24 years.

B. Symptoms: recurrent or chronic infections (because of decreased number of CD4 T cells), including meningitis, pneumonia, and urinary tract infections; fever; weight loss; FTT; anemia; hepatosplenomegaly; persistent lymphadenopathy

C. Diagnosis: abnormal laboratory values, including abnormal T-cell ratio, decreased T lymphocytes, and hypergammaglobulinemia; history of possible exposure to AIDS virus; positive HIV test; and history of recurrent infections

D. Treatment and nursing interventions

1. No cure has been discovered for AIDS; thus treatment and nursing care measures are supportive and designed to prevent and alleviate opportunistic infections.

2. Antiretroviral drugs work to prevent reproduction of new virus particles and delay the progression of the disease (see Chapter 3).

3. Administer antibiotics and antifungal drugs as ordered (see Chapter 3).

4. IV gamma globulin may be helpful in compensating for the deficiency of B lymphocytes.

5. Instruct in adequate nutrition and fluid intake.

6. Use Standard Precautions when caring for the child in the hospital, clinic, or home.

7. Maintain an environment as free from infection as possible.

8. Immunizations against childhood diseases (and the pneumococcal and influenza vaccines) should be given; however, inactivated poliovirus should be given rather than the oral poliovirus.

9. Promote normal development of the child.

10. Provide education and emotional support for the child and family.

E. Prognosis: poor, especially in children with AIDS who are younger than 1 year

BATTERED CHILD SYNDROME

A. Definition: abuse of children by parents or other caregivers. The abuse can be physical, sexual, nutritional, or emotional and can occur at any age.

B. Characteristics of battered children

1. They are often from an unplanned pregnancy.

2. Many of them were premature, had a low birth weight, or had major birth defects.

3. They sometimes resemble a person that the parents disliked.

C. Characteristics of abusive parents

1. One parent often has a previous emotional problem.

2. One parent is usually the abuser; the other parent knows about the abuse but usually does not report it.

3. Abusive parents often have very high expectations of their children; if they do not perform up to these expectations, they are punished.

4. Abusive parents are often substance abusers.

5. The most common characteristic of abusive parents is that often they were abused themselves as children; however, this is not always true.

6. Abusive parents come from all socioeconomic levels.

D. Identifying the battered child

1. The child has many scars, bruises, and injuries that are not consistent with the explanation of the injuries; many of these markings are characteristic of abuse (Figure 8-15).

2. Bone fractures may be seen on x-ray examination at various stages of healing.

3. The child exhibits signs of physical neglect: malnourishment or improper or dirty clothing.

4. The parents' explanations of the child's injury are inconsistent; one parent's explanation differs from the other parent's, or it changes from one time to the next.

5. The child withdraws when approached by the parents, nurse, or physician.

6. The parents' emotional reaction is inconsistent with the extent of the child's injury.

E. Nursing interventions for the battered child and parents

1. Interview the parents calmly regarding the history of the incident; document all information carefully.

2. Nursing personnel must control their own feelings and attitudes toward the parents to work effectively with the family.

3. Provide physical care for the child as needed.

4. Emotional care for the child should include providing a safe environment, explaining all procedures, providing toys and familiar belongings while the child is hospitalized, and providing physical cuddling and holding when appropriate.

5. Referrals should be made to the hospital social worker, the local department of children and family services, the police, and the psychologist as needed. Nurses are considered "mandated reporters" and must report all suspected and confirmed cases of abuse and neglect.

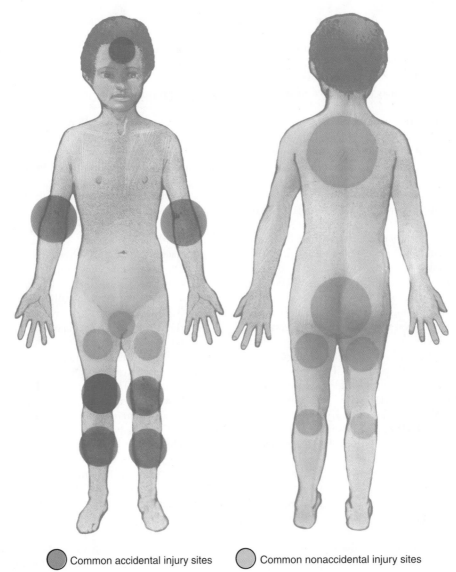

○ Common accidental injury sites   ○ Common nonaccidental injury sites

FIGURE 8-15 Accidents typically cause injuries in specific sites (dark circles). The nurse should suspect physical abuse in children with injuries in nonaccidental sites (light circles). (From Price DL, Gwin JF: *Pediatric nursing: an introductory text,* ed 11, St Louis, 2012, Saunders.)

POISONINGS

A. The most common age for poisoning deaths in young children in the United States is 1 to 4 years. Most poisonings occur as a result of oral ingestion. Children are poisoned by plants, insecticides, household and personal care products, medicines, vitamins, lead, and carbon monoxide.

B. Assessment and treatment begin with an accurate history of the ingestion. Laboratory tests are performed to assess serum levels of the substance involved. Other laboratory tests and x-ray examinations are performed as needed.

C. When a child who has ingested a poison arrives at the hospital, the first step in treatment is to assess the airway, breathing, and circulation (ABC). When the child's condition has been stabilized, the main goals are to remove the poison, prevent further absorption of the poison, and limit complications.

D. Treatment is specific to the type of poison ingested (Table 8-3).

HOSPITALIZATION AND THE CHILD

A. Preparation for hospitalization
1. The rationale for preparing children for hospitalization is based on the theory that fear of the unknown is more severe than fear of the known.
2. Preadmission preparation can be done by both parents and professionals (nurses and physicians) honestly at a level the child can understand.
3. Hospital admission procedures include the admission history, blood tests, chest x-ray studies when necessary, physical examination, and placement in the child's room and bed; these procedures should be explained to the child during preadmission preparation.
4. Establish a good working relationship with the parents by answering their questions honestly. In preparing the child for any hospital procedure, the nurse or parent should include all necessary information regarding the procedure and any necessary preparation. Time should be allowed for questions from the child and parents.

Table 8-3   **Common Poisonous Substances**

SUBSTANCE	PATHOPHYSIOLOGY	CLINICAL MANIFESTATIONS	TREATMENT
ACETAMINOPHEN (TYLENOL, MANY OVER-THE-COUNTER PRODUCTS)			
Toxic dose is uncertain; do not exceed recommended levels. Seriousness of ingestion is determined by amount ingested and length of time before intervention and whether it is an acute or accumulative toxicity. Other factors such as decreased oral intake have been linked with hepatotoxicity.	Metabolic byproducts deplete liver glutathione and cause damage to hepatic cells. Children younger than 6 yr seem to be more resistant to development of hepatotoxicity than do older children and adults.	First stage (first 24 hr): malaise, nausea, vomiting, sweating, pallor, weakness Second stage (24-48 hr): latent period, with a rise in liver enzymes (aspartate and alanine aminotransferase) and bilirubin, right upper quadrant pain, prolonged prothrombin time Third stage (3-7 days): jaundice, liver necrosis, signs of hepatic failure Fourth stage (5-7 days): recovery or progression to death	Administer antidote: *N*-acetylcysteine (Mucomyst) as ordered. IV fluids Sodium-restricted, high-calorie, high-protein diet
SALICYLATES (ASPIRIN, MANY OVER-THE-COUNTER PRODUCTS, OIL OF WINTERGREEN)			
Toxic dose is single dose exceeding 200-280 mg/kg. Peak gastric absorption occurs within 2 hr of ingestion.	First stage: stimulation of respiratory center, leading to respiratory alkalosis Second stage: loss of potassium; increase in metabolic rate; accumulation of ketones, leading to metabolic acidosis, hypokalemia, and dehydration Inhibition of prothrombin formation, decreased platelet levels and adhesiveness, capillary fragility (chronic poisoning)	GI effects: nausea, vomiting, thirst CNS effects: hyperventilation, tinnitus, confusion, seizures, coma, respiratory failure, circulatory collapse Renal effect: oliguria Hematopoietic effects: bleeding tendencies Metabolic effects: sweating, dehydration, fever, hyponatremia, hypokalemia, dehydration, hypoglycemia	IV fluids, sodium bicarbonate (enhances excretion), potassium replacement; volume expanders as needed to support circulation Vitamin K for bleeding tendencies (chronic poisoning) Glucose for hypoglycemia Hemodialysis in severe cases if child unresponsive to therapy
CORROSIVES (TOILET AND DRAIN CLEANERS, BLEACH, AMMONIA)			
Extent of damage depends on causticity of substance and amount ingested.	Severe chemical burns of mouth, throat, esophagus; "splash" burns of eyes and skin Alkali substances can continue to cause damage after initial contact. If damage is severe, long-term care is needed, including gastric button or tube, repeated esophageal dilations, and surgical repair of esophagus, sometimes with colon tissue transplant (done when child is older).	Whitish burns of mouth and pharynx, darkening color (red, swollen, oozing as ulcerations form and tissue erodes) Edema, difficulty swallowing, drooling Respiratory distress, pain Difficulty swallowing; possible esophageal strictures caused by subsequent healing of burns Several burns causing perforation, which can lead to vascular collapse and shock	IV fluids while on NPO status Analgesics, steroids, antibiotics, nasogastric tube feedings
HYDROCARBONS (GASOLINE, KEROSENE, PAINT THINNER, LIGHTER FLUID, TURPENTINE, FURNITURE POLISH)			
Extent of damage depends on amount of substance ingested.	Chemical pneumonitis from aspiration of hydrocarbon Pneumonia and acute hemorrhagic necrotizing disease, usually in 24 hr	Burning sensation in mouth and pharynx Characteristic petroleum breath odor Nausea, vomiting, anorexia, CNS depression, fever Respiratory distress, wheezing	Prevent vomiting. Support ventilation; administer oxygen. IV fluids

Continued

Table 8-3 Common Poisonous Substances—cont'd

SUBSTANCE	PATHOPHYSIOLOGY	CLINICAL MANIFESTATIONS	TREATMENT
LEAD (PAINT CHIPS FROM OLDER HOMES, SOIL CONTAMINATED WITH LEAD, LEAD SOLDER USED IN PLUMBING, VINYL MINI BLINDS, IMPROPERLY GLAZED POTTERY, TOYS)			
Diet high in fat and low in iron and calcium increases lead absorption. Serum lead level >10 mcg/dL: considered harmful 10-15 mcg/dL: more frequent screening indicated 15-20 mcg/dL: nutritional and educational interventions and environmental investigation >20 mcg/dL: possible removal and treatment	GI tract is a major route of absorption. Lead is deposited in blood, bone, and soft tissue. Major toxic effects occur in bone marrow, nervous system, and kidney. Amount of lead ingested, size of particle, and repeated ingestion over time contribute to severity of lead poisoning.	Symptoms may be vague with insidious onset. CNS effects: irritability, lethargy, hyperactivity, cognitive and perceptual-motor difficulties, clumsiness, seizures, coma, and death (associated with blood level of 100 mcg/dL) Hematopoietic effect: anemia GI effects: anorexia, nausea, vomiting, constipation, lead line along gums Skeletal effects: increased density of long bones, lead line in long bones Renal effects: glycosuria, proteinuria, possible acute or chronic renal failure Although kidney damage is reversible early in the disease, with continued lead exposure permanent kidney damage may occur.	Level >25 mcg/dL: remove child from lead source, hospitalize if level is significantly higher. Administer chelating agents: succimer orally for lead level 35-45 mcg/dL; EDTA for level >70 mcg/dL given intravenously over several hours for 5 days (causes lead to be deposited in bone and excreted by kidneys); bronchoalveolar lavage every 4 hr for six doses for level >70 mcg/dL. Monitor kidney function because EDTA is nephrotoxic; monitor calcium levels because EDTA enhances excretion of calcium. Provide adequate hydration. Calcium, phosphorus, and vitamins C and D Anticonvulsants Oral or intramuscular iron for anemia Follow-up of lead levels to monitor progress (lead is excreted more slowly than it accumulates in the body)
CARBON MONOXIDE			
Most often from improperly ventilated heaters; also from poorly ventilated vehicles Cause of exposure should be determined and eliminated.	An odorless, colorless gas that binds to receptors on hemoglobin more effectively than does oxygen, thereby causing hypoxia	Headache, visual disturbances Altered level of consciousness, cherry-red lips and cheeks, nausea, and vomiting	100% oxygen by rebreathing mask Serum carboxyhemoglobin levels; possible need for hyperbaric chamber treatment for patients with high carboxyhemoglobin levels Other interventions based on signs and symptoms

From James SR, Neslon KA, Ashwill JW: *Nursing care of children: principles and practice,* ed 4, St Louis, 2013, Saunders.
CNS, Central nervous system; *EDTA,* ethylenediaminetetraacetic acid; *GI,* gastrointestinal; *IV,* intravenous; *NPO,* nothing by mouth.

B. Hospitalization as a crisis
  1. Children are more vulnerable to the crisis of illness and hospitalization because stress is a change from their usual state of health and routine and they have a limited number of coping mechanisms to deal with stressful events.
  2. The reactions to stress differ in each developmental age group.
    a. Infants and toddlers: A major stress is separation anxiety (fear of being separated from their parents and family).
    b. Preschoolers: Major stresses and fears are separation anxiety, loss of body control, and body injury and pain.
    c. School-aged children: Major stresses and fears are separation (sometimes more from peers than from family); loss of body control; and body injury, mutilation, pain, and death.
    d. Adolescents: Major stresses and fears are separation from their peer group; loss of body control, independence, and identity; and body injury and pain, especially concerning sexual changes.

3. Nursing measures can be used to minimize the hospitalized child's fears and stresses.
   a. Provide open visiting for parents and siblings. Visiting by peers in the school-age and adolescent groups should be encouraged.
   b. Explain procedures or preparation for procedures at the child's age level (medical play).
   c. Allow the child to have favorite toys and games from home.
   d. Nursing personnel should not use parents' visits as rewards or as something to be withheld if the child does not cooperate or behave.
   e. Allow the child as much physical freedom as his or her condition will allow.
   f. Allow the child to participate in decision making as much as possible, especially regarding treatments and procedures; this allows him or her some control in the situation.
   g. Encourage the parents to visit as much as possible; explain all procedures to them and encourage them to assist in their child's care if they are comfortable in doing so.
   h. Instruct the parents not to lie to the child; lying only sets up a sense of mistrust among the child, the parents, and the hospital staff.
   i. Administer pain medications as ordered whenever necessary; a child's pain response is affected by developmental level.
   j. Expect some regressive behavior during the child's hospital stay; tell the parents that this is normal during stressful periods.
C. Use of play during hospitalization
   1. Play in the hospital helps relieve tension and anxiety, lessens the stress of separation and feelings of homesickness, and helps the child relax and feel more secure.
   2. Play activities should be based on the child's age, interests, and limitations.
   3. Play can be used for diversion, for recreation, and to play out the child's fears and anxieties over his or her illness and treatment.
   4. Toys can come from home or the hospital play area; they can even be adapted from hospital "stock" supplies.
   5. Play therapy can be used to teach the child about procedures and surgery and help him or her work through fears and anxieties about hospitalization.
D. Preparation and teaching for discharge
   1. Preparation for discharge should begin during the admission by setting long-term goals concerning discharge.
   2. Discharge planning should include several areas.
      a. Parent-child teaching regarding home-care procedures and medication regimen
      b. Follow-up care, including physician appointments and the importance of keeping them
      c. Referrals to community agencies, public health nurses, and other resources as needed

NURSING CARE OF THE HOSPITALIZED CHILD

A. Safety factors
   1. Side rails should be kept up at all times when the child is in bed; if the bed is adjustable, it should be kept in the low position.
   2. When restraints are used, they should be applied securely to the child. Extremities should be checked frequently for impaired circulation caused by tight restraints. Appropriate charting should be done.
   3. Small toys, game pieces, and other small objects should be kept away from infants and toddlers, who may swallow them.
   4. Toddlers and young children should not be left unattended in their rooms or hallways; if they are out of bed, they should be observed continuously to avoid accidents and injuries.
   5. Medications, needles, and syringes should be kept out of the reach of all children.
B. Medication administration
   1. General guidelines in giving medications to children
      a. Approach the child with a cheerful, positive attitude and explain what the nurse is going to do.
      b. Be honest when talking to the child; tell the child that it is medicine, not "juice" or "candy."
      c. When necessary, use foods or liquids to disguise the taste of bad-tasting medications.
      d. Oral syringes or syringes without needles may be used to deliver oral medications to infants and young children.
      e. Allow the child some control in the situation; make sure that the question the nurse asks the child is appropriate to his or her age level and the situation.
      f. Intramuscular (IM) injections are safer and easier to give to a young child if a second person helps to restrain the child.
      g. Tell the child that it is all right to cry if the shot "hurts"; offer a bandage strip.
      h. Teach the child to "say no" to street drugs but that the medicines received in the hospital are okay to take.
   2. Safe IM injection technique includes the same steps used for IM injections in adults.
      a. In infants the lateral thigh (vastus lateralis muscle) should be used.
      b. In toddlers and preschoolers the ventrogluteal area is the preferred site (lateral thigh can also be used).
      c. In older children and adolescents other regularly used injection sites may be used (ventrogluteal muscle is the safest; deltoid and dorsogluteal muscles may also be used) (Figure 8-16).
C. Assisting with treatments and procedures
   1. All tests and procedures should be explained to the child in an honest, simple manner. Older children and adolescents should be allowed to ask questions and receive answers.
   2. All children should be allowed to say "ouch" or cry if the procedure is a painful one; rewards are often given after a painful procedure (a reward sticker, toy, or special food treat).
   3. The child may need to be held or restrained in certain positions for procedures; all equipment should be assembled before the procedure is started so the nurse can stay with the child as much as possible.
D. Preoperative teaching
   1. Patient teaching in pediatrics should include the child (preschool age and older) and the parents; both should be involved in the teaching and preparation for surgery.

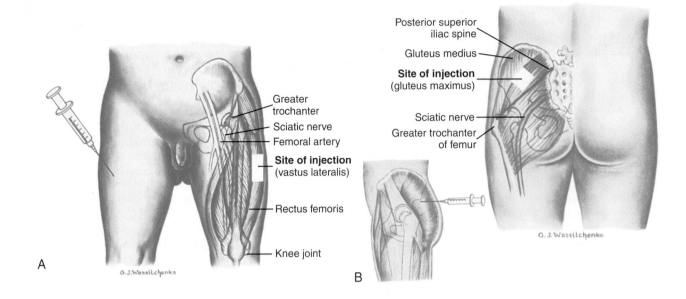

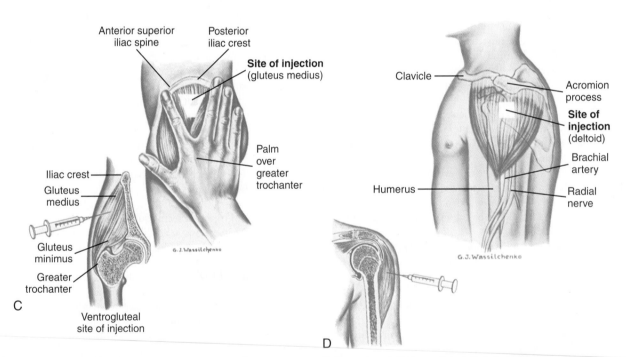

FIGURE 8-16 Acceptable intramuscular sites in children. **A,** Vastus lateralis. **B,** Dorsogluteal. **C,** Ventrogluteal. **D,** Deltoid. (From Hockenberry MJ, Wilson D: *Wong's nursing care of infants and children,* ed 9, St Louis, 2011, Mosby.)

2. Use words that the child can understand. Audiovisual aids (pictures, dolls, puppets, bandages) are extremely useful in helping the child understand the procedure or surgery.
3. Be honest with the child, especially regarding procedures or treatments that may be uncomfortable or painful.
4. Tell the child that he or she will not feel any pain during the surgery because of the "special sleep" of anesthesia and that he or she will wake up after surgery in the recovery room.
5. Include details specific to the child's surgery such as dressings, tubes, IV fluids, medications, the specific site of the pain or discomfort, and the diet restrictions before and after surgery.

E. General postoperative care
1. Basic postoperative care is similar to nursing care of adult postoperative patients.
   a. Frequent vital signs; pulse oximetry as needed
   b. Observation of the incision or dressings
   c. Level of consciousness
   d. I&O, IV fluids, Foley catheter, NG tube
   e. Administration of pain medications as needed (IV, PO, epidurals; IM route may be used but should be avoided)
2. Allow the child's parents to assist in the child's care if they desire to do so.
3. Explain all postoperative procedures before doing them.

F. Care of the child in a cast
1. The child should be repositioned every 2 hours to allow the cast to dry completely.
2. Observe and record the condition of the skin at the edges of the cast for color, warmth, irritation, sensation, and edema; the cast should be handled lightly with open palms while it is still damp to avoid indentations.
3. Check the color of the nail beds below the cast. Check the pulse in the area below the cast if it is in an accessible area (radial or pedal pulse).
4. Teach the child not to put anything inside the cast or to "scratch" the skin beneath the cast.
5. Check the cast for drainage or discoloration; any drainage should be marked, timed, dated, and documented.

6. Observe for signs of osteomyelitis (most commonly seen after injury, surgery to a long bone): pain, tenderness at site of infection, fever, irritability. Osteomyelitis is most often caused by the *Staphylococcus aureus* organism.
7. Protect the cast from water, urine, and stool.
8. "Petal" the edges of the cast before the patient goes home. (If cast is damp, teach parents the proper way to do it.)
9. Before discharge, talk to the parents regarding a safe method for restraining the child with a cast while in the car; infants and children in long leg and hip spica casts need adapted car seats, safety belts, or both.
G. Care of the child in traction
1. Types of traction
a. Skeletal: uses pins, wires, and tongs (Table 8-4)
b. Skin: uses tapes, plastic, and bandages attached to the skin (Table 8-5)

Table 8-4   **Types of Skeletal Traction**

TYPES	ILLUSTRATION	USES	NURSING CONSIDERATIONS
Cervical (Crutchfield) skeletal tongs		Preoperative spine distraction Fractures or dislocations of cervical or high thoracic vertebrae	A special bed may be used to assist with turning patient. Logroll patient while maintaining straight body alignment.
Halo cast or vest		Postoperative immobilization after cervical fusion Fracture or dislocation of cervical or high thoracic vertebrae	Balance is altered with a halo cast; patients ambulating need close supervision. Cast may need to be sawed in case of emergency; front panel of brace may need to be removed in case of emergency.
Dunlop (side-arm 90-90)		Fracture of upper arm	Turn patient toward the affected side only. Hand may feel cool despite intact neurovascular status; cover hand with mitten or sock if desired.
90-90 femoral traction		Femur fractures	Encourage child to dorsiflex foot often to prevent footdrop, or lower leg may be casted. Ensure that weights do not catch on bottom of the bed.
Thomas ring with Pearson attachment (balanced suspension)		Femur fracture Hip fracture Tibial fracture	Avoid pressure to area behind the knee, which could cause popliteal nerve injury. If system is truly balanced, splint can be placed at any height and will remain there.

Modified from Bowden V, Dickey S, Greenberg C: *Children and their families: the continuum of care,* Philadelphia, 1998, Saunders; and McKinney E et al: *Maternal-child nursing,* ed 2, St Louis, 2005, Saunders.

Table 8-5   Types of Skin Traction

TYPES	ILLUSTRATION	USES	NURSING CONSIDERATIONS
Cervical		Neck sprains or strains Torticollis Cervical nerve trauma Nerve root compression	Limit to weights of 5-7 pounds. Avoid compressing the throat or ears with the chin strap.
Side-arm 90-90		Fractures and dislocations of the upper arm or shoulder	Hand may feel cool because of its elevation. Hand can be covered with sock or mitten if desired.
Dunlop		Supracondylar elbow fracture of the humerus	Avoid pressure over bony prominences or nerves.
Buck extension traction		Hip and knee contracture Legg-Calvé-Perthes disease	Remove boot every 8 hours and assess skin. Leg may be slightly abducted.
Russell traction		Supracondylar femur fracture	Sling may need to be repositioned often; mark leg to ensure proper placement. Stabilize fractured femur until callus forms.
Split Russell		Femur fracture Legg-Calve-Perthes disease	Avoid pressure over bony prominences or nerves. Weights are not added or removed without a physician's order.

Modified from Bowden V, Dickey S, Greenberg C: *Children and their families: the continuum of care,* Philadelphia, 1998, Saunders; and McKinney E et al: *Maternal-child nursing,* ed 2, St Louis, 2005, Saunders.

2. Nursing care measures for the child in traction
   a. Explain the traction apparatus to the child; allow the child to participate in his or her care as much as possible.
   b. Maintain traction alignment; be sure that all ropes are in the center tracks of the pulleys and that the weights are hanging freely.
   c. Provide proper skin care; observe for reddened, irritated areas at the edges of the tape and elastic bandages and at other pressure sites.
   d. Observe skeletal pin sites for bleeding, inflammation, and signs of infection; provide pin-site care as ordered.
   e. Observe affected extremity for skin color, nail bed color, and changes in sensation and mobility.
   f. Administer pain medications as ordered and keep the child as comfortable as possible.
   g. Provide range-of-motion exercises to the unaffected body parts to help prevent contractures and muscle atrophy.
   h. Provide toys and activities appropriate to the child's age level and limited mobility.

Bibliography

Emergency Nurse's Association: *Sheehy's manual of emergency care*, ed 7, St Louis, 2013, Mosby.

James SR, Nelson K, Ashwill JW: *Nursing care of children: principles and practice*, ed 4, St Louis, 2013, Saunders.

James SR, White J: *Study guide for nursing care of children: principles and practice*, ed 4, St Louis, 2013, Saunders.

Hockenberry MJ, Wilson D: *Wong's nursing care of infants and children*, ed 9, St Louis, 2011, Mosby.

McCance KL, Huether SE: *Pathophysiology: the biologic basis for disease in adults and children*, ed 6, St Louis, 2010, Mosby.

Price DL, Gwin JF: *Pediatric nursing: an introductory text*, ed 11, St Louis, 2012, Saunders.

REVIEW QUESTIONS

1. Hospitalized adolescents have the most difficulty with:
   1. Dependence versus independence.
   2. Trust versus autonomy.
   3. Reality versus fantasy.
   4. Initiative versus guilt

2. The nurse would be accurate when giving information to the parent of a child with cystic fibrosis by explaining that the pathophysiology responsible for respiratory alterations is:
   1. Decreased ciliary action, causing stasis of mucus in lungs.
   2. Edema of the epiglottis, causing upper airway occlusion.
   3. Excessive production of thick mucus, leading to airway obstruction.
   4. Laryngeal stricture, leading to bronchospasm.

3. The child with cystic fibrosis (CF) takes pancreatic enzymes with each meal. The nurse is accurate when explaining to the parents that this therapy is aimed at facilitating:
   1. Absorption of vitamins A, C, and K.
   2. Increased carbohydrate metabolism for growth.
   3. Digestion and absorption of fats and proteins.
   4. Sodium excretion and electrolyte balance.

4. The nurse knows that, to prevent injury, the safest place to administer an intramuscular (IM) injection to an infant is in the:
   1. Deltoid muscle.
   2. Vastus lateralis muscle.
   3. Ventrogluteal muscle.
   4. Dorsogluteal muscle.

5. The nurse notices a 2-year-old female patient having a complex febrile seizure in her crib. The nurse knows that the most important intervention at this time is to:
   1. Place a seizure stick between her jaws.
   2. Prepare the suction equipment.
   3. Observe the seizure and protect her from harm.
   4. Restrain her to prevent injury.

6. During the assessment of a child with asthma, the nurse would be most observant for signs of airway narrowing typically caused by:
   1. Laryngeal edema, dehydration, anxiety.
   2. Bronchospasm, edema, increased accumulation of mucus.
   3. Increased negative pleural pressure, laryngospasm, mucous plugging.
   4. Carbon dioxide retention, pharyngeal hyperemia, alveolar collapse.

7. A 3-month-old infant is admitted to the pediatric unit for treatment of bronchiolitis. Oxygen therapy is ordered for the infant primarily to:
   1. Reduce fever.
   2. Allay anxiety and restlessness.
   3. Liquefy secretions.
   4. Relieve dyspnea and hypoxemia.

8. Although times of administration may differ slightly, recommended immunizations for an infant, usually before or by the age of 2 months, are:
   1. DPT only.
   2. PPD, IPV, first hepatitis B vaccines.
   3. DTP, IPV, MMR.
   4. DTP, IPV, Hib, second hepatitis B vaccine, and PCV.

9. In caring for a 6-year-old child in a full leg cast, which finding should the nurse report to the physician immediately?
   1. The cast is still damp after 4 hours.
   2. The child's pedal pulse is 110 beats/min.
   3. The child complains of pain in his leg.
   4. The child is unable to move his toes.

10. The most important criterion on which to base the decision to report suspected child abuse is:
    1. Inappropriate parental concern for the degree of injury.
    2. Absence of the parents for questioning about the child's injuries.
    3. A complaint other than the one associated with the signs of abuse.
    4. Incompatibility between the history given and the injury observed.

11. The nurse would recognize the typical signs of sickle cell crisis as being:
    1. Fever, seizures, coma.
    2. Abdominal pain, swollen painful joints.
    3. Polycythemia, tachycardia.
    4. Severe itching, vomiting.

12. The treatment of a child with nephrotic syndrome includes administration of corticosteroids to:
    1. Decrease the amount of proteinuria.
    2. Increase the amount of albumin in the blood.
    3. Help control hypertension.
    4. Reduce edema of the face, extremities, and abdomen.

13. A child with asthma would most likely present with which symptoms?
    1. Laryngitis, sore throat, productive cough
    2. Fever, rhinorrhea, coarse breath sounds
    3. Tightness in the chest, nonproductive cough, wheezing
    4. Rapid respiratory rate, difficulty swallowing, fever

14. The two main types of medication used to treat asthma are:
    1. Antiinflammatory agents, immunosuppressants.
    2. Bronchodilators, antiinflammatory agents.
    3. Antibiotics, bronchodilators.
    4. Decongestants, antihistamines.

15. A 5-month-old infant with chronic lung disease is admitted with a severe case of respiratory syncytial virus (RSV). Treatment for this child includes:
    1. Cromolyn (Intal) nebulizer treatments, intravenous (IV) fluids.
    2. Ribavirin (Virazole), humidified oxygen.
    3. Amoxicillin, intravenous fluids.
    4. Prednisone (Liquid Pred), oxygen.

16. At the time of delivery, an infant is born with its abdominal organs covered by a sac, protruding through an abnormal opening in the umbilical ring. This condition is known as:
    1. Intussusception.
    2. Diaphragmatic hernia.
    3. Omphalocele.
    4. Gastroschisis.

17. The recommended dose of medication for a 10-year-old is 60 mg/kg of body weight in 24 hours. The safe dose for administration to a 66-pound child would be:
    Answer: _____ mg in 24 hours

18. If intravenous fluids are ordered for administration at 40 mL/hr, using mini/micro drip tubing, the drip rate per minute will be:
    Answer: _____ drops/min

19. The symptoms of croup are caused by:
    1. A bacterial infection of the larynx.
    2. Inflammation of the trachea and esophagus.
    3. Spasms of the larynx.
    4. Inflammation of the lungs.

20. A fungal infection of the skin that can occur on the scalp, body, and feet is:
    1. Ringworm.
    2. Pediculosis.
    3. Herpes type 2.
    4. Urticaria.

21. The pediatrician ordered aspirin gr. v PO. The nurse has aspirin, 325-mg tablets, on hand. The nurse should give:
    1. ½ tablet.
    2. 1 tablet.
    3. 1½ tablets.
    4. 2 tablets.

22. To ensure proper administration of eardrops in the left ear of a 2-year-old child, the nurse recognizes that the correct position for installation would be pulling the:
    1. Outer ear up and toward the back of the head.
    2. Outer ear down and toward the back of the head.
    3. Earlobe down and toward the chin.
    4. Earlobe up and toward the nose.

23. The nurse completes her assessment of an 18-month-old boy. Which finding would the nurse report as being abnormal for an 18-month-old?
    1. Cannot throw a ball without falling
    2. Likes to do everything for himself
    3. Says 10 or more words
    4. Builds tower of three or four blocks

24. A mother of an otherwise healthy 18-month-old tells the nurse that the child has had two diarrhea stools. When she asks what fluids and foods she can safely give the child, the nurse tells her to:
    1. Not give the child anything until 24 hours after the diarrhea stops.
    2. Continue to offer normal diet items but substitute foods the child especially likes.
    3. Encourage fluids (diluted juice, soda, Pedialyte) and offer small crackers.
    4. Offer constipating foods such as cheese with each meal and decrease fluid intake.

25. The nurse is assigned to care for a 3-year-old boy on the pediatric unit who has a Wilms tumor. Which nursing intervention is appropriate?
    1. Encourage the child to choose his own activities, but tell him that he must accept responsibility for his own safety
    2. Avoid manipulation or pressure on the child's abdomen, which can increase the possibility of metastasis
    3. Palpate the tumor each shift to determine any change in size or configuration
    4. At regular intervals position the child appropriately and perform postural drainage techniques

26. The desired clinical outcome for a child experiencing respiratory distress from epiglottitis is:
    1. The child remains asleep for 8 hours each night.
    2. The child is in no pain or discomfort.
    3. The airway remains patent.
    4. Oral mucous membranes remain moist and pink.

27. A 6-year-old child with a 3-year history of celiac disease is brought into the clinic for a checkup. If the child and his family have been in compliance with the necessary diet regimen, the nurse should expect to see:
    1. Slow, steady weight loss.
    2. Increase in appetite.
    3. Hemoglobin level above 12 g/dL.
    4. Decrease in steatorrhea.

28. When caring for a child with glomerulonephritis, nursing priorities would include observing for:
    1. Color, motion, and sensation of lower extremities.
    2. Severity of abdominal pain, bowel sounds.
    3. Rise in blood pressure, observation for facial edema.
    4. Neurological checks, level of consciousness.

29. What is the nurse's legal responsibility regarding the reporting of suspected child abuse or neglect?
    1. None; nurses can be sued if they report suspected child abuse or neglect.

2. Nurses must report abuse and neglect to the child's pediatrician before calling a child abuse center.

3. Only physicians are legally required to report abuse or neglect.

4. Nurses must report all suspected and confirmed abuse or neglect.

30. A 3-month-old infant is receiving continuous intravenous (IV) fluids because of dehydration. In providing nursing care for her, the nurse's priority should be to:
    1. Help the infant adjust to restricted activities.
    2. Relieve the infant's anxiety.
    3. Promote fluid elimination.
    4. Prevent interference with the IV therapy.

31. During the physical assessment of a 1-month-old infant, which of the findings by the nurse would be reported to the pediatrician immediately?
    1. Patent anterior fontanel
    2. Can lift the head slightly when lying on the abdomen
    3. Weight loss of 1½ pounds
    4. Head lag occurs when pulled from lying to sitting position

32. An infant begins to differentiate between stranger and familiar faces thus showing "stranger anxiety" at age:
    1. 4 to 5 months.
    2. 6 to 7 months.
    3. 8 to 9 months.
    4. 10 to 11 months.

33. When asked to explain the pathophysiology of respiratory syncytial virus (RSV) to an infant's caregiver, the nurse should tell her that RSV is:
    1. A bacterial infection of the lungs similar to pneumonia.
    2. A viral infection of the lungs and trachea that causes inflammation.
    3. An inflammation of the pleural cavity that can be prevented with ribavirin (Virazole).
    4. A viral infection that causes the bronchioles to become plugged with mucus.

34. Ribavirin (Virazole), an antiviral agent given in the treatment of respiratory syncytial virus (RSV), is administered:
    1. Via slow intravenous infusion.
    2. Via an oxygen hood or mask.
    3. Via intramuscular injection.
    4. Orally; can be given with juice or formula.

35. A newborn with Hirschsprung disease (aganglionic megacolon) often exhibits classic signs and symptoms, including:
    1. Respiratory distress, wheezing.
    2. Pallor, bruising, low hemoglobin.
    3. An olive-shaped mass in the abdomen, projectile vomiting.
    4. Lack of meconium stool, bile-stained emesis.

36. Treatment for an infant newly diagnosed with esophageal atresia should include:
    1. Liquid diet, monitoring of vital signs, accurate intake and output.
    2. Nothing by mouth (NPO), intravenous (IV) fluids, suctioning of mouth and nose as needed.
    3. Oxygen via nasal cannula, bronchodilators.
    4. Half-strength formula in small, frequent amounts; IV fluids.

37. Tetralogy of Fallot consists of four separate cardiac defects:
    1. Atrial septal defect (ASD), ventricular septal defect (VSD), coarctation of the aorta, patent ductus arteriosus (PDA)
    2. VSD, pulmonary stenosis, overriding of the aorta, right ventricular hypertrophy
    3. Coarctation of the aorta, pulmonary stenosis, ASD, right ventricular hypertrophy
    4. VSD, left ventricular hypertrophy, PDA, overriding of the aorta

38. A 1-year-old child is admitted with a diagnosis of spastic cerebral palsy (CP). What would the admitting nurse expect to note on admission? Select all that apply.
    1. _____ Mental retardation, wide-based gait, and flexion contractures
    2. _____ Disintegration of movements of the upper extremities, hypertonicity of the lower extremities
    3. _____ Abnormal involuntary movement; athetosis; and slow, writhing movements
    4. _____ Hypertonicity of muscles and tendon reflexes, poor coordination, contractures
    5. _____ Difficulty eating, walking, and accomplishing other coordinated movements

39. The nurse would report to the surgeon immediately all assessments made on a child 3 hours after a tonsillectomy *except:*
    1. The child is restless and pale.
    2. The blood pressure is low, heart rate increased.
    3. The child is swallowing frequently.
    4. The child is complaining of a sore throat.

40. The nurse would be alert for the following three main consequences of bone marrow dysfunction in a patient diagnosed with leukemia:
    1. Anemia, increased blood clotting, infection
    2. Infection, anemia, bleeding
    3. Decreased clotting, increased hemoglobin, sickling of the red blood cells
    4. Prolonged bleeding time, decreased white blood cells, increased coagulation

41. Epileptic seizures are also known as *tonic-clonic (grand-mal) seizures.* They may also be classified as:
    1. Simple partial seizures.
    2. Complex partial seizures.
    3. Unilateral seizures.
    4. Generalized seizures.

42. Care of the child with pediculosis includes:
    1. Antifungal oral medication, pediculicide shampoo.
    2. Corticosteroids, antifungal ointment.
    3. Pediculicide shampoo, removal of eggs with comb.
    4. Antibiotic shampoo, ointment, and destruction of linens.

43. Which statement by the nurse conveys accurate information to parents and a school-aged child recently diagnosed with type 1 diabetes mellitus?
    1. "Blood sugar monitoring will be required every 1 to 2 days."
    2. "Symptoms of hypoglycemia include glycosuria, blood sugar above 120 mg/dL, and dizziness."
    3. "Insulin injections will be required, and you and your parents should be taught how to administer injections."
    4. "Your diet will remain the same as long as you exercise daily."

44. The nurse would be correct in instructing the parent of a child with acquired immunodeficiency syndrome (AIDS) that antiretroviral agents slow progression of the disease by:
    1. Killing the bacteria that lead to the development of AIDS.
    2. Working to prevent the reproduction of new virus particles.
    3. Decreasing inflammation and promoting formation of healthy T cells.
    4. Compensating for the deficiency of B lymphocytes in the body.

45. The rationale for preparing children for hospitalization is based on the theory that:
    1. Children have a right to know what is going to happen to them.
    2. Leaving their child in the hospital overnight will be easier for the parents.
    3. Fear of the unknown is more severe than fear of the known.
    4. If children are well prepared, parents will not have to visit as often.

46. Russell traction, used as part of the treatment of fractured femur in children, is a type of:
    1. Skin traction.
    2. Skeletal traction.
    3. Wire traction.
    4. Pelvic traction.

47. An adolescent is brought to the pediatrician's office with symptoms of mononucleosis: malaise, sore throat, fever, and lack of energy. A common symptom in the early stages of mononucleosis that the nurse would observe for is:
    1. Acute otitis media.
    2. Red, flat rash on the body.
    3. Cardiac enlargement.
    4. Edema in the lower extremities.

48. Select all of the correct responses related to iron deficiency anemia.
    _____ 1. It is the most common anemia in children.
    _____ 2. There is a decrease in the size and number of red blood cells.
    _____ 3. It can result in severe hemorrhage in children.
    _____ 4. It results in decreased oxygen-carrying capacity of the blood.
    _____ 5. It is caused by a nutritional deficiency.

49. A 12-year-old requires medication based on body weight. The child weighs 110 pounds. The nurse correctly calculates that the child weighs:
    Answer: _____ kg

50. Treatment and nursing interventions for an infant with symptoms of colic include:
    1. Changing from formula to cow's milk.
    2. Taking a thorough history of the infant's diet and activities.
    3. Feeding the infant large amounts of formula every 4 hours.
    4. Following each feeding with a small amount of rice cereal.

51. A nurse's daughter, age 8 years, has developed a red, raised rash on her face, neck, and trunk. She also has a temperature of 101.6° F (38.5° C) and whitish spots on the back of her throat. The nurse would know that these are symptoms of:
    1. Chickenpox.
    2. Measles (rubeola).
    3. Eczema.
    4. German measles (rubella).

52. A 3-year-old has an order for sulfisoxazole (Gantrisin), 600 mg by mouth (PO) every morning. The nurse has sulfisoxazole, 0.5 g/5 mL, on hand. The nurse would administer:
    Answer: _____ mL

53. One type of treatment that is contraindicated for infants and young children with gastroenteritis is:
    1. Intravenous (IV) fluids with electrolytes.
    2. Oral rehydration with Pedialyte.
    3. Age-appropriate solid foods when tolerated.
    4. Antidiarrheal drug therapy.

54. A patient, age 3 years, was admitted with a diagnosis of possible epiglottitis. If the nurse suspects that the patient has epiglottitis, the nurse should:
    1. Check her throat carefully with a flashlight.
    2. Increase her oral intake.
    3. Have the child lie flat in bed.
    4. Have emergency tracheostomy equipment immediately available.

55. Acute bacterial meningitis is:
    1. Easily treated with oral antibiotics.
    2. More common in adults than it is in children.
    3. A medical emergency requiring immediate treatment.
    4. Diagnosed by blood culture and computed tomography (CT) scan.

56. The pediatrician has ordered acetaminophen, 600 mg PO, for a 15-year-old with fever. Available is acetaminophen, gr. v per tablet. The nurse would administer:
    Answer: _____ tablet(s)

57. Rheumatic fever is caused by:
    1. A virus.
    2. *Streptococcus* bacteria.
    3. *Escherichia coli* bacteria.
    4. A fungus.

58. Before surgery an infant with Hirschsprung disease may require:
    1. Total parenteral nutrition (TPN) for malnutrition.
    2. Small, frequent nasogastric feedings.
    3. Diagnostic ultrasound of the stomach.
    4. Intravenous (IV) antibiotics.

59. A 6-month-old is brought to the emergency department with symptoms of dehydration. The nurse would expect to see the following symptoms of moderate dehydration. Select all that apply.
    _____ 1. Decreased urine output
    _____ 2. Cool, moist skin
    _____ 3. Absence of tears
    _____ 4. Dry mucous membranes of the mouth
    _____ 5. Sunken anterior fontanel

60. Symptoms of celiac disease include:
    1. Constipation, anorexia, malnutrition.
    2. Malnutrition, severe thirst, weight loss.
    3. Distended abdomen, constipation, anorexia.
    4. Bulky, greasy stools; distended abdomen; malnutrition.

61. The initial treatment of choice for an intussusception is:
    1. Reduction by manual abdominal pressure.
    2. Surgical bowel resection.
    3. Temporary colostomy.
    4. Hydrostatic reduction with water-soluble contrast.

62. The most common signs and symptoms of leukemia related to bone marrow involvement are:
    1. Headache, papilledema, irritability.
    2. Muscle wasting, weight loss, fatigue.
    3. Decreased intracranial pressure, seizures, confusion.
    4. Anemia, infection, bleeding.
63. An 18-month-old patient is admitted to day surgery for a bilateral myringotomy because of frequent occurrences of otitis media. The nurse would be correct in instructing the parent that otitis media occurs more frequently in young children than it does in older children because of the different position and shape of the young child's:
    1. Epiglottis.
    2. Tympanic membranes.
    3. External ear canals.
    4. Eustachian tubes.
64. Surgical repair of cryptorchidism is known as:
    1. Epispadias.
    2. Cystotomy.
    3. Orchiopexy.
    4. Removal of the testes.
65. The nurse is caring for a child who weighs 45 pounds. The usual dose of ampicillin for children is 100 mg/kg/day. What would be a safe and appropriate dose for this child?
    1. Ampicillin, 250 mg every 4 hours
    2. Ampicillin, 500 mg four times daily
    3. Ampicillin, 200 mg every 6 hours
    4. Ampicillin, 300 mg four times daily
66. The most effective chemotherapy agents for the treatment of nephroblastoma are:
    1. Vancomycin, methotrexate.
    2. Actinomycin D, vincristine.
    3. Cyclophosphamide, dexamethasone.
    4. doxorubicin, cyclophosphamide.
67. The childhood disease that causes elevated erythrocyte sedimentation rate, polyarthritis, fever, and subcutaneous nodules and may be seen after a streptococcal infection is:
    1. Leukemia.
    2. Muscular dystrophy.
    3. Cystic fibrosis.
    4. Rheumatic fever.
68. During a physical examination a 1-month-old infant has limited abduction of the hip and asymmetrical gluteal folds. These are classic signs of:
    1. Talipes equinovarus.
    2. Osteosarcoma.
    3. Cerebral palsy (CP).
    4. Hip dysplasia.
69. Fluids by mouth are initially contraindicated for an infant with bronchiolitis because of feeding difficulty caused by:
    1. Tachypnea.
    2. Nausea.
    3. Irritability.
    4. Fever.
70. The disorder characterized by a malfunction of the motor centers of the brain because of oxygen deprivation before, during, or immediately after delivery is:
    1. Down syndrome.
    2. Hydrocephalus.
    3. Osteomyelitis.
    4. Cerebral palsy

71. The primary goals in the initial treatment of major burns in a child are:
    1. Maintaining an airway and preventing shock.
    2. Inserting an indwelling catheter and monitoring intake and output.
    3. Controlling pain and reducing the risk of infection.
    4. Preventing malnutrition and dehydration.
72. A disorder caused by an obstruction of cerebrospinal fluid (CSF) drainage is:
    1. Opisthotonos.
    2. Hirschsprung disease.
    3. Hydrocephalus.
    4. Meningitis.
73. Normal annual weight gain for toddlers should be approximately:
    1. 4 to 6 pounds.
    2. 8 to 9 pounds.
    3. 11 to 12 pounds.
    4. 13 to 14 pounds.
74. The reference text states that the normal dose of amoxicillin is 30 mg/kg of body weight. The dose for a 99-pound child would be:
    Answer: _____ mg
75. Select all of the characteristics of a 1-year-old infant diagnosed with failure to thrive (FTT).
    _____ 1. Hypertonia and developmental delay
    _____ 2. Hypertonicity, alertness, and a social smile
    _____ 3. Apathy and disinterest in playing with toys
    _____ 4. Weight below the fifth percentile
    _____ 5. Wariness of health care workers and caretakers
76. Symptoms that are typically seen in infants with cystic fibrosis (CF) include:
    1. Abdominal pain.
    2. Loose, congested cough.
    3. Greasy, foul-smelling stools.
    4. Hypertension, dyspnea.
77. A 4-week-old infant is brought to the pediatrician's office with symptoms of weight loss, irritability, and projectile vomiting. On physical examination the infant appears dehydrated. From these symptoms the nurse suspects that the infant probably has:
    1. Tetralogy of Fallot.
    2. Pyloric stenosis.
    3. Esophageal atresia.
    4. Intussusception.
78. Select all of the types of traction used for fracture or dislocation of a lower extremity of a school-aged child.
    _____ 1. Dunlop traction
    _____ 2. Buck traction
    _____ 3. Russell traction
    _____ 4. Thomas ring
79. An 18-month-old infant with developmental dysplasia of her right hip is being hospitalized for surgery and application of a hip spica cast. Which measure is necessary in caring for her?
    1. Avoid giving her pain medication as much as possible to prevent addiction.
    2. Limit fluids so she will be less likely to get the cast wet when she voids.
    3. Instruct the parents that they can take her home in the car propped up on pillows, with her legs down.
    4. Assess sensation, circulation, and motion of her feet and toes.

80. During a routine physical examination the parents of a 2-year-old child tell the nurse they feel that something is wrong with their child, but they can't figure out what it is. The nurse inquires as to the toddler's general behavior. Which comment by the parents should be of concern to the nurse?
    1. "Joey is extremely social and enjoys contact with people."
    2. "Joey exhibits really bizarre behavior at times and seems to be in a world of his own."
    3. "Joey displays appropriate development of language and motor skills for his age."
    4. "Joey appears even-tempered and may display exceptional talent in certain areas."

81. Research has shown that sudden infant death syndrome (SIDS) may be related to a brainstem abnormality in the regulation of cardiorespiratory control. Recent studies have demonstrated that the risk of SIDS is increased in infants who:
    1. Breast-feed rather than bottle-feed.
    2. Have a history of apnea requiring vigorous stimulation.
    3. Are over 10 months of age.
    4. Use a pacifier while they sleep on their back.

82. The nurse accurately describes that the medication used to decrease fever and the incidence of coronary artery damage in Kawasaki disease (KD) is:
    1. Dexamethasone (Decadron).
    2. Ibuprofen (Advil).
    3. IV immune globulin (IVIG).
    4. Sulfasalazine (Azulfidine).

83. A ketogenic diet is sometimes used in the treatment of:
    1. Epilepsy.
    2. Crohn disease.
    3. Hirschsprung disease.
    4. Acute glomerulonephritis.

84. A 2-month-old male infant is brought to the pediatrician's office with a 2-week history of paroxysmal abdominal cramping. The mother states that he is "very fussy" and cries as if he is in pain. He is tolerating his normal amounts of formula well and has gained weight since his last visit. These signs and symptoms indicate that he most likely has:
    1. Intussusception.
    2. Colic.
    3. Pyloric stenosis.
    4. Gastroenteritis.

85. The nurse knows that to prevent injury to the infant during an accident, the car seat should be placed in the:
    1. Front seat passenger side, facing the rear of the car.
    2. Back seat passenger side, facing the front.
    3. Middle of the back seat, facing the rear of the car.
    4. Back seat, driver side, facing the front.

86. Which statement about respiratory syncytial virus (RSV) and bronchiolitis is true?
    1. RSV causes the bronchioles to plug with mucus, trapping air in the lungs.
    2. Peak incidence for RSV infection is 4 to 6 years of age.
    3. RSV occurs primarily in summer and winter.
    4. RSV can be spread only through a bloodborne pathway.

87. According to Kohlberg's theory of moral development, preschoolers conform to rules to:
    1. Please all persons.
    2. Avoid punishment.
    3. Do the right thing.
    4. Follow personal conscience.

88. After a tonsillectomy an early sign of postoperative bleeding is:
    1. Brown-tinged mucus.
    2. Low blood pressure.
    3. Fever.
    4. Frequent swallowing.

89. The nurse receives an order for a preoperative injection: meperidine (Demerol), 40 mg, and atropine, 0.1 mg IM. The meperidine is supplied at 50 mg/mL, and the atropine at 0.2 mg/mL. What volume of meperidine and what volume of atropine should the nurse give?
    1. Meperidine 0.35 mL, atropine 0.5 mL
    2. Meperidine 0.6 mL, atropine 0.4 mL
    3. Meperidine 0.8 mL, atropine 0.5 mL
    4. Meperidine 0.85 mL, atropine 0.1 mL

90. A patient experiencing symptoms of nephrotic syndrome would have which of the following? Select all that apply.
    _____ 1. Proteinuria.
    _____ 2. Hyperlipidemia.
    _____ 3. Hypoproteinemia.
    _____ 4. Hyperglycemia.

91. The nurse has an order to administer ampicillin, 600 mg intravenous piggyback. Ampicillin is supplied as 1 g/4 mL. What volume of ampicillin should the nurse draw from the vial?
    1. 1.25 mL
    2. 1.7 mL
    3. 1.9 mL
    4. 2.4 mL

92. Symptoms of acute glomerulonephritis include:
    1. Frequent, painful urination.
    2. Respiratory distress.
    3. Edema in the extremities.
    4. Dark, tea-colored urine.

93. The order is 25 mg meperidine (Demerol) IM for pain. Available is meperidine 100 mg/mL. The correct amount of fluid to draw into the syringe would be:
    Answer: _____ mL

94. Because no cure has been discovered for muscular dystrophy (MD), the primary goal of treatment is to:
    1. Prevent involvement of the respiratory muscles.
    2. Maintain function in unaffected muscles as long as possible.
    3. Limit the child's food intake to avoid weight gain.
    4. Avoid physical activity whenever possible.

95. A child has an order for intravenous dextrose (D) 5% in 0.25% normal saline (NS) to be infused at 50 mL/hr. If the IV tubing delivers 10 gtt/mL, at what rate should the nurse infuse the IV fluid?
    1. 8 gtt/min
    2. 13 gtt/min
    3. 16 gtt/min
    4. 21 gtt/min

96. The foul-smelling, frothy stools seen in children with cystic fibrosis (CF) results from the presence of large amounts of:
    1. Proteins and enzymes.
    2. Bacteria and mucus.
    3. Sodium and glucose.
    4. Undigested fats.

97. The organ of the digestive system most commonly involved in cystic fibrosis (CF) is the:
    1. Pancreas.
    2. Small intestine.
    3. Esophagus.
    4. Stomach.

98. If a school-aged child is in Kohlberg's stage of conventional morality (level 2), the child would conform to rules:
    1. To avoid punishment.
    2. To obtain rewards.
    3. To please others.
    4. Out of concern for others.

99. Which food is contraindicated in the diet of the child with celiac disease?
    1. Rye breads
    2. Lean meats
    3. Fresh fruits
    4. Broccoli

100. An 18-year-old girl is seen in the clinic and is diagnosed with anorexia nervosa. Her symptoms would most likely include:
    1. Constipation.
    2. Dysmenorrhea.
    3. Abdominal distention.
    4. Tachycardia.

101. Select all of the symptoms that indicate respiratory distress in a premature infant.
    _____ 1. Tachypnea
    _____ 2. Flaring nostrils
    _____ 3. Flushed skin
    _____ 4. Generalized cyanosis
    _____ 5. Sternal retractions

102. A 2-week-old newborn has been admitted to the hospital with a diagnosis of possible hydrocephalus. Which assessment would be most important for the nurse to make?
    1. Fasting blood sugar checks each morning
    2. Frequent neurovascular checks
    3. Specific gravity on all urine output
    4. Daily head circumference measurement

103. The medication of choice for treatment of school-aged children with pinworms is:
    1. Mebendazole (Vermox).
    2. Antifungal ointment.
    3. Pediculicide cream.
    4. Ribavirin (Virazole).

104. The nurse is admitting a child with a diagnosis of trisomy 21. Another term for this genetic problem is:
    1. Marfan syndrome.
    2. Cri du chat syndrome.
    3. Turner syndrome.
    4. Down syndrome.

105. An infant is expected to triple his birth weight at what age?
    1. 9 months
    2. 12 months
    3. 18 months
    4. 24 months

106. Hirschsprung disease is caused by:
    1. An autoimmune reaction that causes damage to the muscles of the large intestine.
    2. Damage to the bowel from a birth injury or accident.
    3. A congenital absence of the ganglion nerve cells in the lower colon.
    4. An infectious organism that causes inflammation and swelling in the lower bowel.

107. The nurse would be correct in educating the parent of a child with asthma that one of the tests frequently used to diagnose asthma is the:
    1. Chest x-ray examination.
    2. Peak expiratory flow rate.
    3. Sweat chloride test.
    4. Sputum culture.

108. What would the nurse recognize as being specific to otitis media (OM)? Select all that apply.
    _____ 1. There are two types of otitis media.
    _____ 2. Symptoms include sucking, pain, and high fever.
    _____ 3. Acute otitis media (AOM) is caused by *Streptococcus pneumoniae* and *Haemophilus influenzae*.
    _____ 4. It affects the inner ear.

109. A 9-year-old boy is admitted to the pediatric unit complaining of localized abdominal tenderness, rigidity, and a fever. He has rebound abdominal tenderness and decreased bowel sounds. These are characteristic signs of:
    1. Meckel diverticulum.
    2. Acute appendicitis.
    3. Bulimia.
    4. Ulcerative colitis.

110. During the initial assessment of a 7-year-old boy with nephrotic syndrome, the nurse should expect to see:
    1. Absence of tears.
    2. Increased urine output.
    3. Jaundice.
    4. Edema of eyes and ankles.

111. The blood test result that is often elevated in inflammatory diseases such as rheumatic fever is:
    1. Red blood cell count.
    2. Clotting time.
    3. Erythrocyte sedimentation rate (ESR).
    4. Blood urea nitrogen.

112. A 12-year-old has just been diagnosed with type 1 diabetes. Which is a classic symptom of the onset of this disease?
    1. Hypoglycemic episodes throughout the day
    2. Excessive thirst and frequent urination
    3. Nausea before meals
    4. History of increased appetite and weight gain

113. Prednisone is often used in the treatment of rheumatic fever because it:
    1. Prevents cardiac damage.
    2. Cures the disease.
    3. Suppresses inflammation.
    4. Takes the place of antibiotic prophylaxis.

114. Moro reflex of a newborn disappears by:
    1. 1 to 2 weeks.
    2. 3 months.
    3. 5 months.
    4. 8 months.

115. An adolescent asks his physician what is required to keep his type 1 diabetes under control. The physician tells him he will be required to:
    1. Limit his activity, eat a regular diet, and take insulin.
    2. Check his blood sugar regularly and take an oral hypoglycemic drug.
    3. Exercise regularly, take insulin, and limit his carbohydrates.
    4. Take insulin three times per day and limit his diet to 1000 calories per day.

116. The last dose of the hepatitis B series should not be administered before:
    1. 6 months of age.
    2. 9 months of age.
    3. 12 months of age.
    4. 18 months of age.
117. Kohlberg's theory of moral development states that adolescents are at the stage where their focus is on:
    1. Following the rules to please others.
    2. Seeking rewards for a job well done.
    3. Behaving in a manner that does not displease others.
    4. Individual rights and principles of conscience.
118. Infectious gastroenteritis in the infant is most often caused by:
    1. Rotavirus infection.
    2. Respiratory syncytial virus infection.
    3. *Escherichia coli* infection.
    4. Staphylococcal infection.
119. The nurse is providing postoperative care for an infant who has had a pyloromyotomy for pyloric stenosis. The first feeding of breast milk or formula is most likely given:
    1. Immediately after surgery.
    2. 4 hours after surgery.
    3. Via nasogastric (NG) tube 12 hours after surgery.
    4. On the second day after surgery.
120. Abuse of the drug ecstasy (3,4-methylenedioxy-*N*-methylamphetamine [MDMA]) has increased in adolescents. This drug is classified as a(n):
    1. Stimulant.
    2. Opiate.
    3. Hallucinogen.
    4. Depressant.
121. A 12-year-old is diagnosed with *Haemophilus influenzae* type B meningitis. What would the nurse anticipate to be included in the treatment plan ordered by the physician? Select all that apply.
    _____ 1. Antibiotics
    _____ 2. Narcotic analgesics
    _____ 3. Antipyretics
    _____ 4. Antiemetics
122. Symptoms of Crohn (regional enteritis) disease include:
    1. Hypertension, headache, nausea.
    2. Abdominal pain, diarrhea, weight loss.
    3. Sore throat, swollen joints, fever.
    4. Bronchial infections, malnutrition, peripheral edema.
123. The principal cause of human immunodeficiency virus (HIV) is:
    1. A virus that targets the T lymphocytes.
    2. A streptococcal infection.
    3. The Epstein-Barr virus.
    4. An autoimmune response.
124. Daily head circumference measurements are important nursing interventions after surgery for the child with:
    1. Wilms tumor.
    2. An omphalocele.
    3. A ventriculoperitoneal shunt.
    4. A spinal cord injury.
125. Adolescents with severe cases of acne vulgaris are often treated with:
    1. Cortisone ointment (Hycort).
    2. Retinoic acid (Accutane).
    3. Sulfasalazine (Azulfidine).
    4. Cromolyn sodium.

126. Diagnosis of nephrotic syndrome in a child is based on:
    1. Symptoms of edema, hyperalbuminemia, orange urine.
    2. Results of renal ultrasound, proteinuria, increased levels of protein in the blood.
    3. Increased proteinuria, edema, decreased serum protein, renal biopsy findings.
    4. Edema of face and abdomen, positive renal computed tomography scan, increased serum protein.
127. Antiretroviral drugs are used in the treatment of human immunodeficiency virus (HIV) infection to:
    1. Compensate for the deficiency of B lymphocytes.
    2. Decrease joint pain and fever.
    3. Prevent reproduction of new virus particles.
    4. Promote an increase in T cells.
128. A bleeding disorder resulting from a congenital deficiency in certain coagulation proteins is:
    1. Sickle cell anemia.
    2. Thalassemia major.
    3. Hemophilia.
    4. Leukemia.
129. A hereditary musculoskeletal disorder that causes symptoms of gradual muscle weakness, a "waddle gait," and difficulty standing and sitting is known as:
    1. Multiple sclerosis.
    2. Cerebral palsy.
    3. Talipes equinovarus.
    4. Muscular dystrophy.
130. Major areas of stress experienced by the hospitalized adolescent are:
    1. Separation from family.
    2. Fear of death.
    3. Loss of control, independence, and identity.
    4. Worry about missing classes and getting behind in school.
131. An adolescent who exhibits changes in behavior patterns, an increase in school absences, and a decrease in academic performance and who starts to spend time with people other than his regular friends may be showing signs of:
    1. Manic-depression.
    2. Schizophrenia.
    3. Drug abuse.
    4. Obsessive-compulsive disorder.
132. The cancer that is seen most often in children is:
    1. Lymphoma.
    2. Leukemia.
    3. Wilms tumor.
    4. Osteosarcoma.
133. The diagnosis of Hirschsprung disease is usually confirmed by:
    1. A rectal biopsy and barium enema.
    2. An upper gastrointestinal series.
    3. An abdominal ultrasound.
    4. A gastroscopy.
134. Projectile vomiting in an infant is a classic sign of:
    1. Intussusception.
    2. Viral gastroenteritis.
    3. Tracheoesophageal fistula.
    4. Pyloric stenosis.
135. An example of a cyanotic congenital heart defect is:
    1. Tetralogy of Fallot.
    2. Coarctation of the aorta.
    3. Atrial septal defect (ASD).
    4. Patent ductus arteriosus (PDA).

136. An infant weighing 15 pounds has been ordered to receive morphine sulfate, 0.7 mg subcutaneously, for postoperative pain. The normal dose of morphine is 0.1 mg/kg. The ordered dose of IV morphine is:
    1. Too low, based on the weight of the infant.
    2. Twice the appropriate dose, based on the weight of the infant.
    3. Inappropriate; morphine should not be given subcutaneously.
    4. Correct, based on the weight of the infant.

137. Aminophylline is ordered for a 55-pound 6-year-old with asthma. The normal dose is 7.5 mg/kg of body weight. The nurse would expect the child to receive:
    Answer: _____ mg

138. A 1-year-old is brought to the pediatrician for a well-baby check. The birth weight was 6 pounds, 11 ounces. If on schedule, the infant should weigh approximately:
    1. 12 pounds.
    2. 15½ pounds.
    3. 18 pounds.
    4. 20 pounds.

139. A complication that commonly occurs in the child with cleft palate is:
    1. Chronic otitis media.
    2. Failure to thrive.
    3. Inability to taste formula and foods.
    4. Gastroenteritis.

140. Bulimia is an eating disorder that is characterized by:
    1. Self-imposed starvation with weight loss and body-image disturbance.
    2. Episodes of binge eating, purging, and dissatisfaction with body size.
    3. Abnormal glandular function, resulting in accumulation of excessive body fat.
    4. Compulsive overeating to satisfy emotional rather than physical needs.

141. Children with sickle cell disease are more prone to infection and sepsis because:
    1. They have poor eating habits and often develop malnutrition.
    2. They do not have a properly functioning spleen.
    3. They are frequently taking antibiotics, which makes them resistant to treatment of infection.
    4. The side effects of the Sickledex medication that they often take decrease their resistance to infection.

142. The most important interventions during tracheostomy suctioning of a 5-year-old would be to do what? Select all that apply.
    _____ 1. Apply suction for 15 to 20 seconds.
    _____ 2. Use a catheter one half the diameter of the tracheostomy tube.
    _____ 3. Maintain sterile technique.
    _____ 4. Pass the suction catheter only the length of the tracheostomy tube.
    _____ 5. Position the child flat in bed.

143. What would be reported to the physician immediately if discovered during an initial assessment of a newborn?
    1. Head circumference of 33 cm
    2. Cyanosis of the hands and feet
    3. Apical heart rate of 145 beats/min
    4. Grunting respirations, flaring nostrils, and mottled skin color

144. The best indicator of possible esophageal atresia during feeding of a newborn would be:
    1. Respiratory rate of 36 respirations per minute.
    2. Poor sucking reflex.
    3. Swallowing sound heard during feeding.
    4. Excessive oral secretions, coughing, and choking during feeding.

145. Potential health problems in a newborn of a 15-year-old mother would include which of the following? Select all that apply.
    _____ 1. A baby having low birth weight
    _____ 2. A baby with good muscle tone
    _____ 3. A baby with bleeding into the brain
    _____ 4. A baby with respiratory difficulty and breathing problems

146. The following is true regarding head lice (pediculosis capitis):
    1. They are transmitted from person to person or from contaminated articles such as combs, hairbrushes, and hats.
    2. They live off of the skin cells of the scalp.
    3. The eggs (nits) attach to the distal end of the hair.
    4. Infestation is treated with antifungal medications.

147. Select all of the appropriate signs of hip dysplasia in a 2-week-old newborn.
    _____ 1. Abduction of the leg is limited on the affected side.
    _____ 2. Skinfolds of the affected thigh are deeper and asymmetrical.
    _____ 3. An Ortolani click is heard and felt as the femoral head slips into the acetabulum under gentle pressure.
    _____ 4. The knee heights are equal bilaterally.

148. Which of the following indicate possible appendicitis? Select all that apply.
    _____ 1. Tightening or rigidity of the abdominal muscles when the abdomen is palpated (guarding)
    _____ 2. When pressure is placed on the right lower quadrant of the abdomen, quick release results in severe pain (rebound tenderness).
    _____ 3. The child lying on the side with knees flexed toward the abdomen
    _____ 4. Oral temperature of 97.6° F (36.4° C)

149. A perfect Glasgow coma score is:
    1. 10.
    2. 3.
    3. 15.
    4. 25.

150. Select all that apply to the postoperative care of a neonate undergoing surgical repair of a cleft lip.
    _____ 1. Prevent crying and sucking.
    _____ 2. Position on the abdomen.
    _____ 3. Cuddle and hold infant.
    _____ 4. Keep suture line clean and free of crusts.

ANSWERS AND RATIONALES

1. Comprehension, assessment, health promotion and maintenance, (a).

    1. Adolescents are at the stage when they are constantly struggling to develop a positive self-image and their own identity and independence. They have a strong desire to remain dependent on parents while trying to detach.

2. These are the developmental skills developed during infancy and toddlerhood.

3, 4. These occur during the preschool stage.

2. Application, implementation, physiological integrity, (a).

   3. Large amounts of abnormally thick mucus are produced in the lungs, the pancreas, and the liver.

   1. Ciliary action is decreased with edema of the airway.

   2. This occurs in epiglottitis.

   4. These symptoms occur with laryngitis and asthma.

3. Application, implementation, physiological integrity, (b).

   3. Pancreatic enzymes are given regularly with food to improve the digestion and absorption of proteins and fats in the small intestine.

   1. Pancreatic enzymes do not directly affect vitamin absorption.

   2. Pancreatic enzymes do not affect carbohydrate metabolism.

   4. Although sodium levels are a problem in the child with CF, pancreatic enzymes do not affect them.

4. Analysis, implementation, physiological integrity, (a).

   2. This is the best-developed muscle in infants and therefore is the safest for IM injections.

   1. This muscle is not well developed in infants, toddlers, or young children.

   3. This muscle is not used until after 3 years of age.

   4. This muscle should not be used until the child has been walking for at least 2 years.

5. Analysis, implementation, safe and effective care environment, (b).

   3. Observing the length and type of seizure is important, as is preventing the child from injuring herself.

   1. This can injure the child's mouth.

   2. Suctioning may be needed, but it would not be feasible until the seizure was over.

   4. Restraints can lead to severe injury.

6. Analysis, assessment, physiological integrity, (b).

   2. These changes in the respiratory system lead to narrowing of the child's airway.

   1. These symptoms may be seen with laryngitis

   3. These symptoms might be seen with bronchitis.

   4. These symptoms do not occur in asthma.

7. Comprehension, assessment, physiological integrity, (b).

   4. The infant with bronchiolitis needs oxygen to maintain a pulse oximetry greater than 92% to relieve his extreme dyspnea and resultant hypoxemia.

   1. Oxygen would not reduce a fever.

   2. Although restlessness can be a result of hypoxia, this is not the primary reason for oxygen therapy.

   3. Oxygen would not liquefy secretions. Fluids and mucolytic medications liquefy secretions.

8. Comprehension, assessment, health promotion and maintenance, (b).

   4. These are the immunizations normally given at 2 months of age.

   1. The IPV is also given.

   2. The PPD is not given.

   3. The MMR vaccine is not given until 12 to 15 months of age.

9. Analysis, evaluation, physiological integrity, (b).

   4. This may indicate nerve damage at the fracture site or pressure from a tight cast and should be reported immediately.

   1. Plaster casts may take up to 24 hours to dry completely.

   2. This is a normal pulse rate. Pulse rate for a 6-year-old is 75 to 111 beats/min.

   3. This is usually a normal finding; any sudden increase in pain or severe muscle spasms should be reported to the physician.

10. Application, implementation, psychosocial integrity, (b).

    4. In cases of child abuse, the history given by the caregiver does not fit with the severity or type of injury.

    1. This may occur with other types of injury and child abuse.

    2, 3. These are not indications of abuse.

11. Analysis, assessment, physiological integrity, (a).

    2. A child in sickle cell crisis often experiences abdominal pain; swollen, painful joints; and fever.

    1. These do not occur in sickle cell crisis.

    3, 4. These are not symptoms of sickle cell crisis.

12. Comprehension, planning, physiological integrity, (b).

    4. The antiinflammatory effects of corticosteroids decrease the edema commonly seen with nephrotic syndrome.

    1. Steroids have no effect on proteinuria.

    2. Steroids have no effect on increased albumin levels.

    3. Steroids are not antihypertensive drugs.

13. Comprehension, assessment, physiological integrity, (c).

    3. The bronchoconstriction and inflammation of the airways seen in asthma cause these symptoms.

    1. These are symptoms of a cold; a child with asthma has a nonproductive cough.

    2. Asthma does not produce a fever or rhinorrhea.

    4. These are symptoms of epiglottitis.

14. Comprehension, planning, physiological integrity, (c).

    2. Bronchodilators (to relieve bronchial constriction) and antiinflammatory agents (to relieve inflammation of bronchial mucosa) are most often used together to treat asthma.

    1. Immunosuppressants are not regularly used to treat asthma.

    3. Antibiotics are not used to treat asthma. They may be ordered to prevent secondary bacterial infection.

    4. Decongestants and antihistamines are not effective in relieving the bronchoconstriction and inflammation seen in asthma.

15. Application, planning, physiological integrity, (c).

    2. Ribavirin (Virazole), an antiviral agent, is used specifically for RSV infection, especially in children with chronic conditions; humidified oxygen relieves the dyspnea and hypoxia seen with RSV disease.

    1. Cromolyn (Intal), a nonsteroidal antiinflammatory agent, is used in the treatment of asthma.

    3. Antibiotics are not used to treat viral infections such as respiratory syncytial virus (RSV).

    4. Prednisone (Liquid Pred) is not used for RSV infection.

16. Knowledge, assessment, physiological integrity, (b).

    3. An omphalocele is a defect in which the abdominal contents protrude through the abdominal wall in an intact sac.

    1. Intussusception is a telescoping of the bowel and occurs within the abdomen.

2. A diaphragmatic hernia is a congenital defect in the diaphragm that allows the abdominal contents to enter the thoracic cavity.
4. Gastroschisis is a herniation of the abdominal contents not covered by a peritoneal sac that herniates lateral to the umbilical ring.
17. Application, implementation, physiological integrity, (b).
Answer: 1800 mg/24 hr
1 lb=2.2 kg
66 lb ÷ 2.2 kg=30 kg
30 kg×60 mg=1800 mg over 24 hours
18. Application, implementation, physiological integrity, (b).
Answer: 40 drops/min
40×60 gtt/mL=2400 gtt/hr ÷ 60 min=40 gtt/min
19. Comprehension, assessment, physiological integrity, (c).
3. Croup is also known as spasmodic laryngitis.
1. Croup is usually of viral origin.
2. The esophagus is not involved in croup.
4. This would be pneumonia or pneumonitis.
20. Comprehension, assessment, physiological integrity, (a).
1. Ringworm is caused by a fungus and can occur on the scalp (tinea capitis), body (tinea corporis), or feet (tinea pedis).
2. This is an infestation of lice.
3. This is caused by a virus.
4. This is hives, often caused by allergies to foods or animal fur.
21. Application, implementation, physiological integrity, (b).
2. gr. v equals 325 mg; one tablet is the correct answer.
1, 3, 4. These are not correct answers.
22. Application, implementation, physiological integrity, (b).
2. In a 2-year-old, pulling the outer ear down and back straightens the ear canal so the drops can be instilled properly.
1. This is the correct position for children over 3 years of age.
3, 4. These are not the correct ear positions for medication administration.
23. Analysis, assessment, health promotion and maintenance, (b).
1. This is abnormal behavior for toddlers at this age level.
2, 3, 4. These are normal behaviors for a 3-year-old toddler.
24. Application, implementation, physiological integrity, (b).
3. These are appropriate fluids and food for a child with mild diarrhea.
1. This can lead to dehydration.
2, 4. These are inappropriate choices for a child with diarrhea.
25. Application, planning, physiological integrity, (b).
2. Palpation of the tumor is to be avoided to decrease the chance of cancer metastasis.
1. A 3-year-old cannot be held responsible for his or her own safety.
3, 4. These are not part of the care of a child with Wilms tumor.
26. Analysis, evaluation, physiological integrity, (c).
3. The most important clinical outcome for a child in respiratory distress is that the airway remains patent.
1. Remaining asleep for 8 hours is not a priority of need.
2. Pain relief is not the most important clinical outcome.
4. Although this is a positive outcome, it is not the most important clinical outcome for a child in respiratory distress.

27. Analysis, evaluation, physiological integrity, (c).
4. A child who follows the appropriate diet should have less fat in the stools (less steatorrhea).
1. The goal should be a slow, steady weight gain.
2. Anorexia is a clinical symptom of celiac disease.
3. This is not related to children with celiac disease who follow their diet.
28. Application, assessment, physiological integrity, (b).
3. Blood pressure measurement and observation for edema are assessment priorities when caring for a child with glomerulonephritis.
1. Assessment of color, motion, and sensation of the lower extremities is not a nursing priority for a child with glomerulonephritis.
2. Alteration of bowel sounds is not usually experienced with glomerulonephritis.
4. Level of consciousness is usually not altered in glomerulonephritis.
29. Application, implementation, psychosocial integrity, (b).
4. Nurses are considered mandated reporters of actual and suspected child abuse and neglect.
1. Because nurses are mandated reporters, they are legally bound to report abuse and neglect, regardless of possible legal consequences.
2. Nurses are not required to report abuse to a physician before calling a child abuse center.
3. Nurses are also required to report abuse.
30. Application, planning, physiological integrity, (b).
4. In an infant receiving IV therapy, special attention should be paid to maintaining the IV line and infusion of IV fluids.
1, 2. These are part of the infant's care but are not a priority.
3. This is not generally a necessary part of the infant's care.
31. Analysis, assessment, health promotion and maintenance, (c).
3. This is a normal characteristic for a healthy 1-month-old infant.
1, 2, 4. These are normal characteristics for a healthy 2- to 3-month-old infant.
32. Comprehension, assessment, health promotion and maintenance, (b).
2. Infants at this age first begin to differentiate between familiar faces and strangers and begin to demonstrate fear of strangers.
1. Fear of strangers has not developed at this age.
3. The infant at this age will show anxiety more consistently with strangers by turning or pushing away and crying.
4. The infant continues to be fearful of strangers; demonstration of anxiety begins earlier.
33. Application, implementation, physiological integrity, (c).
4. RSV bronchiolitis is a viral infection that causes the bronchioles to swell and become plugged with mucus. The trapped mucus makes expelling air difficult for the infant.
1, 2, 3. These are not the pathophysiology seen with RSV.
34. Application, implementation, physiological integrity, (b).
2. Ribavirin is administered by nebulization via an oxygen hood, tent, or mask for 12 to 20 hours per day for 1 to 7 days.
1, 3, 4. These are inappropriate ways to administer ribavirin.

35. Comprehension, assessment, physiological integrity, (b).
    4. An infant with Hirschsprung disease caused by a congenital lack of nerve cells in the wall of the colon exhibits these symptoms during the first several hours of life.
    1, 2. These are not signs of Hirschsprung disease.
    3. These are symptoms of pyloric stenosis.
36. Comprehension, planning, physiological integrity, (c).
    2. The infant with esophageal atresia must be kept on NPO status and on IV fluids until after surgery is completed to correct the defects. Suctioning of excess mucus is often necessary.
    1, 4. The infant must be on NPO status.
    3. This is not the treatment for esophageal atresia.
37. Comprehension, assessment, physiological integrity, (c).
    2. These are the four separate cardiac defects known as tetralogy of Fallot.
    1, 3, 4. These conditions do not make up the condition of tetralogy of Fallot.
38. Analysis, assessment, physiological integrity, (c).
    __X__ **1. These are characteristic signs of the spastic type of CP.**
    __X__ **2. These are characteristic signs of the spastic type of CP.**
    _____ 3. These are signs of athetoid or dyskinetic CP.
    _____ 4. These are signs of athetoid or dyskinetic CP.
    __X__ **5. These are characteristic signs of the spastic type of CP.**
39. Analysis, implementation, physiological integrity, (c).
    4. A sore throat is normal after a tonsillectomy, and the child is uncomfortable for a short period of time. An ice collar or ice popsicles (other than red) can be given to decrease the discomfort.
    1, 2, 3. These are all signs of postoperative bleeding after a tonsillectomy.
40. Analysis, assessment, physiological integrity, (c).
    2. These are the three main consequences of bone marrow dysfunction seen in leukemia.
    1, 3, 4. Blood clotting function is not a consequence of bone marrow dysfunction in leukemia.
41. Comprehension, assessment, physiological integrity, (b).
    4. Generalized seizures are bilaterally symmetrical and accompanied by impaired consciousness; grand mal seizures are one type of generalized seizure.
    1. Simple partial seizures consist of muscle movements involving face, neck, or extremities, with motor activity being the most common symptom.
    2. Complex partial seizure begins with a partial seizure with or without an aura, decreased consciousness, and repetitive movements such as lip smacking.
    3. Unilateral seizures are movements occurring on one side of the body.
42. Application, planning, physiological integrity, (a).
    3. This is the appropriate treatment for pediculosis.
    1. Antifungal oral medications are not used in the treatment of pediculosis.
    2, 4. These are not used in the treatment of pediculosis.
43. Application, implementation, psychosocial integrity, (c).
    3. The child with insulin-dependent diabetes, along with his or her parents (or other caregivers), should be taught how to give insulin injections.

1. Blood sugar (glucose) monitoring will most likely be required more than once each day.
2. Symptoms of hypoglycemia include low blood sugar and a normal glucose in the urine.
4. The child's diet will be different from before the diagnosis; he or she will also be required to exercise to help maintain a regular blood sugar level.
44. Application, planning, physiological integrity, (c).
    2. This is the action of antiretroviral agents in the treatment of HIV.
    1, 3, 4. These are not the actions of antiretroviral agents.
45. Application, implementation, psychosocial integrity, (b).
    3. This is the rationale for preparing children for hospitalization.
    1. This is true, but it is not the rationale for preparing children for hospitalization.
    2, 4. These are not the rationales for preparing children for hospitalization.
46. Comprehension, implementation, physiological integrity, (b).
    1. Russell traction is a type of skin traction.
    2, 3. These are not used for a fractured femur.
    4. Pelvic traction is another type of skin traction, but it is not the type used for a fractured femur.
47. Analysis, assessment, physiological integrity, (b).
    2. A red, flat rash is normally seen on the body of an adolescent with mononucleosis.
    1, 3, 4. These are not common symptoms of mononucleosis.
48. Comprehension, assessment, health promotion, (b).
    __X__ **1. This is true of iron deficiency anemia.**
    __X__ **2. This is true of iron deficiency anemia.**
    _____ 3. Decreased platelet count can result in severe hemorrhage in children.
    __X__ **4. This is true of iron deficiency anemia.**
    __X__ **5. This is true of iron-deficiency anemia.**
49. Application, implementation, physiological integrity, (a).
    Answer: 50 kg
    2.2 lb = 1 kg
    110 ÷ 2.2 = 50
50. Application, implementation, physiological integrity, (b).
    2. Colic, or paroxysmal abdominal pain, usually disappears after 3 months of age. Placing the baby prone over a covered hot water bottle, avoiding overstimulation, and using a pacifier, a swing, or a music box may reduce symptoms of colic.
    1. This does not relieve colic and may worsen symptoms.
    3. Large amounts of formula may increase symptoms.
    4. Ingestion of rice cereal may or may not relieve symptoms of colic.
51. Analysis, assessment, physiological integrity, (c).
    2. These are symptoms of measles (rubeola).
    1. Signs and symptoms include macules, papules, vesicles, and crusts.
    3. Symptoms include redness, intradermal vesicles, weeping, and coarsening of the skin.
    4. Symptoms include a small, pink or pale red rash.
52. Application, implementation, physiological integrity, (b).
    Answer: 6 mL
    0.5 g = 500 mg (500/5 mL)
    600 (DD)/500 (DH) × 5 = 6 mL

53. Comprehension, planning, physiological integrity, (c).

    4. Needs for antidiarrheal medications differ based on the type and severity of dehydration and the age and body size.

    1. IV fluids and electrolyte replacement are required.

    2. Oral rehydration with Pedialyte can be initiated as soon as the child can tolerate PO fluid administration.

    3. Solid foods should be introduced as soon as tolerated.

54. Application, implementation, physiological integrity, (a).

    4. This equipment may be necessary because the enlarged epiglottis may lead to obstruction in a period of hours. It is a life-threatening medical emergency.

    1. Any examination of the throat can lead to laryngospasm.

    2. The child with epiglottitis has difficulty swallowing.

    3. The child should be upright, in a position of comfort.

55. Comprehension, planning, physiological integrity, (b).

    3. Prompt diagnosis and treatment are required to prevent serious side effects and death.

    1. Bacterial meningitis is treated with IV antibiotics.

    2. This disease is more commonly seen in children.

    4. Diagnosis is made by analysis of spinal fluid and symptoms.

56. Application, implementation, health promotion and maintenance, (a).

    Answer: 2 tablets

    gr. v per tablet=5 grains per tablet, 60 mg in 1 grain, 5 grains=300 mg, 10 grains=600 mg, or two tablets

57. Knowledge, assessment, physiological integrity, (b).

    2. Rheumatic fever is an autoimmune response that follows a streptococcal infection.

    1. It is not caused by a virus.

    3. It is not caused by the *E. coli* bacterium.

    4. It is not caused by a fungus.

58. Application, implementation, physiological integrity, (c).

    1. Because of malabsorption, an infant with Hirschsprung disease often needs TPN before surgery to replace nutrients, fluids, and electrolytes.

    2. The child would be on NPO status before surgery.

    3. Hirschsprung disease affects the intestine, not the stomach.

    4. IV antibiotics are not necessary. The disorder is not bacterial.

59. Comprehension, assessment, physiological integrity, (b).

    __X__ **1. This would be a sign of dehydration in an infant.**

    _____ 2. The skin would be warm and dry.

    __X__ **3. This would be a sign of dehydration in an infant.**

    __X__ **4. This would be a sign of dehydration in an infant.**

    __X__ **5. This would be a sign of dehydration in an infant.**

60. Comprehension, assessment, physiological integrity, (b).

    4. These are all common symptoms of celiac disease.

    1, 3. Chronic diarrhea, not constipation, is a classic symptom.

    2. Thirst is not a common symptom of celiac disease.

61. Comprehension, planning, physiological integrity, (b).

    4. This is the safest, most effective method for reducing an intussusception.

    1. This does not reduce an intussusception.

2. Surgery may be necessary if hydrostatic reduction is not successful.

3. This is not necessary for reducing an intussusception.

62. Comprehension, assessment, physiological integrity, (b).

    4. These symptoms of leukemia result directly from changes in the bone marrow.

    1. These symptoms are caused by leukemic effects on the nervous system that lead to increased intracranial pressure.

    2. These symptoms result from the increasing need of the body to meet the metabolic needs of the leukemic cells.

    3. Usually intracranial pressure is increased, leading to seizures and altered mental status.

63. Application, implementation, health promotion and maintenance, (b).

    4. Eustachian tubes are shorter and wider in the young child than they are in the older child, which allows for easier introduction of bacteria.

    1. The epiglottis is in the throat area.

    2. The eardrum separates the external from the middle ear.

    3. The external ear canals are basically the same shape and in the same position in young and older children.

64. Knowledge, implementation, physiological integrity, (a).

    3. This is the correct term for this surgery.

    1. Epispadias is an opening of the urethral meatus on the top of the penis.

    2. Cystotomy is a surgical opening in the bladder.

    4. Removal of the testes is an orchiectomy.

65. Application, implementation, physiological integrity, (b).

    2. Appropriate order is ampicillin 500 mg four times daily.

    44 lb ÷ 2.2=20 kg

    100 mg/kg/day×20=2000 mg/day

    2000 mg ÷ 4 doses=500 mg

    1, 3, 4. These are incorrect doses for this child.

66. Comprehension, planning, physiological integrity, (c).

    2. These two chemotherapy drugs are used in effective treatment of nephroblastoma (Wilms tumor).

    1, 3, 4. These two drugs are not commonly used in treating nephroblastoma.

67. Comprehension, assessment, physiological integrity, (a).

    4. The Jones criteria are used only to diagnose rheumatic fever.

    1. Leukemia is diagnosed by evaluation of blood count levels and physical symptoms.

    2, 3. These are hereditary, not inflammatory, diseases. These symptoms would not apply.

68. Comprehension, assessment, physiological integrity, (b).

    4. These are symptoms commonly seen in developmental dysplasia of the hip.

    1. Classic signs of clubfoot (talipes equinovarus) include feet that are turned inward; the child walks on the toes and outer border of the feet.

    2. Signs of bone cancer (osteosarcoma) include insidious intermittent pain, a palpable mass, limping, limited range of motion, and fracture at tumor site.

    3. Classic signs of CP depend on the type of CP and can include toe walking; jerky movements; and slow, uncontrolled writhing movements.

69. Comprehension, assessment, physiological integrity, (b).

    1. Severe tachypnea seen in bronchiolitis is a contraindication for oral feedings because of the risk of aspiration.

2. An infant with bronchiolitis cannot verbalize complaints of nausea.

3, 4. These are not contraindications for oral fluids.

70. Comprehension, assessment, physiological integrity, (b).

   4. Cerebral palsy is a disorder that affects the motor centers of the brain; it is usually caused by birth trauma or head trauma.

   1. This is a chromosomal abnormality.

   2. This is excess cerebrospinal fluid around the brain.

   3. This is an infection in a bone.

71. Application, implementation, physiological integrity, (b).

   1. Patency of the airway and preventing shock are the initial primary goals after a burn.

   2, 3, 4. Although all of these are important, they are secondary to airway patency and shock.

72. Knowledge, assessment, physiological integrity, (a).

   3. Hydrocephalus occurs when an obstruction of the CSF drainage pathways is present.

   1. Opisthotonos (arching of the back) is a sign of increased intracranial pressure.

   2. It does not cause Hirschsprung disease, a gastrointestinal disorder.

   4. It does not cause infection or inflammation of the meninges, called *meningitis.*

73. Comprehension, assessment, health promotion and maintenance, (b).

   1. This is the amount of weight a toddler should gain each year.

   2, 3, 4. These amounts are higher than the normal annual weight gain for toddlers.

74. Application, implementation, physiological integrity, (b).
   Answer: 1350 mg

   99 lb ÷ 2.2 kg = 45 kg

   30 mg/kg × 45 kg = 1350 mg

75. Comprehension, assessment, physiological integrity, (b).

   __X__ **1. These are classic symptoms of an infant with FTT.**

   _____ 2. The infant would have a rag-doll limpness.

   __X__ **3. These are classic symptoms of an infant with FTT.**

   __X__ **4. These are classic symptoms of an infant with FTT.**

   __X__ **5. These are classic symptoms of an infant with FTT.**

76. Knowledge, assessment, physiological integrity, (b).

   3. Physiological changes in the child with CF cause this symptom.

   1, 2, 4. These are not commonly seen in children with CF.

77. Analysis, assessment, physiological integrity, (b).

   2. These are classic symptoms of an infant with pyloric stenosis.

   1. These are not symptoms of tetralogy of Fallot, which consists of four defects in heart structure.

   3. These are not symptoms of esophageal atresia, a congenital defect in which the esophagus fails to connect to the stomach.

   4. These are not symptoms of intussusception, which is a slipping of one part of the intestine into another part just below it. A classic symptom is currant jelly stools.

78. Comprehension, assessment, physiological integrity, (b).

   _____ 1. Dunlop traction is used for fracture or dislocation of the upper extremity.

   __X__ **2. Buck traction is a type of skin traction used for lower extremity dislocation or fracture.**

   __X__ **3. Russell traction is a type of skin traction used for lower extremity dislocation or fracture.**

   __X__ **4. Thomas ring is a type of skin traction used for lower extremity dislocation or fracture.**

79. Application, planning, physiological integrity, (b).

   4. Assessing sensation, circulation, and motion in affected extremities is necessary for all children in a cast.

   1. Pain management is a primary intervention of care.

   2. Fluids should be encouraged because of the adverse effects of immobility; the cast can be kept dry by careful diapering and padding of the cast.

   3. The legs would be elevated to promote venous return and prevent edema.

80. Analysis, assessment, physiological integrity, (c).

   2. Symptoms of a child with autism include bizarre behavior, temper tantrums, delayed language and development, inability to maintain eye contact, and the appearance of living in a world of their own.

   1, 3. These are considered normal behaviors for a child of this age.

   4. The child with autism is not even-tempered and is prone to temper tantrums. There may be some degree of mental retardation, but some children do show exceptional talent in certain areas.

81. Comprehension, evaluation, physiological integrity, (b).

   2. Several studies have demonstrated that infants with this history are at a greater risk of SIDS.

   1. This is not applicable to SIDS.

   3. The peak age for SIDS is 2 to 4 months.

   4. This is not applicable to SIDS.

82. Analysis, implementation, physiological integrity, (c).

   3. This medication is used in the treatment of these symptoms of KD.

   1, 2, 4. These medications are not used in treating KD.

83. Application, planning, physiological integrity, (b).

   1. In epileptic children with poorly controlled seizures, a ketogenic diet is often suggested as a method of treatment.

   2. Children with Crohn disease are usually on a soft, low-fiber diet.

   3. Children with Hirschsprung disease are not placed on a ketogenic diet.

   4. Children with acute glomerulonephritis are usually on a low-sodium diet.

84. Analysis, assessment, physiological integrity, (b).

   2. The infant with colic demonstrates these signs and symptoms.

   1. Signs and symptoms of intussusception begin suddenly and include vomiting and bloody stools.

   3. Signs and symptoms of pyloric stenosis include projectile vomiting and weight loss.

   4. Signs and symptoms of gastroenteritis include dehydration, irritability, vomiting, and weight loss.

85. Analysis, implementation, physiological integrity, (b).

   3. According to several studies, this is the safest place to position an infant in a car seat.

   1, 2, 4. These car seat positions are more dangerous than the correct answer.

86. Comprehension, assessment, physiological integrity, (b).
    1. **This is the pathophysiology of RSV bronchiolitis.**
    2. Peak incidence for RSV infection is 2 to 5 months of age.
    3. RSV occurs primarily in the winter and spring.
    4. Children are exposed through family members with upper respiratory infections.

87. Knowledge, assessment, health promotion and maintenance, (c).
    1. **Kohlberg's theory states that preschoolers conform to rules to obtain rewards.**
    2. Toddlers follow rules to avoid punishment.
    3, 4. School-aged children follow rules to please others and avoid disapproval.

88. Application, evaluation, physiological integrity, (b).
    4. **This is a common sign of bleeding in the early postoperative period.**
    1. This is normally seen after tonsillectomy.
    2. This is a late sign of blood loss and hypovolemic shock.
    3. This is not a sign of early bleeding.

89. Application, implementation, physiological integrity, (c).
    3. **Meperidine 0.8 mL, atropine 0.5 mL**
    Meperidine: Desired dose (DD)=40 mg
    Dose on hand (DH)=50 mg, volume (V)=1 mL
    DD/DH=40 mg/50 mg×1 mL=0.8 mL
    Atropine: DD=0.1 mg
    DH=0.2 mg, V=1 mL
    DD/DH=0.1 mg/0.2 mg×1 mL=0.5 mL
    1, 2, 4. These are not the correct doses.

90. Analysis, assessment, physiological integrity, (c).
    __X__ 1. **This occurs as the glomeruli fail to filter blood and allow albumin and protein to enter urine. A fall in the level of protein in the blood is seen.**
    __X__ 2. **This occurs as the glomeruli fail to filter blood and allow albumin and protein to enter urine. A fall in the level of protein in the blood is seen.**
    __X__ 3. **This occurs as the glomeruli fail to filter blood and allow albumin and protein to enter urine. A fall in the level of protein in the blood is seen.**
    _____ 4. This is not a sign of nephrotic syndrome.

91. Application, implementation, physiological integrity, (b).
    4. **2.4 mL**
    Desired dose (DD)=600 mg
    Dose on hand (DH)=1 g (1000 mg), volume (V)=4 mL
    DD/DH=600 mg/1000 mg×4 mL=2.4 mL
    1, 2, 3. These are not correct doses.

92. Comprehension, assessment, physiological integrity, (b).
    4. **The urine is dark in color in the early morning in children with acute glomerulonephritis.**
    1. Frequent, painful urination can be a sign of a urinary tract infection.
    2. This is not a symptom of glomerulonephritis.
    3. Although edema can occur, it is not a sign seen early in the morning with acute glomerulonephritis.

93. Application, implementation, physiological integrity, (c).
    Answer: 0.25 mL, or 1/4 mL
    DD/DH×V
    25/100×1=0.25 mL, or 1/4 mL

94. Application, planning, psychosocial integrity, (b).
    2. **This is the main treatment goal for children with MD.**
    1. The respiratory system is usually not involved in early stages of MD.

3. This is not a goal of MD treatment.
    4. Physical activity should be encouraged to promote muscular function.

95. Application, implementation, physiological integrity, (b).
    1. **This is the correct rate of infusion.**
    50 mL×10 gtt/mL=500 gtt/hr
    500 gtt ÷ 60 min=8.3 gtt/min, or 8 gtt/min
    2, 3, 4. These rates are too fast.

96. Comprehension, assessment, physiological integrity, (a).
    4. **Fats are not completely digested in a child with CF because of the lack of the enzyme lipase. These fats are excreted with the stool, making it frothy and foul smelling.**
    1, 2, 3. These do not cause the abnormal stools seen in CF.

97. Knowledge, assessment, physiological integrity, (b).
    1. **The pancreas is the organ most severely affected by CF.**
    2, 3, 4. These organs are not directly affected by CF.

98. Analysis, assessment, health promotion and maintenance, (c).
    3. **Kohlberg's theory states that school-aged children follow rules to please others.**
    1. Toddlers follow rules to avoid punishment.
    2. Preschoolers follow rules to obtain rewards.
    4. Adolescents follow rules out of concern for others.

99. Comprehension, planning, physiological integrity, (b).
    1. **Celiac syndrome is a metabolic defect precipitated by the ingestion of rye or wheat gluten.**
    2, 3, 4. These are not contraindicated for children with celiac disease.

100. Comprehension, assessment, physiological integrity, (b).
    1. **Constipation is a symptom of anorexia nervosa.**
    2. Amenorrhea, not painful menses (dysmenorrhea), may appear with anorexia nervosa.
    3. Abdominal distention is not often seen in these patients.
    4. Bradycardia and hypotension are common, probably because of the state of starvation.

101. Analysis, assessment, physiological integrity, (b).
    __X__ 1. **Tachypnea is a symptom of respiratory distress syndrome.**
    __X__ 2. **Flaring nostrils are a symptom of respiratory distress syndrome.**
    _____ 3. Flushed skin is not a sign of respiratory distress.
    __X__ 4. **Generalized cyanosis is a symptom of respiratory distress syndrome.**
    __X__ 5. **Sternal retractions are a symptom of respiratory distress syndrome.**

102. Application, assessment, physiological integrity, (b).
    4. **This is the most important assessment to make on a child with hydrocephalus.**
    1, 3. These are not important assessments to make on this child.
    2. Frequent neurological checks may be necessary but not neurovascular checks.

103. Application, implementation, physiological integrity, (b).
    1. **This is the medication used to treat pinworms effectively.**
    2, 3, 4. These are not used to treat pinworms.

104. Knowledge, assessment, physiological integrity, (a).
    4. **This is another name for trisomy 21.**
    1, 2, 3. These are other types of genetic syndromes.

105. Knowledge, assessment, health promotion and maintenance, (b).
    2. An infant normally triples his or her birth weight at 12 months of age.
    1. This is too early to expect birth weight to triple.
    3, 4. By this age the birth weight of the infant should be more than tripled.
106. Comprehension, assessment, physiological integrity, (b).
    3. Hirschsprung disease is a congenital anomaly (absence of the ganglion nerve cells) that results in a mechanical obstruction of the colon.
    1, 2, 4. These are not the causes of Hirschsprung disease.
107. Analysis, assessment, health promotion and maintenance, (b).
    2. This is the test most commonly used in diagnosing asthma.
    1. A chest x-ray examination may be ordered, but it alone cannot diagnose asthma.
    3. This test is used to diagnose cystic fibrosis.
    4. This test is not used in the diagnosis of asthma.
108. Comprehension, assessment, health promotion and maintenance, (b).
    __X__ **1. The two types of OM are AOM, also called suppurative or purulent OM, and serous or nonsuppurative OM with effusion (OME).**
    __X__ **2. Sucking, chewing, and high fever (104° F, or 40° C) accompanied by headache, vomiting, and diarrhea are common symptoms of AOM.**
    __X__ **3. The most common cause of AOM is S. pneumonia or H. influenzae infection. The cause of OME is unknown.**
    _____ 4. OM affects the middle ear.
109. Analysis, assessment, physiological integrity, (b).
    2. These are classic symptoms of acute appendicitis.
    1, 3, 4. These are not signs of this disease.
110. Comprehension, assessment, physiological integrity, (b).
    4. Scrotal edema, along with edema to the face, extremities, and abdomen, is a common sign of nephrotic syndrome.
    1. This is a sign of severe dehydration.
    2. Urinary output is decreased in a child with nephrotic syndrome.
    3. The child with nephrotic syndrome is not jaundiced.
111. Comprehension, assessment, health promotion and maintenance, (b).
    3. Inflammation causes the ESR to be elevated.
    1, 2, 4. These levels are not usually affected by inflammation caused by rheumatic fever.
112. Comprehension, assessment, physiological integrity, (b).
    2. The elevated blood glucose and ketones cause thirst and frequency in urination.
    1. A newly diagnosed, untreated person with diabetes is hyperglycemic.
    3. This is not a common symptom of type 1 diabetes.
    4. A child with newly diagnosed diabetes may be hungry but experiences weight loss.
113. Comprehension, evaluation, physiological integrity, (c).
    3. Prednisone is given to decrease inflammation.
    1, 2, 4. These would not be expected actions of prednisone used for rheumatic fever.

114. Comprehension, assessment, health promotion and maintenance, (b).
    3. Primitive reflexes (grasp, tonic neck) disappear by 5 months of age.
    1, 2. Primitive reflexes remain strong at these ages.
    4. Primitive reflexes have disappeared earlier than this age.
115. Application, implementation, physiological integrity, (c).
    3. These are required for the adolescent to maintain control of his diabetes.
    1. Activity should not be limited.
    2. Oral hypoglycemics are not effective for type 1 diabetes.
    4. This would be too few calories and probably too much insulin for the adolescent.
116. Knowledge, implementation, health promotion and maintenance, (b).
    1. The American Academy of Pediatrics has advised that the last dose should not be administered before 6 months of age.
    2, 3, 4. The third dose might be given before these ages.
117. Comprehension, assessment, health promotion and maintenance, (b).
    4. Adolescents are guided by their conscience and focused on their rights as a person.
    1. School-aged children follow rules to please others.
    2. Preschoolers follow rules to obtain rewards.
    3. Avoiding punishment is the reason that toddlers follow rules.
118. Comprehension, assessment, physiological integrity, (b).
    1. The most common cause of infectious gastroenteritis in infants is the rotavirus.
    2, 4. These are not common causes of infectious gastroenteritis.
    3. *E. coli* is normally found in the stool and is usually not a cause of infectious gastroenteritis in infants.
119. Application, planning, physiological integrity, (b).
    2. Normally the first breast-feeding or bottle-feeding is given 4 hours after surgery.
    1. This is too early for oral feedings to begin.
    3. NG feedings are not used after this surgery.
    4. This is usually when formula is started after surgery.
120. Knowledge, assessment, physiological integrity, (b).
    1. Ecstasy is classified as a stimulant.
    2, 3, 4. These are incorrect classifications for ecstasy.
121. Application, implementation, physiological integrity, (b).
    __X__ **1. Antibiotics are used, and the patient is placed in isolation until antibiotics have been given for at least 24 hours.**
    _____ 2. Narcotic analgesics are not used because they will alter the level of consciousness.
    __X__ **3. Antipyretics are ordered to aid in decreasing the high fever.**
    __X__ **4. Antiemetics are ordered to decrease the vomiting that accompanies the condition.**
122. Knowledge, assessment, physiological integrity, (a).
    2. These are commonly seen in children with Crohn disease.
    1, 3, 4. These are not symptoms of Crohn disease.
123. Comprehension, assessment, physiological integrity, (b).
    1. This is the virus that causes HIV.
    2. Strep throat is an example of an infection caused by the streptococcal organism.

3. Mononucleosis is caused by the Epstein-Barr virus.

4. Rheumatoid arthritis is an example of an autoimmune response.

124. Application, implementation, physiological integrity, (b).

   3. Nursing care of the child after ventriculoperitoneal shunt insertion should include head circumference measurements to help determine if the shunt is draining cerebrospinal fluid properly.

   1. Wilms tumor is a tumor of the kidney.

   2. Omphalocele is a protrusion into the umbilical region.

   4. This is not a necessary postoperative nursing intervention for spinal cord injury.

125. Application, implementation, physiological integrity, (c).

   2. Severe acne can often be successfully treated with application of retinoic acid.

   1, 3, 4. These medications are not used in treating severe acne.

126. Comprehension, assessment, physiological integrity, (c).

   3. These are signs and symptoms of nephrotic syndrome.

   1. Nephrotic syndrome includes hypoalbuminemia and dark urine.

   2, 4. Nephrotic syndrome is diagnosed via renal biopsy; levels of protein in the blood are decreased.

127. Analysis, implementation, physiological integrity, (c).

   3. Antiviral drugs help to prevent the development of acquired immunodeficiency syndrome in patients who are HIV-positive by decreasing the replication of virus particles.

   1, 2, 4. These are not the actions of antiretroviral drugs.

128. Comprehension, assessment, physiological integrity, (b).

   3. This bleeding disorder is known as hemophilia.

   1. Sickle cell anemia is an inherited defect in the formation of hemoglobin.

   2. Thalassemia is a form of anemia.

   4. Leukemia is a malignant disease of blood-forming organs.

129. Comprehension, assessment, physiological integrity, (b).

   4. These are all characteristic signs of muscular dystrophy.

   1, 2, 3. These are not characteristic signs of this disease.

130. Analysis, evaluation, health promotion and maintenance, (b).

   3. Along with separation from peers, these are major issues causing stress in hospitalized adolescents.

   1. This is a major stressor for toddlers.

   2. This is a major stressor for preschoolers.

   4. This is usually not a major stressor for most adolescents.

131. Comprehension, assessment, health promotion and maintenance, (b).

   3. These are typical signs of an adolescent who is abusing drugs or alcohol.

   1, 2, 4. These are not all typical signs of this disorder.

132. Knowledge, assessment, physiological integrity, (b).

   2. Leukemia is the most common cancer seen in children.

   1. This type of cancer is seen in children, but it is not as common as leukemia. Lymphoma is cancer of lymphoid tissue.

   3. This type of cancer is seen in children, but it is not as common as leukemia. Wilms tumor is a tumor of the kidneys.

   4. This type of cancer is seen in children, but it is not as common as leukemia. Osteosarcoma is cancer of the bone.

133. Comprehension, implementation, health promotion and maintenance, (b).

   1. This test, along with a barium enema, is used to confirm Hirschsprung disease.

   2, 3, 4. These tests are not used to confirm Hirschsprung disease.

134. Comprehension, assessment, physiological integrity, (b).

   4. Projectile vomiting is a classic sign of pyloric stenosis.

   1. Intussusception is a slipping of one part of the intestine into another.

   2. This is a viral infection of the gastrointestinal tract.

   3. This is an abnormal connection between the esophagus and the trachea.

135. Analysis, assessment, physiological integrity, (c).

   1. Tetralogy of Fallot is a cyanotic heart defect consisting of four separate congenital defects.

   2. Coarctation is a constricting or narrowing of the aortic arch. It is an acyanotic heart defect.

   3. ASD is an abnormal opening between the right and left atria. It is an acyanotic heart defect.

   4. PDA allows blood to pass from the aorta to the pulmonary artery. It is an acyanotic heart defect.

136. Application, implementation, physiological integrity, (c).

   4. This is the correct dose based on the weight of the infant.

   2.2 lb = 1 kg

   15 lb ÷ 2.2 = 6.8 kg

   Desired dose (DD) = 0.1 mg/kg

   6.8 kg × 0.1 mg = 0.68 mg (rounded to 0.7 mg)

   1, 2. These are incorrect doses.

   3. Morphine can be given via subcutaneous, intramuscular, intravenous, and epidural routes.

137. Application, implementation, physiological integrity, (b).

   Answer: 187.5 mg

   1 lb = 2.2 kg

   55 lb ÷ 2.2 = 25 kg

   25 kg × 7.5 mg = 187.5 mg

138. Comprehension, assessment, physiological integrity, (b).

   4. With normal growth and development, the infant's weight triples by 12 months. This infant should weigh approximately 20 pounds.

   1, 2, 3. These weights are below what a 6-pound 11-ounce infant should weigh at 1 year of age.

139. Analysis, assessment, physiological integrity, (c).

   1. The opening in the palate allows formula to enter the nose, airway, and ear canal.

   2, 3, 4. These are not common complications of cleft palate.

140. Knowledge, assessment, physiological integrity, (b).

   2. Bulimia is characterized by episodes of binge eating (eating large amounts in a small amount of time), and purging, vomiting, or taking laxatives.

   1. This is the definition of anorexia nervosa.

   3, 4. These are related to and define obesity.

141. Comprehension, assessment, physiological integrity, (b).

   2. A malfunctioning spleen causes the child with sickle cell disease to be immunocompromised.

   1. Malnutrition is not a common characteristic of children with sickle cell disease.

   3. These children are given antibiotics only if an infection develops.

   4. Sickledex is a laboratory test, not a medication.

142. Application, implementation, physiological integrity, (b).
_____ 1. Suction should be no longer than 5 seconds for this age.
__X__ 2. *This is a basic fundamental of suctioning a tracheostomy of a 5-year-old.*
__X__ 3. *This is a basic fundamental of suctioning a tracheostomy of a 5-year-old.*
__X__ 4. *This is a basic fundamental of suctioning a tracheostomy of a 5-year-old.*
_____ 5. The head should be elevated during tracheal suctioning.

143. Application, implementation, physiological integrity, (b).
4. These signs would indicate respiratory distress.
1. This is a normal circumference of the head (13 to 15 inches [33 to 35 cm]).
2. Acrocyanosis related to an immature circulatory system is normal in a newborn.
3. Normal heart rate for a newborn is 120 to 160 beats/min.

144. Comprehension, assessment, physiological integrity, (a).
4. These are indicators of aspiration from the esophagus into the trachea.
1. Normal respiratory rate is 30 to 50 breaths/min.
2. Poor sucking can be related to hypoglycemia and immaturity of the nervous system.
3. Swallowing heard during eating is an expected finding.

145. Comprehension, assessment, physiological integrity, (a).
__X__ 1. *Low birth weight is seen more commonly in newborns of teenage mothers.*
_____ 2. This is a normal finding.
__X__ 3. *Brain bleeds are seen more commonly in newborns of teenage mothers.*
__X__ 4. *Respiratory difficulty is seen more commonly in newborns of teenage mothers.*

146. Knowledge, assessment, health promotion and maintenance, (b).
1. Head lice (pediculosis capitis) are transmitted from person to person or by contaminated articles.
2. Head lice survive from the blood extracted from the infested person.

3. Head lice affect the scalp and hair. The adult attaches numerous eggs (nits) ⅛ inch from the scalp.
4. Antifungal medications do not kill adult lice. Antiparasitic medications are used.

147. Analysis, assessment, physiological integrity, (a).
__X__ 1. *Limited abduction of the affected thigh is a classic sign of hip dysplasia.*
__X__ 2. *Skinfold of the affected thigh is a classic sign of hip dysplasia.*
__X__ 3. *Audible click (Ortolani click) is a classic sign of hip dysplasia.*
_____ 4. Knee heights are classically unequal in hip dysplasia

148. Comprehension, assessment, physiological integrity, (c).
__X__ 1. *Guarding is characterized by tightening of the abdomen and is seen in a child with appendicitis.*
__X__ 2. *Rebound tenderness is a symptom seen in children with appendicitis.*
__X__ 3. *Side-lying, knee-flexed position is a symptom seen in children with appendicitis.*
_____ 4. Fever is usually seen as a symptom of appendicitis.

149. Analysis, assessment, physiological integrity, (a).
3. Glasgow coma score consists of three parts—eye opening (4 points), motor response (6 points), and verbal response (5 points). A perfect score is 15.
1. A score of 10 points indicates serious neurological deficits.
2. A score of 3 points is the lowest achieved on a Glasgow coma score.
4. A score of 25 points is beyond the maximum achieved on a Glasgow coma score.

150. Application, planning, physiological integrity, (b).
__X__ 1. *Crying and sucking cause tension on the suture line.*
_____ 2. Position with care, never on abdomen, which could cause injury to suture line.
__X__ 3. *Cuddling meets the emotional needs of the infant.*
__X__ 4. *Crusts could result in scarring.*

Nursing Care of the Aging Adult

Objectives

After studying this chapter, the student should be able to:

1. Differentiate between physiological and psychosocial theories of aging.
2. Describe the changes of aging on each body system, including how these normal changes differ from disease processes.
3. Identify important techniques for effective therapeutic communications with older adults.
4. Explain how nursing care and anticipatory teaching can positively affect older adults.
5. Discuss important factors to consider when administering medications to older adults.
6. List assessment techniques and adaptations appropriate for older adults.
7. Describe specific diseases that affect each body system and effective nursing care for older adults.

The percentage of the American population over age 65 years is increasing, and life expectancy is lengthening. By the year 2030 nurses will be challenged to care for an aging adult population that constitutes 22% of the total population. In addition, minority populations will be an increasing percentage of the elderly population in 2030. Maintaining health and wellness and caring for increasingly older adults will be the tasks in future years.

The nursing challenge is to meet the care needs of our older adults. Nurses have an opportunity to play a significant role in determining whether these will be years of continued growth and development, happiness, and accomplishment or years of forced shame, illness, and neglect.

This chapter focuses on aging as a normal process of growth and development. Maslow's hierarchy of needs continues to provide a structure for understanding care of the older adult.

GOVERNMENT RESOURCES FOR THE OLDER ADULT

INCOME

A. Social Security (Old-Age, Survivors, and Disability Insurance [OASDI]): a federal program first adopted in 1935
   1. Funded by employee and employer payroll taxes
   2. Entitlement is determined by U.S. Social Security Administration; benefits are granted in accordance with:
      a. Age.
      b. Lifetime earnings record; retirement age is steadily increasing.
      c. Free earnings credits for active military service.
      d. Whether the required number of work credits has been earned (work credits are measured in quarters).
   3. There is a specific maximum benefit amount with cost-of-living protection against inflation.
   4. Minimum retirement benefits begin at 62 years of age.
   5. Railroad workers have a separate retirement system; workers who have fewer than 10 years of railroad service may transfer earnings to Social Security to be counted toward Social Security benefits.
   6. Federal employees are covered under the Civil Service Retirement System, the Federal Employees Retirement System, and the Thrift Savings Plan.
   7. Social Security benefits are reduced according to money earned over a stated maximum annual allowable income.
   8. Social Security benefits are not reduced for full-time employees over the age of 70 years.
   9. Payments are indexed according to inflation rate.
B. Supplemental Security Income (SSI); established in 1972
   1. Funded from general tax revenues
   2. Cash-assistance program
   3. Administered by the Social Security Administration
   4. Designed to provide for disabled, blind, or aged with limited incomes and resources
   5. Medicaid eligibility in many states is based on SSI eligibility.

HEALTH

A. Medicare (Title XVIII of Social Security Act): established in 1965
   1. Administered by the Centers for Medicare and Medicaid Services (CMS) (www.cms.gov), a branch of the U.S. Department of Health and Human Services
   2. Designed to help people over 65 years of age, certain disabled people under 65 years of age who are eligible under Social Security, and people of any age with permanent kidney failure to meet medical care costs regardless of income
   3. Claims handled by major insurance companies in each state (e.g., Travelers Insurance Company in New York)
   4. Pays for only limited time in long-term care
   5. Do not have to be retired to receive benefits
   6. Financed by employer and employee payroll taxes and self-employment tax money

7. Everyone over 65 years of age who is entitled to Social Security benefits receives hospital insurance without paying premium charges.
8. Automatic hospital insurance is provided to disabled persons who have been entitled to Social Security disability benefits for 24 consecutive months.
9. Initial enrollment period begins 3 months before the month in which the individual will become 65 years of age and continues for 4 months after individual turns 65 years of age.
10. The annual enrollment period is January 1 through March 31.
11. Premiums generally increase if people do not apply when they are eligible.
12. The deductible is applied to each benefit period.
13. Three parts
    a. Part A is designed as hospital insurance that has certain exclusions.
    b. Part B covers physician services and outpatient services.
    c. Part D covers prescription drug costs.
    d. If subscribing to part A, the person is automatically enrolled in part B unless it is declined.
    e. Part A is free; there is a cost for Part B and Part D; premiums can be withheld from the Social Security benefit.
B. Medicaid (Title XIX of Social Security Act); established in 1965
    1. Purposes
       a. To cover specific expenses not provided for by Medicare
       b. To reduce expenses of individuals who have exhausted their Medicare benefits
       c. To defray medical expenses of persons who cannot afford Medicare premiums
    2. Funded by federal and state contributions
    3. State-operated programs
    4. Funds the majority of long-term care after Medicare and personal funds are depleted
    5. Other programs
       a. Qualified Medicare Beneficiary (QMB) Program
          (1) Annual income must be at or below the national poverty level; 12% of older adults fall below the poverty line.
          (2) Functions similar to a Medigap policy
          (3) State Medicaid program helps pay
          (4) Pays Medicare Part B premium
          (5) Pays Medicare Part A premiums for eligible older adults and disabled persons, Medicare deductible, and coinsurance fees
       b. Specified Low-Income Medicare Beneficiary (SLMB)
          (1) Income cannot be more than 20% above the national poverty level.
          (2) The person must be eligible for Medicare Part A.
          (3) Medicare Part B premiums are paid by the individual.
          (4) Medicare coinsurance or deductibles are not paid.
C. Private health insurance
    1. Medigap
       a. Medicare supplement insurance
       b. Regulated by state and federal law
       c. Ten standard plans
       d. Lifetime maximums established

e. Not government sponsored
f. Policies of choice may be purchased from any insurer providing Medigap policies in the state of residency for a 6-month period from date enrolled in Medicare Part B and for those age 65 years or older.
g. Plans pay all or most medical coinsurance amounts; some policies pay for Medicare deductibles.
h. Medicare Part D, effective January 1, 2006, is optional to assist with medication cost.
    2. Medicare Select
       a. Medigap insurance
       b. Supplements Medicare benefits
       c. Sold by insurance companies and health maintenance organizations (HMOs)
       d. Difference between Medicare Select and Medigap is that specific physicians and certain hospitals must be used for nonemergency care to qualify for full benefits.
       e. Federally approved in all states
       f. Assistance for medications now available

HOUSING

A. U.S. Department of Housing and Urban Development
    1. Rent Supplement Program: rent-subsidized apartments for older adults, disabled individuals, or low-income families
       a. Utility and rent costs in existing buildings
       b. Renovations of existing units
       c. Building of new units
    2. Provides home improvement loans
    3. Provides mortgage insurance
    4. Has age, asset, income eligibility requirements
B. Older adult and handicapped housing (Housing Act of 1959)
    1. Provides funding to private, nonprofit organizations for renovation or building of units for the older adult and handicapped
    2. Provides low-interest federal loans for same
C. National Housing Act (Housing and Urban Development Act, 1968): provides funding to private corporations for construction of low- and middle-income housing
D. National Housing Act of 1952: provides funding to private, profit, or nonprofit groups for nursing home construction or renovation

TITLE XX OF THE SOCIAL SECURITY ACT

A. Federal money for social programs is available and appropriate for the older adult.
B. Program is administered by the state.
C. Individual must be eligible for SSI (supplemental security income).

FOOD STAMP PROGRAM

A. Program is administered by U.S. Department of Agriculture.
B. The recipient must meet income requirements.
C. The welfare department of each state determines eligibility.
D. Components
    1. Home-delivered meals
    2. Grocery store food purchases

ADMINISTRATION ON AGING

A. State, regional, area, and local units: Area units are responsible for providing program coordination and development expertise.

B. Major services
  1. Nutrition programs
     a. On-site meals
     b. Home-delivered meals
  2. Senior centers
     a. Services
     b. Programs
  3. Home care
     a. Homemaker
     b. Home health aide
     c. Home visits
     d. Telephone calls
     e. Chore maintenance
  4. Information and referral
  5. Transportation
     a. Urban Mass Transit Act
     b. Area agencies on aging

LEGISLATION AFFECTING THE OLDER ADULT

A. Social Security: established in 1935. Some legislators predict that benefits may soon be depleted. Timelines vary but, viability of Social Security is being closely monitored.
B. Medicare and Medicaid programs: developed in 1965. Programs have been through many reforms.
C. Older Americans Act: first initiated in 1987 and revised in 1992. It established standards for safeguarding the rights of the older adult.
D. The Omnibus Budget Reconciliation Act (OBRA) of 1990: established to improve the lives of individuals residing in nursing homes. It attached stringent guidelines for the use of physical and chemical restraints and established education and training guidelines for the staffs of long-term care facilities.
E. The Patient Self-Determination Act (PSDA): established in 1991. It was developed in an effort to allow individuals to control end-of-life care.
  1. Living wills: completed while the individual is well and outlines what the individual may or may not want done if unable to make decisions regarding end-of-life care
  2. Health care proxy: The individual designates a person to make end-of-life care decisions for him or her should he or she become incapacitated.

NURSING ROLES AND THE CARE OF THE OLDER ADULT

A. Care provider: Nurses are in the unique position to meet the health care needs of the older adult.
  1. Nursing goals focus on positive outcomes to assist the older adult in attaining and maintaining an optimal state of health.
  2. Nursing care focuses on prevention of acute and chronic health problems, promotion of a healthy lifestyle, and management of the symptoms of chronic health problems.
B. Educator
  1. Nurses educate the older adult concerning health promotion and maintenance of acute and chronic health problems.
  2. Nurses increase public awareness of problems affecting the older adult.
C. Data collection
  1. Nurses must assess the older adult's need for services.
  2. Area agencies on aging are the best resource regarding services for older adults in the community.

Box 9-1 | **Cultural Considerations**

Chinese: Achieving old age is a blessing. The family is expected to take care of the older adult. They use alternative medicine such as herbs, acupressure, and acupuncture and may be hesitant to seek out services for the older adult.

Japanese: Older adults are viewed with respect; close family bonds are established. Many Japanese men wed younger women; the proportion of widows is higher. They may reject modern medicine in favor of traditional practices.

Hispanic: Hispanic individuals are from Spain, Cuba, Mexico, and Puerto Rico. They view illness as an act of God. Old age is viewed as a positive time. Families avoid long-term care, and this ethnic group has the lowest rate of institutionalization.

Native American: Older adults are respected as leaders in the community. Illness and health are viewed as good and evil, and evil actions are punished by illness. Many elders believe that the questions used by nurses are too probing and inappropriate. They are strong believers in traditional herbal medicines.

African American: Many African Americans never reach old age; therefore old age is viewed as a goal. The rate of institutionalization among this ethnic group is low. Older adults look to family members for advice and care before contacting service agencies.

Jewish Americans: Although not actually a particular culture, the Jewish religion dictates the customs and practices of these people. Illness typically draws the family together; and this group, with its normally highly educated members, does not hesitate to seek out modern medicine as needed.

D. Patient advocate
  1. Nurses act as patient advocates to ensure that the rights of the older adult are preserved with regard to health care practices, treatment modalities, and end-of-life care.
  2. The American Nurses Association's Council on Gerontological Nursing has established Nursing Standards of Gerontological Practice.
  3. Nurses recognize the older adult as a unique individual, shaped by life experience, family, society, religion, and culture (Box 9-1).

THEORIES OF AGING

SOCIOLOGICAL THEORIES

A. Disengagement
  1. Controversial
  2. Mutual withdrawal from social interaction by older adult and society
  3. Describes engagement as active occupation and devotion
  4. Supports leisure as a form of activity
  5. Respects individual-initiated withdrawal
B. Activity
  1. Remains active and interacts with society and its events
  2. Pursues new interests, friends, and roles to substitute for lost roles
  3. Supports social activity as beneficial to life satisfaction, morale, and mental health

C. Continuity or development
   1. Lifelong personality characteristics and coping strategies continue.
   2. Sense of inferiority develops when continuity is disrupted.
   3. Supportive network of relationships is established.
D. Passages: Life cycle changes can be identified, predicted, planned for, and managed.

BIOLOGICAL THEORIES

A. Wear and tear
   1. Stress and use deplete the body cells of repair ability. Aging results from accumulated stress and damage, not chronological age.
   2. Coping mechanisms decline because of the decrease in available energy.
B. Collagen
   1. Collagen is the most abundant body protein.
   2. Collagen molecules are held together by bonds.
   3. Chemical reactions cause a switching of bonds between collagen molecules, resulting in structural changes characteristic of the aging process.
C. Lipofuscin accumulation (one type of free radical)
   1. Lipofuscin granules or age pigments are insoluble end products of cell metabolism.
   2. Lipofuscins accumulate in the cell, altering the ability of the cell to function normally.
D. Immunological responses
   1. Aging is an autoimmune disease process.
   2. Cells change, and the body does not recognize its own cells.
   3. Autoimmune responses damage the cells, causing cell death.
E. Cell death of genetic programming
   1. Cell reproduction is programmed; "biological clock" is ticking.

2. Programming determines the rate and time at which a member of a given species ages and dies.
F. Free radical
   1. Molecules that have an extra electron are free radicals.
   2. Free radicals attach to other molecules, altering function or structure, causing damage and aging.
   3. Free radicals come from internal and external sources.
   4. The belief is that the free radicals damage membrane function and structure. Antioxidants such as vitamins A, C, and E; carotenoids; selenium; and phytochemicals are thought to reduce free-radical activity.
G. Mutation and error
   1. Cell division errors occur progressively over time; radiation is cited as a contributing factor.
   2. Mutated cells are altered in their function and effectiveness.
   3. Error theory expands mutation theory to include errors in interpretation of cell messages.

PSYCHOLOGICAL THEORIES

A. Freud: did not recommend psychoanalysis for the older adult population (see Chapter 6)
B. Sullivan: See Chapter 6.
C. Maslow: See Chapter 2.
D. Erikson: See Chapter 6.
   1. Eighth stage (65 to 100 years of age) identified as "integrity versus despair" (Table 9-1)
   2. The older adult who views his or her own life as having no meaning ends the stages of life in despair; the older adult who can review his or her accomplishments and errors derives a sense of integrity.
E. Peck
   1. Expanded Erikson's developmental theory of the eighth stage of humankind
   2. Focuses on alternatives to preoccupation with body changes and illness, thereby achieving life satisfaction (Table 9-1)

Table 9-1	Erikson's Stages of Psychosocial Development in the Adult			
DEVELOPMENTAL STAGE	**AGE**	**CORE TASK AND ASSOCIATED QUALITY**	**DESCRIPTION**	
Young adulthood	18-25 yr	Intimacy and isolation Associated quality: love	If strong sense of identity, is willing and able to unite own identity with another; develops devotion; commits to relationships, career If weak sense of identity, has impersonal, short-term relationships; shows prejudice; becomes socially isolated	
Middle adulthood	25-65 yr	Generativity and stagnation Associated quality: caring	Strives to actualize identity that was formed in earlier stages; generates or produces children, ideas, products, services; is creative, productive, concerned for others; demonstrates caring through parenting, teaching, guiding others; adults who do not care become stagnant, self-indulgent, absorbed in themselves	
Maturity	65 yr-death	Integrity and despair Associated quality: wisdom (to accept one's life and value the contribution that one has made)	Adjusts to changes; senses flow of time—past, present, and future; accepts worth and uniqueness of own life as it was and is; finds order and meaning in own life; despairs when life is viewed as waste; adults who focus on what "might have been" blame others, feel a sense of loss and contempt for others	

From Morrison-Valfre M: *Foundations of mental health care,* ed 5, St Louis, 2013, Mosby.

ROLE CHANGES

A. Types
1. Crisis
   a. Sudden, unplanned, stress producing
   b. No readily available substitute
2. Gradual
   a. Develops slowly
   b. Time available for preparation, which eases transition
   c. Control over whether to develop a substitute
B. Sufficient preparation and adequate support determine adjustment success or failure.
C. Role changes that occur in the life of the older adult are predominantly crisis oriented, both sudden and gradual.
1. Forced retirement
2. Alteration in income
3. Loss of spouse
4. Illness
5. Friends who move away or die
6. Family members who relocate, assume new roles, have increasingly less time for relationships
7. Society's assigned role of decreased psychological and physiological functioning
D. Role losses
1. Work
   a. Income
   b. Job-related companionship
   c. Usefulness, competence, identity
   d. Sense of purpose
   e. Self-esteem
2. Family
   a. May no longer be the decision maker
   b. May not be held in the same esteem
   c. Loss of independence; reversal of roles with children
E. Role gains
1. Grandparenthood or great-grandparenthood
2. Family support roles assumed
   a. Economic
   b. Child care
   c. Caring role in illness
   d. Care of the home
3. Community activities
4. Religious activities
5. Recreational activities
6. Clubs, organizations, and associations
7. Advisory roles
8. New friends
9. Adult education
10. Volunteerism

ALTERATIONS IN LIFESTYLE

EMPLOYMENT

A. Society emphasizes the employed as valuable and the unemployed as useless.
B. The number of older women working has increased.
C. The number of older men working has decreased.
D. Part-time employment is more common.
E. The trend is toward early retirement, although much depends on the state of the economy at any given time.
F. Serial careers are emerging in keeping with interest changes.

G. More women are joining the work force at a time when men are winding down their working lives.
H. The older worker possesses involuntary limitations.
1. Health problems
2. Sensory or perceptual alterations (e.g., in vision and auditory acuity)
3. Decline in physical strength, endurance, and speed
I. Older workers possess innumerable strengths.
1. Reliability
2. Dependability
3. Knowledge
4. Expertise
5. Experience

RETIREMENT

A. Mandatory retirement in federal employment has been eliminated.
B. Mandatory retirement age may be 70 years of age in private employment, depending on occupation.
C. Changes in the economy are leading to forced retirements.
D. More people are taking advantage of early retirement because of incentives by companies to retire older workers either to replace them with younger workers or to simply decrease the overall size of the workforce. Pension plans are changing.
E. Health problems are the primary reason for voluntary retirement.
F. Leisure time is increased.
G. Tremendous anxiety may be created for some older adults.
H. Some older adults derive an initial feeling of relief; however, for most it is a loss that comes at a time of meaningful productivity.
I. Adjustment depends on previously established patterns of adjustment, degree of financial security, state of health, and future outlook.
J. For many older adults, retirement creates an additional series of losses and problems at a time in life when coping and problem-solving abilities are fragile.
K. Job loss
1. Loss of daily routine
   a. Alters household routine
   b. Alters lifestyle
   c. Creates discouragement, depression, and loneliness
   d. Alters family relationships; may increase marital stress
   e. May result in alcohol abuse from drinking as a reaction to a loss
2. Loss of income
   a. Relocation
   b. Daily decision making determined by economics
   c. Decreases self-esteem
   d. Increases fear and anxiety
   e. Increases insecurity
L. Welcome changes can result if retired adult remains socially engaged.
1. New friends
2. New activities
3. New interests and time to devote to established interests
4. Renewal of marriage
5. Seeking new and different employment
6. Finding purpose and opportunity
7. Rest and relaxation

ECONOMIC CHANGES

A. Most older adults live on fixed incomes.
B. Of older adult persons, 1 out of 10 lives below the U.S. poverty level.
C. Independence declines as costs increase and buying power decreases.
D. For many older adults Social Security is the sole source of income.
E. Many older adults are not receiving the assistance to which they are entitled.
 1. Lack of resource knowledge
 2. Inability to find out about resources
  a. Lack of mobility
  b. Health problems
F. SSI: may qualify for this in addition to or instead of Social Security benefits
G. Economic penalties: limit on the amount a Social Security beneficiary can earn annually without losing some monthly payments
H. Income tax reforms (e.g., once-in-a-lifetime capital gains tax exemption on sale of personal residence for person over 55 years of age)
I. Income sources
 1. Public
  a. Social Security—OASDI (Old-Age, Survivors, and Disability Insurance)
  b. SSI (Supplemental Security Income)
 2. Private (e.g., pensions, investments)
 3. Other (e.g., Railroad Retirement System, Federal Employees Retirement System, Civil Service Retirement System)

HEALTH

A. Most older adults have more than one chronic disease.
B. Health care needs increase with age.
C. Cost of health care is increasing as financial income is either decreasing or fixed.
D. Older adults account for one third of U.S. health care costs.

HOUSING

A. Most older adults prefer to remain independent as long as family and friends live nearby.
B. Most older adults live with spouse, alone, or with family.
C. A large percentage of older adults continue to own their home and prefer this lifestyle because it provides:
 1. Security.
 2. Privacy.
 3. Independence.
 4. Sense of purpose.
 5. Familiarity.
 6. Household activities.
 7. Pride.
 8. Socialization.
D. Other housing alternatives
 1. Mobile homes
  a. Convenient
  b. Economical
 2. Retirement communities
  a. Minimum age requirement
  b. Different cost levels (e.g., houses, apartments, and condominiums)
 3. Foster home
 4. Life care facilities: living, recreational, medical facilities on the premises
 5. Nursing homes: Of individuals aged 65 to 85 years, 5% live in nursing homes. After the age of 85 years, 25% live in nursing homes. The typical nursing home resident is a woman over 80 years of age; the terms *extended-care facility* (ECF), *skilled nursing facility* (SNF), and *long-term care facility* (LTCF) may be used interchangeably with the term *nursing home.*
 6. Assisted-living facilities are increasing to meet the needs of older adults with minor-to-moderate health care problems.
 7. House sharing
 8. Public housing
 9. Rooming houses
 10. Hotels: single room occupancy
E. Special assistance needs of older adults enable them to remain in their own homes longer.
 1. Transportation
  a. Reliable
  b. Nearby
  c. Inexpensive
  d. Safe
 2. Meals are available in the event of illness or disability.
 3. Health hotlines: When older adults are institutionalized, it is usually because of health needs and lack of convenient community health services.
 4. Housecleaning services
 5. Homemaker services
 6. Social services
 7. Home care services
 8. Neighborhood safety programs

RECREATION

A. Although older adults have more time for recreation, limiting factors exist.
 1. Cost
  a. Transportation
  b. Special equipment
  c. Special clothing
  d. Fees for membership and use of facilities
 2. Health problems
 3. Diminished energy level
 4. Lack of incentive
 5. Sensory losses
 6. Lack of environmental aids
 7. Lack of conveniently located facilities (e.g., restrooms)
 8. Lack of handicapped facilities
B. Most older adults depend on family as the major source of activity and interaction.
C. Alternatives
 1. Religious activities
 2. Community activities (e.g., volunteerism)
 3. Adult day care
 4. Senior citizen centers
 5. Clubs, organizations, and associations
 6. Recreation centers
 7. Adult education
 8. Shopping
 9. Cultural events
 10. Elder hostel

SOCIAL ISOLATION

A. Four classifications
  1. Attitudinal: isolation that is self-imposed and isolation that is imposed by society
    a. Self-imposed aloneness, loneliness
    b. Society imposes myths about the aged and perceptions of aging.
  2. Presentational: set apart or sets one apart
  3. Behavioral: exhibits behaviors that are not acceptable to a youth-oriented society (e.g., confusion, eccentricity)
  4. Geographical
    a. Lack of resources to relocate
    b. Psychological safety and security at present location
    c. Fear of being victims of crime
    d. Distance from family and friends who have moved away
B. Rural areas have a higher proportion of older adults.

? Critical Thinking Challenge

An 85-year-old woman has recently been diagnosed with atrial fibrillation and has been seeing her physician regularly for the past several months. On a recent follow-up visit to the clinic she tells the nurse that she started taking aspirin on a daily basis because she heard on TV about the many benefits of taking a daily aspirin. Currently she is on a daily regimen of atenolol (a beta-blocker), verapamil (a calcium channel blocker), and warfarin (an anticoagulant). How should the nurse react in response to what the patient has just told her?

SUGGESTION/RECOMMENDATION:

The nurse should see a red flag with this situation and should immediately begin educating the patient about the dangers involved. The patient is already on a controlled dose of an anticoagulant prescribed by her physician. Adding a daily dose of aspirin, also considered a medication with anticoagulant properties, could lead to serious consequences (hemorrhaging) since the anticoagulant effect will undoubtedly be increased. The physician needs to be notified and arrangements made to meet with the physician so appropriate testing can be ordered to determine the patient's clotting time. The nurse should strongly recommend that the patient stop taking the aspirin until she (the patient) discusses the matter with her physician.

MEDICATION USE

A. The largest users of prescription medications are those over 65 years of age.
B. The tendency is to self-medicate; use of over-the-counter remedies, herbal products, and supplements is common.
C. The frequency of hospital admissions that are drug related is higher than that for other age groups.
D. Self-administration errors are common.
E. Absorption of the drug into the system is slower as a result of a decline in gastric acid secretion and decreased gastric motility.
F. Circulatory alterations affect drug distribution to body tissues.
G. Drug metabolism is altered by factors such as a diminished rate of body metabolism and diminished liver function.
H. Drug excretion time is delayed by illness, disease, and the aging process, especially decreased renal blood flow.
I. Management
  1. Patient education
  2. Medication administration times more compatible with lifestyle
  3. Color coding
  4. Larger print on labels
  5. Easily removable bottle and vial caps
  6. Monitoring of drug effectiveness and compatibility
  7. Drug holidays (periods of drug withdrawal to reverse the ineffectiveness of a drug resulting from chronic use).
  8. Daily or weekly medication containers
  9. Cost of medications frequently the reason for noncompliance (i.e., either not taking the medication or not taking it as ordered)

ALCOHOL ABUSE

A. High-risk group for alcoholism
  1. A significant number of alcohol abusers are over 60 years of age.
  2. Adult men have a higher incidence of abuse than do adult women.
  3. Statistics are inaccurate because of protection by family members.
B. Tolerance to alcohol decreases with age because the body systems do not excrete and detoxify as rapidly as those of a younger adult (diminished liver and kidney function).
C. Alcohol is a substitution for unmet psychological needs and untreated physiological problems. Drinking frequently increases after a loss such as the death of a spouse or retirement.
D. Alcohol abuse is the cause of accidents, nutrition deficiencies, drug incompatibilities, self-neglect, alterations in self-esteem, and psychosocial and physiological health care problems.

ELDER ABUSE

A. Physical (Box 9-2)
  1. Battering
  2. Neglect
  3. Sexual abuse
  4. Confinement or restraint
  5. Abandonment

Box 9-2   Signs that May Indicate Elder Abuse

- Demonstrates excessive agreement or compliance with the caregiver
- Shows signs of poor hygiene such as body odor, uncleanness, or soiled clothing or undergarments
- Shows signs of malnutrition or dehydration
- Has evidence of burns or pressure sores
- Shows signs of bruises, particularly clustered on the trunk or upper arms
- Has evidence of bruises in various stages of healing that may indicate repeated injury
- Lacks adequate clothing or footwear
- Has had inadequate medical attention
- Verbalizes lack of food, medication, or care
- Verbalizes being left alone or isolated in some way
- Verbalizes fear of the caregiver
- Verbalizes his or her lack of control in personal activities or finances

Adapted from Wold GH: *Basic geriatric nursing*, ed 5, St Louis, 2012, Mosby.

B. Psychological: threatened or forced
  1. Relinquishment of assets (financial)
  2. Institutionalization
  3. Loss of control over independent functioning
  4. Social isolation
  5. Sensory deprivation
C. Prevention
  1. Acquire knowledge of family abuse and patterns of violence.
  2. Identify predisposing factors.
  3. Incorporate assessment tools into interviewing and counseling strategies; if abuse is suspected, interview alone.
  4. Increase public awareness and education.
  5. Identify actual and potential sources of emergency protection.
  6. Acquire knowledge of community resources.

HEALTHY OLDER ADULT

A. Although older adults are sometimes plagued by chronic health problems, most live in the community.
B. The focus of education for the older adult regarding healthy living includes:
  1. Disease prevention: prevention of acute or chronic health problems.
    a. Self-maintenance: taking responsibility for own health practices.
    b. Maintenance of activity: engaging in moderate physical activity at least three times every week.
    c. Dietary practices: eating a varied diet that includes adequate amounts of carbohydrates, proteins, and fats.
    d. Diagnostic testing: regularly undergoing examinations for the detection and early treatment of disease (mammograms, prostate examination, colorectal screening).
    e. Influenza and pneumonia vaccines: as recommended by a physician.
    f. Management of stress.
  2. Health promotion: maintenance for chronic health problems
    a. Regularly visiting physician for examinations
    b. Engaging in healthy lifestyle practices
    c. Taking prescribed medications

PHYSIOLOGICAL ALTERATIONS (NORMAL AGING PROCESS) AND SELECTED DISORDERS (ABNORMAL)

A. Normal aging changes are gradual and begin in early middle age.
B. Specific changes of aging do not alter the older adult's ability to cope on a day-to-day basis.
C. Because of specific changes of aging, the older adult has a decreased capacity to bounce back from stress or illness, known as a *decreased physiological reserve.*

Integumentary System
A. Alterations
  1. Moisture loss, dryness
  2. Epithelial layer thinning; fragility
  3. Shrinkage and rigidity of elastic collagen fibers: sagging and wrinkling

  4. Decrease of sweat glands in number, activity, and size: less efficient body cooling system
  5. Subcutaneous fat loss, deepening of hollows, and more prominent contours; less efficient in maintaining body temperature
  6. Loss of capillaries and melanocytes: sallow skin
  7. Skin pigmentation increases: keratosis (scaly, raised area), senile lentigo (liver spots—brown or yellow spots).
  8. Changes in hair color (gray, white), changes in texture (becomes fine or coarse), and thinning (balding)
  9. Appearance of facial hair for women; decrease in facial hair for men
B. Factors contributing to problems of the integumentary system
  1. Peripheral circulation diminishes, causing thick brittle nails.
  2. Cardiovascular changes cause decreased healing of wounds.
  3. Immune system decreases ability to overcome disease.
C. Resulting problems
  1. Skin tears
  2. Pressure ulcers, also known as *decubitus ulcers*
D. Nursing management of the dependent older adult
  1. Use extra lotions or creams on dry skin; use less soap.
  2. Handle gently when moving. Position to prevent pressure; reposition every 2 hours.
  3. Use extra care when performing venipunctures.
  4. Assess and document condition of skin. Intervene to prevent the development of pressure ulcers. Document new lesions or changes in existing lesions. Older adults are at risk for basal cell carcinoma.

See Chapter 5 for additional information on integumentary system issues.

Musculoskeletal System
A. Alterations
  1. Loss of lean muscle mass and muscle cells: decreased muscle strength, size, and tone
  2. Loss of elastic fibers in muscle tissue: increased stiffness and decreased flexibility
  3. Thinning of long bones: brittle, porous bones
  4. Thinning of intervertebral disks: height loss and changes in posture
B. Factors contributing to general musculoskeletal problems
  1. Poor nutrition patterns
  2. Endocrine system changes: decreased estrogen and testosterone
  3. Gastrointestinal system changes: decreased absorption of vitamins and minerals
  4. Cardiovascular system changes: poor circulation
  5. Neurological deficits that cause safety hazards
  6. Decreased level of activity and periods of prolonged bed rest
  7. Side effects of medications (e.g., steroids)
C. Resulting problems
  1. Susceptibility to fractures is increased, especially in the postmenopausal woman who develops osteoporosis.
  2. Risk factors for osteoporosis include early menopause; Caucasian or Asian heritage; thin, sedentary lifestyle; cigarette smoking; caffeine usage; and low calcium intake.

3. Altered body image
4. Pain and discomfort
5. Decreased mobility
6. Impaired ability to perform activities of daily living (ADLs)
7. Increasing feelings of dependency
8. Calcium deposits in blood vessels and renal structures
9. Weakened muscles affecting other systems
   a. Diaphragm
   b. Bladder
   c. Myocardium
   d. Abdominal wall
D. Nursing management of the dependent older adult
   1. Handle patient gently.
   2. Reduce environmental safety hazards.
   3. Encourage mobility and exercise; weight-bearing and weight-lifting exercises are effective in reducing the progression of bone and muscle loss.
   4. Allow extra time for performing activities.
   5. Assist with ADLs and exercises as needed.
   6. Provide encouragement and support for accomplishments.
   7. Prevent deformities.
      a. Proper positioning; support for extremities in each position
      b. Range-of-motion (ROM) exercises
   8. Alleviate pain.
      a. Rest periods
      b. Positioning
   9. Encourage liberal fluid intake.
See Chapter 5 for additional information regarding musculoskeletal system issues.

Respiratory System
A. Alterations
   1. Structural alterations (scoliosis, kyphosis, osteoporosis): decrease in lung expansion
   2. Alveoli that enlarge and thin out: decreased oxygen and carbon dioxide diffusion
   3. Loss of bronchiole elasticity: decreased breathing capacity, increased residual air
   4. Diaphragm fibrotic and weakened; diminished efficiency
   5. Respiratory muscle structure and function decreased: diminished strength for breathing and coughing
   6. Changes in larynx: weaker, higher-pitched voice
   7. Decrease in ciliary function: increased susceptibility to upper respiratory tract infection
B. Factors contributing to respiratory problems
   1. Decreased resistance to infection
   2. Musculoskeletal system changes: weakened muscles and postural changes
   3. Long history of smoking and exposure to pollutants
   4. Periods of prolonged bed rest
   5. Cardiovascular system changes
   6. Side effects of medications (e.g., sedatives and hypnotics)
C. Resulting problems
   1. Dyspnea
   2. Chronic cough
   3. Fatigue and debilitation
   4. Cerebral hypoxia
      a. Confusion
      b. Restlessness
      c. Behavioral changes

5. Decreased activity tolerance
6. Cardiovascular problems (e.g., congestive heart failure)
7. Anorexia
D. Nursing management of the dependent older adult
   1. Assist with ADLs as necessary.
   2. Encourage breathing exercises; activities such as singing and those that create laughter are excellent for increasing air exchange.
   3. Administer oxygen therapy as prescribed.
   4. Change position frequently.
   5. Encourage liberal fluid intake.
   6. Discourage smoking.
   7. Position for maximum comfort and efficiency of respiration (e.g., extra pillows, Fowler position).
   8. Allow rest periods.
   9. Assess pulmonary status when assessing behavioral changes.
See Chapter 5 for additional information on respiratory system issues.

Cardiovascular System
A. Alterations
   1. Decrease in enzymatic stimulation: longer and less forceful contractions
   2. Increase in fat and collagen amounts: decline in cardiac output
   3. Increase in oxygen demands of coronary arteries and brain: decreased peripheral circulation
   4. Loss of elasticity of vessel walls; decrease in contraction and recoiling responses; collateral circulation developed by the heart to compensate for coronary artery
   5. Reduced or unaltered heart rate at rest
   6. Mild tachycardia on activity
   7. Slow increase in serum cholesterol
B. Factors contributing to problems of the cardiovascular system
   1. Poor nutrition patterns
   2. Anxiety and stress
   3. Decreased activity level
   4. Arteriosclerosis, hypertension
   5. Pulmonary system changes
   6. Side effects of medications
C. Resulting problems
   1. Fatigue and decreased activity tolerance
   2. Increased anxiety
   3. Edema
   4. Hypertension: increased risk of cerebrovascular accident (CVA)
   5. Behavioral changes
   6. Poor circulation to other systems and extremities: delayed healing, decreased efficiency of kidneys
   7. Potential risk for coronary artery disease, heart failure
D. Nursing management of the dependent older adult
   1. Assist with ADLs as necessary.
   2. Encourage moderate activity and exercise.
   3. Provide patient teaching considerations regarding:
      a. Confusion.
      b. Forgetfulness.
      c. Resistance to change.
   4. Avoid excess pressure on the skin.
   5. Assess cardiovascular status when assessing behavioral changes.
   6. Avoid tight, constrictive clothing and shoes.

7. Provide special foot care.
   a. Prevent trauma.
   b. Prevent infection.

See Chapter 5 for additional information on cardiovascular system issues.

Gastrointestinal System

A. Alterations
   1. Muscle atrophy in the tongue, cheeks, mouth
   2. Esophageal wall thinning, increased incidence of gastroesophageal reflux disease (GERD)
   3. Decrease in ptyalin and amylase secretion by salivary gland: alkaline saliva
   4. Decrease in saliva secretion: thicker mucus and dryness
   5. Oral sensitivity loss, loss of taste discrimination
   6. Ill-fitting dentures, periodontal disease, lack of teeth: nutrition deficiencies
   7. Shrinkage of bony structures of mouth
   8. Shrinkage of gastric mucosa: decline in digestive enzyme secretion leading to delayed digestion
   9. Decrease in lipase secretion: fat intolerance
   10. Decrease in gastric acid: diminished ability to use calcium
   11. Decrease in intrinsic factor: pernicious anemia
   12. Decrease in iron absorption: iron deficiency anemia
   13. Internal sphincter muscle tone loss: alterations in bowel evacuation
B. Factors contributing to problems of the gastrointestinal system
   1. Decreased level of activity
   2. Dental problems
   3. Poor nutrition patterns
   4. Weakened muscles
   5. Nervous system changes
   6. Overuse of laxative and enemas
   7. Anorexia, which may be related to depression
   8. Side effects of medications (e.g., opiates and steroids)
   9. Dehydration
C. Resulting problems
   1. Discomfort (e.g., heartburn and bloating)
   2. Constipation and impaction
   3. Fecal incontinence
   4. Anorexia
   5. Increased risk of aspiration
D. Nursing management of the dependent older adult
   1. Promote nutrition intake.
      a. Consistency of food
      b. Ability to manage utensils
      c. Extra time for feeding (oral and tube)
      d. Smaller, more frequent meals
   2. Provide good oral hygiene.
   3. Encourage mobility and exercise.
   4. Provide adequate fluid intake.
   5. Educate patient regarding constipation and laxative abuse.
   6. Check bowel habits regularly.
   7. Give prompt assistance to bathroom or with bedpan.
   8. Prevent skin and mucosal breakdown.
      a. Prompt, thorough cleansing of anal area
      b. Extra gentleness when inserting rectal and feeding tubes

See Chapter 5 for additional information on gastrointestinal system issues.

Renal System

A. Alterations
   1. Decrease in kidney size
   2. Decline in renal blood flow
   3. Reduced ability of nephron to filter urine: decreased clearance
   4. Reduced ability of tubule cells to selectively secrete and reabsorb: fluid and electrolyte alterations
   5. Decreased bladder capacity: frequency and urgency
   6. Loss of muscle tone of bladder and uterus
   7. Loss of pelvic muscle tone
   8. Decreased urine concentration ability
   9. Prostate gland enlargement
B. Factors contributing to problems of the renal system
   1. Periods of prolonged bed rest
      a. Increased urinary stasis, increased urinary tract infections (UTIs)
      b. Renal calculi formation
   2. Cardiovascular system change (e.g., decreased renal perfusion)
   3. Nervous system changes
   4. Decreased fluid intake
   5. Muscle weakness
   6. Social withdrawal and apathy (e.g., sensory deprivation)
   7. Side effects of medication (e.g., diuretics, antiparkinsonian drugs)
C. Resulting problems
   1. Hyperglycemia
   2. Behavioral changes (e.g., confusion may be caused by electrolyte imbalance or problems with liver or kidney function)
   3. Interference with sleep and recreational patterns
      a. Urinary frequency
      b. Urinary urgency
      c. Nocturia
   4. Increased chance of skin breakdown (e.g., incontinence)
   5. Feelings of embarrassment, rejection, and withdrawal
D. Nursing management of the dependent older adult
   1. Prevent urinary stasis.
      a. Encourage liberal fluid intake.
      b. Encourage frequent change of position.
      c. Encourage ambulation.
   2. Prevent skin breakdown: prompt and thorough cleansing.
   3. Retrain bladder. Scheduling toileting may be helpful. See Chapter 2 for additional measures to assist in meeting elimination needs.
   4. Promptly respond to call for bathroom or bedpan.
   5. Leave night-light on if patient is experiencing nocturia.
   6. Assess renal status when assessing behavioral changes.
   7. Recognize UTI early; first sign may be a change in mental status.
   8. Alter clothing for ease in using toilet.

See Chapter 5 for additional information on renal system issues.

Neurological System

A. Alterations
   1. Decrease in weight and size of brain
   2. Decline in number of neurons
   3. Diminished nerve conduction speed
      a. Voluntary movement slower

b. Decreased reaction time

c. Delayed decisions

4. Alterations in sleep-wake cycle

a. Less rapid eye movement (REM) sleep

b. Less deep sleep: tendency to catnap

c. Easily awakened

d. Difficulty falling asleep

e. Average 5 to 7 hours sleep at night

f. Need less sleep at night but require more rest periods during the day

5. Brain tissue atrophy and meningeal thickening: short-term memory loss

B. Factors contributing to problems of the neurological system

1. Poor nutrition patterns

2. Cardiovascular system changes (e.g., decreased circulation)

3. Pulmonary system changes (e.g., cerebral hypoxia)

4. Sensory deprivation; may be physiological or environmental

5. Side effects of medications (e.g., sedatives)

C. Resulting problems

1. Safety hazards

a. Impaired senses (e.g., vision, hearing, pain, and temperature)

b. Forgetfulness and confusion

2. Anorexia (e.g., decreased number of taste buds, resulting in changes of taste, flavor, and smell)

3. Social isolation and rejection

4. Impaired ability to perform ADLs

a. Decreased coordination

b. Decreased ability to concentrate

c. Safety hazards

5. Increased sense of dependency

6. Incontinence

7. Altered self-image and declining confidence

8. Behavioral changes (e.g., forgetfulness and confusion)

D. Nursing management of the dependent older adult

1. Provide for safety.

2. Establish means of communication if patient has hearing impairment.

3. Assess all systems when assessing behavioral changes, especially with acute changes.

4. Maintain sense of independence when possible.

5. Assist with ADLs only when necessary; allow extra time.

6. Encourage socialization.

7. Provide sensory stimulation.

8. Consider educational level, hearing or visual deficits, forgetfulness, and confusion when teaching.

a. Be consistent.

b. Repeat when necessary.

c. Be patient.

d. Provide positive reinforcement and encouragement.

e. Use diagrams, illustrations, and visual cues to assist memory.

9. Assess other symptoms carefully when assessing for infection and trauma: decreased temperature control and pain perception mask these symptoms.

10. Carefully check temperature of bath water and forms of heat therapy to avoid burns: There is a discrepancy in sensation of heat and cold.

11. Maximize use of environmental aids.

See Chapter 5 for additional information on neurological system issues.

Endocrine System

A. Alterations

1. Decline in growth hormone secretion

2. Diminished estrogen secretion

3. Decreased size of the uterus

4. Decreased size and motility of fallopian tubes

5. Loss of elasticity of vagina

6. Shrinking vulva and external genitalia with loss of subcutaneous fat

7. Diminished vaginal secretions

8. Increased time required to respond to sexual stimulation

9. Reduced elasticity of breast tissue

10. Decreased testosterone secretion

11. Decreased size and firmness of testes

12. Decreased production of sperm

13. Increased time required to achieve an erection; subsides more rapidly

14. Development of drug, sildenafil (Viagra); treats erectile dysfunction in some men; tadalafil (Cialis) also used

15. Shorter and less forceful ejaculation

16. Increasing time between erection and orgasm

17. Decreased basal metabolic rate

18. Diminished glucose metabolism

19. Decreased pancreatic secretions

B. Factors contributing to problems of the endocrine system: related changes in other body systems

C. Resulting problems

1. Adult-onset diabetes mellitus (type 2)

2. Musculoskeletal system changes

3. Hypothyroidism

4. Sexual dysfunction

D. Nursing management of diabetes mellitus: special considerations

1. Poor vision: diabetic retinopathy a common complication

2. Lack of coordination

3. Poor nutrition patterns

4. Forgetfulness and confusion

5. Greater resistance to change

6. Masking of symptoms by physiological changes of aging and disease

7. Insulin requirements increased with decreased activity level, decreased with exercise

8. Stress and anxiety

9. Increased susceptibility to complications, including nephropathy, neuropathy, peripheral vascular disease, coronary artery disease, diabetic foot ulcers

10. Development of complications reduced by proper management of blood sugar

See Chapter 5 for additional information on endocrine system issues.

Immune System

A. Alterations

1. Diminished immune serum globulin production

2. Weakened antibody response

3. Atypical signs and symptoms frequently a response to infection (e.g., subnormal temperature, behavioral changes, and decreased pain sensation)

4. Recommend immunizations for shingles (herpes zoster), pneumonia, booster for tetanus and pertussis. Annual influenza vaccine recommended.

B. Factors contributing to problems in the immune system
   1. Weakened antibody response
   2. Reduced immune serum globulin production
      a. Thymus gland shrinking
      b. Reticuloendothelial system alterations

C. Resulting problems
   1. Self-destructive autoaggressive phenomenon
   2. Increased susceptibility to infection (e.g., occurrence of herpes zoster [shingles], a reactivation of the chickenpox virus along the nerve route, more frequently after the age of 50 years)
   3. Increased susceptibility to disease
   4. Misdiagnosis may lead to incorrect treatment

D. Nursing management of the dependent older adult
   1. Be careful in observation and assessment. Knowing what is normal for each older adult is especially important. Any change is suspect.
   2. Be aware that atypical symptoms of infection are common among older adults; for example, with pneumonia, an early symptom is a change in the level of consciousness rather than the symptoms of productive cough and fever noted in a younger adult.
   3. Use early nursing interventions.
   4. Educate regarding available vaccines. The use of the influenza and pneumococcal vaccines is recommended for the high-risk older adult and all adults residing in group living facilities.

Sense Organs

A. Vision
   1. Alterations
      a. Diminished pupil size: loss of responsiveness to light
      b. Decline in peripheral vision
      c. Decreased accommodation ability, causing presbyopia (farsightedness)
      d. Decreased tear production
      e. Decrease in lens transparency and elasticity
      f. Decline in ability to focus quickly
      g. Decline in color discrimination
      h. Difficulty adjusting to dark-light changes
      i. Altered depth perception
   2. Selected disorders
      a. Cataracts affect 70% of adults over age 75 year. They appear to be related to metabolic changes in the eye and exposure to ultraviolet light and radiation. They can be accelerated by chronic diseases and steroid use. Intake of antioxidants may help reduce their development. Primary symptoms are a gradual loss of vision and seeing halos around objects. Treatment is surgical.
      b. Glaucoma has been described as a thief in the night because symptoms are subtle until vision is lost. Open-angle glaucoma is the most common type. Intraocular pressure is increased, leading to damage of the optic nerve and irreversible blindness. Increased age, family history, African-American or Chinese background, and female gender are risk factors. Intraocular pressure and visual field assessments are the primary monitoring tools. Loss of peripheral vision is the primary symptom. Treatment for glaucoma begins with ophthalmic medications to lower intraocular pressure; if medications are unsuccessful, surgical intervention may be an option.
      c. Senile macular degeneration is the leading cause of blindness in older adults. The retina and the layers below the retina are affected, leading to a loss of central vision. Tasks requiring close focus become difficult, and objects—especially lines—may appear wavy and distorted. Treatment options are limited; laser surgery may reduce the amount of distortion.

B. Auditory alterations
   1. Progressive loss of hearing, starting with high-frequency tones
      a. Presbycusis (loss of sound perception): a type of sensorineural hearing loss. The primary cause is aging.
      b. Otosclerosis (bone cell overgrowth): a form of conductive hearing loss that results from the reduction in sound passage to the cochlea
      c. Cerumen accumulation is a cause of conductive hearing loss. Older adults are at risk for cerumen impaction because of the thicker cerumen produced by the aging glands. The use of hearing aids is an additional factor for cerumen impaction. Cerumen buildup can be viewed with an otoscope. The older adult may experience dizziness, pain, pruritus, pressure in the ear, and a decrease in hearing.
   2. Thickened and more opaque eardrum

C. Taste bud alterations
   1. Declining number of taste buds
   2. Declining taste sensation
   3. Taste buds possibly affected by medication side effects
   4. Declining taste bud function can cause oversweetening or oversalting of foods.

D. Olfactory alterations
   1. Decrease in olfactory nerve fibers
   2. Diminished sense of smell
   3. Decreased olfactory and taste sensations can affect appetite.
   4. Decreased olfactory sensation can cause an inability to smell smoke fumes or spoiled food.

E. Tactile alterations
   1. Dulled sense of touch
   2. Higher pain threshold
   3. Diminished sense of vibration
   4. Declining heat or cold discrimination
   5. Decreased tactile sensation can increase the risk of injury.

F. Vestibular or kinesthetic alterations
   1. Diminished proprioception
   2. Decrease in coordination
   3. Decline in equilibrium
   See Chapter 5 for additional information on sensory issues.

SPECIAL CONSIDERATIONS

NUTRITION

A. Diet
   1. Nutrition needs of older adults are the same as those of other adults.
   2. The need for calories decreases.
   3. Older adults need adequate protein to prevent muscle wasting and weakness.

4. They need adequate fats for padding, insulation, and energy. Low saturated fat intake is recommended by physicians. Low trans fat ingestion is important.
5. They need adequate carbohydrates from unprocessed foods for energy. The tendency is to buy high-carbohydrate, empty-calorie foods because they:
   a. Are less costly.
   b. Are filling.
   c. Are easy to chew.
   d. Require minimal preparation and no refrigeration.
6. Ethnic, cultural, and lifestyle preferences should be encouraged for identity reinforcement and appetite stimulation.
7. Fluid intake should be 1500 to 2000 mL/day. The tendency is to reduce intake because of urinary frequency, urgency, and incontinence.
8. Older adults may need vitamin supplements to prevent deficiencies. Women should continue with increased intake of calcium supplements with vitamin D.
9. Lactose deficiency is common. Calcium can be obtained from other sources (e.g., spinach, asparagus, broccoli, and sardines).
10. Older adults need fiber, roughage, and bulk to aid elimination.
11. Consistency and preparation are dictated by chewing, swallowing, and digestive abilities.
12. Small, frequent meals are easier to digest and conserve energy.
13. Older adults need to pay attention to cholesterol and fat intakes.
14. They need to be aware of food-drug and food-food interactions (e.g., warfarin [Coumadin] and foods high in vitamin K; antibiotics and antacids; levodopa and vitamin B_6; monoamine oxidase inhibitors [MAOIs] and aged cheese and certain alcoholic drinks).

B. Provide unhurried atmosphere to increase appetite and incentive to eat.
C. Caution against food fads and megavitamin therapy.
D. Assess facilities for appropriateness.
   1. Storage
   2. Cooking
   3. Refrigeration
E. Encourage financial assistance and planning.
F. Arrange for transportation to and from grocery store.
G. Provide assistance with packages because of weakness and physical disabilities or limitations.
H. Provide mealtime socialization.
I. Provide assistance for the confused, forgetful, and ill person.
J. Encourage regular meals; older adults have a tendency to skip meals.
K. Provide education classes on purchasing healthful foods on limited income.
L. Identify factors that increase risk of nutrition problems in the older adult (Box 9-3).
M. Refer to community agencies for food stamps, senior center meals, Meals on Wheels, or other community assistance.

Box 9-3   **The Nutrition Checklist**

The Nutrition Checklist is based on the following warning signs. Use the word *DETERMINE* to remind you of the warning signs.

DISEASE
Any disease, illness, or chronic condition that causes you to change the way you eat, or makes it hard for you to eat, puts your nutritional health at risk. Four in five adults have chronic diseases that are affected by diet. Confusion or memory loss that keeps getting worse is estimated to affect at least one in five older adults. This can make it hard to remember what, when, or if you've eaten. Feeling sad or depressed, which happens to about one in eight older adults, can cause big changes in appetite, digestion, energy level, weight, and well-being.

EATING POORLY
Eating too little and eating too much both lead to poor health. Eating the same foods day after day or not eating fruit, vegetables, and milk products daily will also cause poor nutritional health. One in five adults skip meals daily. Only 13% of adults eat the minimum amount of fruit and vegetables needed. One in four older adults drink too much alcohol. Many health problems become worse if you drink more than one or two alcoholic beverages per day.

TOOTH LOSS OR MOUTH PAIN
A healthy mouth, teeth, and gums are needed to eat. Missing, loose, or rotten teeth or dentures that do not fit well or cause mouth sores make it hard to eat.

ECONOMIC HARDSHIP
As many as 40% of older Americans have incomes of less than $6000 per year. Having less—or choosing to spend less—than $25 to $30 per week for food makes it very hard to get the foods you need to stay healthy.

REDUCED SOCIAL CONTACT
One third of all older people live alone. Being with people daily has a positive effect on morale, well-being, and eating.

MULTIPLE MEDICINES
Many older Americans must take medicines for health problems. Almost half of older Americans take multiple medicines daily. Growing old may change the way we respond to drugs. The more medicines you take, the greater the chance for side effects such as increased or decreased appetite, change in taste, constipation, weakness, drowsiness, diarrhea, nausea, and others. Vitamins or minerals, when taken in large doses, act like drugs and can cause harm. Alert your doctor to everything you take.

INVOLUNTARY WEIGHT LOSS OR GAIN
Losing or gaining a lot of weight when you are not trying to do so is an important warning sign that must not be ignored. Being overweight or underweight also increases your chance of poor health.

NEEDS ASSISTANCE IN SELF-CARE
Although most older people are able to eat, one in every five has trouble walking, shopping, and buying and cooking food, especially as age increases.

ELDER YEARS ABOVE AGE 80
Most older people lead full and productive lives. But as age increases, risk of frailty and health problems increase. Checking your nutritional health regularly makes good sense.

From Bagley B: Nutrition and health, *Am Fam Physician* 57:934, 1998.

HYGIENE

A. Skin
1. Water temperature 100° to 105° F (37.7° to 40.5° C)
2. Daily baths not necessary
3. Oil-based or emollient lotion. Safety is a priority if oil is added to bath water.
4. Alcohol and dusting powder not appropriate because they dry out the skin (dusting powder can be inhaled)
5. Avoidance of friction
6. Avoidance of pressure
7. Neutral-reaction or oil-based soap
8. Susceptible to bruising and skin tears

B. Nose: blunt-end scissors to trim nasal hairs that extend beyond nares

C. Oral hygiene
1. Dentures
   a. Remove dentures at night and reinsert the next morning to prevent tissue swelling unless contraindicated by dentist.
   b. Provide frequent cleaning.
   c. Encourage proper storage.
   d. If patient is institutionalized, make sure that dentures are labeled.
2. Use soft nylon toothbrush, electric toothbrush, or adaptive toothbrush.
3. Mouthwash is optional.
4. Apply lanolin to lips.
5. Schedule semiannual dental visits.
6. Inspect mouth frequently for food accumulation, injury, disease, and infection (tendency to cheek or pouch food can lead to infection).

D. Ears
1. Clean with warm, soapy water and dry with towel.
2. Do not use cotton swabs because they force cerumen back against the tympanum.
3. Trim ear hair growth in men.
4. Provide hearing aid maintenance.
   a. Wash mold and receiver with mild soap and warm water.
   b. Check cannula for patency and clean and dry with pipe cleaner.
   c. Remove batteries when aid is not in use.
   d. Store traditional batteries in refrigerator to retain freshness; new lithium batteries should be stored at room temperature.
   e. Turn aid to "off" position when inserting in patient's ear.
   f. Turn aid "on" to adjust volume.
   g. Store aid in its original box away from cold, heat, and sunlight.
   h. Be familiar with components, styles, nursing care (Box 9-4).

E. Eyes
1. Decreased tear production may necessitate use of artificial tears.
2. Provide eyeglass care. Use lint-free cotton towel to dry. Tissues and paper towels are wood products and may scratch protective coatings.
   a. More frequent cleaning of eyeglasses is required.
   b. Use warm water to clean eyeglasses.
   c. Store only in eyeglass case.
   d. If patient is institutionalized, make sure that glasses are labeled.

Box **9-4**	Hearing Aids

- Hearing aids require care and maintenance.
- Clean the ear mold regularly and carefully with a damp cloth.
- Check for cracks or rough edges.
- Batteries should be checked and changed regularly. Without a good power source, the hearing aid will not function properly. To save battery life the hearing aid should be turned off when not in use.
- If hearing aid does not seem to be working, check the batteries, check the connection between aid parts, and clean cerumen from the ear mold.
- Reassure patients that adjustment to a hearing aid takes time.

Modified from Wold G: *Basic geriatric nursing*, ed 5, St Louis, 2012, Mosby.

F. Nails
1. Provide daily care.
2. Use moisturizer on nails and cuticles.
3. Encourage circulation with buffing of nails.
4. File with emery board (cutting makes them more brittle and risks injury).

G. Hair
1. Use mild shampoo that is not irritating to the eyes.
2. Remove facial hair from women with tweezers or waxing as requested.
3. Use of a shaving brush is recommended for men.
4. Moisturizers are beneficial for men's facial hair.

H. Feet: The older adult is often unable to care for the feet adequately because of limitation of movement or visual difficulties.
1. Give daily care (washing, inspection, skin care).
2. Inspect between and under toes for abrasions, cracking, lacerations, and scaling.
3. Clip toenails straight across.
4. Pumice stone should be used to remove dry, hard skin.
5. Discourage use of irritants.
6. Avoid elastic-top socks or knee-high stockings that put pressure on popliteal space.
7. Recommend properly fitting shoes with low, broad, rubber heels for safety, comfort, and fatigue reduction.
8. Persons with diabetes need especially attentive assessment of feet. A person with newly diagnosed diabetes should be evaluated initially by a podiatrist and as necessary thereafter.

SAFETY

A. Susceptibility to accidents is increased by:
1. Decline in sensory acuity.
2. Decreased ability to interpret environment.
3. Increased reflex time.
4. Postural change sensitivity.
5. Gait disturbances.
6. Muscular weakness.
7. Urinary urgency and frequency.
8. Confusion.
9. Judgment alterations.
10. Forgetfulness.
11. Proprioceptive inadequacies.
12. Improper footwear.

13. Depression.
14. Environmental hazards.
15. Medications that cause drowsiness.
B. Accident prevention
   1. Attire
      a. Provide short or three-quarter-length sleeves rather than long, loose-fitting sleeves.
      b. Avoid long garments.
      c. Provide fastening-tape (Velcro) closures.
      d. Provide properly fitted shoes with rubber, nonslip soles.
   2. Furniture
      a. Proper height
      b. Chairs with arms
   3. Floors
      a. No-slip wax
      b. No scatter rugs or deep-pile carpeting
      c. No clutter
      d. Rubber tips on ambulation aids
   4. Kitchen
      a. Tong reachers should be used instead of climbing on footstools, chairs, and stepladders.
      b. Temperature-controlled faucets
      c. Electric rather than gas stoves
      d. Stoves with controls on the front
      e. Shelves within comfortable reach
      f. Wall cabinets at comfortable height instead of floor-based cabinets to avoid bending and stooping
      g. No accumulation of trash
      h. Easy-grip utensils; ergonomic handles
   5. Bathroom
      a. Nonskid strips or rubber mats in tub and shower
      b. Temperature-controlled faucets
      c. Convenient soap containers
      d. Tub and toilet handrails
      e. Bathtub seats
      f. Shower chairs
      g. Chair-height toilet seats
      h. Colored toilet seats
      i. Night-light
   6. Bedroom
      a. Bedside commode
      b. Side rails
         c. Night-light
         d. Telephone next to bed (amplifier; dial enlarger; lighted)
   7. General
      a. Proper lighting
      b. Railings on stairways
      c. Safe electric appliances
      d. No overloading of electric outlets
      e. No frayed wiring or extension cords
      f. Securely taped cords
      g. Emergency telephone numbers readily available at telephone
      h. Smoke detectors; carbon monoxide detectors
      i. Crime-prevention assessment and implementation
      j. Medications
         (1) Separated from those of other household members
         (2) Internal and external medications in different locations
         (3) Large-print labels
         (4) Color-coded labels
         (5) Daily supply containers
         (6) Calendar or alarm clock reminders
         (7) Outdated medications and prescriptions discarded
      k. Medical emergency alarm system
   8. Mobility aids (Table 9-2)

VISION

A. Bright, diffused light is best.
B. Place items on better-vision side.
C. Avoid glare.
D. Strips on stairs improve depth perception.
E. Eyeglasses should be kept clean (older adults frequently forget or ignore this).
F. Use bright colors that increase visual acuity (e.g., red, orange, and yellow).
G. Avoid night driving.
H. Use resources and aids for visually handicapped persons.
I. Preserve independence.
J. Visual losses increase susceptibility to delusions, disorientation, confusion, isolation.
K. Place objects directly in front of individual with decreased peripheral vision.
L. Stimulate other senses.

Table 9-2	Mobility Aids		
AID	**CHARACTERISTICS**	**FIT**	**USE**
Cane	Most commonly used canes are standard (one point) and quad (four point). A quad cane stands by itself.	Hand grip is at hip level, and the person's elbow is bent at a 15- to 30-degree angle when he or she places weight on the cane.	Use cane on unaffected side. Intact rubber tip is important.
Walker	Rectangular tubular metal frames are at least waist high and open on one side. There are hand grips on the crossbars. They may have rubber-capped tips or wheels.	Height is correct if elbow is bent at a 15- to 30-degree angle while the user is standing upright and grasping the hand grips. Individual must have use of both hands and arms and at least one leg. Generalized weakness may still allow person to use a walker effectively.	It was frequently the first aid used when training an individual to walk after a loss of function. It is helpful for individuals who are weak or tend to lose their balance because it offers a wide base of support.

Continued

Table 9-2	Mobility Aids—cont'd		
AID	**CHARACTERISTICS**	**FIT**	**USE**
Wheelchair	It is used when individuals are not able to ambulate independently or with other aids such as crutches, canes, or walkers.	It is individually fitted based on height, weight, limb use, arm strength, and ability to move the wheelchair.	Environment may need to be adapted for wheelchair use: doorways may need to be widened, access to toilet changed, furniture rearranged to avoid use of stairs. Throw rugs should be eliminated. Mirrors, sinks, appliances may need to be lowered or adapted. Ramps are necessary to enter buildings. Special pads and cushions can reduce pressure areas; reposition frequently.
Crutches	Use of crutches may follow the use of a walker or be the first aid to ambulation Crutches are frequently difficult for older person to use because of inadequate upper body strength, arthritis, and balance problems. They are not as stable as other mobility aids.	They are individually sized for padded axillary bar to be 1½ to 2 inches below the axilla. Elbow should be flexed 15 to 20 degrees when palms are resting on hand grips. Resting the body's weight on the axillary bar puts pressure on vital nerves and can occlude blood vessels in the axilla, causing temporary or permanent damage, including paralysis.	Use of crutches for walking is usually taught by a physical therapist. The hands, not the axillae, support the weight of the body. Good posture is important, with the head held up and the eyes looking ahead as in normal walking. For safety, eliminate obstacles such as the following: • Waxed floors • Throw rugs • Extension cords • Uneven surfaces • Clutter

Modified from deWit S: *Fundamental concepts and skills for nursing,* ed 3, St Louis, 2009, Saunders.

HEARING

A. Older adults usually do poorly on hearing tests because of cautious responsiveness (fear need for a hearing aid).
B. Reduce distractions.
C. Do not tire them with unnecessary noise and talk.
D. Speak in a normal tone of voice; shouting is misinterpreted by persons who have normal hearing.
E. Observe for signs of developing hearing loss.
   1. Leaning forward
   2. Inappropriate responses
   3. Cupping ear when listening
   4. Loud speaking voice
   5. Requests to repeat what has been said
F. Reduce background noise (e.g., television and radio) before speaking.
G. Hearing deficits increase social isolation, suspiciousness, and fears.
H. Speak toward the better ear.
I. Be sure to have the person's attention before speaking.
J. Use resources and aids for the hearing-impaired population (e.g., television and telephone amplifiers, sound lamps, and alarm clocks that shake the bed).
K. Keep hands and objects away from mouth when speaking.

ACTIVITIES OF DAILY LIVING

A. Older adults may ignore appearance because of fatigue, unawareness, or lack of incentive.
B. Clean clothing is essential for maintaining pride and dignity.
C. Choosing what to wear provides a source of control over one's life, fosters independence, and increases self-confidence and self-esteem.
D. Lifelong habits of sleeping attire or lack of attire should be encouraged to be maintained.
   1. Reinforces individuality
   2. Reduces sleep interference
E. Standard clothing sizes no longer fit; loose-fitting, comfortable clothing should be encouraged.
F. Front closures are more easily managed.
G. Cotton socks absorb perspiration.
H. Zippers, fastening tape (Velcro), and large buttons make dressing easier.
I. Layering and sweat suits provide warmth in cold weather.
J. Daily exercise should be encouraged and paced.
K. Increase self-awareness with mirrors.
L. Use ADL resources and aids.
   1. Zipper aids
   2. Extra-long shoehorns
   3. Shoelace tiers, Velcro fasteners
   4. Adaptive utensils
M. Encourage functional independence: ability to perform ADLs and instrumental activities of daily living (IADLs). Examples of IADLs include shopping, using the telephone, paying bills, obtaining meals, and obtaining transportation.

SEXUALITY

A. Cultural stereotypes deny freedom of sexual expression for the older adult.
B. Lifelong sexual adjustment determines how the older adult deals with sexual needs.
C. Partner availability is made difficult.
   1. Older adult women outnumber men.
   2. Social and business roles change.

Encouraging Intimacy in the Older Adult

- Educate others, including family members, concerning need for intimacy in old age.
- If sexual intimacy is not possible, promote expression of intimacy in other ways (hugging, cuddling, spending time together).
- Avoid belittling the older person's desire for intimacy.
- Provide education for the older adult concerning intimacy, because it is not always comfortable for him or her to inquire about this subject.
- Older adults may need detailed instruction after life-altering events such as myocardial infarction, cerebrovascular accident, or other acute or chronic illness.

D. Physiological alterations affect self-image and foster nonparticipation.
E. Families of older adults tend to discourage sexual relationships because of stereotypes and inheritance threats.
F. Sexual focus shifts to companionship.
G. Older persons continue to enjoy sexual activity. Decrease is primarily a result of declining health or lack of available partner (Box 9-5).

SPEECH

A. Older adults tend to rely more on the words of caregivers than on actions, but at times it may be a combination of both.
B. Speak slowly and clearly.
C. Allow sufficient time for comprehension and response.
D. Speak directly to the adult; treat him or her as an individual.
E. Explanations reduce fear.
F. Recovery of speech is influenced by multiple impairments and dependency.

NEUROLOGICAL SYSTEM (SELECTED DISORDERS)

ORGANIC MENTAL SYNDROMES (ALZHEIMER DISEASE AND OTHERS)

A. Onset may be rapid or progressive.
B. Cognitive function alterations
   1. Judgment
   2. Memory
   3. Intellect
   4. Orientation
   5. Affect
C. Associated factors (Figure 9-1)
D. Cognitive dysfunction dementia

DEMENTIA

A. Alzheimer disease: Progressive, deteriorating, chronic dementia is the most common form of dementia. Incidence increases with age. Cause is unknown, but theories include genetic, chemical, environmental, and viral factors; family history and the presence of the apolipoprotein E gene appear to indicate increased risk.
   1. Types
      a. Senile dementia—Alzheimer type (SDAT): onset over age 65 years
      b. Presenile dementia: onset between ages 40 and 60 years
   2. Cerebral pathophysiology
      a. Senile plaques
      b. Neurofibrillary tangles
      c. Neurotransmitter abnormalities
      d. Atrophy
   3. Diagnosis confirmed only on autopsy
   4. Assessment: Mini-Mental State Examination (MMSE) is used as assessment tool; scores below 24 generally indicate dementia.
      a. Personality changes
      b. Memory changes

Delirium
- Acute onset
- Causes: metabolic disorders, diseases: infections, fever, dehydration, pain, drug reactions, lack of oxygen to the brain
- Reversible if treated early

Damage
- Acute onset
- Causes: stroke, head injury, disease, exposure to chemicals
- Sometimes reversible

Dementia
- Slow onset
- Causes: cardiovascular disease, HIV, metabolic problems, Alzheimer disease; more than 60 causes
- Usually not reversible

Depression
- Causes: loss, drugs, inner sadness, metabolic imbalances
- Subacute onset
- Usually reversible

Deprivation
- Variable onset
- Causes: sensory impairments, poor hearing, poor vision, loss of touch, lack of social interaction
- Sometimes reversible

FIGURE 9-1 The five "Ds" of confusion. *HIV,* Human immunodeficiency virus. (From Morrison-Valfre M: *Foundations of mental health care,* ed 5, St Louis, 2013, Mosby.)

c. Aphasia (language difficulties), apraxia (impaired ability to perform purposeful tasks), and agnosia (impaired ability to recognize persons or objects)

d. Behavioral changes; subtle behavioral changes possibly the first sign

e. Impaired cognition

f. Late-stage physical alterations affecting mobility and swallowing

5. Nursing interventions and management
   a. Support independence with ADLs: do not rush; focus on one task at a time.
   b. Provide structured, consistent environment.
   c. Facilitate sleep-activity balance. Plan quiet, non-stimulating events in the evening.
   d. Promote bowel and bladder continence. Toilet every 2 hours, reduce fluid intake after evening meal, and encourage fluids before noon.
   e. Provide reality orientation, remotivation, and reminiscence.
   f. Provide patient safety. Reduce environmental dangers. Use visual barriers such as half doors, red lines, stop signs. Manipulate environment to help control behavior.
      (1) At risk for wandering
      (2) Becomes lost easily
      (3) Fails to recognize environmental hazards
   g. Encourage socialization because withdrawal and social isolation are common.
   h. Reduce anxiety-provoking situations: do not argue or try to reason.
   i. Provide nutrition needs; high-calorie, easily managed finger food can be offered to the wandering, restless patient.
   j. Recognize self-concept needs.
   k. Encourage verbal communications; use validation techniques to focus.
   l. Monitor effectiveness of medications; cholinesterase inhibitors such as tacrine (Cognex), donepezil (Aricept), and rivastigmine (Exelon) slow the progression of symptoms of Alzheimer disease.

B. Multi-infarct dementia: Cognitive impairment caused by cerebrovascular disease is the second leading cause of dementia in older adults. Often a history of transient ischemic attacks (TIAs) and hypertension symptoms are similar to Alzheimer disease, but onset is more abrupt. Changes in functioning fluctuate rather than progressing slowly as in Alzheimer disease. Treatment is aimed at the vascular cause.

C. Psychoactive substance-induced mental disorders: These are chemically induced organic disorders, frequently accompanied by delirium. In many cases delirium can be reversed.

PARKINSONIAN SYNDROME

Parkinsonian syndrome is a progressive, degenerative neurological movement disorder.

A. Primary
   1. Parkinson disease
   2. Paralysis agitans

B. Secondary
   1. Tumors
   2. Drugs
   3. Infection, especially UTIs and upper respiratory infections (URIs)

C. Assessment
   1. Slowness of movement
   2. Waxlike rigidity of extremities
   3. Facial masking
   4. Tremors while at rest; characteristic pill-rolling motion
   5. Muscular weakness
   6. Shuffling gait
   7. Stature alterations
   8. Drooling; swallowing difficulties
   9. Cognitive impairment
   10. Mood swings

D. Nursing interventions and management
   1. Foster independence with ADLs.
   2. Maintain physical mobility.
   3. Provide adequate nutrition.
      a. Keep swallowing difficulties in mind.
      b. Person may require suction and is prone to aspiration.
      c. Monitor weight weekly.
      d. Provide adaptive eating devices.
      e. Provide thickened liquids to assist in swallowing.
   4. Prevent constipation.
   5. Provide good skin care.
   6. Encourage communication.
      a. Be attentive; speech is soft and low pitched.
      b. Allow time; speech is slow and monotonous.
   7. Enhance self-concept.
      a. Focus on patient's strengths.
      b. Encourage activities that foster success.
      c. Give positive feedback.
      d. Establish realistic goals.
      e. Encourage verbalization of feelings.
      f. Maintain intellectual activity stimulation.
   8. Monitor effectiveness of medications in controlling tremors and rigidity and alleviating characteristic depression.
      a. Tricyclic antidepressants, MAOIs
      b. Antihistamines
      c. Anticholinergics
      d. Levodopa (eliminate vitamin B_6 from diet)
      e. Catechol-O-methyltransferase (e.g., tolcapone inhibitors)
      f. Nonergot dopamine agonists
   9. Provide safety.
   10. Decrease stress.

See Chapter 5 for additional information on parkinsonian syndrome. See Chapter 2 for information regarding living wills and legal issues, end-of-life care, and hospice.

PSYCHOLOGICAL CHANGES (NORMAL AGING PROCESS)

SELF-IMAGE

A. Physiological alterations
B. Youth-oriented society
C. Retirement
D. Income alterations
E. Role changes
F. Sexual expression alterations

INTELLIGENCE

A. Verbal ability and retained information remain unchanged.
B. Abstract thinking and performance response decline.

C. Performance of activities involving neuromuscular learning declines.

D. Attention span shortens.

E. Literal approach to problem solving affects ability.

F. Fluid intelligence declines after adolescence.

G. Crystallized intelligence continues to increase throughout life.

H. Learning capacity continues.

MEMORY

A. Short term: Concentration and retention decline.

B. Long term: Minimal impairment occurs.

C. Remote
1. Remote memory is better than short-term memory.
2. Remote memory is involved in reminiscence.

MOTIVATION—A HIGHLY INDIVIDUAL RESPONSE TO AGING

A. Less likely to take risks with decision making; not risk takers

B. Do not actively seek change

C. May have a fear of failure

D. Self-fulfilling prophecies

E. Decline of competitiveness

F. Decline of energy levels

ATTITUDES, BELIEFS, INTERESTS

A. General attitude realignment

B. Either narrow or expanded interests

C. Generally tend to keep lifelong beliefs amid rapidly changing society

PERSONALITY

A. Personality is basically unchanged.

B. Some exaggeration of behavioral responses may be evident.

C. Adaptive capacities may be diminished.

D. The ability to handle physiological and psychological stress is reduced.

PSYCHOLOGICAL DISORDERS (ABNORMAL)

DEPRESSION

A. Reaction to loss of:
1. Independence
2. Status
3. Spouse, relatives, friends
4. Possessions
5. Income
6. Mobility

B. Many commonly prescribed medications can cause depression (e.g., digitalis, propranolol [Inderal], beta-adrenergic blockers such as atenolol, levodopa, oxycodone [OxyContin], zolpidem [Ambien]).

C. Physical illness and changes can be intensified by existing depression or can be a contributing factor to depression or both.
1. Lowered self-esteem
2. Self-concept alterations
3. Feelings of hopelessness and worthlessness

D. Types
1. Exogenous

a. Referred to as *neurotic;* external; caused by outside events

b. Common in the older adult

c. Usually a reaction to losses

2. Endogenous

a. Referred to as *psychotic;* caused by internal events

b. Characterized by:
(1) Guilt
(2) Reduced self-esteem
(3) Early-morning awakening
(4) Slowing of thought, verbalization, and level of activity

c. Classifications
(1) Unipolar: life history of depression
(2) Bipolar: manic-depressive psychosis
(a) Mood swings from depression to euphoria
(b) May have hallucinations and delusions

E. Symptoms of depression (Box 9-6)

F. Nursing interventions
1. Encourage self-expression; increase self-esteem.
2. Improve appearance.
3. Provide structure and routine.
4. Assist with maintaining or regaining control.
5. Have kind, understanding attitude.
6. Provide physical care as needed. Encourage independence.
7. Provide safety and security.
8. Reduce environmental stimuli and stress.
9. Continuously test reality perception.
10. Ascertain emotional support network.

Box 9-6 Signs and Symptoms of Depression in Older Adults

PHYSICAL
Muscle aches
Abdominal pain, nausea or vomiting
Dry mouth
Headache

COGNITIVE (INTELLECTUAL)
Decreased or slowed memory
Slowing intellectual functions
Agitation
Paranoia
Focus on the past
Thoughts of death and suicide

EMOTIONAL
Fatigue
Lack of interest
Increased anxiety or dependence
Inability to experience pleasure or laughter
Feelings of uselessness, hopelessness, helplessness

BEHAVIORAL
Activities of daily living become difficult
Changes in appetite
Changes in sleeping patterns
Lowered energy levels
Poor grooming
Withdrawal from people and activities

From Morrison-Valfre M: *Foundations of mental health care,* ed 5, St Louis, 2013, Mosby.

11. Prevent isolation and avoidance.
12. Realize that potential for suicide exists.
    a. Suicide is an act that may stem from depression.
    b. Approximately 25% of suicides occur in persons over age 65 years.
    c. Caucasian men over age 75 years have the highest rate of suicide.
    d. Refer to Chapter 6 for suicidal risk assessment, crisis intervention, and nursing interventions.
13. Teach about medications and evaluate understanding.

AGGRESSIVE BEHAVIOR

A. Abnormal anger, rage, or hostility, which if turned inward would lead to depression and if turned outward would lead to aggressiveness
B. Response to:
   1. Anxiety
   2. Stress
   3. Guilt
   4. Insecurity
   5. Loss of self-esteem
   6. Loss of control of destiny
   7. Forced dependency
C. Clinical manifestations
   1. Lack of cooperation
   2. Irritability
   3. Demanding
   4. Hostility
   5. Demonstration of coping mechanisms characteristically used to decrease stress (e.g., rationalization and repression)
   6. Altered interpersonal relationships
   7. Altered reality testing
D. Nursing interventions
   1. Reduce stress source and sensory overload.
   2. Encourage verbalization.
   3. Set realistic, reachable goals.
   4. Respond to questions directly and briefly.
   5. Allow ample time for task completion.
   6. Meet physical needs as necessary. Determine if acute behavioral changes are a result of illness.
   7. Encourage environmental participation and activity involvement.
   8. Positively recognize attainments.
   9. Set limits on activities.
   10. Anticipate hostile, demanding behavior.
   11. Allow only the degree of independence that can be handled successfully.
   12. Avoid responses and action that might lead to guilt, feelings of rejection, bother, or dislike.
   13. Increase feeling of self-worth.
   14. Administer medication.
   15. Provide therapy if indicated.

REGRESSION

The display of regressive behavior, an ego defense mechanism, is not an uncommon response in the older adult to external stressors. This return to an earlier behavioral stage (e.g., temper tantrums, rocking, incontinence) requires prevention, early detection, and prompt intervention (remove the source of stress and reverse the behavior).

PARANOID BEHAVIOR

A. Inappropriate attempt to cope with stress
B. Response to:
   1. Physical impairments
   2. Sensory deprivation
   3. Loss
   4. Loneliness
   5. Medications
   6. Environmental changes
   7. Isolation
   8. Vision alterations
   9. Auditory alterations
C. Clinical manifestations
   1. Secretiveness
   2. Mistrust
   3. Mood disturbances
   4. Oversensitivity
   5. Insecurity
   6. Superiority attitude
   7. Alterations in behavior
   8. Delusions
   9. Withdrawal
   10. Fearfulness
   11. Aloofness
   12. Refusal to take medications, eat, or carry out normal self-care activities
D. Nursing interventions
   1. Attempt to allay anxiety.
   2. Allow patient to refuse treatments.
   3. Do not argue with patient.
   4. Try not to take patient's anger personally.
   5. Administer medication.
   6. Do not make promises to patient.
   7. Look for alterations in ADLs as cues to whether the patient's verbalizations are of real concern or are for attention.
   8. Be aware of events precipitated by environment.
   9. Use stress-management techniques.
   10. Point out patient-predicted events that do not occur to patient.
   11. Encourage independence.
   12. Monitor impact on hygiene and nutrition.
   13. Encourage socialization.

See Chapter 6 for additional information on mental health issues.

REHABILITATION AND MAINTENANCE OF COGNITIVE FUNCTION

REALITY ORIENTATION (TABLE 9-3)

A. A total approach to keeping individuals oriented; small groups that emphasize time, place, and person; weather; holidays; and daily schedule
B. First used with disoriented, confused older adults at Veterans Administration Hospital in Tuscaloosa, Alabama, in 1965
C. Orientation boards may be used to provide contact with reality.
D. Program success depends on total staff commitment and 24-hour implementation.
E. Many facilities that care for the older adult have implemented modified programs.

Table 9-3   Psychosocial Approaches for Confusion and Disorientation

APPROACH	PURPOSE	ACTIVITIES
Reality orientation	Orient patient to person, place, and time.	Consistent 24 hr/day interaction with staff or family Continual reminders of day, year, time Consistent mealtimes, activities of daily living, treatment Memory aids such as TV, radio, newspaper, clock, calendar
Validation therapy	Decrease stress, promote self-esteem and communication, reduce use of chemical and physical restraints, and delay institutionalization.	Group support to encourage respect for the feelings of the individual from his or her perspective Sample activities include singing favorite songs, reminiscing, sharing a memento or family photo
Reminiscence	Reexamine past to promote socialization and mental stimulation; wrap up unresolved issues.	Individual or group sharing of information about past life experiences
Remotivation therapy	Stimulate senses and provide new motivation in life through factual information rather than feelings.	Introduce pictures, plants, animals, or sounds to encourage interaction
Resocialization	Encourage socialization patterns within a group.	Assign socialization roles in a group such as serving one another refreshments

From deWit S: *Fundamental concepts and skills for nursing,* ed 3, St Louis, 2009, Saunders.

F. Program implementation is not limited to an institutional setting.

G. Components
  1. Small groups
  2. Formal classroom sessions
    a. 20 to 30 minutes
    b. Morning sessions recommended (older adults are more alert in the morning)
    c. Reality orientation board, calendars, clocks, and other materials used according to instructor plan
    d. Positive verbal feedback emphasized
    e. Confusion never reinforced

H. All personnel who come in contact with patients participating in the program are expected to use reality orientation.
  1. Address patient by name and title.
  2. Orient patient to time, place, and person.
  3. Give positive verbal feedback.
  4. Do not reinforce confusion.

REMOTIVATION

A. Similar to reality orientation
B. Normal behavior is reinforced through structured group program.
C. Stimulation of participation and interest in the environment is a key component.
D. Sessions average 20 to 60 minutes.
E. Visual aids (e.g., items that stimulate sensory responses) are used.
F. Patient behavior is recorded.
G. Staff support and involvement are essential.

REMINISCENCE

A. Small-group sessions
B. Based on life-review process
C. Older adults with cognitive dysfunction retain long-term memory and through reminiscence can adapt to the aging process.

D. Purposes
  1. Resolving conflict
  2. Sharing memories
  3. Achieving sense of identity and self-importance
  4. Focusing on a life that has meaning rather than one viewed as a waste of time
  5. Natural for older adult
    a. They feel comfortable.
    b. They are good at it.
    c. It reinforces sense of belonging (everyone talks about trials and tribulations of life).
  6. Therapeutic relationship with leader is more likely to develop as patients realize that their memories are important and valued.
  7. Depressed patients find a caring listener and an opportunity to externalize their anger.
  8. Psychologically disturbed patients receive acceptance, group validation, and a forum for expression. Encourage active exploration of past strengths.
  9. Strive to change outlook on the past rather than establishing new future directions.
  10. Reminiscence is a psychological assessment tool (e.g., insight into past coping mechanisms).
  11. It reduces isolation, insecurity, and negative self-esteem.
  12. Confused patients can be assisted in exploring a memory that stimulates latent thoughts, becomes more oriented, and improves ability to focus.
  13. Current circumstances are often reflected through memories.

E. If patients have difficulty focusing their thoughts, assist by selecting a specific memory.

F. Stimulating dormant thoughts to the surface decreases disorientation.

G. Patients who are reluctant to talk usually can be stimulated with topics such as food, movies, and music.

H. Program implementation is not limited to institutional settings.

COGNITIVE TRAINING

A. Memory exercises, problem-solving situations, and memory training are used.
B. Leader must be familiar with the patient's past leisure time use, hobbies, and occupations.
C. Individual, small, or large groups are used.
D. The purpose is to maintain mental activity.

PET THERAPY

A. Carefully chosen pets as part of a pet therapy program for a facility or as personal pets
B. Benefits: decreases tension, stimulates interest in surroundings, provides emotional support, encourages activity, and comforts with touch

MUSIC THERAPY

A. May reach patients when other methods fail
B. Uses
  1. Calms and reduces agitation in patients with Alzheimer disease
  2. Promotes attention span and expression of feelings
  3. Provides motivation for exercise and socialization
  4. Sing-a-longs to enhance cognitive function and foster contact with reality

RELAXATION THERAPY

A. Promotes sense of physical well-being, reduces stress, releases tension
B. Uses small groups
C. Involves rhythmical breathing, tension-relaxation exercises, and altered state of consciousness

VALIDATION THERAPY

A. It is useful for persons with permanent cognitive loss.
B. The nurse accepts the patient's feeling to give him or her a sense of dignity and self-worth.
C. Validation therapy provides comfort to patient and enables nurse to find the meaning in patient's behavior.

BLADDER RETRAINING: URINARY INCONTINENCE

A. Causes: Maintaining a log of incontinence events for 24 to 48 hours may assist in determining cause or issue.
  1. Physiological changes
    a. Decline in muscle support of pelvis
    b. Reduction in capacity of bladder to hold urine
    c. Sphincter weakness
  2. Behavioral alterations
    a. Regression
    b. Insecurity
    c. Rebellion
    d. Attention seeking
    e. Dependency
    f. Sensory deprivation
  3. Drugs
  4. Consciousness alterations
  5. Disease
  6. Obstruction
  7. Trauma
  8. Immobility
  9. Bedpans and urinals
  10. Lack of privacy
  11. Lack of time

B. Types
  1. Stress or passive
    a. Bladder outlet weakness
    b. Involuntary
    c. Frequency when sneezing, coughing, laughing, lifting
  2. Paradoxical or overflow
    a. Uncontrollable contraction waves
    b. Bladder that does not empty
    c. Frequency accompanied by retention
    d. At risk for UTI
  3. Total
    a. Constant dribbling
    b. Storage problem
C. Older adults susceptible to:
  1. UTIs
  2. Urgency
  3. Frequency
D. Patient reactions to incontinence
  1. Insecurity
    a. Social withdrawal
    b. Isolation
    c. Sensory deprivation
    d. Avoidance of previously developed relationships
  2. Depression
    a. Embarrassment
    b. Guilt
    c. Shame
E. Interventions
  1. Pelvic exercises
    a. Bearing down
    b. Push-ups from a chair
  2. Indwelling catheter only as a last resort if skin integrity is threatened
  3. Condom drainage
  4. Absorbent, waterproof underpants
  5. Keep patient clean and dry
  6. Skin care; handwashing
  7. Retraining
    a. Assess and record voiding pattern for minimum of 72 hours.
      (1) Time
      (2) Place
      (3) Quantity
      (4) Activity
      (5) Patient awareness
      (6) Significant medications
      (7) Character of urine
      (8) Presence or absence of constipation or discharge
      (9) Problems (e.g., clothing and ambulation hindrances)
    b. Reestablish voiding pattern.
      (1) First scheduled voiding of the day should be attempted immediately after awakening in the morning even if bed is wet.
      (2) Voiding should be attempted at intervals determined from the assessment period (usually at 1-, 2-, or 3-hour periods; goal is every 4 hours).
      (3) Patient takes one or two 8-oz (240-mL) glasses of fluid 1 hour before attempting to urinate.
      (4) No fluids should be taken between 6:00 PM and 6:00 AM if no urinating is desired.
      (5) Fluid intake should be at least 2000 mL/day.
      (6) Alcoholic drinks are contraindicated.

(7) Soft drinks, tea, and coffee should be avoided.

(8) All fluid intake should be measured and recorded.

(9) All urine output should be measured and recorded.

BOWEL RETRAINING: FECAL INCONTINENCE

A. Causes
1. Physiological changes
   a. External anal sphincter relaxation
   b. Perineal relaxation
   c. Muscle atony
2. Behavioral alterations
   a. Regression
   b. Rebellion
   c. Dependency
   d. Sensory deprivation
3. Central nervous system injury
4. Obstruction
5. Impaction
6. Consciousness alterations
7. Immobility
8. Trauma
B. Interventions
1. Keep patient clean and dry.
2. Provide absorbent, waterproof underpants.
3. Provide skin care.
4. Provide retraining.
   a. Bowel retraining is easier than bladder retraining. If patient is incontinent of urine and stool, start a bowel-retraining program first.
   b. Use no laxatives.
   c. Ensure adequate fluid intake (2 L/day).
   d. Fluids and solids that promote patient's bowel movements (e.g., bran, orange juice) and roughage should be included in the diet.
   e. Encourage physical activity.
   f. Obtain bowel history.
   g. Procedure
      (1) Establish regular day and time to assist patient to the toilet for evacuation, preferably after a meal.
      (2) After 20 minutes, if patient has not had a bowel movement, insert a lubricated glycerin suppository.
         (a) Do not use directly from refrigerator.
         (b) Do not insert into a bolus of stool (ineffective).
         (c) After ascertaining that patient requires the suppository for training, it can be inserted 1 to 2 hours before the scheduled training time and after a meal.
      (3) Take the patient to the bathroom at the scheduled time daily even if he or she has had a bowel movement between scheduled times.

Bibliography

Christensen BL, Kockrow EO: *Foundations and adult health nursing*, ed 6, St Louis, 2010, Mosby.

deWit SC: *Fundamental concepts and skills for nursing*, ed 4, St Louis, 2014, Saunders.

Edmunds MW: *Introduction to clinical pharmacology*, ed 7, St Louis, 2013, Mosby.

Emergency Nurse's Association: *Sheehy's manual of emergency care*, ed 7, St Louis, 2013, Mosby.

Feldman RS: *Development across the life span*, ed 6, Englewood Cliffs, 2011, Prentice Hall.

Hogstel MO, Curry LC: *Practical guide to health assessment through the life span*, ed 4, Philadelphia, 2005, FA Davis.

Meiner SE: *Gerontologic nursing*, ed 4, St Louis, 2011, Mosby.

Morrison-Valfre M: *Foundations of mental health care*, ed 5, St Louis, 2013, Mosby.

Polan E, Taylor DC: *Journey across the life span: human development and health promotion*, ed 4, Philadelphia, 2011, FA Davis.

Nix S: *Williams' basic nutrition and diet therapy*, ed 14, St Louis, 2013, Mosby.

Thibodeau GA, Patton KP: *Structure and function of the body*, ed 14, St Louis, 2012, Mosby.

Timby BK: *Fundamental nursing skills and concepts*, ed 10, Philadelphia, 2010, Lippincott Williams & Wilkins.

Wold GH: *Basic geriatric nursing*, ed 5, St Louis, 2012, Mosby.

REVIEW QUESTIONS

1. A patient with Parkinson disease has difficulty swallowing. The patient is able to meet dietary requirements when he can do which of the following? Select all that apply.
   _____ 1. Eat solid food
   _____ 2. Drink thin liquids
   _____ 3. Eat a meal in 20 minutes
   _____ 4. Swallow without choking
   _____ 5. Drink thickened liquids

2. A 67-year-old patient is admitted to a nursing home with a diagnosis of senile dementia—Alzheimer type (SDAT). The nurse observes the resident moving toward the exit door. The nurse meets the resident at the door and volunteers assistance. The resident responds, "You can leave me alone. I'm going home." Which nursing action is most appropriate?
   1. Going with the resident
   2. Engaging him in an activity
   3. Calling the security department
   4. Physically preventing him from leaving

3. An 89-year-old nursing home resident with a history of dementia and poor nutrition intake eats a few mouthfuls of dinner and then gets up and leaves the table. Which nursing approach is most appropriate?
   1. Applying a vest restraint during meals
   2. Offering five or six small feedings daily
   3. Having a staff member feed him his meals
   4. Providing him with a variety of finger foods

4. A patient diagnosed with Parkinson disease is placed on carbidopa-levodopa (Sinemet), 10/100 orally three times daily, by his physician. As he is leaving the physician's office, he asks the nurse what the drug will do. Which explanation by the nurse is most correct?
   1. "You'll have to discuss that with the physician."
   2. "It can decrease your tremors and improve your gait."
   3. "It's the carbidopa/levodopa content ratio of the drug."
   4. "It's really very complicated and not necessary for you to know."

5. A patient taking carbidopa-levodopa (Sinemet) reports to the nurse that he really does not want to eat and occasionally vomits when he does eat. To reduce the gastrointestinal side effects of Sinemet and enhance its

absorption, which instructions should the nurse give the patient?
1. Take the medication before meals
2. Take the medication after meals
3. Crush the medication and mix it with food
4. If any problems exist, call the physician to lower the dosage

6. A 73-year-old nursing home resident reports that the staff ignores her needs but takes care of all the other patients. Which response by the nurse is most therapeutic?
1. "That's not true. We take care of you."
2. "I think you are imagining things. I'm here to help you."
3. "What do you need?"
4. "How can I help you?"

7. A 78-year-old widow is brought to the local emergency department by the police, who found her wandering aimlessly about the street. She is confused and disoriented and later admitted with pneumonia. The nurse suspects that the cause of her confusion and disorientation is:
1. Infection.
2. Unknown pathology.
3. Arteriosclerosis.
4. Organic brain syndrome.

8. An older man is hospitalized with pneumonia and has a poor nutrition intake. The patient's appetite may improve if:
1. His food is pureed.
2. All liquids are served warm.
3. A roll is served with each meal.
4. He is served small meals frequently.

9. The night staff members in a nursing home express concern about an older resident who is awake most of the night. During a team meeting, what would be the most appropriate response by the nurse?
1. "Let's try to increase his daytime activities."
2. "He needs rest. I'll get a physician's order for a sedative."
3. "As people get older, they require less sleep."
4. "Older adults require less sleep at night but more rest periods during the day."

10. During the initial assessment for admission to the long-term care facility, the nurse notes that the patient has a loss of subcutaneous tissue. The nurse should be alert for which manifestation of this normal aging phenomenon?
1. Foot pain with ambulation
2. Muscle cramps at night
3. Increased urination at night
4. Increased susceptibility to infection

11. Given the normal aging changes in the sensory system, which color would be most effective when color coding the door to the room of an older nursing home resident?
1. Red
2. Pink
3. Blue
4. Green

12. An 80-year-old patient with diabetes mellitus is hospitalized and scheduled for a right below-the-knee amputation (BKA). On the fifth postoperative day, the nurse notices that the residual limb is edematous. The nurse should plan to:
1. Elevate the limb on a pillow.
2. See if the patient has an order for a diuretic.

3. Instruct the patient to sit on the edge of the bed and dangle.
4. Ensure proper application of the elastic bandage to the residual limb.

13. The nurse is caring for an older adult with partial-thickness burns from a kitchen accident. After nutrition teaching, which breakfast choices by the patient would indicate she understands her nutritional needs?
1. Two poached eggs, toast with jam, whole milk, coffee
2. Dry cereal with skim milk, orange juice, coffee
3. Pancakes with syrup, two strips of bacon, apple juice
4. Oatmeal with skim milk, orange juice, coffee

14. When attempting to teach a patient with dementia, an important point for the nurse to remember is to:
1. Speak quickly and repeat several times in succession.
2. Talk in a very animated, loud voice so the patient can hear what is being said.
3. Eliminate background noise by shutting doors and turning off the television.
4. Talk to the patient when he or she is stress free, such as while watching television.

15. The nurse is administering medications via a nasogastric (NG) feeding tube to a 68-year-old patient. What is the correct sequence of administration?
1. Aspirate stomach contents (5 to 10 mL), give medication, flush with at least 150 mL of water.
2. Check tube placement, flush with water, give medication, aspirate stomach contents (5 to 10 mL).
3. Flush tube with water, aspirate stomach contents (5 to 10 mL), give medication, flush with water again.
4. Check tube placement, flush with water, give medication, flush with water again.

16. One day after open reduction internal fixation (ORIF) of the right hip, an 80-year-old patient is exhibiting extremely restless behavior. What is the first nursing action at this time?
1. Medicate him for pain
2. Ask his wife what is wrong with him
3. Assess his cardiac and respiratory status
4. Call the physician from the nurses' station to see him

17. A nurse is instructing an older adult concerning the Patient Self-Determination Act. Which statement by the nurse accurately describes a health care proxy or durable power of attorney?
1. The health care proxy makes financial decisions for the patient.
2. The state appoints a guardian who is given the power to make health care decisions for the patient.
3. The patient forms a list of activities that he does not want done if he should become incapacitated.
4. The patient appoints an individual who is given power of attorney to make medical decisions for the patient.

18. A nurse is presenting a seminar on culture to a group of nursing assistants. The nurse relates that the culture most likely to use traditional or alternative therapies before accessing health care is:
1. African Americans.
2. Jewish Americans.
3. Chinese Americans.
4. Hispanic Americans.

19. When caring for a patient receiving radiation therapy for cancer, which tasks can be safely assigned to a nursing assistant? Select all that apply.
    _____ 1. Exploring the patient's coping mechanisms for the cancer therapy.
    _____ 2. Helping the patient ambulate.
    _____ 3. Monitoring how the patient manages fatigue during the shift.
    _____ 4. Observing the skin after a treatment session.
    _____ 5. Documenting intake from meals and bedside water pitcher.

20. As adults age, they frequently experience multiple health problems. Which of these topics should the nurse emphasize in her teaching of the older adult?
    1. Prevention of acute illness
    2. Prevention of chronic illness
    3. Health maintenance with acute illnesses
    4. Symptom management with chronic illnesses

21. An 81-year-old patient visits the physician's office with a fractured right ankle. A family member states that the individual fell down the stairs. Which additional assessment most strongly suggests elder abuse?
    1. Anorexia, ill-fitting dentures
    2. Chronic cough, shortness of breath
    3. Confusion, abrasions in various stages of healing
    4. Fatigue, extreme pain on palpation of the right ankle

22. An older patient asks the nurse if the new drug sildenafil citrate (Viagra) would be something that would help him resume sexual relations with his wife. The most correct response by the nurse would be:
    1. "Viagra allows for a more intimate sexual experience."
    2. "It is best that you put that part of your life behind you."
    3. "Viagra assists some individuals in achieving an erection."
    4. "Viagra helps some people become more sexually excited."

23. A nursing assistant asks the nurse why some older residents fail to fill in all the responses to a multiple-choice survey concerning nutrition. The nurse responds that older adults:
    1. Have brain atrophy that affects intelligence.
    2. Do not care about surveys concerning nutrition.
    3. May be afraid to take the risk of answering "wrong."
    4. Were probably unable to see the small circles on the paper.

24. The nurse is teaching a nursing assistant to put in a patient's hearing aid. The nurse instructs the assistant to turn the hearing aid on:
    1. Before placing it in the ear.
    2. While inserting it in the ear canal.
    3. Only after the aid is in the ear canal.
    4. When the person decides to turn it on.

25. The nurse is evaluating the best possible mobility aid for a patient with vertigo. Which mobility aid would be the most stable for this patient?
    1. Cane
    2. Walker
    3. Crutches
    4. Wheelchair

26. One factor that is considered when determining if negligence has occurred is the:
    1. Policy of the facility.
    2. Age of the nurse.
    3. Gender of the resident.
    4. Severity of the injury.

27. After knocking on the resident's door, the nurse enters the room and observes a male resident masturbating. The most appropriate action by the nurse is to:
    1. Distract the resident in a conversation about the weather.
    2. Get the resident out of bed and walk with him to the day room.
    3. Quietly leave the room, making sure to close the door.
    4. Tell the resident to stop.

28. The best way to help the resident of an Alzheimer unit identify his or her room is to:
    1. Put the resident's name on the door.
    2. Post a picture of the resident taken 15 to 20 years earlier on the door of his or her room.
    3. Post a very recent picture of the resident on the door of the resident's room.
    4. Color code the door of the room to match the resident's identification bracelet.

29. A nurse observes a resident with a diagnosis of senile dementia buttering her napkin and using it to soak up sauce from her dinner plate. This resident is exhibiting symptoms of:
    1. Aphasia.
    2. Agnosia.
    3. Vertigo.
    4. Akinesia.

30. The term *tunnel vision* describes the vision changes that occur with:
    1. Cataracts.
    2. Night blindness.
    3. Glaucoma.
    4. Macular degeneration.

31. An older adult with type 2 (non–insulin-dependent) diabetes mellitus who develops pneumonia is at the greatest risk for developing:
    1. Diabetic coma.
    2. Hyperglycemic hyperosmolar nonketotic coma.
    3. Urinary tract infection.
    4. Hypoglycemia.

32. An appropriate intervention for a resident who is at risk for falls is:
    1. A 2-hour toileting schedule while the resident is awake.
    2. Keeping side rails up at all times while the resident is in bed.
    3. Obtaining an order for a vest restraint as needed.
    4. Dressing the resident in heavy clothing.

33. A patient's wife died 4 years ago. The patient has kept all of her personal belongings and cries every time he speaks of her. The patient is exhibiting symptoms of:
    1. Dysfunctional grief.
    2. Depression.
    3. Anticipatory grief.
    4. Paranoia.

34. Validation therapy is a valuable therapy for:
    1. Residents with dementia.
    2. Any resident, because it accepts feelings and provides comfort.
    3. Maintaining mental activity.
    4. Life review.

35. An 81-year-old patient tells the nurse, "I don't know why I bother; life just isn't worth living anymore." The most appropriate response by the nurse is:
    1. "Life is good; smile."

2. "You sound upset; let's sit down and talk."
3. "Don't be silly; you have a lot of friends."
4. "Surely you're not thinking about killing yourself."

36. A patient suspected to have senile macular degeneration will experience:
    1. Loss of central vision.
    2. Loss of peripheral vision.
    3. Hemianopsia.
    4. Aphakia.

37. When a patient asks how he or she can prevent cataracts, the nurse's most therapeutic response is:
    1. "Cataract development is related to vitamin B_6 deficiency. Increase your intake of this vitamin by taking daily supplements."
    2. "Cataract development is related to exposure to ultraviolet light. Wear sunglasses and protect your eyes from glare."
    3. "Cataract development is related the ingestion of alcohol. Cut down on alcohol intake."
    4. "Cataracts are more common in men. Your risk is not as great as a woman."

38. During the admission assessment, a patient states she takes several herbal preparations daily. Because the patient has warfarin sodium (Coumadin) ordered, the nurse will plan to report to the doctor the use of which herbal preparation?
    1. Ginkgo biloba
    2. Chamomile
    3. Basil
    4. Saw palmetto

39. The nurse knows that a patient needs additional teaching regarding alendronate sodium (Fosamax) when she says:
    1. "I'll take this with water right before bed."
    2. "I'll sit up for at least 30 minutes after I take it."
    3. "I'll take it with water in the morning."
    4. "If I forget to take it in the morning, I'll just skip it for that day."

40. When teaching a patient to use calcitonin-salmon (Miacalcin), the nurse must:
    1. Establish the patient's baseline bone density.
    2. Instruct the patient to wear a MedicAlert tag.
    3. Instruct the patient to alternate nostrils for administration.
    4. Instruct the patient to sit up for at least 20 minutes after using it.

41. The nurse is admitting four new patients to the long-term care facility. She assesses their risk for osteoporosis and is most concerned about the patient with which of the following characteristics?
    1. Late menopause, 10 pounds under ideal body weight, square dances three times per week
    2. Early menopause, coffee drinker, sedentary lifestyle
    3. Late menopause, vegetarian diet, walks 2 miles daily
    4. Late menopause, 25 pounds above ideal body weight, employed as a housekeeper

42. A 70-year-old patient is to receive amphotericin B. This drug has been mixed in a 500-mL bag of normal saline. If the drug is to be infused over 5 hours, what is the flow rate? _____ mL/hr

43. Wernicke encephalopathy and Korsakoff syndrome are associated with a deficiency of:
    1. Vitamin C.

2. Vitamin B_{12}.
3. Vitamin K.
4. Vitamin B_1.

44. Pill rolling is a movement sometimes seen in:
    1. Huntington chorea.
    2. Tardive dyskinesia.
    3. Parkinson disease.
    4. Diabetic retinopathy.

45. After interviewing a 70-year-old patient during the admission assessment, the nurse identifies which factor as significant for development of bronchogenic carcinoma?
    1. Exposure to air pollution in the factory where he worked for 35 years
    2. Smoking cigarettes since age 18
    3. Development of COPD at age 50
    4. Use of chewing tobacco for 5 years

46. When assessing a patient who states he has herpes zoster, the nurse will expect to observe:
    1. Red welts that ooze serous fluid.
    2. Vesicular eruption along a nerve route.
    3. Dry scaly skin on one side of the body.
    4. Redness and pruritus in the axillary folds.

47. The nurse knows that the caregiver understands an important aspect of caring for the family member with Alzheimer dementia when the caregiver says:
    1. "I will avoid arguing or trying to reason with him."
    2. "I'll keep him busy all evening."
    3. "He can listen to radio talk shows."
    4. "It's important that he wear incontinent products at all times."

48. An undesirable physiological adaptation to atherosclerosis is:
    1. Increased cardiac output.
    2. Collateral circulation.
    3. Coronary artery disease.
    4. Coronary artery bypass.

49. Right-sided neglect or right-sided body blindness is related to:
    1. Seizure disorders.
    2. Myocardial infarctions.
    3. A cerebrovascular accident (CVA) affecting the right side of the brain.
    4. A CVA affecting the left side of the brain.

50. The most appropriate way to enhance sexuality in a long-term care facility is to:
    1. Routinely assign men and women as roommates.
    2. Provide sexually explicit reading materials.
    3. Plan group activities that encourage socialization.
    4. Serve alcoholic beverages with the evening meal.

51. A resident is showing changes in behavior, including confusion. The nurse should first:
    1. Review the resident's medication orders.
    2. Obtain a urine specimen for culture and sensitivity.
    3. Administer the ordered analgesic.
    4. Assess the resident completely.

52. A 78-year-old resident wanders from room to room looking for Dora, his deceased wife. The nurse says to the resident, "You loved your wife very much." This therapeutic response is an example of:
    1. Reality orientation.
    2. Validation.
    3. Reminiscence.
    4. Life review.

53. Decreased cardiac output is most directly responsible for:
    1. Mitral regurgitation.
    2. Cardiac enlargement.
    3. Deceased coronary circulation.
    4. Reduced renal blood flow.
54. When music therapy is used with a restless resident exhibiting acting-out behaviors, a successful outcome is that the:
    1. Resident is comforted; behavior is calm.
    2. Resident is reoriented to self.
    3. Resident is free of injury.
    4. Resident's functional level improves.
55. An 80-year-old resident has frequent complaints of a dry mouth despite adequate fluid intake. The nurse should:
    1. Check the resident's blood sugar.
    2. Request a dental consultation.
    3. Review the medication orders.
    4. Apply petroleum jelly to his lips.
56. A family is planning a surprise birthday party for their father's eighty-sixth birthday. The music that would best encourage socialization in this age group is:
    1. Big bands of the 1940s.
    2. Classical piano concertos.
    3. Gospel hymns.
    4. Folk ballads.
57. One advantage of employing the older worker is that he or she:
    1. Increases employee morale.
    2. Can orient new employees.
    3. Has a better memory than young employees have.
    4. Has an established work ethic.
58. Assessing for pain in the older adult is important because older adults:
    1. Have lower pain thresholds.
    2. Exhibit more pain behaviors than younger people do.
    3. Are easily addicted to pain medications.
    4. Have a higher pain threshold.
59. A 70-year-old Jewish woman is scheduled for a bowel resection. The best time to schedule this procedure would be:
    1. 8:00 AM Friday.
    2. 8:00 AM Thursday.
    3. 4:00 PM Friday.
    4. 8:00 AM Saturday.
60. A thin, elderly woman of Asian heritage is at risk for:
    1. Hashimoto disease.
    2. Osteoporosis.
    3. Herpes zoster.
    4. Glaucoma.
61. An older adult woman with osteoarthritis of her hands is compliant with her medication regimen. She asks the nurse for suggestions to help relieve the morning stiffness of her hands. An appropriate response by the nurse is:
    1. "Gentle range-of-motion exercises of your hands and fingers can be useful."
    2. "Try using ice packs on your hands."
    3. "Soak your hands in Epsom saltwater."
    4. "Massage your hands with cortisone cream."
62. A 59-year-old woman visits her family doctor to request updates on her immunizations. She says the school district requires some additional immunizations because she is getting involved in a volunteer mentoring program for junior high school students. She states, "It's about time I started getting involved in my community!" The nurse realizes the patient is in which developmental stage?
    1. Industry versus inferiority
    2. Generativity versus stagnation
    3. Ego integrity versus despair
    4. Identity versus role confusion
63. A mentally stimulating activity for older adults that uses remote memory is:
    1. Reality orientation.
    2. Reminiscence.
    3. Spelling bee competition.
    4. Scrabble.
64. A 75-year-old male patient has been diagnosed with inoperable pancreatic cancer. The nurse observes that his wife is melancholy and is devoting much of her time to scrapbooking and compiling family photo albums. The wife's behavior is best described as:
    1. Situational depression.
    2. Denial.
    3. Anticipatory grieving.
    4. Social withdrawal.
65. An older patient is complaining of inability to sleep through the night. He says he is restless and tosses and turns. Interventions that are helpful in promoting restful sleep include:
    1. Wearing earplugs, exercising 1 hour before bedtime.
    2. Drinking 8 oz of red wine 1 hour before bedtime, practicing controlled relaxation.
    3. Maintaining a regular bedtime, wearing an herbal sleep mask.
    4. Using a fan for white noise, limiting fluids in the evening.
66. A 72-year-old patient is admitted with an acute exacerbation of chronic obstructive pulmonary disease (COPD). The most appropriate nursing diagnosis for this patient is:
    1. Deficient knowledge of treatment regimen.
    2. Anxiety.
    3. Risk for infection.
    4. Ineffective breathing pattern.
67. An older patient tells the nurse that constipation has become a real problem and asks for suggestions that might help. The most appropriate response by the nurse is:
    1. "Most people have trouble with their bowels as they get older; you should talk to your doctor about it."
    2. "Changes in what you eat and drink can often help. Tell me what kinds of foods you usually eat."
    3. "Many medications are available that can help. What have you tried so far?"
    4. "That can be serious; how are you feeling? Have you had any blood from your rectum or abdominal pain?"
68. An older adult receives a prescription for metronidazole (Flagyl). Which complementary therapy would be contraindicated with this medication?
    1. St John's wort
    2. Gin-soaked raisins
    3. Chamomile tea
    4. Acupuncture

69. An older adult has a purified protein derivative (PPD) (Mantoux) test result of 12-mm induration at 48 hours. The nurse should anticipate that the follow-up will be:
    1. Second-step PPD in 4 weeks.
    2. Bronchoscopy.
    3. Computed tomography (CT) scan of the chest.
    4. Chest x-ray examination.

70. Identify and put in order the five stages of grief as described by Dr. Kübler-Ross.
    1. Denial
    2. Resolution
    3. Bargaining
    4. Peace
    5. Anger
    6. Acceptance
    7. Bartering
    8. Depression

71. A medication order reads, "Infuse 1000 mL of normal saline IV over 12 hours." Calculate the number of milliliters to be infused in 1 hour based on this order.
    _____ mL/hr

72. Select all factors that contribute to the increase in human immunodeficiency virus and acquired immunodeficiency syndrome (HIV/AIDS) in older adults.
    _____ 1. Past blood transfusions
    _____ 2. Lack of need regarding birth control
    _____ 3. Increase in the number of sexual partners
    _____ 4. Aging immune system
    _____ 5. Knowledge deficit regarding safe sex
    _____ 6. Poor muscle control for safe injection technique

73. Communication with unlicensed assistive personnel is critical for patient care. The best way for a charge nurse to communicate a procedure change to nursing assistants is to:
    1. E-mail them on their home computers.
    2. Post a notice at the time clock.
    3. Tell the nursing assistant who arrives first about the change; have her tell the other assistants.
    4. Have a brief meeting with everyone involved at the start of the shift to explain the change.

74. When a 70-year-old Chinese woman is hesitant to undress for an examination, the nurse will assess her symptoms by asking the patient to:
    1. Write a detailed description of her symptoms.
    2. Draw a picture of her symptoms.
    3. Point out the symptoms on the nurse.
    4. Point out the symptoms on a model doll.

75. A nurse has the following responsibilities immediately after receiving a change-of-shift report at 7 AM. Prioritize these tasks from highest priority through lowest priority.
    1. Neurological checks on a resident who fell during the night
    2. Insulin administration for two residents
    3. Routine vital signs for three residents
    4. Eyedrops for four residents

76. A diet of 2400 calories via continuous tube feeding is ordered for a resident. The feeding formula has a concentration of 1.3 calories/mL. The nurse should set the feeding pump for:
    Answer: _____ mL/hr

77. When assessing an older woman, the nurse must recognize that older female relatives are highly esteemed and frequently consulted for advice by:
    1. African Americans.
    2. Italian Americans.
    3. Native Americans.
    4. Chinese Americans.

78. A resident of a nursing home has a new medication order for ceftriaxone sodium (Rocephin). This order should be questioned if the resident is allergic to:
    1. Penicillin.
    2. Sulfa.
    3. Aspirin.
    4. Shellfish.

79. A nursing assistant asks the charge nurse what to do with the religious-looking object that a resident is wearing around his neck. The best response by the nurse is:
    1. "Call the family, and ask them."
    2. "Put it in the bedside stand for now."
    3. "Take it off, and I'll lock it in the medication cart."
    4. "Leave it on unless the resident asks for it to be removed."

80. In developing a teaching plan for a patient diagnosed with osteoporosis, the nurse includes information about risk factors, including:
    1. Cigarette smoking.
    2. Low caffeine intake.
    3. Too much calcium.
    4. An active lifestyle.

81. When a patient dies, the nurse should use which communication technique when talking with the family?
    1. Saying "I know just how you feel."
    2. Saying "Her death was for the best."
    3. Never crying in front of family members
    4. Talking quietly and encouraging family members to share their feelings

82. Good bowel hygiene for an 85-year-old adult includes:
    1. A regular, nonhurried time for bowel movements.
    2. Occasional exercise before lunch.
    3. A diet low in fiber and high in carbohydrates.
    4. Taking laxatives regularly to promote bowel movements.

83. Which statement would help a grieving family member express feelings?
    1. "Tell me how you're feeling."
    2. "You're just afraid to be alone."
    3. "Things will get better."
    4. "Time heals all wounds."

84. When teaching an older adult about medications, the nurse must be certain that the person:
    1. Knows about the actions and side effects of the drugs and how to take them.
    2. Understands the actions and contraindications of the drugs.
    3. Keeps the physician informed about the medication schedule.
    4. Takes the medications on a flexible schedule with meals.

85. One of the earliest signs of drug toxicity is usually:
    1. Incontinence.
    2. Belligerence.
    3. Confusion.
    4. Dementia.

86. Which assessment of the older adult should be reported to the charge nurse?
    1. The integumentary system has lost elasticity, and the epidermis is thin.
    2. There is a gradual loss of weight caused by loss of muscle tissue and fluid.
    3. There is decreased resistance to infections, resulting in pneumonia.
    4. There is increasing incidence of choking and aspiration.

87. When administering medications to older adults, it is important to remember that absorption, distribution, metabolism, and excretion tend to decrease with age:
    1. Because of altered liver and kidney function and decreased circulation.
    2. And doses may need to be increased to achieve desired results.
    3. So brain receptors become less sensitive to drugs.
    4. And older persons use over-the-counter medications to enhance excretion of other drugs.

88. When instituting a bladder retraining program, the nurse includes:
    1. An established elimination time of every 2 hours.
    2. A fluid restriction of 1800 to 2000 mL in 24 hours.
    3. The elimination of diuretic medications.
    4. Scheduling voiding times around the schedule of the facility.

89. Which statement regarding health care given in a long-term care facility is correct?
    1. Assessment is performed on every resident every week.
    2. Residents' rights and choices are important considerations in planning care.
    3. A goal is to provide care for the older adult in the most restrictive environment.
    4. Functional status is not assessed after initial admission.

90. When using laxatives for older adults, the nurse should always:
    1. Start with the strongest ones and move down to the gentlest ones that work for the person.
    2. Start with the gentlest ones and move up to the stronger ones until one is effective.
    3. Start with a moderately irritating one and move in either direction, depending on the person's need.
    4. Start and stay with the ones that achieve the quickest results.

91. For a patient to be physically mobile after a fall, which nursing goal takes priority?
    1. Preventing contractures
    2. Preventing edema
    3. Preventing pain
    4. Preventing depression

92. Urinary calculi in the older person can be prevented by:
    1. Encouraging fluids.
    2. A low-calcium diet.
    3. Weight-bearing exercise.
    4. Medications.

93. On admission assessment, the nurse is concerned about the limited joint movement of an 87-year-old woman. The nurse is aware that this finding is not unusual since most older adults have some degree of:
    1. Osteoarthritis.
    2. Rheumatoid arthritis.
    3. Ankylosing spondylitis.
    4. Gouty arthritis.

94. If the physician orders acetylsalicylic acid (aspirin) for an older adult, the nurse should administer it:
    1. With food.
    2. In the morning and afternoon.
    3. By mixing it with fruit juice.
    4. Subcutaneously.

95. When attempting to defuse a confrontation between nursing assistants in the hallway, the nurse will:
    1. Tell the nursing assistants to talk about this issue in private.
    2. Reprimand both of them and put a note in their personnel file
    3. Discuss their behavior with the nursing supervisor at the end of the shift
    4. Speak calmly and take the nursing assistants into the conference room for further discussion.

96. Adequate circulation is present if the nail beds:
    1. Blanch on pressure and color returns rapidly.
    2. Do not blanch with pressure.
    3. Blanch and refill slowly.
    4. Blanch and do not refill.

97. Which statement would suggest a positive coping mechanism for a patient with rheumatoid arthritis?
    1. "This disease will go away once treated."
    2. "The pain medication will make me well."
    3. "This is going to be difficult. What do I need to know?"
    4. "I think I'll wear a copper bracelet."

98. Calculate the kilocalorie intake for a patient with diabetes eating 50 g of carbohydrate, 10 g of fat, and 20 g of protein for lunch.
    Answer: _____ Kcal

99. At 8 PM (2000) the nurse assesses a finger-stick blood glucose reading as 139 mg/dL. According to the following sliding scale, which dose of insulin will the nurse administer?

SLIDING INSULIN SCALE		
Blood sugar	below 80 mg/dL =	No insulin
Blood sugar	81-120 mg/dL =	2 units regular insulin
Blood sugar	121-150 mg/dL =	5 units regular insulin
Blood sugar	over 151 mg/dL =	8 units regular insulin

    1. The nurse will not administer insulin.
    2. 2 units
    3. 5 units
    4. 8 units

100. Using the data given during shift report, the night nurse prioritizes patient assessments. Put these patients in correct order of assessment priority from highest to lowest.
    1. Patient with chronic obstructive pulmonary disease scheduled for herniorrhaphy at 8 AM, vital signs (VS) T 98.8° F (37.1° C), P 82, R 22, BP 138/82
    2. Patient with diabetes, finger-stick blood glucose reading of 210 mg/dL at 9:30 PM (2130), 15 units regular insulin administered at 10 PM (2200)

3. Patient with congestive heart failure and 1 ankle edema, 8-hour intake 1150 mL, 8-hour output 900 mL

4. Patient with suspected coronary artery disease scheduled for angiogram at 7 AM (0700), VS T 99 °F (37.2 °C), P 72, R 16, BP 140/76 at 8 PM (2000)

ANSWERS AND RATIONALES

1. Analysis, evaluation, physiological integrity, (b).
   _____ 1. Feeding a patient who has difficulty swallowing any type of solid food is inappropriate.
   _____ 2. Thin liquids are very difficult to swallow for individuals who have dysphagia.
   _____ 3. This patient may take much longer to eat because special precautions must be taken.
   __X__ 4. *When the patient swallows without choking and takes his time eating, he is safely able to meet dietary requirements.*
   __X__ 5. *Thickened liquids may be a part of this diet.*

2. Application, implementation, safe and effective care environment, (b).
   2. *The nurse uses the short-term memory loss to her advantage; this produces little anxiety in the resident.*
   1. Accompanying the resident may be appropriate if diversion does not work.
   3. Show of force only further agitates the resident.
   4. Agitation increases if the resident is confronted.

3. Application, implementation, physiological integrity, (b).
   4. *This is the best choice for the resident who does not sit at mealtime; it ensures proper nutrition intake.*
   1. Restraints should be used for resident safety only.
   2. Normally this would be a good choice; however, the resident does not sit at the table.
   3. This is inappropriate because it promotes dependence.

4. Application, implementation, physiological integrity, (b).
   2. *This is the only response that answers the patient's question.*
   1. This does not acknowledge the patient's question.
   3. This response does not answer the patient's question.
   4. This is demeaning to the patient.

5. Application, implementation, physiological integrity, (b).
   2. *Administering the drug after meals enhances absorption and decreases gastrointestinal irritation.*
   1. This increases gastrointestinal irritation.
   3. This is inappropriate; medications should not be mixed with the patient's food.
   4. No indication exists that this may be necessary; the physician determines this.

6. Analysis, evaluation, psychosocial integrity, (c).
   4. *This addresses the person's needs.*
   1. This is judgmental and does not address the needs of the resident.
   2. This belittles the resident.
   3. This is an abrupt statement and will block communication.

7. Analysis, assessment, physiological integrity, (b).
   2. *Not enough information is given to arrive at a diagnosis.*
   1. This may be the cause; however, further evaluation is necessary.

3. No indication exists that this may be the cause of the episode.
4. Further testing is required before this diagnosis can be made.

8. Comprehension, planning, physiological integrity, (b).
   4. *Frequent small meals are easier to digest and not as overwhelming to the patient.*
   1. No indication exists for pureed foods.
   2. There is no reason to believe that warm liquids would increase his appetite.
   3. Rolls would most likely not stimulate his appetite.

9. Analysis, planning, health promotion and maintenance, (b).
   4. *This is a normal aging change.*
   1. This would not be compatible with the rest needs of the patient.
   2. A more thorough assessment is needed before medication is given.
   3. The quality and continuity of sleep patterns change with aging.

10. Analysis, assessment, physiological integrity, (c).
    1. *Loss of fat tissue on the soles of the feet, coupled with the trauma of walking, places the patient at risk for foot problems.*
    2. With the decrease in muscle mass, tendons shrink and sclerose.
    3. Changes in the kidney predispose the patient to nocturia.
    4. Respiratory system changes alter the ability of the body to handle foreign particles and secretions, which increases susceptibility to infection.

11. Application, planning, safe and effective care environment, (b).
    1. *Because of the yellowing of the lens of the eye, older adults can see reds, oranges, and yellows best.*
    2. This is a lower color tone, which is not seen well by older adults.
    3. Blue is difficult for older adults to differentiate.
    4. Green is difficult for older adults to distinguish from other colors.

12. Application, planning, physiological integrity, (c).
    4. *A properly applied elastic bandage (Ace wrap) reduces edema and shapes the limb in preparation for prosthesis application.*
    1. The residual limb is elevated for the first 24 hours after surgery; after that it is not elevated to prevent hip flexion contractures.
    2. A diuretic is not indicated in this situation.
    3. This does not decrease the amount of edema in the residual limb; it creates further edema.

13. Analysis, evaluation, physiological integrity, (b).
    1. *Eggs and whole milk provide needed protein and calories.*
    2. Cereal, juice, and skim milk will provide carbohydrates and vitamins but little protein and few calories.
    3. Pancakes are carbohydrates for increased calories but bacon is a fat, not a protein.
    4. Oatmeal provides carbohydrates and fiber, orange provides vitamins, but protein is low.

14. Application, implementation, psychosocial integrity, (b).
    3. *This is the best way to get the patient's attention.*
    1. Speaking too quickly confuses the patient.

2. Talking loudly may agitate the individual.

4. Watching television would provide too much distraction.

15. Application, implementation, physiological integrity, (c).

    4. This is the proper sequence to administer medications through a nasogastric (NG) feeding tube.

    1. The tube should be flushed with a small amount of water (unless otherwise directed by physician) before and after the medication.

    2. Checking residual amount after giving the medication results in withdrawing some of the medication from the tube; the nurse will not get a true residual amount.

    3. Residual amounts (stomach contents) should be checked before flushing with water.

16. Application, planning, physiological integrity, (c).

    3. Any restless and confused behavior necessitates a cardiac and respiratory assessment; the patient may be hypoxic.

    1. The patient is not complaining of pain; a thorough assessment must be made before any intervention can be done.

    2. The spouse may provide valuable information about her husband's former cognitive status; however, the nurse needs to perform an assessment.

    4. This may be appropriate if an emergency problem is found with the patient, but the nurse should first assess the patient.

17. Application, implementation, safe and effective care environment, (b).

    4. The patient appoints an individual to make medical decisions for the patient should the patient become incapacitated.

    1. The health care proxy makes medical decisions for the patient.

    2. The patient usually chooses the individual; if the state makes the decision, a family member may or may not be chosen.

    3. This more accurately describes a living will.

18. Comprehension, implementation, health promotion and maintenance, (b).

    3. Chinese Americans are most likely to access alternative or traditional therapies before contacting the modern medical establishment.

    1. African Americans use community and family resources readily and are likely to access health care in a short period.

    2. Jewish Americans are likely to readily access modern health care.

    4. Hispanic Americans tend to access health care after consulting community and family relations.

19. Analysis, implementation, safe and effective care environment, (b).

    _____ 1. Exploring coping with the patient is the responsibility of the nurse.

    __X__ **2. Assisting with ambulation is an appropriate task.**

    _____ 3. Monitoring fatigue will be the responsibility of the nurse.

    _____ 4. Observing skin is the responsibility of the nurse; nursing assistants may report variations but should not be responsible for examining the skin after treatment.

    __X__ **5. Documenting intake is an appropriate task.**

20. Application, implementation, health promotion and maintenance, (b).

    4. The focus of care for most of the older adult population encompasses the management of the symptoms of chronic illness.

    1. Although prevention is important, older adults have many chronic illnesses that must be managed.

    2. Prevention is always important; however, older adults have many chronic illnesses that need symptom management.

    3. Health maintenance is not usually associated with acute illnesses.

21. Application, assessment, safe and effective care environment, (b).

    3. These assessment data most strongly indicate that elder abuse may be a problem. The confusion might be caused by excessive stress, and individuals who have had repeated abuse may have wounds in various stages of healing.

    1. These assessment data indicate changes in the patient's gastrointestinal system and can signify weight loss.

    2. Chronic cough and shortness of breath are symptoms associated with aging changes in the respiratory system.

    4. Fatigue can be caused by a variety of factors; pain on movement and palpation of the ankle are to be expected with a fracture.

22. Application, implementation, physiological integrity, (b).

    3. This is the most correct statement. Sildenafil is used to treat erectile dysfunction.

    1. This may not be true; sildenafil does not promote a more intimate experience.

    2. This is judgmental; the individual obviously wishes to resume sex with his wife.

    4. This is not a true statement.

23. Application, implementation, health promotion and maintenance, (b).

    3. Older adults do not take risks and will not fill in answers to multiple-choice tests if they think they will get them "wrong."

    1. The slight brain shrinkage that older adults experience does not result in loss of intelligence.

    2. The nurse cannot generalize that all older adults do not care about nutrition.

    4. This assumes that all older adults have a profound loss of vision.

24. Comprehension, implementation, physiological integrity, (a).

    3. The hearing aid should be turned on only when it is in the ear canal to decrease unpleasant noise from the aid.

    1. This results in squealing and pain as it is inserted.

    2. Air flow causes a high-pitched squeal, which is annoying and painful to the patient.

    4. The patient should be encouraged to turn the aid on when it is safely in the ear canal so the nursing assistant can help adjust the volume.

25. Comprehension, planning, safe and effective care environment, (b).

    2. A walker would provide a stable mobility aid while fostering as much independent movement as possible.

1. A cane is not as stable as a walker.
3. Crutches are a very dangerous mobility aid for a patient with vertigo.
4. Although a wheelchair is very stable, this patient needs to have as much independent movement as possible.

26. Application, implementation, safe and effective care environment, (b).
    1. **This is the guideline for employee actions.**
    2. This is not a factor; all nurses, regardless of age, must comply with facility policies and procedures.
    3. Gender of the patient is not an issue in providing safe care.
    4. Although this may affect the final outcome, the severity of the injury is purely incidental.

27. Application, implementation, health promotion and maintenance, (b).
    3. **The sexual self-gratification of the resident is a private matter and should be respected.**
    1. This denies the resident's needs.
    2. This infringes on the resident's rights.
    4. This is judgmental and disrespectful.

28. Comprehension, implementation, psychosocial integrity, (a).
    2. **Persons with Alzheimer disease relate to themselves at an earlier stage in their life.**
    1. The ability to read and understand is frequently impaired.
    3. Frequently the person with Alzheimer disease is unable to recognize himself or herself.
    4. This is too complicated for the resident to understand.

29. Comprehension, assessment, psychosocial integrity, (a).
    2. **The resident is not recognizing the napkin as a napkin.**
    1. This is a disturbance in speaking or understanding speech.
    3. This is dizziness.
    4. This is inability to sit still.

30. Knowledge, assessment, physiological integrity, (a).
    3. **Glaucoma results in narrowing of the visual field.**
    1. Cataracts result in decreased visual acuity.
    2. This is decreased ability to see at night.
    4. Macular degeneration results in central vision loss.

31. Comprehension, assessment, physiological integrity, (b).
    2. **The stress of infection is a major precipitating factor for hyperosmolar hyperglycemic nonketotic coma.**
    1. This is more likely to occur in the person with insulin-dependent diabetes.
    3. Other factors not included would be necessary for this to occur.
    4. Low blood sugar is unlikely with the stress of an infection.

32. Application, implementation, safe and effective care environment, (b).
    1. **This avoids a sudden need for the resident to ambulate to the bathroom or impatiently attempt to manage for himself or herself.**
    2. Side rails are very ineffective in preventing a fall.
    3. Order for a vest restraint is inappropriate.
    4. This might help prevent injury but not the fall itself.

33. Analysis, assessment, psychosocial integrity, (c).
    1. **The extended time frame and the inability to let go and move on with life are characteristic of dysfunctional grief.**

2. This may be a component but does not directly answer the question.
3. This occurs before the loss.
4. No indication exists of the patient feeling suspicious or persecuted.

34. Application, implementation, psychosocial integrity, (b).
    2. **Validation therapy identifies and focuses on the feelings and meaning of the behavior.**
    1. This does not usually work with dementia.
    3. This is the function of cognitive training.
    4. This describes reminiscence.

35. Application, planning, psychosocial integrity, (b).
    2. **This response provides opportunity to explore the patient's feelings.**
    1. This denies the patient's feelings.
    3. This offers false reassurance and denies feelings.
    4. This is a negative response and shuts down communication.

36. Analysis, assessment, physiological integrity, (c).
    1. **This describes the usual visual field loss with macular degeneration.**
    2. This occurs with glaucoma.
    3. This describes loss of one half of the usual field.
    4. This is the absence of the lens of the eye.

37. Application, implementation, physiological integrity, (c).
    2. **Ultraviolet light contributes to the crystallization, clouding, and decreased flexibility of the lens of the eye.**
    1. A specific vitamin deficiency is not related to cataract development.
    3. Alcohol abuse is not related to cataract development.
    4. Men and women are both affected by cataracts.

38. Analysis, planning, physiological integrity, (b).
    1. **Ginkgo biloba increases the anticoagulant effect of sodium warfarin.**
    2. Chamomile is usually consumed as a tea and has no effect on warfarin.
    3. Basil is an herb used for flavoring and has no effect on warfarin.
    4. Saw palmetto is an herbal remedy sometimes used for benign prostatic hypertrophy and has no effect on warfarin.

39. Analysis, evaluation, physiological integrity, (c).
    1. **She must remain upright for at least 30 minutes after taking alendronate.**
    2. Sitting or standing for 30 minutes is an appropriate action after taking alendronate.
    3. Taking the medication in the morning helps to keep the person upright for 30 minutes after taking alendronate.
    4. Skipping doses of a medication interferes with efficacy of the drug.

40. Application, implementation, physiological integrity, (b).
    3. **This is the proper method for administering calcitonin-salmon.**
    1. Bone density studies are nice but not a necessity.
    2. This is not necessary.
    4. This does not affect the absorption or use.

41. Analysis, assessment, health promotion and maintenance, (c).
    2. **These are risk factors for osteoporosis.**
    1. Square dancing is weight-bearing exercise, which is not a risk factor.
    3. None of these are risk factors.
    4. None of these are risk factors.

42. Analysis, implementation, safe and effective care environment, (b).
    Answer: 100 mL/hr
    Calculated by dividing the volume by the time for infusion.
43. Comprehension, assessment, physiological integrity, (b).
    4. Vitamin B$_1$ (thiamine deficiency) is typically seen in chronic alcoholism and is associated with these neurological disturbances.
    1. Vitamin C deficiency results in scurvy.
    2. Vitamin B$_{12}$ deficiency results in anemia.
    3. Vitamin K deficiency results in bleeding disorders.
44. Knowledge, evaluation, physiological integrity, (a).
    3. The repetitive grasping, rolling movements of the fingers is most often seen with Parkinson disease.
    1. Movements associated with Huntington disease are related to disturbances in large muscle groups and are generally "jerky."
    2. Tardive dyskinesia movements are usually associated with side effects of antipsychotic medications.
    4. Diabetic retinopathy is a vision disorder.
45. Analysis, assessment, health maintenance and promotion, (c).
    2. Smoking is a significant risk factor.
    1. Air pollution is not as important a risk factor.
    3. COPD may contribute but is not a causative factor.
    4. Chewing tobacco is a risk factor for oral cancer.
46. Application, assessment, physiological integrity, (b).
    2. This describes the typical herpes zoster outbreak.
    1. This describes a large number of conditions.
    3. This is not indicative of any particular process.
    4. This may describe an allergic response.
47. Analysis, evaluation, psychosocial integrity, (b).
    1. This response reduces the confrontation and stress and permits redirection.
    2. Excessive evening activity increases agitation and sleeping disturbances.
    3. Radio talk shows may contribute to disorientation.
    4. Incontinence is not always a problem; a toileting schedule may delay its onset.
48. Comprehension, implementation, physiological integrity, (c).
    2. Additional blood vessels develop to compensate for loss of flow because of the atherosclerotic process.
    1. Cardiac output may decrease.
    3. Coronary artery disease may result but is not an adaptation.
    4. This is a surgical treatment.
49. Comprehension, assessment, physiological integrity, (a).
    4. Left-sided brain damage results in disturbance of the right side of the body.
    1. Seizure disorders may result from CVAs.
    2. This is not a factor.
    3. This might result in left-sided neglect.
50. Application, implementation, psychosocial integrity, (b).
    3. Mixer activities that encourage interaction enhance sexuality.
    1. This is contraindicated unless mutually acceptable to both roommates.
    2. This may be offensive to some residents.
    4. Alcohol metabolism is slowed in older adults; routine serving of alcoholic beverages is contraindicated. Alcohol may be ordered on an individual basis.
51. Analysis, assessment, health promotion and maintenance, (b).
    4. All pertinent data regarding the resident need to be collected before proceeding.
    1. This is important but is not the first thing that should be completed.
    2. This may be indicated after the assessment.
    3. The assessment needs to be completed before this determination is made.
52. Application, implementation, psychosocial integrity, (b).
    2. Validation affirms and accepts the resident's feelings.
    1. Reality orientation focuses on the present.
    3. Reminiscence focuses on life review and its meaning.
    4. This is part of reminiscence therapy.
53. Application, evaluation, physiological integrity, (b).
    4. Cardiac output is directly related to renal blood perfusion.
    1. This may be a cause of decreased cardiac output.
    2. This may be a physiological impediment to reduced cardiac output.
    3. This is a cause of angina.
54. Analysis, evaluation, psychosocial integrity, (c).
    1. This is the most appropriate goal for this therapy with this specific behavior.
    2. No indication exists that this resident is not oriented to self.
    3. This is an ongoing goal for all residents.
    4. This is not specific for the targeted behavior described.
55. Application, planning, physiological integrity, (c).
    3. Dry mouth is a frequent side effect of many medications; this may be the cause of the resident's discomfort.
    1. No indication exists that the resident has diabetes. Elevated blood sugar may cause increased thirst; it is not usually described as dry mouth.
    2. This may be an appropriate intervention, but it is not the first intervention.
    4. Dry lips do not necessarily accompany dry mouth; further assessment is necessary to determine if this intervention is appropriate.
56. Analysis, implementation, psychosocial integrity, (b).
    1. This music was popular dance music of their young adult years and will encourage the social feelings associated with life at that time.
    2. Classical music is a personal choice and may not encourage socialization.
    3. Gospel music is a personal choice and may not be suitable for a party.
    4. Folk ballads are a later phenomenon of the 1960s and not necessarily appropriate for this age group.
57. Comprehension, planning, psychosocial integrity, (b).
    4. The older adult has a known work history.
    1. No evidence exists of this effect on morale.
    2. Being older does not necessarily mean that the employee will be good at orientation.
    3. Memory may not be better or worse.
58. Comprehension, implementation, health promotion and maintenance, (b).
    4. Research has shown this to be true, and older adults are less likely to offer complaints of pain.
    1. Older adults usually have a higher pain threshold.
    2. Older adults usually exhibit fewer manifestations of pain than younger patients.
    3. Age does not affect addictions.

59. Application, implementation, psychosocial integrity, (b).
    2. Of the choices available, 8:00 AM Thursday is the least likely to cause interference with the Jewish Sabbath, which lasts from sundown Friday through sundown Saturday.
    1. This would be the second choice.
    3. This time would interfere with the Sabbath.
    4. Surgery should not be scheduled during the Sabbath observance.

60. Application, assessment, health promotion and maintenance, (b).
    2. All four characteristics are risk factors for osteoporosis.
    1. This is a thyroid condition more common in women.
    3. Herpes zoster is most common in older adults.
    4. Glaucoma is not related to the other factors listed.

61. Application, planning, physiological integrity, (b).
    1. Morning pain and stiffness are common with arthritis. Gently moving the involved joints helps to prevent further restriction and relieve pain.
    2. Although cold reduces inflammation, it may aggravate the restriction of movement associated with arthritis.
    3. This may be effective, but Epsom salts might be irritating for some skin types.
    4. Cortisone cream should not be used over large areas and is not effective for arthritis pain relief.

62. Analysis, assessment, psychosocial integrity, (c).
    2. This statement reflects the contributions and accomplishments of the person's life and the realization that she wants to give more to her community and share her life experiences.
    1. This is the fourth stage of development as described by Erickson and is typically faced by school-aged children as they experience new social and academic demands.
    3. This is the eighth stage described by Erikson and has more to do with a reflection of one's own life and is typically faced by those over age 65.
    4. Identity versus role confusion is the fifth stage described by Erickson and is typically faced in adolescence.

63. Comprehension, implementation, psychosocial integrity, (b).
    3. The spelling bee uses information and social interaction patterns learned during grade school years.
    1. Reality therapy focuses on the present.
    2. Reminiscence is a life-review process, not necessarily using remote memory.
    4. Scrabble is mentally challenging but does not use remote memory to the extent of a spelling bee.

64. Comprehension, assessment, psychosocial integrity, (b).
    3. The wife is preparing for the loss of her spouse and has started the grieving and remembering process.
    1. No indication of depression exists.
    2. The wife is working on accepting, not denial.
    4. No indication exists that she has withdrawn from social contacts.

65. Application, implementation, physiological integrity, (c).
    4. These interventions can be helpful in promoting restful sleep by eliminating distractions.
    1. Exercising close to bedtime can raise metabolic rate, which makes sleeping peacefully more difficult.

2. Alcohol may make falling asleep easier but frequently interferes with sleep patterns.
3. Herbal sleep masks may be distracting and uncomfortable.

66. Analysis, assessment, physiological integrity, (b).
    4. An exacerbation of COPD by its very definition is an ineffective breathing pattern.
    1. Deficient knowledge may affect discharge planning, but the ineffective breathing is a more immediate concern.
    2. The person may be anxious, but decreased oxygenation is the more critical issue.
    3. There may be a risk for infection, but oxygenation is the most critical need on admission.

67. Application, assessment, physiological integrity, (c).
    2. This gathers the information needed to make suggestions.
    1. This may be an appropriate response after additional information has been gathered.
    3. Dietary habits must be assessed first.
    4. Although this may be an issue, the priority should be data collection for specific details.

68. Application, implementation, physiological integrity, (b).
    2. The alcohol in this complementary arthritis therapy would cause a disulfiram-type reaction with the metronidazole.
    1. St John's wort is noted for its photosensitization.
    3. No indication exists of drug interaction with chamomile.
    4. Acupuncture would not be contraindicated with metronidazole.

69. Comprehension, planning, physiological integrity, (c).
    4. This is the next step after a significant reaction to a tuberculosis skin test.
    1. This is contraindicated after a significant positive reaction.
    2. This is not indicated at this time.
    3. After the results of the patient's x-ray examination are known, a CT scan may be ordered.

70. Comprehension, planning, psychosocial integrity, (a).
    Correct order: 13586
    1. Denial
    3. Anger
    5. Bargaining
    8. Depression
    6. Acceptance
    These are the correct stages in order as described by Dr. Kübler-Ross
    2, 4, 7 are not stages of grieving as described by Dr. Kübler-Ross

71. Analysis, implementation, safe and effective care environment, (b).
    Answer: 83.3 mL/hr
    Calculate infusion rate by dividing the volume by the hours of infusion.

72. Comprehension, assessment, health promotion and maintenance, (b).
    __X__ **1. Past blood transfusions are a factor in the increase in AIDS/HIV infection in the older adult.**
    __X__ **2. Lack of concern regarding birth control is a factor in the increase in AIDS/HIV infection in the older adult.**

_**X**_ 3. *Increase in the number of sexual partners is a factor in the increase in AIDS/HIV infection in the older adult.*

_**X**_ 4. *Aging immune system is a factor in the increase in AIDS/HIV infection in the older adult.*

_**X**_ 5. *Deficient knowledge of safe sex is a factor in the increase in AIDS/HIV infection in the older adult.*

_____ 6. Sterility of needles is a factor in HIV/AIDS infections; injection technique is not a factor.

73. Application, implementation, safe and effective care environment, (b).
    4. This permits explanation and clarification of the change.
    1. E-mail is unreliable.
    2. This may breach confidentiality.
    3. This is not within the responsibility of a nursing assistant.

74. Application, implementation, psychosocial integrity, (c).
    4. This is a nonthreatening, neutral method of assessing symptoms for reluctant patients.
    1. The nurse is not certain of this patient's verbal ability.
    2. Many patients are reluctant and embarrassed to draw pictures.
    3. For the patient to point at or touch the nurse may be inappropriate.

75. Application, implementation, physiological integrity, (b).
    Correct order: 1243.
    1. This is the most critical.
    2. Insulin needs to be given before breakfast and is a priority.
    4. Routine medication administration comes after giving the priority medications.
    3. Routine vital signs can be delegated to a nursing assistant.

76. Application, implementation, physiological integrity, (b).
    Answer: 77 mL/hr
    2400 cal ÷ 24 hr = 100 cal/hr
    100 cal/hr ÷ 1.3 cal/mL = 77 mL/hr

77. Application, implementation, safe and effective care environment, (b).
    1. Older African-American women are highly regarded and frequently consulted in the primarily matriarchal group.
    2. The Italian-American culture is more patriarchal.
    3. Native-American cultures vary according to tribal origin.
    4. The Chinese-American culture is more patriarchal than matriarchal.

78. Application, implementation, physiological integrity, (b).
    1. Ceftriaxone sodium is a third-generation cephalosporin; a degree of cross-sensitivity to penicillin exists.
    2, 3, 4. None of these allergies interferes with this medication being administered as ordered.

79. Application, implementation, safe and effective care environment, (b).
    4. If unsure about a significant object, it is best not to disturb it unless directed by the resident; this respects the resident's rights.

1. The family may not be of the same belief system, unless a specific designee has been appointed; this can confuse the issue.
2. This may be disrespectful.
3. The resident's belongings should not be locked in medication carts. Each facility has a policy for checking valuables that the resident does not want to keep in his or her possession.

80. Application, implementation, health promotion and maintenance, (a).
    1. Cigarette smoking is a recognized risk for osteoporosis.
    2. Low caffeine intake is a positive change of lifestyle, not a risk.
    3. An increase in calcium may be beneficial.
    4. Weight-bearing exercise is important.

81. Application, implementation, health promotion and maintenance, (a).
    4. Silence can be an effective listening technique; encouraging the family to talk is therapeutic.
    1. This is sympathy and can be demeaning.
    2. Using a cliché is a block to therapeutic communication.
    3. Nonverbal communication can be very powerful.

82. Application, implementation, physiological integrity, (b).
    1. Allowing sufficient time for bowel evacuation encourages good bowel hygiene.
    2. Regular exercise is important for normal bowel function.
    3. A diet high in fiber and moderate in carbohydrates assists bowel function.
    4. Laxatives disrupt bowel hygiene and should be avoided.

83. Application, implementation, health promotion and maintenance, (b).
    1. Encouraging family members to express their feelings is therapeutic.
    2. A false assumption is a block to communication.
    3. False reassurance is a block to communication.
    4. Using a cliché is a block to communication.

84. Analysis, planning, physiological integrity, (c).
    1. Every patient should know the action, side effects, and correct administration for each of his or her medications.
    2. This is true, but answer No. 1 is more complete.
    3. Keep the physician informed of side effects.
    4. The blood level of medications can be maintained with a specific administration schedule.

85. Application, implementation, physiological integrity, (b).
    3. A change in mental status may indicate a drug toxicity.
    1. Incontinence may be connected with confusion and drug toxicity.
    2. Belligerence may be related to delirium or toxicity.
    4. Delirium, not dementia, is related to drug toxicity.

86. Analysis, assessment, physiological integrity, (c).
    4. Difficulty swallowing can have many causes, including a stroke or neurological impairment, local trauma, or obstruction.
    1. Loss of skin elasticity and thinning epidermis are normal effects of aging.
    2. A gradual weight loss is a normal response to loss of body mass.
    3. Resistance to infections is not applicable to this question.

87. Comprehension, implementation, physiological integrity, (b).
    1. *Liver and kidney functions along with circulation decrease with age.*
    2. Toxicity may result with increased doses.
    3. This may be true in some individuals, but option No. 1 is a more complete answer.
    4. Over-the-counter medications may interact with many prescription medications.

88. Application, planning, physiological integrity, (b).
    1. *A strict routine of voiding helps to avoid incontinence during bladder retraining.*
    2. Fluid intake should be at least 2000 mL/day for adequate kidney perfusion.
    3. Eliminating diuretic medications is not a nursing function.
    4. The patient's needs take precedence over the needs of the facility.

89. Knowledge, implementation, safe and effective care environment, (a).
    2. *Residents' rights and their ability to make choices are of paramount importance in long-term care facilities.*
    1. Individual needs specify the frequency of assessment.
    3. The Omnibus Budget Reconciliation Act (OBRA) specifies the "least restrictive environment."
    4. Frequency of assessments is determined as appropriate for individual needs.

90. Application, planning, physiological integrity, (b).
    2. *Using the gentlest laxative first helps to preserve normal bowel function.*
    1. The goal is to promote good bowel hygiene with gentle stimulation; this would not meet that goal.
    3. This may be too harsh.
    4. Quickest is not necessarily safest.

91. Analysis, planning, physiological integrity, (c).
    1. *Maintaining mobility means that joints are functional.*
    2. Maintaining mobility may help decrease edema.
    3. Pain may need to be treated so exercise is possible.
    4. Treating depression increases the quality of life.

92. Application, implementation, physiological integrity, (b).
    1. *Adequate fluids increase kidney perfusion and help clear the urine solutes.*
    2. A low-calcium diet affects calculi only if the composition of the calculi is calcium.
    3. Exercise affects general health and circulation.
    4. Diuretics may have some effect on urinary output but not directly on calculi.

93. Application, assessment, health promotion and maintenance, (b).
    1. *Most adults over 40 years of age have some degree of osteoarthritis.*
    2. Rheumatoid arthritis has the highest incidence in women of childbearing age.
    3. Ankylosing spondylitis usually affects young men.
    4. *Gouty arthritis* refers specifically to the presence of uric acid crystals and a problem with purine metabolism.

94. Application, implementation, physiological integrity, (b).
    1. *Administering aspirin with food or milk helps to decrease gastric irritation.*
    2. The medication should be administered as ordered.
    3. Chemical composition of the drug may change when it is dissolved in juice.
    4. Aspirin is an oral medication.

95. Application, implementation, safe and effective care environment, (b).
    4. *Discussion should be private and confidential and away from the patients.*
    1. Without follow-through by the nurse, the confrontation may escalate.
    2. Reprimands do not immediately address the issue.
    3. Although discussion with the nursing supervisor may occur, it does not assist with the confrontation.

96. Comprehension, assessment, physiological integrity, (a).
    1. *Brisk blood return after blanching is an important indication of cardiovascular status in extremities.*
    2. This is a sign of circulatory impairment.
    3. This is a sign of sluggish digital circulation.
    4. This is an abnormal sign.

97. Analysis, evaluation, psychosocial integrity, (b).
    3. *Recognition that information is important for managing the illness is a positive coping mechanism.*
    1, 2. Rheumatoid arthritis is not curable.
    4. This is a common myth for treatment.

98. Application, implementation, physiological integrity, (b).
    Answer: 370 Kcal
    Carbohydrates supply 4 Kcal/g consumed. Fats supply 9 Kcal/g consumed. Proteins supply 4 Kcal/g consumed. Then calculate:
    (50g ÷ 4Kcal/g)+(10g ÷ 9Kcal/g)+(20g×4Kcal/g) =370 Kcal

99. Analysis, implementation, physiological integrity, (a).
    3. *Correctly interpreting the sliding scale, the nurse will administer 5 units.*
    1, 2, 4. These insulin amounts interpret the sliding scale incorrectly.

100. Analysis, planning, safe and effective care environment, (c).
    Correct order: 2341.
    2. *Patient with diabetes should be assessed first because of risk of hypoglycemia 1 hour after regular insulin administration.*
    3. *Patient with congestive heart failure should be assessed second to ascertain change of edema status and intake/output.*
    4. *Patient with suspected coronary artery disease should be assessed third because of timing of surgery at 7 AM (0700).*
    1. *Patient with chronic obstructive pulmonary disease should be assessed fourth because of timing of surgery at 8 AM (0800).*

Emergency Preparedness

Objectives

After studying this chapter, the student should be able to:

1. Identify emergent interventions for a patient with respiratory compromise.
2. Recognize the common signs of poor circulatory perfusion.
3. Describe the basic steps of cardiac resuscitation.
4. List three abnormal findings observed with an inadequate cerebral blood flow.
5. List data to be included in the nursing assessment of a patient with an emergent digestive disorder.

This chapter emphasizes the nursing assessments and interventions that are essential to preserving the lives of victims of acute illness or injury. Rapid clinical assessment emphasizing circulation, airway, and breathing; establishment of care priorities; and implementation of lifesaving measures should be instituted until emergency medical care is available. The most serious and life-threatening injuries should be treated first, and all first-aid measures should be carried out before transporting the victim or victims.

Concurrent with emergency management of physical needs is the practitioner's recognition and understanding of the victim's emotional state. The feelings of the victim's significant others should also be acknowledged and responded to as realistically, gently, and expeditiously as possible.

Nurses should be familiar with the extent of protection and legal limitations of practice under the Nurse Practice Act and Good Samaritan Act, which vary from state to state.

The high incidence of acquired immunodeficiency syndrome (AIDS), hepatitis B virus (HBV), and hepatitis C virus (HCV) necessitates that nurses consider all patients to be potentially infected; have access to equipment that minimizes the need for mouth-to-mouth, mouth-to-nose, and mouth-to-stoma resuscitation; and use Standard Precautions for Infection Control.

BASIC LIFE SUPPORT

ARTIFICIAL RESPIRATION

A. Simultaneously shake victim and shout to check for response; look for signs of breathing.
B. After determining unresponsiveness, look for signs of breathing (do not listen for breaths or feel for breaths).
C. If no response (breathing is absent or inadequate [gasping]) call for help (even if you do not see anyone in the immediate vicinity). Activate the emergency medical system (EMS) (call 911) and get automated external defibrillator (AED) if available.
   1. Do so immediately if the victim is an adult, if the victim is a child (1 year to puberty), or if the victim is an infant (birth to 1 year) who experiences sudden *witnessed* collapse.

2. If you are alone and the victim is a child or infant whose arrest was *not* witnessed, provide 2 minutes (five cycles) of cardiopulmonary resuscitation (CPR) before activating EMS.
D. Quickly place victim in supine position.
E. Check for pulse; if present, begin rescue breathing.
   1. If the victim is an adult, child, or infant and no pulse is detected, provide 2 minutes of CPR (five cycles).
   2. If the victim is a child or infant and the pulse rate is less than 60 beats/min with signs of poor perfusion, begin CPR.
F. Establish airway using the head tilt–chin lift maneuver (Figure 10-1) or jaw thrust maneuver. For patients with possible neck or spine injuries, use only the jaw-thrust maneuver; if unsuccessful, switch to head tilt–chin lift maneuver.
   1. Infant: Maintain neck in neutral position.
   2. Child: Maintain neck slightly further back than neutral position.
   3. For patients with a stoma, use mouth-to-stoma breathing.
G. Begin rescue breathing by delivering one breath (delivered over 1 second) at the lowest possible pressure using the bag-mask technique. If a mask or bag is not available, begin mouth-to-mouth, mouth-to-nose, or mouth-to-stoma resuscitation.
   1. Victim's chest should rise with each ventilation provided.
   2. In the adult victim, deliver one breath every 5 to 6 seconds (10 to 12 per minute).
   3. In the child or infant victim, deliver one breath every 3 to 5 seconds (12 to 20 per minute).
H. Pause between breaths to allow for victim's exhalation.
I. Check the carotid pulse (brachial pulse for infant) every 2 minutes for 5 to 10 seconds.
J. If pulse is present, continue until breathing is restored (rescue breathing).
K. If victim is child or infant and pulse is less than 60 beats/min with signs of poor perfusion, begin CPR.
L. If pulse is absent, begin CPR.
M. If breathing resumes, stay with victim until EMS arrives (American Heart Association Guidelines, 2011).

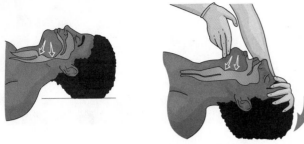

FIGURE 10-1 Head tilt–chin lift maneuver. One hand is on the person's forehead. Pressure is applied to tilt the head back. The chin is lifted with the fingers of the other hand. (From Sorrentino SA, Remmert LN: *Mosby's textbook for nursing assistants,* ed 8, St Louis, 2012, Mosby.)

CARDIOPULMONARY RESUSCITATION

A. Follow previously mentioned steps A to D. Be sure victim is supine and on a firm surface for the compression activities.

B. In the absence of a pulse, place the heel of one hand in the center of the victim's chest, toward the lower half of the breastbone, with the other hand on top (Figure 10-2).

1. Child (age 1 year to puberty): Rescuer may use one hand with heel placed in the center of the chest toward the lower half of the breastbone and deliver at rate of at least 100 compressions per minute.

2. Infant (younger than 1 year) for one rescuer: Place two fingers in the center of the chest, just below the infant's nipple line (do not compress bottom of breastbone) and

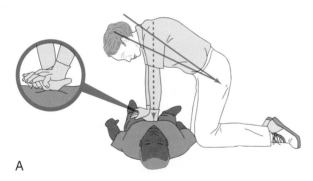

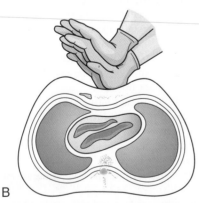

FIGURE 10-2 Body and hand position for cardiopulmonary resuscitation. **A,** The rescuer should be kneeling, with knees slightly separated and elbows in straight, locked position over the hands. **B,** The rescuer's fingers are extended or interlaced and kept off the chest. (From Sorrentino SA, Remmert LN: *Mosby's textbook for nursing assistants,* ed 8, St Louis, 2012, Mosby.)

deliver compressions at the rate of at least 100 compressions per minute.

3. Infant when two rescuers are available: Use the two thumb–encircling hand chest compression technique.

C. Compress the adult sternum at least 2 inches for 30 compressions at the rate of at least 100 compressions per minute; then deliver two breaths.

D. Complete approximately 2 minutes (five cycles of compressions and breaths); recheck carotid pulse and switch positions with second rescuer (if available).

E. Compress the sternum of the child approximately 2 inches or one third the chest depth.

1. Single-rescuer child CPR: Compress the sternum for 30 compressions, then deliver two breaths.

2. Two-rescuer child CPR: Compress the sternum for 15 compressions, and deliver two breaths.

F. Compress infant sternum approximately 1½ inches or one third the depth of the chest.

1. Single-rescuer, infant CPR: compress sternum for 30 compressions and deliver two breaths.

2. Two-rescuer, infant CPR: compress the sternum for 15 compressions and deliver two breaths.

G. For adult, child, and infant, push hard and fast (100 compressions per minute). Minimize interruptions in compressions (American Heart Association, 2011 guidelines).

HEIMLICH MANEUVER

The Heimlich maneuver is used for management of foreign body airway obstruction (FBAO). Do not interfere if the victim can cough, speak, or breathe.

A. Conscious adult or child victim

1. Stand or kneel behind the victim, encircle his or her waist with your arms, place the thumb side of your fist slightly above the umbilicus and well below the sternum. Place your other hand around your fist and apply pressure in a quick inward and upward motion (Figure 10-3).

2. Repeat the thrusts until the obstruction is expelled or the victim loses consciousness.

B. Unconscious adult or child victim with FBAO or conscious victim who becomes unconscious

1. Place victim in supine position, call for help, and activate EMS.

2. Begin CPR; begin with compressions (do not check for pulse).

3. When preparing to deliver breaths using head tilt–chin lift, open victim's mouth and inspect for obstruction. If obstruction can be easily removed, do so with your fingers. If you cannot see cause of obstruction, continue CPR.

4. Perform five cycles or 2 minutes of CPR.

5. Call EMS (911) if not already done.

6. Continue repeating chest compressions, airway check, and breathing attempts in rapid sequence (American Heart Association, 2011 guidelines).

C. Unconscious adult victim

1. Simultaneously shake victim and shout to establish unconsciousness.

2. Activate EMS.

3. Quickly place victim in supine position.

4. Begin CPR sequence (compressions followed by ventilations).

5. After first set of compressions, if unable to ventilate, reposition head and again attempt to deliver two breaths.

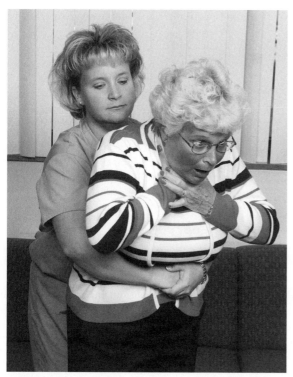

FIGURE 10-3 Heimlich maneuver. Abdominal thrusts with the person standing. (From Sorrentino SA: *Mosby's textbook for nursing assistants,* ed 6, St Louis, 2004, Mosby.)

6. If still unable to deliver breaths, continue with compressions.
7. Repeat steps C1 to C6 for conscious adult victim who loses consciousness until effective.

D. Child
1. Same as adult, except:
   a. Provide 2 minutes of rescue support and then activate EMS.
   b. Do not perform blind finger sweeps as they may cause object to become further lodged.

E. Obese victim and later stages of pregnancy
1. Conscious victim: deliver chest thrusts (place thumb side of fist on middle of breastbone) until foreign body is expelled or victim becomes unconscious.
2. Unconscious victim
   a. Deliver chest compressions with victim in supine position by placing heel of hand on lower half of sternum with other hand on top (CPR position).
   b. Follow CPR maneuver with head tilt–chin lift. Look in mouth and remove foreign object if seen. Give rescue breaths.

F. Conscious infant
1. Place infant in your lap while in a sitting or kneeling position.
2. Supporting head and neck, position infant face down with head lower than trunk along rescuer's forearm. Forearm should be resting on your thigh for support.
3. With heel of hand, administer five back blows between the shoulder blades.
4. Continue to support head, turn infant over onto other forearm, keeping head lower than trunk. Infant will now be face up.
5. Using two fingers, administer five chest thrusts.

6. Compression location is directly below the point where the sternum is bisected by an imaginary line between the nipples.
7. Continue to administer back blows and chest thrusts until airway is cleared or infant becomes unconscious.

G. Conscious infant who loses consciousness
1. Place in supine position and call for help; if someone responds, instruct that individual to activate EMS.
2. Begin steps of CPR (compressions and ventilations).
   a. If alone, compression rate is 30:2.
   b. If a second rescuer is present, compression rate is 15:2.
3. After each set of compressions, perform head tilt–chin lift in neutral position. Inspect airway. Remove object only if you see it (do not perform blind finger sweeps).
   a. Airway inspection should occur after each set of compressions. If object can be seen and easily removed, remove it.
4. Establish airway using the head tilt–chin lift maneuver.
5. Attempt to deliver two breaths; if unable to ventilate, reposition head and repeat.
6. If second attempt to ventilate fails, continue with CPR.
7. After five cycles of CPR or approximately 2 minutes, activate EMS if not already done.
8. Continue CPR until EMS arrives.

H. Unconscious infant
1. Simultaneously shake and tap victim to establish unconsciousness.
2. Repeat steps G1 to G8 for unconscious infant victim (American Heart Association, 2011 guidelines).

HEMORRHAGE

A. Description: loss of a large amount of blood in a short period; may be external or internal
B. Types
1. Venous: dark red color; steady flow
2. Arterial: bright red color; spurting flow
3. Capillary: red; oozing flow
C. Assessment for shock
1. Restlessness
2. Anxiety
3. Rapid, weak pulse
4. Cool, clammy, pale skin
5. Shortness of breath
6. Thirst
7. Nausea and vomiting
8. Alteration in level of consciousness (LOC)
9. Hypotension
10. If bleeding is internal (within a cavity or joint), pain develops because the cavity is stretched by increasing blood volume.
    a. May also develop hematemesis
D. Interventions: external
1. Remove any clothing covering the injury for direct visualization of hemorrhage.
2. If possible, place victim in supine position.
3. Apply firm, direct pressure to the injury (use gloves if available).
   a. Apply pressure with heel of hand using a clean, thick bandage or cloth.
   b. Pressure should be maintained for at least 10 minutes

c. Place cold compress over the bandage (not under) to further support vasoconstriction.
4. Elevate injured part above heart level.
5. If bleeding continues, apply more dressings to the first and apply more pressure.
6. If arterial bleeding does not respond to direct pressure, attempt to control by applying direct pressure on supply artery (Figure 10-4).
7. Tourniquets are not recommended unless bleeding is life-threatening and should be applied only by an experienced individual.
  a. Leave tourniquet exposed (visible).
  b. Apply approximately 2 inches above wound if possible.
  c. Tourniquet should be tightened until bleeding is stopped.
  d. Time tourniquet was applied should be noted.
  e. Tourniquet should be removed only by someone with advanced training.

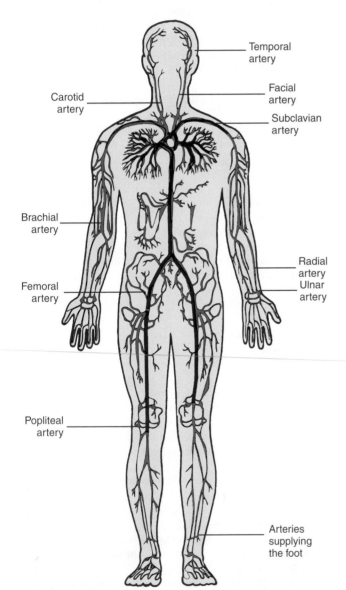

FIGURE 10-4 Pressure points for bleeding control. (From Fultz J, Sturt PA: *Mosby's emergency nursing reference,* ed 3, St Louis, 2005, Mosby.)

8. Cover victim to maintain body temperature; maintain supine position.
9. Treat for shock and transport immediately.
E. Interventions: internal
  1. Cover victim to maintain body temperature.
  2. Keep victim in supine position.
  3. Monitor vital signs.
  4. Treat for shock and transport immediately.
F. Usual medical care
  1. Monitor vital signs.
  2. Replace fluids intravenously to expand blood volume.
  3. Give blood transfusions.
  4. Locate source of hemorrhage and stop it.

EPISTAXIS (NOSEBLEED)

A. Description: bleeding from the nose caused by trauma, local irritation, violent sneezing, or chronic conditions such as hypertension
B. Assessment: obvious bleeding from one or both nares (most often unilateral)
C. Interventions
  1. Sit victim upright, head slightly forward, to prevent aspiration of blood.
  2. Apply firm, continuous pressure by using thumb and forefinger to pinch nose for 15 minutes.
  3. Apply ice compress to nose.
  4. Limit activity.
  5. Monitor vital signs.
D. Usual medical care
  1. Apply nasal pack soaked in a topical vasoconstrictor.
  2. Cauterize (silver nitrate or electrocautery).

ANAPHYLACTIC REACTION

A. Description: type of vasogenic or distributive shock (see section on shock)
B. Assessment
  1. Pallor
  2. Diaphoresis
  3. Tachycardia or bradycardia
  4. Hypotension
  5. Wheezing, dyspnea
  6. Anxiety, restlessness
  7. Urticaria
  8. Edema
  9. Pruritus
  10. Rash
  11. Possible respiratory distress
  12. Diffuse erythema
C. Interventions
  1. Ensure adequate airway and ventilation.
  2. Elevate feet slightly (about 12 inches) unless contraindicated (e.g., head, neck, back, or leg injury)
D. Usual medical care
  1. Oxygen
  2. Epinephrine
  3. Antihistamines
  4. Steroids
  5. Intravenous (IV) fluids
  6. Drug therapy for cardiovascular support
  7. Bronchodilators

E. Preventive measures
1. Allergy history
2. Medical identification tag for high-risk individuals
3. Insect (sting) emergency medical kits
4. Skin testing when possible
5. Ask about previous allergic reactions before administering medications.

SHOCK

A. Description: condition in which organs of the body are not meeting metabolic demands because of insufficient blood supply.
B. Three basic types (Box 10-1)
1. Hypovolemic: primarily a fluid problem caused by a loss of blood or fluid volume (e.g., hemorrhage, severe burns, trauma, dehydration)
2. Cardiogenic: reduced cardiac output that is the result of faulty pumping action (e.g., myocardial infarction, cardiomyopathy, diseases of the heart valves)
3. Vasogenic or distributive: a vascular problem or disturbance in tissue perfusion caused by alteration in circulating blood volumes (vascular dilation); may be one of three types
   a. Septic: massive bacterial infection resulting in release of endotoxin that causes vasodilation (e.g., gramnegative organisms)
   b. Neurogenic or spinal: disruption of arterioles and venules, resulting in a decrease of circulating blood volume (e.g., spinal cord injury)

Box 10-1   Causes of Shock

HYPOVOLEMIC
- Ascites
- Burns
- Excessive diuretic use
- External major bleeding
- Fluid loss from diabetes
- Fractures
- Gastrointestinal bleeding
- Hemoperitoneum
- Hemothorax
- Major diaphoresis
- Major diarrhea
- Major vomiting
- Renal failure

CARDIOGENIC
- Arrhythmia
- Cardiac contusion
- Cardiomyopathy
- Diseases of heart valve
- Myocardial infarction

VASOGENIC OR DISTRIBUTIVE
- Anoxia
- Anaphylaxis
- Overdose
- Sepsis
- Spinal cord injury

Modified from Emergency Nurses Association: *Sheehy's emergency nursing: principles and practice,* ed 5, St Louis, 2005, Mosby.

---

c. Anaphylaxis: severe sensitivity reaction resulting in histamine release and increased capillary permeability with eventual dilation of arterioles and venules
C. Assessment: Determination of the exact cause is vital to patient survival.
1. Shallow, rapid respirations
2. Cool, pale, clammy skin
3. Weak, thready pulse
4. Tachycardia
5. Decreased blood pressure
6. Possible confusion or disorientation
7. Restlessness
8. Thirst
9. Decreased urine output
10. Urinary or stool incontinence
D. Interventions: Order of priority may differ based on situation; therefore isolation of cause determines specific intervention strategies, which include the following:
1. Ensure adequate airway and ventilation.
2. Control bleeding if present.
3. Place in supine position with legs elevated unless contraindicated (e.g., head, neck, back, or leg injuries).
4. Monitor vital signs.
5. Cover victim to conserve body heat.
6. Insert urinary catheter.
7. Remain with victim if possible.
E. Usual medical care
1. Oxygen
2. IV fluids
3. Medications specific to the type of shock

HEAD INJURIES

Head injuries are traumatic damage to the head from blunt or penetrating trauma, resulting in scalp, skull, and brain injuries.

SCALP INJURY (TYPE AND INTERVENTION)

A. Abrasion: Wash with soap and water.
B. Hematoma: Apply ice.
C. Laceration
1. Stop bleeding by compression (only if no depression is present).
2. Shave around laceration.
3. Cleanse wound.
4. Suture.

SKULL FRACTURE

A. Simple: linear crack in surface of skull with no displacement of bone
1. Observation for alteration of respiration, vision, LOC, pupils (dilated, fixed, pinpoint), motor strength, and speech
2. X-ray examination
B. Depressed: skull fracture with depressed bone fragments, resulting in a concave appearance
1. Interventions
   a. Ensure adequate airway and ventilation.
   b. Administer oxygen.
   c. Control bleeding.
   d. Treat for shock.

e. Observe for alteration of respiration, vision, LOC, pupils (dilated, fixed, pinpoint), motor strength, and speech.

f. Maintain body temperature.

g. Protect cervical spine.

h. Monitor vital signs.

2. Usual medical care

a. X-ray examination

b. Antibiotic therapy

c. Surgical intervention

C. Basilar: fracture located along base of skull

1. Assessment

a. Periorbital ecchymoses (black eyes)

b. Cerebrospinal fluid (CSF) leak from nose or ear

c. Ecchymosis behind ears (Battle sign)

d. Blood behind eardrum (hemotympanum)

2. Interventions

a. Observe for alterations of respiration, vision, LOC, pupils (dilated, fixed, pinpoint), motor strength, and speech. Monitor vital signs.

b. If CSF leak is noted, do not attempt to stop; apply a loose, bulky dressing over area. Protect cervical spine.

3. Usual medical care

a. X-ray examination (although usually not visible)

b. Antibiotic therapy if CSF leak occurs

BRAIN INJURY

A. Concussion: temporary alteration of neurological functioning caused by a blow to the head, which results in jarring of the brain

1. Assessment

a. Nausea and vomiting

b. Headache

c. Possible brief period of unconsciousness and memory loss

d. Possible skull fracture

e. Confusion

2. Interventions

a. Observe for alteration of respiration, vision, LOC, pupils (dilated, fixed, pinpoint), and motor strength.

b. Administer nonnarcotic analgesics as ordered.

c. Maintain hydration.

d. Protect cervical spine.

B. Contusion: brain surface bruise resulting in structural alteration

1. Assessment

a. Nausea and vomiting

b. Visual alterations (diplopia)

c. Neurological alterations (ataxia, confusion)

2. Interventions

a. Maintain adequate airway and ventilation.

b. Close observation.

c. Protect cervical spine.

d. Monitor vital signs.

3. Usual medical care

a. Hospitalization

b. Antiemetics

C. Intracranial bleeding: hemorrhage or bleeding within the cranial vault

1. Assessment

a. Epidural (extradural) hematoma: bleeding between skull and dura mater; short period of unconsciousness followed by consciousness; severe headache, hemiparesis if conscious, bradycardia, increased blood pressure

b. Subdural hematoma: bleeding between dura mater and arachnoid membrane; can be acute or chronic; change of LOC from baseline; loss of consciousness, fixed dilated pupils, hemiparesis, positive Babinski sign

c. Subarachnoid hematoma: bleeding between arachnoid membrane and pia mater; severe headache, nausea and vomiting, delirium, syncope, or coma

2. Interventions

a. Maintain adequate airway and ventilation.

b. Administer oxygen.

c. Monitor vital signs.

d. Protect cervical spine.

e. Observe for alterations of respiration, vision, LOC, pupils (dilated, fixed, pinpoint), and decreased motor strength (signs of increased intracranial pressure [IICP]).

f. Maintain body temperature.

g. Treat for shock.

3. Usual medical care

a. Hospitalization

b. Computed tomography (CT) scan

c. Possible surgery

Cerebrovascular Accident

A. Definition: abnormal condition of the blood vessels of the brain characterized by hemorrhage into the brain or formation of an embolus or thrombus that occludes a cerebral artery

B. Clinical manifestations

1. May have effect on many body functions

a. Motor activity

b. Elimination

c. Intelligence

d. Spatial-perceptual alterations

C. Medical management

1. Thrombolytics (for ischemic stroke)

2. Drugs to reduce intracranial pressure (dexamethasone [Decadron])

3. CT or magnetic resonance imaging (MRI)

4. Blood tests for coagulation disorders

D. Interventions

1. Vital signs

2. Elevate head of bed at least 30 degrees.

3. Neurological assessment

4. IV therapy

5. Assessment of swallowing (nothing by mouth [NPO])

6. Oxygen

Seizure Disorders

A. Definition: transitory disturbance in consciousness or in motor, sensory, or autonomic function with or without loss of consciousness

B. Classification of seizures with signs or symptoms

1. Generalized tonic-clonic (grand mal)

a. Loss of consciousness

b. Falling to floor or ground

c. Stiffening (tonic phase for 10 to 20 seconds)

d. Jerking of extremities (clonic phase for 30 to 40 seconds)

e. May have aura

f. Incontinence, cyanosis, salivation, biting tongue or cheek

2. Absence (petit mal)
   a. Sudden loss of consciousness with little or no tonic-clonic movement
   b. Blank stare lasting only a few seconds
   c. Rarely continues beyond childhood
3. Psychomotor (automatisms)
   a. Sudden change in awareness
   b. Lip smacking, repetitive movements, shivering
   c. May exhibit antisocial behavior such as exposing self or violent acts
4. Jacksonian—focal (local-partial)
   a. Depends on site of focus
   b. Seizure may begin on hand, foot, face
   c. May manifest as a tonic-clonic seizure that "marches" on one side of body
5. Myoclonic
   a. Possible mild or rapid forceful movements
   b. Sudden jerk of body or extremities
   c. Brief seizures that occur in clusters

C. Diagnosis
1. Based on evidence of seizure
2. Differentiation of seizure type by physical examination

D. Treatment
1. Maintenance of patent airway
2. Anticonvulsant medications (see Chapter 3)
3. Patient education

E. Status epilepticus: most common type of seizure in emergency department visits
1. Ensure patent airway.
2. Protect from injury, particularly cervical spine.
3. Administer lorazepam (Ativan); diazepam (Valium) may also be used; monitor patient.
4. Administer IV fluids.
5. Insert indwelling urinary catheter.
6. Monitor closely for recurrent seizures.

? Critical Thinking Challenge Box

The nurse enters the room of a 45-year-old female patient who was admitted 2 hours ago for vertigo. While the nurse begins the assessment process, she notes the patient begins to demonstrate a sudden jerking movement of her arms and legs. The patient is unable to respond to the nurse's questions. The nurse also notes excessive salivation when suddenly the patient becomes incontinent of urine. What nursing interventions take precedence in this situation and which takes priority?

RECOMMENDATION

The priority nursing intervention in this situation is to ensure and maintain a patent airway for this patient. Assessing respiratory status and breathing of the patient throughout the event will determine patency of the airway. Removing anything that may incur harm and placing pillows around patient to protect head and extremities from injury, administering medications as ordered by the physician, and remaining with the patient throughout and following the seizure are all important nursing interventions. Upon awakening the patient will be disoriented and will need the support of the nurse.

EYE INJURIES

FOREIGN BODY IN EYE

A. Evert eyelid (Figure 10-5).
B. Touch particle gently with sterile swab moistened in sterile saline solution or water (do not remove if particle is on the cornea or eyeball penetration has occurred).
C. Apply an eye patch after ensuring that the eye is closed.

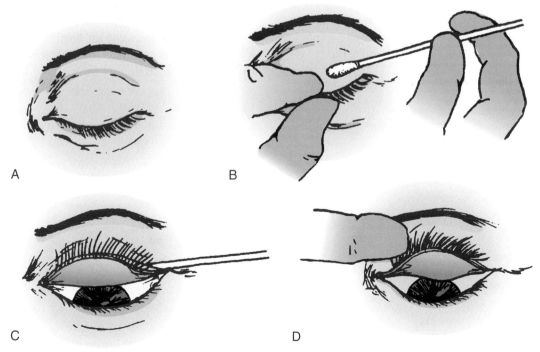

FIGURE 10-5 Steps in everting eyelid. **A,** Eyelid. **B,** Placement of cotton swab (eyelashes are pulled down and back over swab). **C,** Eyelid everted over swab. **D,** Examination of inside of eyelid and eye. (From Emergency Nurses Association: *Sheehy's emergency nursing: principles and practice,* ed 5, St Louis, 2005, Mosby.)

FOREIGN BODY IN CONJUNCTIVA

A. Evert eyelid.
B. Remove particle as previously described.
C. Irrigate with saline solution or water.
D. Eye patch may be applied.

EYELID CONTUSION (BLACK EYE)

A. Cold compresses or ice pack intermittently for the first 24 hours
B. Warm compresses after 48 hours
C. Bilateral eye patches if intraocular hemorrhage is present

CORNEAL ABRASION

A. Assessment
   1. Pain
   2. Photosensitivity
   3. Spasms of the eyelid
   4. Excessive tear production
B. Intervention: Apply eye patch to injured eye.
C. Usual medical care: local ophthalmic antibiotics

PENETRATING EYE INJURIES

A. Do not remove object.
B. Place a protective shield such as a paper cup over the eye to prevent further damage by pressure.
C. Apply eye patch to the uninjured eye.
D. Patient should see an ophthalmologist immediately.

BURNS

A. Chemical
   1. If in respiratory distress, maintain airway and administer oxygen.
   2. Remove any jewelry or clothes that are nonadherent.
   3. If the action of the chemical is not enhanced by water, immediately flush area with copious amounts of normal saline solution or tap water for 20 minutes (damage increases with length of chemical contact).
   4. Usual medical care: topical application of antibiotics, administration of cycloplegic agents or corticosteroids (alkali burns)
   5. The following solutions neutralize the following types of burns:
      a. Acid: sodium bicarbonate 2% solution
      b. Lime: ammonium tartrate 5% solution
      c. Alkali: boric or citric acid solution
B. Thermal (usually occurs with facial burns)
   1. Evaluate for respiratory distress; maintain airway and administer oxygen.
   2. Irrigate with cool normal saline solution or tap water for 2 to 5 minutes.
   3. Remove any jewelry or clothes that have not adhered to the skin.
   4. Apply bilateral eye patches.
   5. Administer usual medical care: analgesia, sedation, antibiotics, cycloplegics.
   6. Apply a clean, dry dressing.
C. Radiation
   1. Types
      a. Ultraviolet (sun). Severity depends on period of exposure.
      b. Infrared (x-rays). Severity depends on wavelength and period of exposure (may cause loss of vision).

2. Assessment
   a. Excessive blinking
   b. Excessive tear production
   c. Feeling that something is in the eye
   d. Pain
3. Interventions
   a. Cold compresses
   b. Bilateral eye patches
4. Usual medical care
   a. Topical antibiotics
   b. Cycloplegics
   c. Analgesics

SPINAL CORD INJURIES (TABLE 10-1)

A. Assessment
   1. Pain, tenderness
   2. Numbness, tingling, paralysis
   3. Weakness of extremities
   4. Alterations of sensation and motor function below level of injury
   5. Possible signs and symptoms of shock
B. Interventions
   1. Ensure adequate airway and ventilation. If helmet is on victim, leave it in place if airway is accessible; never attempt to remove helmet alone.
   2. Treat for shock.
   3. Immobilize (movement may cause further damage).
   4. Maintain body temperature.
   5. When help (EMS) arrives, place victim on board without flexing neck or back.
   6. Transport immediately (via EMS).

Table 10-1	Cervical Spine and Spinal Cord Lesions and Resultant Physiological Function
LESION	**RESULTANT FUNCTION**
C3, C4, or above	Respiratory arrest; flaccid paralysis; quadriplegia (tetraplegia)
C5, C6	Reduced respiratory effort; almost total dependence; flaccid paralysis; quadriplegia (tetraplegia)
C7	Reduced respiratory effort; almost total dependence; splints necessary for functioning of forearms; quadriplegia (tetraplegia)
T1	Reduced respiratory effort; partial dependence; paraplegia
T1, T2	Reduced respiratory effort; complete independence; paraplegia
T7	Complete independence; walking with long-leg braces; paraplegia
L4	Complete independence; walking with foot braces; paraplegia

From Emergency Nurses Association: *Sheehy's manual of emergency care,* ed 6, St Louis, 2006, Mosby.

SOFT-TISSUE NECK INJURIES

FRACTURED LARYNX

A. Assessment
1. Hoarse voice
2. Cough with hemoptysis
3. Difficulty breathing; respiratory distress
4. Subcutaneous emphysema

B. Interventions
1. Administer oxygen.
2. Observe closely for respiratory difficulties.

C. Usual medical care
1. Emergency cricothyrotomy or tracheostomy
2. Broad-spectrum antibiotics

PENETRATING NECK WOUNDS

A. Assessment
1. Noticeable penetrating wound
2. Airway obstruction
3. Signs and symptoms of hypovolemia, hemothorax, or shock

B. Interventions
1. Ensure adequate airway and ventilation.
2. Control bleeding.
3. Surgery is necessary.

CHEST INJURIES

FRACTURED RIB (SIMPLE, UNDISPLACED)

A. Assessment
1. Chest pain (increases on inspiration), tenderness
2. Shortness of breath, shallow breathing
3. Tachycardia
4. Hypotension
5. Ecchymosis

B. Interventions (individualized)
1. Rest.
2. Apply intermittent ice for first 24 hours, then heat.
3. Observe for signs and symptoms of pneumothorax by monitoring breathing patterns and lung sounds.
4. Encourage deep breathing.
5. Administer analgesics sparingly.
6. Observe for signs and symptoms of hemorrhage caused by possible laceration of spleen or liver.

FLAIL CHEST

A. Fracture of several ribs resulting in loss of chest wall stability. Pulmonary or myocardial contusion may also be present because of force of injury. May be life-threatening.

B. Assessment
1. Pain
2. Difficulty breathing
3. Shallow, rapid, noisy respirations
4. Chest movement opposite from normal direction: moves in on inspiration, out on expiration
5. Tachycardia and cyanosis
6. Possible bruising

C. Interventions
1. Ensure adequate airway and ventilation.
2. Stabilize chest wall.
3. Apply pressure dressing.
4. Position victim on affected side in semi-Fowler position.
5. Monitor vital signs and lung sounds.

D. Usual medical care
1. Pain control
2. Possible intubation and ventilation with severe flail
3. Possible traction

SIMPLE PNEUMOTHORAX

A. Description: entrance of air into the pleural cavity; loss of negative pressure, resulting in partial or total lung collapse

B. Assessment
1. Chest pain
2. Dyspnea, tachypnea
3. Decreased breath sounds

C. Interventions
1. Ensure adequate airway and ventilation.
2. Place victim in semi-Fowler position.
3. Administer oxygen.

D. Usual medical care: possible chest tube placement

TENSION PNEUMOTHORAX

A. Description: air that enters the pleural cavity on inspiration and is trapped during exhalation, creating pressure that causes eventual collapse of the lung (same side), resulting in a life-threatening condition in which mediastinal shift occurs, compressing the heart, great vessels, trachea, and the opposite lung

B. Assessment
1. Extreme shortness of breath
2. Observed tracheal deviation
3. Paradoxical movement of the chest
4. Neck vein distention
5. Hypotension
6. Tachycardia
7. Restlessness
8. Cyanosis
9. Distant breath sounds
10. History of chest trauma

C. Interventions
1. Ensure adequate airway, breathing, and circulation.
2. Administer oxygen.

D. Usual medical care
1. Needle thoracotomy
2. Chest tube placement
3. IV fluids

OPEN PNEUMOTHORAX (SUCKING CHEST WOUND)

A. Description: presence of air in the chest resulting from an open wound in the chest wall
1. One-way flap: Air enters pleural space but cannot escape (tension pneumothorax).
2. Two-way flap: Air enters and leaves pleural space.

B. Assessment
1. Audible sucking noise
2. Shortness of breath
3. Chest pain
4. Cyanosis
5. Shock
6. Possible signs and symptoms of tension pneumothorax

C. Interventions
1. Ensure adequate airway, breathing, and circulation.
2. Cover wound with airtight dressing (depends on size of wound).

3. Administer oxygen.
4. CPR may be necessary.
D. Usual medical care
1. Chest tube placement
2. Treatment with antibiotics
3. Treatment for shock

SPONTANEOUS PNEUMOTHORAX

A. Description: presence of air in the intrapleural space resulting from rupture of lung tissue and visceral pleura with no evidence of trauma; can occur during periods of strenuous physical activity
B. Assessment
1. Sudden, sharp chest pain
2. Shortness of breath
3. Diaphoresis
4. Anxiety
5. Hypotension
6. Tachycardia
7. Cessation of normal chest movement on affected side
C. Interventions
1. Ensure adequate airway and ventilation.
2. Keep victim quiet.
3. Place in semi- or high-Fowler position.
D. Usual medical care
1. Needle aspiration
2. Chest tube
3. IV fluids
4. Oxygen

HEMOTHORAX

A. Description: blood in the pleural space from traumatic injury (stabbing) or rupture of congenital blebs
B. Assessment
1. Chest pain
2. Shortness of breath
3. Distant breath sounds
4. Anxiety
5. Shock
6. Cyanosis
C. Interventions
1. Ensure adequate airway and ventilation.
2. Treat for shock.
D. Usual medical care: chest tube placement; thoracentesis

PULMONARY EMBOLISM

A. Description: Thrombus becomes detached and lodges in a branch of the pulmonary artery, causing a partial or total occlusion and resulting in a pulmonary infarct; commonly seen in women taking oral contraceptives, smokers, and those who have sustained trauma or undergone surgery or those with long-bone fractures.
B. Assessment
1. Sudden, sharp chest pain (may be worse on inspiration)
2. Shortness of breath
3. Pallor, possible cyanosis
4. Anxiety
5. Tachycardia
6. Rapid, shallow respirations (tachypnea)
7. Possible hypotension
8. Possible cough, wheeze, hemoptysis
9. Possible sudden death if large blood vessel is blocked

10. Elevated body temperature caused by lung inflammation
C. Interventions
1. Ensure adequate airway, breathing, and circulation.
2. Treat for shock.
3. Administer oxygen.
4. Keep victim quiet.
5. Place patient in semi- to high-Fowler position if vital signs permit.
D. Usual medical care
1. Anticoagulant therapy
2. IV fluids
3. Surgical intervention in cases of profound shock or cardiovascular collapse

INTRAABDOMINAL INJURIES

PENETRATING WOUND

A. Description: wounds resulting from stabbings, shootings, impalement
B. Assessment
1. Hypotension
2. Shock
3. Diminished bowel sounds
4. Pain
5. Tenderness
6. Progressive abdominal distention
7. Nausea or vomiting
C. Interventions
1. Do not move victim.
2. Ensure adequate airway, breathing, and circulation.
3. Control bleeding.
   a. Look for entrance and exit wounds.
   b. Apply compression for external bleeding.
   c. Look for chest injuries.
4. Cover wounds with wet, sterile, or nonadhesive dressings (e.g., saline or plastic wrap). Leave impaled objects in place to control bleeding.
5. Monitor vital signs.
6. Treat for shock.
7. Keep on NPO status.
D. Usual medical care: Follow Maslow's hierarchy of needs.
1. Oxygen
2. Analgesics
3. Nasogastric tube
4. IV fluids
5. Indwelling catheter
6. Antibiotics
7. Tetanus prophylaxis
8. X-ray examination
9. Possible surgery

BLUNT WOUND

A. Description: wound resulting from a motor vehicle accident (MVA), a contact-sport injury, a fall, or physical abuse (e.g., domestic violence)
B. Assessment
1. Observable bruises and abrasions
2. Abdominal pain, rigidity, palpable masses, or distention
3. Signs and symptoms of shock
4. Guarding
5. Diminished bowel sounds

C. Interventions
1. Do not move victim.
2. Ensure adequate airway, breathing, and circulation.
3. Observe for hemorrhage.
4. Observe for chest injuries.
5. Monitor vital signs.
6. Treat for shock.
D. Usual medical care
1. Oxygen
2. Nasogastric tube
3. X-ray examination
4. Peritoneal lavage
5. Possible surgery

BURNS

A. Depth of burn classification (Table 10-2)
B. Surface area classification
1. The greater the body surface area (BSA) affected, the more serious is the damage.
2. Use the rule of nines (Figure 10-6) to estimate the percentage of BSA affected.

MAJOR BURNS

A. Burns are considered major or critical if they fulfill the following criteria:
1. Deep partial-thickness burns: more than 25% of BSA in adults or more than 20% in children under 10 years of age and adults over 40 years of age
2. Full-thickness burns: more than 10% of BSA in adults and children
3. Electrical burns
4. Burns involving face, eyes, ears, hands, feet, and perineum
5. Burns in victims with preexisting chronic conditions (diabetes, cardiac conditions, renal failure)
B. Interventions
1. Lay victim flat (standing forces him or her to breathe flames and smoke; running fans flames).
2. Roll victim in carpet or blankets or use water to extinguish fire.
3. Remove any smoldering or tight-fitting clothing that is nonadherent.
4. Ensure adequate airway and ventilation.

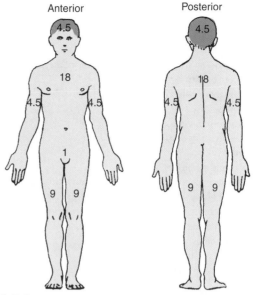

FIGURE 10-6 Rule of nines is used to estimate amount of body surface area burned. (From Monahan FD, et al: *Phipps' medical-surgical nursing: health and illness perspectives,* ed 8, St Louis, 2007, Mosby.)

5. Administer oxygen.
6. Assess for inhalation burns.
7. Remove jewelry.
8. Apply cold soaks.
9. Cover burns with moist, sterile dressings or clean cloth.
10. Elevate affected parts if possible.
11. Cover victim.
12. Insert indwelling catheter.
13. Treat burned areas as ordered by physician.
C. Usual medical care: Follow Maslow's hierarchy.
1. Standard Precautions
2. IV therapy
3. Pain management
4. Central venous pressure line
5. Nasogastric tube
6. Antibiotic therapy
7. Tetanus prophylaxis
D. Warnings
1. Do not use salves, ointments, or oils.
2. Do not soak large burns unless you can maintain body warmth.
3. Do not use ice or ice water on deep partial-thickness or full-thickness burns; causes further injury and promotes hypothermia.
4. Monitor urine for myoglobin, a sign of tissue damage especially common in electrical burns.

CHEMICAL BURNS

A. Powdered chemicals: Sweep off skin.
B. Nonpowdered chemicals: Irrigate with copious amounts of water or saline solution.
C. Cover loosely with a clean cloth.
D. Usual medical care: Treat as thermal burns (cleanse wound, open blisters and remove outer layer, apply topical antibacterial agent).

Table 10-2	Burn Classification	
DEPTH	**DEGREE**	**ASSESSMENT**
Superficial, partial thickness (involves only the epidermis)	First	Pain; red; minimal or no edema
Deep partial thickness (involves epidermis and part of the dermis)	Second	Pain; mottled color; blistering; wet appearance
Full thickness (involves epidermis and damage to subcutaneous layer, muscle, and bone)	Third	Gray, white, brown, leathery, or charred appearance; edema; minimal or no pain

ELECTRICAL BURNS

A. Assessment
1. Discoloration
2. Edema
3. Cardiac dysrhythmias as a result of heart stress from electrical current
4. Entrance and exit sites of current visible
5. Confusion
6. Unconsciousness
7. Respiratory distress
B. Interventions
1. Do not touch the victim.
2. Remove electrical source with a nonconductor (i.e., nonmetal object), shut off current source, or both.
3. If victim has no pulse and is not breathing, begin CPR.
4. Extremities should be handled minimally and with extreme caution.
5. Check victim for other injuries.
6. Monitor cardiac and renal function.

RADIATION BURNS

A. Interventions
1. Remove contaminated clothing.
2. Apply cool, moist compresses.
B. Usual medical care
1. Analgesics
2. Antipyretics
3. Eye patches

SMOKE INHALATION

A. Assessment
1. History of exposure
2. Singed hair in nares
3. Mouth burns
4. Brassy cough
5. Respiratory distress
6. Rales, rhonchi, or wheezes
7. Restlessness
8. Cyanosis
B. Interventions
1. Ensure adequate airway and ventilation.
2. Administer oxygen.
3. Be prepared to initiate CPR.
C. Usual medical care
1. Hospitalization for 24 to 48 hours
2. IV fluids
3. Chest physical therapy
4. Possible endotracheal intubation or tracheostomy
5. Bronchodilators, steroids
6. Nasogastric tube

WOUNDS

A. Open (break in skin integrity)
1. Laceration: jagged cut through the skin and underlying tissue
2. Abrasion: skin scrape or "brush burn"
3. Avulsion: flap of skin and subcutaneous tissue torn loose
4. Puncture: tissue penetration by a sharp object
5. Abscess: localized pus formation
B. Closed (no break in skin integrity [e.g., contusion]): injury to underlying tissue by blunt object

C. General management
1. Stop bleeding.
   a. Apply pressure dressing.
   b. Elevate affected part.
   c. Use digital pressure on supply artery.
   d. Apply tourniquet only as a lifesaving measure and leave tourniquet visible.
2. Treat for shock.
3. Control infection.
   a. Wounds requiring medical care: It is generally recommended not to clean them until they have been seen by a physician.
   b. Cover open wounds with a clean, nonadhesive dressing; use moist dressing if an evisceration is present.
   c. Apply ice during the first 24 to 48 hours for closed wounds.
   d. Minor wounds being treated at home: Clean well with soap and water; thoroughly rinse. Approximate wound edges with adhesive. Cover with a clean dressing. Seek medical care for signs of infection.
4. Puncture wounds
   a. Stabilize impaled object and leave in place.
   b. Seek medical attention.
   c. Assess tetanus toxoid status.
D. Special wounds
1. Human bites
   a. May be self-inflicted or inflicted by another person; evidenced by teeth marks and often by knuckle lacerations (occurs when fist hits another person's teeth during a fight)
   b. Interventions
      (1) Clean with soap and water.
      (2) Rinse thoroughly.
      (3) Apply clean dressing.
      (4) Keep injured part elevated.
   c. Usual medical care
      (1) Administer tetanus prophylaxis.
      (2) Administer antibiotic therapy.
      (3) Observe closely for systemic responses to bite—toxic shock syndrome, hepatitis, or human immunodeficiency virus (HIV)—which can occur after the injury or during the healing process.
2. Animal bites: potential for contracting rabies; must be considered seriously with any animal bite.
   a. Dog bites are most common, causing crushing injury to skin and underlying tissue or avulsion injuries should the victim attempt to pull away.
   b. Cat bites are more likely to cause puncture wounds.
   c. Interventions
      (1) Obtain history of bite.
      (2) Clean minor wounds with soap and water.
      (3) Rinse thoroughly.
      (4) Flush with povidone-iodine (Betadine) or other cleansing solutions if victim is allergic to povidone-iodine.
      (5) Apply clean dressing.
   Note: Major wounds (severe bleeding) require control of bleeding and medical attention.
   d. Usual medical care
      (1) Antibiotic therapy for large, contaminated bites
      (2) Tetanus prophylaxis
      (3) Rabies prophylaxis if necessary

3. Snakebites
   a. Assessment
      (1) Teeth marks; possibly fang marks
      (2) Edema
      (3) Pain
      (4) Ecchymosis
      (5) Bleeding
      (6) Numbness of affected part
   b. Interventions
      (1) Have victim limit movement and remain calm.
      (2) Remove tight-fitting jewelry and clothes.
      (3) Clean wound with fresh water and soap.
      (4) Apply clean dressing.
      (5) Immobilize affected limb.
      (6) Affected limb should be in dependent position.
      Note: **Do Not** *use mouth suction or a snakebite kit as they can cause additional complications.*
   c. Usual medical care
      (1) Analgesics
      (2) IV fluids
      (3) Tetanus prophylaxis
      (4) Antivenin therapy
4. Insect (bees, wasps, hornets)
   a. Assessment
      (1) Obtain detailed medical and activity history.
      (2) Assess for pruritus.
      (3) Assess for burning sensation.
      (4) Observe for swelling.
      (5) Monitor for anaphylaxis.
   b. Interventions
      (1) Remove the stinger and venom sac by scraping. Use of forceps or tweezers releases more toxin and is not advised.
      (2) Clean with soap and water.
      (3) Apply ice (do not apply heat).
      (4) Apply ammonia diluted with warm water if available.
   c. Usual medical care
      (1) Epinephrine
      (2) Antihistamines
      (3) Steroids
5. Tick
   a. It attaches to host with its teeth.
   b. It releases a toxin that may cause tick paralysis or Lyme disease.
   c. Squeezing it releases more toxin.
   d. If paralysis progresses, respiratory failure and subsequent death may occur.
   e. Paralysis disappears after the tick is removed.
   f. Interventions
      (1) Grasp tick with tweezers and pull slowly and steadily to remove with head intact.
      (2) Wash area with soap and water.
      (3) Seek medical treatment.

MUSCULOSKELETAL INJURIES

FRACTURE

A. Description: complete or incomplete break in bone continuity
   1. Fracture without displacement presents normal alignment despite the fracture.
   2. Fracture with displacement presents a separation of bone fragments at fracture site.
   3. Compound or open: There is bone protrusion through the skin.
   4. Simple or closed: There is no bone protrusion through the skin.
   5. Incomplete: Part of bone is broken.
   6. Complete: Breakage produces two fragments.
B. Types of fractures (Box 10-2)
C. Assessment
   1. Five *P*s (pain, pallor, pulses, paresthesia, paralysis)
   2. Discoloration, ecchymosis
   3. Swelling
   4. Deformity, possible limb shortening and external rotation
   5. Crepitus (characteristic grating sound)
   6. Possible bone snap heard by victim
   7. External bleeding from associated wounds
   8. Tenderness (pain) relative to specific area of the body (sacrum, hip, symphysis pubis)
D. Interventions
   1. Control bleeding if necessary.
   2. If wound is open, apply a clean gauze or cloth.
   3. Treat for shock.
   4. Immobilize affected part.

Box 10-2 Types of Fractures

TYPICAL COMPLETE FRACTURES
- Closed (simple) fracture: noncommunicating wound between bone and skin
- Open (compound) fracture: communicating wound between bone and skin
- Comminuted fracture: multiple bone fragments
- Linear fracture: fracture line parallel to long axis of bone
- Oblique fracture: fracture line at 45-degree angle to long axis of bone
- Spiral fracture: fracture line encircling bone
- Transverse fracture: fracture line perpendicular to long axis of bone
- Impacted fracture: fracture fragments pushed into each other
- Pathological fracture: fracture at a point in the bone weakened by disease (e.g., with tumors or osteoporosis)
- Avulsion: fragment of bone connected to a ligament breaks off from the main bone
- Extracapsular: fracture close to the joint but remains outside the joint capsule
- Intracapsular: fracture within the joint capsule

TYPICAL INCOMPLETE FRACTURES
- Greenstick fracture: break on one cortex of bone with splintering of inner bone surface
- Torus fracture: buckling of cortex
- Bowing fracture: bending of bone
- Stress fracture: microfracture
- Transchondral fracture: separation of cartilaginous joint surface (articular cartilage) from main shaft of bone

Modified from McCance KL, Huether SE: *Pathophysiology: the biological basis for disease in adults and children,* ed 6, St Louis, 2010, Mosby.

5. Apply splint so it extends above and below the fracture. If affected limb is bent or deformed, maintain position while splint is applied.
6. Apply ice.
7. Elevate affected part if possible.
8. Observe for changes in sensation, temperature, and color (indicate nerve injury or circulation interference).
9. Remove jewelry from extremities to reduce risk of further injury if swelling should occur.

E. Usual medical care
1. X-ray examination
2. Possible cast application
3. Possible surgery
4. Analgesics
5. Traction

DISLOCATION

A. Description: joint injury and bone displacement
B. Assessment
1. Pain, tenderness
2. Swelling
3. Deformity
4. Alterations in function
5. Discoloration
C. Interventions
1. Control hemorrhage if present (not usually seen with a simple dislocation).
2. Immobilize the affected part.
3. Apply sterile dressing to any open wounds.
4. Apply splint extending above and below the site in the position found.
5. Apply ice.
6. Elevate affected part, if possible.
7. Check for fractures.
8. Monitor neurological status (check pulses distal to the injury).

SPRAIN

A. Description: stretched or ruptured ligaments. Sprain should be considered a fracture until proven otherwise by x-ray examination.
B. Assessment
1. Pain, tenderness
2. Discoloration
3. Swelling
4. Alterations in function
C. Interventions
1. Immobilize affected part.
2. Apply ice intermittently for 72 hours.
3. Apply elastic (Ace) bandages.
4. Elevate affected part.

STRAIN

A. Description: muscle or tendon damage caused by excessive physical use
B. Assessment
1. Pain
2. Discoloration
C. Interventions
1. Elevate affected part.
2. Apply ice intermittently for 72 hours.
3. Apply elastic (Ace) bandages.

4. Immobilize affected part.
5. Limit activity to no weight bearing.

HYPERTHERMIA

HEAT STROKE

A. Description: life-threatening emergency; breakdown of bodily mechanism for heat regulation and retention of excessive body heat; occurs with overexposure to high environmental temperatures, especially those accompanied by high relative humidity and low wind
B. Assessment
1. Hyperpyrexia to 106° or 107° F (41.1° to 41.6° C)
2. Skin flushed, hot, and dry or clammy and diaphoretic
3. Dizziness
4. Headache
5. Confusion
6. Nausea
7. Tachycardia
8. Hypotension
9. Fixed and diluted pupils
10. Seizures
11. Possible altered LOC
12. Shallow, rapid breathing
13. Delirium
C. Predisposing factors
1. Age (older adults and infants)
2. Obesity
3. Alcoholism
4. Preexisting illness (cardiovascular or neurological dysfunction)
5. Prescription medications that decrease perspiration (anticholinergics such as antihistamines and antispasmodics; diuretics and beta blockers such as propranolol [Inderal])
6. Excessive strenuous exercise
D. Interventions
1. Activate EMS (911).
2. Ensure adequate circulation, airway, and breathing.
3. Move victim out of sun.
4. Loosen or remove clothing.
5. Provide rapid cooling (e.g., immerse in cold water to neckline if possible); apply towels soaked in cold water; use air conditioning, fanning, and cool-water sponge. Discontinue cooling actions if victim's behavior returns to normal (continued cooling can lead to hypothermia)
6. If conscious, provide cool water to drink.
7. Reassess victim's core body temperature every 5-10 minutes.
8. Advise victim to avoid reexposure and warn of possible lowered tolerance to heat for a long time or possibly indefinitely.
E. Usual medical care
1. Oxygen
2. IV therapy

HEAT EXHAUSTION

A. Description: ineffective circulating blood volume caused by excessive fluid loss and exposure to heat without sufficient fluid and electrolyte replenishment; increased risk for heat stroke

B. Assessment
1. Headache
2. Dizziness, faintness
3. Nausea and vomiting
4. Marked diaphoresis
5. Cool, pale, damp skin
6. Muscle cramps
7. Possible temperature elevation
8. Orthostatic hypotension
9. Tachycardia
10. Dehydration
11. Anxiety
12. Anorexia, thirst
C. Especially at risk
1. Older adults.
2. Very young children.
D. Interventions
1. Move victim to cool, quiet area.
2. Loosen or remove constricting clothing.
3. Cool victim with water (towels soaked in cold water; use air conditioning, fanning, and cool-water sponge).
4. Rehydrate victim (juice, sports drinks, water).
5. Provide rest.
6. Advise victim of preventive measures: drink plenty of fluids and curtail activity on hot days.

COLD INJURIES

FROSTBITE

A. Classification
1. Superficial: Superficial tissue below the skin freezes.
2. Deep: Deep subcutaneous tissue freezes, and temperature of affected part is lowered.
B. Most frequently affected areas: ears, nose, cheeks, fingers, and toes
C. Assessment
1. Superficial
a. Numbness, tingling, burning
b. Gray-white appearance of affected parts
2. Deep
a. Hyperemic skin
b. Edema
c. Blister formation
d. Discoloration
e. Numbness
D. Interventions
1. Superficial
a. Remove wet, constricting clothing.
b. Give warm-water soaks.
c. Advise victim of preventive measures.
2. Deep
a. Remove wet, constricting clothing and jewelry.
b. Give warm-water soaks only if continuously available; otherwise keep area dry, place sterile gauze between affected fingers and toes, cover, and elevate frozen part.
c. Use a blanket to cover victim.
d. If victim is conscious, give warm liquids.
e. Do not allow use of frostbitten part.
3. Usual medical care
a. Tetanus prophylaxis
b. Analgesics
c. Antibiotic therapy
d. Administration of warm fluids

E. Warnings
1. Do not rub area with snow or ice.
2. Do not touch frostbitten area unless necessary to avoid further damage.

IMMERSION FOOT

A. Cause: wet foot in continuous contact with cold temperatures
B. Assessment
1. Foot is cold and damp.
2. Foot appears shriveled.
3. Gangrene can result (if conditions are prolonged and repeated).
C. Interventions
1. Dry footwear
2. Warm-water soaks
D. Warnings
1. Do not rub area with snow or ice.
2. Do not massage.

CHILBLAIN

A. Description: localized redness and swelling of the skin resulting from excessive exposure to cold
B. Commonly affected areas: fingers, toes, and earlobes
C. Assessment: possible burning, itching, blistering, and ulceration (similar to thermal burn)
D. Interventions
1. Protect part from cold and further injury.
2. Warm gently.
3. Avoid use of tobacco products.

HYPOTHERMIA

A. Description: exposure to cold resulting in heat loss and reduction in body temperature below the average normal range
B. Assessment (Table 10-3)

Table 10-3	Stages, Signs, and Symptoms of Hypothermia	
STAGE	**CORE TEMPERATURE**	**SYMPTOMS**
Mild	90°-95° F (32°-35° C)	Tachypnea, tachycardia, ataxia, shivering, lethargy, confusion, occasional atrial fibrillation
Moderate	86°-90° F (30.0°-32.2° C)	Rigidity, hypoventilation, decreased level of consciousness, increased myocardial irritability, hypovolemia, blood sludging with metabolic acidosis, Osborne or J wave (positive deflection in the RT segment)
Severe	Under 86° F (30° C)	Loss of reflexes, coma, hypotension, acidosis, apnea, cyanosis, ventricular fibrillation, asystole

From Fultz J, Sturt PA: *Mosby's emergency nursing reference*, ed 3, St Louis, 2005, Mosby.

C. Interventions
1. Ensure adequate airway and ventilation.
2. Administer oxygen.
3. Remove wet clothing and cover victim.
4. Give warm beverages high in sugar content.
5. Warm body gradually.
   a. Passive rewarming: warm room, blankets, and draft prevention (mild hypothermia)
   b. Active external rewarming: heat packs, warming blankets, and overhead radiant warmers (mild-to-moderate hypothermia)
D. Usual medical care (moderate-to-severe hypothermia): active internal warming
1. Warmed humidified oxygen
2. Warmed gastric and peritoneal lavage
3. Warmed IV fluids
E. Warning: Do not rub or massage the skin.

POISONING

FOOD

A. Cause: pathogenic organisms transferred to victim from contaminated food; illness caused by toxins produced by the organism
B. Botulism (*Clostridium botulinum* infection)
1. Causes
   a. Improperly canned food
   b. Improperly cured food
2. Assessment
   a. Headache
   b. Fatigue
   c. Nausea and vomiting
   d. Double vision (diplopia)
   e. Muscle incoordination
   f. Difficulty swallowing, talking, and breathing
3. Interventions
   a. Ensure adequate airway and ventilation.
   b. Be prepared to administer CPR.
   c. Induce vomiting if consumption was recent or if victim has clinical and neurological symptoms, no seizure activity, and no alterations in LOC.
4. Usual medical care
   a. Antitoxin
   b. IV fluids
C. *Staphylococcus aureus* infection
1. Causes
   a. Secretions from respiratory tract and skin of food handlers
   b. Unrefrigerated cream-filled foods
   c. Fish
   d. Meat
2. Assessment
   a. Nausea and vomiting
   b. Diarrhea
   c. Abdominal cramps
   d. Weakness
3. Interventions
   a. Fluids
   b. Bed rest
4. Usual medical care
   a. Possible IV therapy

b. Antiemetics
c. Antidiarrheals
D. *Salmonella* infection
1. Causes: inadequately cooked meat, poultry, and eggs
2. Assessment
   a. Nausea and vomiting
   b. Diarrhea
   c. Weakness
   d. Abdominal pain
   e. Elevated temperature
   f. Chills
3. Interventions
   a. Bed rest
   b. Fluids
4. Usual medical care
   a. Possible IV therapy
   b. Antiemetics
   c. Antidiarrheals

ACCIDENTAL POISONING

A. Description: ingestion, inhalation, or absorption of toxic substances or other substances such as drugs that, when taken in large amounts, are toxic to the body
B. Assessment: Signs and symptoms vary according to cause.
1. General
   a. Nausea and vomiting
   b. Abdominal pain
   c. Convulsions
   d. Change in LOC
   e. Decreased pulse and respirations
2. Drug poisoning: coma; flaccid muscles; hypotension (symptoms vary depending on drug)
3. Chemical poisoning
   a. Burns around lips and mouth
   b. Excessive salivation
   c. Difficulty swallowing
   d. Breath odor (from cleaning or petroleum products)
4. Inhalation poisoning
   a. Coughing and choking
   b. Headache; bright red skin (carbon monoxide—late indicator)
5. Absorption poisoning: localized itching and burning (poison)
C. Interventions (Box 10-3)
D. Usual medical care
1. IV fluids (severe cases)
2. Hyperbaric oxygenation (carbon monoxide poisoning)

DIABETES MELLITUS AND HYPOGLYCEMIA

A. Ketoacidosis: Life-threatening condition caused by acute insulin deficiency (develops over a period of 2 to 3 days); severe hyperglycemia and acidosis
1. Assessment
   a. Polydipsia
   b. Weak, rapid pulse
   c. Hypotension
   d. Dry, warm, flushed skin
   e. Pallor
   f. Diaphoresis
   g. Acetone odor on breath

| Box 10-3 | Guidelines to Stop Absorption of Poisons |

INHALED POISON
- Remove victim from source of toxic gas.
- Assess cardiopulmonary status and give artificial ventilation if possible.
- Give oxygen if available.

CONTACT POISON
- Rinse skin with copious amounts of water.
- Remove garments and rinse skin again.

INGESTED POISON
- If person is conscious, call physician or poison control center for assistance.
- Substances other than caustics or hydrocarbons: Induce emesis by giving 15 to 30 mL syrup of ipecac; follow with full glass of warm water.
- Inactivate poison by giving activated charcoal (especially after drug ingestion).
- Caustics or hydrocarbons (petroleum products): Give nothing by mouth.
- Seek immediate medical attention.
- Do not induce emesis.
- If person is unconscious, transport without delay to medical facility.

From Phipps WJ, et al: *Medical-surgical nursing: health and illness perspectives,* ed 5, St Louis, 1995, Mosby.

h. Kussmaul respirations
i. Nausea and vomiting
j. Alterations in consciousness
k. Dehydration
l. Weakness
m. Headache
n. Abdominal tenderness

2. Interventions
   a. Ensure adequate airway and ventilation.
   b. Monitor vital signs, fluid intake and output, and LOC.
   c. Provide fluids if conscious (e.g., broth).

3. Usual medical care
   a. Regular insulin
   b. Administer IV therapy: normal saline solution or 0.45% saline solution.
   c. Monitor blood sugar and serum potassium levels.

B. Hypoglycemia (low blood sugar; insulin reaction)
   1. Assessment
      a. Sudden onset of symptoms
      b. Weakness
      c. Pallor
      d. Hunger
      e. Nervousness, irritability
      f. Cool, moist skin
      g. Tachycardia
      h. Tremors
      i. Dizziness, syncope
      j. Headache
      k. Visual disturbances
      l. Drowsiness
      m. Confusion

2. Interventions
   a. Ensure adequate airway and ventilation.
   b. Administer quick-acting sugar (e.g., orange juice with sugar, honey, lump sugar, cola beverage, hard candy, glucose tablets).
   c. If symptoms remain after 15 minutes, repeat treatment.
   d. When crisis resolves, encourage consumption of protein and complex carbohydrate snack (crackers with peanut butter or cheese, milk and crackers).

3. Usual medical care if unconscious
   a. Administer IV therapy: 50% glucose.
   b. Monitor blood sugar.

DROWNING

A. Description: asphyxiation that results from aspiration of fluid into the lungs, which is inhaled as the individual panics or gasps for breath
B. Causes
   1. Accidental (e.g., exhaustion, inability to swim, panic, injury, medical incident such as a seizure)
   2. Intentional: suicide attempt
C. Interventions
   1. Remove victim from water.
   2. If victim is not breathing, initiate CPR beginning with compressions.
   3. Observe for pulmonary edema.
D. Usual medical care
   1. IV fluids
   2. Oxygen under pressure

DRUG ABUSE

A. Description: use of a substance in a manner, amounts, or situations in which the drug use causes problems or greatly increases the chance of problems occurring
B. Assessment
   1. Needle marks on the body along the veins (many addicts wear long-sleeved shirts to conceal evidence of mainlining)
   2. Anorexia
   3. Abdominal cramping
   4. Constipation
   5. Nutritional deficiencies
   6. Watery, reddened eyes
   7. Runny nose
   8. Dilated or constricted pupils
   9. Central nervous system (CNS) alterations (agitation, euphoria, seizures)
   10. Poor personal hygiene
   11. History of difficulty in school, on job, with interpersonal relationships
   12. Accident-prone
   13. History of personality change
   14. Possible hepatitis
C. Clinical manifestations and treatment (Table 10-4)
D. Interventions
   1. Ensure circulation, airway, and breathing.
   2. Administer oxygen.

3. Insert indwelling catheter.
4. Monitor vital functions and neurological status.
5. Take seizure precautions.
E. Usual medical care
    1. Arterial blood gases
    2. Specific drug antagonist (e.g., naloxone hydrochloride [Narcan])
    3. IV therapy
    4. Central venous pressure line

5. Possible dialysis
6. High-protein, high-calorie diet
7. Vitamin supplements
8. Psychotherapy
9. Withdrawal treatment: methadone hydrochloride (Dolophine); usually used for heroin addiction
    a. Legal synthetic drug addiction
    b. Supervised administration
10. Rehabilitation

| Table 10-4 | Clinical Manifestations and Treatment of Acute Intoxication and Withdrawal of Mind-Altering Drugs |

DRUG GROUP	CLINICAL MANIFESTATIONS OF ACUTE INTOXICATION	TREATMENT	CLINICAL MANIFESTATIONS OF WITHDRAWAL
Narcotics	Respiratory depression, bradycardia, hypotension, cold clammy skin, decreased body temperature; deep sleep, stupor, or coma; pinpoint pupils	Maintain ventilation; provide oxygen Give narcotic antagonist: naloxone (Narcan), 0.4 mg IV Monitor vital signs every 15-30 min until patient is conscious Treat for shock	Not life-threatening Early: restlessness, irritability, drug craving, yawning, lacrimation, diaphoresis, rhinorrhea, followed by "yen" sleep (intense desire to sleep; sleeps restlessly) Later: awakens with more severe symptoms, nausea, vomiting, anorexia, abdominal cramps, bone and muscle pain, tremors, piloerection (gooseflesh)
Other CNS depressants	Same as for narcotics	Lavage if recent oral ingestion with possible tremors, activated charcoal treatment Maintain ventilation: provide oxygen Monitor vital signs every 15-30 min until patient is conscious Position patient side-lying or prone, not supine Treat for shock Hemodialysis for renal shutdown	May be life-threatening Insomnia, restlessness, anorexia, followed by convulsions and symptoms similar to DTs (confusion, visual and auditory hallucinations), dehydration
CNS stimulants	Labile cardiovascular symptoms (flushing or pallor, pulse and blood pressure changes, arrhythmias), hyperpyrexia, mental disturbances (agitation, paranoia, hallucinations), convulsions, circulatory collapse	Give chlorpromazine (Thorazine, 25-50 mg IM Provide a quiet environment Orient patient to reality Monitor vital signs until stable	Withdrawal is not severe Somnolence, apathy, irritability, depression, fatigue
Hallucinogens	Physiological toxicity low at doses that produce strong psychological effects Acute panic reaction ("bad trip") may lead to suicide "Flashback" episodes Prolonged psychotic disorders (paranoia, depression) Phencyclidine: CNS depression or stimulation may lead to death	Provide quiet, supportive environment and constant attention Give diazepam (Valium; 2-10 mg IM), major tranquilizers (chlorpromazine [Thorazine] IM), or both, for severe anxiety	No evidence of withdrawal symptoms
Cannabis	Adverse reactions infrequent Simple depression, paranoid ideation, confusion, disorientation, hallucinations	Provide support and reassurance Give tranquilizer for agitation	Withdrawal symptoms rare Insomnia, anorexia

Table 10-4	Clinical Manifestations and Treatment of Acute Intoxication and Withdrawal of Mind-Altering Drugs—cont'd		
DRUG GROUP	**CLINICAL MANIFESTATIONS OF ACUTE INTOXICATION**	**TREATMENT**	**CLINICAL MANIFESTATIONS OF WITHDRAWAL**
Deliriants	Slowing of heart rate, brain activity, and breathing Slurred speech, blurred vision, inflamed mucous membranes, excessive tearing, nasal secretions With high doses loss of consciousness and seizures may occur Brain damage may occur (memory loss, depression, paranoia, hostility) Feeling of stimulation and energy Death may occur from suffocation or cardiac arrest	Maintain respirations Provide quiet environment and support Monitor vital signs Orient patient to reality	Chills, hallucination, pains, cramps, DTs

From Phipps WJ, et al: *Medical-surgical nursing: health and illness perspectives,* ed 6, St Louis, 1999, Mosby.
CNS, Central nervous system; *DTs,* delirium tremens; *IM,* intramuscularly; *IV,* intravenously.

ACUTE ALCOHOLISM

A. Description: large alcohol intake in a short time
B. Assessment
   1. Alcohol on breath
   2. Slurring of speech
   3. Ataxia
   4. Agitation
   5. Belligerence
   6. Vomiting
   7. Drowsiness to stuporous state to unconsciousness
   8. Respiratory failure
   9. Death
C. Interventions
   1. Protect airway.
   2. Observe for respiratory depression.
   3. Monitor cardiac status.
   4. Assess for head injury.
D. Usual medical care
   1. Hydration
   2. Vitamin supplements
   3. High-protein diet
   4. Anticonvulsants to control or prevent seizures

MILD ALCOHOL WITHDRAWAL

A. Assessment
   1. Nausea and vomiting
   2. Shaking
   3. Headache
   4. Ataxia
B. Interventions
   1. Rest
   2. Quiet environment
C. Usual medical care
   1. Analgesics
   2. Hydration

DELIRIUM TREMENS

A. Assessment
   1. Tachycardia
   2. Insomnia
   3. Hypertension
   4. Tremors
   5. Anxiety
   6. Hallucinations (auditory, visual, tactile, [rarely] olfactory)
   7. Disorientation
   8. Amnesia
   9. Seizures
B. Interventions
   1. Ensure adequate airway and ventilation.
   2. Treat for shock.
   3. Hydrate.
   4. Monitor vital signs.
   5. Provide crisis counseling.
C. Usual medical care
   1. Treatment for seizures
   2. Anticonvulsant drugs
   3. IV therapy
   4. Sedation
   5. Vitamin therapy
   6. High-protein diet

DISULFIRAM (ANTABUSE) REACTIONS

A. Assessment
   1. Nausea and vomiting
   2. Diaphoresis
   3. Hypotension
   4. Consciousness alterations
   5. Tachycardia
   6. Headache
   7. Facial flushing
   8. Reddened conjunctiva
B. Interventions
   1. Ensure adequate circulation, airway, and breathing.
   2. Administer oxygen.
C. Usual medical care
   1. IV therapy
   2. Diphenhydramine hydrochloride (Benadryl)
   3. Chlorpheniramine maleate (Chlor-Trimeton)
   4. Ascorbic acid

SEXUAL ASSAULT

A. Examine and treat victim as quickly as possible.
B. Notify law enforcement.
C. Do not leave victim alone.
D. Ask victim who he or she wishes to have stay with him or her; offer to call family member, friend, or rape crisis center advocate.
E. Provide immediate privacy.
F. Kindness and support are crucial.
G. Obtain history.
H. Assess acuteness of physical and psychological needs.
I. Assess victim's readiness for physical examination.
J. Explain all procedures and encourage questions.
K. Obtain necessary written permissions, including consent to take photographs.
L. Assist victim in undressing.
M. Observe for and ask about other possible injuries.
N. Assist with physician's examination.
  1. A water-moistened speculum is used.
  2. History indicates the body orifices from which specimens for semen analysis are required.
  3. Pubic hair is combed for foreign hairs.
  4. Clothing is usually saved for analysis, and replacement clothing is necessary; save in paper rather than plastic bags, which retain moisture that can cause evidence to deteriorate.
  5. Follow protocol for collection of specimens that will be used as evidence.
  6. Testing is done for sexually transmitted diseases (STDs), including HIV; follow-up testing is done at appropriate intervals.
  7. Administer STD prophylaxis.
  8. Administer pregnancy prophylaxis if contraception was not in effect at time of attack. The "morning after" pill (norgestrel [Ovral]), a combination of estrogen and progesterone, is given within 72 hours of sexual assault; treatment and side effects should be explained thoroughly.
  9. If possible and desired, offer accommodations for bathing and douching.
  10. Care for tissue trauma: immediate and follow-up.
  11. Care for psychological trauma: immediate and follow-up.
  12. If present, family and friends often require assistance and counseling.

DISASTER

A. Definition: catastrophic event
  1. Natural (e.g., flood, earthquake, hurricane)
  2. Man-made (e.g., riot, fire, train accident, terrorist attack; bioterrorism with anthrax or sarin)
B. May involve as few as 10 or more than 100 victims
C. Prevention
  1. Community planning
  2. Public education
D. Assessment
  1. Civilian triage: care priority to people whose lives are threatened
  2. Military triage: care priority to people most likely to survive

E. Planning: most capable person designated to sort casualties
F. Interventions
  1. First aid should be rendered before victims are transported.
  2. Care priorities
    a. Ensure airway, breathing, and circulation.
    b. Control bleeding.
    c. Treat for shock.
  3. Medical interventions
    a. Whole blood
    b. IV fluids
    c. Parenteral medications; treatment of bioterrorism dependent on causative agent
    d. Pain relief
    e. Emergency wound care
      (1) Preserve motor and sensory functioning.
      (2) Provide psychological support.
      (3) Treat and transport.
G. The purpose of medical and nursing care during a disaster is to assess the injured, provide immediate treatment to stabilize the patient, and transport to a medical facility for further intervention.

Bibliography

American Heart Association: *BLS for Healthcare Providers*, Dallas, TX, 2011, American Heart Association.

American Heart Association: *Heartsaver First Aid CPR AED*, Dallas, TX, 2011, American Heart Association.

Christensen BL, Kockrow EO: *Foundations and adult health nursing*, ed 6, St Louis, 2010, Mosby.

Emergency Nurse's Association: *Sheehy's manual of emergency care*, ed 7, St Louis, 2013, Mosby.

Fultz J, Sturt PA: *Mosby's emergency nursing reference*, ed 3, St Louis, 2005, Mosby.

Monahan FD, et al: *Phipps' medical-surgical nursing: health and illness perspectives*, ed 8, St Louis, 2007, Mosby.

Monahan FD, Green C, Neighbors M: *Swearingen's manual of medical-surgical nursing: a care planning resource*, ed 7, 2011, Mosby.

Mosby's dictionary of medicine, nursing, and health professions, ed 9, St Louis, 2013, Mosby.

Potter PA, et al: *Fundamentals of nursing*, ed 8, St Louis, 2013, Mosby.

Price DL, Gwin JF: *Pediatric nursing: an introductory text*, ed 11, St Louis, 2012, Saunders.

Proehl J: *Emergency nursing procedures*, ed 4, St Louis, 2009, Saunders.

Roth J, Berman S: *Status epilepticus treatment and management*, Available at: http://emedicine.medscape.com/article/1164462-treatment#a1126. Retrieved July 17, 2012.

Skidmore-Roth L: *Mosby's 2013 nursing drug reference*, St Louis, 2013, Mosby.

REVIEW QUESTIONS

1. An individual developed an airway obstruction while eating dinner at a restaurant. After attempts to dislodge the obstruction failed, the victim became unconscious. As a nurse, you know the next action to take is:
  1. Open the airway and attempt to deliver two breaths.
  2. Check for pulse and if absent, begin compressions.
  3. Place individual in supine position and begin compressions.
  4. Straddle the individual's body and begin abdominal thrusts.

2. The nurse knows that a patient with epistaxis could have respiratory compromise caused by aspirated blood. To avoid this complication, the nurse would position the patient:
   1. In a prone position with the head elevated.
   2. Leaning forward with direct pressure on the nose.
   3. Sitting straight up with the head tilted backward.
   4. On the side with ice compresses to the back of the neck.

3. The mother of a pediatric patient states that the child began to have difficulty breathing after eating a peanut butter sandwich. The child is now hypotensive, dyspneic, and restless. The nurse recognizes these as symptoms of:
   1. Folic acid deficiency.
   2. Anaphylaxis.
   3. Electrolyte imbalance.
   4. Inborn error of metabolism.

4. A patient is brought to the emergency department after falling from a ladder and sustaining a fracture of the left leg. The nurse observes that the skin is broken and part of the bone fragment is visible. The appropriate intervention is to:
   1. Immobilize the leg and cover the open wound.
   2. Apply traction to the leg to attempt to reduce the fracture.
   3. Elevate the leg as high as possible with pillows.
   4. Apply an adduction pillow between the patient's knees.

5. The nurse receives a telephone call from a neighbor whose husband collapsed while mowing the lawn. He is described as being dizzy, confused, clammy, and nauseated. The nurse should instruct the wife to:
   1. Encourage the patient to ambulate vigorously to stimulate circulation.
   2. Have the patient drink saltwater to replace fluids lost through vomiting and diaphoresis.
   3. Leave the patient in the position in which he was found and apply blankets.
   4. Move the patient to a cool, quiet area, and loosen his clothing.

6. A man who was rescued from drowning was brought to the emergency department for follow-up. The nurse should assess and observe for:
   1. Pulmonary edema.
   2. Ketoacidosis.
   3. Fluid and electrolyte imbalance.
   4. Left shift.

7. A patient who is being evaluated and treated for delirium tremens should undergo:
   1. Nutritional assessment.
   2. Seizure Precautions.
   3. Range-of-motion activities.
   4. Universal Precautions.

8. A firefighter who was brought to the emergency department for evaluation after an accident in a factory insists that he is not injured and wants to wait until other victims are treated before being seen by the physician. The nurse observes that he has singed nasal hair and a brassy cough and recognizes that he is at risk now for:
   1. Pulmonary edema as a result of smoke inhalation.
   2. Respiratory infection caused by exposure to toxic chemicals.
   3. Esophageal reflux as a result of irritation of the oropharynx.
   4. Increased sputum production related to oxygen deprivation.

9. A marathoner comes to the emergency department reporting the sudden onset of sharp chest pain and difficulty breathing during his usual daily workout. Chest excursion on the affected side is reduced. The nurse assesses him for:
   1. Muscle strain.
   2. Respiratory infection.
   3. Spontaneous pneumothorax.
   4. Myocardial infarction.

10. To preserve possible evidence, clothing from a sexual assault victim is stored in:
    1. Airtight plastic bags.
    2. Cloth bags with drawstrings.
    3. Nonconductive plastic bags.
    4. Paper bags sealed with tape.

11. An individual arrives in the emergency room after having been found in hypovolemic shock. Emergency medical technicians (EMTs) arrive at the scene and intubate the patient, start an intravenous infusion, and obtain an electrocardiogram (ECG). The receiving nurse in the emergency department knows that one of the first tests to be performed is/are which of the following?
    1. Complete blood count (CBC) to rule out leukopenia.
    2. Liver function tests (LFTs) to rule out cirrhosis.
    3. Hemoglobin and hematocrit (H&H) and electrolytes to rule out anemia and dehydration.
    4. Glucose to rule out hypoglycemia.

12. A patient who has been in a motorcycle accident states that he is experiencing pain in his neck, numbness and tingling in his legs, and weakness on his left side. The nurse should:
    1. Remove his helmet as quickly as possible.
    2. Ask him to remove his helmet.
    3. Leave his helmet in place until assistance is available to remove it.
    4. Secure the helmet in place with adhesive tape.

13. A patient is brought to the emergency department after experiencing a sudden onset of sharp chest pain at home. He is now pale and tachycardic, and he is wheezing and coughing up small amounts of blood. The nurse assesses him for:
    1. Myocardial infarction.
    2. Pulmonary embolus.
    3. Tension pneumothorax.
    4. Pneumonia.

14. A nurse sees a motorcycle rider struck by a car and stops at the scene. The patient is alert, complains of inability to move his legs, and has his helmet still in place. The nurse's next action should be to:
    1. Assess the patient and call 911.
    2. Elevate his legs with his helmet after carefully removing it from his head.
    3. Refrain from helping because of legal concerns.
    4. Begin CPR.

15. A patient on a medical unit complains of sudden chest pain. She has shortness of breath and a heart rate of 110 beats/min. The nurse hears no breath sounds on the patient's right side. The patient, who appears to have a simple pneumothorax, should be placed:
    1. On her affected side with pillows to support her.
    2. Supine with her feet elevated 30 degrees.
    3. Prone with her arms raised over her head.
    4. In semi-Fowler position.

16. A motor vehicle accident (MVA) victim has a hoarse voice, subcutaneous emphysema, cough with hemoptysis, and respiratory distress. The nurse should prepare him for an immediate:
    1. Blood transfusion.
    2. Computed tomography or magnetic resonance imaging scan.
    3. Cricothyrotomy or tracheostomy.
    4. Intubation.

17. A patient in the emergency room is having an anaphylactic reaction to an antibiotic she took approximately 1 hour ago. She is awake and alert but in clear respiratory distress. Her BP is 170/98, pulse is 110, and respirations are 24 with audible wheezing. The nurse knows the first intervention is to:
    1. Apply oxygen
    2. Administer albuterol inhaler
    3. Administer Benadryl PO
    4. Administer adrenaline

18. While shopping for groceries, the nurse witnesses an adult shopper fall to the ground. The patient is assessed and found to be without pulse or respirations. The nurse begins CPR by placing his hands on the sternum to begin compressions at a depth of:
    1. Approximately 1 inch.
    2. Approximately $1\frac{1}{2}$ inches.
    3. Approximately 2 inches.
    4. Minimum of 2 inches.

19. A 36-year-old man is brought to the emergency department with a diagnosis of morphine overdose. The first medication the nurse would expect to administer in his treatment should be:
    1. Disulfiram (Antabuse).
    2. Epinephrine (Adrenalin).
    3. Methylprednisolone (Solu-Medrol).
    4. Naloxone (Narcan).

20. A 23-year-old patient is brought to the hospital in an agitated state and is hyperventilating. She has an elevated blood pressure and a temperature of 100.1 ° F (37.8 ° C). She is hallucinating. The nurse should suspect that the patient has taken:
    1. Inhalants.
    2. Stimulants.
    3. Depressants.
    4. Cannabis.

21. An older woman with diabetes is brought to the hospital by a neighbor who is concerned about a change in her level of consciousness and activity. The patient admits that she does not remember when she last ate or took her insulin. In addition to measuring her blood glucose, the nurse should also check the patient's level of:
    1. Potassium.
    2. Hemoglobin.
    3. Protein.
    4. Estrogen.

22. A man is brought to the hospital after having been in a house fire. He is burned over all of his chest and his right leg. Using the rule of nines, the nurse estimates that the burned percentage of his body is:
    1. 25% to 30%.
    2. 1% to 5%.
    3. 0% to 15%.
    4. 75% to 80%.

23. A patient arrives in the emergency department with a fractured left wrist. The complaint that is the most likely to indicate serious injury and must be addressed first is:
    1. Pain in the affected wrist.
    2. Swelling in the fingers.
    3. Bruising in the hand and arm.
    4. Numbness in the fingers.

24. A firefighter is brought to the hospital by ambulance from the scene of a factory explosion where he was burned and also sustained a severe laceration to his lower right leg. His heart rate is 112 beats/min, respirations are 78 and shallow, and blood pressure is 72/40 mm Hg. The nurse recognizes that the patient is in:
    1. Hypovolemic shock.
    2. Neurogenic shock.
    3. Septic shock.
    4. Cardiogenic shock.

25. The usual medical intervention for an orally ingested drug overdose is:
    1. Lavage with normal saline.
    2. Gavage with activated charcoal.
    3. Emesis induced by paregoric.
    4. Intravenous (IV) normal saline by bolus.

26. A patient with a history of alcohol abuse is brought to the emergency department with vomiting, hypotension, and facial flushing. The nurse prepares to administer:
    1. Diphenhydramine (Benadryl) to sedate the patient, who is having delirium tremens.
    2. Naloxone (Narcan) to reverse the narcotic effect of ethanol ingestion.
    3. Normal saline fluid challenge because the patient is dehydrated from vomiting.
    4. Chlorpheniramine maleate (Chlor-Trimeton) to counteract the reaction to disulfiram (Antabuse).

27. A surgical patient who has been in the hospital for 3 days begins to have symptoms of tremors, anxiety, and hallucinations. The nurse institutes precautions for:
    1. Aspiration of emesis.
    2. Seizures related to alcohol withdrawal.
    3. Falling caused by unstable gait.
    4. Elopement caused by anxiety and disorientation.

28. A patient with insulin-dependent diabetes is brought to the emergency department with a blood glucose of 680 mg/dL. The nurse prepares an IV infusion of:
    1. 50% glucose.
    2. Normal saline.
    3. 5% dextrose.
    4. Mannitol.

29. A hiker is brought to the emergency department after having been bitten on his lower leg by a snake. The nurse immobilizes the affected limb and:
    1. Places it in a dependent position.
    2. Elevates it on two pillows.
    3. Places warm moist packs on it.
    4. Cleans it vigorously with antimicrobial soap.

30. A spill of powdered chemicals occurs at a factory, and one of the employees is contaminated with the substance. Before he is transported to the emergency department, the contaminant should be:
    1. Flushed from his skin with running water for at least 10 minutes.
    2. Contained by applying dry dressings to the affected skin.

3. Swept from the skin with a dry dressing.

4. Neutralized with petroleum jelly.

31. A man who was involved in an MVA insists that he is "only bruised" and does not want to be admitted to the hospital for observation. The nurse observes that he has decreased chest wall stability and suspects several fractured ribs. She tells him:
   1. "You can go home if you promise to come back if you start having trouble breathing."
   2. "You may have injuries to your lungs or heart as a result of rib fractures. Staying here would provide you with critical immediate treatment should problems with pain or breathing occur."
   3. "You probably don't have anything seriously wrong, but it would be a good idea to stay anyway."
   4. "You will have to sign this form stating that you are leaving against medical advice."

32. A patient who was severely injured in a fall from a scaffold is concerned about how much of his independent function he will be able to regain. The nurse knows that his injury is at the T7 level. She would expect that the patient may:
   1. Be ventilator dependent for life.
   2. Have paraplegia and partial loss of independence.
   3. Not have any problems because the injury is so low in the spinal cord.
   4. Have flaccid paralysis in all extremities.

33. A patient with a myocardial infarction is clammy, tachycardic, and disoriented. The nurse recognizes that he has shock that is described as:
   1. Vasogenic.
   2. Cardiogenic.
   3. Distributive.
   4. Hypovolemic.

34. A 10-year-old boy is stabbed on the school playground. By the time the school nurse reaches him, he is pale, cyanotic, and diaphoretic and has a pulse of 120 beats/min. The nurse's highest priority action is to:
   1. Administer fluid boluses to maintain blood pressure.
   2. Cover him with a blanket or jacket to maintain his body temperature.
   3. Establish and maintain a patent airway.
   4. Apply pressure to the bleeding wound.

35. A 3-year-old boy was bitten by another child at his daycare center. In giving discharge instructions, the nurse includes information about:
   1. Contacting an attorney.
   2. Administering the full dose of the prescribed antibiotic.
   3. Waking the child every hour through the night to make sure he can be roused.
   4. Making sure that the child has a fluid intake of at least 700 mL over the next 24 hours.

36. A 26-year-old woman is being examined for complaints of right lower-quadrant abdominal pain. She is febrile and has a white blood cell count of $26,000/mm^3$. In responding to her request for something cold to drink, the nurse replies:
   1. "It would be better for you to have a hot beverage right now."
   2. "You can have plain water but no ice."
   3. "Given that you may go to surgery in the very near future, you must refrain from drinking anything right now."
   4. "How about a nice cold soft drink?"

37. A 36-year-old sexual assault survivor is brought to the emergency department for examination and treatment. For the prevention of pregnancy, the nurse prepares to administer:
   1. Cefixime (Suprax).
   2. Norethindrone and mestranol (Ortho-Novum).
   3. Estrogen and progesterone (Ovral).
   4. Doxycycline (Vibramycin).

38. The police brought a 43-year-old man who is having tremors, intestinal cramps, chills, and sweating to the emergency department. His eyes are watery, and his nose is runny. The nurse suspects:
   1. Overdose of narcotics.
   2. Withdrawal from narcotics.
   3. Overdose of stimulants.
   4. Withdrawal from stimulants.

39. A 2-year-old boy is brought to the emergency department after a bee sting. He is wheezing and has urticaria and diffuse erythema. The nurse, recognizing that an allergic reaction can progress rapidly, should:
   1. Ensure adequate airway and ventilation.
   2. Apply cold packs to the affected area for comfort.
   3. Administer antibiotics to prevent infection.
   4. Administer steroids and antihistamines to counteract swelling.

40. A 46-year-old man diagnosed with a pulmonary embolus is waiting for treatment. The nurse should prepare to administer what type of medication?
   1. Antiarrhythmic
   2. Anticonvulsant
   3. Anticoagulant
   4. Antipsychotic

41. A 36-year-old woman receiving antibiotic therapy for a gram-negative infection comes to the emergency department complaining of weakness, restlessness, and thirst. The vital sign assessment reveals a temperature of 103.8° F (39.9° C). The nurse recognizes that this patient is likely experiencing:
   1. Anaphylactic shock
   2. Neurogenic shock.
   3. Septic shock.
   4. Anxiety reaction.

42. Assessment of a trauma patient reveals that his chest moves inward with inhalation and outward with exhalation. The nurse recognizes this as a sign of:
   1. Flail chest.
   2. Pulmonary embolus.
   3. Simple rib fracture.
   4. Tension pneumothorax.

43. The nurse knows that she has been successful in teaching a patient admitted for treatment of chilblain when the patient states:
   1. "I should rub my toes and fingers until they warm up."
   2. "I should avoid cigarettes because of the effects on circulation."
   3. "This will spread to my whole body if I'm not careful."
   4. "I inherited this tendency from my father."

44. A trauma patient with an abdominal stab wound is brought by ambulance to the emergency department. Inspection reveals that a loop of bowel is protruding from the wound. The nurse's priority action is to:
   1. Administer oxygen by nasal mask.
   2. Administer tetanus toxoid injection.

3. Apply wet dressings to the wound site.
4. Apply a pressure dressing to the wound after replacing the bowel.

45. The wife of a patient who is being treated for burns is alarmed that his urine appears reddish brown in the drainage bag. The nurse explains to her that this is most likely the result of damage to his:
   1. Kidney.
   2. Muscle tissue.
   3. Skin.
   4. Urethra.

46. A mother reports that she allowed her two small children to eat raw dough containing eggs when she was making cookies yesterday. Last night they began to have severe stomach cramps, headaches, and fever. The nurse tells the mother:
   1. "This may be *Salmonella* poisoning from eating uncooked eggs."
   2. "This may be an allergic reaction to an ingredient in the recipe."
   3. "This is probably the flu that has been going around."
   4. "This sounds like trichinosis poisoning from eating undercooked dough."

47. After an earthquake the victim who would be triaged with the highest priority is a(n):
   1. Crying 4-year-old boy with a bleeding head laceration.
   2. Dazed 26-year-old woman with a broken right arm.
   3. Unresponsive 48-year-old man with contusions of the head.
   4. Alert 70-year-old woman with diabetes who has burns of both arms.

48. A 52-year-old dockworker comes to the emergency department complaining of severe crushing chest pain radiating to his left arm. He is cool, pale, and diaphoretic. The nurse recognizes that these might be signs of a myocardial infarction. The first intervention would be to:
   1. Apply electrodes for the cardiac monitor.
   2. Administer nitroglycerin sublingually.
   3. Administer oxygen at 5 L/min by mask.
   4. Insert a large-bore IV line and begin a normal saline infusion.

49. The victim of a motor vehicle accident is brought to the emergency department and diagnosed with an unstable fracture of the pelvis. The nurse should report to the physician the presence of:
   1. Nausea and vomiting.
   2. External rotation of the lower extremities.
   3. Pain in the lower extremities.
   4. Increasing tenderness over the symphysis pubis.

50. A construction worker without a hardhat on was injured when he was hit on the head by falling lumber. He is bleeding profusely from the laceration on his scalp. The nurse's priority is to:
   1. Flush the wound with normal saline until it appears to be free of debris.
   2. Scrub the wound with 4×4 gauze dressings and antiseptic skin cleanser.
   3. Control bleeding and cover the open wound with a clean, nonadhesive dressing until it is examined by a physician.
   4. Apply antibiotic ointment to the wound and apply a pressure dressing.

51. A vital nursing intervention for a patient who was burned over 70% of the body with second- and third-degree injury would be to:
   1. Establish and maintain an airway.
   2. Establish and maintain vascular access.
   3. Establish and maintain a sterile environment.
   4. Establish a medical history.

52. A short-term goal for a rape survivor who is being treated in the emergency department would be to:
   1. Initiate social interaction with friends and co-workers.
   2. Express feelings about the event.
   3. Return to pretrauma level of functioning.
   4. Verbalize two methods of stress management.

53. A 32-year-old person with insulin-dependent diabetes comes to the emergency department with a blood-glucose-by-finger stick of 46 mg/dL. The nurse expects to see which symptom?
   1. Fruity acetone breath
   2. Complaints of hunger
   3. Dry, warm skin
   4. Kussmaul respirations

54. On the way to work a nurse encounters a motor vehicle accident with multiple trauma victims. The nurse would know to provide immediate care to the individual experiencing:
   1. Hemorrhage.
   2. Altered level of consciousness.
   3. Cyanosis of nail beds.
   4. Obvious fracture of the femur.

55. A patient called 911 after falling down with a headache, dizziness, and nausea. The ambulance personnel found him unconscious but breathing. They suspect that the victim was overcome by carbon monoxide from a faulty furnace. Initial treatment for this patient may include oxygen administration at:
   1. 2 L/min via nasal cannula.
   2. 5 L/min via nasal cannula.
   3. 40% by face mask.
   4. 100% by face mask.

56. For the first 24 hours after sustaining an eyelid contusion (black eye), the patient should apply:
   1. Continuous warm, moist packs.
   2. Intermittent cold packs.
   3. Continuous cold packs.
   4. Intermittent warm, moist packs.

57. To establish an airway in a patient with possible neck or spine injuries, the nurse uses the:
   1. Head tilt–chin lift.
   2. Head tilt–jaw thrust.
   3. Chin lift only.
   4. Jaw thrust only.

58. A patient who hit her head on the windshield in a motor vehicle accident has fixed, dilated pupils and a positive Babinski sign. The nurse recognizes that these signs indicate:
   1. Intracranial bleeding.
   2. Internal bleeding.
   3. Spinal cord injury.
   4. Meningitis.

59. A lineman sustained electrical burns on both hands when he fell from a utility pole. His wife says that his burns do

not appear to be too serious. The nurse should explain to her why these burns are considered to be:
1. Superficial.
2. Minor.
3. Moderate.
4. Major.

60. In addition to inspecting the site of a penetrating wound, the nurse should also assess for a(n):
1. Foreign body such as a bullet.
2. Exit wound.
3. Medical information tag.
4. Concealed weapon.

61. Which are considered to be major or critical burns? Select all that apply.
_____1. Burns caused by electrical trauma
_____2. Full-thickness burns that are less than 10% of body surface area (BSA)
_____3. Burns in patients with preexisting chronic conditions
_____4. Partial-thickness burns that are greater than 20% of BSA in children younger than 10 years
_____5. Burns on face, hands, or perineum

62. The nurse notes that the patient admitted with burns has the following areas indicated on the rule of nines diagram:
Frontal aspect of the right arm
Frontal aspect of the left arm
Right anterior chest wall
The approximate amount of body surface area involved in this injury is:
Answer: _____ %

63. In performing one-rescuer CPR on an adult, the rate of chest compressions per minute is a minimum of:
1. 70
2. 80.
3. 90.
4. 100.

64. A patient caught the sleeve of her robe on fire while cooking breakfast. She is an 85-year-old woman with insulin-dependent diabetes. She has superficial burns over 5% of her arm. This injury is classified as:
1. Minor.
2. Moderate.
3. Major.
4. Superficial.

65. A young man has been diagnosed with a strain to his left ankle sustained when he tripped on a rock while he was jogging. The nurse should instruct him to do which of the following? Select all that apply.
_____1. Place his foot on the floor to stabilize the ankle.
_____2. Soak his ankle in warm water with Epsom salts.
_____3. Use crutches to avoid weight bearing.
_____4. Exercise the foot to reduce the chance for stiffening of the joints.
_____5. Ice the affected area, and elevate.

66. What does the nurse focus on when assessing a recent fracture? Select all that apply.
_____1. Pain
_____2. Purulence
_____3. Pallor
_____4. Pulses
_____5. Paresthesia

67. A patient who has been hemorrhaging from a severe injury is becoming restless, anxious, and clammy. The nurse recognizes that this indicates possible progression to:
1. Shock.
2. Sepsis.
3. Sedation.
4. Syndactyly.

68. A 14-year-old football player arrives at the doctor's office with his mother. The mother states she was contacted by the coach because the teenager was tackled during practice and hit his head. In addition to a neurological assessment, the nurse would expect the physician to:
1. Instruct the mother to wake her son every 2 hours to prevent concussion.
2. Administer ibuprofen for pain control.
3. Instruct the patient and mother to avoid strenuous activity for 2 weeks, including reading, playing video games, and watching television.
4. Administer Decadron to decrease risk of intracranial swelling.

69. A 34-year-old man was working in his garage when he accidentally impaled his hand on a screwdriver. He was brought to the emergency room with a towel wrapped around his hand, and the towel is now soaked in blood. The nurse should treat the wound by:
1. Removing the screwdriver immediately to prevent further tissue damage.
2. Removing the screwdriver after flushing the area with normal saline for 5 minutes.
3. Leaving the screwdriver in place to control bleeding.
4. Leaving the screwdriver in place as long as the patient is not in pain.

70. A 76-year-old man is admitted to the hospital with a cerebrovascular accident. The patient's wife is concerned because his daily aspirin regimen has not been included in his medication orders. As you review the patient's testing, the nurse should expect to find:
1. The patient had an ischemic stroke.
2. The patient had a hemorrhagic stroke.
3. The patient developed a paralytic ileus.
4. The patient developed diplopia.

71. A patient with a tension pneumothorax complains of increased pain and dyspnea; his heart rate has increased to 100 beats/min. The nurse recognizes that this may be the result of:
1. Coarctation of the aorta.
2. Cardiac tamponade.
3. Vasovagal response.
4. Mediastinal shift.

72. An elderly woman who was brought to the emergency department from her nursing home experienced sudden, sharp chest pain with shortness of breath and pallor. She is very anxious; her heart rate is 112 beats/min, and her respiratory rate is 28 breaths/min. The nurse should explain to her that, to confirm the physician's diagnosis of possible pulmonary embolism, she will have a:
1. Chest x-ray examination.
2. Bronchoscopy.
3. Ventilation-perfusion ($\dot{V}/\dot{Q}$) scan.
4. Lung biopsy.

73. A child is brought to the emergency department by his mother after he lacerated his scalp in a fall. She is very

anxious about the amount of blood that is oozing from his head. The nurse explains to the mother that bright red blood signals that this type of bleeding is:
1. Capillary.
2. Venous.
3. Arterial.
4. Afferent.

74. In a conscious infant who loses consciousness, removing a foreign body from his airway should entail:
1. Shining an examination light into the mouth to visualize the object.
2. Vigorous finger sweeps to palpate the object.
3. Removing the object only if it is visible.
4. Applying pressure on the cricoid cartilage to expel the object.

75. In triage of a disaster event, the civilian priority is care to the victims who:
1. Are most likely to survive.
2. Have children.
3. Have the least serious wounds and can be cared for quickly.
4. Have the most serious, life-threatening injuries.

76. A 3-year-old child is brought to the emergency department after a motor vehicle accident. She has a scalp laceration that is oozing blood; pain, discoloration, and swelling of her right lower arm; and right-sided chest pain that increases on inspiration. The nursing actions with the highest priority are:
1. Administration of analgesic medication and tetanus toxoid.
2. Immobilization and elevation of the right arm.
3. Assessment and maintenance of airway and adequate ventilation.
4. Application of ice packs and pressure dressings to the scalp laceration.

77. A victim of domestic violence is brought to the emergency department by the police. She is complaining of abdominal pain where she was struck forcibly with a baseball bat. On examination, she is found to have guarding, diminished bowel sounds, and bruising on the abdomen. The nurse explains to her that she may undergo which procedure?
1. Peritoneal lavage
2. Gastric lavage
3. Barium enema
4. Abdominal MRI

78. A nurse arrives at the scene of a motor vehicle accident and quickly assesses the injured parties. The priority care should be given to the:
1. Driver with a head laceration and severe knee pain.
2. Passenger with a bleeding nose who is complaining of a headache.
3. Driver with a hoarse voice who is coughing blood.
4. Passenger with an arm laceration who is crying hysterically.

79. During afternoon rounds the nurse discovers a 60-year-old patient with diabetes unconscious on the floor near his bed. The nurse's immediate action should be to:
1. Call the physician and prepare intravenous glucose.
2. Assess for breathing and circulation.
3. Check the blood glucose and administer regular insulin.
4. Check for medical alert identification and call the family.

80. A 79-year-old woman comes to the urgent care clinic complaining of nausea, headache, and muscle cramping. She reports that she was in the garden all afternoon weeding. She is anxious and pale. The nurse's first action should be to:
1. Move the patient to a cool, quiet room.
2. Administer a bolus of normal saline intravenously.
3. Encourage the patient to drink 1 L of water with 2 tablespoons of table salt dissolved in it.
4. Apply ice packs to facilitate rapid cooling.

81. A 46-year-old man who was shoveling his driveway all morning is brought to the urgent care clinic by his wife. The nurse notes that his toes are numb, discolored, and blistered. She explains to them that these signs indicate:
1. Immersion foot.
2. Chilblain.
3. Frostbite.
4. Hypothermia.

82. What would care of the patient with a gunshot injury include? Select all that apply.
_____1. Documenting the exact location of the wound
_____2. Recording the number of wounds
_____3. Placing the patient's clothing in a paper or plastic bag and securing it for the police
_____4. Placing paper bags over hands to protect evidence of gunshot residue

83. An ambulatory patient enters the emergency department after exposure to a toxic substance. Place the steps in the process of decontamination of the victim in order of priority from first step to last.
1. Place the patient's valuables in a plastic zipper bag, label, and give to the patient.
2. Brush off visible dry material from the patient or patient's clothing.
3. Remove patient's clothing.
4. Use a paper towel or diaper to absorb blistering agents.

84. A 49-year-old patient was brought to the emergency department by a friend. The patient was complaining of cough, dyspnea, and aching chest pain. On auscultation the nurse notes a grating sound on inspiration that is similar to pieces of leather rubbing together. The nurse recognizes this to be an abnormal breath sound called:
1. Egophony.
2. Bronchovesicular.
3. Pleural friction rub.
4. Crackles.

85. The goal of pulmonary edema management is to increase oxygenation, decrease cardiac workload, and optimize cardiac function. The nursing interventions that can meet this goal include:
1. Keeping the patient supine and elevating the lower extremities 12 inches.
2. Placing the patient in high-Fowler position and administering oxygen therapy.
3. Giving a chewable children's aspirin.
4. Offering the patient a hot beverage such as coffee or tea.

86. A 72-year-old biker is brought into the urgent care center after complaining of headache pain and vertigo. The nurse assesses the patient and finds unequal hand grips, with the left hand weaker than the right and an unequal

smile. The patient cannot puff out his cheeks bilaterally. The nurse knows that these may be symptoms of:
1. Hyperglycemic reaction.
2. Pulmonary emboli.
3. Cerebrovascular accident.
4. Rheumatoid arthritis.

87. A 22-month-old is brought to the emergency department with multiple white pustules covering the chest and face. The physician has made the diagnosis of smallpox. The nurse would follow which bioterrorism infection control practices for patient management? Select all that apply.
_____1. Contact Precautions
_____2. Semiprivate room with the door opened
_____3. Airborne precautions with an N95 mask
_____4. Discharge of the toddler after 72 hours of antibiotic therapy
_____5. No restrictions relating to patient transport

88. That further education of a new staff member is necessary regarding assessment of breath sounds is indicated by which statement?
1. "A wheeze can indicate partial obstruction of the bronchi."
2. "Crackles may be caused by early congestive heart failure."
3. "Rhonchi suggest a pneumothorax."
4. "I will auscultate the breath sounds using the diaphragm of the stethoscope."

89. Select all clinical manifestations of intestinal trauma.
_____1. Rebound tenderness
_____2. Hypoactive bowel sounds
_____3. Joint pain
_____4. Abdominal guarding
_____5. Hemiparesis

90. Rabies is transmitted to humans through a bite from an infected animal. The causative agent is a:
1. Bacterium.
2. Fungus.
3. Virus.
4. Helminth.

91. Select all that apply to anaphylactic shock.
_____1. It is a severe allergic reaction.
_____2. It is a profound antibody response to an antigen.
_____3. It causes increased capillary permeability and angioedema.
_____4. It is caused by an overwhelming bacterial infection.
_____5. It causes bloody stools.

92. Acidosis is indicated on arterial blood gas (ABG) measurement by a pH of:
1. 7.40.
2. 7.55.
3. 7.1.
4. 7.36.

93. Select all that apply to cardiogenic shock.
_____1. It often leads to death within 24 hours.
_____2. It decreases cardiac output.
_____3. It lowers blood pressure.
_____4. It results in decreased oxygen to the tissues.
_____5. It causes an increase in urinary output.

94. Which sign or symptom should the nurse look for in a patient diagnosed with diazepam (Valium) overdose?
1. Pinpoint pupils
2. Respiratory depression

3. Convulsions
4. Acute psychosis

95. A nurse who works in the emergency department administers 4 units of Humulin (human) regular insulin to a patient with a blood glucose of 368 mg/dL. The nurse explains to the patient that the onset of action of regular insulin is:
1. 4 to 8 hours.
2. 2 to 5 hours.
3. 10 to 12 hours.
4. ½ to 1 hour.

96. Hemophilia is a congenital disorder that can result in:
1. Bleeding into the tissue spaces.
2. Blood clotting in the peripheral vessels.
3. Fluid entering the pleura.
4. Deformity of the spine.

97. A bite from a brown recluse spider produces the following local reactions. Select all that apply.
_____1. A blue ring around the bite site
_____2. Edema and blistering 2 to 8 hours after the bite
_____3. A stinging sensation that may go unnoticed
_____4. Muscle spasms
_____5. Seizures

98. The nurse knows that the hepatitis C virus attacks the liver and can cause cancer and death. Transmission of hepatitis C can occur through which of the following? Select all that apply.
_____1. Needle sharing
_____2. Kissing and hugging
_____3. Body piercing with a contaminated needle
_____4. Drinking glass
_____5. Uncooked meat

99. A 90-year-old patient who resides in a nursing home falls and sustains a left hip fracture of the acetabulum, greater trochanter, and femoral head. The nurse knows that the symptoms of hip fracture may include which of the following? Select all that apply.
_____1. Trousseau sign
_____2. Severe pain with movement of the limb
_____3. External rotation of the limb
_____4. Fever and night sweats
_____5. Lengthening of the affected limb

100. A symptom of hyperkalemia may include:
1. Abdominal cramping with diarrhea.
2. Hypothermia.
3. Polydipsia.
4. Polyphagia.

ANSWERS AND RATIONALES

1. Comprehension, implementation, safe and effective care environment, (a).
   3. According to American Heart Association 2011 guidelines, relieving choking in an individual who is conscious and becomes unconscious dictates the initiation of compressions without checking for a pulse.
   1, 2, 4. These are not in accordance with current American Heart Association guidelines.

2. Analysis, implementation, safe and effective care environment, (a).
   2. This position reduces the risk of aspiration of blood.
   1, 3, 4. These positions would increase the risk of aspiration of blood from the nasal hemorrhage.

3. Comprehension, assessment, safe and effective care environment, (b).
   2. *This is characteristic of an anaphylactic reaction, which suggests an allergy to peanuts.*
   1. This is characterized by weakness and confusion.
   3. This is characterized by weakness, confusion, and electrocardiographic changes.
   4. This condition is not characterized by the symptoms the child is having.

4. Comprehension, planning, physiological integrity, (b).
   1. *The bone ends may cause further injury to the surrounding tissue, and this patient has an increased risk of infection.*
   2. Reduction of the fracture will be undertaken later, possibly in surgery.
   3. Moving the leg to elevate it can cause further injury.
   4. Proper immobilization would require the use of splints above and below the fracture site.

5. Comprehension, planning, safe and effective care environment, (b).
   4. *The patient should be removed from the heat and made as comfortable as possible to reduce further illness caused by heat and exertion.*
   1, 3. The patient should not exert himself or be subjected to any more heat.
   2. If the patient is vomiting, nothing should be given by mouth, to prevent aspiration or gastric distention.

6. Analysis, evaluation, physiological integrity, (c).
   1. *The patient is at risk of developing pulmonary edema as a result of the trauma of near drowning.*
   2. Alteration in glucose metabolism is less likely to occur compared with the risk of respiratory distress and pulmonary edema.
   3. Alteration in fluid imbalance is less likely to occur compared with the risk of respiratory distress and pulmonary edema.
   4. Alterations in blood counts are less likely to occur compared with the risk of respiratory distress and pulmonary edema.

7. Application, implementation, safe and effective care environment, (b).
   2. *Seizures are an important risk for the patient in delirium tremens.*
   1, 3, 4. These interventions have low priority for the patient compared with the need for a safe and effective care environment.

8. Comprehension, assessment, physiological integrity, (c).
   1. *Smoke inhalation, as evidenced by brassy cough, singed nasal hairs, and respiratory distress, is a serious complication that can lead to death if left untreated.*
   2. Infection is not an immediate risk.
   3. Gastric distress is not an immediate risk.
   4. Sputum production is not related to oxygen deprivation.

9. Comprehension, assessment, physiological integrity, (b)
   3. *Spontaneous pneumothorax can occur during periods of strenuous activity.*
   1. Muscle strain does not commonly cause sudden pain in the chest.
   2. Infection does not commonly cause sudden pain in the chest.
   4. Myocardial infarction does not typically produce alterations in chest excursion.

10. Comprehension, planning, psychosocial integrity, (b).
    4. *Clothing is placed in paper bags because they do not retain moisture and subsequently cause evidence to deteriorate.*
    1. Plastic can cause moisture to be retained.
    2. Cloth bags are not easy to write on for labeling purposes.
    3. Plastic can cause moisture to be retained.

11. Application, planning, physiological integrity, (b).
    3. *Hemoglobin and hematocrit and electrolytes can identify severe anemia and hypernatremia, which can cause hypovolemic shock.*
    1, 2, 4. These are not causes of hypovolemic shock.

12. Application, implementation, safe and effective care environment, (b).
    3. *To reduce risk of further injury to the patient's cervical spine, the helmet should be removed only when assistance is available to stabilize his neck.*
    1, 2, 4. These actions would increase the risk of further injury to the patient.

13. Analysis, assessment, physiological integrity, (b).
    2. *Pulmonary embolism is characterized by sudden chest pain, hemoptysis, and wheezing. The patient may proceed rapidly to shock and even death if a large blood vessel is blocked.*
    1. Myocardial infarction does not usually produce sharp chest pain and hemoptysis.
    3. Pneumothorax usually produces pain on one side of the chest unless bilateral involvement occurs; it does not usually produce hemoptysis.
    4. Pneumonia usually features chest pain associated with coughing. Hemoptysis is not usually sudden in onset and is related to the trauma of coughing.

14. Application, planning, physiological integrity, (b).
    1. *Rapid entry into the emergency response system is indicated.*
    2. The helmet should not be removed, and the legs should not be moved until qualified medical assistance with proper equipment arrives on the scene.
    3. Rapid entry into the emergency response system is delayed.
    4. If the patient is awake and talking, resuscitation is not a requirement.

15. Application, implementation, physiological integrity, (b).
    4. *The patient has less difficulty breathing in a semi-Fowler position. Oxygen should be administered as soon as possible.*
    1, 2, 3. These positions increase the difficulty of breathing for this patient.

16. Application, implementation, physiological integrity, (b).
    3. *The patient with a fractured larynx must be prepared for immediate surgical intervention to establish an airway.*
    1. Blood loss is a secondary risk in comparison with the compromised airway.
    2. Without a patent airway the patient would likely have a respiratory arrest during a radiological assessment examination.
    4. Because of the injuries to the neck, establishing an airway through traditional vertical access most likely is not possible.

17. Analysis, implementation, physiological integrity, (b).

    4. The first intervention is the administration of adrenaline intravenously or subcutaneously to promote vasoconstriction and decrease bronchoconstriction.

    1, 2, 3. Although these are appropriate interventions, they are not the first intervention taken.

18. Knowledge, implementation, physiological integrity, (b).

    4. This is the correct depth of compressions for an adult victim according to the American Heart Association guidelines.

    1. This is an inappropriate depth for any compressions in any age group.

    2. This is the correct depth for compressions in an infant.

    3. This is the correct depth for compressions in a child.

19. Comprehension, implementation, physiological integrity, (b).

    4. Naloxone is a narcotic antagonist and reverses the adverse effects of an overdose.

    1. Disulfiram is prescribed for alcohol dependency.

    2. Epinephrine is not indicated for initial treatment of narcotic overdose.

    3. Methylprednisolone is not indicated for initial treatment of narcotic overdose.

20. Analysis, assessment, physiological integrity, (b).

    2. Effects of stimulant overdose include agitation, increased body temperature and blood pressure, hallucinations, and possibly death.

    1. Inhalant overdose is characterized by anxiety; respirations are likely depressed.

    3. Depressants produce decreased heart rate and respirations, stupor, and coma.

    4. Cannabis intoxication is characterized by confusion and disorientation but usually not agitation and increased heart and respiratory rates.

21. Application, assessment, physiological integrity, (b).

    1. Because potassium is given along with glucose and insulin to patients with hypoglycemia, a baseline level of this electrolyte is needed to monitor the effectiveness of treatment and avoid causing cardiac problems for the patient.

    2, 3, 4. These laboratory values do not play an important role in the management of hypoglycemia and ketoacidosis.

22. Comprehension, assessment, physiological integrity, (a).

    1. The chest is estimated at 18% of the body, and the leg is estimated at 9%; therefore the combined area would be approximately 27%.

    2. This percentage is equal to less than the area of one arm.

    3. This percentage is approximately equal to the area of one arm.

    4. This is a much larger area than is indicated on the patient's chart.

23. Application, assessment, physiological integrity, (b).

    4. Numbness in the fingers can signal nerve damage.

    1. Pain is an expected symptom in a fracture.

    2. Swelling is an expected symptom in a fracture.

    3. Bruising is a common symptom in a fracture.

24. Comprehension, assessment, physiological integrity, (b).

    1. Hypovolemic shock is primarily a fluid problem caused by loss of blood or fluid volume.

2. Neurogenic shock results from widespread dilation of blood vessels caused by an imbalance in autonomic stimulation of the smooth muscles in vessel walls. It is usually associated with spinal cord injury.

    3. Septic shock results from complications of massive bacterial infection in which toxins released into the blood cause vasodilation.

    4. Cardiogenic shock is the result of faulty pumping action, an unlikely condition in a firefighter in good physical condition.

25. Comprehension, implementation, physiological integrity, (b).

    2. Gavage with activated charcoal is implemented for substances other than caustics or hydrocarbons.

    1. Lavage is useful only in limited circumstances, usually within 2 hours of ingestion of most drugs.

    3. Emesis is induced with ipecac, not paregoric.

    4. IV infusion has limited usefulness in diluting gastrointestinal contents.

26. Analysis, implementation, physiological integrity, (c).

    4. The symptoms indicate a reaction to disulfiram (Antabuse), and the antihistamine is indicated to control the symptoms.

    1. The patient is not having symptoms of delirium tremens. Diphenhydramine, although indicated in the treatment of disulfiram reactions, is not administered for its sedative effect but rather its antihistamine activity.

    2. Naloxone, not ethanol or disulfiram, is indicated for the treatment of opioid ingestion.

    3. Fluid challenges are administered for hypotension caused by hypovolemia.

27. Comprehension, planning, physiological integrity, (c).

    2. The patient is exhibiting symptoms of delirium tremens and is at risk for seizures.

    1. Aspiration is a less likely complication than seizures.

    3. Falling is a less likely and a less serious complication than seizures.

    4. The patient is not exhibiting signs of nausea or vomiting, ataxia, or risk of elopement.

28. Application, planning, physiological integrity, (b).

    2. Normal saline contains no dextrose and is used as a maintenance fluid for the patient with hyperglycemia.

    1, 3. These are contraindicated in a patient with hyperglycemia.

    4. This would exacerbate the patient's hyperglycemia.

29. Application, implementation, physiological integrity, (b).

    1. The affected limb is placed in a dependent position to minimize circulation of toxins.

    2. Elevation would facilitate circulation of the toxin.

    3. Heat and increased circulation would facilitate circulation of the toxin.

    4. Cleaning and increased circulation would facilitate circulation of the toxin.

30. Application, implementation, physiological integrity, (b).

    3. The powder should be carefully swept from the skin, making sure not to contaminate anyone else in the process.

    1. Diluting with water increases the volume of the contaminant and increases the risk of tissue injury.

    2. The contaminant should be removed from the skin immediately.

    4. Petroleum jelly is ineffective in neutralizing powdered chemicals.

31. Application, implementation, physiological integrity, (c).
    2. The patient has a flail chest and may have cardiorespiratory problems as a result. Explaining the risks to him increases his understanding of the situation and makes his compliance with admission more likely.
    1. If the patient develops respiratory difficulty, he may not be able to return to the hospital in time to receive assistance.
    3. The nurse should not dismiss the risks of complications and must inform the patient of the situation and its possible outcomes.
    4. The nurse must inform the patient of the risks involved and not encourage him to leave against medical advice.
32. Comprehension, assessment, physiological integrity, (b).
    2. This injury is often characterized by paraplegia, but the individual may be able to rehabilitate to walk with support.
    1. This outcome is characteristic of an injury at the cervical spine level.
    3. Advising the patient that he will have no problems in the case of any spinal injury is unrealistic.
    4. This outcome is characteristic of injury at higher levels (cervical and upper thoracic spine).
33. Comprehension, assessment, physiological integrity, (b).
    2. Cardiogenic shock is the result of faulty pumping action that results in reduced cardiac output.
    1. Vasogenic shock is the result of sepsis, spinal cord injuries, or anaphylaxis.
    3. Distributive shock is the result of sepsis, spinal cord injuries, or anaphylaxis.
    4. Hypovolemic shock is the result of blood or fluid loss associated with thermal or other injury.
34. Application, implementation, physiological integrity, (b).
    3. Establishing and maintaining an airway are the highest priorities.
    1. Fluid balance is a lesser priority compared with maintaining the airway.
    2. Body temperature is a lesser priority compared with maintaining the airway.
    4. This intervention, although appropriate for treatment of a penetrating wound, is a lesser priority compared with maintaining the airway.
35. Application, implementation, physiological integrity, (b).
    2. To treat or prevent infection in the wound, all of the antibiotic must be administered as ordered.
    1. Discussing legal matters with the parents regarding the event is inappropriate for the nurse.
    3. Checking levels of consciousness is indicated for head injuries.
    4. Forcing fluids is not indicated for treatment of human bites.
36. Application, planning, safe and effective care environment, (b).
    3. The patient should be on NPO status before surgery for appendicitis.
    1, 2, 4. The patient should have no oral intake before surgery.
37. Application, implementation, physiological integrity, (b).
    3. This medication is used after sexual contact to prevent pregnancy.
    2. This contraceptive is prescribed for administration on an ongoing basis before sexual contact.

1, 4. These are antibiotics that have no contraceptive activity.
38. Comprehension, assessment, physiological integrity, (b).
    2. Watery eyes and a runny nose are characteristic of narcotic withdrawal.
    1. Overdose of narcotics does not produce chills, sweating, or intestinal cramps. In addition, the patient would most likely be comatose.
    3, 4. Stimulants do not produce these symptoms, either in overdose or withdrawal.
39. Analysis, implementation, physiological integrity, (b).
    1. Anaphylactic shock can easily progress to respiratory arrest or compromised airway. The priority actions are to establish and maintain the airway.
    2. Although the application of cold may provide comfort and decrease swelling, it is not a priority action.
    3. Administration of antibiotics is a lesser priority compared with establishing and maintaining an airway.
    4. Administration of medications is a lesser priority compared with establishing and maintaining an airway.
40. Application, planning, physiological integrity, (b).
    3. Anticoagulant therapy is indicated to decrease clotting and control further embolization.
    1. This patient does not have a cardiac arrhythmia at this time.
    2. No indication exists that this patient is at risk for seizures.
    4. This medication is not indicated in the treatment of pulmonary embolus.
41. Comprehension, assessment, physiological integrity, (c).
    3. Septic shock results from the release of endotoxin that causes vasodilation.
    1. Although the patient might be allergic to antibiotics, a reaction would not be characterized by these symptoms.
    2. Neurogenic shock is the result of a decrease in circulating blood volume caused by an injury such as spinal cord trauma.
    4. The patient's fever indicates that her experience is not psychogenic.
42. Application, assessment, physiological integrity, (b).
    1. Paradoxical breathing results from instability of the chest wall in flail chest.
    2. Pulmonary embolus is characterized by sudden chest pain, dyspnea, and cyanosis.
    3. Symptoms of a simple rib fracture include pain on inspiration and rapid, shallow breathing.
    4. Tension pneumothorax is characterized by neck vein distention, tracheal deviation, and distant breath sounds on the affected side, in addition to paradoxical breathing.
43. Analysis, evaluation, physiological integrity, (b).
    2. Nicotine causes vasoconstriction that worsens the symptoms of chilblain.
    1. Friction worsens the symptoms of burning, itching, and blistering.
    3. Chilblain is a localized reaction to excessive exposure to cold.
    4. Although the patient may have underlying risks for compromised circulation in the extremities such as Raynaud disease or diabetes mellitus, chilblain is the result of excessive exposure to cold.

44. Application, implementation, physiological integrity, (b).
    3. *Tissue death takes place if the exposed bowel dries.*
    1. This is not a priority action for exposed bowel tissue.
    2. After ascertaining that the patient has had a primary tetanus immunization, the nurse should prepare to administer a booster. However, this is not a priority action for exposed bowel tissue.
    4. The bowel should be replaced by a physician, possibly in a surgical procedure; this is not within the scope of the nurse's practice.

45. Application, assessment, physiological integrity, (c).
    2. *The presence of myoglobin in the urine indicates muscle damage.*
    1. Renal tissue damage is not necessarily indicated by the color of urine.
    3. Epithelial tissue damage is not demonstrated by urine color.
    4. Internal injuries do usually occur with burns.

46. Application, assessment, safe and effective care environment, (b).
    1. *Food poisoning such as this is caused by eating raw eggs that are contaminated with Salmonella bacteria.*
    2. Allergic reactions are not characterized by these symptoms.
    3. This history of eating raw eggs points to another probable cause for the illness.
    4. Trichinosis is caused by eating undercooked contaminated meat such as pork.

47. Analysis, evaluation, physiological integrity, (c).
    3. *The unconscious victim must be monitored for airway management.*
    1. The crying child appears to have superficial injuries and can be treated later.
    2. The fractured arm is not as much of a treatment priority as is the head injury with loss of consciousness.
    4. Although the age and underlying disease state of this patient make her a high risk for complications, this is not as high a priority as is the head injury with loss of consciousness.

48. Analysis, implementation, physiological integrity, (b).
    3. *Immediate administration of oxygen may prevent more severe pain and tissue damage.*
    1. Comfort and preservation of tissue integrity are higher priorities.
    2. Further assessment must be done before administering medication.
    4. Comfort and preservation of tissue integrity are higher priorities.

49. Comprehension, assessment, physiological integrity, (c).
    4. *Hemorrhage related to internal injuries can produce life-threatening complications in the patient with a pelvic fracture.*
    1. Nausea and vomiting are common in patients who have pain and injury.
    2. External rotation is characteristic of pelvic fracture.
    3. Pain in the back and lower extremities is common in patients with pelvic fracture.

50. Comprehension, implementation, safe and effective care environment, (b).
    3. *The wound should not be cleaned until after it has been examined by a physician who then treats it accordingly.*
    1. Flushing the wound can cause alterations in its appearance or damage tissue by dislodging clots that have formed.
    2. Scrubbing would change the appearance of the wound and might cause tissue damage and further bleeding.
    4. Applying ointment would change the appearance of the wound.

51. Analysis, implementation, physiological integrity, (b).
    1. *Establishing and maintaining an airway is always a priority for the burn patient. Because of the possible complications of smoke inhalation, the respiratory status must be monitored continually.*
    2. Although this is a very important aspect of burn care, it is a priority that is secondary to maintaining an airway.
    3. This is not as high a priority as is maintaining an airway.
    4. This has the lowest priority of the interventions mentioned.

52. Comprehension, planning, psychosocial integrity, (b).
    2. *This is the only appropriate short-term goal for this situation. All the other options are long-term goals.*
    1. This goal may take weeks to months to achieve.
    3. This long-term goal may take months to achieve.
    4. The patient may not be able to achieve this goal for days or weeks.

53. Knowledge, assessment, physiological integrity, (a).
    2. *This is a symptom of hypoglycemia.*
    1. This symptom of ketoacidosis is the result of the insulin deficiency.
    3. The patient with hypoglycemia is likely to have cool, moist skin.
    4. Air hunger is a symptom of ketoacidosis or severe hyperglycemia.

54. Analysis, planning, physiological integrity, (b).
    3. *Cyanosis is a distinct sign of compromised oxygenation and is the highest priority of the situations listed.*
    1. Hemorrhage may produce compromised oxygenation but is a lesser priority than cyanosis.
    2. Altered level of consciousness is less life-threatening than cyanosis or hemorrhage.
    4. This fracture is not a life-threatening emergency.

55. Application, implementation, physiological integrity, (b).
    4. *Saturating the blood with oxygen may allow the tissues in the body to remain oxygenated.*
    1. This rate of flow does not provide adequate oxygenation.
    2. This rate of flow allows carboxyhemoglobin to remain in place.
    3. This rate of flow does not break the affinity of hemoglobin for carbon monoxide.

56. Knowledge, implementation, physiological integrity, (a).
    2. *Intermittent cold packs help reduce swelling and discoloration.*
    1. Warm packs cause vasodilation and increase swelling and discoloration.
    3. Continuous application of cold packs would be uncomfortable and possibly cause tissue damage resulting from prolonged vasoconstriction.
    4. Warm compresses are appropriate after the first 48 hours.

57. Comprehension, implementation, physiological integrity, (a).

    4. Tilting the head may cause further injury if the patient has trauma to the neck or spine.

    1. This is the first method to be used for a patient who does not have suspected neck or spine injury.

    2. This is the method to use in the case of a patient who does not have suspected neck or spine injury if additional jaw displacement is required.

    3. Lifting only the chin does not open the airway; it is likely to further occlude it.

58. Comprehension, assessment, physiological integrity, (b).

    1. These are signs of a subdural hematoma.

    2. *Internal bleeding* refers to the abdominal organs and does not produce these symptoms.

    3. Spinal cord injuries do not produce these symptoms.

    4. Meningitis, which would take several days to develop, does not produce these symptoms.

59. Application, implementation, physiological integrity, (b).

    4. All electrical burns are considered to be major because of the possibility of internal damage to tissue.

    1. Superficial burns involve only the epidermal layer of tissue.

    2. Minor burns involve 15% or less of body surface area (BSA).

    3. Moderate burns involve 15% to 25% of BSA.

60. Application, assessment, physiological integrity, (a).

    2. Penetrating wounds often have an entrance and an exit and must be inspected thoroughly to assess the extent of the trauma.

    1. Internal inspection of a wound should be conducted by the physician.

    3. Information about conditions is a lesser priority compared with determining the extent of the injury.

    4. Although the patient may be armed, this information is a lesser priority compared with determining the extent of the injury.

61. Comprehension, assessment, safe and effective care environment, (b).

    __X__ **1. Electrical burns can produce tissue damage based on conductivity through the body.**

    _____ 2. Full-thickness burns are considered major when they involve more than 10% of BSA.

    __X__ **3. Chronic conditions such as diabetes or renal failure can cause life-threatening complications for burn patients.**

    __X__ **4. Because of the ratio of body mass to BSA, the amount of involvement for partial-thickness burns in children (20%) is less than in adults (25%).**

    __X__ **5. Burns of the face, hands, or perineum are more likely to produce complications compared with other areas of the body and are always considered to be major injuries.**

62. Application, assessment, safe and effective care environment, (c).

    Answer: 18%

    Each aspect of the arm is estimated at 4.5%, and the right anterior chest is approximately 9%.

63. Knowledge, implementation, physiological integrity, (a).

    4. This rate of compressions promotes optimum blood flow and blood pressure.

    1. This is not sufficient to provide adequate blood flow and blood pressure.

    2. This rate is not sufficient to allow adequate blood flow and blood pressure.

    3. This rate is not rapid enough to promote adequate blood flow and blood pressure in resuscitation.

64. Application, assessment, physiological integrity, (b).

    3. Because of the age of the patient and her underlying chronic condition, this burn is considered a major injury.

    1, 2, 4. Although the burn is superficial, her age and underlying condition escalate the classification of the burn.

65. Application, implementation, physiological integrity, (b).

    _____ 1. The extremity should be elevated to reduce swelling.

    _____ 2. Ice is recommended to reduce pain and swelling. Warm packs or soaks will increase swelling.

    __X__ **3. Treatment for sprains includes immobilization and limited weight bearing.**

    _____ 4. The foot should be immobilized until it has recovered from the damage resulting from excessive physical use.

    __X__ **5. Ice is recommended to reduce pain and swelling. Elevating the affected part will also aid in controlling edema.**

66. Application, assessment, physiological integrity, (b).

    __X__ **1. The periosteum is richly supplied with nerve endings, producing significant pain in a fractured bone.**

    _____ 2. Purulence is a sign of infection, which would not be evident in the early stages of recovery from a fracture.

    __X__ **3. Compromised circulation may be evidenced by pallor resulting from impaired blood flow to the injured tissue.**

    __X__ **4. Vascular compromise may result from compression by bone fragments, swelling, or other tissue injury. Assessing for pulses on an ongoing basis is necessary to detect changes as early as possible.**

    __X__ **5. Paresthesia may result from compromise to the neurological function of the injured tissue.**

67. Analysis, assessment, physiological integrity, (b).

    1. Restlessness, anxiety, and clammy skin are signs of shock in the bleeding patient.

    2. Although sepsis may produce shock in a bleeding patient, these are not symptoms of infection.

    3. Sedation is produced by the administration of medications.

    4. Syndactyly is a congenital webbing of fingers or toes.

68. Comprehension, assessment, physiological integrity, (a).

    3. A concussion is a brain injury requiring rest and decreased activity to heal, including decreasing activities that require concentration.

    1. Waking an individual routinely will not change progression of an injury.

    2. Ibuprofen can promote bleeding, thus increasing risk of intracranial bleed.

    4. Decadron would not be administered without confirmation of intracranial swelling and increased intracranial pressure (IICP).

69. Application, implementation, physiological integrity, (b).
    3. *An impaled object should be left in place to control possible bleeding and to avoid further injury to the tissue.*
    1. Removing the screwdriver can cause further trauma to the hand and severe bleeding.
    2. Cleaning the surrounding area does not diminish the possible damage that removing the screwdriver might cause.
    4. The patient is likely to experience pain either way, but removing the screwdriver can cause further complications.

70. Comprehension, implementation, physiological integrity, (a).
    2. *Aspirin is an antiplatelet that will increase the effects of a hemorrhagic stroke.*
    1. Antiplatelets may be prescribed for an ischemic stroke to reduce the chance of recurrence.
    3, 4. These diagnoses would not influence the decision to discontinue aspirin therapy.

71. Comprehension, assessment, physiological integrity, (b).
    4. *Mediastinal shift is a life-threatening condition that occurs when pressure within the intrapleural space increases and the heart and mediastinal structures are pushed to the contralateral side.*
    1. Coarctation of the aorta is a congenital condition characterized by stenosis of the vessel.
    2. Cardiac tamponade results from the accumulation of fluid in the pericardium.
    3. When the vagus nerve is activated, heart rate and blood pressure decrease.

72. Application, implementation, physiological integrity, (b).
    3. *Nuclear scintigraphic V̇/Q̇ scanning of the lung is the diagnostic modality for detecting pulmonary thromboembolism.*
    1. A chest x-ray examination would not necessarily demonstrate the pathology of a pulmonary embolism.
    2. Bronchoscopy is used to evaluate tissue within the bronchial tubes.
    4. A biopsy would be contraindicated for a patient with a diagnosis related to blood clotting.

73. Application, implementation, safe and effective care environment, (b).
    1. *Capillary blood is bright red and oozes from a wound.*
    2. Venous bleeding is dark in color and flows steadily.
    3. Arterial blood is bright, but it spurts.
    4. *Afferent* describes the direction that blood is flowing in a vessel and can be used in reference to both arteries and veins, depending on their function.

74. Comprehension, implementation, physiological integrity, (b).
    3. *The object should be removed only if it is clearly visible and can be grasped.*
    1. If the object is not readily visible, no further efforts toward examination should be made because they will delay the rescue.
    2. Finger sweeps may force the object further into the airway.
    4. Locating this anatomical landmark on the neck of an infant would be difficult, and pressure on the neck or throat area would not facilitate removal of a foreign body in the airway.

75. Comprehension, assessment, physiological integrity, (a).
    4. *The civilian priority is for the care of patients whose lives are threatened.*
    1. The military priority is for those who are most likely to survive.
    2. Triage is done on the basis of risk to the patient, not to survivors or family members.
    3. This choice places people already at the greatest risk in further danger of morbidity or mortality.

76. Application, assessment, physiological integrity, (b).
    3. *Assessing and maintaining an airway and adequate ventilation are always the highest priorities.*
    1. Administering medication is not as high a priority as maintaining an airway and ventilation.
    2. A fractured arm is a lesser priority compared with airway and ventilation.
    4. Given that the scalp laceration is oozing and not bleeding freely, it is not as great a priority compared with airway and ventilation.

77. Application, planning, physiological integrity, (b).
    1. *Diagnostic peritoneal lavage helps determine whether an intraabdominal injury exists and whether surgery is required.*
    2. Gastric lavage is indicated in cases of ingestion of drugs or poisons.
    3. As a radiological examination of the lower intestine, the barium enema would not be the best way to obtain information about possible internal injuries to the abdomen.
    4. Although abdominal MRI would show information about abdominal trauma, peritoneal lavage provides a method of intervention and treatment as well, and it is much more economical.

78. Application, evaluation, physiological integrity, (c).
    3. *The victim who is hoarse and coughing blood may have serious injuries to the throat that can compromise the airway.*
    1. This victim has no apparent injuries that would compromise his or her airway or circulation.
    2. This victim should be leaned forward to prevent aspiration of blood but is not a treatment priority.
    4. This victim may have the least serious injury and is not the greatest priority.

79. Application, implementation, physiological integrity, (c).
    2. *The priority for any unconscious victim is to assess for breathing and circulation.*
    1. This assumes that the patient is unconscious because of insulin shock.
    3. This assumes that the patient is unconscious because of hypoglycemia.
    4. Notification of the family is a lower priority than patient interventions.

80. Application, implementation, physiological integrity, (b).
    1. *Removing one of the causes of heat exhaustion is important in preventing the progression of the condition.*
    2. Fluid replacement is a lesser priority compared with controlling the progression of the condition.
    3. The patient is nauseated and might vomit if she drinks large quantities of saltwater.
    4. Rapid cooling is an appropriate treatment for heat stroke.

81. Application, implementation, physiological integrity, (b).
    3. Deep frostbite is characterized by hyperemic skin, numbness, blister formation, and edema.
    1. Immersion foot gives the extremity a shriveled appearance.
    2. Burning, itching, and ulcerations characterize chilblain.
    4. Hypothermia is a generalized condition characterized by tachypnea, tachycardia, and confusion. Frostbite is a localized condition.

82. Comprehension, assessment, physiological integrity, (a).
    __X__ 1. Documenting exact location of wounds is an appropriate intervention.
    __X__ 2. Recording the number of wounds is an appropriate intervention.
    __X__ 3. Placing the clothing of the victim in a paper bag for authorities is an appropriate intervention.
    _____ 4. Specific testing would reveal evidence of gunshot residue; no special precautions are necessary.

83. Comprehension, assessment, physiological integrity, (a).
    Correct order: 2431.
    2. Brush off particles.
    4. Use paper towel to absorb blistering agents.
    3. Remove clothing.
    1. Place valuables in plastic bag.
    The nurse's interventions in order of priority are to brush off particles, use a paper towel to absorb blistering agents, remove clothing, and place valuables in plastic bag.

84. Analysis, implementation, physiological integrity, (b).
    3. A pleural friction rub is the sound heard when there is a collection of fluid in the pleura.
    1. *Egophony* is a symptom of pleural effusion, but it is not a grating sound.
    2. Bronchovesicular sounds are normal breath sounds.
    4. Crackles have a popping sound.

85. Knowledge, implementation, physiological integrity, (c).
    2. High-Fowler position promotes lung expansion and oxygenation.
    1. Keeping the patient supine with lower legs elevated is a treatment for shock.
    3, 4. Chewing a children's aspirin and drinking a hot beverage are not appropriate interventions for pulmonary edema.

86. Application, assessment, physiological integrity, (c).
    3. Unequal hand grips and smile are indicators of cerebrovascular accident.
    1. Unequal hand grips and smile are not indicators of hyperglycemic reaction.
    2. Chest pain and dyspnea indicate pulmonary emboli.
    4. Joint pain and deformity are more commonly seen in rheumatoid arthritis.

87. Application, implementation, safe and effective care environment, (c).
    __X__ 1. Contact Precautions are an appropriate intervention.
    _____ 2. A private room with door closed is appropriate.
    __X__ 3. Airborne Precautions with an N95 mask are an appropriate intervention.
    _____ 4. Discharge would not occur after 72 hours of antibiotic therapy.
    _____ 5. Patient must wear mask and be gowned or wrapped in a sheet so rash is fully covered when he or she is outside of isolation room.

88. Analysis evaluation, physiological integrity, (b).
    3. Rhonchi are not a symptom of pneumothorax; they are heard over fluid-filled larger airways.
    1. Wheezes are caused by partial obstruction of the airway by spasm or mucus.
    2. Crackles are popping noises that can be heard in early stages of congestive heart failure.
    4. Breath sounds are heard best by using the diaphragm of the stethoscope.

89. Comprehension, assessment, physiological integrity, (a).
    __X__ 1. Rebound tenderness is a typical symptom of intestinal trauma that a patient would exhibit, depending on the trauma.
    __X__ 2. Hypoactive bowel sounds are a typical symptom of intestinal trauma that a patient would exhibit, depending on the trauma.
    _____ 3. Joint pain is commonly noted in arthritis such as osteoarthritis and rheumatoid arthritis.
    __X__ 4. Abdominal guarding is a typical sign of intestinal trauma that a patient would exhibit, depending on the trauma.
    _____ 5. Hemiparesis is a muscular weakness of one half (one side) of the body.

90. Knowledge, assessment, physiological integrity, (a).
    3. Rabies is a viral infection.
    1. Bacteria are small unicellular microorganisms that vary in shape; they can be spherical (cocci), rod-shaped (bacilli), spiral (spirochete), or comma-shaped (vibrios). Bacteria do not cause rabies.
    2. Fungus does not cause rabies. Fungi may be saprophytes or parasites. Yeasts reproduce by budding, and molds reproduce by spore formation.
    4. Helminths are worms of the pathogenic parasite division such as tapeworms and roundworms.

91. Comprehension, assessment, physiological integrity, (c).
    __X__ 1. Anaphylactic shock is a severe allergic reaction.
    __X__ 2. Anaphylactic shock is a profound antigen-antibody response.
    __X__ 3. Capillary permeability and angioedema are symptoms of anaphylactic shock.
    _____ 4. A bacterial infection does not apply to anaphylactic shock.
    _____ 5. Anaphylactic shock does not cause bloody stools.

92. Analysis, evaluation, physiological integrity, (c).
    3. pH less than 7.35 is acidosis.
    2. pH greater than 7.45 is alkalosis.
    1, 4. Normal pH is 7.35 to 7.45.

93. Comprehension, assessment, physiological integrity, (b).
    _____ 1. Cardiogenic shock can occur within 24 hours after an acute myocardial infarction in patients with severely impaired pumping action of the heart.
    __X__ 2. Cardiogenic shock decreases cardiac output.
    __X__ 3. Cardiogenic shock lowers blood pressure.
    __X__ 4. Cardiogenic shock decreases blood flow to tissues, resulting in decreased oxygen to the tissues.
    _____ 5. Urinary output is decreased in cardiogenic shock.

94. Application, assessment, physiological integrity, (b).
    2. Benzodiazepines have the adverse effect of respiratory depression.
    1. Pinpoint (constricted) pupils can occur with an overdose of opiates.

3. Convulsions can occur with an overdose of central nervous system stimulants.
4. Acute psychotic episodes are noted with hallucinogens such as lysergic acid diethylamide (LSD) and phencyclidine (PCP).

95. Application, implementation, physiological integrity, (b).
4. Regular insulin has an onset of action in ½ to 1 hour.
1. Long-acting insulin has an onset of action of 4 to 8 hours.
2. Regular insulin has its peak of action in 2 to 5 hours.
3. Intermediate insulin has a peak of action in 4 to 12 hours.

96. Comprehension, assessment, physiological integrity, (a).
1. This is caused by a lack of clotting factors, which results in bleeding into the tissue spaces, muscles, and weight-bearing joints.
2. Emboli resulting from peripheral vascular disease in conjunction with bacterial endocarditis can occur, producing gangrenous infarctions of distal parts of the body.
3. Pleural effusion results from abnormal buildup of fluid in the intrapleural spaces of the lungs.
4. This condition is scoliosis, which is a lateral curvature of the spine.

97. Comprehension, assessment, physiological integrity, (b).
__X__ **1. A blue ring around the bite site is symptomatic of a brown recluse spider bite.**
__X__ **2. Edema and blistering are symptomatic of a brown recluse spider bite.**
__X__ **3. A stinging sensation that goes unnoticed is symptomatic of a brown recluse spider bite.**

_____ 4. Muscle spasms are typically noted from the bite of a black widow spider.
_____ 5. Seizures are typically noted from the bite of a black widow spider.

98. Comprehension, assessment, physiological integrity, (b).
__X__ **1. Needle sharing is a common mode of transmission of hepatitis C.**
_____ 2. Kissing and hugging do not transmit hepatitis C.
__X__ **3. Body piercing with a contaminated needle is a mode of transmission of hepatitis C.**
_____ 4. Hepatitis B, C, D, and G are transmitted by a blood or sexual transmission route.
_____ 5. Hepatitis B, C, D, and G are transmitted by a blood or sexual transmission route.

99. Comprehension, assessment, physiological integrity, (b).
_____ 1. Trousseau sign is an indicator of brachial blood flow.
__X__ **2. Severe pain with movement is a symptom of fractured hip.**
__X__ **3. External rotation of the affected limb is a symptom of a fractured hip.**
_____ 4. Fever is noted in the early stages of tuberculosis, and night sweats occur as the disease progresses.
_____ 5. Shortening, not lengthening, of the affected limb is seen in a fractured hip.

100. Knowledge, assessment, physiological integrity, (a).
1. Abdominal cramping with diarrhea is a symptom of hyperkalemia (a serum potassium level greater than 5 mEq/L).
2. This is an indicator of low body temperature.
3, 4. These are symptoms of diabetes mellitus.

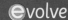
Comprehensive Examinations

COMPREHENSIVE EXAMINATION 1: PART 1

This examination contains individual questions, the majority of which relate to clinical situations. Read all questions carefully. Most questions have only one best answer, but several questions reflect the multiple-response alternate format that requires more than one answer. Answers and Rationales begin on p. 549.

TEST TIME ALLOTMENT (PART 1): APPROXIMATELY 2 HOURS

1. The nurse observes peaked T waves on the heart monitor of a patient with renal disease. The nurse should review the patient's labs for an increase in which of these electrolytes?
   1. Calcium
   2. Chloride
   3. Sodium
   4. Potassium
2. A dark-skinned patient is at high risk for a pressure ulcer. The nurse assesses for skin blanching by looking for which skin color?
   1. Pale
   2. Grayish
   3. Hyperemic
   4. Pinkish
3. The nurse observes frequent, greasy stools in a patient with celiac disease as a result of malabsorption of:
   1. Proteins.
   2. Carbohydrates.
   3. Vitamins.
   4. Fats.
4. A patient who has diabetes mellitus fell on the ice and sustained a skin abrasion. She asks the nurse to apply an ice wrap to her ankle. The nurse hesitates based on the understanding that:
   1. The open area will become infected.
   2. She will first have to get an x-ray examination of her ankle.
   3. Rebound swelling may occur once the ice is removed.
   4. People with diabetes have a greater potential for injury related to cold.
5. The nurse is preparing to ambulate a postoperative patient for the first time. Prioritize from highest to lowest priority the following actions the nurse should take to maintain patient safety.
   1. Assist patient to sitting position.
   2. Give pain medication if needed 15 minutes before ambulation.
   3. Raise head of bed to facilitate ease of getting out of bed.
   4. Use two-person assist.
   5. Encourage the patient to dangle for 5 minutes before ambulation.

6. Fluids by mouth are initially contraindicated for an infant with bronchiolitis because of feeding difficulty caused by:
   1. Tachypnea.
   2. Bradycardia.
   3. Irritability.
   4. Fever.
7. The purpose for recommending that a patient stop smoking when diagnosed with peripheral vascular disease is that:
   1. Smoke causes hypotension.
   2. Nicotine constricts blood vessels.
   3. Smoke irritates the lungs.
   4. The tars in smoke decrease the red blood cell (RBC) count.
8. When assessing a patient who is in kidney failure, the nurse suspects potassium imbalance based on the patient's symptoms. Which are signs of potassium imbalance and should be reported to the physician? Select all that apply.
   _____ 1. Nausea and vomiting
   _____ 2. Anxiety
   _____ 3. Irregular heartbeat
   _____ 4. Crackles
   _____ 5. Abdominal cramps
   _____ 6. Dark amber urine
9. The nurse is caring for a patient who has had a subtotal thyroidectomy. The nurse is aware that accidental removal of the parathyroid glands can occur and closely monitors the patient for:
   1. Tetany.
   2. Seizures.
   3. Renal shutdown.
   4. Loss of the gag reflex.
10. During a patient's annual physical, the physician notes an enlarged, boggy prostate. Which data from the patient's history should the nurse report to the physician?
    1. Hesitancy, change in urine stream
    2. Color and odor of urine
    3. Constipation, smoking history
    4. Type and amount of fluids taken daily
11. During routine morning rounds the nurse notes that a patient with chronic pulmonary disease is more forgetful today. The nurse also notes an unusual odor on the patient's breath while assessing lung sounds. The nurse must evaluate the patient within the hour because the patient:
    1. May need to be oriented to her environment more today.
    2. May be developing a respiratory infection.
    3. May need more encouragement to eat today.
    4. Is at risk for developing acidosis.

12. A patient scheduled for an open reduction and internal fixation of the left hip resulting from a fracture should be taught that the immediate expected postoperative outcome of this surgery relative to activity is:
    1. Bed rest only.
    2. Pivoting into a chair.
    3. Ambulating with full weight bearing.
    4. Confinement in bed with skeletal traction.

13. A patient with severe degenerative joint disease has been scheduled for arthroscopy of the left knee. The patient asks the nurse what to expect after the surgery. What is the nurse's best response?
    1. "You may need to ask your surgeon that question."
    2. "You should not need a knee replacement in the future."
    3. "You should have less pain and improved joint function."
    4. "The procedure will virtually cure your degenerative joint disease."

14. After a thyroidectomy a patient develops carpopedal spasms and tingling of the lips. Which complication would the nurse consider as the most likely to occur?
    1. Hyperglycemia
    2. Hypocalcemia
    3. Hyperkalemia
    4. Thyroid storm

15. A nurse is caring for an overweight patient with osteoarthritis. What would the nurse suggest to the patient to help control joint strain?
    1. Exercising the involved joint
    2. Reducing and maintaining weight
    3. Applying intermittent heat
    4. Taking medication at the onset of pain

16. The nurse assesses an unconscious patient injured in a fall from a horse in which sequence?
    1. Breathing, airway, circulation
    2. Airway, breathing, circulation
    3. Circulation, airway, breathing
    4. Breathing, circulation, airway

17. The nursing assistant asks the nurse about the turning schedule for a patient who underwent a right pneumonectomy yesterday. The nurse explains that the patient should be turned every hour from:
    1. Back to left side to right side.
    2. Back to left side to back.
    3. Left side to right side to left side.
    4. Back to right side to back.

18. After assessment of baseline vital signs, the next priority nursing assessment or intervention for a patient about to undergo dialysis is to:
    1. Administer diphenhydramine (Benadryl).
    2. Weigh the patient.
    3. Do a urinalysis.
    4. Keep the patient on nothing by mouth (NPO) status.

19. The disorder characterized by a malfunction of the motor centers of the brain caused by a lack of oxygen to the brain is:
    1. Down syndrome.
    2. Scoliosis.
    3. Osteomyelitis.
    4. Cerebral palsy.

20. When caring for a comatose patient, the nurse knows that discussing the patient's condition with the family at the patient's bedside is inappropriate because:
    1. It may confuse the patient.
    2. It may upset the family.
    3. It may speed up the dying process.
    4. Hearing is one of the last senses lost.

21. The nurse knows that family members assisting in the care of a dying loved one is beneficial because this:
    1. Prolongs the dying process.
    2. Lessens the nurse's workload.
    3. Helps to prevent the family from feeling helpless.
    4. Causes too much work for a grieving family.

22. What would a nurse consider a normal assessment finding in the urine of a newly admitted patient?
    1. Lack of odor
    2. Clear yellow liquid
    3. Presence of a high specific gravity
    4. Presence of red blood cells (RBCs) in the urine

23. When caring for a patient with a tracheostomy, the nurse observes that the tube appears to be filled with dry mucus. Which action is appropriate for the nurse to implement at this time?
    1. Remove the inner cannula and clean with alcohol-soaked cotton swabs.
    2. Remove the inner cannula and clean with hydrogen peroxide.
    3. Remove the outer cannula and clean with hot water.
    4. Remove the outer cannula and suction the trachea.

24. A 7-year-old child has developed a red, raised rash on her face, neck, and trunk; a temperature of 101.4°F (38.5°C); and whitish spots on the back of her throat. The nurse suspects that the child has:
    1. Chickenpox.
    2. Measles (rubeola).
    3. Mumps.
    4. German measles (rubella).

25. A patient is being discharged after a suprapubic prostatic resection. What is an appropriate discharge instruction for this patient?
    1. "Use daily laxatives to avoid straining to have a bowel movement."
    2. "Limit fluid intake to what you had in the hospital to prevent stretching the bladder."
    3. "If dribbling or incontinence occurs, use Kegel exercises 10 to 20 times per hour."
    4. "Don't worry if your urine turns a bright red; this is caused by passing clots."

26. An older patient who states that she has "always been healthy" is being treated for a respiratory tract infection. The nurse observes that the patient uses her diaphragm during inspiration and plans to teach her pursed-lip breathing, based on the understanding that:
    1. Older adults need to consciously think about taking deep breaths.
    2. The older a person becomes, the more likely it is that he or she will develop chronic obstructive pulmonary disease (COPD).
    3. Age-related changes from loss of elastic recoil of the lungs occur.
    4. Older adults lose the use of their intercostal muscles.

27. Wilms tumor is an adenosarcoma found in the:
    1. Bladder.
    2. Ureters.
    3. Kidney.
    4. Urethra.

28. A nurse obtains a positive result of a Hemoccult test on a patient's stool. Which statement made by the patient would lead the nurse to question the validity of the test results?
    1. "I love my coffee. I drink four or five cups every day."
    2. "I wish they would stop giving me that blue gelatin; I'm sick of it!"
    3. "I really enjoyed the steaks I've had on my tray the past two evenings."
    4. "The hospital must have its own garden, judging by the amount of vegetables they feed you."

29. A newly admitted clinic patient complains of extreme fatigue, weight loss, and anorexia. One of her nursing diagnoses is imbalanced nutrition: less than body requirements. Which nursing intervention is most appropriate for this patient?
    1. Suggesting use of hard candy, chewing gum, or artificial saliva to increase moisture in the mouth
    2. Discussing benefits of adequate moisture in the environment
    3. Keeping a dietary record of amount, type, and frequency of food intake
    4. Planning low-calorie snacks in daily routine

30. A 5-week-old infant is brought to the pediatrician's office with symptoms of irritability, weight loss, and projectile vomiting. Physical examination reveals signs of dehydration. From these symptoms the nurse suspects that the infant has:
    1. Hirschsprung disease.
    2. Pyloric stenosis.
    3. Esophageal atresia.
    4. Intussusception.

31. While collecting a 24-hour urine specimen, the nurse should:
    1. Discard every other voided specimen.
    2. Save all urine that the patient voids.
    3. Insert a retention catheter for 24 hours.
    4. Send each void to the laboratory separately.

32. A nurse is caring for a patient who has a diagnosis of dysphagia. What is the priority intervention to include in the plan of care for this patient?
    1. Facial exercises
    2. Special feeding precautions
    3. Allowing extra time for formation of words
    4. Referral to an occupational therapist for assessment

33. The nurse makes a diagnosis of disturbed sensory perception related to hemianopsia. Which nursing intervention is appropriate?
    1. Covering the eyes with a blindfold
    2. Approaching the patient on the right side
    3. Teaching the patient to scan the environment
    4. Using artificial tears to prevent drying of the corneas

34. Which nursing activity occurs during the assessment phase of the nursing process?
    1. Observing the patient's skin integrity.
    2. Teaching the patient deep-breathing exercises.
    3. Determining the priority patient care problem.
    4. Collaborating with the patient to determine a realistic diet plan.

35. A patient has a p.r.n. order for a straight catheter. Which observation by the nurse might best indicate that the order needs to be implemented?
    1. The patient has not voided in 4 hours.
    2. The patient has consumed 2000 mL of fluid in 6 hours.
    3. The patient had an incontinence episode 30 minutes ago.
    4. The patient voids 5 to 10 mL of amber-colored urine every hour.

36. What would the nurse expect the drug of choice to be for treating a hypertensive crisis?
    1. Propranolol hydrochloride (Inderal)
    2. Enalapril maleate (Vasotec)
    3. Nifedipine (Procardia)
    4. Nitroprusside (Nipride)

37. A nurse is caring for a patient with a hearing impairment. Which measure should the nurse do first?
    1. Call the hospital's American Sign Language practitioner.
    2. Ask significant others how the patient communicates at home.
    3. Arrange for a family member to stay with the patient continually.
    4. Arrange for a social worker to visit with the patient and family members.

38. A patient asks the nurse why his eyes water and his nose runs during episodes of hay fever, especially in the spring. Which response by the nurse best answers the patient's concerns?
    1. The body is attempting to flush out the irritant.
    2. The hay fever response is an autoimmune reaction.
    3. These are normal reflexes that the body uses in times of stress.
    4. The hay fever is actually an allergic response to grass and tree pollen.

39. The physician orders meperidine sulfate (Demerol), 75 mg IM, every 4 hours p.r.n. postoperatively. On hand is Demerol 50 mg/mL. How many milliliters should be administered?
    Answer: _____ mL

40. A patient has decided to decrease her intake of red meat, but she is concerned that she will also be decreasing her intake of iron. The nurse suggests that she can increase her intake of iron by eating additional:
    1. Milk and dairy products.
    2. Refined cereal products.
    3. Dried fruits such as apricots
    4. Yellow vegetables such as carrots.

41. A patient, diagnosed with left ventricular heart failure, is being treated with dobutamine hydrochloride (Dobutrex). The nurse knows that this medication is classified as an adrenergic and serves to:
    1. Decrease cardiac contractility.
    2. Increase peripheral resistance.
    3. Decrease cardiac output.
    4. Increase cardiac contractility.

42. A patient has been diagnosed with a peptic ulcer and has been placed on medication therapy. Which instructions would be most beneficial concerning diet therapy?
    1. "Include a lot of dairy products in your diet."
    2. "Eat a very bland diet, eliminating all caffeine and spicy foods."
    3. "Eat a well-balanced diet while taking your medications."
    4. "Eat six small meals each day to decrease your stomach discomfort."

43. A patient is admitted to the rehabilitation unit after a cerebrovascular accident (CVA) with residual dysphagia. To better assist him during mealtimes, the nurse should put him in which position?
    1. Sitting in an upright position with head slightly forward
    2. Standing with legs abducted for 2 minutes and then adducted for 1 minute
    3. Sitting in a comfortable position to promote speaking
    4. Turning him every 2 hours to a different position

44. Which arrhythmia is the most dangerous and life-threatening?
    1. A sinus arrhythmia
    2. An atrial arrhythmia
    3. An atrioventricular (AV) nodal arrhythmia
    4. A ventricular arrhythmia

45. An outbreak of *Escherichia coli*–related illness is noted in the community. When providing information to the public, the nurse is knowledgeable that *E. coli*–related illness can be prevented by which of the following? Select all that apply.
    _____ 1. Proper home canning of food.
    _____ 2. Ensuring that red meats are well done.
    _____ 3. Heating food to at least 140° F (60° C) for 10 minutes.
    _____ 4. Making sure that eggs are used quickly after purchase.
    _____ 5. Thorough washing of all fruits and vegetables.

46. After a seizure, the nurse knows to place the patient in which position?
    1. Lateral
    2. Prone
    3. Supine
    4. High Fowler

47. A patient tells the nurse that she is going on a strict vegetarian diet that includes no meat or dairy products. In which nutrient will this patient be particularly deficient if she continues on this diet?
    1. Iron
    2. Protein
    3. B-complex vitamins
    4. Fat-soluble vitamins

48. A patient with Parkinson disease experiences posture and gait changes. Which statement best reflects how gait is affected in this disease?
    1. Patient displays muscle rigidity and brief, jerky motor movements.
    2. Patient displays limp, fidgeting movement of legs when walking.
    3. Tremors cause the patient's ambulation to appear spastic.
    4. Patient is bedridden; ambulation is not possible.

49. A patient asks the nurse what information is available concerning omega-3 fatty acids. Which statement by the nurse is most correct?
    1. "No fatty acids are good for you."
    2. "Why don't I make an appointment for you with the dietitian?"
    3. "Physicians believe that omega-3 fatty acids may actually prevent cancer."
    4. "Some research suggests that these fatty acids may help prevent heart disease."

50. A patient tells the nurse that she uses mineral oil as a base for her salad dressing. The nurse's best response to this statement should be:
    1. "That's a good idea! It even fits into your mother's bland diet."
    2. "That's a good idea! Mineral oil doesn't add calories to your diet."
    3. "I would use another type of oil. Mineral oil is high in calories with very few vitamins."
    4. "I would suggest using vegetable oil. Mineral oil hinders absorption of important vitamins."

51. A 76-year-old female is admitted to the surgical unit after hip replacement surgery. The nurse administers meperidine (Demerol), 20 mg IV, as ordered for pain. The patient sleeps for 3 hours and awakens confused, drowsy, and lethargic. The nurse should:
    1. Call the physician and report the patient's condition.
    2. Not call the physician but chart the patient's response to the medication.
    3. Keep reminding the patient of where she is, the day, and the time.
    4. Observe the patient because older adults metabolize drugs at a slower rate.

52. A patient 4 years of age was admitted with a diagnosis of positive epiglottitis. The nurse caring for this patient should include which of the following in her plan of care?
    1. Checking the patient's throat with a flashlight
    2. Increasing the patient's oral intake
    3. Directing warm steam toward the patient
    4. Having tracheostomy equipment available

53. A nurse is counseling a 23-year-old woman who is trying to eat a healthier diet. She says she is trying to quit smoking but is having a hard time doing so. Which vitamin should the nurse recommend as a supplement?
    1. Vitamin A
    2. Vitamin K
    3. Vitamin C
    4. Vitamin B

54. A woman brings her father into the clinic because he has been lost and was unable to remember his address. Which question should the nurse ask first to identify a possible cause of the problem?
    1. "What medications are you taking?"
    2. "When did you move to this address?"
    3. "Have you had trouble sleeping lately?"
    4. "Are you eating balanced meals daily?"

55. A 30-year-old patient was admitted to the neurosurgical unit 2 days ago after surgery for a brain tumor. When out of bed for the first time, she reports to the nurse that she is seeing zigzag lines in front of her face and hears singing voices. The nurse should first:
    1. Note her comments in the chart, and refer the patient to her psychiatrist.
    2. Have the patient lie down.
    3. Start an intravenous (IV) line and administer IV diazepam (Valium).
    4. Call the patient's physician.

56. Which statement should indicate to the nurse that a mother understands the dietary needs of her teenage daughter with diabetes?
    1. "Lots of fruit is good because fruit has natural sugar."
    2. "She can eat my baked goods if I use a sugar substitute."

3. "I am definitely going to start serving more pasta and whole grains."

4. "I am definitely not going to let her go with her friends to fast-food places."

57. A home–health care nurse is interviewing and assessing a family with a newborn. Two toddlers are also living in the household. Which food on the kitchen counter would be of most concern to the nurse?
1. Apples
2. Whole milk
3. Chocolate cake
4. Bag of popcorn

58. A patient who underwent a transurethral resection of the prostate has had his catheter removed and is placed on the four-bottle technique. He has just voided for the fifth time today. The nurse knows to discard the:
1. Bottle contents on the left and place the newest specimen bottle to the right.
2. Bottle contents on the right and place the newest specimen bottle to the left.
3. Number 2 bottle contents and place the newest specimen bottle to the right.
4. Number 3 bottle contents and place the newest specimen bottle to the left.

59. Which statement made by the nurse fosters feelings that would bolster a patient's self-esteem?
1. "Mr. Jones, you are always so negative."
2. "How nice of you to accept Charles into your group, Sally."
3. "Remember, Peter, you must leave the past behind and focus only on changing behavior."
4. "Steve, you are to do exactly as I say."

60. A 19-year-old patient who has type 1 diabetes mellitus is taking Ortho-Novum for birth control. She comes to the physician's office complaining of an upper respiratory infection and is subsequently prescribed ampicillin for 1 week. The nurse should instruct her to:
1. Use another means of birth control.
2. Perform a urine test to check her blood sugar.
3. Take ampicillin until she feels better.
4. Expect a rash from the ampicillin.

61. Which would be the most therapeutic response for the nurse to make to a patient who complains of feeling "blue"?
1. "You have been so successful."
2. "Don't be blue; put this out of your mind."
3. "Don't let your feelings get the best of you."
4. "Is there something in particular that is worrying you?"

62. The nurse is caring for a patient recently diagnosed with breast cancer. While discussing the new diagnosis with her, the patient tells the nurse, "You must have me confused with someone else; I have polycystic disease." What defense mechanism is the patient using?
1. Repression
2. Denial
3. Fantasy
4. Rationalization

63. The nurse assigned to a neurology floor is assessing a 21-year-old male patient admitted with facial trauma. The nurse asks the patient to occlude each nostril separately and close his eyes while she presents sources of familiar odors. Which cranial nerve is being assessed?
1. I
2. II

3. III
4. VII

64. The nurse just received a call from the emergency department that a patient diagnosed with acquired immunodeficiency syndrome (AIDS) is coming to the unit. Which action should the nurse take first?
1. Prepare the patient's room for isolation.
2. Face her own feelings about AIDS.
3. Orient the patient to his or her room.
4. Explain unit policies to the patient.

65. A 16-year-old patient is admitted to the neurology floor after being involved in a motor vehicle accident (MVA). His head hit the windshield, and he is being admitted for observation. During the afternoon he begins to complain of a headache, has two episodes of vomiting, and is more difficult to arouse. The initial nursing intervention is to:
1. Do nothing; he needs his rest.
2. Place him in a recumbent position, administer oxygen, and notify the physician immediately.
3. Prepare him for emergency surgery.
4. Assess his neurological status, elevate the head of the bed slightly, and notify the physician immediately.

66. A nurse who is providing discharge teaching for patients receiving antidepressant therapy should tell them that generally they can expect to feel better in:
1. 2 to 3 days.
2. 5 to 7 days.
3. 2 to 4 weeks.
4. 4 to 6 weeks.

67. Prednisone is often used in the treatment of rheumatic fever because it:
1. Prevents infection.
2. Cures the disease.
3. Suppresses inflammation.
4. Takes the place of antibiotic prophylaxis.

68. An infant can be expected to triple his or her birth weight at:
1. 6 months of age.
2. 9 months of age.
3. 12 months of age.
4. 15 months of age.

69. An individual with a seizure disorder is being evaluated in the primary care center. Gathering appropriate assessment data would include questioning the patient regarding:
1. Events that occurred before or after the seizure.
2. Diet and exercise history.
3. Social and educational levels.
4. Work history.

70. A priority teaching strategy for the nurse to include for the individual diagnosed with epilepsy is to:
1. Control seizure activity and prevent injury.
2. Wear a medical identification (MedicAlert) bracelet and avoid situations known to trigger seizures.
3. Follow up with the primary care physician on an annual basis.
4. Refrain from going into crowded areas.

71. The nurse is admitting a patient who is delusional; a priority nursing measure should be to:
1. Encourage the patient to talk about the delusions.
2. Explain the delusion to the patient.
3. Place the patient in seclusion.
4. Explain to the patient that he is wrong and the delusion is not real.

72. A nurse has just received a laboratory report on a patient with a bipolar disorder. The patient's lithium level is 1.9 mEq/L. What should the nurse do first?
    1. Administer the next dose of lithium.
    2. Hold the lithium and call the physician.
    3. Double the lithium dose.
    4. Hold the lithium and administer alprazolam (Xanax).

73. A nurse is caring for a patient who is receiving total parenteral nutrition (TPN). Appropriate nursing interventions for this patient include:
    1. Weighing daily, monitoring blood glucose levels, and weaning from TPN gradually.
    2. Assessing for degree of hunger every shift.
    3. Monitoring liver, renal, and cardiovascular function.
    4. Weighing every week, monitoring for glycosuria, and discontinuing TPN on the third day.

74. A nurse is preparing a patient for discharge. Because the patient is taking a monoamine oxidase inhibitor (MAOI), the nurse emphasizes which instructions?
    1. "Avoid aged cheeses."
    2. "Take the medication with food."
    3. "Take the medication at bedtime."
    4. "Limit caffeine intake."

75. A patient with a personality disorder is brought to the outpatient clinic by her mother, who states that her daughter is out of control. The nurse should begin to foster trust with the patient by:
    1. Telling her that she is available, regardless of the patient's behavior.
    2. Telling her that she cares about her but may not always approve of her behavior.
    3. Avoiding an establishment of trust because the relationship will eventually be terminated.
    4. Letting the patient know that she can call the nurse day or night.

76. The patient tells the nurse to leave her alone; she says, "I'm no good to anyone. Why don't you attend to someone else?" Which response by the nurse would be the most therapeutic?
    1. "I will stay with you for 15 minutes."
    2. "I am responsible for you, so I will stay with you."
    3. "You are a good person."
    4. "Why do you say you are no good to anyone?"

77. A 12-year-old patient is in the emergency department with a dislocated shoulder after a playground accident. The physician orders midazolam (Versed), 0.5 mg IV, before performing a closed reduction of the shoulder. Which nursing diagnosis is a priority for this patient?
    1. Ineffective airway clearance
    2. Pain related to trauma
    3. Ineffective health maintenance
    4. Risk for infection related to trauma

78. During the termination phase of the nurse-patient relationship, the patient abruptly gets up and leaves. The most appropriate nursing action should be to:
    1. Go after the patient and bring him back.
    2. Remain at the interaction site until the end of the contracted time.
    3. Resume the patient's regularly scheduled activities.
    4. Speak with the head nurse about assigning another nurse to the patient.

79. A patient was admitted 3 days ago for depression and attempted suicide. Her depression seems to have lifted. The nurse knows that this means her risk for suicide:
    1. Is less than it was when she was severely depressed.
    2. Is more than it was when she was severely depressed.
    3. Does not exist anymore because she is no longer depressed.
    4. Needs to be reevaluated.

80. Which of the following are characteristic of the average 3-month-old? Select all that apply.
    _____ 1. Babbles
    _____ 2. Is now considered an infant
    _____ 3. Has a closed posterior fontanel
    _____ 4. Has one lower incisor
    _____ 5. Stays awake for longer periods of time
    _____ 6. Has a budding personality

81. A patient's injuries sustained in a motor vehicle accident have resulted in cerebral edema. Which position is the most appropriate for this patient?
    1. Supine
    2. Prone
    3. Low to mid Fowler
    4. Mid to high Fowler

82. After a myocardial infarction, a patient receives warfarin (Coumadin). Which symptom would alert the nurse to a possible adverse effect to the warfarin?
    1. Vomiting
    2. Epistaxis
    3. Back pain
    4. Blurred vision

83. A 72-year-old patient is taking diuretics for congestive heart failure. As part of his home-care directions, the nurse should instruct him to weigh himself:
    1. Each morning on arising.
    2. 1 hour after taking his medication.
    3. If he notices an increase in pedal edema.
    4. Whenever he develops shortness of breath.

84. Which instruction is most appropriate for a patient with chronic obstructive pulmonary disease (COPD) who has copious bronchial secretions?
    1. "Decrease your fluid intake to solidify bronchial secretions."
    2. "Tracheal suctioning is the best method for removing heavy secretions."
    3. "Try to drink several glasses of juice or water daily to loosen secretions."
    4. "You'll find it easier to breathe if you sit up straight during postural drainage treatments."

85. A patient diagnosed with a seizure disorder is being treated with phenytoin (Dilantin) and valproic acid (Depakene). Which statement should the nurse consider to be the priority teaching need for this patient?
    1. Practice good oral hygiene.
    2. Increase intake of green, leafy vegetables.
    3. Carry a padded tongue blade at all times.
    4. Sleep 6 to 8 hours each night.

86. A patient is being transferred to the unit where he is to be observed after a 2-day stay in coronary care for a possible myocardial infarction. The patient is receiving several medications and is complaining of a headache. Which

medication taken by the patient commonly causes the side effect of headache?
1. Acetaminophen (Tylenol)
2. Digoxin (Lanoxin)
3. Nitroglycerin
4. Potassium chloride

87. After thoracentesis the patient is monitored closely for:
1. Increased respiratory rate, chest tightness, hypoxemia.
2. Decreased respiratory rate, low blood pressure, decreased pulse rate.
3. Bradycardia, dry hacking cough, hypotension.
4. Normal sinus rhythm, normotension, ventilation.

88. A concern for a patient who has experienced a recent myocardial infarction is the development of cardiogenic shock. Which are signs of cardiogenic shock? Select all that apply.
_____ 1. Bounding pulses
_____ 2. Hypotension
_____ 3. Hypertension
_____ 4. Hot, dry skin
_____ 5. Weak pulses
_____ 6. Clammy skin

89. A nurse arrives at the scene of an accident and finds a man lying on the ground with his eyes closed. The nurse's first action should be to:
1. Notify emergency personnel.
2. Open the airway with the head tilt–chin lift maneuver.
3. Attempt to arouse the person.
4. Start cardiopulmonary resuscitation.

90. A patient has been experiencing intermittent episodes of mild chest pain and shortness of breath, particularly with exertion but also at rest. The physician wants to assess whether the symptoms are aggravated or precipitated by activity. The nurse anticipates counseling the patient in the use of:
1. A glucometer.
2. Urine collection equipment.
3. A Holter monitor.
4. A Doppler flow study.

91. A patient sustained an injury to his spinal cord at the C5 level. For a spinal cord injury at this level, the nurse would most likely expect the patient to have loss of:
1. Emotions.
2. Sexual desires.
3. Speaking ability.
4. Movement of all extremities.

92. A child with *Haemophilus influenzae* type B meningitis is usually treated with intravenous (IV) fluids, antibiotics, and:
1. IV furosemide (Lasix).
2. IV dexamethasone (Decadron).
3. Oral diphenhydramine (Benadryl).
4. Intramuscular ribavirin.

93. In planning care for a patient with arteriosclerosis obliterans, the nurse would consider:
1. Direct application of heat to improve circulation to the affected area.
2. Giving instructions in avoiding injury and maintaining circulation.
3. Elevating the foot of the bed to increase arterial circulation.
4. Massaging the extremities several times per day to improve circulation.

94. A competitive racer had a near-drowning accident when the canoe she was paddling tipped over and struck her on the head. Her lips and nails are cyanotic. Immediate emergency care for this patient's hypoxia includes:
1. Bag-valve-mask resuscitation.
2. Inserting chest tubes to drain the water.
3. Cricothyroid puncture to ensure a patent airway.
4. Placing her in Trendelenburg position to facilitate fluid drainage.

95. Which early signs of hypoxemia should the nurse watch for in a patient with chronic bronchitis? Select all that apply.
_____ 1. Yawning
_____ 2. Bradycardia
_____ 3. Tachycardia
_____ 4. Restlessness
_____ 5. Dyspnea
_____ 6. Confusion

96. The nurse needs to obtain a sterile urine specimen for culture and sensitivity. The best way to obtain this specimen in a patient with an indwelling Foley catheter is to:
1. Remove the old Foley, and recatheterize with a straight catheter.
2. Place a towel under the bag and open the drainage valve at the bottom of the drainage bag.
3. Disconnect the catheter from the drainage tubing and let the urine drip into a sterile bottle.
4. Use a needle and syringe to withdraw urine from the tubing port and inject the specimen into a sterile tube.

97. A patient is to receive acetylsalicylic acid (ASA), 600 mg. The label reads, "gr. V." How many tablets should be given?
Answer: _____ tablet(s)

98. A patient's wife is concerned because her husband, who had a cerebrovascular accident (CVA) 3 days ago, laughs and cries inappropriately. The nurse's best reply is:
1. "I would ignore him when he starts acting like that."
2. "Men your husband's age like to tease us by acting this way."
3. "This is a normal healing sign for someone who has had a stroke."
4. "He has what is called *emotional lability,* which may occur after a stroke."

99. A patient who grows her own fruits and vegetables is concerned that her urine, which is red, indicates that she is bleeding. The most appropriate response from the nurse is:
1. "You must increase your milk intake to about 8 to 10 glasses per day."
2. "This is nothing to be concerned about. Let me know if it is still happening next week."
3. "Do you feel any pain or pass flatus when you urinate?"
4. "What types of vegetables and fruits have you been eating?"

100. A nurse instructs a nursing assistant not to fully bathe a resident with extremely dry skin every day. What is the best reason older adults do not need to have a complete bath every day?
1. Body odor is diminished.
2. Activity level is decreased.
3. Interest in hygiene is diminished.
4. Sweat and oil glands are less active.

101. A patient entered the clinic with symptoms of nervousness and weight loss. A tentative diagnosis of hyperthyroidism was made. Which additional assessment data would support the diagnosis?
    1. Constipation, depression, brittle hair
    2. Increased sweating, hand tremors, palpitations
    3. Dry skin, intolerance to cold, slowed response time
    4. Urinary frequency, blurred vision, frequent infections

102. A patient has a radioactive device implanted to treat carcinoma of the bladder. Which approach would best address the safety of the nurse in performing daily care?
    1. Perform nursing measures as quickly and completely as possible.
    2. Enter the patient's room frequently to assess the implanted device.
    3. Perform skills slowly to facilitate discussion of the patient's disease.
    4. Spend as much time with the patient as possible to decrease his or her feelings of loneliness.

103. The nurse is to administer eye medications to a group of six patients, all of whom have glaucoma and are receiving cholinergic agents (miotics) such as pilocarpine (Salagen). The nurse knows that these medications must be given as ordered based on the understanding that:
    1. Giving medications on time is part of the nurse's job.
    2. These medications keep the pupil constricted to permit better aqueous humor drainage.
    3. Glaucoma is a leading cause of blindness.
    4. The patient will experience severe eye pain if a dose is late.

104. While bathing a patient, the nurse notes a reddened area on the right hip. The appropriate nursing action is to:
    1. Massage around the reddened area every 2 hours, turning frequently.
    2. Clean with alcohol and apply a sterile dressing.
    3. Apply warm, moist compresses intermittently.
    4. Apply lotion and powder before turning the patient on the right side.

105. Which foods should be suggested to combat constipation in older adults?
    1. Fruit juices and dairy products
    2. Meats, cheeses, and poultry products
    3. Processed carbohydrates and milk products
    4. Whole-grain cereals, fresh vegetables, and water

106. The presence of human immunodeficiency virus (HIV) infection is increasing. Which measure is essential for the nurse to incorporate into care?
    1. Ask the patient his or her HIV status.
    2. Adhere strictly to Standard Precautions.
    3. Have an HIV-positive health care worker care for the patient.
    4. Observe Standard Precautions only if exposure to blood or body fluids is obvious.

107. Rheumatic fever is caused by:
    1. A virus.
    2. A fungus.
    3. *Streptococcus* bacteria.
    4. *Staphylococcus* bacteria.

108. A 42-year-old man has ingested 18 diazepam (Valium) tablets and 18 unidentified capsules. He is in the emergency department and is now alert after gastric lavage. He is calling his son to come and take him home. He is exhibiting which defense mechanisms?
    1. Denial
    2. Projection
    3. Regression
    4. Sublimation

109. A 78-year-old man is returning home with his daughter. The daughter is concerned that her home is not safe for her father. What may indicate a possible safety hazard?
    1. Electric stoves
    2. Hardwood floors
    3. Nonglare lighting
    4. Elevated toilet seats

110. What is a reason that adverse drug reactions occur in older adults?
    1. Older adults excrete drugs more effectively.
    2. Older adults have a higher percentage of muscle tissue.
    3. Increased gastric motility causes changes in the absorption of drugs.
    4. Older adults have altered drug distribution caused by circulatory changes.

111. A patient who has been receiving antipsychotic drugs reports that he has a dry mouth, tight throat, and mouth movements. The nurse should consider that:
    1. These may be somatic delusions.
    2. These are transitory reactions that will disappear.
    3. The patient is probably manipulating for more medication.
    4. These may be extrapyramidal reactions that require intervention.

112. A 21-year-old unconscious man is brought to the emergency department by a friend. His breath smells of alcohol, and the friend reports that they were at a fraternity party where everyone was drinking quite heavily. The nurse should:
    1. Treat the patient for shock.
    2. Ensure adequate airway and ventilation.
    3. Recommend rest in a quiet environment.
    4. Administer disulfiram (Antabuse) immediately.

113. Which nursing intervention would be appropriate when giving an older adult oral medications?
    1. Elevate head of bed 15 degrees.
    2. Give fluids before and after medications.
    3. Give all medications at one time to enhance absorption.
    4. Crush the medications and mix them with the patient's food.

114. An 80-year-old patient asks the nurse what is included in an advance directive. Which of the following contains accurate information concerning advance directives?
    1. Guardianships and living wills
    2. Organ procurement and donation
    3. Living wills and health care proxies
    4. Active and passive acts of euthanasia

115. Cardiopulmonary resuscitation (CPR) recommendations for calling for help suggest "phone first" for an adult and "phone fast" for a child. The best explanation for this rule is that:
    1. Children can go longer without oxygen.
    2. An arrest in a child is usually caused by an obstructed airway.

3. An arrest in an adult is usually caused by cardiac arrhythmias.

4. It is usually too late by the time the first responder finds an adult.

116. An 18-month-old infant is to have a long-acting antibiotic given intramuscularly. The nurse selects the best muscle or site to use, which is the:
    1. Deltoid.
    2. Vastus lateralis.
    3. Gluteus maximus.
    4. Ventrogluteal area.

117. Which eye condition is the most common reason for blindness in the older adult?
    1. Glaucoma
    2. Cataracts
    3. Presbyopia
    4. Macular degeneration

118. The nurse should anticipate that patients with early Alzheimer disease would have difficulty:
    1. Remembering how to operate an automobile.
    2. Remembering that they have put a meal in the oven.
    3. Remembering where they put the house keys the evening before.
    4. Recalling a telephone conversation right after hanging up the telephone.

119. A patient has sustained burns on the front and back of both legs and her right arm. What percentage of her body would the nurse estimate is involved?
    1. 18%
    2. 45%
    3. 54%
    4. 72%

120. The normal inflammatory response is not always a reliable indicator of disease in the older adult because:
    1. Aging changes heighten the older adult's pain perception.
    2. Cardiovascular changes heighten the erythema that develops around infection sites.
    3. Changes in the hypothalamus diminish the ability of the older adult to produce a fever.
    4. Changes in the hypothalamus grossly elevate temperature changes in the older adult.

121. Within the first few hours after treating a severely burned patient, the nurse should observe for:
    1. Absence of pain
    2. Eschar formation
    3. Leathery appearance to skin
    4. Laryngeal and tracheal edema

122. The nurse is the first to arrive on the scene of a motorcycle accident and observes that a bone is protruding through the skin of the victim's leg. The nurse's first action would be to:
    1. Cover the area with a dressing.
    2. Apply a splint to the victim's leg.
    3. Push the bone back through the skin.
    4. Apply antibiotic ointment to the skin.

123. The nurse should encourage family members of a confused, demented patient to bring personal items along to a long-term care facility. The purpose of doing this is to:
    1. Increase attention span.
    2. Decrease dementia behaviors.
    3. Facilitate short-term memory.
    4. Foster recognition in the environment.

124. A patient complains of tenderness at her intravenous (IV) puncture site. On assessment the nurse notes redness and swelling. The nurse should first:
    1. Notify the physician and fill out an incident report.
    2. Stop the flow of the IV fluids and report this to the head nurse.
    3. Elevate the arm and apply warm compresses to the puncture site.
    4. Change the dressing over the puncture site using sterile technique.

125. While the nurse's 14-year-old neighbor boy is mowing her lawn, he is stung by a bee. He starts wheezing and complaining of difficulty breathing. The nurse takes him to the emergency department, where he is diagnosed as having:
    1. Asthma.
    2. Hay fever.
    3. Pneumonia.
    4. Anaphylaxis.

COMPREHENSIVE EXAMINATION 1: PART 2

This examination contains individual questions, the majority of which relate to clinical situations. Read all questions carefully. Most questions have only one best answer, but several questions reflect the multiple-response alternate format that requires more than one answer. Answers and Rationales begin on p. 558.

TEST TIME ALLOTMENT (PART 2): APPROXIMATELY 2 HOURS

1. A patient who has had frequent bouts of pneumonia spends most of her time in bed, insisting that the head of the bed remain at 90 degrees. Because she has reddened areas on her coccyx, the nurse teaches her that:
    1. She needs to stay off her back for the next 24 hours.
    2. The head of the bed should be kept at 15 to 30 degrees.
    3. Her buttocks hurt because the skin over the bones is dying.
    4. She keeps getting pneumonia because of the moisture that forms on her skin.

2. The nurse has taught an elderly patient with type 2 diabetes mellitus the importance of maintaining good glucose control. The nurse knows that learning has occurred when the patient states:
    1. "My fasting blood sugar should be 100 to 140 mg/dL and between 120 and 180 mg/dL after eating."
    2. "My fasting blood sugar should be 180 to 240 mg/dL and between 250 and 300 mg/dL after eating."
    3. "My fasting blood sugar should be between 75 and 100 mg/dL and between 150 and 275 mg/dL after eating."
    4. "My fasting blood sugar should be between 225 and 275 mg/dL and between 276 and 375 mg/dL after eating."

3. Symptoms of hypertension are vague and subtle. When assessing patients diagnosed with hypertension, the nurse may expect the patient to complain of which symptoms? Select all that apply.
    _____ 1. Nausea and vomiting
    _____ 2. Blurred vision
    _____ 3. Shortness of breath
    _____ 4. Irritability

_____ 5. Nervousness

_____ 6. Occipital headaches

4. A patient who has had lung surgery is having difficulty doing deep-breathing and productive-coughing exercises, even with the use of an incentive spirometer. Nursing notes indicate that the patient's cough is weak and dry and that he tires easily. The most appropriate plan of action the nurse should consider is to:
   1. Encourage the patient to drink 8 to 10 glasses of water each day.
   2. Ask the physician to order "as needed" (p.r.n.) throat lozenges and cough demulcent.
   3. Report to the physician and ask if aerosol treatments may help.
   4. Increase the room temperature to 70° F (21° C) and humidity to 70%.

5. Digoxin, a water-soluble drug, should be administered cautiously in the older adult for which reason?
   1. Digoxin is less likely to accumulate to toxic levels.
   2. Digoxin is distributed in larger compartments in older adults.
   3. Digoxin is distributed in smaller compartments in older adults.
   4. Digoxin administration is the same in the older adult as it is in the younger adult.

6. Two patients are admitted to the cardiac unit, one with a diagnosis of mitral stenosis and the other with a diagnosis of mitral insufficiency. Which symptom would the nurse find common in both of these conditions?
   1. Angina
   2. Murmur
   3. Syncope
   4. High blood pressure

7. A patient's sputum has suddenly become pink and frothy. Which assessment finding is significant and needs to be reported and documented?
   1. Decreased appetite
   2. Coughing when supine
   3. Complaints of dull headache
   4. Respirations 16, regular, easy

8. A patient with hypertension wants the nurse to tell him the name of the recommended annual eye examination he is to have. The best response by the nurse would be to explain that the examination is called a:
   1. Vision screen.
   2. Tonometer test.
   3. Funduscopic examination.
   4. Visual fields examination.

9. When external cardiac compression is performed, the victim must be positioned on a firm surface because:
   1. Palpation of landmarks is easier.
   2. The risk of breaking the xiphoid process is reduced.
   3. The heart is compressed between the sternum and spine.
   4. This position enables the rescuer to deliver more compressions.

10. A patient confides to a nurse that she is desperate to lose 10 pounds before going to her class reunion in 2 weeks. She tells the nurse that she plans to eat only fruits and drink a lot of water. The most appropriate response by the nurse should be:
    1. "All nutrients are needed in a healthy diet."
    2. "It is all right for a short period, but be sure to take plenty of vitamins."
    3. "The fruit will supply you with energy, and the water will help circulation."
    4. "Eat a variety of foods from all levels of the "MyPlate food guide" and increase exercise."

11. The nutritional requirements of older adults differ from those of younger people. In particular, older adults require:
    1. Increased fats.
    2. Fewer calories.
    3. Decreased fluid intake.
    4. Fewer vitamins and minerals.

12. A 75-year-old patient is recovering from a right total hip replacement. The nurse has identified a diagnosis of impaired physical mobility related to decreased muscle strength and should plan to:
    1. Provide active range of motion (ROM) to the right ankle.
    2. Encourage quadriceps-setting exercises.
    3. Keep the right leg in extension and abduction.
    4. Provide passive ROM to the right ankle.

13. A patient is known to be lactose intolerant. When teaching dietary adjustments to the patient, the nurse advises her to avoid:
    1. Citrus fruits.
    2. Highly seasoned foods.
    3. Milk and milk products.
    4. Foods containing seeds and nuts.

14. When cleansing an open wound, the nurse should:
    1. Apply constant pressure.
    2. Forcefully irrigate all wound areas.
    3. Scrub encrusted areas thoroughly.
    4. Work from cleanest to dirtiest areas.

15. The nurse established a nursing diagnosis of excess fluid volume related to decreased glomerular filtration caused by acute glomerulonephritis. Clinical data that support this nursing diagnosis include:
    1. Fever
    2. Thirst
    3. Polyuria
    4. Periorbital edema

16. A patient receiving an initial dose of intravenous (IV) ampicillin begins complaining of itching during infusion of the drug. The nurse notes that her back and abdomen are covered by red wheals. The nurse's next course of action is to:
    1. Discontinue the IV line immediately and notify the physician.
    2. Discontinue the IV line and set up for a restart in the opposite arm.
    3. Reassure her regarding this normal reaction and apply ointment to the rash.
    4. Discontinue the piggyback unit, restart original fluid, and notify the physician.

17. A patient has undergone complicated abdominal surgery and is now receiving total parenteral nutrition (TPN) via a central venous catheter. During the morning bath the patient suddenly becomes dyspneic, anxious, and cyanotic. The nurse finds that the TPN is disconnected from the central line. The nurse should first:
    1. Initiate hospital protocol for respiratory emergency.
    2. Reconnect the TPN ports after swabbing them with alcohol.

3. Place the patient on his left side with his head below chest level.
4. Place the patient in high-Fowler position to assist respiratory efforts.

18. When preparing to administer oxygen via nasal cannula, the nurse attaches the oxygen flow meter to a container of sterile distilled water to:
    1. Decrease the danger of oxygen combustion.
    2. Increase the patient's level of oxygen absorption.
    3. Remove any particle contaminants from the tubing.
    4. Prevent drying of the patient's naso-oropharyngeal mucosa.

19. The best criteria for evaluating the care given based on the nursing diagnosis of imbalanced nutrition: less than body requirements related to anorexia, nausea, and vomiting include:
    1. Stable body weight.
    2. Absence of diarrhea.
    3. Normal body temperature.
    4. Moist mucous membranes.

20. When preparing a feeding pump for a patient's tube feeding, the nurse knows that the pump should be filled with:
    1. The full day's supply of formula.
    2. One full can of formula each time.
    3. 8 hours' worth of feeding each time.
    4. No more than a 2-hour supply each time.

21. What is a critical nursing measure when caring for patients undergoing nasogastric suctioning?
    1. Mouth care every 2 hours
    2. Thorough skin care to the nares
    3. Turn and position every 2 hours
    4. Maintain accurate intake and output record

22. A patient has been taking a diuretic for the last 3 months. Which statement made by the patient would alert the nurse to a possible dietary deficiency caused by the diuretic?
    1. "I seem to bruise so easily these days."
    2. "My eyes seem especially sensitive to light."
    3. "Every once in a while, my heart feels like it's skipping beats."
    4. "I feel so terribly nervous. Do you think I need a tranquilizer?"

23. The physician has determined that a patient has increased intracranial pressure (IICP). The nurse positions her in which position?
    1. Elevation of the head of the bed to 20 degrees
    2. Elevation of the head of the bed to 30 degrees
    3. Elevation of the head of the bed to 60 degrees
    4. Elevation of the head of the bed to 90 degrees

24. An 84-year-old woman is in the health care provider's office complaining of fatigue, anorexia, and indigestion. Which group of vitamins might be prescribed if the health care provider suspects a deficiency?
    1. C and B_{12}
    2. B_6 and B_{12}
    3. A, D, and E
    4. C and B complex

25. When monitoring a patient receiving intravenous therapy, which observations may indicate infiltration? Select all that apply.
    _____ 1. Poor skin turgor
    _____ 2. Redness at insertion site
    _____ 3. Warmth at insertion site
    _____ 4. Swollen area above the catheter
    _____ 5. Coolness at the insertion site
    _____ 6. Area at insertion site painful to touch

26. According to the history of maternity care in the United States, the single greatest deterrent to maternal complications, particularly gestational hypertension (GH), has been:
    1. Prenatal care.
    2. A salt-free diet.
    3. The age of the mother.
    4. Discovery and use of antihypertensive drugs.

27. A patient is concerned with edema that develops in her feet throughout the day. Which food choice made by the individual most likely contributed to edema formation?
    1. Eggs and toast
    2. Tuna fish and cantaloupe
    3. Hamburger and French fries
    4. Salami sandwich and potato chips

28. The nurse is gathering data related to the growth and development of a 3-week-old infant. The nurse should expect to observe which behavior in the infant?
    1. Holding head erect
    2. Moro "startle" reflex
    3. Cooing and babbling
    4. Recognizing a familiar face

29. A patient in her sixth month of pregnancy is complaining of insomnia. The intervention that the nurse might suggest includes:
    1. Elevating the hips.
    2. A balanced diet.
    3. Warm milk at bedtime.
    4. Keeping legs uncrossed.

30. A patient with cancer is experiencing anorexia. Which recommendation made by the nurse should assist the patient in increasing oral intake?
    1. "Try to eat three large meals every day."
    2. "Take pain medication after your meals."
    3. "Try to supplement your meals with nutritious milk shakes."
    4. "Eat as many fruits and vegetables as you can instead of protein foods."

31. A prenatal patient is complaining of low back pain. What might the clinic nurse suggest for some relief of the discomfort the patient is experiencing?
    1. Sitz baths
    2. Pelvic rock-tilt exercise
    3. Visits to the chiropractor
    4. Heating pads to the back

32. What is the most appropriate nursing action when caring for a patient with streptococcal meningitis?
    1. Wound Precautions
    2. Respiratory Precautions
    3. Judicious handwashing
    4. Strict Isolation Precautions

33. Which assessment would be of most concern to the nurse during examination of a 2-week-old newborn?
    1. Babinski reflex is present.
    2. A cephalhematoma is present.
    3. The infant is waking up twice during the night.
    4. A small red pin dot is present in the white of the sclera.

34. The nurse should explain to the patient that the contraction stress test (CST) is an invasive test because medication is given in the veins and it:
    1. Is not painful at all.
    2. Is uncomfortable for a short while.
    3. Will take a few minutes to complete.
    4. Is a routine procedure for all pregnant women.

35. When discussing nutrition with a patient who is a 3-month pregnant gravida 1, para 0, the nurse explains that the most important consideration in her prenatal diet is to provide:
    1. A low-calorie diet to maintain the mother's weight.
    2. A diet high in protein for nourishment of the fetus.
    3. An adequate diet to ensure optimum nutrition for mother and fetus.
    4. Limited fluid intake to prevent edema in the body tissues of both the mother and the fetus.

36. Because of her history of diabetes, a patient is classified as having a high-risk pregnancy. The health care provider knows that her prenatal visits will be scheduled approximately as follows:
    1. On a week-to-week basis
    2. Two times per month for the first 28 weeks
    3. Every 2 weeks after the thirty-eighth week
    4. Every week from the thirty-sixth week and thereafter

37. The nurse should caution a patient who drinks alcohol while taking chlorpropamide (Diabinese) to expect what specific type of reaction?
    1. Reverse reaction
    2. Anaphylactic reaction
    3. Antigen-antibody reaction
    4. Disulfiram (Antabuse)-type reaction

38. A gravida 2, para 1 goes into labor at 24 weeks and gives birth prematurely. Physically the infant's appearance would most closely resemble which description?
    1. 7 inches long, 6 oz, and covered with lanugo
    2. 12 inches long, 1½ pounds, and covered with vernix caseosa
    3. 19 inches long, 7 pounds, and small amount of vernix caseosa
    4. 10 inches long, 1 pound, and covered with vernix caseosa

39. The nurse in a local nursing home assigns a certified nursing assistant (CNA) to an 87-year-old resident. The nurse instructs the CNA to help the resident with his total bath:
    1. Once each week using hot water.
    2. Every other day using cold water.
    3. Every other week using tepid water.
    4. Three times each week using tepid water.

40. A charge nurse has the following tasks to perform at 9:00 AM: taking vital signs for two residents, administering medications to four residents, attending an interdisciplinary care team meeting, and performing documentation regarding four residents. Which of these tasks would be most appropriate to assign to a nursing assistant?
    1. The documentation
    2. Taking the vital signs
    3. Administering medications
    4. Attending the care planning meeting

41. The physician prescribes oral acyclovir (Zovirax) for a patient with genital herpes lesions. The nurse should include which statement when teaching the patient about this medication?
    1. "Once the lesions disappear, you will be cured of genital herpes."
    2. "You may stop taking this drug once the pain and itching subside."
    3. "You should drink at least 3 quarts of water every day while you are taking this medication."
    4. "As long as you are taking the medication, your sexual partner will be protected from contracting the virus."

42. Which nursing intervention should be the priority after a fall has occurred?
    1. Moving the patient to a bed or stretcher
    2. Checking the extremities for symmetry and alignment
    3. Assessing for skin intactness and any bruises or swelling
    4. Assessing the patient's airway and any difficulty breathing

43. The physician prescribes propranolol (Inderal), a nonselective beta-adrenergic blocking agent, to treat a patient's hypertension. The nurse should monitor the patient for which side effect?
    1. Dyspnea
    2. Tachycardia
    3. Photophobia
    4. Nervousness

44. A patient states that he has difficulty climbing stairs. What would be the best way for the nurse to validate this claim?
    1. Ask a family member if it is true
    2. Watch the patient as he climbs the stairs
    3. Ask for a physical therapy referral for the patient
    4. Ask the patient what happens when he climbs the stairs

45. In caring for an unconscious individual suspected of having an airway obstruction, put in priority order the following actions the nurse should take when rendering assistance to this individual.
    1. Start cardiopulmonary resuscitation (CPR)
    2. Remove any foreign object obstructing the airway
    3. Place victim in supine position on a firm, flat surface
    4. Open the airway using the head tilt–chin lift maneuver

46. A licensed practical/vocational nurse is assisting a registered nurse in counseling an older couple concerning finances and long-term care. The couple indicates that they thought that Medicare would cover all nursing home expenses. The nurse advises the couple that:
    1. Medicare should cover all of the expenses of long-term care.
    2. Medicare covers only 1 or 2 years of long-term care expenses.
    3. Social Security covers the expenses incurred during nursing home stays.
    4. Medicare covers many of the expenses incurred in nursing home care.

47. To best assist a patient who has been on bed rest to prepare for ambulation, the nurse should:
    1. Perform passive range-of-motion (PROM) exercises three times daily.
    2. Dangle the patient's legs and swing them back and forth daily.

3. Have him or her perform push-ups and use the bed trapeze bar as much as possible.

4. Have him or her push his popliteal space against the bed to the count of five several times daily.

48. A conscious person with diabetes arrives at the emergency department with a blood glucose level of 378 mg/dL. The nurse should expect the treatment of choice would be to:
    1. Administer regular insulin.
    2. Administer 50% glucose intravenously.
    3. Initiate an intravenous (IV) dextrose infusion.
    4. Monitor the potassium level.

49. When a patient in diabetic ketoacidosis comes to the emergency department, blood electrolyte levels should be monitored. The nurse is aware that the most important electrolyte to monitor in this patient is:
    1. Calcium.
    2. Chloride.
    3. Potassium.
    4. Sodium.

50. What would be a priority emergency nursing concern for a victim with severe burns?
    1. Relieving pain
    2. Tetanus prophylaxis
    3. Hemodynamic stability
    4. Administering cardiopulmonary resuscitation

51. A 36-year-old woman has undergone a total hip replacement. The postoperative orders include aspirin, 5 grains (325 mg) by mouth (PO) daily. The nurse is aware that the rationale for this treatment is to:
    1. Prevent joint inflammation.
    2. Provide better pain control.
    3. Maintain normal body temperature.
    4. Produce a mild anticoagulant effect.

52. The nurse is caring for a rape trauma survivor. The initial assessment indicates that the patient appears calm and very much in control. Which psychological reaction best describes the patient's behavior?
    1. Denial
    2. Disorganization
    3. Hyperalertness
    4. Reorganization

53. When performing passive range of motion (PROM) for a patient, the nurse should:
    1. Exercise the joint just past the point of stiffness to gradually increase joint motion.
    2. Perform no more than five repetitions for each exercise to avoid tiring the patient.
    3. Watch the patient's nonverbal communication to help evaluate the response to the exercise.
    4. Vary the order in which the exercises are performed so the patient does not become bored.

54. A patient is in the clinic waiting room awaiting results of the biopsy of his prostate gland. He is laughing and cracking jokes. The nurse should:
    1. Ask the patient to be quiet.
    2. Ignore the patient's behavior.
    3. Overlook the patient's different behavior.
    4. Know the patient is manifesting anxiety.

55. A patient is admitted for possible obstructive urinary retention caused by an enlarged prostate gland. During the assessment the nurse would expect the patient to complain of:
    1. Nausea.
    2. Burning on urination.
    3. Hesitancy in initiating voiding.
    4. Hematuria.

56. The nurse is caring for a patient with bipolar disorder who is currently in the manic phase. The nurse is trying to get the patient involved in a diversional activity. What would be the most appropriate activity?
    1. Bridge
    2. Table tennis
    3. Exercise class
    4. Jigsaw puzzle

57. When receiving a physician's orders by telephone, the nurse must:
    1. Write the physician's name on the order sheet.
    2. Write the patient's name, next of kin, and date on the order sheet.
    3. Repeat the orders and then write them on the physician's order sheet.
    4. Write the order as the physician gives it, repeating it back to the physician for immediate verification.

58. The nurse is interacting with a patient with obsessive-compulsive disorder. What statement by the patient may validate that certain activities help her deal with her anxiety?
    1. "I have a stupid problem, don't I?"
    2. "I am willing to take medication if necessary."
    3. "I worry about dirt and germs, and I clean a lot."
    4. "I worry about the health of my aging parents."

59. When caring for a patient with chronic obstructive pulmonary disease (COPD), the nurse notes that the patient is more comfortable after:
    1. Fluids are restricted.
    2. Having postural drainage.
    3. He has provided all his own care.
    4. Being placed in low-Fowler position.

60. A nurse is caring for a patient taking haloperidol (Haldol). What is a common side effect the nurse should observe for in this patient?
    1. Sedation
    2. Weight loss
    3. Dry mouth
    4. Anxiety

61. Frequent assessment of a patient with a fractured left leg would include maintaining proper alignment and:
    1. Taking the apical pulse every 2 hours.
    2. Checking sensation and circulation in the leg.
    3. Checking temperature and performing range of motion (ROM) in the right leg.
    4. Increasing the weight of traction as ordered to maintain countertraction.

62. To facilitate proper positioning of the patient's arm after a modified radical mastectomy, the nurse should take which action?
    1. Flex the arm on the affected side across the chest and assist to semi-Fowler position.
    2. Abduct the affected arm at least 8 inches and suspend it from a trapeze or IV pole.
    3. Place the affected arm on pillows with the elbow higher than the shoulders and the wrist higher than the elbow.
    4. Keep the patient in high-Fowler position with the hand of the affected side positioned on one pillow.

63. The nurse administering medications should adhere to the gold standard for administering medications. What conforms to that accepted standard?
    1. Use of computerized guidelines as defined by the pharmacist
    2. Use of the five rights of medication administration: right drug, dose, route, patient, time
    3. Use of the five rights of medication administration: right drug, hospital policy, dose, patient, route
    4. Use of the six rights of medication administration: right drug, dose, route, patient, time, room number

64. A patient is hearing voices that are telling him to do harmful things to himself. Which nursing diagnosis should be included on this patient's plan of care?
    1. Dressing self-care deficit
    2. Risk for self-directed violence
    3. Impaired verbal communication
    4. Ineffective impulse control

65. The nurse is gathering objective data about a patient who is experiencing "kidney problems." The nurse reviews the laboratory results, knowing that the glomerular filtration rate (GFR) can be measured by evaluating the:
    1. Hemoglobin.
    2. White blood cells (WBCs).
    3. Creatinine clearance.
    4. Blood urea nitrogen (BUN).

66. An individual known to be taking lithium and currently under psychiatric care has taken cocaine. She telephones the hospital with abdominal cramps and extreme anxiety. The nurse's best response would be to:
    1. Refer her to her psychiatrist.
    2. Give her the cocaine hotline number.
    3. Have her come to the emergency department immediately.
    4. Put her on hold and get another nurse to take the call.

67. A patient with a spinal cord injury complains of a severe headache and profuse sweating. Vital signs reveal bradycardia and severe hypertension. The nurse suspects the manifestation of autonomic hyperreflexia and assesses for which possible causes? Select all that apply.
    _____ 1. Visitors
    _____ 2. Full bladder
    _____ 3. Taking an apical pulse
    _____ 4. Full bowel
    _____ 5. Taking tympanic temperatures
    _____ 6. Wrinkled sheets

68. A patient has shallow respirations at 8 to 10 times per minute. This hypoventilation results in acidosis by:
    1. Retention of carbon dioxide (CO_2).
    2. Excretion of needed CO_2.
    3. Excretion of oxygen (O_2).
    4. Retention of too much O_2.

69. A 32-year-old patient is being admitted to the medical floor with a diagnosis of bronchiectasis. She has a chronic cough with expectoration of copious amounts of purulent sputum and hemoptysis. An appropriate outcome criterion is that the:
    1. Patient demonstrates improved ventilation and adequate oxygenation.
    2. Nurse encourages alternating rest and activity.
    3. Patient may have activity intolerance related to fatigue.
    4. Patient's arterial blood gases are improved.

70. When two rescuers are performing adult cardiopulmonary resuscitation (CPR), the ratio of compressions to respirations is:
    1. 15:2.
    2. 30:2.
    3. 15:1.
    4. 30:1.

71. A nurse assessing motor function in a patient who has had a stroke includes assessment of:
    1. Cranial nerves VIII through XII.
    2. Intellectual function and speech pattern.
    3. Muscle movement, strength, and coordination.
    4. Body position, level of consciousness, and mental status.

72. A patient with diabetes mellitus is going to engage in a strenuous activity. Which snack would the nurse suggest that the patient consume before engaging in the activity?
    1. An orange
    2. A candy bar
    3. A can of soda
    4. Cheese and crackers

73. A 60-year-old patient is being discharged after having undergone cardiac catheterization. What important instructions should the nurse include at the time of discharge?
    1. Drive a car that has an automatic transmission.
    2. Tub baths are allowed after 24 hours.
    3. Rest and avoid heavy lifting or strenuous activity.
    4. Do not change the bandage for 48 hours and report site soreness to the physician.

74. A resident in long-term care has a diagnosis of elevated ammonia levels related to cirrhosis. Which food would the nurse advise the nursing assistant to eliminate as a possible snack for the resident?
    1. Pretzels
    2. Crackers and cheese
    3. Chicken salad sandwich
    4. A bowl of vanilla ice cream

75. A 72-year-old patient is admitted to the cardiac floor with a diagnosis of acute myocardial infarction. Which blood test is the most reliable in detecting heart muscle damage?
    1. Fibrin split products
    2. Complete blood cell count
    3. Lactic dehydrogenase (LDH)
    4. Creatinine kinase myoglobin (CK-MB)

76. In which position should a nurse assist the patient after a thyroidectomy?
    1. Supine
    2. Left Sims
    3. Semi-Fowler
    4. Trendelenburg

77. A patient had a myocardial infarction 2 days ago. Which finding might suggest that the patient may be experiencing left-sided heart failure?
    1. Nausea
    2. Heart murmur
    3. Crackles in the lungs
    4. Edema in feet and legs

78. The nurse is aware that oral hypoglycemic agents may be used for patients with diabetes mellitus who have:
    1. Obesity.
    2. Liver disease.

3. Type 1 diabetes.

4. Some insulin production.

79. A new mother asks the nurse at what age it is best to hang a new, colorful mobile for her newborn baby boy. The nurse answers that newborns are able to follow bright and colorful objects:
    1. At 1 year of age.
    2. During the first week of life.
    3. At 2 or 3 weeks of life.
    4. At 9 to 10 months of life.

80. Patients with sensory dysfunction such as people with paraplegia have many teaching needs. What is a high-priority teaching need?
    1. Importance of decreasing calcium intake
    2. Importance of avoiding cold or very hot foods
    3. Importance of adequate fluid intake of 2000 mL/day
    4. Importance of doing 5-minute weight shifts every hour

81. In a patient receiving continuous bladder irrigations after a transurethral prostatectomy, the nurse assesses that the catheter may be blocked. The most appropriate instruction the nurse should give the patient is to:
    1. Try to void around the catheter.
    2. Increase fluid intake to 4000 mL/day.
    3. Deep breathe, cough, and remain still until the physician arrives.
    4. Notify the nurse if he notices a change in the color of the drainage in the bag.

82. A patient receiving chlorpromazine (Thorazine) should be instructed to:
    1. Avoid certain foods containing tyramine.
    2. Use a sunscreen when outdoors.
    3. Take medication with milk.
    4. Use a prophylactic antacid.

83. The nurse on the previous shift charted that the patient was drowsy. Which behavior would support this description of the patient's level of consciousness?
    1. Appropriate response when aroused
    2. Absence of response even to painful stimuli
    3. Incomplete arousal to painful stimuli
    4. Response to verbal command inconsistent and vague

84. When preparing a patient for a bowel-retraining program, the nurse should understand that the most important factor for a successful retraining program is:
    1. Regular administration of a mild laxative.
    2. Making sure that the patient understands the purpose of the program.
    3. Establishing regular day or days and time to assist the patient to the toilet.
    4. Skipping a day in the program if the patient had more than one bowel movement the day before.

85. A patient is being observed for increased intracranial pressure. Which classification of medications, other than anticonvulsants and corticosteroids, would the nurse expect the physician to order?
    1. Antibiotics
    2. Antiemetics
    3. Osmotic diuretics
    4. Narcotic analgesics

86. In a patient with head trauma being treated for increased intracranial pressure, which would be least likely to cause complications?
    1. Isometric exercises

2. Aerobic exercises

3. Passive range-of-motion exercises

4. High-Fowler position

87. Which nursing action is the most appropriate to stop the bleeding from an occipital laceration?
    1. Applying ice to the site
    2. Elevating the extremities
    3. Applying pressure to the site
    4. Elevating the head of the bed

88. A nurse is working in the newborn nursery when a baby being fed by a colleague begins to choke on the formula. Immediately the nurse assesses the situation and begins the procedure for severe obstructed airway in a conscious infant. To perform the procedure correctly, the nurse knows to administer:
    1. Eight back blows and eight chest thrusts.
    2. Six back blows and six chest thrusts.
    3. Five back blows and five chest thrusts.
    4. Four back blows and four chest thrusts.

89. A patient is being instructed on postlumbar puncture care and is apprehensive about getting "sick with a terrible headache like her neighbor did when she had the same test done." The nurse's most appropriate response is:
    1. "Moving about after the test is the best way to prevent a headache."
    2. "You will need to remain flat on your stomach after the test. This will prevent getting a headache."
    3. "You will be able to drink fluids after the test. This, as well as lying flat, helps most people."
    4. "With all the advances in medicine, these types of headaches are not common anymore."

90. Which one special precaution will the nurse incorporate into the plan of care for an 82-year-old patient who has undergone an open reduction and internal fixation (ORIF) of the hip?
    1. Monitoring for nutritional problems
    2. Maintaining proper alignment of the extremity
    3. Keeping the side rails in an elevated position
    4. Observing linen and dressings for drainage

91. Immediate physical observations of a burn patient by emergency personnel would include which of the following as the most important?
    1. Quality of respirations
    2. Physical development
    3. Height and weight
    4. Head circumference

92. The nurse is determining an asthmatic patient's achievement of the goals for the nursing diagnosis of activity intolerance related to imbalance between oxygen supply and demand. Which expected outcome is appropriate?
    1. No evidence of anxiety
    2. Demonstrated knowledge of disease process
    3. Ability to perform activities of daily living
    4. Clear breath sounds

93. During a major snowstorm a 51-year-old man sustains frostbite of both hands. Because continuous warm-water soaks are not available, the nurse would:
    1. Rub the hands with snow.
    2. Massage the hands vigorously.
    3. Do aggressive range of motion to both hands.
    4. Apply a dry dressing with gauze between the fingers.

94. The nurse's neighbor fell from a ladder and is complaining of pain in his right arm. The nurse notes deformity between the wrist and the elbow. The first action for the nurse would be to:
    1. Assess for additional injuries.
    2. Observe for bleeding from the site.
    3. Apply a splint from the wrist to the elbow.
    4. Have him lie flat with his right arm elevated.

95. A nurse witnesses a motorcycle accident in which the victim is thrown forcefully from the vehicle to the pavement. On initial assessment of the patient, the nurse notes a crack in the helmet. In administering care to this accident victim, which of the following should receive priority?
    1. Maintaining an open airway
    2. Maintaining normal body temperature
    3. Minimizing movement of the individual's head
    4. Monitoring pulse and respiratory rate every 15 minutes

96. A 70-year-old woman has been hospitalized several times in the last year with complications from chemotherapy for metastatic breast cancer. She is placed on an antidepressant medication the day of her discharge. Discharge teaching for the patient should include:
    1. Three or more (even up to 12) weeks may be required before symptoms improve.
    2. Fluids should be limited to three glasses per day while taking the antidepressant.
    3. Call the physician immediately if dry mouth or orthostatic hypotension occurs.
    4. If this antidepressant fails to control depression, others would not be effective.

97. A patient who wears a hearing aid in her left ear has disturbed sensory perception: auditory, related to decreased hearing secondary to cerumen buildup. The most appropriate plan is to encourage:
    1. Periodic ear washing in the clinic.
    2. Increasing fluid intake to 2000 mL/day.
    3. Cleaning the hearing aid with hydrogen peroxide.
    4. Chewing motions and daily washing of the external parts of the ears.

98. The nurse must recognize which of the following as a recommendation made by the U.S. Food and Drug Administration (FDA) and The Joint Commission (TJC) about restraints?
    1. Restraints can be used indefinitely once the need for them has been documented.
    2. Alternatives to restraints should be developed and implemented before restraints are used.
    3. Restraints should be removed every 4 hours to allow for activities of daily living.
    4. Restraints should be tied with a square knot to the immovable part of the bed.

99. One important complication to avoid after a cesarean delivery is a pelvic thrombosis. The nursing care plan would therefore include:
    1. Teaching good perineal care.
    2. Encouraging early ambulation.
    3. Splinting the lower abdomen when coughing.
    4. Forcing fluids and offering stool softeners.

100. In planning preoperative care for a patient who is about to undergo a below-the-knee amputation (BKA), the nurse may focus on postoperative care by explaining:
    1. Elements of the exercise program.
    2. Postoperative measures to control pain.
    3. Visiting hours immediately after surgery.
    4. Turning, coughing, and deep-breathing maneuvers.

101. If the amniotic sac is to be ruptured by the physician, what is the priority nursing responsibility after the procedure?
    1. Noting time, checking contractions afterward, and reporting
    2. Noting time and amount of fluid and placing pad on perineum
    3. Noting time and characteristics of fluid and checking fetal heart tone after the procedure
    4. Noting amount of fluid and instrument used, testing with Nitrazine, and reporting

102. A patient with diabetes is being treated for pneumonia. She received 22 units of regular insulin at 6:30 AM and was unable to eat her breakfast. The nurse should be alert for signs of:
    1. Polydipsia.
    2. Somnolence.
    3. Diaphoresis.
    4. Increased urine output.

103. A patient with a diagnosis of myocardial infarction has been admitted to the coronary care unit. The nurse assesses the patient's breath sounds and hears fine crackles in the lower lung bases. This symptom may indicate:
    1. Pneumonia.
    2. Arrhythmias.
    3. Lung congestion from heart failure.
    4. An extension of the myocardial infarction.

104. A nurse who is observing a 2-day-old, full-term infant girl in the nursery notes that her hands and feet are cyanotic but her body and cheeks are pink. She has passed greenish-black stool and has lost several ounces since birth. This baby is:
    1. Premature.
    2. Immature.
    3. Normal.
    4. Slightly abnormal.

105. A patient has chronic respiratory disease and is newly diagnosed with Alzheimer disease. In planning his care the nurse should prioritize it based on which aspect of care?
    1. Safety, pain relief, cueing
    2. Safety, physiological assessment, comfort
    3. Psychological care, personal integrity, comfort
    4. Physiological assessment, reorientation, cueing

106. A 9-year-old child was admitted to the hospital in sickle cell anemia crisis. Symptoms of sickle cell crisis include which of the following? Select all that apply.
    _____ 1. Constant or recurrent joint pain
    _____ 2. Elevated temperature
    _____ 3. Elevated hemoglobin
    _____ 4. Acute abdominal pain
    _____ 5. Edema of the hands and feet
    _____ 6. Headache, dizziness, and convulsions

107. A patient has started receiving a xanthine-derivative bronchodilator (aminophylline). When checking for adverse (side) effects, the nurse should observe for which of the following? Select all that apply.
    _____ 1. Abdominal cramping
    _____ 2. Restlessness
    _____ 3. Anorexia
    _____ 4. Tachycardia

_____ 5. Blurred vision

_____ 6. Insomnia

108. During a home visit, the wife of a 78-year-old patient with diabetes tells the nurse that he has been "crankier than usual" the last few days. He is also "moody and hungry as a horse." Which statement tells the nurse that she needs to check his blood sugar?
   1. He refuses to take a bath and stinks.
   2. He has had a cough the last 3 or 4 days.
   3. He had diarrhea once last week in the middle of the night.
   4. He has been in the bathroom off and on all morning urinating.

109. A patient is being evaluated because of complaints of cervical neck pain. As part of the evaluation, the intent is to rule out the possibility of a ruptured disk. What is a common symptom of cervical disk involvement?
   1. Stiff neck
   2. Difficulty walking
   3. Numbness of the lower extremities
   4. Atrophy of the gastrocnemius muscle group

110. A patient with a diagnosis of heart failure is being treated with furosemide (Lasix). The patient has begun to experience tinnitus. The nurse advises her that:
   1. She will not be able to drive.
   2. The sounds she hears are normal.
   3. This symptom is caused by nerve deafness.
   4. This may be related to her diuretic medication.

111. A patient with multiple sclerosis has a neurogenic bladder. When evaluating the patient's response to medical therapy, the nurse would expect which medication to be therapeutic for this bladder condition?
   1. Oxybutynin (Ditropan)
   2. Bethanechol (Urecholine)
   3. Propantheline bromide (Pro-Banthine)
   4. Trimethoprim-sulfamethoxazole (Bactrim, Septra)

112. An elderly patient who is going to undergo gastrointestinal testing has hematuria. The nurse needs to take a complete medication history because this condition can be caused by:
   1. Diuretics.
   2. Phenazopyridine (Pyridium).
   3. Nitrofurantoin (Macrodantin).
   4. Anticoagulants.

113. While sitting in the park in the middle of the afternoon, the nurse hears cries for help from a young mother whose infant is not breathing and has no pulse. To begin cardiopulmonary resuscitation, the nurse places two fingers:
   1. At the nipple level.
   2. On the top half of the sternum.
   3. On the breastbone just below the nipple line.
   4. Two finger widths above the xiphoid process.

114. A patient is admitted with the diagnosis of ruptured appendix. The nurse is alert for the development of the complication of peritonitis. What data would necessitate immediate documentation and reporting to alert the physician of this complication?
   1. Fever, nervousness
   2. Fever, reduced urine output
   3. Increased bowel motility accompanied by fever
   4. Abdominal muscle rigidity accompanied by fever

115. A retired schoolteacher whose husband is on a low-cholesterol diet after a heart attack says that she is totally confused about cholesterol and its importance in the diet. Which statement about cholesterol should the nurse know to be true?
   1. It is best to be totally eliminated from the diet.
   2. It is a normal component of blood and all body cells.
   3. It is not necessary for normal body functions.
   4. It is found in increased amounts in grain products.

116. When a patient returns from dialysis, the nurse notes that she is diaphoretic, restless, and vomiting and has tachycardia. Which action by the nurse is most appropriate initially?
   1. Applying a cool washcloth to the patient's forehead and monitoring vital signs
   2. Encouraging frequent sips of water and elevating the foot of the bed
   3. Lowering the head or elevating the foot of the bed and turning the patient on her side
   4. Decreasing the temperature in the room and turning the patient on her side

117. A 14-year-old girl had spina bifida corrected at birth. She has since developed marked scoliosis and is now admitted to the hospital for spinal fusion and instrumentation. During her admission procedure the primary goal is to provide:
   1. Privacy.
   2. Orientation to the ward.
   3. Her mother's presence.
   4. Introduction to her roommates.

118. A patient is in the emergency department after an automobile accident. Which problem would the nurse consider the most emergent?
   1. The blood glucose level is high at 396 mg/dL.
   2. The patient has a 3-cm laceration of his left eye.
   3. The patient is complaining of shortness of breath.
   4. A distraught family member is crying in the hallway.

119. The primary reason that adverse drug reactions occur frequently in older patients is because older adults have a:
   1. Higher percentage of body water.
   2. Higher percentage of lean muscle.
   3. Lower percentage of body fat.
   4. Higher percentage of body fat.

120. A nurse is evaluating the effectiveness of a patient's intravenous (IV) therapy. Which symptoms would lead the nurse to suspect that the patient may have circulatory overload? Select all that apply.
   _____ 1. Bounding pulse
   _____ 2. Erythema at the infusion site
   _____ 3. Dyspnea
   _____ 4. Cough
   _____ 5. A palpable venous cord at the infusion site
   _____ 6. Chills

121. The nurse is in the process of putting on sterile gloves and must be careful to:
   1. Handle only the outside of each glove.
   2. Pick the first glove up by the inside of the cuff.
   3. Keep the gloves on the sterile field throughout the procedure.
   4. Insert fingers under the outside cuff to apply the first glove.

122. While preparing to administer digitalis to a newly admitted patient, the nurse counts an apical pulse rate of 52 beats/min. The nurse would be correct to:
1. Give the drug as usual.
2. Omit the drug and report the finding to the physician.
3. Give the patient one half the dose.
4. Give the drug but with twice as much water as usual.

123. When moving a patient with a newly inserted chest tube from the stretcher to the bed, the most appropriate action is to:
1. "Strip" the tube to enhance drainage.
2. Mark the time of measurement and the fluid level.
3. Raise the drainage container to chest height to check for air bubbles.
4. Place the drainage system at the foot of the bed.

124. An 11-year-old female patient has an order for prochlorperazine (Compazine), 4 mg intramuscularly. On hand is prochlorperazine, 10 mg/mL. The nurse gives the patient how many milliliters?
Answer: _____ mL

125. Using Clark's rule, calculate the appropriate dose for this child.
Child's weight: 30 pounds
Average adult dose: 10 mg
Clark's rule: Weight in pounds × Adult dose/150
Answer: _____ mg

ANSWERS AND RATIONALES

COMPREHENSIVE EXAMINATION 1: PART 1

1. Application, assessment, physiological integrity, (b).
   4. An increase in potassium can result in cardiac irregularities. Patients are usually on diets low in potassium, phosphorus, and sodium.
   1. An increase in calcium has side effects, but they are not as serious as is an increase in potassium.
   2. An increase in chloride does not have significant side effects.
   3. An increase in sodium has side effects, but they are not as serious as is an increase in potassium. Patients are carefully monitored regarding sodium and potassium.

2. Comprehension, assessment, physiological integrity, (a).
   2. This is true. In dark-skinned people, pressure areas appear darker. With blanching these areas appear gray.
   1. This is descriptive of light-skinned people.
   3. This is a sign of pressure, not blanching.
   4. This may be a sign of pressure.

3. Knowledge, assessment, physiological integrity, (a).
   4. Celiac disease is a basic defect of metabolism, leading to impaired fat absorption.
   1. Celiac disease does not affect absorption of proteins.
   2. Celiac disease does not affect absorption of carbohydrates.
   3. Celiac disease does not affect absorption of vitamins.

4. Application, implementation, physiological integrity, (b).
   4. Because of the neuropathy that can occur in patients with diabetes, they are more sensitive to the cold and can get frostbite more easily.
   1. This is an abrasion and, if cared for properly, should not become infected.

2. Substantial data are not given to warrant the need for an x-ray examination at this time.
3. Rebound swelling should not occur if the time of the cold application is no longer than 20 to 30 minutes.

5. Application, implementation, safe and effective care environment, (a).
   Correct order: 23541.
   2. Give pain medication if needed 15 minutes before ambulation.
   3. Raise head of bed to facilitate ease of getting out of bed.
   5. Encourage the patient to dangle for 5 minutes before ambulation.
   4. Use two-person assist.
   1. Assist patient to sitting position.
   Lowering the height and raising the head of the bed facilitate assisting the patient to a sitting position. Having two people help the patient dangle for 5 minutes and then ambulate maintains safety and provides assistance should the patient complain of feeling dizzy. Pain medication may be necessary but should be given well in advance of any attempt to ambulate to avoid potential falls. Some patients may request pain medication after ambulation.

6. Comprehension, assessment, physiological integrity, (b).
   1. Severe tachypnea seen in bronchiolitis is a contraindication to oral feedings.
   2. Bronchiolitis normally causes tachycardia.
   3, 4. These are not contraindications for oral fluids.

7. Comprehension, planning, health promotion and maintenance, (a).
   2. Nicotine is a potent vasoconstrictor, and further narrowing of the arterial walls worsens peripheral vascular disease.
   1. Smoking causes hypertension, not hypotension.
   3. Smoking does irritate the lungs, but this is not the mechanism by which it worsens peripheral vascular disease.
   4. Smoking does not decrease the RBC count.

8. Analysis, assessment, physiological integrity, (b).
   _____ 1. This is a vague, generalized sign noted in many conditions.
   X 2. This is a sign of hyperkalemia.
   X 3. This is a sign of hyperkalemia.
   _____ 4. This is a sign of fluid imbalance.
   X 5. This is a sign of hyperkalemia.
   _____ 6. This is a sign of a fluid deficit.

9. Application, assessment, physiological integrity, (b).
   1. Accidental removal of the parathyroid glands can lead to tetany because the glands secrete a hormone that regulates calcium balance.
   2. A seizure is possible in tetany but is not one of the initial symptoms.
   3. This is not associated with parathyroid removal.
   4. Although respiratory compromise is a potential problem with a thyroidectomy, loss of the gag reflex is not associated with parathyroid removal.

10. Analysis, assessment, physiological integrity, (b).
    1. These are the early symptoms of prostatitis.
    2. This is related and may indicate a urinary tract infection.
    3, 4. This is a routine part of any general health history.

11. Application, planning, physiological integrity, (b).
    4. People with pulmonary disease are at risk for acidosis secondary to CO_2 retention.
    1. This does not warrant checking within the next hour.
    2, 3. Data are insufficient to support this assumption.

12. Application, implementation, safe and effective care environment, (b).
    2. The patient will be able to get out of bed and pivot into a chair with no weight bearing on the affected leg.
    1. Bed rest is not needed and increases the risk of deep vein thrombosis.
    3. Full weight bearing is not appropriate immediately after surgery.
    4. No skeletal traction is used for this type of procedure.

13. Application, implementation, psychosocial integrity, (b).
    3. The purpose of arthroscopy is to improve joint function and limit the amount of pain.
    1. This does not alleviate the patient's anxiety; and, although a surgeon may need to speak to the patient, the nurse should answer the patient's question to the best of his or her ability.
    2. Undergoing arthroscopy will most likely postpone the need for a knee replacement, but it may not eliminate the need for a knee replacement at a later time.
    4. This procedure does not cure degenerative joint disease, but it will alleviate some of the symptoms.

14. Analysis, assessment, physiological integrity, (b).
    2. Hypocalcemia can occur after thyroidectomy as a result of inadvertent removal of parathyroid tissue. The signs and symptoms of this complication are numbness and tingling of fingertips, toes, and lips; carpopedal spasms; tachycardia; tachypnea; and hypertension.
    1. Hyperglycemia is not a usual consequence of thyroid surgery; the signs and symptoms of hyperglycemia are polydipsia, polyuria, and polyphagia.
    3. Hyperkalemia is not a usual consequence of thyroid surgery; the signs and symptoms of hyperkalemia would include cardiac rhythm disturbances.
    4. Thyroid storm can occur after surgery, but it is characterized by severe tachycardia, severe hypertension, and hyperthermia.

15. Application, implementation, health promotion and maintenance, (b).
    2. Obesity increases strain on weight-bearing joints; reduction of weight minimizes some of the presenting symptoms.
    1. This does not reduce joint strain but does maintain existing range of motion.
    3. This provides comfort but does not reduce strain.
    4. This does not control strain but aids in pain control.

16. Application, assessment, physiological integrity, (a).
    3. The standard assessment model for a CPR emergency situation is CAB—circulation, airway, and breathing. These changes are based on the 2011 AHA Guidelines for CPR and ECC. Change in sequence allowed for starting compressions sooner and minimal delay in giving breaths.
    1, 2, 4. These sequences are incorrect according to the latest guidelines.

17. Application, implementation, physiological integrity, (b).
    4. This direction allows the fluid left in the space to consolidate and lessens the possibility of mediastinal shift.
    1, 2, 3. These are inappropriate; they increase the risk of mediastinal shift when the patient is placed on the unaffected side.

18. Application, assessment, physiological integrity, (a).
    2. Fluid balance and removal of excess fluids are two of the primary goals of dialysis. Comparing predialysis and postdialysis weights measures the effectiveness of therapy.
    1. Diphenhydramine is not routinely given for dialysis.
    3. Urinalysis is not necessary because blood tests are used to measure kidney function.
    4. Patients do not need to be on NPO status.

19. Knowledge, assessment, physiological integrity, (b).
    4. Cerebral palsy is a disorder that affects the motor centers of the brain; it is usually caused by birth trauma or head trauma.
    1. This is a chromosome abnormality.
    2. This is an S-shaped curvature of the spine.
    3. This is an infection of the bone.

20. Application, planning, physiological integrity, (a).
    4. Comatose patients can still hear what is being said and may react physiologically.
    1, 3. No data are available to support these.
    2. The family may be upset by bad news, but that is not the reason to avoid bedside conversation.

21. Comprehension, planning, psychosocial integrity, (a).
    3. It aids in family grieving and allows the family to feel useful.
    1. No evidence exists that this prolongs the dying process.
    2. Actually it increases the workload because the nurse must assist the family members and their psychosocial needs.
    4. Family members often want to help and do not view it as work.

22. Comprehension, assessment, physiological integrity, (b).
    2. Normal urine should be a clear yellow liquid. Differences in color and clarity may signify body fluid imbalance.
    1. Normally urine is slightly aromatic.
    3. The specific gravity of urine is normally low.
    4. The presence of RBCs in a urine sample would signify kidney disease.

23. Application, implementation, physiological integrity, (a).
    2. The inner cannula is removed, and hydrogen peroxide is used to break up the dried mucus.
    1. Cotton swabs are never used because they can leave behind tiny cotton fibers, which can be inhaled.
    3, 4. The outer cannula is never removed.

24. Analysis, assessment, physiological integrity, (c).
    2. These are symptoms of rubeola.
    1. Symptoms of chickenpox include a clear, vesicular rash; fever; irritability; and pruritus.
    3. Symptoms of mumps include enlarged parotid glands and fever with no rash.
    4. Symptoms of rubella do not include a high fever or white spots at the back of the throat.

25. Application, planning, physiological integrity, (b).
    3. *This is an appropriate discharge instruction; Kegel exercises help strengthen the perineal floor muscles.*
    1. This is an unsafe instruction that may cause further bleeding.
    2. This is an unsafe instruction; fluids should be encouraged to 10 to 12 glasses per day.
    4. This is an unsafe instruction; any increased redness of the urine should be reported because it may indicate hemorrhage.

26. Application, planning, physiological integrity, (a).
    3. *It takes longer to inspire or expire air because of age-related physiological changes.*
    1. This is not a proven fact for older adults.
    2. This is not a proven correlation.
    4. Overall respiratory muscle structure and function decrease in older adults.

27. Knowledge, assessment, physiological integrity, (b).
    3. *Wilms tumor is found only in the kidney and kidney area (lymph nodes, renal vein, or vena cava).*
    1. Although part of the genitourinary (GU) system, the bladder is not part of the kidney area.
    2. Although part of the GU system, the ureters are not part of the kidney area.
    4. Although part of the GU system, the urethra is not part of the kidney area.

28. Analysis, evaluation, physiological integrity, (b).
    3. *The presence of meat in this patient's system will cause the Hemoccult test result to be positive, whether or not blood is actually in his stool. The patient should be free of red meat for 2 to 3 days for the test result to be considered accurate.*
    1. Ingestion of coffee should have no bearing on the test results.
    2. The gelatin should not cause the developer slide to turn blue, which would indicate the presence of blood.
    4. Lots of fiber should not have any bearing on the results of the test.

29. Application, implementation, physiological integrity, (b).
    3. *A dietary record assists the nurse in determining problem areas.*
    1. This intervention promotes salivation but does not affect food or caloric intake.
    2. This intervention promotes elasticity of the skin but does not affect food or caloric intake.
    4. This is an appropriate intervention for the diagnosis of imbalanced nutrition: more than body requirements.

30. Analysis, assessment, physiological integrity, (b).
    2. *These are classic symptoms of an infant with pyloric stenosis.*
    1. Symptoms of Hirschsprung disease include constipation, abdominal distention, bile-stained mucus and emesis, and inadequate weight gain.
    3. Symptoms of esophageal atresia include excessive salivation and drooling, coughing and choking during feedings, and regurgitation of all feedings.
    4. Symptoms of intussusception appear suddenly and include pallor, vomiting, stools with blood and mucus, drawing up of the legs and crying out caused by sharp colicky pain, and signs of shock.

31. Application, implementation, physiological integrity, (b).
    2. *For the proper laboratory tests to be completed, all voided urine must be collected.*
    1. In a 24-hour urine specimen all urine that the patient voids in a 24-hour period is collected.
    3. No discernible reason exists to insert a retention catheter unless the patient is incontinent.
    4. All urine is sent to the laboratory in one large, dark container.

32. Application, planning, physiological integrity, (b).
    2. *The patient has difficulty swallowing and needs to have special feeding precautions taken.*
    1. Facial exercises do not help the patient swallow.
    3. The patient may or may not have difficulty forming words; however, if dysphagia is present, then special feeding precautions must be instituted.
    4. This may be necessary and needs to be determined, but the plan of care needs to address the swallowing difficulty.

33. Application, implementation, physiological integrity, (b).
    3. *Hemianopsia is blindness of one half of the visual field. For the patient to maximize eyesight, scanning the environment is necessary.*
    1. This further blinds the patient.
    2. Both eyes have lost one half the vision.
    4. The problem is not dry corneas.

34. Comprehension, assessment, physiological integrity, (a).
    1. *In the assessment phase the nurse observes the physiological, psychosocial, health, and safety needs of patients.*
    2. Teaching is part of nursing intervention.
    3. Prioritizing problems is part of the planning phase.
    4. Collaborating to determine a plan of care is part of the planning phase.

35. Application, assessment, physiological integrity, (b).
    4. *The patient may be unable to expel all urine fully from the bladder. Further assessment is indicated to assess the fullness of the urinary bladder, but this response is the best indicator that the patient may need the catheter.*
    1. Without further data this would not indicate that the patient needs the catheter.
    2. The urinary bladder should be palpated to assess fullness. Consuming large amounts of fluids is not an indication that the catheterization is necessary.
    3. The patient's bladder is most likely empty if the incontinent episode occurred. Further assessment is necessary.

36. Analysis, planning, physiological integrity, (c).
    4. *Nitroprusside is preferred because of its quick vasoactivity and short half-life.*
    1. Propranolol hydrochloride is a maintenance drug for hypertension.
    2. Enalapril maleate is primarily used for maintenance therapy for hypertension.
    3. Nifedipine is used as a maintenance drug for hypertension.

37. Application, assessment, psychosocial integrity, (b).
    2. *Collecting data concerning normal home practices allows the nurse to plan care effectively for the patient and is a priority.*
    1. Whether this is necessary has not been ascertained.

3. This may not be possible, and the nurse must communicate effectively with the patient.

4. This is appropriate; however, the nurse must first establish communication with the patient.

38. Application, implementation, physiological integrity, (c).

   1. *This response best describes the reason for the runny nose and watery eyes, which is the question posed by the patient.*

   2. This is not clearly established, and it does not answer the patient's question.

   3. This may be a normal reflex; however, the patient is asking why it happens during a specific time.

   4. This is true, but it does not describe the reason for the watery eyes and runny nose.

39. Application, implementation, physiological integrity, (b).

   Answer: 1.5 mL
   Dose desired (DD) = 75 mg
   Dose on hand (DH) = 50 mg
   Volume (V) = 1 mL
   DD/DH = 75 mg/50 mg × (V) 1 mL = 1.5 × 1 = 1.5 mL

40. Application, planning, physiological integrity, (b).

   3. *Dried fruits are excellent sources of iron.*

   1. Milk and dairy products contain very little iron.

   2. Refined cereals have had many of the valuable nutrients removed.

   4. These are good sources of vitamin A, not iron.

41. Comprehension, planning, physiological integrity, (c).

   4. *Dobutamine stimulates beta₁ receptors to increase cardiac contractility and stroke volume. At therapeutic dosages the drug increases cardiac output by decreasing peripheral vascular resistance, reducing ventricular filling pressure, and facilitating AV node conduction.*

   1. Decreased cardiac contractility is the basic mechanism of heart failure.

   2. Peripheral resistance is decreased, not increased.

   3. Cardiac output is increased, not decreased.

42. Application, implementation, physiological integrity, (b).

   3. *Newer medications decrease gastric acid secretion. A well-balanced diet provides nutrients for healing.*

   1. Dairy products provide only temporary relief and have a high fat content.

   2. A bland diet is no longer indicated.

   4. Eating three full meals is better. Any food intake produces acid.

43. Analysis, implementation, physiological integrity, (c).

   1. *Because the patient is having difficulty swallowing, this position creates a gravity force for downward motion of food.*

   2. This position would put him in danger of injury if he should fall.

   3. This position would not help his dysphagia.

   4. Position changes every 2 hours would not help the patient's swallowing difficulty.

44. Comprehension, assessment, physiological integrity, (c).

   4. *In general, ventricular arrhythmias are the most dangerous and potentially life-threatening.*

   1. A sinus arrhythmia may cause difficulty, but it is generally not life-threatening.

   2. An atrial arrhythmia is not as dangerous as a ventricular arrhythmia.

3. An AV nodal arrhythmia can cause serious consequences but is not as dangerous as a ventricular arrhythmia.

45. Comprehension, planning, safe and effective care environment, (b).

   _____ 1. Botulism is prevalent in improperly canned foods.

   X 2. **E. coli*–related illness is prevented by ensuring that red meats are thoroughly cooked.***

   _____ 3. This may prevent infection; however, it is indicated in preventing salmonellosis.

   _____ 4. Eggs contribute to infections caused by *Salmonella.*

   X 5. **E. coli*–related illness is also prevented by ensuring proper and thorough washing of fruits and vegetables.***

46. Application, implementation, physiological integrity, (a).

   1. *Positioning the patient on his or her side (laterally) lessens the danger of aspiration of secretions.*

   2, 3, 4. These are not practical and might cause injury to the patient in a postictal state.

47. Analysis, assessment, physiological integrity, (b).

   2. *Meat and dairy products are the main source of protein in the diet.*

   1. Green, leafy vegetables and dried fruits can be good sources of iron.

   3. Bread and cereals can provide many B-complex vitamins.

   4. Many fruits and vegetables are good sources of vitamins A, D, E, and K.

48. Comprehension, evaluation, physiological integrity, (b).

   1. *The muscle rigidity caused by the involuntary contraction of striated muscles may inhibit fluid voluntary movement. This results in the "cogwheel" jerking motor contractions that are a characteristic manifestation of this disease.*

   2. Movement may appear weak, especially when the patient is tired.

   3. The tremors associated with Parkinson disease usually lessen with voluntary movement.

   4. The goal is to get and keep the patient as physically active as long as possible.

49. Application, implementation, physiological integrity, (b).

   4. *Research studies have indicated that a link may exist between omega-3 fatty acids and a low incidence of heart disease.*

   1. This is not a true statement. Fatty acids are essential to the diet.

   2. No evidence exists that this is necessary. The patient merely requires information from the nurse.

   3. No evidence exists to support this.

50. Application, implementation, physiological integrity, (b).

   4. *Mineral oil is indigestible and carries fat-soluble vitamins with it as it leaves the body.*

   1. Mineral oil is not irritating, but it is also not a good idea, as previously indicated.

   2. It does not add calories, but it is indigestible, and its action on fat-soluble vitamins makes it a poor choice.

   3. Mineral oil has no calories because it is not digested by the body.

51. Analysis, evaluation, physiological integrity, (b).

   1. *An unexpected change has occurred in the patient's condition, especially with the confusion; the physician must therefore be notified.*

2. This would be negligent.

3. Reality orientation is in order but is not a priority.

4. Older adults do not absorb drugs in the same manner as younger adults do. However, simply observing would be negligent given that the physician has to be kept current; the medication may not be causing the confusion.

52. Application, implementation, physiological integrity, (b).

4. This equipment may be necessary if the enlarged epiglottis completely obstructs the airway.

1. Any examination of the throat may lead to laryngospasm.

2. The child with epiglottis has difficulty swallowing.

3. Warm steam is not a method of treatment in epiglottis.

53. Comprehension, implementation, physiological integrity, (b).

3. Recommendations are that smokers increase their vitamin C by 100 mg/day.

1. Vitamin A is fat soluble and can be toxic in megadoses.

2. Vitamin K is synthesized by the body.

4. Vitamin B has not been shown to be deficient in smokers.

54. Analysis, assessment, safe and effective care environment, (b).

1. This is the first priority question.

2, 3, 4. These questions ask for information that is not important at this time.

55. Analysis, assessment, physiological integrity, (c).

2. The patient is experiencing an aura, which can appear as any sensory sensation. An aura is a precursor to a seizure. The nurse has her lie down immediately to protect her from injury should she fall.

1. The nurse would note her comments later but needs to stay with her at this point; a psychiatrist need not be contacted.

3. IV diazepam would probably be given but only with an order.

4. Her physician would be called to inform him or her of the seizure, but this would be done later.

56. Analysis, evaluation, physiological integrity, (b).

3. Approximately 60% of the total calories in the diet should come from carbohydrates. Of this amount 40% should come from complex forms such as pastas and whole grains. They break down more slowly than do simple sugars, thus providing a steadier blood level.

1. Approximately 15% of carbohydrates come from simple sugars such as those found in fruit or milk.

2. Artificial sweeteners should be used only in moderation.

4. Adolescents find support with peers, and they must spend time with them. Healthy choices can be made at most fast-food restaurants.

57. Application, planning, safe and effective care environment, (b).

4. Popcorn is a choking hazard for young children.

1. Apples are appropriate for toddlers.

2. Toddlers should drink whole milk to help promote growth and energy metabolism.

3. Chocolate cake is not a hazard, although it is not very nutritious.

58. Analysis, evaluation, physiological integrity, (c).

1. One of the purposes of the four-bottle technique is to observe the color changes in the urine to assess

for blood over time. Normally the urine lightens in color as bleeding decreases. Therefore the oldest specimen is discarded, which would be the one to the left.

2, 3, 4. These choices do not follow proper procedure for such a technique; refer to the rationale for the correct answer.

59. Application, implementation, psychosocial integrity, (b).

2. This is the most therapeutic.

1. This has a negative effect.

3. Previous unacceptable behavior should be challenged and integrated into current behavioral activities.

4. This is not therapeutic.

60. Application, implementation, physiological integrity, (b).

1. Many antibiotics, including ampicillin, decrease the effects of Ortho-Novum 1/50 and other oral contraceptives.

2. Blood sugar is checked routinely because ampicillin can cause a false-positive urine sugar result; focus of question is the contraception.

3. The full course of antibiotics should be completed to decrease the chances of a superinfection.

4. A rash indicates an allergic reaction and is to be observed for but is not an expected effect of treatment.

61. Application, implementation, psychosocial integrity, (b).

4. Additional information is needed to provide the necessary care for this patient.

1. This does not help the current situation.

2. This is false reassurance.

3. This does not help solve the situation.

62. Comprehension, assessment, psychosocial integrity, (b).

2. Denial is common when an individual is diagnosed with a potentially fatal disease.

1. Repression is a response to a painful experience.

3. Fantasy is unacceptable behavior.

4. Rationalization is using a "good" reason to explain behavior.

63. Comprehension, implementation, physiological integrity, (c).

1. Cranial nerve I (olfactory) is assessed by following the technique described. A normal finding occurs when the person correctly identifies odors presented.

2. Cranial nerve II (optic) is the nerve that controls sight.

3. Cranial nerve III (otic) is the oculomotor nerve.

4. Cranial nerve VII (facial) is the facial nerve and provides symmetry of facial movement.

64. Analysis, evaluation, psychosocial integrity, (b).

2. The nurse must be able to deal with his or her own feelings first.

1. Standard Precautions are all that are required.

3. This is not a priority.

4. This is not the first thing to do.

65. Analysis, implementation, physiological integrity, (c).

4. A change in neurological status may indicate increased intracranial pressure (IICP). A thorough neurological assessment is indicated. Placing the head of bed in a slightly elevated position aids in decreasing the pressure rise. The physician should be notified immediately in case emergency interventions are required.

1. This is an inappropriate and negligent action.

2. In suspected IICP, the head of the bed is elevated slightly to decrease intracranial pressure.

3. Preparing the patient for emergency surgery may be indicated, but the nurse must begin with assessment of the patient's status and subsequent notification of the physician.

66. Application, evaluation, physiological integrity, (a).
    3. Patients usually show improvement in 2 to 4 weeks.
    1, 2. This is not long enough to see the desired effect.
    4. Seeing improvement should not take this long.

67. Knowledge, planning, physiological integrity, (b).
    3. Prednisone is given to decrease inflammation.
    1, 2, 4. Prednisone is not used for these reasons in the treatment of rheumatic fever.

68. Knowledge, assessment, health promotion and maintenance, (b).
    3. An infant normally triples his or her birth weight by 12 months of age.
    1, 2. Six and 9 months are too short a time frame to triple birth weight; weight doubles during these months.
    4. At 15 months a normal infant weighs more than he or she did at 12 months.

69. Application, assessment, physiological integrity, (a).
    1. Assessment data relevant to seizure disorder include a complete history, medication history, and allergy history. Data collection should be specific to the seizure disorder such as onset, duration, behavior before and after, type of body movements, loss of consciousness, incontinence, and awareness of seizure afterward.
    2. Diet and exercise history is not specific to the seizure disorder.
    3. Social and educational levels are not relative to this disorder.
    4. Work history is not relative to this disorder.

70. Application, implementation, physiological integrity, (b).
    2. Patient teaching should include the importance of wearing a medical identification (MedicAlert) bracelet or tag or other means of medical identification. The patient should also be taught to avoid situations known to trigger seizures, such as flashing or blinking lights, stress, or lack of sleep and to be particularly aware of situations that may act as triggers specifically for them.
    1. This response is an expected outcome of the nursing and medical treatment plan.
    3. People with a diagnosis of seizure disorders are frequently evaluated many times throughout the year and should be encouraged to keep follow-up medical appointments and appointments to have blood drawn for laboratory work.
    4. This response supports social stigmas associated with epilepsy. Individuals in the community need education regarding seizure disorders. Individuals with a seizure disorder are encouraged to live normal lives.

71. Application, implementation, psychosocial integrity, (b).
    1. This helps identify the content of the delusion.
    2. Logic cannot be used to explain delusions.
    3. Do not leave the patient alone.
    4. Do not imply that the patient is wrong.

72. Analysis, implementation, physiological integrity, (b).
    2. This is a toxic level. The dose should be held and the physician notified.
    1, 3. The level is already toxic.
    4. Alprazolam is an antianxiety medication and does not substitute for lithium.

73. Application, implementation, physiological integrity, (b).
    1. An appropriate nursing action in the administration of TPN is to weigh the patient daily, monitor blood glucose levels regularly to assess the patient's ability to metabolize concentrated glucose, and wean gradually to avoid a sudden drop in blood sugar.
    2. This response reflects a lack of knowledge relevant to the rationale for administering TPN. The patient may express hunger sensations but be physiologically compromised, requiring TPN for nutritional support.
    3. Monitoring liver, renal, and cardiovascular function is required of any patient receiving fluids but is not specific to the administration of TPN.
    4. This response is incorrect; refer to No. 1.

74. Application, implementation, physiological integrity, (b).
    1. This can cause hypertensive crisis.
    2. The medicine can be taken on an empty stomach.
    3. It is taken in the morning or may be taken in multiple doses.
    4. This is not necessary.

75. Application, implementation, psychosocial integrity, (b).
    2. This is a realistic, feasible approach.
    1. Blanket approval is unrealistic.
    3. She should begin to learn to tolerate separation.
    4. This is unrealistic and leads to mistrust.

76. Application, implementation, psychosocial integrity, (b).
    1. This is the best response; it helps develop trust.
    2. This is not a good reason to stay. In this response the nurse rather than the patient is the focus. This does not foster trust.
    3. This is false reassurance.
    4. This puts the patient on the defensive.

77. Application, planning, physiological integrity, (b).
    1. The effect of conscious sedation requires careful monitoring of the airway; therefore the risk for ineffective airway clearance is appropriate.
    2. Although a concern and an appropriate nursing diagnosis for the patient, it is not a priority.
    3. This nursing diagnosis is appropriate after the procedure when discussing physical limitations with the patient.
    4. This is inappropriate because the procedure being done is noninvasive.

78. Application, implementation, psychosocial integrity, (c).
    2. Being dependable is necessary for the patient to trust and feel secure. Contracted time with the patient is for that patient only. Terminating a session early is a patient response that the nurse should understand and anticipate.
    1. This is inappropriate; the patient has to assume responsibility for his or her behavior.
    3. Contracted time with the patient is time for that patient only; the nurse should remain for the duration of the contracted time.
    4. This is inappropriate; the focus is always the patient, not the nurse.

79. Analysis, evaluation, psychosocial integrity, (b).

   2. Patients who are less depressed have more energy to commit suicide.

   1, 3. The opposite is true.

   4. Patients may not verbalize suicide plans.

80. Knowledge, assessment, physiological integrity, (a).

   _____ 1. Babbling develops at 6 to 7 months of age.

   X   2. The newborn has reached a milestone and is now considered an infant.

   X   3. The posterior fontanel closes by this age.

   _____ 4. Lower incisor is apparent at 7 to 8 months of age.

   X   5. The infant now stays awake for longer periods of time.

   X   6. A budding personality is beginning to develop at this age.

81. Application, implementation, physiological integrity, (a).

   3. This position promotes venous return.

   1, 2. These positions may increase intracranial pressure.

   4. This position causes flexion of the hips and perhaps the neck.

82. Analysis, evaluation, physiological integrity, (b).

   2. Bleeding is a serious side effect of anticoagulant therapy. Nursing measures focus on monitoring for signs of active bleeding.

   1. This is a common side effect of any medication. Hematemesis would be of serious concern.

   3. This is not a common side effect of this class of medications and does not suggest bleeding.

   4. This is a common side effect of many medications.

83. Application, implementation, physiological integrity, (b).

   1. Weight should be measured at the same time each day in the same clothing.

   2. Not enough information is given to assume this. The patient may be taking medication several times per day or at irregular intervals.

   3. Daily weights are a more accurate measurement of fluid retention.

   4. Daily weights indicate early fluid retention, avoiding symptoms of advancing congestive heart failure.

84. Application, implementation, health promotion and maintenance, (b).

   3. Increased fluid intake decreases the tenacity of respiratory secretions, making sputum removal easier.

   1. Low hydration makes respiratory secretions tenacious and difficult to expel.

   2. Tracheal suctioning is invasive and should be used only if the patient is unable to expel secretions independently.

   4. Postural drainage relies on gravity to assist with expulsion of secretions. Affected lung areas vary and must be vertical for this to occur.

85. Application, implementation, physiological integrity, (a).

   1. People taking this anticonvulsant are especially prone to developing gingival hyperplasia.

   2. This is inappropriate and is not relative to the situation presented; see No. 4.

   3. This is inappropriate and is not a patient responsibility.

   4. Adequate rest and diet are important. Answer No. 1 is individualized to the situation and is the better choice.

86. Analysis, evaluation, physiological integrity, (b).

   3. Nitroglycerin has a vasodilating effect and is often the cause of headaches, at least in the initial period of therapy.

   1. Acetaminophen normally alleviates headache discomfort.

   2. Digoxin is a cardiotonic and does not normally cause headache.

   4. Potassium chloride is used to counter the side effect of hypokalemia and does not cause headaches.

87. Application, evaluation, physiological integrity, (b).

   1. Increased respiratory rate, chest tightness, and hypoxemia are signs of complications following a thoracentesis and should be reported to the physician immediately.

   2. Respiratory rate would be increased, as would the pulse; hypotension would be noted.

   3. Bradycardia is not an early sign of respiratory distress. Low blood pressure may occur secondary to removing a volume of fluid and should be monitored. A dry, hacking cough usually does not indicate respiratory distress.

   4. A normal sinus rhythm indicates adequate cardiac function, normotension reflects blood pressure within normal limits, and ventilation is the act of moving air into and out of the lungs.

88. Comprehension, assessment, health promotion and maintenance, (b).

   _____ 1. A bounding pulse normally is not seen in patients with cardiogenic shock.

   X   2. This is a classic sign of cardiogenic shock.

   _____ 3. Hypertension is not a usual symptom of cardiogenic shock.

   _____ 4. Hot, dry skin normally is not seen in a patient diagnosed with cardiogenic shock.

   X   5. Weak pulses and rapid respirations are classic signs of cardiogenic shock.

   X   6. Clammy skin and chest pain are classic signs of cardiogenic shock.

89. Application, assessment, physiological integrity, (a).

   3. Assessment begins with first determining responsiveness.

   1. Activation of the emergency medical system occurs after responsiveness is determined.

   2, 4. These actions are initiated only after determining responsiveness.

90. Application, implementation, physiological integrity, (b).

   3. The Holter monitor records a heart tracing during various activities and is compared with activities that the patient is also documenting.

   1. A glucometer evaluates capillary blood sugar levels.

   2. Urine tests are used to evaluate various conditions but not heart activity during exertion.

   4. This study evaluates blood flow through a carotid artery or extremity.

91. Comprehension, assessment, physiological integrity, (a).

   4. Injuries at or above C5 result in quadriplegia.

   1. Emotions remain intact; however, grief and mourning reactions and depression frequently occur.

   2. Desire remains; however, it may be affected by emotional reactions to the trauma and its effects.

   3. Speaking ability remains intact.

92. Comprehension, implementation, physiological integrity, (b).
    2. *This steroidal medication is usually used for this specific type of meningitis.*
    1, 3, 4. These drugs are not used for treating *H. influenzae* type B meningitis.

93. Application, planning, health promotion and maintenance, (b).
    2. *Injury can lead to infection. The tissues are already compromised with regard to oxygen and nutrients; certain positions (legs crossed, knees flexed) hamper circulation.*
    1, 3, 4. These measures can lead to greater compromise in circulation and burns.

94. Application, implementation, physiological integrity, (b).
    1. *Bag-valve-mask or Ambu ventilation provides oxygen to correct the hypoxia.*
    2. Chest tubes only drain the pleural space.
    3. Cricothyroid puncture would be indicated if injury to the upper airway has occurred.
    4. Trendelenburg position may assist with fluid drainage but does not help to correct hypoxia; it may also cause dyspnea.

95. Application, assessment, physiological integrity, (b).
    __X__ 1. *Yawning is the body's way of taking deep breaths to increase oxygen to the brain.*
    _____ 2. Bradycardia is a later sign.
    __X__ 3. *Tachycardia is an early sign reflecting the attempt of the heart to compensate.*
    __X__ 4. *Restlessness is an early sign reflecting the attempt of the heart to compensate through tachycardia.*
    _____ 5. Dyspnea is a sign of prolonged or severe oxygen deprivation.
    _____ 6. Confusion is a later sign.

96. Application, implementation, safe and effective care environment, (a).
    4. *This maintains an intact drainage system. The urine specimen will not likely become contaminated.*
    1. These are unnecessary actions and increase risk to the patient of acquiring trauma or infection or both.
    2. Urine collecting in the drainage bag is likely to have organisms present, thereby giving inaccurate test results.
    3. This disrupts the patency of the system and increases likelihood of contamination and a urinary tract infection.

97. Application, implementation, physiological integrity, (a).
    Answer: 2 tablets
    60 mg = 1 gr.
    60 × 5 = 300 mg/tablet
    300 mg × 2 tablets = 600 mg (dose desired) = 2 tablets

98. Application, implementation, psychosocial integrity, (a).
    4. *This is an emotional change that is common after a CVA. Emotional lability may or may not be appropriate to the situation.*
    1. This is inappropriate and encourages a negative behavior-modification technique. The patient has emotional lability.
    2. This is inappropriate. The patient is not acting this way on purpose.
    3. This is common but not a normal sign of healing.

99. Analysis, assessment, physiological integrity, (b).
    4. *This question seeks more data and demonstrates attentive listening. Beets, blackberries, rhubarb, and some medications may turn the urine red or orange.*
    1. Milk increase is unnecessary. Liquids normally should be approximately 2000 mL/day. This response gives a quick fix.
    2. This response offers false reassurance and belittles the patient's concern.
    3. This response does show that the nurse is listening and seeking more data; however, No. 4 is individualized and therefore a better choice.

100. Comprehension, planning, health promotion and maintenance, (b).
    4. *As individuals age, the action of the sweat and oil glands becomes less active; therefore daily bathing is not required.*
    1. Body odor may not diminish, although perspiration does.
    2. This may not be true of all older adults.
    3. This is not a true statement.

101. Application, assessment, health promotion and maintenance, (b).
    2. *These are the classic symptoms of hyperthyroidism.*
    1. These symptoms are typical of hypothyroidism.
    3. These symptoms are caused by a slowed metabolic rate and are seen in hypothyroidism.
    4. These do not indicate thyroid disease.

102. Application, planning, safe and effective care environment, (b).
    1. *This allows the nurse to perform skills completely yet decreases the amount of time that he or she must spend in the radioactive environment.*
    2. Entering the patient's room frequently exposes the nurse to the radioactive environment. The implant should not be visible for the nurse to assess.
    3. This increases the amount of time the nurse spends in the radioactive environment.
    4. Although decreasing the loneliness of an isolated patient is important, this measure would increase the amount of time the nurse is in the radioactive environment.

103. Comprehension, planning, physiological integrity, (b).
    2. *This is the physiological action of the pharmacological therapy.*
    1. This is true of any medication.
    3. This is true, but it is not the appropriate rationale.
    4. This may occur after multiple consecutive missed doses.

104. Application, implementation, physiological integrity, (a).
    1. *Massaging the area around the reddened area and avoiding repeated pressure by turning frequently from left side to back enhances circulation to the right side.*
    2, 3, 4. These are inappropriate nursing actions for pressure areas.

105. Application, implementation, safe and effective care environment, (b).
    4. *These foods increase the amount of bulk and fiber in the diet.*

1. Although fruit juices contain some fiber, dairy products will constipate the individual.
2. Meat, cheese, and poultry products do not increase fiber in the diet.
3. Processed carbohydrates and milk products do not combat constipation.

106. Application, planning, safe and effective care environment, (b).
    2. The Centers for Disease Control and Prevention recommends using Standard Precautions at all times.
    1. In emergency situations patients often are not able to provide accurate information.
    3. This is highly impractical and inappropriate.
    4. Relying only on the obvious is inappropriate.

107. Knowledge, assessment, physiological integrity, (a).
    3. Rheumatic fever is a chronic disease caused by a streptococcal infection.
    1. It is not caused by a virus.
    2. It is not caused by a fungus.
    4. It is not caused by *Staphylococcus* bacteria.

108. Application, assessment, psychosocial integrity, (b).
    1. Denial is indicated by the patient's inability to recognize the seriousness of his act and his belief that he can go home.
    2. Projection is placing unacceptable impulses onto another person.
    3. Regression is moving back to an earlier time or developmental level during periods of stress.
    4. Sublimation is the process by which negative impulses are channeled into more acceptable outlets.

109. Comprehension, evaluation, safe and effective care environment, (a).
    2. Hardwood floors may pose a risk for slippage, especially if scatter rugs are used.
    1. An electric stove is safer than a gas stove.
    3. Nonglare lighting helps older adults to read.
    4. Elevated toilet seats may help older adults transfer to and from the toilet.

110. Comprehension, evaluation, health promotion and maintenance, (b).
    4. Circulatory changes cause drug distribution in older adults to be altered, thereby increasing the chances for adverse drug reactions.
    1. Older adults do not excrete drugs more effectively.
    2. This statement is not true; some muscle wasting occurs.
    3. Absorption is altered, but it is the result of decreased gastric motility.

111. Analysis, assessment, physiological integrity, (a).
    4. This is a correct assessment.
    1. These are not likely to be delusions.
    2. This is incorrect; symptoms may worsen.
    3. This is unlikely.

112. Application, implementation, physiological integrity, (a).
    2. Vomiting from acute alcoholism can cause aspiration, and the depressed central nervous system can lead to respiratory arrest.
    1. Shock is associated with delirium tremens, not acute alcoholism.
    3. This is appropriate for mild alcohol withdrawal; acute alcoholism requires observation.

4. Disulfiram may be recommended as part of an aftercare program for the person with alcoholism who has already undergone withdrawal.

113. Application, implementation, physiological integrity, (b).
    2. This allows the older adult, who may have dry mucous membranes, to swallow the medications more easily.
    1. The head of the bed should be at 60 to 90 degrees.
    3. Medications given in this manner may not be compatible and may be overwhelming.
    4. Medications should never be mixed with the patient's food.

114. Comprehension, planning, safe and effective care environment, (b).
    3. Advance directives include living wills and health care proxies (durable power of attorney).
    1. Guardianship is established by the courts.
    2. Organ donation is not included under advance directives.
    4. Active euthanasia is currently illegal in the United States, and passive euthanasia includes "do not resuscitate" (DNR) orders.

115. Application, implementation, physiological integrity, (b).
    3. An arrest in an adult is usually caused by a cardiac arrhythmia such as ventricular fibrillation. Early defibrillation is necessary to revive the patient.
    1. Prolonged lack of oxygen in either the child or the adult causes brain damage; this is not the correct explanation.
    2. Children need to be ventilated as quickly as possible because an arrest in a child usually results from choking or suffocation. The child may revive quickly after CPR is initiated.
    4. Adults can be resuscitated many times, especially if defibrillation is done early. The rescuer must always try, unless the patient has obviously been without oxygen for a long time.

116. Application, implementation, physiological integrity, (b).
    2. The vastus lateralis is the recommended muscle and site to be used for a patient this age.
    1. The deltoid muscle is not developed enough to safely give an intramuscular injection in a patient this age.
    3. The gluteus maximus should not be used because it is not developed enough, and the sciatic nerve and artery are in this area.
    4. The patient should be older than 2 years of age if the ventrogluteal area is to be used.

117. Knowledge, assessment, health promotion and maintenance, (b).
    2. Cataracts, which are easily removed, cause more blindness than any other disorder.
    1. Glaucoma can cause blindness if not treated.
    3. Presbyopia is the result of the normal changes of aging.
    4. Macular degeneration causes blindness; however, more individuals have cataracts.

118. Comprehension, assessment, psychosocial integrity, (b).
    2. In early Alzheimer disease, short-term memory, which spans a few minutes or hours, is impaired.
    1. This is long-term memory, which is usually preserved in early Alzheimer disease.

3. This is benign forgetfulness, which is usually limited to trivial matters and tends to occur in all individuals at some time in their life.

4. This is an example of immediate memory, which is not impaired in early Alzheimer disease.

119. Application, assessment, physiological integrity, (b).
    2. Follow the rule of nines:
    Left leg = 18%
    Right leg = 18%
    Right arm = 9%
    Total = 45%
    1, 3, 4. These do not follow the rule of nines.

120. Comprehension, assessment, health promotion and maintenance, (b).
    3. The changes in this portion of the brain diminish the ability of older adults to produce a fever in response to an inflammatory agent.
    1. Aging changes normally increase the older adult's pain threshold.
    2. Cardiovascular aging changes do not increase erythema.
    4. Older adults generally have normal-to-subnormal temperature levels.

121. Analysis, evaluation, physiological integrity, (b).
    4. Victim should be observed for laryngeal and tracheal edema because the degree of inhalation burns is unknown.
    1, 2, 3. These are characteristic of third-degree burns; it was previously determined that the victim has second-degree burns.

122. Application, implementation, physiological integrity, (b).
    1. The area should be covered with a dressing to reduce the risk of infection until it can be evaluated.
    2. A splint can put pressure on the fracture site, causing further injury.
    3. Attempting to return the bone would cause further injury.
    4. Although this is not totally inappropriate, the victim might be allergic to the ointment The best action is to apply a dressing.

123. Application, planning, psychosocial integrity, (b).
    4. Surrounding the patient with familiar objects increases a feeling of recognition in the new facility.
    1. Bringing along familiar objects does not increase the attention span of the individual.
    2. Although the familiar objects are calming, they do not decrease dementia behaviors.
    3. The objects would most likely facilitate long-term memory if they facilitate memory at all.

124. Application, implementation, physiological integrity, (a).
    2. Stop the flow of the IV fluids to prevent further swelling, and report to the charge nurse.
    1, 3, 4. These are inappropriate responses that do not correct the stated situation.

125. Application, assessment, physiological integrity, (b).
    4. Wheezing and respiratory distress are symptoms of an anaphylactic reaction to the bee sting.
    1, 2, 3. Although wheezing and respiratory distress are common with these disorders, the precipitating event was the bee sting.

COMPREHENSIVE EXAMINATION 1: PART 2

1. Application, implementation, physiological integrity, (b).
    2. Keeping the head of the bed below 30 degrees reduces shearing of the skin.
    1. A turning schedule that is adhered to is most effective.
    3. This is inappropriately stated; in addition, nerve endings may be compromised, and pain may not be present.
    4. Incorrect information is being given.

2. Analysis, evaluation, physiological integrity, (c).
    1. Health care professionals generally agree that elderly people with diabetes are best managed by maintaining a fasting blood glucose in the 100 to 140 mg/dL range and postprandial glucose in the 120 to 180 mg/dL range.
    2, 3, 4. This information is incorrect; therefore learning has not occurred.

3. Analysis, assessment, health promotion and maintenance, (b).
    _____ 1. Nausea and vomiting are not common symptoms of hypertension.
    X   2. Blurred vision is a common manifestation of hypertension.
    _____ 3. Shortness of breath is not a common symptom noted in patients with hypertension.
    X   4. Irritability is commonly noted in patients diagnosed with hypertension.
    _____ 5. Nervousness is not commonly seen as a specific symptom of hypertension.
    X   6. Occipital headaches are a common complaint of patients diagnosed with hypertension.

4. Application, planning, physiological integrity, (b).
    3. If mucus is too thick for the patient to expectorate, aerosol treatments would help.
    1. This is appropriate but may not be as effective or act as quickly as No. 3.
    2. These actions would relieve the throat irritation but would not assist in making his cough productive.
    4. This is inappropriate. The high humidity may make breathing more difficult.

5. Application, planning, physiological integrity, (c).
    3. Normal changes of aging include reduction in total body water and muscle mass, which results in a greater risk of adverse drug reactions. Digoxin is a water-soluble drug and is distributed in smaller compartments, placing the older adult at risk for drug toxicity.
    1. In the older adult digoxin is more likely to accumulate to toxic levels in association with physiological changes.
    2. In the older adult a water-soluble drug is distributed into smaller compartments, causing an increased risk of drug toxicity.
    4. Digoxin dose in the older adult is usually smaller than the dose prescribed for the younger adult because of a decrease in total body water and muscle mass and an increase in total body fat.

6. Application, assessment, health promotion and maintenance, (b).
    2. Both of these conditions create regurgitation of blood back through the mitral valve, causing murmurs.

1. Angina is not a common assessment finding in valvular disease.
3. Syncope is not a finding in these types of valvular disease.
4. Hypertension may be an underlying condition, but it is not specifically associated with either of these diseases.

7. Analysis, assessment, physiological integrity, (c).
   2. Coughing when supine may be associated with left-sided heart failure.
   1. Decreased appetite may be caused by a variety of factors.
   3. This may have a variety of causes.
   4. Respirations should be documented, although easy, regular respirations are normal.

8. Application, implementation, physiological integrity, (b).
   3. The funduscopic examination is useful in examining the retina of the eye for changes that are suggestive of those accompanying hypertension.
   1. A vision screen tests only visual acuity.
   2. A tonometer test evaluates pressure within the eye and is useful in monitoring glaucoma.
   4. A visual fields examination evaluates peripheral vision and is useful in monitoring glaucoma and evaluating neurological problems.

9. Application, implementation, physiological integrity, (b).
   3. A firm surface provides support so the heart is adequately compressed between the sternum and spine.
   1. Palpation of landmarks is not affected by the surface composition.
   2. The risk of breaking the xiphoid process depends on the hand position on the chest wall.
   4. The speed of compressions is not affected by the surface composition.

10. Application, implementation, physiological integrity, (b).
    4. A healthy weight-loss diet should include a variety of foods and exercise.
    1. This is true, but it does not completely answer the question.
    2. A variety of nutrients is needed for a healthy diet.
    3. This is true, but it does not completely answer the question.

11. Comprehension, assessment, health promotion and maintenance, (b).
    2. Metabolism slows in the older adult; therefore fewer calories are needed.
    1. Frequently the tolerance to fat is lower, and it is harder to digest.
    3. Fluid intake should be increased to help eliminate waste products.
    4. Vitamin and mineral intake should be maintained and perhaps increased to account for decreased absorption.

12. Application, planning, physiological integrity, (b).
    2. Quadriceps muscles must be strengthened to allow for ambulation.
    1. Active ROM to the ankle prevents joint freezing but does not strengthen muscles.
    3. Extension and abduction should prevent possible dislocation of the prosthesis but do not strengthen muscles.
    4. Passive ROM to the ankle prevents joint freezing but does not strengthen muscles.

13. Application, implementation, physiological integrity, (b).
    3. Lactose intolerance refers to the inability to digest milk sugar (lactose) because of a deficiency of the enzyme lactase.
    1. These contain no lactose.
    2. These do not contain lactose and thus do not need to be avoided.
    4. These foods contain no lactose.

14. Application, implementation, physiological integrity, (b).
    4. This prevents bacterial spread into the wound.
    1. Pressure on a wound diminishes bleeding; it would interfere with wound cleansing.
    2. Forceful wound irrigation disrupts healing tissue.
    3. Scrubbing disrupts healing tissue.

15. Application, assessment, physiological integrity, (b).
    4. In acute glomerulonephritis an immune response occurs, which damages the kidney and reduces glomerular filtration. This results in fluid volume excess, which is characterized by periorbital edema, lung crackles, distention of neck veins, and weight gain.
    1. Typically fever is characteristic of inflammation, infection, or injury. A person with glomerulonephritis can exhibit a fever, but this is not the result of the decreased glomerular filtration rate (GFR).
    2. Thirst is characteristic of deficient fluid volume, not excess.
    3. Polyuria is urination of large volumes, which does not occur with decreased GFR.

16. Analysis, evaluation, physiological integrity, (c).
    4. These are symptoms of an allergic reaction; this action removes the allergen while preserving the IV line.
    1. This causes the patient pain and undue risk if the IV line must be restarted.
    2. This causes the patient undue risk and pain; it does not correct the problem. Also, if the allergic reaction worsens, an IV line may be needed quickly.
    3. This is not a normal reaction, and the nurse cannot apply medication without an order.

17. Analysis, implementation, physiological integrity, (c).
    3. The symptoms indicate air embolism. Placing the patient in this position prevents the embolism from moving from the right atrium.
    1. Despite the respiratory symptoms, this is a circulatory emergency, and the patient needs to be positioned to prevent further injury.
    2. TPN ports should be reconnected after the patient is positioned.
    4. Placing the patient in high-Fowler position allows embolism dispersal to vital organs and does not diminish the patient's distress.

18. Application, implementation, physiological integrity, (b).
    4. Oxygen has a drying effect on mucous membranes.
    1. Ventilating oxygen through water does not reduce its combustibility.
    2. The patient's level of oxygen absorption is related to liter flow, not humidity.
    3. Particle contamination is not a factor in oxygen therapy.

19. Analysis, evaluation, physiological integrity, (b).
    1. The outcome of care related to imbalanced nutrition: less than body requirements would be stable body weight, indicating maintenance of nutritional status.

2. Absence of diarrhea would be an appropriate outcome of care for diarrhea related to infection or gastrointestinal disorders.

3. Normal body temperature would be an appropriate outcome of care for imbalanced body temperature: higher than normal.

4. Moist mucous membranes would be an appropriate outcome of care for dehydration.

20. Comprehension, implementation, safe and effective care environment, (a).

    3. Formula hang time should not exceed 8 hours because bacteria multiply in the feeding once it has been opened and kept at room temperature.

    1. One day's supply of formula may require 16 to 20 hours of infusion time, providing an environment for bacteria growth.

    2. More than one can of formula can be hung for efficiency, as long as the solution is not open at room temperature for more than 8 hours.

    4. A 2-hour time frame is inefficient and unnecessary.

21. Application, implementation, physiological integrity, (b).

    4. An accurate intake and output record is necessary for correct calculation of the patient's fluid replacement needs.

    1. Mouth care is an important comfort measure for the patient undergoing gastrointestinal suction, but it is not as critical compared with intake and output amounts.

    2. Thorough skin care of the nares is important for skin integrity, but fluid balance is more critical.

    3. Turning and positioning the patient may promote better gastrointestinal drainage and will prevent decubitus formation, but fluid balance is more critical.

22. Analysis, evaluation, physiological integrity, (c).

    3. Cardiac arrhythmias are a serious consequence of potassium deficiency. Diuretics can cause hypokalemia.

    1. This can indicate a deficiency of vitamin C.

    2. This can be caused by a deficiency of riboflavin.

    4. This can indicate a deficiency of niacin or B-complex vitamins.

23. Application, implementation, physiological integrity, (b).

    2. This degree allows for the best circulation and drainage of central nervous system fluid.

    1. This is not enough elevation.

    3. This is too much elevation.

    4. This would be uncomfortable and may promote flexion of the neck, which would increase pressure.

24. Comprehension, assessment, health promotion and maintenance, (b).

    1. These are symptoms of deficiency of vitamins C and B$_{12}$. The aging process may increase the need for these nutrients because of impaired absorption and decreased intake.

    2. Symptoms are not typical of these deficiencies; deficiency of B$_6$ can include hyperirritability, neuritis, and possible convulsions; a deficiency of B$_{12}$ leads to anemia.

    3. These are fat-soluble vitamins stored in the liver; deficiency can result in night blindness, rickets, and bleeding tendencies.

4. The symptoms are not typical of these vitamin deficiencies, which include deficiency diseases such as scurvy, beriberi, pellagra, and anemia.

25. Application, evaluation, physiological integrity, (b).

    _____ 1. Poor skin turgor is a symptom of dehydration.

    _____ 2. Redness at the site is a symptom of infection or phlebitis.

    _____ 3. Warmth at the insertion site indicates infection or phlebitis.

    __X__ **4. Edema found above the catheter indicates infiltration.**

    __X__ **5. Coolness at site of insertion is usually a sign of infiltration.**

    __X__ **6. Patient may complain of discomfort at insertion site caused by infiltration.**

26. Comprehension, planning, health promotion and maintenance, (a).

    2. Absence of prenatal care precludes early detection so the condition can be watched and controlled.

    1. This is controversial; recent studies reveal that it may have no effect.

    3. GH may occur at any age; the number of pregnancies is of more concern (i.e., whether this is the first baby). Although GH is more likely in adolescents or older women, this is not the best possible answer.

    4. Hypertensive drugs were discovered and used for primary hypertension and were adopted for use by obstetricians; this is a poor answer.

27. Comprehension, assessment, physiological integrity, (a).

    4. The high salt content in the lunch meat and potato chips would contribute to edema formation.

    1. Although eggs contain salt, this food choice would not be as likely to contribute to edema.

    2. Tuna fish and cantaloupe are low-salt food choices that should not contribute to edema.

    3. Although the French fries may be salted, this food choice is less likely to contribute to edema than the salami and potato chips.

28. Application, assessment, health promotion and maintenance, (b).

    2. The primitive Moro reflex is still present at 3 weeks of age.

    1, 3. Vocalizations and holding the head erect are behaviors that can be observed in the 2-month-old infant. This infant does not have the neuromuscular development to perform these behaviors.

    4. Recognizing familiar faces occurs at approximately 3 months. Before this time younger infants may start to recognize familiar voices.

29. Application, implementation, physiological integrity, (a).

    3. This helps prevent muscle cramping.

    1. This relieves urinary incontinence.

    2. This prevents anemia.

    4. This promotes circulation and helps prevent thrombophlebitis.

30. Application, planning, physiological integrity, (b).

    3. Milk shakes or nutritional supplements can supply the patient experiencing anorexia with additional calories and nutrients without overwhelming the person.

    1. This overwhelms the person, makes him or her feel too full, and is not encouraged for patients with anorexia.

2. Taking pain medication before meals allows a pain-free dining experience that may encourage the patient to eat more.

4. Fruits and vegetables are nutritious but should not be eaten in exclusion of protein or other foods.

31. Application, implementation, physiological integrity, (b).
   2. **This is the best answer.**
   1. These relieve perineal discomfort.
   3. This is improper advice.
   4. These provide temporary relief at best.

32. Application, implementation, safe and effective care environment, (b).
   3. **Streptococcus pneumoniae *is the most common cause of meningitis and a common cause of upper respiratory infections. It may result in meningitis caused by extension of the infection into the central nervous system. Only good handwashing is needed.***
   1. Meningitis transmission usually does not occur through wounds.
   2. Respiratory Precautions are necessary only as a part of Strict Isolation for meningococcal meningitis.
   4. Strict Isolation is not required for the streptococcal organism but is for meningococcal meningitis to prevent transmission of the organism.

33. Application, assessment, health promotion and maintenance, (b).
   4. **This should resolve in 5 days.**
   1. This plantar reflex is normal for 1 year.
   2. This should disappear in 3 to 4 weeks.
   3. This is normal; sleep patterns vary widely.

34. Application, implementation, health promotion and maintenance, (c).
   2. **This provides reassurance and an explanation.**
   1. Levels of perception of pain differ; therefore the nurse does not promise that "no pain" will occur.
   3. This test takes from 20 minutes to more than 1 hour.
   4. This is untrue; most women will never need this test.

35. Application, planning, health promotion and maintenance, (b).
   3. **A balance of all nutrients provides a favorable environment for the developing fetus.**
   1. An adequate amount of calories is needed for protein use and fat metabolism.
   2. A well-balanced diet is recommended for adequate metabolism.
   4. Fluid intake facilitates the clearance of creatinine, urea, and other waste products of fetal and maternal metabolism.

36. Analysis, planning, physiological integrity, (b).
   1. **Evaluating each pregnancy individually will be necessary.**
   2. This would be possible but not guaranteed.
   3. Pregnancy lasts only approximately 40 weeks.
   4. A high-risk pregnancy would generally require starting weekly visits sooner.

37. Application, planning, safe and effective care environment, (c).
   4. **A disulfiram-type reaction can occur, causing severe nausea and vomiting.**
   1. The two substances should not be taken together, therefore making this an incorrect response.
   2, 3. No significant literature reports this occurring.

38. Comprehension, assessment, health promotion and maintenance, (b).
   2. **This is appropriate for an infant at 24 weeks.**
   1. This is appropriate at 16 weeks.
   3. This is appropriate for a full-term infant.
   4. This is appropriate at 20 weeks.

39. Application, planning, physiological integrity, (a).
   4. **Because glandular function of the skin in older adults is decreased, they have dryer, thinner, and extremely fragile skin. They also tolerate extreme heat and extreme cold poorly.**
   1. Hot water can damage the skin, causing scalds.
   2. Cold water would cause chilling and discomfort.
   3. This is not frequent enough.

40. Application, planning, safe and effective care environment, (b).
   2. **Monitoring vital signs is within the nursing assistant's scope of practice.**
   1. Documentation should be done by the individual who cared for the residents, presumably the nurse.
   3. Administering medications is not within the scope of practice of the nursing assistant.
   4. The nurse should provide the input concerning the resident's care.

41. Application, implementation, physiological integrity, (c).
   3. **Fluid intake of at least 2400 mL should be encouraged to prevent crystalluria. The nurse should use terms that the patient understands ("3 quarts" rather than "3 liters" or "3000 mL").**
   1. Acyclovir helps reduce the duration of the lesions but does not eradicate the virus.
   2. The patient should be encouraged to complete the full prescribed course of the medication.
   4. The medication does not protect a sexual partner from contracting the virus. The patient should be instructed to use condoms for or abstain from sexual intercourse.

42. Application, implementation, safe and effective care environment, (b).
   4. **This is priority emergency care; the patient must have an intact airway before any other assessment can begin.**
   1. This may cause injury before the assessment.
   2, 3. These are done after the patient's airway is secured.

43. Analysis, evaluation, physiological integrity, (b).
   1. **Nonselective beta-adrenergic blocking agents may affect the beta$_1$ receptors, leading to bronchoconstriction or bronchospasm, producing dyspnea.**
   2. An increase in heart rate is caused by the stimulation, rather than the blocking, of adrenergic receptors.
   3. Photophobia is a result of pupil dilation, such as occurs with adrenergic stimulation, not blocking.
   4. Stimulation rather than blocking of the adrenergic receptors causes nervousness.

44. Application, assessment, physiological integrity, (b).
   2. **The best way to assess for this patient problem is to actually watch the patient perform the activity.**
   1. Although helpful, this does not provide as much information as would watching the patient perform the activity.
   3. This is an assessment that the nurse is capable of making.

4. This is descriptive, but it still does not provide as much information as would watching him perform the task.

45. Application, implementation, physiological integrity, (c).
Correct order: 3241
3. Place victim in supine position on a firm, flat surface
2. Remove any foreign object obstructing the airway
4. Open the airway using the head tilt–chin lift maneuver
1. Start cardiopulmonary resuscitation (CPR)
With an unconscious victim, the priority is always the airway. To open the airway, the victim must first be positioned correctly, which is in a supine position on a firm, flat surface. This action is followed by opening the airway using the head tilt–chin lift maneuver and checking for and removing any foreign object that may be obstructing the airway. It may be necessary to initiate CPR if breathing and circulation are absent.

46. Application, planning, safe and effective care environment, (b).
4. Medicare covers many of the expenses related to care in a nursing home; costs not covered by Medicare are covered by the individual's supplemental insurance and/or personal resources.
1. Medicare covers only some of the expenses such as those that would necessitate highly skilled care.
2. Medicare generally covers skilled nursing services, some of which do not last 1 or 2 years.
3. Social Security payments assist in paying for long-term care, but Medicaid pays for most of the care once the individual has used all of his or her personal resources.

47. Application, planning, physiological integrity, (b).
2. Quadriceps-setting exercises improve the strength of muscles needed for walking.
1, 3, 4. These actions do not strengthen muscles as indicated in No. 2 because they do not target the quadriceps muscles critical to walking.

48. Application, implementation, physiological integrity, (b).
1. Regular insulin is administered either intravenously or subcutaneously to treat the elevated blood glucose.
2. This is the recommended treatment for hypoglycemia.
3. An IV infusion should be initiated with a normal saline solution, not a dextrose solution.
4. Blood potassium levels should be monitored, but this is not a treatment.

49. Comprehension, evaluation, physiological integrity, (c).
3. Potassium is needed to allow the body to use insulin to metabolize glucose.
1, 2, 4. These electrolytes do not work with metabolism of glucose and insulin.

50. Application, implementation, physiological integrity, (a).
3. The hemodynamic instability that follows burn injury must be stopped to proceed with airway, breathing, and circulation and prevent further trauma to the victim.
1, 2. These are appropriate but not priorities.
4. The situation does not indicate that CPR is necessary.

51. Comprehension, planning, physiological integrity, (a).
4. Thromboembolic problems are a postoperative complication of hip surgery. Low-dose aspirin reduces the risks of this complication.
1. This dose is too low for an antiinflammatory effect.
2, 3. These are not the primary purpose behind such an order for this patient.

52. Comprehension, assessment, psychosocial integrity, (b).
2. The acute stage, disorganization, immediately follows sexual assault and is either verbally expressed or hidden. Regardless of the manner of expression, the survivor experiences feelings of shock, restlessness, anger, guilt, confusion, and fear.
1, 3. These usually follow acute disorganization and precede reorganization.
4. Reorganization indicates that the survivor has put the event in perspective and moves toward some degree of recovery.

53. Application, implementation, physiological integrity, (a).
3. The patient's nonverbal responses may indicate pain or discomfort associated with the exercise.
1. The joint should not be exercised past the point of pain or stiffness to prevent joint injury.
2. Each exercise should be repeated at least two to five times; the number of repetitions varies among patients.
4. The exercises should be performed in a consistent order to prevent overlooking a joint.

54. Application, implementation, psychosocial integrity, (b).
4. This behavior can be caused by anxiety over the unknown biopsy results.
1. This would be insulting to the patient.
2. The nurse needs to acknowledge the behavior.
3. The nurse needs to address the behavior.

55. Analysis, assessment, physiological integrity, (b).
3. Hesitancy in initiating voiding is a frequent symptom associated with prostate enlargement.
1. Nausea is a vague symptom and may occur with various disease states.
2. Burning on urination is more common with a urinary tract infection.
4. Hematuria is more common with bladder carcinoma or upper urinary tract infection.

56. Application, planning, psychosocial integrity, (b).
3. Exercise helps the patient burn calories and use energy.
1, 4. These require the patient to be still and concentrate.
2. This is not as good a choice and may be too focused.

57. Application, implementation, safe and effective care environment, (a).
4. Nurses always write the orders as the physician gives them and then repeat them for verification (a Joint Commission requirement). The nurse then signs the order using the physician's name and also signs his or her name to the order. The physician must countersign the order within a specified time period.
1. Telephone orders are signed by the nurse receiving the order along with the name of the physician giving the order. The physician must countersign the order within a specified time period.
2. The steps are to write the orders as the physician is giving them, verify the orders, and make sure that the

patient's name appears on the order sheet. The next of kin is not information that is found on the order sheet.

3. Orders are written as given and then repeated for verification.

58. Comprehension, assessment, psychosocial integrity, (b).

3. Compulsive behavior helps the patient cope with the anxiety.

1, 2. These do not address specific activities.

4. This is normal, not an obsession.

59. Application, evaluation, physiological integrity, (b).

2. Postural drainage helps drain sections of the lung, aids in coughing and removing secretions, and improves breathing.

1. Fluids should be forced to liquefy secretions.

3. The patient should have rest and conserve energy.

4. High-Fowler position (45- to 90-degree elevation) is most effective in relieving dyspnea.

60. Application, evaluation, physiological integrity, (b).

1. Sedation is a common side effect of haloperidol.

2. Weight gain is more common.

3. Dry mouth is not a common side effect.

4. Agitation is seen with an overdose.

61. Application, assessment, physiological integrity, (a).

2. Circulation and sensation are assessed periodically to determine the presence of pressure areas that may obstruct circulation and nerve pathways.

1. Circulation is assessed in the lower extremities by taking the pedal pulse.

3. The left leg is fractured, not the right leg. Checking temperature and performing ROM on the right leg are not appropriate actions.

4. No data are given indicating that the patient is in traction; also, this is not an appropriate action for assessing circulation and sensation.

62. Application, implementation, physiological integrity, (b).

3. This position elevates the extremity high enough to prevent lymphedema.

1. Abduction and adduction of the affected arm are contraindicated after a mastectomy.

2. Abduction and adduction of the affected arm are contraindicated after a mastectomy. The arm should not be suspended.

4. The patient's arm is not elevated high enough in this position.

63. Comprehension, planning, safe and effective care environment, (a).

2. The gold standard for administering medications is the five rights: the right drug, dose, patient, route, and time. Today, many institutions include documentation as the sixth right of medication administration.

1. This is an inaccurate response.

3. Hospital policy should be followed but is not considered one of the components in the standard.

4. Five rights are presented in this response, although many consider documentation as the sixth right; room number is not included in the standards.

64. Application, planning, psychosocial integrity, (b).

2. Safety is always a number one priority.

1. Ability to perform self-care is unknown.

3. He is hearing voices, but safety is more important.

4. This is a problem but not as much a priority as safety.

65. Analysis, planning, physiological integrity, (b).

3. This is correct. The creatinine clearance increases as renal function diminishes.

1, 2, 4. These may be indications of renal function (BUN), anemia (decreased hemoglobin), or infection (increased WBCs) but not glomerular filtration rate (GFR).

66. Application, implementation, safe and effective care environment, (b).

3. This victim requires immediate medical care.

1. This is appropriate but not the first priority.

2. This is inappropriate; the victim needs immediate medical care.

4. Referring a victim to a physician for emergency care does not put the nurse at legal risk; not referring a victim to a physician can result in legal action being initiated against the nurse.

67. Analysis, assessment, physiological integrity, (b).

_____ 1. Visitors may unknowingly cause a draft, which may stimulate this reaction; however, this is not considered a common cause of autonomic dysreflexia.

__X__ 2. **A full bladder is a common cause of this phenomenon.**

_____ 3. Skin stimulation may be a stimulus, although not common, and needs to be done gently such as when taking an apical pulse.

__X__ 4. **A full bowel is also a common cause of autonomic dysreflexia.**

_____ 5. Taking a tympanic temperature could stimulate this reaction, but again is not a common cause of the phenomenon.

__X__ 6. **Wrinkled sheets have also been noted as a common cause of autonomic dysreflexia.**

68. Comprehension, assessment, physiological integrity, (b).

1. Hypoventilation reduces O_2 to the alveoli and reduces CO_2 elimination. The retained CO_2 then combines with water to form an excess of carbonic acid (H_2CO_3), decreasing the blood pH. As a result, concentration of hydrogen ions in body fluids, which directly reflects acidity, increases.

2. The lungs excrete CO_2 and water. The rate of excretion of CO_2 is controlled by the respiratory center in the medulla of the brain. If increased amounts of CO_2 or hydrogen ions are present, the respiratory center stimulates an increased rate and depth of breathing.

3, 4. The lungs excrete CO_2 and water, which are byproducts of cellular metabolism.

69. Application, planning, physiological integrity, (c).

1. This is an outcome-criteria statement.

2. This is a nursing intervention.

3. This is an appropriate nursing diagnosis.

4. This is an appropriate evaluation statement.

70. Comprehension, planning, physiological integrity, (a).

2. 30:2 is correct for two-rescuer adult CPR.

1. 15:2 is correct for two-rescuer CPR for infants and children.

3. This would be too few compressions for two-rescuer CPR for infant and child.

4. This would be too few ventilations for two-rescuer adult CPR.

71. Application, assessment, physiological integrity, (c).
    3. Assessment of motor function includes muscle movement, size, tone, strength, and coordination of muscle groups.
    1. Cranial nerve VIII is responsible for hearing; cranial nerves IX and X are responsible for the gag reflex and ability to speak. Cranial nerve XI allows the person to raise the shoulders, and cranial nerve XII allows movement of the tongue.
    2. Intellectual functions and speech patterns are components of a neurological examination but are not included in the motor function assessment.
    4. Body positioning is evaluated during the inspection portion of the assessment; mental status and level of consciousness are assessed throughout the examination and are not specific to motor function.

72. Application, planning, physiological integrity, (b).
    4. Cheese and crackers provide enough complex carbohydrates to sustain the person through the activity.
    1. This provides a rapid form of glucose that would not sustain the person.
    2. This rapidly acting form of glucose is best taken during a hypoglycemic episode.
    3. A can of soda, sweetened, would not sustain the person through the activity.

73. Application, implementation, physiological integrity, (b).
    3. Rest and avoidance of heavy lifting or strenuous activity promote healing and decrease intraabdominal pressures to the puncture site. Heavy lifting or strenuous exercise may precipitate a bleeding episode. Large volumes of blood can be lost should bleeding occur; therefore prompt medical attention is required.
    1. Driving and climbing stairs are contraindicated for 24 hours after catheterization because of an increased risk of bleeding.
    2. Tub baths are contraindicated until the puncture site is healed because of placing undue stress at the puncture site.
    4. The bandage can be changed in 24 hours; the puncture is expected to be sore for several days, no matter how healing is progressing.

74. Application, planning, safe and effective care environment, (b).
    3. Chicken salad is a protein food and would be restricted in someone with elevated ammonia levels.
    1. Pretzels would not be restricted for a person with this diagnosis.
    2. Although cheese does contain some protein, chicken salad would more likely be restricted.
    4. A bowl of ice cream is mostly fat and carbohydrates and would not be restricted.

75. Comprehension, assessment, physiological integrity, (b).
    4. CK-MB is found mainly in cardiac muscle and rises 4 to 12 hours after infarction, peaks in 24 hours, and returns to normal in 3 to 4 days.
    1. This is a test used primarily to screen for disseminated intravascular coagulation (DIC).
    2. The white blood cell count may be elevated by the third day because of the inflammatory response. However, this test is not specific to myocardial infarction.

3. This is a test useful in the diagnosis of several disorders: anemia, cardiomyopathy, congestive heart failure, delirium tremens, hypothyroidism, inflammation, leukemia, muscle injury, myxedema, pulmonary infarction, and renal infarction. LDH is elevated 24 to 48 hours after infarction, peaks in 3 to 6 days, and returns to normal in 7 to 14 days.

76. Application, implementation, physiological integrity, (b).
    3. The patient should be placed in low- or semi-Fowler position to decrease strain on the sutures.
    1. The supine position would lead to increased edema of the neck, which would compromise the patient's airway.
    2. Placing the patient in left lateral Sims position has no benefit.
    4. Trendelenburg position would compromise the airway and place undue strain on the suture line.

77. Analysis, assessment, physiological integrity, (c).
    3. With left-sided heart failure blood becomes backed up in the lungs, causing crackles or fluid in the lungs.
    1. Nausea normally is not associated with heart failure.
    2. An extra heart sound (S3) may be heard, but it is not the sound of a murmur.
    4. Right ventricular heart failure would result in peripheral edema.

78. Comprehension, planning, physiological integrity, (b).
    4. Oral agents are useful in treating diabetes when some beta cell function still exists.
    1. Obesity is not a measurement for beta cell function.
    2. The liver clears most agents, but this fact is unrelated to the need for functioning beta cells.
    3. Type 1 diabetes usually is associated with no beta-cell function.

79. Application, implementation, health promotion and maintenance, (a).
    3. At this age the baby should be able to follow bright lights and moving objects.
    1. Vision is 20/100 at 1 year of age. Because vision is not yet normal, this is the age at which babies keep bumping into things.
    2. Visual acuity is approximately 20/300, and babies can see only at a very close range.
    4. By 9 to 10 months of age depth perception is developing.

80. Application, planning, physiological integrity, (b).
    4. The patient is at high risk for a decubitus ulcer. Sensory loss prevents perception of pain and pressure, the warning signs of tissue injury. If the patient is able, encourage patient involvement.
    1. This is inappropriate; adequate calcium intake is essential for all individuals.
    2. This is inappropriate and is not relative to the situation.
    3. This is not individualized to people with sensory or motor loss.

81. Application, implementation, physiological integrity, (b).
    4. The clot may dislodge itself; bright red or darker color may indicate hemorrhage.
    1. This would cause painful bladder spasms.
    2. This may increase the patient's discomfort. He is already at risk for fluid and electrolyte imbalance because of absorption of the irrigation fluid.

3. This may increase the patient's anxiety. The coughing may also increase the patient's discomfort.

82. Application, implementation, safe and effective care environment, (a).

   2. Chlorpromazine makes skin sensitive to sunlight.

   1. This is related to monoamine oxidase inhibitors (MAOIs).

   3, 4. These are not related.

83. Application, assessment, physiological integrity, (b).

   1. This answer is accurate. Other behaviors include sleepiness and very short attention span, and the person is able to respond verbally. The patient fends off painful stimuli with purposeful movement.

   2. This describes a deep coma state.

   3, 4. These answers describe a stuporous state.

84. Comprehension, planning, physiological integrity, (a).

   3. Pattern is essential with retraining.

   1. Laxatives are never used with bowel retraining.

   2. The patient need not understand the program for the program to be successful.

   4. Regular days and times must be followed strictly to establish a pattern.

85. Comprehension, implementation, physiological integrity, (a).

   3. These are known as hyperosmolar drugs. Mannitol (Osmitrol) is an example. These agents draw water from the edematous brain.

   1. These may be ordered if an open wound is caused by trauma.

   2. These may be ordered if nausea is present.

   4. These should be used carefully; they may mask level of consciousness or cause respiratory distress.

86. Application, implementation, physiological integrity, (b).

   3. These do not increase systemic blood pressure because they are not resistive.

   1, 2. These are unsafe; they cause a sudden increase in blood pressure and intracranial pressure.

   4. This is unsafe and may cause flexion of hips or neck or both. Both of these positions may cause a sudden increase in intracranial pressure.

87. Application, implementation, physiological integrity, (b).

   3. The first step in treating hemorrhage is to apply pressure for at least 6 minutes.

   1. Application of ice is not an emergency measure.

   2. This action would have no effect on occipital bleeding.

   4. Elevating the affected part aids in controlling the bleeding but would not stop it.

88. Application, implementation, safe and effective care environment, (b).

   3. This is correct according to the 2011 guidelines instituted by the American Heart Association for severe foreign body airway obstruction (FBAO).

   1. This is incorrect; eight back blows and eight chest thrusts were never a recommended sequence for obstructed airway in an infant.

   2. This is incorrect; six back blows and six chest thrusts were never a recommended sequence for obstructed airway in an infant.

   4. This is incorrect; four back blows and four chest thrusts were the recommended sequence for obstructed airway in an infant before 1993.

89. Application, implementation, physiological integrity, (a).

   3. Hydration and lying flat for 4 to 6 hours help individuals who may develop a spinal headache. This response addresses her concerns and offers a plan of action.

   1. This is not a proven fact. Some individuals develop a headache.

   2. Staying prone versus supine does not give any additional benefit. It may increase the patient's apprehension because she may be fearful of moving. This is not a comfortable position to maintain.

   4. Although advances have occurred in medicine, this response does not allay the individual's apprehension about getting a headache after the procedure.

90. Application, planning, physiological integrity, (b).

   1. Delayed wound healing is common in older adults because of nutritional problems.

   2, 3, 4. These interventions are appropriate regardless of the patient's age.

91. Comprehension, assessment, physiological integrity, (a).

   1. An immediate physical observation of any burn patient, especially a person burned in the area of the face, is assessment of respiration (difficulty, rate, sound).

   2, 3, 4. These are not immediate physical observations during an emergency.

92. Analysis, evaluation, physiological integrity, (b).

   3. Being able to perform activities of daily living indicates that activity tolerance is increasing.

   1. Anxiety is most likely related to being unable to breathe.

   2. This is related to a deficient knowledge diagnosis.

   4. This is related to an ineffective airway clearance problem.

93. Application, implementation, physiological integrity, (c).

   4. This action prevents further injury to the fingers.

   1, 2. These actions are contraindicated.

   3. The frostbitten parts should not be used.

94. Application, implementation, physiological integrity, (a).

   3. The splint should be applied above and below the fracture.

   1, 2. Although these are important, no indications of the problems exist.

   4. Although the fracture should be elevated, lying flat is unnecessary.

95. Application, implementation, physiological integrity, (c).

   1. The priority is always circulation, airway, and breathing.

   2. Although important, this is not the priority.

   3. This is necessary and important but not the priority.

   4. A person cannot breathe unless the airway is patent.

96. Application, implementation, physiological integrity, (b).

   1. As long as 12 weeks may be required for antidepressants to achieve their full therapeutic effect.

   2. Fluids need not be limited while taking antidepressants.

   3. Dry mouth and orthostatic hypotension are common, bothersome side effects of antidepressants.

   4. If the first antidepressant fails to control depression, other effective medications are available.

97. Comprehension, planning, physiological integrity, (b).

   4. Chewing and daily ear hygiene aid in the removal of cerumen.

1. This may be necessary; however, it subjects the patient to a procedure that can be prevented through health-promoting habits.
2. This allows for hydration, but it is not directly related to cerumen buildup.
3. This may damage the hearing aid.

98. Application, planning, safe and effective care environment, (b).

    2. Alternatives should be tried before resorting to restraints.

    1. Restraints are to be used only for a specific period.
    3. Restraints should be removed at least every 2 hours to allow for activities of daily living.
    4. Restraints should be tied with knots that can be released quickly and secured to parts of the bed that move with the patient.

99. Comprehension, planning, physiological integrity, (b).

    2. Ambulation stimulates circulation and prevents the formation of thrombi, in addition to aiding in breaking up clots.

    1. This is to relieve pain, promote healing, and prevent infection.
    3. Splinting helps to diminish pain and discomfort.
    4. Keeping urinary functions at a maximum aids in promoting involution, and offering stool softeners relieves initial pain and discomfort during the postpartum period.

100. Application, planning, physiological integrity, (c).

    1. Focusing specifically on rehabilitation, the elements involved, and the rationale for those elements should expedite recovery by gaining the patient's cooperation.

    2. This is common in normal preoperative teaching.
    3. This information would be given to any individual before surgery.
    4. This is common information for any individual before surgery.

101. Application, implementation, physiological integrity, (b).

    3. This is the first priority.

    1. This is not first priority.
    2. Pads are not used during labor and delivery.
    4. The physician knows the instrument used; it is not necessary to do a test unless asked to do so.

102. Application, evaluation, physiological integrity, (b).

    3. Diaphoresis is one of the first symptoms of hypoglycemia. Hypoglycemia would result when taking insulin without eating or from a sudden increase in activity or body demands such as during illness, surgery, or stress.

    1. Polydipsia is a symptom of hyperglycemia.
    2. This is a late sign of both hyperglycemia and hypoglycemia. The nurse needs to assess for early signs to intervene before this occurs.
    4. This is a symptom of hyperglycemia.

103. Application, assessment, physiological integrity, (b).

    3. As the heart fails, circulating blood backs up into the pulmonary tree; a sign of congestion is crackles in the lung bases.

    1. Although fluid does build up in pneumonia, given the patient's history, the crackles most likely signify the beginning of heart failure.

2. Arrhythmias are not assessed by listening to lung sounds. A heart monitor, change in vital signs, or patient symptoms will alert the nurse to this complication.
4. This normally does not manifest itself as crackles in the lungs. Increased complaints of chest pain or changes in vital signs would alert the nurse to an extension of the myocardial infarction.

104. Analysis, assessment, physiological integrity, (b).

    3. These signs are normal for a 2-day-old newborn.

    1. This is a full-term infant; thus she cannot be premature.
    2. No indication in the situation suggests that the infant is immature.
    4. Nothing abnormal is reported in the situation.

105. Application, planning, physiological integrity, (b).

    2. Safety should come first. In this patient's case use of Maslow's hierarchy of needs is appropriate.

    1. Answer No. 2 is the better choice. The situation did not indicate that pain was present. Assessment of respiratory function would be more appropriate and more individualized.
    3. Safety should always be the first priority; psychological care, comfort, and personal integrity are important, but safety is critical.
    4. Safety should always be the first priority; reorientation and cueing, along with physical assessment, cannot precede safety issues.

106. Comprehension, assessment, physiological integrity, (b).

    ___X___ **1. This is a common symptom of sickle cell crisis.**
    ___X___ **2. Sickle cell crisis is usually preceded by an upper respiratory or gastrointestinal infection.**
    _____ 3. Hemoglobin is decreased, not increased.
    ___X___ **4. Acute abdominal pain is the result of visceral hypoxia.**
    ___X___ **5. Painful swelling of the soft tissue of the hands and feet, known as hand-foot syndrome, occurs.**
    ___X___ **6. Headache, dizziness, and convulsions can occur if the central nervous system is affected.**

107. Application, evaluation, physiological integrity, (b).

    _____ 1. Abdominal cramping is not a typical side effect of bronchodilators.
    ___X___ **2. Restlessness is a typical side effect of these medications; excessive use can result in seizures and delirium; adjustment of dosage necessary.**
    _____ 3. Anorexia is not a typical side effect of these medications.
    ___X___ **4. Tachycardia is a typical adverse effect of these medications.**
    _____ 5. Blurred vision is not a typical side effect noted with these medications.
    ___X___ **6. Insomnia is a typical adverse effect of these medications; overdose can also cause serious adverse reactions (confusion, respiratory failure, hyperthermia).**

108. Application, assessment, physiological integrity, (b).

    4. Excessive urination is one of the classic signs and symptoms that blood sugar levels may be abnormal.

    1. Refusing to bathe is no indication that diabetes is out of control.

2. A cough does not indicate that the blood sugar needs to be checked.

3. One diarrheal stool last week does not need further assessment.

109. Application, assessment, health promotion and maintenance, (b).

    1. Neck pain, decreased neck mobility caused by pain, and upper extremity motor or sensory changes are common symptoms.

    2. This may be a symptom of lumbar involvement.

    3. This may also be a symptom of lumbar involvement.

    4. Muscle atrophy of this group is not a finding when the cervical region is involved.

110. Application, implementation, physiological integrity, (b).

    4. Some diuretics such as furosemide are ototoxic and can cause tinnitus and dizziness.

    1. This is most unlikely; the tinnitus should not affect her ability to drive.

    2. This would not alleviate the patient's concern and is an untrue statement.

    3. The tinnitus is caused by the ototoxicity of the diuretic.

111. Application, evaluation, physiological integrity, (b).

    1. Oxybutynin acts by exerting a direct antispasmodic effect on smooth-muscle tissue, such as that found in the bladder.

    2. Cholinergic drugs are helpful with an atonic bladder.

    3. Propantheline bromide is used for complaints of urinary frequency and urgency.

    4. Trimethoprim-sulfamethoxazole is an antiinfective.

112. Comprehension, assessment, physiological integrity, (b).

    4. Anticoagulants can cause blood to be present in urine.

    1. Diuretics alter the urine quantity output.

    2. Pyridium alters the urine color to red or orange but does not test positive for blood.

    3. Nitrofurantoin alters the color of urine to a harmless brown.

113. Knowledge, implementation, physiological integrity, (a).

    3. Sternal compression is performed on the breastbone (sternum) just below the nipple line.

    1, 2. These positions are too high.

    4. This is the position for adults.

114. Analysis, assessment, health promotion and maintenance, (b).

    4. These are common assessment findings in peritonitis.

    1. This symptom is common in several conditions but not in peritonitis.

    2. Reduced urine output may occur as a late symptom if the infection is not controlled.

    3. Frequent stool or diarrhea is not a common assessment finding.

115. Comprehension, assessment, physiological integrity, (a).

    2. Cholesterol is found in blood and body cells, especially brain and nerve tissue.

    1. It should not nor can it be eliminated totally from the diet.

    3. It is necessary for normal body functioning.

    4. It is mainly through animal sources—meat, eggs, saturated fats.

116. Application, implementation, physiological integrity, (b).

    3. The patient is displaying signs of hypovolemia. Initial measures would be those for treating shock. Turning the patient on the side helps prevent aspiration.

    1. Monitoring vital signs is important; application of a cool cloth is a later measure.

    2. Sips of water are inappropriate if the patient is going into shock.

    4. Decreasing the room temperature is not relative to the situation; turning the patient on the side helps prevent aspiration.

117. Application, planning, psychosocial integrity, (c).

    1. Modesty and sensitivity are of prime importance to patients in this age group.

    2, 4. These are part of the normal admission procedure for patients in any age group.

    3. This is not the case for this age group.

118. Application, assessment, physiological integrity, (b).

    3. This complaint can be life-threatening and is a priority.

    1. This blood glucose level does need to be corrected; however, respiratory status takes priority.

    2. This small laceration needs to be attended to at some time; however, the shortness of breath is of primary importance.

    4. Although it is important to keep the family calm and informed, the patient's complaints of "shortness of breath" are priority.

119. Comprehension, assessment, physiological integrity, (b).

    4. Older adults have a higher percentage of body fat, which affects the metabolism and storage of medications.

    1. Older adults have a lower percentage of body water.

    2. Older adults have a decrease in lean muscle mass.

    3. Older adults have a higher percentage of body fat.

120. Analysis, evaluation, physiological integrity, (c).

    X   1. A bounding pulse is a symptom of heart failure caused by the inability of the heart to pump excessive IV fluid volume.

    _____ 2. This is symptom of IV infiltration.

    X   3. Dyspnea is a symptom of heart failure caused by the inability of the heart to pump excessive IV fluid volume.

    X   4. A cough is also a symptom of heart failure when noted with dyspnea and a bounding pulse caused by the inability of the heart to pump excessive fluid volume.

    _____ 5. A palpable venous cord at the infusion site is a symptom of phlebitis.

    _____ 6. Chills may also indicate a systemic infection.

121. Application, implementation, safe and effective care environment, (b).

    2. Handling the glove on the inside guarantees that the nurse's bare, nonsterile hand will not contaminate the sterile exterior of the glove.

    1. Contamination occurs if the nurse's nonsterile hand touches the sterile exterior of the glove.

    3. Keeping the gloves on the sterile field throughout the gloving procedure risks contamination of the field.

    4. Contamination occurs if the nonsterile hand touches the outside of the glove.

122. Application, assessment, safe and effective care environment, (a).
    2. **This is proper procedure because the pulse rate is below 60 beats/min.**
    1, 3, 4. These can lead to adverse reactions.
123. Application, implementation, physiological integrity, (c).
    2. **Marking the level of drainage and noting the time should be done according to prescribed protocol. Changes in the amount or characteristics of drainage can also be noted and reported.**
    1. The practice of "stripping" chest tubes is controversial and needs a specific order. It is not usually necessary when chest tubes are used to drain air.
    3. Lifting the drainage container would allow air or fluid (or both) to be pulled back into the pleural cavity.

4. The drainage system should be placed below the level of the patient's chest so air or fluid (or both) is not pulled back into the pleural cavity. Drainage is also facilitated. Placing the drainage system at the foot of the bed would be inappropriate.

124. Application, implementation, physiological integrity, (a).
    Answer: 0.4 mL
    Dose desired (DD) = 4 mg
    Dose on hand (DH) = 10 mg
    Volume (V) = 1 mL
    DD/DH = 4 mg/10 mg × 1 mL = 0.4 mL
125. Application, implementation, safe and effective care environment, (b).
    Answer: 2 mg
    Weight in pounds (30) × Adult dose (10 mg)/150 = 300/150 = 2 mg

Standards of Practice and Educational Competencies of Graduates of Practical/Vocational Nursing Programs

These standards and competencies are intended to better define the range of capabilities, responsibilities, rights, and relationship to other health care providers for scope and content of practical/vocational nursing education programs. The guidelines will assist:

- Educators in development, implementation, and evaluation of practical, vocational nursing curricula
- Students in understanding expectations of their competencies on completion of the educational program
- Prospective employers in appropriate utilization of the practical/vocational nurse
- Consumers in understanding the scope of practice and level of responsibility of the practical/vocational nurse.

A. PROFESSIONAL BEHAVIORS

Professional behaviors, within the scope of nursing practice for a licensed practical nurse/licensed vocational nurse (LPN/LVN), are characterized by adherence to standards of care, accountability for one's own actions and behaviors, and use of legal and ethical principles in nursing practice. Professionalism includes a commitment to nursing and a concern for others demonstrated by an attitude of caring. Professionalism also involves participation in lifelong self-development activities to enhance and maintain current knowledge and skills for continuing competency in the practice of nursing for the LPN/LVN, as well as individual group, community, and societal endeavors to improve health care.

Upon completion of the practical/vocational nursing program, the graduate will display the following program outcome: *Demonstrate professional behaviors of accountability and professionalism according to the legal and ethical standards for a competent LPN/LVN.* The following competencies demonstrate that this outcome has been attained:

1. Comply with the ethical, legal, and regulatory frameworks of nursing and the scope of practice as outlined in the LPN/LVN nurse practice act of the specific state in which licensed.
2. Utilize educational opportunities for lifelong learning and maintenance of competence.
3. Identify personal capabilities and consider career mobility options.
4. Identify own LPN/LVN strengths and limitations for the purpose of improving nursing performance.
5. Demonstrate accountability for nursing care provided by self and/or directed to others.
6. Function as an advocate for the health care consumer, maintaining confidentiality as required.
7. Identify the impact of economic, political, social, cultural, spiritual, and demographic forces on the role of the LPN/LVN in the delivery of health care.
8. Serve as a positive role model within health care settings and the community.
9. Participate as a member of a practical/vocational nursing organization.

B. COMMUNICATION

Communication is the process by which information is exchanged between individuals verbally, nonverbally, and/or in writing or through information technology. Communication abilities are integral and essential to the nursing process. Those who are included in the nursing process are the LPN/LVN and other members of the nursing and health care team, client, and significant support person(s). Effective communication demonstrates caring, compassion, and cultural awareness and is directed toward promoting positive outcomes and establishing a trusting relationship.

Upon completion of the practical/vocational nursing program, the graduate will display the following program outcome: *Effectively communicate with patients, significant support person(s), and members of the interdisciplinary health care team, incorporating interpersonal and therapeutic communication skills.* The following competencies demonstrate that this outcome has been attained:

1. Utilize effective communication skills when interacting with clients, significant others, and members of the interdisciplinary health care team.
2. Communicate relevant, accurate, and complete information.
3. Report to appropriate health care personnel and document assessments, interventions, and progress or impediments toward achieving client outcomes.
4. Maintain organizational and patient confidentiality.
5. Utilize information technology to support and communicate the planning and provision of client care.
6. Utilize appropriate channels of communication.

C. ASSESSMENT

Assessment is the collection and processing of relevant data for the purpose of appraising the client's health status. Assessment provides a holistic view of the client that includes physical, developmental, emotional, psychosocial, cultural, spiritual, and functional status. Assessment involves the collection of information from multiple sources to provide the foundation for nursing care. Initial assessment provides the baseline for future comparisons to individualize client care. Ongoing assessment is required to meet the client's changing needs.

Upon completion of the practical/vocational nursing program, the graduate will display the following program outcome: *Collect holistic assessment data from multiple sources, communicate the data to appropriate health care providers, and evaluate client responses to interventions.* The following competencies demonstrate that this outcome has been attained:

1. Assess data related to basic physical, developmental, spiritual, cultural, functional, and psychosocial needs of the client.
2. Collect data within established protocols and guidelines from various sources, including client interviews; observations and measurements; health care team members; family; significant other(s); and review of health records.
3. Assess data related to the client's health status, identify impediments to client progress, and evaluate response to interventions.
4. Document data collection and assessment, and communicate findings to appropriate members of the health care team.

D. PLANNING

Planning encompasses the collection of health status information, the use of multiple methods to access information, and the analysis and integration of knowledge and information to formulate nursing care plans and care actions. The nursing care plan provides direction for individualized care and ensures the delivery of accurate, safe care through a definitive pathway that promotes the clients' and support persons' progress toward positive outcomes.

Upon completion of the practical/vocational nursing program, the graduate will display the following program outcome: *Collaborate with the registered nurse or other members of the health care team to organize and incorporate assessment data to plan and revise patient care and actions based on established nursing diagnoses, nursing protocols, and assessment and evaluation data.* The following competencies demonstrate that this outcome has been attained:

1. Utilize knowledge of normal values to identify deviation in health status to plan care.
2. Contribute to formulation of a nursing care plan for clients with noncomplex conditions and in a stable state, in consultation with the registered nurse and, as appropriate, in collaboration with the client or support person(s) as well as members of the interdisciplinary health care team, utilizing established nursing diagnoses and nursing protocols.
3. Prioritize nursing care needs of clients.
4. Assist in the review and revision of nursing care plans with the registered nurse to meet the changing needs of clients.
5. Modify client care as indicated by the evaluation of stated outcomes.
6. Provide information to client about aspects of the care plan within the LPN/LVN scope of practice.
7. Refer client as appropriate to other members of the health care team about care outside the scope of practice of the LPN/LVN.

E. CARING INTERVENTIONS

Caring interventions are nursing behaviors and actions that assist clients and significant others in meeting their needs and the identified outcomes of the plan of care. These interventions are based on a knowledge of the natural sciences, behavioral sciences, and past nursing experiences. Caring is the "being with" and "doing for" that help clients achieve the desired outcomes. Caring behaviors are nurturing, protective, compassionate, and person centered. Caring creates an environment of hope and trust in which client choices related to cultural, religious, and spiritual values, beliefs, and lifestyles are respected.

Upon completion of the practical/vocational nursing program, the graduate will display the following program outcome: *Demonstrate a caring and empathic approach to the safe, therapeutic, and individualized care of each client.* The following competencies demonstrate that this outcome has been attained:

1. Provide and promote the client's dignity.
2. Identify and honor the emotional, cultural, religious, and spiritual influences on the client's health.
3. Demonstrate caring behaviors toward the client and significant support person(s).
4. Provide competent, safe, therapeutic, and individualized nursing care in a variety of settings.
5. Provide a safe physical and psychosocial environment for the client and significant other(s).
6. Implement the prescribed care regimen within the legal, ethical, and regulatory framework of practical/vocational nursing practice.
7. Assist the client and significant support person(s) to cope with and adapt to stressful events and changes in health status.
8. Assist the client and significant other(s) to achieve optimum comfort and functioning.
9. Instruct the client regarding individualized health needs in keeping with the LPN/LVN's knowledge, competence, and scope of practice.
10. Recognize the client's right to access information, and refer requests to appropriate person(s).
11. Act in an advocacy role to protect client rights.

F. MANAGING

Managing care is the effective use of human, physical, financial, and technological resources to achieve the client-identified outcomes while supporting organizational outcomes. The LPN/LVN manages care through the process of planning, organizing, and directing.

Upon completion of the practical/vocational nursing program, the graduate will display the following program outcome: *Implement patient care at the direction of a registered nurse, licensed physician, or dentist through performance of nursing interventions or directing aspects of care, as appropriate, to unlicensed assistive personnel (UAP).* The following competencies demonstrate that this outcome has been attained:

1. Assist in the coordination and implementation of an individualized plan of care for clients and significant support person(s).
2. Direct aspects of client care to qualified UAPs commensurate with abilities and level of preparation and in a manner that is consistent with the state's legal and regulatory framework for the scope of practice for the LPN/LVN.
3. Supervise and evaluate the activities of UAPs and other personnel as appropriate within the state's legal and

regulatory framework for the scope of practice for the LPN/LVN, as well as facility policy.

4. Maintain accountability for outcomes of care directed to qualified UAPs.

5. Organize nursing activities in a meaningful and cost-effective manner when providing nursing care for individuals or groups.

6. Assist the client and significant support person(s) to access available resources and services.

7. Demonstrate competence with current technologies.

8. Function within the defined scope of practice for the LPN/LVN in the health care delivery system at the direction of a registered nurse, licensed physician, or dentist.

From National Association for Practical Nurse Education and Service (NAPNES): *Standards of practice and educational competencies of graduates of practical/vocational nursing programs.* Approved and adopted by NAPNES Board of Directors May 6, 2007, NAPNES, Alexandria, Virginia.

Table B-1   Communicable Diseases

DISEASE	COMMUNICABILITY PERIOD AND ROUTE	CLINICAL MANIFESTATIONS	TREATMENT AND NURSING CARE	COMPLICATIONS
Chickenpox (varicella) *Incubation period:* 10-21 days *Causative agent:* Varicella-zoster virus	5 days after onset of rash and until all lesions are crusted *Route:* Airborne, droplet infection; direct or indirect contact Dry scabs are not infectious	General malaise, slight fever, anorexia, headache. Successive crops of macules, papules, vesicles, crusts. These may all be present at the same time. Itching of the skin. Generalized lymphadenopathy.	Oral acyclovir should be considered for otherwise healthy people at increased risk (e.g., people older than 12 yr, individuals with pulmonary disorders). Intravenous (IV) antiviral therapy is recommended for immunocompromised children. Symptomatic. Prevent child from scratching. Keep fingernails short and clean. Sedation may be necessary. Use soothing lotions to allay itching. If secondary infections occur, antimicrobials may be given. Do not give aspirin because of high risk for Reye syndrome. Salicylate therapy should be stopped in a child who has been exposed to varicella.	Bacterial superinfection; thrombocytopenia, arthritis, encephalitis, nephritis, Reye syndrome (with aspirin use).
Diphtheria *Incubation period:* 2-7 days or longer *Causative agent:* *Corynebacterium diphtheriae*	In untreated persons, organisms can be present in discharges from the nose and throat and from eye and skin lesions for 2-6 wk after infection *Route:* Droplets from respiratory tract of infected person or carrier; contact with discharges from skin lesions	Local and systemic manifestations. Membrane over tissue in nose or throat at site of bacterial invasion. Hoarse, brassy cough with stridor. Toxin from organism produces malaise and fever. Toxin has affinity for renal, nervous, and cardiac tissue.	A single dose (IV preferred) of equine antitoxin should be administered on the basis of clinical diagnosis, even before culture results are available (test for sensitivity to horse serum). Antimicrobial therapy with erythromycin or penicillin G procaine is given for 14 days in addition to antitoxin. Strict bed rest. Prevent exertion. Cleansing throat gargles may be ordered. Liquid or soft diet. Gavage or parenteral administration of fluids may become necessary. Observe for respiratory obstruction. Equipment for suctioning should be available. Oxygen and emergency tracheostomy may be necessary. Isolate.	Local infections: Low-grade fever with gradual onset. Serious complications include severe neck swelling (bull neck), upper airway obstruction, myocarditis, and peripheral neuropathies.

Table B-1 Communicable Diseases—cont'd

DISEASE	COMMUNICABILITY PERIOD AND ROUTE	CLINICAL MANIFESTATIONS	TREATMENT AND NURSING CARE	COMPLICATIONS
Epidemic influenza *Incubation period:* 1-4 days *Causative agent:* Influenza virus types A, B, and C	*Route:* Airborne, droplet infection; direct contact	Manifestations in respiratory tract. Sudden onset with chills, fever, muscle pains, cough. If infection is severe and spreads to lower respiratory tract, air hunger may develop.	Symptomatic. Provide bed rest and increased fluid intake. Antimicrobials and sulfonamides may prevent secondary infection. Acetaminophen (antipyretic), drugs to control cough, and analgesics for pain may be given. Do not give aspirin because of high risk for Reye syndrome. Amantadine, rimantadine, zanamivir, and oseltamivir (antiviral medication) are approved for treatment in children 1 yr of age and older, but different strains have developed some resistance.	In severe cases, pulmonary edema and cardiac failure. Secondary invaders may produce bacterial infections of respiratory tract.
Erythema infectiosum (fifth disease) *Incubation period:* 4-14 days or longer *Causative agent:* Parvovirus B19	Uncertain *Route:* Droplet; infected persons	Three-stage rash: Erythema on face, mostly on cheeks (disappears in 1-4 days). One day after face rash, maculopapular red spots appear on upper and lower extremities, progressing proximally to distally; lacy appearance. Rash subsides but reappears if skin is irritated (sun, heat, cold); may last 1-3 wk. Child not contagious after rash appears.	Reinforce benign nature of the condition to parents. No treatment indicated. Exposed pregnant women should notify their obstetrician. Avoid exposing immunosuppressed children and children with sickle cell disease.	Aplastic crisis in children with sickle cell anemia.
Exanthema subitum (roseola) *Incubation period:* 9-10 days *Causative agent:* Human herpesvirus type 6	Unknown *Route:* Droplet; primarily affects children younger than 2 yr of age	Persistent high fever for 3-4 days in child who appears well. Precipitous drop in fever to normal temperature with appearance of rash. Rash: discrete rose-pink macules appearing first on trunk, then spreading to neck, face, and extremities. Nonpruritic, fades on pressure, lasts 1-2 days.	Antipyretics to control fever. Anticonvulsants for child who has history of febrile seizures. Teach parents measures for combating high temperature. Reinforce benign nature of illness.	Febrile seizures during febrile period. Bulging fontanel.

Continued

| Table B-1 | Communicable Diseases—cont'd |

DISEASE	COMMUNICABILITY PERIOD AND ROUTE	CLINICAL MANIFESTATIONS	TREATMENT AND NURSING CARE	COMPLICATIONS
Hepatitis type A *Incubation period:* 15-50 days (average 28 days) *Causative agent:* Hepatitis A virus (HAV)	1-2 weeks before onset of jaundice or elevation of liver enzymes *Route:* Oral contamination by intestinal excretions; contaminated food, milk, or water Hepatitis A is a major potential health problem in day-care centers	Manifestations occur rapidly and vary from mild to severe, from mild fever, anorexia, generalized malaise, nausea, vomiting, unpleasant taste in mouth, abdominal discomfort, and nonexistent or mild jaundice to severe jaundice, coma, and death. Early leukopenia is seen. Bile may be detected in urine; bowel movements are clay-colored. Liver function tests are useful for diagnosis.	Symptomatic. No specific therapy for uncomplicated HAV infection. Enteric precautions are necessary for 1 wk after onset of jaundice. Persons caring for those who are not toilet-trained, have diarrhea, or are incontinent should use disposable gloves when carrying fecal waste. Prevention: In day-care centers, practice thorough hand hygiene after changing diapers and before preparing and serving food. Because HAV may survive on objects in the environment for weeks (e.g., infant changing tables), adequate environmental hygiene is essential. Children should be immunized at 1 yr of age (12-23 mo). Administer immunoglobulin to contacts of affected child younger than 1 yr in a day-care setting.	Usually benign in children. Liver damage, recurrence of symptoms. May be a source of chromosomal damage.
Hepatitis type B *Incubation period:* 45-160 days (average 90 days) *Causative agent:* Hepatitis B virus (HBV)	Few days before to 1 mo or more after onset *Route:* Person-to-person by percutaneous introduction of blood; direct contact with secretions or blood contaminated with HBV. Routine preexposure immunization recommended for all infants; appropriate immunoprophylaxis of infants born to hepatitis B surface antigen (HBsAg)–positive women and of infants born to women with unknown HBsAg status; some risk in children on hemodialysis, children receiving blood or blood products (including those with hemophilia), and IV drug users	Manifestations occur slowly. See hepatitis A for clinical manifestations.	Symptomatic. Children should be allowed to regulate own activity. Diet should be high protein, high calorie, high carbohydrate, and low fat. Food should be served in small, attractive, frequent feedings. Chief reasons for hospitalization are persistent vomiting and toxicity. Fluids may be given parenterally. Prevention: Universal immunization of infants and preteen children not immunized during infancy. Careful handling of blood and secretions; Universal Precautions. No specific therapy for acute HBV vaccine is available. Hepatitis B immune globulin (HBIG) and corticosteroids are not effective.	Acute fulminating hepatitis characterized by rapidly rising bilirubin, encephalopathy, edema, ascites, and hepatic coma. Chronic HBV-infected persons are at risk for serious liver disease including primary hepatocellular carcinoma (HCC) with advancing age.

| Table B-1 | Communicable Diseases—cont'd |

DISEASE	COMMUNICABILITY PERIOD AND ROUTE	CLINICAL MANIFESTATIONS	TREATMENT AND NURSING CARE	COMPLICATIONS

Lyme disease
Incubation period:
  1-32 days but
  up to months or
  years
Causative agent:
  Borrelia
  burgdorferi
	Not communicable from person to person; persons with active disease should not donate blood
	Route: Spread by ticks; most common hosts are white-tailed deer and white-footed mice
		Begins with a skin lesion at the site of a recent tick bite. The painless red macule expands to form a large papule with a raised border and a clear center. Systemic manifestations include malaise, lethargy, fever, headache, arthralgias, stiff neck, myalgias, and lymphadenopathy. Late manifestations involve the joints and the cardiac and neurologic systems. Often first appears as single joint redness, swelling, and limitation.	Early treatment is doxycycline for children 8 yr of age and older. All ages: amoxicillin or cefuroxime. Later-stage disease is treated with high-dose IV ceftriaxone or penicillin. Prevention by teaching parents to observe for signs of disease during tick season. Protective clothing should be worn in areas where tick exposure is likely. Ticks should be removed.	Neurologic complications, carditis, and chronic arthritis may develop.
				Transplacental infection has resulted in fetal death, prematurity, and congenital anomalies.

Measles (rubeola)
Incubation period:
  8-12 days
Causative agent:
  RNA virus
	From 4 days before to 5 days after rash appears
	Route: Direct contact; airborne by droplets and contaminated dust
		Coryza, conjunctivitis, and photophobia are present before rash. Koplik spots in mouth, hacking cough, high fever, rash, and enlarged lymph nodes. Rash consists of small reddish brown or pink macules changing to papules; fades on pressure. Rash begins behind ears, on forehead, or on cheeks, progresses to extremities, and lasts about 5 days.	Symptomatic. Keep child in bed until fever and cough have subsided. Light in room should be dimmed. Keep hands from eyes. Irrigate eyes with physiologic saline solution to relieve itching. Tepid baths and soothing lotion relieve itching of skin. Encourage fluids during fever. Humidify the child's room. Antimicrobial therapy given for complications.
			Vitamin A supplementation is recommended once daily for 2 days to reduce mortality. Immunoglobulin (IG) can help prevent or modify measles within 6 days of exposure.
				Vary with severity of disease: otitis media, pneumonia, tracheobronchitis, nephritis. Encephalitis with permanent brain damage may occur. Death from respiratory and neurologic complications.
				Subacute sclerosing panencephalitis (SSPE), a rare degenerative central nervous system (CNS) disease, may occur. The mean incubation period is 7 yr after measles illness.

Continued

| Table B-1 | Communicable Diseases—cont'd |

DISEASE	COMMUNICABILITY PERIOD AND ROUTE	CLINICAL MANIFESTATIONS	TREATMENT AND NURSING CARE	COMPLICATIONS
Measles, German (rubella) *Incubation period:* 14-23 days *Causative agent:* Virus	During prodromal period and for 5 days after appearance of rash *Route:* Direct contact with secretions of nose and throat of infected person; airborne by contaminated dust particles	Fetus may contract rubella in utero if mother has the disease; slight fever, mild coryza. Rash consists of small pink or pale red macules closely grouped to appear as scarlet blush that fades on pressure. Rash fades in 3 days. Swelling of posterior cervical and occipital lymph nodes. No Koplik spots or photophobia as in measles.	Symptomatic. Bed rest until fever subsides. Children should be excluded from school or daycare for 7 days after onset of rash. Infants with congenital rubella should be considered contagious until 1 yr of age unless cultures are repeatedly negative.	Chief danger of disease is damage to fetus if mother contracts infection during first trimester of pregnancy. Neonate may have congenital rubella syndrome with permanent defects (e.g., cataracts, cardiovascular anomalies, deafness, microcephaly, mental retardation). Virus can be isolated from blood, urine, throat, cerebrospinal fluid, lens, and other involved organs. Infants may shed virus for 12-18 mo. Severe complications are rare. Encephalitis may occur.
Mumps (infectious parotitis) *Incubation period:* 16-18 days *Causative agent:* Rubulavirus in the Paramyxoviridae family	1-2 days before swelling to 5 days after onset of swelling *Route:* Direct or indirect contact with salivary secretions of infected person; droplet	Salivary glands are chiefly affected. Parotid, sublingual, and submaxillary glands may be involved. Swelling and pain occur in these glands either unilaterally or bilaterally. Child may have difficulty swallowing, headache, fever, and malaise.	Local application of heat or cold to salivary glands to reduce discomfort. Liquids or soft foods are given. Foods containing acid may increase pain. Bed rest until swelling subsides. Children are excluded from school or daycare for 9 days from onset of parotid gland swelling. Mumps vaccine should be given at least 2 wk before or 3 mo after administration of IG or blood transfusion.	Complications are less frequent in children than in adults. Meningoencephalitis, inflammation of ovaries or testes, or deafness may occur.

| Table B-1 | Communicable Diseases—cont'd |

DISEASE	COMMUNICABILITY PERIOD AND ROUTE	CLINICAL MANIFESTATIONS	TREATMENT AND NURSING CARE	COMPLICATIONS
Pertussis (whooping cough) *Incubation period:* 7-10 days *Causative agent:* *Bordetella pertussis*	4-6 wk from onset *Route:* Direct contact; airborne by droplet spread from infected person	Begins with symptoms of upper respiratory tract infection. Coryza, dry cough, which is worse at night. Cough occurs in paroxysms of several sharp coughs in one expiration, then a rapid deep inspiration, followed by a whoop. Dyspnea and fever may be present. Vomiting may occur after coughing. Lymphocytosis occurs. Duration of illness is 6-10 wk.	Symptomatic. Azithromycin is the drug of choice for treatment or prophylaxis of pertussis in infants younger than 1 mo. Erythromycin may limit communicability. Protect child from secondary infection. Erythromycin for household and day-care contacts. Primary or booster vaccination of exposed children younger than 7 yr. Provide mental and physical rest to prevent paroxysms of coughing. Provide warm, humid air. Oxygen may be necessary. Avoid chilling. Offer small, frequent feedings to maintain nutritional status. Refeed if child vomits. Small amounts of sedatives may be given to quiet the child. Most infants younger than 6 mo of age are hospitalized; intensive care may be required.	Very serious disease during infancy because of complication of bronchopneumonia. Otitis media, marasmus, bronchiectasis, and atelectasis may occur. Hemorrhage may occur during paroxysms of coughing. Encephalitis may occur.
Poliovirus infection (poliomyelitis) *Incubation period:* 3-6 days *Causative agent:* Enteroviruses	During period of infection, latter part of incubation period, and first week of acute illness *Route:* Oral contamination by pharyngeal and intestinal excretions, respiratory route	Acute illness. Initial symptoms of upper respiratory tract infection, headache, fever, vomiting. Nonparalytic: Previous symptoms plus sore or stiff muscles of neck, trunk, and extremities. Nuchal rigidity. Paralytic: Includes muscular paralysis. Clinical manifestations may vary from mild to very severe following symptomless period after initial symptoms.	Both parents and child need support and reassurance, for they are fearful of the term *polio.* Treatment and nursing care are symptomatic. Because oral polio vaccine is no longer available in the United States, the chance for exposure to vaccine-type polio is remote.	Emotional disturbances, gastric dilation, melena, hypertension, or transitory paralysis of bladder may occur. Severe complications of paralytic polio include respiratory failure and permanent muscle deficits.
Rotavirus infection *Incubation period:* 1-3 days *Causative agent:* Rotavirus	*Route:* Fecal-oral	Acute onset of fever and vomiting followed 24-48 hr later by watery diarrhea.	Oral or parenteral fluids and electrolytes are given to prevent and correct dehydration. No antiviral therapy is available. Contact precautions are used when diapering or cleaning incontinent children during illness.	Dehydration, electrolyte abnormalities, and acidosis.

Continued

Table B-1 **Communicable Diseases—cont'd**

DISEASE	COMMUNICABILITY PERIOD AND ROUTE	CLINICAL MANIFESTATIONS	TREATMENT AND NURSING CARE	COMPLICATIONS
Smallpox (variola) *Incubation period:* 7-17 days *Causative agent:* Virus (variola) *Note:* A smallpox vaccination plan has been implemented in the United States; however, the plan does not currently include immunization of children.	Persons are not infectious during the incubation period or febrile prodrome but become infectious with the onset of mucosal lesions, which occur within hours of the rash; the first week of rash illness is the most infectious period, although individuals remain infectious until all scabs have separated *Route:* Droplets (from the oropharynx of infected individuals); may be transmitted from aerosol and direct contact with infected lesions, clothing, or bedding	Severe prodromal illness with high fever (generally 102° F-104° F [38.9° C-40° C]), malaise, severe headache, backache, abdominal pain, and prostration (exhaustion), lasting for 2-5 days. May include vomiting and seizures. Prodromal period is followed by lesions on the mucosa of the mouth or pharynx that last less than 24 hr before the onset of rash. The child is considered infectious once the lesions have appeared. The rash begins on the face and spreads rapidly to the forearms, trunk, and legs in a centrifugal distribution. Many have lesions on the palms and soles. After 8-10 days, lesions begin to crust. Once all lesions have separated (3-4 wk), the child is no longer infectious.	Treatment is supportive. Vaccinia immune globulin (VIG) is used for certain complications of immunizations and has no role in treatment of smallpox. The vaccination may provide some protection against the disease if administered within 3-4 days of exposure. Children are isolated in a private, airborne infection isolation room with negative pressure ventilation. Anyone entering the room must wear an N95 or higher-quality respirator, gloves, and gown even if there is a history of recent successful immunization. If the child leaves the room, he or she should wear a mask and be covered with sheets or gowns to decrease the risk of possible transmission. Cidofovir has been suggested as having a role in smallpox therapy, but no data are available.	Fatality rates reached 30% in the past; death occurred during the second week of illness from overwhelming viremia. The potential for modern supportive therapy in improving outcome is not known.

Table B-1   Communicable Diseases—cont'd

DISEASE	COMMUNICABILITY PERIOD AND ROUTE	CLINICAL MANIFESTATIONS	TREATMENT AND NURSING CARE	COMPLICATIONS
Streptococcal infection, group A beta-hemolytic (streptococcal sore throat, scarlet fever, scarlatina) *Incubation period:* 2-5 days *Causative agent:* Beta-hemolytic streptococci, group A strains	Onset to recovery *Route:* Droplet infection; direct and indirect transmission may occur	Initial symptoms of streptococcal sore throat are seen in the pharynx. The source of this organism may also be in a burn or wound. Toxin from site of infection is absorbed into bloodstream. Typical symptoms of scarlet fever are headache, fever, rapid pulse, rash, thirst, vomiting, lymphadenitis, and delirium. Throat is injected, and cellulitis of throat occurs. White tongue coating desquamates, and red strawberry tongue results. Other manifestations may include otitis media, mastoiditis, and meningitis.	Penicillin G is the drug of choice. Erythromycin is used for penicillin-sensitive individuals. Adequate fluid intake, bed rest, pain-relieving drugs, and mouth care are important. Diet should be given as the child wishes: liquid, soft, or regular. Warm saline throat irrigations may be given to the older child. Increased humidity for severe infection of upper respiratory tract. Cold or hot applications to painful cervical lymph nodes.	Complications are caused by toxins, the streptococci, or secondary infection. Complications of pneumonia, glomerulonephritis, or rheumatic fever may occur.
Tetanus *Incubation period:* 3-21 days (average 8 days) *Causative agent:* Clostridium tetani	*Route:* Wound contaminant; umbilical stump contamination in neonates	Early signs are headache, restlessness, followed by spasm of masticatory muscles (chewing), difficulty opening the mouth, dysphagia. Progresses to opisthotonos (severe arching of back and head bending to back), seizures.	Human tetanus immune globulin is given to neutralize neurotoxins to stop the infectious process. Surgical wound débridement Quiet environment as muscle spasms are aggravated by external stimuli. Metronidazole is the drug of choice for 10-14 days; an alternative is IV penicillin G. Diazepam (Valium) to alleviate muscle spasms.	Respiratory failure requiring support. Seizures.

Modified from Pickering L, et al, eds: *Red book: 2009 Report of the Committee on Infectious Diseases,* ed 28. Elk Grove Village, Ill, 2009, American Academy of Pediatrics. Retrieved November 5, 2010 from http://aapredbook.aappublications.org. InPrice DL, Gwin JF: *Pediatric nursing: an introductory text,* ed 11, St Louis, 2012, Mosby.

Table B-2 | Bacterial Infections

DISORDER AND CAUSATIVE ORGANISM	MANIFESTATIONS	MANAGEMENT	COMMENTS
Impetigo contagiosa— *Staphylococcus*	Begins as a reddish macule Becomes vesicular Ruptures easily, leaving superficial, moist erosion Tends to spread peripherally in sharply marginated irregular outlines Exudate dries to form heavy, honey-colored crusts Pruritus common *Systemic effects*—Minimal or asymptomatic	Careful removal of undermined skin, crusts, and debris by softening with 1:20 Burow solution compresses Topical application of bactericidal ointment Systemic administration of oral or parenteral antibiotics (penicillin) in severe or extensive lesions	Tends to heal without scarring unless secondary infection Autoinoculable and contagious Common in toddlers, preschoolers May be superimposed on eczema
Pyoderma—*Staphylococcus, Streptococcus*	Deeper extension of infection into dermis Tissue reaction more severe *Systemic effects*—Fever, lymphangitis	Soap and water cleansing Wet compresses Bathing with antibacterial soap as prescribed Do not share washcloths or towels Mupirocin to nares and lesions as prescribed Systemic antibiotics	Autoinoculable and contagious May heal with or without scarring
Folliculitis (pimple), furuncle (boil), carbuncle (multiple boils)—*Staphylococcus aureus*	Folliculitis—Infection of hair follicle Furuncle—Larger lesion with more redness and swelling at a single follicle Carbuncle—More extensive lesion with widespread inflammation and "pointing" at several follicular orifices *Systemic effects*—Malaise, if severe	Skin cleanliness Local warm, moist compresses Topical application of antibiotic agents Systemic antibiotics in severe cases Incision and drainage of severe lesions, followed by wound irrigations with antibiotics or suitable drain implantation	Autoinoculable and contagious Furuncle and carbuncle tend to heal with scar formation Never squeeze a lesion
Cellulitis—*Streptococcus, Staphylococcus, Haemophilus influenzae*	Inflammation of skin and subcutaneous tissues with intense redness, swelling, and firm infiltration Lymphangitis "streaking" frequently seen Involvement of regional lymph nodes common May progress to abscess formation *Systemic effects*—Fever, malaise	Oral or parenteral antibiotics Rest and immobilization of both affected area and child Hot, moist compresses to area	Hospitalization may be necessary for child with systemic symptoms Otitis media may be associated with facial cellulitis
Staphylococcal scalded skin syndrome—*S. aureus*	Macular erythema with "sandpaper" texture of involved skin Epidermis becoming wrinkled (in 2 days or less), and appearance of large bullae	Systemic administration of antibiotics Gentle cleansing with saline, Burow solution, or 0.25% silver nitrate compresses	Infant subject to fluid loss, impaired body temperature regulation, and secondary infection, such as pneumonia, cellulitis, and septicemia Heals without scarring

From Hockenberry MJ, Wilson D: *Wong's essentials of pediatric nursing,* ed 9, St Louis, 2013, Mosby.

Table B-3   Viral Infections

INFECTION	MANIFESTATIONS	MANAGEMENT	COMMENTS
Verruca (warts) *Cause*—Human papillomavirus (various types)	Usually well-circumscribed, gray or brown, elevated, firm papules with a roughened, finely papillomatous texture Occur anywhere, but usually appear on exposed areas such as fingers, hands, face, and soles May be single or multiple Asymptomatic	Not uniformly successful Local destructive therapy, individualized according to location, type, and number—surgical removal, electrocautery, curettage, cryotherapy (liquid nitrogen), caustic solutions (lactic acid and salicylic acid in flexible collodion, retinoic acid, salicylic acid plasters), x-ray treatment, laser	Common in children Tend to disappear spontaneously Course unpredictable Most destructive techniques tend to leave scars Autoinoculable Repeated irritation will cause to enlarge Apply topical anesthetic EMLA
Verruca plantaris (plantar wart)	Located on plantar surface of feet and, because of pressure, are practically flat; may be surrounded by a collar of hyperkeratosis	Apply caustic solution to wart, wear foam insole with hole cut to relieve pressure on wart; soak 20 minutes after 2-3 days; repeat until wart comes out	Destructive techniques tend to leave scars, which may cause problems with walking Apply topical anesthetic EMLA
Herpes simplex virus infection Type I (cold sore, fever blister) Type II (genital)	Grouped, burning, and itching vesicles on inflammatory base, usually on or near mucocutaneous junctions (lips, nose, genitalia, buttocks) Vesicles dry, forming a crust, followed by exfoliation and spontaneous healing in 8-10 days May be accompanied by regional lymphadenopathy	Avoidance of secondary infection Burow solution compresses during weeping stages Topical therapy (penciclovir) to shorten duration of cold sores Oral antiviral (acyclovir) for initial infection or to reduce severity in recurrence Valacyclovir (Valtrex), an oral antiviral, used for episodic treatment of recurrent genital herpes; reduces pain, stops viral shedding, and has a more convenient administration schedule than acyclovir	Vesicles heal without scarring unless secondary infection Type I cold sores prevented by use of sunscreens protecting against ultraviolet A (UVA) and ultraviolet B (UVB) light to prevent lip blisters Aggravated by corticosteroids Positive psychological effect from treatment May be fatal in children with depressed immunity
Varicella-zoster virus (herpes zoster; shingles)	Caused by same virus that causes varicella (chickenpox) Virus has affinity for posterior root ganglia, posterior horn of spinal cord, and skin; crops of vesicles usually confined to dermatome following along course of affected nerve Usually preceded by neuralgic pain, hyperesthesias, or itching May be accompanied by constitutional symptoms	Symptomatic Analgesics for pain Mild sedation sometimes helpful Local moist compresses Drying lotions sometimes helpful Ophthalmic variety: use systemic corticotropin (adrenocorticotropic hormone [ACTH]) or corticosteroids Acyclovir Lidocaine (Lidoderm) topical anesthetic	Pain in children usually minimal Postherpetic pain does not occur in children Chickenpox may follow exposure; isolate affected child from other children in a hospital or school May occur in children with depressed immunity; can be fatal

Continued

Table B-3 Viral Infections—cont'd

INFECTION	MANIFESTATIONS	MANAGEMENT	COMMENTS
Molluscum contagiosum *Cause*—Pox virus Small, benign tumors	Flesh-colored papules with a central caseous plug (umbilicated) Usually asymptomatic	Cases in well children resolve spontaneously in about 18 months Treatment reserved for troublesome cases Apply topical anesthetic EMLA and remove with curette Use tretinoin gel 0.01% or cantharidin (Cantharone) liquid* Curettage or cryotherapy	Common in school-aged children Spread by skin-to-skin contact, including autoinoculation and fomite-to-skin contact

From Hockenberry MJ, Wilson D: *Wong's essentials of pediatric nursing,* ed 9, St Louis, 2013, Mosby.
* Not available in the United States, but can be purchased in Canada.

Table B-4 Dermatophytoses (Fungal Infections)

DISEASE AND CAUSATIVE ORGANISM	MANIFESTATIONS	MANAGEMENT	COMMENTS
Tinea capitis—*Trichophyton tonsurans, Microsporum audouinii, Microsporum canis*	Lesions in scalp but may extend to hairline or neck Characteristic configuration of scaly, circumscribed patches or patchy, scaling areas of alopecia Generally asymptomatic, but severe, deep inflammatory reaction may occur that manifests as boggy, encrusted lesions (kerions) Pruritic Microscopic examination of scales is diagnostic	Oral griseofulvin Oral ketoconazole for difficult cases Selenium sulfide shampoos Topical antifungal agents (e.g., clotrimazole, haloprogin, miconazole)	Person-to-person transmission Animal-to-person transmission Rarely, permanent loss of hair *M. audouinii* transmitted from one human being to another directly or from personal items; *M. canis* usually contracted from household pets, especially cats Atopic individuals more susceptible
Tinea corporis—*Trichophyton rubrum, Trichophyton mentagrophytes, M. canis, Epidermophyton*	Generally round or oval, erythematous scaling patch that spreads peripherally and clears centrally; may involve nails (tinea unguium) *Diagnosis*—Direct microscopic examination of scales Usually unilateral	Oral griseofulvin Local application of antifungal preparation such as tolnaftate, haloprogin, miconazole, clotrimazole; apply 1 inch beyond periphery of lesion; continual application 1-2 weeks after no sign of lesion	Usually of animal origin from infected pets Majority of infections in children caused by *M. canis* and *M. audouinii*
Tinea cruris ("jock itch")—*Epidermophyton floccosum, T. rubrum, T. mentagrophytes*	Skin response similar to tinea corporis Localized to medial proximal aspect of thigh and crural fold; may involve scrotum in boys Pruritic *Diagnosis*—Same as for tinea corporis	Local application of tolnaftate liquid Wet compresses or sitz baths may be soothing	Rare in preadolescent children Health education regarding personal hygiene

Table B-4   Dermatophytoses (Fungal Infections)—cont'd

DISEASE AND CAUSATIVE ORGANISM	MANIFESTATIONS	MANAGEMENT	COMMENTS
Tinea pedis ("athlete's foot")—*T. rubrum, Trichophyton interdigitale, E. floccosum*	On intertriginous areas between toes or on plantar surface of feet Lesions vary: Maceration and fissuring between toes Patches with pinhead-sized vesicles on plantar surface Pruritic *Diagnosis*—Direct microscopic examination of scrapings	Oral griseofulvin Local applications of tolnaftate liquid and antifungal powder containing tolnaftate *Acute infections*—Compresses or soaks followed by application of glucocorticoid cream Elimination of conditions of heat and perspiration by clean, light socks and well-ventilated shoes; avoidance of occlusive shoes	Most frequent in adolescents and adults; rare in children, but occurrence increases with wearing of plastic shoes Transmission to other individuals rare despite general opinion to contrary Ointments not successful
Candidiasis (moniliasis)—*Candida albicans*	Grows in chronically moist areas Inflamed areas with white exudate, peeling, and easy bleeding Pruritic *Diagnosis*—Characteristic appearance	Amphotericin B, nystatin ointment, or other antifungal preparations to affected areas	Common form of diaper dermatitis Oral form common in infants Vaginal form in older girls May be disseminated in immunosuppressed children

From Hockenberry MJ, Wilson D: *Wong's essentials of pediatric nursing,* ed 9, St Louis, 2013, Mosby.

Index

Page numbers followed by *f* indicate figures; *t,* tables; *b,* boxes.